SIXTH EDITION

Medical and Psychosocial Aspects of Chronic Illness and Disability

Donna R. Falvo, PhD

Beverley E. Holland, PhD, RN

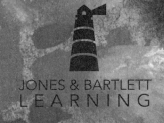

JONES & BARTLETT
LEARNING

World Headquarters
Jones & Bartlett Learning
5 Wall Street
Burlington, MA 01803
978-443-5000
info@jblearning.com
www.jblearning.com

Jones & Bartlett Learning books and products are available through most bookstores and online booksellers. To contact Jones & Bartlett Learning directly, call 800-832-0034, fax 978-443-8000, or visit our website, www.jblearning.com.

Production Credits
VP, Executive Publisher: David D. Cella
Executive Editor: Amanda Martin
Associate Acquisitions Editor: Rebecca Stephenson
Editorial Assistant: Christina Freitas
Vendor Manager: Sara Kelly
Senior Marketing Manager: Jennifer Scherzay
Product Fulfillment Manager: Wendy Kilborn
Composition and Project Management: S4Carlisle
    Publishing Services
Cover Design: Kristin E. Parker
Rights & Media Specialist: Wes DeShano
Media Development Editor: Troy Liston
Cover Image: © Nicolae Popovici/E+/Getty
Printing and Binding: Edwards Brothers
    Malloy
Cover Printing: Edwards Brothers Malloy

Library of Congress Cataloging-in-Publication Data
Names: Falvo, Donna R., author. | Holland, Beverley, author.
Title: Medical and psychosocial aspects of chronic illness and disability / Donna Falvo and Beverley Holland.
Description: Sixth edition. | Burlington, MA : Jones & Bartlett Learning,
    [2018] | Includes bibliographical references and index.
Identifiers: LCCN 2016040476 | ISBN 9781284105407 (casebound)
Subjects: | MESH: Chronic Disease | Disabled Persons--psychology | Disabled
    Persons--rehabilitation | Social Adjustment
Classification: LCC RC108 | NLM WT 500 | DDC 616/.044--dc23 LC record available at https://lccn.loc.gov/2016040476
6048

Printed in the United States of America
21 20 19 18 17   10 9 8 7 6 5 4 3 2 1

Dedication

This book is dedicated to the memory of

Judy Mayer Irick, RN

1945–2015

Dedicated nurse, loving mother, loyal and trusted friend.

Contents

Preface

Each person is unique. Consequently, chronic health conditions are not experienced in exactly the same ways by all individuals. The effects of chronic illness and disability are individual, and encompass not only physical function but also psychological, social, and work function. The extent to which individuals are able to function in their environment is, however, not always a direct result of their chronic health condition but rather may reflect misconceptions, lack of understanding, erroneous attitudes, and prejudice on the part of those persons encountered in the individual's environment or other environmental barriers that impede function. An understanding of chronic illness and disability, their functional implications, and the environmental constraints that may be present can contribute to removal of these barriers and support increased functional capacity.

This text, like the four previous editions, is designed as a reference for nonmedical professionals and as a text for students who have little prior medical knowledge but who work with individuals with chronic illness and disability. Moreover, this edition, like the previous edition, reflects the approach and philosophical underpinnings of the International Classification of Functioning, Disability and Health (ICF), which conceptualizes health as a continuum.

This edition has been revised and updated and, like previous editions, attempt to acquaint the reader with little or no medical background with concepts and medical terminology. In addition to basic information regarding physical aspects of each chronic health condition, the text addresses psychosocial aspects as well as the potential functional impact on activities and participation at home, work, and employment. Focusing on functional capacity in the context of personal goals and individual environment rather than focusing solely on physical effects of chronic health conditions can enable individuals to achieve not only optimal functional capacity but also increased quality of life.

Donna R. Falvo
Beverley E. Holland

About the Authors

Donna R. Falvo, PhD, has more than 35 years of experience as a registered nurse, licensed clinical psychologist, and certified rehabilitation counselor. At Southern Illinois University at Carbondale School of Medicine, she was Director of Behavioral Science in the Department of Family and Community Medicine and later directed the Rehabilitation Counseling Program at the Rehabilitation Institute at SIU. Most recently, she was clinical professor in the Rehabilitation Counseling and Psychology Program at the University of North Carolina at Chapel Hill School of Medicine. Dr. Falvo is past president of the American Rehabilitation Counseling Association and a former Mary Switzer Scholar. She served as Dimension Expert with the National Research Corporation/Picker Institute, Lincoln, Nebraska, from 2005 to 2008.

Beverley Holland, PhD, RN, is a registered nurse and an adult nurse practitioner. She received her PhD in rehabilitation from the Rehabilitation Institute, Southern Illinois University at Carbondale. She is an associate professor of nursing at the School of Nursing, Western Kentucky University in Bowling Green, Kentucky. In addition to teaching graduate students in nursing, she maintains a practice, which includes community wellness visits and working with the geriatric population.

Contributors

Thanks and appreciation to the following people who are responsible for major revisions of selected chapters. Their dedication, expertise, and professionalism are greatly appreciated.

Elizabeth Moran Fitzgerald, EdD, RN, CNS-BC, LMFT, LPCC. Dr. Fitzgerald is an associate professor of clinical nursing at Ohio State University. In addition to clinical teaching she practices as a Child & Adolescent Psychiatric Mental Health Clinical Nurse Specialist.

Kathy K. Hager, DNP, RN, is a family nurse practitioner and diabetes nurse educator and associate professor at Bellarmine University Lansing School of Nursing and Health Sciences, Louisville, KY. She practices at the university clinic and in the community with individuals with diabetes.

Kelly A. Kazukauskas, PhD, LCPC, CRC, CVE is a clinical assistant professor, clinical coordinator, and admissions coordinator with the Division of Counseling and Rehabilitation Science, Lewis College of Human Sciences at the Illinois Institute of Technology, Chicago, IL.

David B. Peterson, PhD, CRC, clinical psychologist, is a professor in rehabilitation education and Coordinator of the Clinical Counseling Certificate Program at California State University, Los Angeles.

Acknowledgments

Special thanks to the following people who generously volunteered their time to read, review, critique, and discuss various sections of the book. Their dedication and commitment to individuals with chronic illness and disability is greatly appreciated by the authors as by the individuals they serve.

Bruce Cairns, MD
Director, NC Jaycee Burn Center
John Stackhouse Distinguished Professor
 of Surgery
University of North Carolina School
 of Medicine
Chapel Hill, NC

Richard Falvo, PhD
Professor Emeritus
Department of Physiology
Southern Illinois University School of Medicine
Carbondale, IL

Travis Meredith, MD
Emeritus Professor and Chair
Department of Opthalmology
University of North Carolina School
 of Medicine
Chapel Hill, NC

Steve Prystowsky, MD
Clinical Associate Professor
Department of Dermatology
New York University School of Medicine
New York, NY

Alfredo C. Rivadeneira, MD
Associate Professor of Medicine
Division of Rheumatology, Allergy and
 Immunology
University of North Carolina
Chapel Hill, NC

Carlo Smirne, MD, PhD
Assistant Professor of Internal Medicine
University of Piemonte Orientale
Department of Translational Medicine
Novara, Italy

Mitchell Mass
Reader, reviewer, and good friend
Chapel Hill, NC

CHAPTER 1

Conceptualizing Functioning, Disability, and Health

Revised by David Peterson

INTRODUCTION

From the time an individual is born, life unfolds in an environment that is both physical and social. Throughout history, attitudes toward health and disability have reflected broad social and cultural values of the time. As social patterns change and evolve, so do concepts of health and disability. As a way to conceptualize disability and its relationship to health, a number of models have emerged throughout history. Each model carries with it fundamental assumptions about health and disability and about these concepts' relationship to the social norm. These assumptions affect the attitudes, expectations, and actions of individuals with disability, as well as individuals within society as a whole, and have the potential to influence social and political policies related to disability issues.

PAST MODELS TO CONCEPTUALIZE HEALTH AND DISABILITY

The Medical Model

In the United States, for many years, the understanding of chronic illness and disability was delineated by the *medical model*, which focused on specific medical conditions that were viewed as "problems" and were intrinsic to the individuals experiencing them (Smart, 2001). The medical profession was considered the authority, central to curing, altering,

or managing the specific medical condition, while the individual with the condition was viewed as the passive recipient of medical care. The medical model was diagnosis driven, emphasizing pathology, defining and characterizing the condition by standardized measures, and focusing on medical treatments and solutions to "eliminate" or control the condition, thereby returning the individual to "normal" (Fowler & Wadsworth, 1991; Longmore, 1995; McCarthy, 1993). The underlying philosophy of the medical model emphasized "normalcy" based on valued societal roles and norms. When an individual deviated from the "norm" in some way, the goal was to return that person to "normal." Given this premise, it followed that anyone who was in need of "cure," yet proved incurable, deviated from the "norm" and was, consequently, considered "abnormal," "dysfunctional," or "disabled." This conceptualization of disability carried with it a notion of social incapacitation that often engulfed an individual's social identity, which was subsumed by medical labels. The medical model emphasized the diagnosis and any corresponding limitation or functional incapacity relative to the societal norm (Stucki, Cieza, & Melvin, 2007).

While there are limitations to the medical model, it bears mentioning that the medical model has benefited health care. Diagnoses developed from this perspective and their health-related presentations have been used to quickly triage services that preserve life and to select appropriate treatments that minimize or ameliorate acute problems following the onset of health conditions. Generally speaking they have allowed us to develop a language that helps us keep track of what makes us sick and ends life, information critical in planning for the use of resources to optimize world health (Peterson & Elliott, 2008).

However, the medical model has difficulty accommodating the types of permanent and chronic long-term care needs that promote optimal health and quality of life for people living with a disability. This is due in part to the context of people dealing with chronic health conditions not adequately addressed by service delivery systems focused on acute, short-term conditions (Peterson & Elliott, 2008).

Further, the medical model relies heavily on measures and tests of the disease process, placing limited value on subjective reports of health and functioning, leading health providers to undervalue patient input concerning their treatment (Peterson & Elliott, 2008).

A growing body of research suggests that diagnostic labels alone, without functional data, may not adequately reflect an individual's health condition (see Peterson & Elliott, 2008). Diagnostic information alone can neither predict nor describe actual functional capacity of the individual within the context of his or her daily life. Emphasis on the medical condition alone not only ignores the individual's function within his or her environment or within the broader context of society but also overlooks the roles that society and the environment play in the individual's ability to function.

The Social Model

The *social model* of disability represented a reaction to the medical model (Paley, 2002). Rather than viewing disability as a condition of the individual to be cured so that the person can conform to social norms, the social model emphasized societal and environmental barriers as primary contributors to disability. A key component of the social model was equality (Hurst, 2003); thus a major focus was not to "cure" the individual but rather to make changes in society and the environment that would provide equality

and opportunity. The social model paralleled the civil rights/human rights movements, which were the catalyst for the development of a number of social policies and legislative actions. In the United States, the Americans with Disabilities Act, enacted in 1990, established the right of individuals with disability to receive reasonable accommodations that would enable them to function in the environment and prohibited discrimination based on their disability.

In accordance with the social model, disability was viewed not as a specific medical condition but rather as the result of the restrictions imposed through society's lack of attention and accommodation to the needs of individuals with disability. The social and physical environments within which individuals live and interact can either enhance their ability to function or exaggerate a disability. Consequently, social and physical environments can determine the extent and type of function that individuals experience (Pledger, 2003). Although it recognized that individuals with disability may experience functional limitations as a direct result of their condition, the social model emphasized society's failure to take these limitations into account as the major contributor to disabling effects of the condition.

The social model, as with the medical model is not without its limitations. In contrast with the specific information defining what comprise diagnoses in the medical model, the social model has not historically distinguished who qualifies as a person with a disability, or how disability is measured or determined. Proponents of this tradition have not established a distinct body of research that systematically posits empirically testable and potentially falsifiable hypotheses. Complicating matters further, some proponents appear to regard such research as a continuation of a medical model that equates disability with person-based pathology that is largely independent of environmental and social factors (see Olkin & Pledger, 2003; Peterson & Elliott, 2008).

The Biopsychosocial Model

The *biopsychosocial model* was proposed as an alternative to prevailing medical and social models, which were perceived as being excessively narrow (Engel, 1977). The biopsychosocial model uses useful aspects from both the medical model and the social model of disability (Peterson & Rosenthal, 2005a; Simeonsson et al., 2003; Ueda & Okawa, 2003). Philosophically, rather than focusing solely on the medical condition or solely on the societal or environmental barriers as contributors to disability, the biopsychosocial model posits that it is the complex interaction of biological, psychological, and social factors in combination that play a significant role in an individual's ability to function. Consequently, the effects of any one health condition would be dependent on the individual involved and the social context and circumstances surrounding that person. The biopsychosocial model implies that many variables, not simply the chronic illness or disability itself, determine the extent and type of function that individuals with a health condition experience. Conceptualizing chronic illness and disability as *health conditions* in terms of functional capacity rather than as a medical diagnosis permits a greater understanding of the individual's subjective experience of his or her health condition.

THE EXPERIENCE OF DISABILITY

The experience of disability is individual, is dynamic, and varies in different circumstances and in different environments. The term *experience* implies that not all individuals—even those with the same medical condition—are affected by disability in the same way. How individuals perceive disability and the impact such disability has on function are not only the result of the condition itself, but also the result of personal factors and the circumstances that the individual encounters within his or her own particular social and physical environment (Imrie, 2004).

Personal factors can relate to gender, race, age, fitness, religion, lifestyle, habits, upbringing, coping styles, social background, education, profession, past and current experience, overall behavior pattern and character, individual psychological assets, other health conditions, or any number of other factors that contribute to an individual's experience of disability (WHO, 2001). Social environments

exist at many levels, extending from the insular level of family and friends, to the larger social environment of community and work, and finally to the broader level that encompasses cultural, economic, and political environments. Physical environments include not only physical barriers within the immediate environment but also other factors such as climate, weather, housing, and transportation (WHO, 2001).

Developmental factors also affect an individual's experience of disability. Each age group and each life stage present new challenges associated with that particular stage of life, which would occur whether or not an individual had a disability. These life-stage challenges, in turn, influence individuals' experience with disability. For instance, the experience of disability during childhood is different from the experience of the same condition in adulthood. The experience of disability in adolescence is different from what would be experienced with the same disability in later years of life.

Social environments also affect a person's experience with disability. The degree to which an individual has strong social support in terms of family or friends, the beliefs and attitudes of the community, and cultural expectations and norms of the individual's social group all influence how the affected person will experience disability.

The experience of disability also varies with the environment. The experience of disability at home may differ significantly from the experience in the workplace. The experience of disability while conducting household tasks may be much different than the experience of disability during recreational activities.

In short, there is a dynamic interaction between individuals' experience with disability and their consequent functional capacity within a given context. The experience of disability is multidimensional and unique to each individual. Individuals with the same disability do not experience disability in the same way.

CLASSIFYING DISABILITY

The concept of disability is complex and has been interpreted in a variety of ways. As the concept evolved from an emphasis on a cure to an emphasis on the individual experience and functional capacity within the context of the environment, it became evident that a medical diagnosis alone revealed little about how an individual would experience a health condition in terms of functional outcomes. Likewise, a medical diagnosis alone was insufficient to determine the types of accommodations needed to enhance an individual's ability to function in his or her environment. It became evident that there was a need to develop a common language by which consequences of health conditions and individual outcomes could be measured.

In response to these changes in perception, the World Health Organization (WHO) worked to develop a unified, standard classification of consequences of health conditions. The result was a classification system entitled the International Classification of Impairments, Disabilities, and Handicaps (ICIDH) (WHO, 1980). A complement to the International Statistical Classification of Diseases and Related Health Problems (ICD, now in its 10th revision (WHO, 1992)), the ICIDH was intended to provide a classification of function that complemented the diagnostic and mortality information historically classified by the ICD.

The ICIDH was influenced by the medical model but defined consequences of medical conditions with classifications related to function. The terms *impairment*, *disability*, and *handicap* were used to indicate the level and type of impact that the medical condition had on the individual's function. *Impairment* was defined as an abnormality in body structure or appearance; *disability* was defined as a restriction or lack of ability to perform an activity; and *handicap* was defined as a disadvantage the individual experienced as result of the impairment or disability.

As concepts continued to evolve and the medical model fell increasingly out of favor, the ICIDH was revised (De Kleijin-De Vrankrijker, 2003). In 2001, WHO adopted a new model to conceptualize functioning, disability, and health. The revised classification system, called the International Classification of Functioning, Disability and Health (ICF), was developed through a process of international consensus building including 652 individuals from 18 countries over a 7-year period (see Peterson, 2011; WHO, 2001).

PHILOSOPHICAL UNDERPINNINGS OF THE INTERNATIONAL CLASSIFICATION OF FUNCTIONING, DISABILITY AND HEALTH (ICF)

The ICF (WHO, 2001) presents a different way of conceptualizing chronic illness and disability; that is, it is a classification of *health and functioning* rather than *disease*. In the past, from the perspective of the medical model, the focus was on diagnostic labels and causes of disability, with emphasis on deficits and limitations and medical interventions to treat them. This perspective had the potential to overshadow the individual's potential and abilities, failed to recognize the degree to which his or her potential and abilities were hampered or enhanced by the social and physical environment, and did not typically seek out or value the individual's perspective on his or her health and functioning. The ICF changed this paradigm by placing a positive focus on function and health, emphasizing the integration of health conditions (disease, injury, or other biological factors) and personal, societal, and environmental factors. The ICF places health on a continuum, acknowledging that everyone has the potential to experience a decline in health with some degree of disability. Rather than viewing disability as a personal attribute that is directly caused by disease or injury and that requires medical care to correct the problem, the ICF addresses disability as a social construct that is a synthesis of biological, individual, and social factors and reflects the interaction between the individual and his or her social and physical environment (WHO, 2001). Thus the ICF promotes the concept of disability not as a problem within the person but rather as the result of assets or barriers found within the social or physical environment (Peterson & Kosciulek, 2005). This new conceptualization recognizes that the potential for disability is a universal human experience and not limited to a minority of the population.

Using the ICF classification system, disability is viewed as more than a medical diagnosis or a medical or biological dysfunction; rather, it is seen as a part of the health continuum as it affects function. Consequently, health and disability are viewed as a universal human experience with emphasis on the integration of biological, individual, social, and environmental aspects of a health condition.

GENERAL USES OF THE ICF

The ICF provides an international standard for describing and measuring health domains and is a universal classification of functional status associated with a number of health conditions (Peterson, 2005, 2015; Peterson & Rosenthal, 2005a). Its unified and standard definition of health and disability helps to provide a basis for common understanding.

The uses of the ICF are varied. The ICF can provide a structure to facilitate communication within and between multidisciplinary groups (Steiner et al., 2002); clarify team roles and enhance clinical reasoning (Tempest & McIntyre, 2006); organize service provision (Bruyére & Peterson, 2005; Rauch, Cleza, & Stucki, 2008; Stucki, Bedirhan Ustun, & Melvin, 2005); serve as a catalyst for research (Threats, 2002; Wade & deJong, 2000); and provide a framework for legislative, regulatory, social, and health policy related to disability (Peterson, 2011; WHO, 2001). In addition, it provides a means of comparison for individual experience with disability (Khan, Amatya, & Ng, 2010) and highlights the impact of environmental factors in enhancing or hindering function (Khan & Pallant, 2007).

The ICF classification system serves as a tool not only for standardizing concepts related to functional impact of disability but also for measuring the efficiency and effectiveness of rehabilitation services (Peterson, 2011; Üstün, Okawa, Bickenbach, Kastanjsek, & Schneider, 2003).

CONCEPTUAL FRAMEWORK OF THE ICF

The ICF addresses more than disability; that is, it also classifies health and health-related states with or without disability because the emphasis is on function and health conditions, both of which may be on a continuum. The *experience* of disability focuses on the individual and his or her personal resources, health condition, and individual environment. Health, as portrayed by the ICF, is a dynamic interaction between function and disability

within the context of the individual's environment and personal factors (Stucki & Melvin, 2007).

The ICF (WHO, 2001) defines key terms in its conceptual framework as follows:

- **Health** refers to *components of health* (physical or psychological function) and *components of well-being* (capacity to function within the environment).
- **Function** refers to all body functions, activities, and participation in society.
- **Disability** refers to any impairment, activity limitations, or participation restrictions that result from the health condition or from personal, societal, or environmental factors in the individual's life.
- **Impairment** refers to a deviation from certain generally accepted population standards of function.

Although impairments associated with a number of health conditions cause some degree of disability in most people (e.g., spinal cord injury), the degree to which an impairment results in disability is also determined by an individual's unique circumstances. What may appear to be a relatively minor disruption of function may actually have major consequences for the life of the individual affected. For example, loss of an index finger would be more disabling for a baseball pitcher than it would be for a heavy-equipment operator. Spinal cord injury resulting in paraplegia would have a different impact on someone who is an accountant than it would have on someone who is a construction worker. Rather than imposing preconceived ideas about the extent of a disability associated with a particular health condition, determining the extent of disability requires that consideration be given to the condition in the context of the individual's life, particular circumstances, and goals.

A health condition that results in a disability for one individual may not result in a disability for another individual with the same health condition. Therefore, the degree of disability an individual experiences as a result of a health condition depends on both the individual's goals and those facilitators or barriers that are present in the physical and social environment.

The ICF emphasizes functional capacity in the individual's natural environment. Evaluation and assessment of an individual's functional capacity in a laboratory or testing environment may not be an accurate reflection of his or her level of function. What individuals are able to do in a standardized environment may be quite different from what they are able to do in their natural environment. For example, an individual, after suffering a stroke resulting in hemiplegia, may be able to ambulate to the bathroom in a laboratory setting; in contrast, at home, with no indoor plumbing and only outdoor facilities, the same person may be unable to perform this task. Without assessing function in the context of the individual's everyday life, a realistic view of function may not be obtained. Likewise, there may be a discrepancy between the individual's capacity to function and his or her actual performance. Individuals may have the capacity to perform a task yet lack the motivation or social support to carry it out. For instance, an individual with emphysema may have the ability to carry out household chores but because of overprotective family members may be discouraged from doing so. Function, therefore, is more complex than merely having the ability to carry out a task or action.

STRUCTURE OF THE ICF

The core structure of the ICF is divided into two parts, each with two components (see **Table 1-1**).

The first part, *function and disability*, is divided into two components: *body function and structure* and *activity and participation*. In the first component, *body function* refers to physiological functioning of body systems, such as mental function, sensory function, function of the heart, or function of the immune system; *body structure* refers to anatomical components of the body, such as the structure of the nervous system or the structure of the cardiovascular system.

The second component, *activity and participation*, is conceptualized by qualifiers of *capacity* and *performance*. *Activity* refers to tasks or actions that individuals carry out in daily life, such as reading, writing, managing daily routines, dressing, and bathing. *Participation* refers to the individual's involvement in activities of daily life or in society. It includes the individual's ability to fully participate in activities in the broader social system, such as going to school, holding a job, engaging in recreational activities, or being integrated into the community. The qualifier *capacity* refers to the individual's *actual ability*, or level of function to perform a task or action, whereas *performance* refers to what the individual *actually does* in his or her current environment. For instance, an individual may have the capacity to walk from the front porch to the mailbox, but might not do so because a neighbor brings the mail to the individual's door each day.

The second part of the core structure of the ICF, *contextual factors*, consists of two components: *environmental factors* and *personal factors*. Both components include factors that can be either *facilitators* or *barriers* in helping individuals acquire full participation.

The first component, *environmental factors*, refers to more than the physical environment, such as accessibility of buildings or the availability of accessible transportation. That is, it also includes products and technology (such as telephones or computers), climate (such as dry, humid, hot, or cold), and factors in the social environment (such as social attitudes, norms, services, and political systems). In this context, environmental factors are divided into three levels:

- Individual level: individual systems of support; support network
- Services level: services and resources available
- Cultural/legal systems level: societal and cultural attitudes; political and legal factors (Peterson & Rosenthal, 2005b)

Table 1-1   Core Structure of the International Classification of Functioning, Disability, and Health

Part 1: Function and Disability	Part 2: Contextual Factors
A. Body functions and structures	A. Environmental factors
B. Activities and participation	B. Personal factors

The second component, *personal factors*, is recognized as an important interactive component in defining function, but is not coded in the ICF because of the complexity and highly individualized nature of these factors. Personal factors include gender, race, education, occupation, and difficult-to-quantify human factors, such as past personal experiences, individual temperament, and other intrinsic characteristics, such as state of mind. Although these factors are not coded, they are considered and recognized as contributing to the overall function of the individual.

The core structure of the ICF provides a perspective on health conditions from the standpoint of function. It offers a perspective on how body structure and function affect individuals' ability to function in the context of their particular social and physical environment as well as the direct impact of the social and physical environment on function. The ICF focuses on the dynamic and interactive nature of biological, social, personal, and environmental factors in determining individuals' functional capacity.

OPTIMUM VERSUS MAXIMUM FUNCTION, CAPACITY, AND PERFORMANCE

The domains of the *activities* and *participation* described above are operationalized through the use of the qualifiers *capacity* and *performance*. Capacity "describes an individual's ability to execute a task or an action," or more specifically, "the highest probable level of functioning that a person may reach in a given domain at a given moment" (WHO, 2001, p. 15). One must apply the capacity qualifier in the context of a "uniform" or "standard" environment; a heuristic for capacity could be what a person *can* do. The performance qualifier describes "what a person does in his or her current environment" (p. 15); a heuristic for performance could be what a person *does* do. The gap between capacity and performance can be very useful in intervention targeting, informed by the ICF's conceptual framework. If an individual is not performing at his or her capacity and that is that individual's desired goal, the health professional can explore interventions at the individual and

contextual levels that may increase functioning. Medications and therapy to treat body functions and structures and modifications in the home or work environments can have great effect on helping an individual perform at maximum capacity (Peterson, 2011).

However, for individuals to achieve full functional capacity, there must be an awareness of not only the functional implications of various health conditions but also the implications of the strengths and barriers that are found in the social and physical environment, particularly from the individual's unique perspective. One of the remarkable strengths of the ICF is that it is intended to be used *in collaboration* with the person whose health and functioning is being classified (Peterson & Threats, 2005). This collaborative approach is consistent with the social and biopsychosocial approaches to healthcare and provides the health professional with the benefit of the individual's unique perspective on his or her health and functioning (Peterson, 2011).

It is commonly assumed that achieving *maximum function* is the ideal goal; however, *optimal function* rather than *maximum function* is emphasized in the ICF. Although *maximum* refers to the greatest degree of function possible, defined in the ICF as capacity, maximum function for an individual may not be, in his or her opinion, optimal. *Maximum function* is based on an objective viewpoint, whereas *optimal function* is based on the subjective viewpoint of the individual and derived from his or her own goals and experience. Optimizing function requires a comprehensive understanding of the individual within the context of his or her environment and unique frame of reference. The emphasis is on building and strengthening personal resources, with the goal of helping individuals achieve *optimal functioning* and full *inclusion* and *participation* in all aspects of life. In this context, it is most useful for both strengths and limitations to be identified from both professional and personal, individual perspectives.

CONCLUSIONS

Conceptualizing chronic illness and disability as *health conditions* in the context of the continuum of health and function helps to decrease the stigmatization and isolation that have been associated with chronic illness and disability in the past. By emphasizing functional capacity rather than deficits, and by focusing on personal goals and the ability to perform in the context of the environment, optimal function can be achieved. Greater understanding of health conditions as an experience rather than as a medical condition can help to decrease the discrimination and prejudice that too often accompany chronic illness and disability and that too often are the major barriers to achievement of optimal activity and participation in the broader community, social, and vocational environments (Peterson, 2011).

REFERENCES

Bruyére, S. M., & Peterson, D. B. (2005). Introduction to the special section on the International Classification of Functioning, Disability and Health (ICF): Implications for rehabilitation psychology. *Rehabilitation Psychology, 50*, 103–104.

De Kleijin-De Vrankrijker, M. W. (2003). The long way from the International Classification of Impairments, Disabilities, and Handicaps (ICIDH) to the International Classification of Functioning, Disability, and Health (ICF). *Disability and Rehabilitation, 25*, 561–564.

Engel, G. (1977). The need for a new medical model: A challenge for biomedicine. *Science, 196*, 129–136.

Fowler, C. A., & Wadsworth, J. S. (1991). Individualism and equity: Critical values in North American culture and the impact on disability. *Journal of Applied Rehabilitation Counseling, 22*, 19–23.

Hurst, R. (2003). The international disability rights movement and the ICF. *Disability and Rehabilitation, 25*, 572–576.

Imrie, R. (2004). Demystifying disability: A review of the International Classification of Functioning, Disability and Health. *Sociology of Health and Illness, 26*, 287–305.

Khan, F., Amatya, B., & Ng, L. (2010). Use of International Classification of Functioning, Disability and Health to describe patient reported disability: A comparison of Guillain-Barré syndrome with multiple sclerosis in a community cohort. *Journal of Medical Rehabilitation, 42*(8), 708–714.

Khan, P., & Pallant, J. F. (2007). Use of International Classification of Functioning, Disability, and Health (ICF) to describe patient reported disability in multiple sclerosis and identification of relevant environmental factors. *Journal of Rehabilitation Medicine, 39*(1), 63–70.

Longmore, P. K. (1995). Medical decision-making and people with disabilities: A clash of cultures. *Journal of Law, Medicine, and Ethics, 23*, 82–87.

McCarthy, H. (1993). Learning with Beatrice A. Wright: A breath of fresh air that uncovers the unique virtues and human flaws in us all. *Rehabilitation Education, 10*, 149–166.

Olkin, R., & Pledger, C. (2003). Can disability studies and psychology join hands? *American Psychologist, 58*, 296–304.

Paley, J. (2002). The Cartesian melodrama in nursing. *Nursing Philosophy, 3*(3), 189.

Peterson, D. B. (2005). International Classification of Functioning, Disability and Health (ICF): An introduction for rehabilitation psychologists. *Rehabilitation Psychology, 50*, 105–112.

Peterson, D. B. (2011). *Psychological aspects of functioning, disability and health.* New York, NY: Springer Publishing Company.

Peterson, D. B. (2015). The International Classification of Functioning, Disability & Health: Applications for professional counseling. In I. Marini & M. Stebnicki (Eds.), *The professional counselor's desk reference* (2nd ed.). New York, NY: Springer Publishing Company.

Peterson, D. B., & Elliott, T. R. (2008). Advances in conceptualizing and studying disability. In S. Brown & R. Lent (Eds.), *Handbook of counseling psychology* (4th ed.). Hoboken, NJ: John Wiley & Sons.

Peterson, D. B., & Kosciulek, J. F. (2005). Introduction to the special issue of *Rehabilitation Education*: The International Classification of Functioning, Disability and Health (ICF). *Rehabilitation Education, 19*(2 & 3), 75–80.

Peterson, D. B., & Rosenthal, D. (2005a). The ICF as an historical allegory for history in rehabilitation education. *Rehabilitation Education, 19*, 95–104.

Peterson, D. B., & Rosenthal, D. A. (2005b). The International Classification of Functioning, Disability and Health (ICF): A primer for rehabilitation educators. *Rehabilitation Education, 19*(2 & 3), 81–94.

Peterson, D. B., & Threats, T. T. (2005). Ethical and clinical implications of the International Classification of Functioning, Disability and Health (ICF) in rehabilitation education. *Rehabilitation Education, 19*, 129–138.

Pledger, C. (2003). Discourse on disability and rehabilitation issues: Opportunities for psychology. *American Psychologist, 58*, 279–284.

Rauch, A., Cleza, A., & Stucki, G. (2008). How to apply the International Classification of Functioning, Disability, and Health (ICF) for rehabilitation management in clinical practice. *European Journal of Physical and Rehabilitation Medicine, 44*(3), 329–342.

Simeonsson, R. J., Leonardi, M., Lollar, D., Bjorck-Akesson, E., Hollenweger, J., & Martinuzzi, A. (2003). Applying the International Classification of Functioning, Disability and Health (ICF) to measure childhood disability. *Disability and Rehabilitation, 25*, 602–610.

Smart, J. F. (2001). *Disability, society and the individual.* Austin, TX: Pro-Ed.

Steiner, W., Ryser, L., Huber, E., Uebelhart, D., Aeschlimann, A., & Stucki, G. (2002). Use of the ICF model as a clinical problem-solving tool in physical therapy and rehabilitation medicine. *Physical Therapy, 82*(11), 1098–1107.

Stucki, G., Bedirhan Ustun, T., & Melvin, J. (2005). Applying the ICF for the acute hospital and early post-acute rehabilitation facilities. *Disability and Rehabilitation, 27*(7/8), 349–352.

Stucki, G., Cieza, A., & Melvin, J. (2007). The International Classification of Functioning, Disability and Health: A unifying model for the conceptual description of the rehabilitation strategy. *Journal of Rehabilitation Medicine, 39,* 279–285.

Stucki, G., & Melvin, J. (2007). The International Classification of Functioning, Disability and Health: A unifying model for the conceptual description of physical and rehabilitation medicine. *Journal of Rehabilitation Medicine, 39,* 286–292.

Tempest, S., & McIntyre, A. (2006). Using the ICF to clarify team roles and demonstrate clinical reasoning in stroke rehabilitation. *Disability and Rehabilitation, 28*(10), 663–667.

Threats, T. (2002). Evidence based practice research using the WHO framework. *Journal of Medical Speech-Language Pathology, 10,* 17–24.

Ueda, S., & Okawa, Y. (2003). The subjective dimension of functioning and disability: What is it and what is it for? *Disability and Rehabilitation, 25,* 596–601.

Üstün, S., Okawa, Y., Bickenbach, J., Kastanjsek, N., & Schneider, M. (2003). The International Classification of Functioning, Disability and Health: A new tool for understanding disability and health. *Disability and Rehabilitation, 25,* 565–571.

Wade, D. T., & deJong, B. A. (2000). Recent advances in rehabilitation. *Behavioral Medicine Journal, 320,* 1385–1388.

World Health Organization (WHO). (1980). *International Classification of Impairments, Disabilities, and Handicaps (ICIDH).* Geneva, Switzerland: Author.

World Health Organization (WHO). (1992). *International Statistical Classification of Diseases and Related Health Problems,* 10th revision *(ICD-10).* Geneva, Switzerland: Author.

World Health Organization (WHO). (2001). *ICF: International Classification of Functioning, Disability and Health.* Geneva, Switzerland: Author.

disease — medical model

health conditions — bio psychosocial model

CHAPTER 2

Psychosocial and Functional Aspects of Health Conditions

THE EXPERIENCE OF HEALTH CONDITIONS AND ALTERED FUNCTION

The way individuals experience health conditions with associated alterations in functional capacity encompasses many different areas and is influenced by numerous factors, including the following:

- Personal factors (such as gender, race, age, coping styles, and past experience)
- Social and family relationships and social support
- Socioeconomic status
- Culture
- Environment (physical, social, and political)
- Activities (including those related to daily living, recreation, school, and work)
- Goals of the individual

The extent to which a health condition is "disabling" depends on the interplay between the condition and the factors listed previously. Any alteration in functional capacity experienced with a health condition may not be so much a function of the condition itself as it is a function of elements in the environment. Individual reactions to health conditions vary considerably. The individual with a health condition who has associated alteration in function, for example, may not place as much importance on the condition and its associated features as do members of society.

Social groups establish their own standards with regard to idealized physical and emotional traits, roles, and responsibilities. Individuals with health conditions who do not fit the societal determined "norm" may find that, regardless of their strengths and abilities, society as a whole focuses more on the limitations and "disability" associated with the condition rather than focusing on "ability" and what an individual is actually able to do.

People vary in terms of their personal resources, such as their tolerance of manifestations of a health condition, functional capacity, general ability to cope, and social supports. Consequently, each individual must be considered in the context of all aspects of his or her life, and specifically in terms of the capacity to function within the environment.

Functional capacity goes beyond specific tasks and activities—it also includes significant events and relationships with family, friends, employers, and casual acquaintances. No relationship exists in isolation. Just as individuals' reactions to their health condition influences the reactions of others, so the reactions of others affect individuals' self-concept and perception of their own strengths and abilities.

Participation in family, social, and work events assumes interaction and the capacity to perform a variety of activities. As interactions or capacities change, or as they become limited or restricted, alterations in roles and relationships may also occur. Although some changes and adjustments may be made with relative ease, other changes can have repercussions in many areas of daily life.

The meaning and importance that individuals and their families attach to these associated changes influence their ability to accept the condition and to make necessary adjustments. The health condition itself is merely one factor that determines an individual's ability to function effectively.

DISEASE AND ILLNESS VERSUS HEALTH CONDITION

Words are powerful conveyers of concepts. Using a standard definition of terms facilitates communication and understanding of what each term implies. The term *disease* is derived from the *medical model*, which refers directly to changes in structure or function of body systems and focuses on treatment and elimination of symptoms. The term *illness* refers to individuals' perception of manifestations of their condition and how they and their families respond to it (Morof Lubkin & Larsen, 2002).

The *biopsychosocial model*, which is the basis of the *International Classification of Functioning, Disability, and Health* (ICF), defines *health conditions* by focusing on how biological, psychological, and social factors in combination interact to determine functional capacity. Professionals working with individuals experiencing chronic illness or disability must understand manifestations, functional ability, and progression of a health condition to better understand individuals' experience and to support their ability to achieve optimal functional capacity. Insight into the nature of each individual's health condition helps guide professionals in assessments and interventions as well as in understanding each individual's functional capacity and general experience (Dudgeon, 2002). It is also important for professionals to have insights into individuals' perception of their condition, the personal relevance and meaning that the condition has for them, and their goals so that interventions can be directed toward meeting individual needs and goals (Shaw, Segal, Polatajkos, & Harburn, 2002).

There must be an understanding of the individual's strengths, resources, and abilities, as well as how these attributes affect functional capacity. Professionals should possess an understanding of personal factors, activities, and social and physical environments to effectively assess how the condition will affect an individual's daily life and goals in relationship to functional ability at home, at work, and in the community.

TERMINOLOGY

Although understanding the experience of the individual in regard to his or her health condition is crucial, understanding terms and concepts utilized by the medical community as a whole is also important to facilitate communication and avoid misinterpretation. Two key concepts that influence the management of a health condition by medical personnel are *acute* and *chronic*. **Acute** refers to sudden onset of symptoms that are short term in nature and affect functional capacity on a temporary basis. **Chronic** refers to symptoms that last indefinitely and are attributed to a cause that may or may not be able to be identified. Some conditions begin acutely but are not resolved, thus becoming ongoing and chronic.

When health conditions are chronic, depending on the nature of the condition and the circumstances, *activities* and *participation* may be affected, and changes in activities may be needed to accommodate manifestations of the condition. In some instances, if manifestations of the condition progress or as other personal, social, or environmental factors change, accommodations may be needed to manage the condition. The course of a health condition over time, plus actions taken by individuals and their families to manage or shape the course of the condition, is called a *trajectory* (Corbin, 2001). This concept is important to professionals working with individuals with health conditions because it implies a continuum and emphasizes the social and environmental effects of the condition.

The *course* of the condition refers to the nature or stages of the condition. Some conditions are classified as *stable*, meaning that the condition is being managed, manifestations of the condition are not progressing, and the health status of the individual is not deteriorating. In other instances, conditions are known as *progressive*, meaning that manifestations of the condition continue to progress, while health and functional capacity continue to decline. Other conditions are classified as *episodic*, meaning that manifestations may not always be present, but flare up occasionally. The term *degenerative* refers to conditions characterized by continuing breakdown of structure or function. Some conditions have periods of **exacerbations** (periods when manifestations become worse) and periods of **remissions** (periods of time when symptoms remain stable or do not progress).

The course of a health condition can have a major influence on individuals' experience of the condition as well as on their functional capacity. For instance, individuals who have a progressive condition have continuing adaptation and adjustment as their health and function continue to decline, whereas individuals with a stable condition may have an initial period of adjustment but no ongoing functional loss.

STRESS IN HEALTH CONDITIONS

Change is an unavoidable part of life. Change of job, change of home, change of family composition, or changes brought about through the normal aging process are all events that everyone experiences. Depending on individuals' perceptions and the circumstances involved, change may be positive or negative. Whether positive or negative, change requires some adjustment or adaptation, which produces a certain degree of stress.

Health conditions can produce significant change—and consequently stress associated with both physical imbalance and psychological turmoil as individuals adjust to changes in customary lifestyle, loss of control, disruption of physiological processes, pain or discomfort, and potential change of role, status, independence, and financial stability. When individuals have confidence in their ability to maintain control over their destiny, and when they believe that changes—although inevitable—are manageable, stress is less pronounced. When individuals perceive changes associated with a health condition as insurmountable or beyond their ability to cope, stress can be overwhelming.

Causes of Stress with Health Conditions

The degree of stress associated with health conditions is often related to the degree of threat it represents to individuals. Potential threats posed by health conditions can include the following:

- Threats to life and physical well-being
- Threats to body integrity and comfort as a result of the illness or disability itself, diagnostic procedures, or treatment
- Threats to independence, privacy, autonomy, and control
- Threats to self-concept and fulfillment of customary roles
- Threats to life goals and future plans
- Threats to relationships with family, friends, and colleagues
- Threats to the ability to remain in familiar surroundings
- Threats to economic well-being

In addition to threats associated with health conditions, another source of stress may be the individual's perception of the meaning or purpose of his or her life. If individuals feel that their life has no meaning or that they have already fulfilled their purpose, the stress experienced may be quite different from that experienced by individuals with the same condition who believe they still have a significant role and purpose to fulfill.

Responses to stresses associated with health conditions depend on individuals' perceptions of the impact the condition has on various areas of their life as well as on their capacity to cope. Stress cannot easily be quantified, but it can be interpreted through behaviors or actions. When demands exceed psychological, social, or financial resources, stress may be manifested through a variety of behaviors, such as nonadherence with recommended management strategies, self-destructive behaviors such as substance abuse, and emotional reactions such as irritability, hostility, or depression.

Reactions to and stress related to health conditions are highly individualized. In other words, individuals with the same health condition do not necessarily experience the same degree of stress. The amount of change or adjustment required with a health condition is not necessarily an indicator of the amount of stress an individual experiences. Individuals who are able to adapt and cope effectively and mobilize resources are more successful in managing stress and achieving more stable outcomes than those who have few resources and limited coping skills.

Coping

Coping is not a single entity but rather an individualized constellation of many acts that are constantly changing. Coping skills are learned and developed over time as a way to manage, tolerate, or reduce stress associated with significant life events and to restore psychological equilibrium. Everyone develops a variety of coping skills through life experiences, although each individual relies on a predominant coping style to reduce anxiety and restore equilibrium when confronted with a stressful situation. Coping is manifested through behavior. Coping is *effective* and *adaptive* when it helps individuals reduce stress and enhance potential. It is *ineffective* and *maladaptive* when it inhibits growth or potential or when it contributes to physical or mental deterioration.

Coping skills may be required when individuals first learn about a new health condition, as well as for managing subsequent events associated with that condition. Health conditions that are progressive and accompanied by compounding, ongoing changes in functional capacity necessitate continuing coping and adjustment.

Individuals cope with health conditions in different ways. Some cope by actively confronting their condition, learning new skills, and becoming proactive in management of their health condition. Others defend themselves from stress and the realities of the condition by denying the seriousness of the health condition, ignoring recommendations for management, or refusing to learn new skills or behaviors to enhance functional ability. Still others cope by engaging in self-destructive behavior, such as actively continuing behavior that has detrimental effects on their health status.

Effective coping enables individuals to attain emotional equilibrium, to achieve a positive mental outlook, and to avoid incapacitation from fear, anxiety, anger, or depression. Effective coping must be viewed in the context of each individual's personal background and experiences, life situation, and perception of his or her own circumstances.

Coping strategies that have worked successfully for individuals in the past are more likely to be used in the future. When old strategies are no longer effective or are not appropriate to the new situation, individuals may implement new coping strategies to neutralize stress and adjust to associated changes.

Coping, however, does not occur in a vacuum. The individual's social environment can facilitate or discourage effective coping. In general, an environment that helps individuals gain a sense of control through active participation in decision making and take responsibility for their own destiny as much as possible best enables them to cope effectively with their health condition.

Coping Strategies

Coping strategies are subconscious mechanisms used to cope with stress. Although coping strategies are useful to reduce anxiety and maintain balance and productivity, their overuse can also be detrimental. Examples of some common coping strategies include the following:

- Denial
- Regression
- Compensation
- Rationalization
- Diversion of feelings

Denial

Learning about a new health condition and its associated implications can be anxiety provoking. As a way to deal with anxiety, individuals may subconsciously use *denial* to negate the reality of the situation. Specifically, they may deny that they have the condition by forgoing management recommendations or by rejecting the implications of the condition. In the early stages of adjustment, denial may be beneficial, in that it enables individuals to adjust to the reality of their situation at their own pace, preventing excessive anxiety. When denial continues, however, it can interfere with adequate management of the condition or impede the process of learning new skills that would enhance functional capacity.

Depending on the nature of the health condition, an individual's denial of his or her condition can have a negative impact on others by placing them at risk. For example, if the health condition has an infectious component—as is true for tuberculosis and HIV—individuals in denial may avoid use of proper precautions to prevent the spread of the condition to others. In other situations, individuals may put others in jeopardy by denying limitations in function, such as by continuing to drive even though they are legally blind.

Regression

Regression is a coping strategy in which individuals subconsciously revert to an earlier stage of development, so that they become more dependent, behave more passively, or exhibit more emotionality than would normally be expected at their developmental level. In the acute or early stages of a health condition, returning to a state of dependency experienced in an earlier stage of development can be helpful, especially if management of the condition requires rest and inactivity. When individuals remain in a regressive mode, however, it can interfere with their adjustment and attainment of a level of independence that allows them to reach optimal functional capacity. For example, after a **myocardial infarction** (heart attack), individuals may be encouraged to walk several miles each day to increase their strength and endurance. Individuals continuing to cope with regression, however, may refuse to engage in strength and endurance activities that would enhance their functional capacity and instead remain inactive and dependent on others.

Compensation

Individuals using *compensation* as a coping strategy learn to counteract functional incapacitation in one area by becoming stronger or more proficient in another area. That is, when function is compromised in one area, individuals may find ways to excel in another sphere. Compensatory behavior is generally highly constructive when new behaviors are directed toward positive goals and outcomes. For example, individuals who are unable to maintain their level of activity because of physical manifestations associated with their condition may turn to creative writing or other means of self-expression. Compensation as a

coping strategy can be detrimental, however, if the new behaviors used in compensating for functional changes are self-destructive or socially unacceptable. For example, an individual who experiences disfigurement as a result of a health condition may become promiscuous as a way of compensating for his or her perception of physical unattractiveness.

Rationalization

As a coping strategy, *rationalization* enables individuals to find socially acceptable reasons for their behavior or to excuse themselves for not reaching goals or not accomplishing tasks. Although rationalization can soften the disappointment of dreams unrealized or goals not reached, it can also produce negative effects if it becomes a barrier to adjustment, prevents individuals from reaching their full potential, or interferes with effective management of the health condition itself. For example, an individual with visual impairment who is a student may rationalize that he or she failed the test because of the difficulty with vision rather than admitting that the test failure occurred because he or she went to the beach with friends rather than studying.

Diversion of Feelings

One of the most positive and constructive of all coping strategies can be the *diversion* of unacceptable feelings or ideas into socially acceptable behaviors. Individuals with health conditions may have particularly strong feelings of anger or hostility about their condition or the circumstances surrounding their condition. If their emotional energy can be redefined and diverted into positive activity, the coping strategy can be beneficial, making virtue out of necessity and transforming deficit into gain. As with all coping strategies, diversion of feelings can, however, have negative effects if anger or hostility is channeled into negative behaviors or socially unacceptable activities. For example, an individual with diabetes may have neglected to follow foot care precautions, which resulted in lower leg amputation. Rather than acknowledging self-anger, the individual may instead express hostility and blame toward family members.

POTENTIAL EMOTIONAL REACTIONS TO HEALTH CONDITIONS

Sudden, unexpected, or life-threatening situations related to health conditions can engender a variety of reactions. How individuals view their condition, its causes, and its implications greatly affects what they do in the face of it. They may view their condition as a challenge, an enemy to be fought, a punishment, a sign of weakness, a relief, a strategy for gaining attention, an irreparable loss, or an uplifting spiritual experience. Although emotional reactions vary both in type and in intensity, the following reactions are common. Each emotional reaction is discussed individually, but it is important to note that reactions are often experienced simultaneously.

Grief

Grieving is a natural reaction to loss, albeit one that is dependent on the meaning of the experience to the individual. What is perceived as a loss by one individual may be perceived as a hidden blessing by another. Assumptions regarding the meaning or degree of loss to an individual cannot be made, nor can assumptions be made regarding how, how long, or whether an individual will go through a grieving process. Although health conditions can involve what would appear to be a variety of associated losses, including changes in body composition, function, role, or social status, which could result in a reaction of grief, perceptions of loss and reactions to it are highly individualized.

Some individuals may have an initial reaction to a new health condition and associated implications of shock, disbelief, or numbness; others may accept the loss with little reaction. Whether an initial grieving period is experienced or not, after a period of adaptation, many individuals begin to accept changes resulting from the condition, and make adjustments and adaptations that are necessary to reestablish their place within the everyday world.

In some instances the grief reaction is prolonged, and individuals may develop a pathological grief reaction, which may interfere with functional ability more than the health condition itself.

Fear and Anxiety

Individuals naturally become anxious when confronted with a threat. Health conditions can pose a threat because of the potential loss of function, loss of love, loss of independence, or loss of financial security. Some individuals fear the unknown or unpredictability of the condition, which provokes anxiety. For others, hospitalizations that immerse them in a strange and unfamiliar environment away from home, family, and the security of routine produce anxiety. When conditions are life threatening, fear and anxiety may be associated not only with loss of function, but also with loss of life. Fear and anxiety associated with health conditions may render some individuals psychologically immobile and unable to act.

Assisting individuals to regain a sense of control over their situation through information and shared decision making can be an important step in reducing anxiety and facilitating rehabilitation. Note, however, that fear experienced by individuals may have both rational and irrational aspects. Fear and anxiety are oftentimes future oriented, having to do with perceptions of what could occur rather than being based on what is actually known in the present.

Anger

Individuals with health conditions may experience anger at themselves or at others for perceived injustices or loss associated with their condition. They may believe that their condition was caused by negligence or that their condition could have been avoided. If they perceive themselves as victims, anger may be directed toward the persons or circumstances they blame for the condition or situation. If they believe that their own actions were partly to blame for the health condition, anger may be directed inward.

Anger can also be the result of frustration. Individuals may vent their frustration and anger by displacing hostility toward others, even when those parties have no relationship to the development of the health condition and no influence over its outcome. Anger may also be an expression of the realization of the seriousness of the situation and associated feelings of helplessness. At times, anger may not be openly expressed, but rather hidden in quarreling, arguing, complaining, or being excessively demanding, in an attempt to gain some control. Helping individuals express anger in appropriate ways and enabling them to regain a sense of control over their situation can help to resolve anger that would otherwise be detrimental to successful rehabilitation.

Depression

Some individuals may experience feelings of depression after they realize the implications of their condition (Katon et al., 2010). They may express feelings of helplessness and hopelessness, apathy, or feelings of dejection and discouragement. Signs of depression include sleep disturbances, changes in appetite, difficulty concentrating, and withdrawal from activity. Not all individuals with health conditions experience significant depression, and, in those who do, depression may not be prolonged. The extent to which and whether depression is experienced vary from person to person. Prolonged or unresolved depression can result in self-destructive behaviors, such as substance abuse or attempted suicide. Individuals with prolonged depression should be referred for mental health evaluation and treatment.

Guilt

Guilt can be described as self-criticism or blame. Individuals or family members may feel guilty if they believe they contributed to, or in some way caused, the health condition. For instance, individuals who develop lung cancer or emphysema after years of tobacco use or those who experienced a spinal cord injury owing to an accident that occurred because they were driving while intoxicated, may experience guilt because of the role they played in the development of their condition. In other instances, they may experience guilt because they believe their health condition places a burden on their family or because they are unable to fulfill former roles. Still other scenarios of guilt include the concept of survivor guilt, in which an individual survives a situation when others in the same situation did not. For example, an individual who, although sustaining severe injuries, survives a tornado when none

of his or her family members did may experience intense guilt, questioning why he or she survived when other family members perished.

Family members may also experience guilt because of feelings of anger or resentment they have toward the individual. Guilt may also be associated with blame if family members believe the individual is actively to blame for his or her health condition. For instance, if an individual develops cirrhosis of the liver due to heavy alcohol use, but had been told previously to reduce alcohol consumption because of impending liver failure, family members may actively blame the individual for his or her condition, causing the person to experience more guilt.

Guilt may be expressed or unexpressed and can occur in varying dimensions. It can be an obstacle to successful adjustment to the condition and its implications. Self-blame or blame ascribed by others is detrimental not only to the individual's self-concept but also to rehabilitative efforts as a whole. Guilt that affects rehabilitation potential or well-being is an indication that referral to appropriate professionals for evaluation and treatment may be appropriate.

DEVELOPMENTAL STAGES

Development is neither static nor finite but rather a continuous process from infancy to old age and death. Each developmental stage is associated with certain age-appropriate behaviors, skills, and developmental tasks, which allow for psychological and cognitive transitions from one stage to another. Individuals' age and developmental stage influence their reactions to chronic illness or disability and the problems and consequences they experience.

Each developmental stage of life has its own particular stresses or demands, apart from those experienced as a result of a specific health condition. A health condition at various stages of development can influence the independence and self-control associated with the developmental stages and can impede development of qualities and life skills associated with different developmental stages. The needs, responsibilities, and resources of adults differ from those of children;

as a consequence, the impact of a health condition in later years is different from the impact of a health condition experienced in young adulthood.

Family members and others generally adjust their behavior to accommodate and appropriately interact with individuals as they pass from one developmental stage to the next. When individuals experience a health condition, however, others may modify expectations of age-appropriate behavior. These modified expectations may then interfere with the individual's mastery of the skills required to meet the challenges of future developmental stages.

All aspects of development are related, so each developmental stage must be understood within the context of the individual's past and current experiences. Individuals with a health condition must be considered in the context of their particular developmental stage and the way in which the changes associated with their condition influence attitudes, perceptions, actions, and behaviors characteristic of their stage of development. Individuals' stage of development serves as a guideline not only in assessing their functional capacity but also in determining potential stressors and reactions.

Problems and stresses at different developmental stages are similar whether or not individuals have a specific health condition. Although no clear lines of demarcation separate life stages, and all individuals certainly develop at different rates, some commonalities are nevertheless associated with different life stages.

Ideally, those with a specific health condition should be encouraged to progress through each stage of development as naturally as possible, despite their condition. Individuals whose emotional, social, educational, or occupational development has been thwarted may be more incapacitated by their inability to cope with the subsequent challenges of life than by any limitations experienced because of illness or disability per se.

Childhood

Although the majority of children with a specific health condition and their families adapt successfully, children with a health condition are at increased risk of emotional and behavioral disorders

(Gledhill, Rangel, & Garralda, 2000). In early life, children develop a sense of trust in others, a sense of autonomy, and an awareness and mastery of their environment. During these years, they begin to learn communication and social skills that enable them to interact effectively with others. They also learn that limits are set on their explorations, expressions of autonomy, and behaviors. Important to their development is a balance between encouraging initiative and setting limits consistently.

A health condition in childhood can impede attainment of developmental goals. Repeated or prolonged hospitalizations may deprive children of nurturing by a consistent and loving caregiver. Physical incapacity associated with the condition or management issues may prevent regular activities, socialization, and exploration of the environment. In some cases, overly protective family members may restrict activities or prohibit the child from displaying typical emotional expression. In other instances, overly sympathetic parents may condone inappropriate behaviors rather than correct them.

Conditions affecting development of communication skills may also affect children's interaction with the environment as well as their future development. *Developmental disabilities* (conditions present at birth or occurring during childhood) require adjustments throughout individuals' development. Any incapacity associated with such a developmental disability must be confronted and compensated for with every new aspect of development. Maintaining awareness of developmental needs and facilitating experiences that foster development will enhance children's ability to reach their maximal potential.

For most children, entering school expands their world beyond the scope of their family. Before children attend school, the values, rules, and expectations that they experience are, for the most part, largely those expressed within the family. When they enter school, however, they are exposed to a larger social environment. Not only do they learn social relationships and cooperative interactions but they also begin to develop a sense of initiative and industry. Children gradually become aware of their special strengths. As new skills begin to develop, school-aged children gain the capacity for sustained effort that eventually results in the ability to follow through with tasks to completion. The approval and encouragement of others and acceptance by their peers help children to build self-confidence, further enhancing development.

When children with a health condition enter school, they may not need special education placement, but they may require coordinated school interventions to maximize attendance and facilitate educational and social growth. Children with a health condition may experience school-related problems reflected in their psychological well-being, interactions with other children, or academic performance. When physical or cognitive incapacities affect children's ability to perform skills usually valued at this developmental stage, acceptance by peers may be affected. School attendance may be disrupted by the need for repeated absences, resulting in an inability to interact on a consistent basis within the peer group, which in turn may diminish social interactions.

In an attempt to shield the child from hurt and emotional pain, family members may further isolate the child from social interactions, creating the potential for reduced self-confidence. Reluctance of sympathetic family members to allow the child to participate in activities in which the child may experience failure can interfere with the child's ability to accurately evaluate his or her potential. Encouragement of social interactions and activities to the greatest degree possible allows the child the opportunity to develop the skills and abilities that are needed for later integration into the larger world.

Adolescence

Adolescence, as a period of transition between childhood and adulthood, is a unique developmental period that can influence future health and development. Chronic illness or disability may affect the adolescent's development, or the adolescent's stage of development may affect the adolescent's health condition (Katzman & Neinstein, 2016). Perceptions of and interactions with peers become increasingly important as adolescents further define their identity apart from membership in their family. With the need to establish independence, adolescents begin to emancipate themselves from their parents and may rebel against the authority of parents or others. Physical maturation brings a strong preoccupation with the body and appearance. Adolescents' need to identify themselves as someone attractive to others often becomes paramount. Awareness of and experimentation with sexual feelings present a new dimension with which the adolescent must learn to cope. Dating and expression of sexuality are important aspects of maturation. Any alteration in physical appearance caused by the health condition can influence adolescents' perception of body image and self-concept, thereby thwarting expression of sexual feelings.

Adolescents with a health condition may be at risk for secondary incapacities associated with psychosocial factors. A health condition during adolescence can disrupt relationships with peers, resulting in delayed social and emotional development. Alterations experienced because of the condition, its treatment, or sympathetic and protective reactions by family members may emerge as barriers to the adolescent's attainment of independence and individual identity. Parents may be overprotective to the point of infantilizing the adolescent, which decreases the youth's self-esteem and self-confidence.

In the attempt to become independent, regular characteristics of adolescent development, such as rebellion against authority or the need to be accepted by a peer group, may sometimes interfere with management of the health condition. If adolescents deny alterations associated with their health condition or ignore management recommendations, such behavior can have further detrimental effects on physical and functional capacity.

Young Adulthood

In young adulthood, individuals establish themselves as productive members of society, integrating vocational goals, developing the capacity for intimate relationships, and accepting social responsibility. When a health condition occurs during this stage of the development, associated manifestations—rather than interests or abilities of individuals—may define social, vocational, and occupational goals.

Physical manifestations may also inhibit individuals' efforts to build intimate relationships or to maintain relationships that they have already established. At this developmental stage, established relationships are likely to be recent, and the level of commitment and willingness to make necessary sacrifices may vary. Depending on the nature of the condition, procreation may be difficult or impossible. If the individual already has young children, childcare issues may be the source of additional concerns in light of the functional incapacities inherent in a specific health condition. Young adults who had not fully gained independence or left their family of origin at the time of the onset of the health condition may find gaining independence subsequent to the health condition's emergence more difficult. In some cases, the family's overprotectiveness may prevent individuals from having experiences appropriate to their own age group.

Middle Age

Individuals in middle age are generally established in their careers, have committed relationships, and are often providing guidance to their own children as they leave the family to establish their own careers and families. At the same time, middle-aged individuals may be assuming greater responsibility for their own aging parents, who may be becoming increasingly fragile and dependent. During middle age, individuals may begin to reassess their goals and relationships as they begin to recognize their own mortality and limited remaining time.

A health condition during middle age can interfere with further occupational development and even result in early retirement. Such changes can have a significant impact on the economic well-being of individuals and their families, as well as on individuals' identity, self-concept, and self-esteem. It may be necessary to alter established roles and associated responsibilities within the family. At the same time, individuals' partners, even when the relationship is a long-term one, may be reevaluating their own life goals. They may perceive a health condition as a violation of their own well-being and may choose to leave the relationship. Responsibilities for children and aging parents add more financial and emotional stress to that experienced as a result of a health condition.

Older Adulthood

Ideally, older adults have adapted to the triumphs and disappointments of life and have accepted their own life and imminent death. Although physical manifestations associated with aging are variable, older adults may experience diminished physical strength and stamina, as well as diminishing visual and hearing acuity. A health condition during older adulthood can impose physical or cognitive incapacities in addition to those caused by aging. The spouse or significant others of the same age group may also have decreased physical stamina, making physical care of individuals with a health condition more difficult. When older adults with a health condition are unable to attend to their own needs or when care in the home is unmanageable, they may find it necessary to change their lifestyle and move to another environment for care and supervision. Many individuals in the older age group live on fixed retirement incomes, so the additional expenses associated with a health condition may place a strain on an already tight budget. Not all older individuals, of course, have retirement benefits, savings, or other resources to draw on in times of financial need.

SELF-CONCEPT AND SELF-ESTEEM

Self-concept is tied to self-esteem and personal identity and includes individuals' perceptions and beliefs about their own strengths and weaknesses, as well as others' perceptions of them. *Self-esteem* can be defined as "the evaluative component of an individual's self-concept" (Corwyn, 2000, p. 357). It is often thought of as individuals' assessment of their own self-worth with regard to attained qualities and performance (Gledhill et al., 2000).

Self-concept influences the perceptions of others about an individual. A negative self-concept can produce negative responses in others, just as a positive self-concept can increase the likelihood that others will react in a positive manner. Individuals' self-esteem is related to their self-concept as well as to how others respond to them. Consequently, self-concept has a significant impact on interactions with others and the psychological well-being of the individual.

Social Identity

Social identity refers to an individual's self-concept that is derived from perceived membership in a social group (Tajfel & Turner, 1986). Depending on the social context, individuals may have different social identities at different levels according to their internalized perception of group membership. For example, an individual may identify himself or herself as a medical student but may also identify himself or herself as a member of the Young Republicans or Young Democrats, or according to an ethnic group, such as Native American. Group membership involves defining the self in terms of characteristics of the group rather than as an individual. Group membership can be an aspect of self-concept and can provide grounds for group comparisons. The more individuals view group membership as central to their self-definition, the stronger their social identity with the group (Haslam, 2001).

Social identity can influence how individuals think, act, and feel based on their perception of group inclusion or exclusion. If an individual views a group positively, his or her perception of inclusion in the group can boost self-esteem. Conversely, perceptions of exclusion from the group can have the opposite effect. Likewise, if an individual perceives a group negatively but identifies as part of the group, the person's self-esteem can be negatively affected.

Body Image

Body image, which is an important part of self-concept, involves individuals' mental view of their body with regard to appearance, sexuality, and ability to perform various physical tasks. It is influenced by bodily sensations, social and cultural expectations, and reactions of and experiences with others (White, 2000). Body image is influenced by each individual's personal conception of attractiveness, which is also determined by social and cultural influences and is related to both self-concept and self-esteem.

Body image is influenced by biological, cultural, social, and historical factors. It changes over time as alteration of appearance, capabilities, functional status, and social role occurs over the life cycle.

Individuals' perceptions of their body are associated with more than cosmetic concerns; they also influence individuals' general health, personal relationships and intimacy, and general well-being (Biordi et al., 2002).

Health conditions may modify body image by requiring an alteration of self-view to accommodate the associated changes. The following factors influence the degree of alteration:

- Visibility of the change
- Functional significance of the change
- Speed with which the change occurred
- Importance of the physical change or associated functional limitations to the individual
- Reactions of others

(de Moore, Hennessey, Kunz, Ferrando, & Rabkin, 2000)

Body image is a reflection of individuals' image of themselves and how they believe others see them. Individuals' feelings and thoughts about their body image influence not only social relationships but also psychological characteristics and perceptions of the world. The degree to which the alteration of self-view is perceived by the individual in a negative way influences social and intrapersonal interactions, functional capacity, and success or failure in the workplace (Cusack, 2000).

The extent to which individuals incorporate change into their body image also depends on the meaning and significance of the change to the particular individual. The degree of physical change or disfigurement is not always proportional to the reaction it provokes. Indeed, a change considered minimal by one individual may be considered catastrophic by another.

Changes do not have to be visible to alter body image. Burn scars on parts of the body normally covered by clothing or the introduction of an artificial opening or stoma such as with colostomy, for example, may cause significant alteration in body image even though physical changes are not readily apparent to others.

The concept of body image is complex and individually determined. Body image incorporates not only the way individuals perceive themselves but also the way they perceive others as seeing them. Negative views of body image can be a barrier to psychological well-being, social interactions, functional capacity, and workplace adjustment. Consequently, the ultimate goal is to help individuals adapt to changes brought about by chronic illness or disability, integrating changes into a restructured body image that can be assimilated and incorporated into daily life.

Stigma

Stigma is a socially constructed concept that is a universal phenomenon and has evolved throughout history. This concept is generally associated with individual feelings of shame due to disapproval of others and guilt resulting from being discredited or devalued by others. Stigma may preclude an individual's full social acceptance. The degree of stigma varies from setting to setting, and from person to person. Although the concept of stigma is universal, it is socially constructed. As a consequence, a number of factors within different societies as well as within different cultures may modify what is considered stigmatizing.

Overall, stigma is related to what a certain society considers to be deviations from the norm in a number of different areas. These areas are defined by societally determined categories, which include those attributes, characteristics, and behaviors that individuals exhibit in each category. Because these categories are based on the expectations of the majority, they define what is considered acceptable or the norm based on majority standards. Categories may include age, race, gender, ethnic background or nationality, religion, occupation, or social roles. Individuals who meet the expectations of the majority regarding appearance, behavior, or group association are generally accepted and valued. In contrast, individuals who deviate from the expectations of the majority regarding what is acceptable in these categories are labeled as different from the majority and, therefore, less desirable. Thus individuals deviating from these expectations are often stigmatized. Because stigma is socially defined, it can vary from setting to setting, depending on the views of the majority. What is stigmatizing in one setting may not be stigmatizing in another venue.

Most stigmas are viewed as anxiety provoking and threatening to others. For example, older adults are often stigmatized because aging is a reminder of mortality and vulnerability. Individuals from different ethnic backgrounds, nationalities, or religions may be stigmatized because of lack of understanding by the majority of the meanings of traditions or beliefs in different groups. Individuals with HIV/AIDS are often stigmatized based on moral judgments. Likewise, individuals with health conditions often experience stigma owing to negative value judgments. Stigma results in discrimination, social isolation, disregard, depreciation, devaluation, and, in some instances, threats to safety and well-being.

The power of stigma may overshadow the positive characteristics of individuals who experience stigma. Individuals who are stigmatized may find it difficult to overcome the negative social reactions of others regardless of their positive attributes. For example, individuals with psychiatric disability may face continued stereotypes and prejudices regarding psychiatric disability regardless of their level of success in the workplace or community (Lyons & Ziviani, 1995).

Individuals with health conditions continue to experience stigma. Modern society's emphasis on youth, attractiveness, self-sufficiency, and productivity contribute to the tendency to devalue those who are perceived as deviating from these valued characteristics (Saylor, Yoder, & Mann, 2002). Stigma can have a profound effect on the ability to regain and maintain functional capacity and on the individual's acceptance of his or her health condition. Gender and race or ethnic background may be secondary sources of prejudice and subsequent stigma, causing additional stress and creating additional barriers to effective functioning (Nosek & Hughes, 2003).

Stigma affects not only the individual but also members of his or her family. Family members may experience social isolation and prejudice because of their association with the individual. Family members' ability to cope with their family member's health condition may be severely compromised by societal stigma. If there are unresolved family problems, societal stigma may merely exacerbate shame and guilt they may already feel.

Stigma has an impact on individuals' self-concept and self-esteem and can produce barriers that prohibit them from achieving their maximal potential. In an effort to avoid stigma, individuals may deny, minimize, or ignore their condition or management recommendations. If the condition is not readily discernible, hiding the health condition may be more easily accomplished. As time goes by and the individual's attempt to hide the condition becomes reinforced, he or she may become proficient in concealing the health condition so as to reduce the associated stigma. Although stigma may be reduced, pretending not to have the condition can become detrimental. Not only can denial interfere with needed management of the condition, but it may also delay acceptance and adjustment (Saylor et al., 2002).

Although efforts to reduce or obliterate stigma in society should continue, stigma is most likely to be overcome through positive interactions with individuals. It is possible to reduce negative implications of societal stigma through public education programs and by helping individuals establish a sense of their own intrinsic worth.

Uncertainty

Uncertainty in the lives of individuals with a health conditions can exist for a variety of reasons but is often related to concerns about an unknown future, the erratic nature of manifestations of the condition, the unpredictability of progression of the condition, or the ambiguity of manifestations. Some health conditions have immediate and permanent effects on functional capacity; in other cases, the course of the health condition is more variable. Deterioration may occur slowly over the span of several years or rapidly within months. Some conditions have periods of remission, when manifestations become less noticeable or almost nonexistent, only to be followed by periods of unpredictable exacerbation, when manifestations become worse. In some cases, the same condition progresses at different rates for different individuals—progressing rapidly for some, but slowly for others. With some conditions, it is difficult to determine when or whether the condition will reach the point of severe incapacitation or whether a dramatic change of functional capacity will take place.

Uncertainty of outcome or progression of the condition can make planning and prediction of the future difficult and can sometimes render an individual immobile. The unpredictability of health conditions can be frustrating for both affected individuals and those around them. There may be reluctance to plan for the future at all, so that inability to predict the future becomes more incapacitating than the actual physical manifestations of the condition itself. In other instances, given the unpredictability of their condition, individuals may elect to follow a different life course than they would have otherwise chosen. Decisions not to have children, to cut down on the number of hours spent in the work environment, or to suddenly relocate to a different part of the country may be misinterpreted by those unaware of the individual's condition or its associated unpredictability. For those persons having conditions in which manifestations or residual effects are unapparent to others, such decisions may be met with misunderstanding or criticism. Criticism of such decisions may be particularly distressing to individuals who do not wish to disclose or share intimate details of their condition with the casual observer.

Insecurity about the course of the condition may also be reflected by the attitudes of those closest to the individual, who, in an attempt to protect the person from potential future loss, withdraw emotional interactions or support. Uncertainty about progression of a condition imposes particular challenges on individuals and their families and can be a source of stress. Emphasizing the importance of living in the present, rather than dwelling on events that may or may not occur in the future, can help to reduce the amount of stress and anxiety experienced as well as enhance the quality of life currently experienced.

INVISIBLE HEALTH CONDITIONS

Some chronic illnesses or disabilities have associated physical changes that can be objectively assessed by others or have functional implications that necessitate the use of adaptive devices. The *visibility* of a condition has often been associated with stigmatization and marginality (Livneh & Wilson, 2003). Some conditions, such as diabetes or cardiac conditions, have no outward signs that alert casual observers to individuals' health status. The term *invisible condition* is used to refer to these conditions. Because there are no outward physical signs or other cues to indicate limitations associated with the condition, others have no basis on which to alter expectations with regard to individuals' functional capacity. Although this lack of reaction can be positive (in the sense that it prevents actions by others that are based on prejudice or stereotypes), it can also be negative in the sense that it can enable individuals to deny or avoid acceptance of their condition and its associated implications.

The degree to which a condition remains invisible may be a function of the closeness of the observer's association with the individual. Although casual acquaintances might not notice manifestations or alterations associated with the condition, those more closely involved with the individual in day-to-day activities may more readily observe them. Other conditions under regular circumstances may offer no visible signs or cues, no matter how close the association with the individual.

The unapparent aspect of manifestations in invisible disability may be a unique element related to individuals' adjustment and acceptance of those manifestations and resulting alterations that are needed. Without environmental feedback to create a tangible reality of the condition, individuals with an invisible condition may postpone adaptation or ignore management recommendations necessary for regulating the condition and prevention of further manifestations.

Sexuality

Human sexuality is more than genital acts or sexual function; it is intrinsic to a person's sense of self. It is an ever-changing, lived experience, affecting the way individuals view themselves and their bodies (Hordern & Currow, 2003). Sexuality encompasses the whole person and is reflected in all of the individual's behavior. It is an important part of identity, self-image, and self-concept (Brodwin & Frederick, 2010). Each person is a sexual being with a need for intimacy, physical contact, and love. The effects of health conditions on sexuality are multifactorial and can affect all phases of sexual response (McInnes, 2003).

Expression of sexual urges is one form of sexuality. Health conditions can affect sexual expression through physical manifestations, depression, lack of energy, pain, alterations in self-image, or the reactions of others. In some conditions, the main barrier to sexual expression may be issues of self-concept and body image; with other conditions, physical changes may present physical barriers that affect sexual function directly. In other instances, attitudes of others or of society as a whole can be a major barrier to sexual expression. For example, although there has been increased acceptance of expression of sexuality by adults with intellectual disability, sexual expression that includes marriage or desire to start a family remains contentious (Cuskelly & Bryde, 2004).

Regardless of the types of alterations associated with a health condition, sexual expression remains an important part of function that should be addressed (McBride & Rines, 2000). In some instances, it may be necessary to help individuals overcome their own misperceptions and fears to establish a means for sexual expression. In other instances, individuals may need assistance to overcome barriers or to learn methods of sexual expression different from those used previously. In any case, sexual adjustment is a significant element in the restoration of an individual's optimal functional capacity.

FAMILY ADAPTATION

Family is the social network from which individuals derive identity and with which individuals feel strong psychological bonds. Family has different meanings for different people and is not always defined based on blood relationships or law. Family provides protection, socialization, physical care, support, and love. Each individual within the family structure plays some role that is incorporated into everyday family function.

Health conditions have both emotional and economic impacts on families as well as on individuals. Family reactions to a health condition may be similar to those experienced by the individual and may include shock, denial, anger, guilt, anxiety, and depression. Families must make adaptations, adjustments, and role changes both as a unit and as individual family members. The way in which families react and adapt to a health condition will influence affected individuals' subsequent adjustment. Whether families foster independence or dependence, show acceptance or rejection, or encourage or sabotage adherence with alterations and management recommendations has profound effects on individuals' ultimate functional capacity.

Specific issues for families when a family member develops a health condition are loss related to family functioning and loss related to functioning of the individual. There may be a strong desire to be a "normal" family again. Family members' prior expectations for the individual's future or "what might have been" may lead them to experience anger, resentment, or disappointment if they see the health condition as interfering with achievement of their expectations.

Family members can also act as advocates for the individual. They may need to become more involved with health professionals and service agencies or become increasingly assertive to obtain necessary services. If individuals with a health condition require significant care or interventions to be administered at home, family members may become fatigued because of the extra responsibility and tasks required, especially if respite services are limited.

Families, like individuals, have differing resources, depending on life circumstances, previous experiences, and the personalities involved. Individual family members may be called upon to provide not only emotional support but also physical care, supervision, transportation, or a variety of other services necessitated by the individual's condition. In addition, changes of roles or financial circumstances due to a health condition may alter goals and plans of other family members, such as college plans of a sibling or early retirement plans of a parent. The amount of care and attention required by individuals with a health condition may create emotional strain among family members, resulting in feelings of resentment, antagonism, and frustration. Role change and ambiguity may make it necessary to redefine family relationships as new and unaccustomed duties and responsibilities arise.

QUALITY OF LIFE

Successful rehabilitation entails more than assisting individuals to reach their optimal functional capacity; it also means assisting individuals to achieve and enhance their quality of life. *Quality of life* is subjective in nature, with no universal meaning. No two people define the term in quite the same way. Although quality of life may be viewed by some as optimal functioning at the highest level of independence, others may place greater emphasis on life itself, regardless of level of function. Only the individual can determine the personal meaning of the quality of life. Individual value systems, cultural backgrounds, spiritual perspectives, and the attitudes and reactions of those within the environment all influence the interpretation of quality of life.

Each individual's situation and experience are unique. Perceptions of the same condition and its impact vary from individual to individual (Burker, Carels, Thompson, Rodgers, & Egan, 2000; Crews, Jefferson, Broshek, Barth, & Robbins, 2000). As a consequence, people with similar conditions, symptoms, and limitations may perceive their condition in totally different manners.

The perception of a health condition depends on characteristics of the condition and its management, the age and developmental stage of the affected individual, the degree and extent of alterations needed, and the manner in which manifestations of the condition affect the individual's definition of quality of life. Manifestations or alterations that one individual accepts and to which he or she adapts may be perceived as overwhelming and intolerable to another individual. The impact of a health condition on the overall quality of life often determines daily choices and day-to-day management of the condition.

Assessment of quality of life is made difficult by the ambiguous nature of the concept. Attempts to discover and accurately measure quality of life have caused considerable confusion and resulted in the development of multiple indicators. Indicators of quality of life have ranged from physiologic parameters, to the ability to return to work, to the ability to participate in social activities, to the number of psychological problems experienced by the individual. In addition, studies of quality of life have often identified discrepancies between the judgment of service providers and that of consumers regarding quality-of-life outcomes (Leplege & Hunt, 1997).

Individuals' perception of quality of life is one of the main determinants of demand for services, adherence with management recommendations, and satisfaction with services provided. How some individuals assess the impact of their condition on their quality of life is determined by the degree to which they feel they have control over their life circumstances or destiny. Accurate knowledge about their condition and its management, together with active participation in decision making about the management of the condition, can enable individuals with a health condition to make judgments that will enable them to enhance quality of life in terms of their own needs, goals, and circumstances.

ADHERENCE TO MANAGEMENT RECOMMENDATIONS

Most health conditions require ongoing management, monitoring, or alteration of activity to regulate the condition or to prevent complications. However, many individuals with a health condition fail to follow management recommendations, potentially imperiling their own well-being (Dunbar-Jacob et al., 2000; Graham, 2003). Neglecting to take medications as recommended, resisting alteration of activities, or engaging in behaviors that are likely to cause complications of the condition can significantly influence individuals' outcomes and functional capacity (Dolder, Lacro, Leckband, & Jeste, 2003; Schmaling, Afari, & Blume, 2000; Vergouwen, Bakker, Katon, Verheij, & Koerselman, 2003; Zygmunt, Olfson, Boyer, & Mechanic, 2002). The best rehabilitation plan is of little value if individuals do not follow management plans designed to regulate the condition or to prevent complications or progression from occurring (Kovac, Patel, Peterson, & Kimmel, 2002; Loghman-Adham, 2003).

Although individuals who purposely behave in a way that makes their condition worse seem irrational, a number of explanations for nonadherent behavior are possible. Health conditions elicit many responses from individuals and their families. Different reactions, experiences, and motives direct behavior and can help or hinder adherence to management recommendations.

Individuals' lives are guided by a set of standards and values—both expressed and unexpressed. Each individual has a personal, unique perspective on health, illness, and health care itself. Consequently, a remarkable difference in perceptions of and reactions to apparently similar health conditions is possible. The meaning of a health condition and the significance ascribed to adherence to management recommendations are based mainly on individuals' perceptions of the condition and its associated alterations as well as their perceptions of management recommendations and their implications. While some individuals react mildly to a condition that might devastate another person, others display substantial emotional and physical discomfort with conditions that most people would consider minor. Obviously, various psychosocial factors determine individuals' reactions to a health condition and, consequently, their reactions to the recommendations given.

Health conditions can disrupt the way an individual views his or her self and the world, and can produce distortions in thinking. Most individuals initially experience a feeling of vulnerability and a shattering of the magical belief that they are immune from illness, injury, or even death. With this realization, they may lose their sense of security and cohesiveness. Life may seem a maze of inconveniences, hazards, and alterations. Nonadherence to recommendations may be an attempt to exert self-determination, to regain a sense of autonomy and control, and to claim some mastery over individual destiny. In other instances, resistance to management recommendations may be a denial of the condition itself.

Nonadherence can also reflect the individual's feelings about his or her life circumstances. For some individuals, having a health condition is not a positive role; for others, it may be far preferable to the social role that they held previously. Some persons may vacillate between the wish to be independent and the wish to remain dependent. Health conditions can be a means of legitimizing dependency as well as a means of increasing the amount of attention received. Subsequently, an individual may be reluctant to return to his or her former roles and obligations. The motivation to retain the sick role is at times greater than the motivation to gain optimal function. As a result, rehabilitation may be hampered.

Failure to adhere to recommendations is sometimes a response to guilt that has been incorporated into the reaction to or beliefs about the health condition. If health and well-being are perceived as rewards for a life well lived, onset of a health condition may be viewed as punishment for real or imagined actions of the past. Adherence to management recommendations that helps to regulate the condition may be perceived as interference with a punishment believed to be deserved. In other instances, individuals may feel guilty because they believe that the health condition is a direct result of their own negligence or overt actions.

Guilt or shame at being different may also hinder adherence to management recommendations. Some individuals may attempt to hide their condition from others and, therefore, fail to follow recommendations that they fear may call attention to their condition.

The impact of a health condition on an individual's general economic well-being can also affect his or her ability and willingness to follow management recommendations. While many occupations offer fringe benefits, such as paid sick days or even time off with pay during which to seek health care, other occupations provide no such benefits. In the latter case, days taken off from work because of a health condition or healthcare appointments can decrease income. The economic consequences of health conditions may also cause the opposite reaction. If an individual is receiving disability benefits and has little opportunity to find satisfactory employment, he or she may not follow recommendations that would increase the ability to return to work, thereby decreasing or eliminating benefits.

Finally, quality of life is a relative concept, uniquely defined by each individual. If treatment recommendations, or side effects of treatment, result in pain, discomfort, or inconvenience greater than the benefit perceived by the individual in terms of his or her own subjective definition of the quality of life, adherence with prescribed recommendations may not be perceived as worth the psychological, social, or physical cost. Management recommendations can sometimes—but not always—be adjusted to make adherence to recommendations more palatable. Individuals' right to self-determination must be carefully balanced with assurance that the choice of nonadherence is based on solid information and full understanding of the implications.

Some individuals readily adjust to the challenges and alterations necessitated by a health condition. Other individuals actively subvert management recommendations, to their own detriment. In such instances, professionals' goals should be to attempt to understand the underlying problems and motivations of individuals and to help them make the necessary adjustments and adaptations to optimize functional outcomes. Rather than criticizing individuals with a health condition for disinterest, a lack of motivation, or failure to follow recommendations, it is important to identify the barriers that inhibit adherence and to recognize that such reactions may indicate difficulty in accepting the condition or incorporating recommendations into the individual's own unique way of life. The best way to achieve adherence is to consider the individual's perceptions, goals, environment, and lifestyle, and to tailor recommendations to best meet those needs (Falvo, 2011).

HEALTH INFORMATION

Although health care, support, and auxiliary services are important aspects of helping individuals reach their optimal potential, successful management of health conditions requires considerable individual and family effort. Regardless of the complexity of the condition, many individuals are now expected to carry out management recommendations in their home rather than depend on the assistance of healthcare personnel in healthcare settings. Individuals' understanding of their condition, manifestations, and management recommendations is one of the basic components of self-determination and responsible care. Not only must they understand how to integrate these management recommendations into their daily routines and how to carry out daily care activities, but they must also understand how preventive healthcare measures can help them retain function and avoid further health-related problems (Falvo, 2011). In addition to individuals' motivation to learn and manage their condition, as well as family support, creation of more accessible environments increases the likelihood that individuals will be able to effectively manage their condition (Rimmer, 2005).

Because of increasing public awareness of the need for individuals to accept this greater role of responsibility and self-determination, a number of programs and counseling services have been established to help individuals and their families reach this goal. Patient and family education can take place either on an individual basis or in a group setting, can be formal or informal, and can include ongoing counseling or referral to resources for self-directed learning. Regardless of the type of setting in which educational services are delivered, the most effective education will consider the specific circumstances and goals of the individual (Falvo, 2011).

STAGES OF ADAPTATION AND ADJUSTMENT

A host of personal, social, and environmental experiences, demands, supports and resources, and coping strategies interact to influence adaptation outcomes (Livneh, 2001). The process of adjustment includes a search for meaning in the experience and an attempt to regain control and self-determination over the events that affect one's life. Most individuals with a health condition experience some form of loss—either a direct physical loss or a more indirect loss of the ability to participate in some previously performed activity. Regardless of the nature of the loss, a variety of reactions may take place while individuals attempt to make necessary adaptations and changes.

Stages of adjustment are both individual and varied. The shock of diagnosis and its consequent implications may have a numbing effect, such that initially individuals demonstrate little emotional reaction. As the reality of the situation becomes clear, individuals may experience a sense of hopelessness and despair, mourning for a self, a role, or a function that is lost. They may also experience feelings of anger that alternate with depression. Many individuals go through a period of mourning and bereavement similar to that experienced when a loved one is lost. Mourning is a natural reaction to loss and allows time for reflection and reestablishment of emotional equilibrium. As individuals begin to appraise their condition realistically, examine the alterations that it requires, and adjust to the associated losses, they may gradually seek alternatives and adaptations to achieve their integration into a broader world.

The ultimate outcome of adjustment is acceptance of the condition and its associated alterations, along with a realistic appraisal and implementation of strengths. Acceptance does not mean passivity regarding implications of the condition but rather that individuals are ready to move forward in reaching optimal functional capacity. The amount of time that individuals need to reach acceptance depends on personality, reactions of family and significant others, life circumstances, available resources, and the types of challenges that confront each individual. Some individuals never reach acceptance. Nonacceptance may be characterized by immobility, marked dependency, continued anger and hostility, prolonged mourning, or participation in detrimental or self-destructive activities. Just as coping strategies are vital parts of human nature that protect against stress, reduce anxiety, and facilitate adjustment, so overuse or negative use of coping strategies can postpone or inhibit adjustment.

MULTICULTURAL ISSUES

Culture consists of more than race or ethnicity. It can be defined by a shared system of values, beliefs, and patterns of behavior that is shaped by many factors, including country of origin, language, religion, and sexual orientation (Taylor, 2016). Cultural factors shape individuals' perception of self as well as define views of health and health conditions and their meaning in the context of culture. Concepts related to causes of and reasons for various health conditions, values, and accepted ways of managing a condition are all cultural variables that determine attitude, adjustment, expectations, and outcomes related to chronic illness and disability. Adjustment and adaptation to a health condition are related to a variety of cultural aspects, including race, gender, ethnicity, spiritual or religious beliefs, and sexual orientation.

FUNCTIONAL ASPECTS

Functional effects of health conditions are many and varied. Each individual has different needs, abilities, and circumstances that determine how a health condition affects his or her functional capacity. The extent to which the individual experiences limitation as a result of the condition depends to a great extent on his or her goals and perception of the condition, the environment, and the reactions of family, friends, and the societal and political environment. The severity of the condition as measured by tests is not always an indication of functional capacity. Moreover, individuals' ability to function is not always directly correlated with the severity of the condition. Rather, function is determined by an interaction of factors related to the person and his or her environment. As a consequence, individuals' reactions may differ even though they have similar health conditions.

Professionals working with individuals with health conditions need an understanding of the potential alterations associated with a specific condition or management recommendations to help individuals and their families make appropriate changes to gain optimal functional capacity. The effects of health conditions are far-reaching and include psychological, social, and vocational effects as well as changes and adjustments in both general lifestyle and activities of daily living. The condition per se is not as important as the individual's goals and the degree to which function in each area of the individual's life is affected. The interactive nature of function between each of the areas determines the extent to which individuals can reach their optimal level of function. Thus a focus on any one area without full consideration of the impact of the health condition on all other areas can dilute the effectiveness of rehabilitative efforts. Understanding and working effectively with individuals who have a health condition requires adopting a broad outlook that goes beyond labeling the condition; it requires recognition that the most important factor is individuals' ability to function with the condition within their environment and all areas of their life.

Personal and Psychosocial Issues

Individuals react both cognitively and emotionally to events that involve them. These reactions, in turn, affect the later course of those events. Personal and psychological factors are always present in all aspects of health conditions, and they influence individuals' response to the health condition. Sometimes psychological factors are part of the manifestations of the condition itself. These factors affect not only individuals' adjustment and subsequent functional capacity but also outcomes.

Activities and Participation

Life activities consist of the tasks and activities of daily living within an individual's environment. They include the ability to perform tasks related to grooming, housekeeping, and preparing meals. They also include activities related to transportation, daily schedules, need for rest or activity, recreation, sexuality, and privacy. At times, limitations in performing the activities of daily living may result from environmental considerations that serve as barriers to effective functioning. Modifications such as widening doorways to permit the passage of a wheelchair, placing handrails in a bathroom, or installing more effective lighting may be required to increase functional capacity. Other modifications may be necessary because of the additional tasks and time commitments related to medical treatment of a specific condition. In some instances, alterations of diet or activity, continued treatments, medical appointments, and related activities may require significant changes in the individual's daily schedule.

The social environment can be defined as individuals' perceived involvement in personal, family, group, and community relationships and activities. Interpersonal support has been found to be significant in enabling persons with health conditions to effectively manage their condition (Bisschop, Kriegsman, Beekman, & Deeg, 2004; Chapman, Craven, & Chadwick, 2005; Glasgow,

Strycker, Toobert, & Eakin, 2000). Social well-being is based on emotionally satisfying experiences in social activities involving those within the individual's social group. Health conditions can lead to changes in social status. Individuals with a health condition may find themselves in a socially devalued role. As a result, they may experience changes in social relationships or interactions, or limit the number of social activities; any of these changes can result in social isolation. Even when individuals with a health condition attempt to remain socially active, they may have difficulty entering community facilities because of environmental barriers or because of prejudice or stereotyping. Many factors contribute to an individual's adaptation or adjustment to any social alterations associated with a particular health condition.

In addition, individuals' perception or misperception of the reactions of others in social groups may determine the level of acceptance that they receive. The degree to which individuals are able to adapt, accept, and adjust to their condition is determined in part by their interactions with others in their environment as well as by their interpretation of the reactions of others.

VOCATIONAL ISSUES

The significance of work in the rehabilitation of people with health conditions has been well documented (Cunningham, Wolbert, & Brockmeier, 2000). Work involves more than remuneration for services rendered, and it does not necessarily include only activity related to financial incentives. Work provides a sense of contribution, accomplishment, and meaning to life (Ben-Shlomo, Canfield, & Warner, 2002; Bond et al., 2001; Corrigan, Bogner, Mysiw, Clinchot, & Fugate, 2001). Consequently, loss of ability to work extends beyond financial considerations to social and psychological well-being. Loss of ability to work means more than the loss of income; it also means the loss of a socially valued role. For many individuals, work is not merely a major part of their identity but a source of social interaction, structure, and purpose in life.

The degree to which a health condition affects an individual's ability and willingness to work depends on a variety of factors in addition to the alterations associated with the health condition (Young & Murphy, 2002). These factors include the nature of the work, the physical environment of the work setting, and the attitudes of employers and coworkers. Psychosocial variables may also complicate functional capacity and, therefore, the rehabilitation process. At times, individuals with a health condition may continue to perform the same work they performed before the onset of the condition. At other times, certain work tasks, environmental conditions, or work schedules may need to be modified to accommodate alterations associated with the health condition. If modifications cannot be made in these cases, individuals must change employment. Some individuals must assume disability status because appropriate modifications cannot be made or because manifestations of their condition preclude work in their previous occupation. Job stress and attitudes of employers or coworkers can also significantly interfere with individuals' ability to return to the workforce. Problems with transportation to and from work because of manifestations or alterations associated with a health condition may make a return to work more difficult. In other instances, time required to carry out management recommendations related to the condition may make completing a full day at work virtually impossible.

Individuals' capacity to function at a job can depend on cognitive, psychomotor, and attitudinal factors as well as on the physical aspects of the health condition. Accurate assessment of individuals' capacity to return to work incorporates more than evaluation of physical factors alone; that is, success or failure at work is often determined by factors other than physical skill or ability. Individuals' fear of reinjury, vocational dissatisfaction, or legal issues can hamper return to work. Individuals' ability to relate to and interact with others within the work environment must also be considered. Interests, aptitudes, and abilities are always pivotal factors in determining vocational success, regardless of manifestations or alterations related to the health condition. Effective rehabilitation that enables individuals to function effectively in their job often involves interdisciplinary efforts of many types of professionals to conduct assessment, evaluation, therapy, and offer vocational guidance.

REFERENCES

Ben-Shlomo, Y., Canfield, L., & Warner, T. (2002). What are the determinants of quality of life in people with cervical dystonia? *Journal of Neurology and Neurosurgical Psychiatry, 72,* 608–614.

Biordi, D. L., Boville, D., King, D. S., Knapik, G., Warner, A., Zartman, K. A., & Zwick, D. M. (2002). In: I. Morof Lubkin & P. D. Larsen (Eds.)., *Chronic illness: Impact and interventions* (5th ed., pp. 261–277). Sudbury, MA: Jones and Bartlett.

Bisschop, M. I., Kriegsman, D. M. W., Beekman, A. T. F., & Deeg, D. J. H. (2004). Chronic diseases and depression: The modifying role of psychosocial resources. *Social Science & Medicine, 59,* 721–733.

Bond, G. R., Resnick, S. G., Bebout, R. R., Drake, R. E., Xie, H., & McHugo, G. J. (2001). Does competitive employment improve nonvocational outcomes for people with severe mental illness? *Journal of Consulting Clinical Psychology, 69,* 489–501.

Brodwin, M. G., & Frederick, P. C. (2010). Sexuality and societal beliefs regarding persons living with disabilities. *Journal of Rehabilitation, 76*(4), 37–41.

Burker, E. J., Carels, R. A., Thompson, L. F., Rodgers, L., & Egan, T. (2000). Quality of life in patients awaiting lung transplant: Cystic fibrosis versus other end-stage lung diseases. *Pediatric Pulmonology, 30,* 453–460.

Chapman, J. J., Craven, J. J., & Chadwick, D. D. (2005). Fighting ft? An evaluation of health practitioner input to improve healthy living and reduce obesity for adults with learning disabilities. *Journal of Intellectual Disabilities, 9,* 131–144.

Corbin, J. (2001). Introduction and overview of chronic illness and nursing. In R. Hyman & J. Corbin (Eds.)., *Chronic illness: Research and theory for nursing practice* (pp. 1–15). New York, NY: Springer.

Corrigan, J. D., Bogner, J. A., Mysiw, J. W., Clinchot, D., & Fugate, L. (2001). Life satisfaction after traumatic brain injury. *Journal of Head Trauma Rehabilitation, 16,* 543–555.

Corwyn, R. F. (2000). The factor structure of global self esteem among adolescents and adults. *Journal of Research and Personality, 34,* 357–379.

Crews, W., Jefferson, A., Broshek, D., Barth, J., & Robbins, M. (2000). Neuropsychological sequelae in a series of patients with end-stage cystic fibrosis: Lung transplant evaluation. *Archives of Clinical Neuropsychology, 15,* 59–70.

Cunningham, K., Wolbert, R., & Brockmeier, M. B. (2000). Moving beyond the illness: Factors contributing to gaining and maintaining employment. *American Journal of Community Psychology, 28*(4), 481–493.

Cusack, L. (2000). Perceptions of body image: Implications for the workplace. *Employee Assistance Quarterly, 15*(3), 23–29.

Cuskelly, M., & Bryde, R. (2004). Attitudes toward the sexuality of adults with an intellectual disability: Parents, support staff and a community sample. *Journal of Intellectual and Developmental Disability, 29*(3), 255–264.

de Moore, G. M., Hennessey, P., Kunz, N. M., Ferrando, S., & Rabkin, J. G. (2000). Kaposi's sarcoma: The scarlet letter of AIDS. The psychological effects of a skin disease. *Psychosomatics, 41*(4), 360–363.

Dolder, C. R., Lacro, J. P., Leckband, S., & Jeste, D. V. (2003). Interventions to improve antipsychotic medication adherence: Review of recent literature. *Journal of Clinical Psychopharmacology, 23*(4), 389–399.

Dudgeon, B. J. (2002). Physical disability and the experience of chronic pain. *Archives of Physical Medicine and Rehabilitation, 83*(2), 229–235.

Dunbar-Jacob, J., Erlen, J. A., Schlenk, E. A., Ryan, C. M., Sereika, S. M., & Doswell, W. M. (2000). Adherence in chronic disease. *Annual Review of Nursing Research, 18,* 48–90.

Falvo, D. R. (2011). *Effective patient education: A guide to increased adherence.* Burlington, MA: Jones & Bartlett Learning.

Glasgow, R. E., Strycker, L. A., Toobert, D. J., & Eakin, E. (2000). A social-ecologic approach to assessing support for disease self-management: The Chronic Illness Resources Survey. *Journal of Behavioral Medicine, 23,* 559–583.

Gledhill, J., Rangel, L., & Garralda, E. (2000). Surviving chronic physical illness: Psychosocial outcomes in adult life. *Archives of Disease in Childhood, 83*(2), 104–110.

Graham, H. (2003). A conceptual map for studying long-term exercise adherence in a cardiac population. *Rehabilitation Nursing, 28*(3), 80–86.

Haslam, A. S. (2001). *Psychology in organizations: The social identity approach.* London, England: Sage.

Hordern, A. J., & Currow, D. C. (2003). A patient-centered approach to sexuality in the face of life-limiting illness. *Medical Journal of Australia, 179*(6 Suppl), S8–S11.

Katon, W. J., Lin, E. H. B., Von Korff, M., Ciechanowski, P., Ludman, E. J., Young, B., . . . McCulloch, D. (2010). Collaborative care for patients with depression and chronic illnesses. *New England Journal of Medicine, 363*(27), 2611–2620.

Katzman, D. K, & Neinstein, L. S. (2016). Adolescent medicine. In: L. Goldman & A. I. Schafer (Eds.)., *Goldman-Cecil medicine* (25th ed.). Philadelphia, PA: Elsevier Saunders.

Kovac, J. A., Patel, S. S., Peterson, R. A., & Kimmel, P. L. (2002). Patient satisfaction with care and behavioral compliance in end-stage renal disease patients treated with hemodialysis. *American Journal of Kidney Disease, 39*(6), 1236–1244.

Leplege, A., & Hunt, S. (1997). The problem of quality of life in medicine. *Journal of the American Medical Association, 278*(1), 47–50.

Livneh, H. (2001). Psychosocial adaptation to chronic illness and disability: A conceptual framework. *Rehabilitation Counseling Bulletin, 44*(3), 150–160.

Livneh, H., & Wilson, L. M. (2003). Coping strategies as predictors and mediators of disability-related variables and psychosocial adaptation: An exploratory investigation. *Rehabilitation Counseling Bulletin, 46*(4), 194–208.

Loghman-Adham, M. (2003). Medication noncompliance in patients with chronic disease: Issues in dialysis and renal transplantation. *American Journal of Managed Care, 9*(2), 155–171.

Lyons, M., & Ziviani, H. (1995). Stereotypes, stigma, and mental illness: Learning from fieldwork experiences. *American Journal of Occupational Therapy, 49*(10), 1002–1008.

McBride, K. E., & Rines, B. (2000). Sexuality and spinal cord injury: A road map for nurses. *SCI Nursing, 17*(1), 8–13.

McInnes, R. A. (2003). Chronic illness and sexuality. *Medical Journal of Australia, 179*(5), 263–266.

Morof Lubkin, I., & Larsen, P. D. (Eds.). (2002). *Chronic illness: Impact and interventions* (5th ed.). Sudbury, MA: Jones and Bartlett Publishers.

Nosek, M. A., & Hughes, R. B. (2003). Psychosocial issues of women with physical disabilities: The continuing gender debate. *Rehabilitation Counseling Bulletin, 46*(4), 224–233.

Rimmer, J. H. (2005). The conspicuous absence of people with disabilities in public fitness and recreation facilities: Lack of interest or lack of access? *American Journal of Health Promotion, 19,* 327–329.

Saylor, C., Yoder, M., & Mann, R. J. (2002). Stigma. In I. Morof Lubkin & P. D. Larsen (Eds.)., *Chronic illness: Impact and interventions* (5th ed.). Sudbury, MA: Jones and Bartlett Publishers.

Schmaling, K. B., Afari, N., & Blume, A. W. (2000). Assessment of psychological factors associated with adherence to medication regimens among adult patients with asthma. *Journal of Asthma, 37*(4), 335–343.

Shaw, L., Segal, R., Polatajkos, H., & Harburn, K. (2002). Understanding return to work behaviors: Promoting the importance of individual perceptions in the study of return to work. *Disability & Rehabilitation, 24*(4), 185–195.

Tajfel, H., & Turner, J. C. (1986). The social identity theory of inter-group behavior. In S. Worchel & L. W. Austin (Eds.), *Psychology of intergroup relations.* Chicago, IL: Nelson-Hall.

Taylor, V. M. (2016). Cultural context of medicine. In L. Goldman & A. I. Schafer (Eds.), *Goldman-Cecil medicine* (25th ed.). Philadelphia, PA: Elsevier Saunders.

Vergouwen, A. C., Bakker, A., Katon, W. J., Verheij, T. J., & Koerselman, F. (2003). Improving adherence to antidepressants: A systematic review of interventions. *Journal of Clinical Psychiatry, 64*(12), 1415–1420.

White, C. A. (2000). Body image dimensions and cancer: A heuristic cognitive behavioural model. *Psycho-Oncology, 9,* 183–192.

Young, A., & Murphy, G. A. (2002). A social psychology approach to measuring vocational rehabilitation intervention effectiveness. *Journal of Occupational Rehabilitation, 12,* 175–189.

Zygmunt, A., Olfson, M., Boyer, C. A., & Mechanic, D. (2002). Interventions to improve medication adherence in schizophrenia. *American Journal of Psychiatry, 159*(10), 1653–1654.

CHAPTER 3

Introduction to the Structure and Function of the Nervous System

STRUCTURE AND FUNCTION OF THE NERVOUS SYSTEM

The nervous system is a complex regulatory system that, along with the *endocrine system*, controls and coordinates activities and functions throughout the body, internally and externally, by sending, receiving, and sorting electrical impulses and chemical signals. Disruption of any part of the nervous system affects body function in some way, either internally or externally.

The nervous system consists of the *central nervous system*, which includes the *brain* and *spinal cord*, and the *peripheral nervous system*, which includes *nerve fibers* extending from the brain and spinal cord that carry information between the central nervous system and the rest of the body. The peripheral nervous system is further divided into two parts: the *afferent* (sensory) *system*, which carries messages from other parts of the body *to* the central nervous system, and the *efferent* (motor) *system*, which carries messages *from* the central nervous system to other parts of the body (see **Table 3-1**).

Function of the Nervous System

Functions of the nervous system include the following:

- Organizing and directing motor responses of the *voluntary muscle system*, enabling the body to move more effectively as a whole and to achieve purposeful movement. This coordination of voluntary muscles makes possible complex activities, such as walking, running, playing a piano, and using a computer, as well as simple activities, such as maintaining muscle tone and posture while at rest.
- Monitoring and recognizing stimuli (and information) within the environment, and then directing an appropriate response to the stimuli. This function makes possible reflex actions, such as pulling away one's hand from a hot surface, as well as perceiving music being played in the next room.
- Monitoring and coordinating internal body states so that internal organs function as a unit, internal body constancy (**homeostasis**) is maintained, and protective action is taken. For example, in response to a lack of oxygen, more rapid breathing occurs; the body shivers in response to cold; and when threat or danger is encountered, the heart beats more rapidly.

Other functions, such as display of personality traits, language, speech, learning, remembering, feeling emotion, reasoning, and generating and relaying thoughts, are also controlled by the nervous system—specifically, by the brain.

Table 3-1   The Nervous System (Central and Peripheral)

I.   Central nervous system

   A. Brain

   B. Spinal cord

II. Peripheral nervous system

   A. Afferent (sensory)

   B. Efferent (motor)

      1. Somatic nervous system

      2. Autonomic nervous system

         a. Sympathetic nervous system

         b. Parasympathetic nervous system

Nerve Cells

Specialized cells called **neurons** are the functional units of the nervous system. Neurons transmit messages to and from the brain. They consist of a cell body and processes (*nerve fibers*) that extend beyond the cell body. In most cases, a single long nerve fiber called an *axon* conducts nerve impulses (and information) away from the cell body to other neurons. Smaller, shorter nerve fibers called **dendrites** conduct nerve impulses toward the cell body after receiving information from other neurons. Fibers that carry information from parts of the body to the brain are called **afferent neurons** (sensory neurons). Fibers that carry information from the brain to other parts of the body are called **efferent neurons** (motor neurons).

Surrounding neurons is a fatty sheath called **myelin**, which, much like the covering of electrical cords, provides insulation, ensuring that electrical impulses are able to flow smoothly and reliably. Information is passed from neuron to neuron by both electrical and chemical impulses. The electrical impulse, which has been picked up by the dendrites, is passed through the cell body to the axon. The electrical impulse then moves down the full length of the axon until it reaches its tip. At the tip of the axon are tiny processes, which release chemicals known as **neurotransmitters**. Neurotransmitters, chemically transfer the impulse from one neuron to another across a space between the two neurons called the **synapse**. The electrical impulse, through the vehicle of neurotransmitters, then moves to the next neuron's dendrites and the process begins again (see **Figure 3-1**). After

Figure 3-1   Neurons

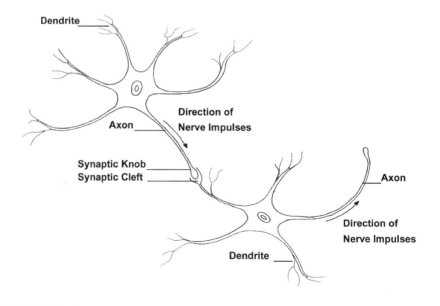

neurotransmitters are released, they are either taken up again by the neuron or destroyed.

Longer axons are generally grouped in bundles. When they are transmitting impulses within the central nervous system, these bundles are referred to as *tracts*. Those bundles located outside the central nervous system are referred to as *nerves*.

The Central Nervous System

The *central nervous system* is made up of the brain and spinal cord. Bony coverings protect both the brain and the spinal cord. On the interior of these bony coverings are three membranes (**meninges**) that provide additional protection:

- The **dura mater** is the outer membrane, lying closest to the bony covering of the brain and spinal cord.
- The **arachnoid membrane** is the middle membrane, a **cobweb**-appearing membrane.
- The **pia mater** is the inner membrane, which lies closest to the brain and spinal cord.

Between each of the membrane layers are spaces. The space between the dura mater and the inner surface of the bony covering is the *epidural space*; the space between the dura mater and the arachnoid membrane is the *subdural space*; and the space between the arachnoid membrane and the pia mater is the *subarachnoid space.*

The central nervous system is also protected and cushioned by **cerebrospinal fluid** (CSF), which is formed by specialized capillaries called the *choroid plexus* in inner chambers within the brain called **ventricles**. The cerebrospinal fluid bathes the brain and spinal cord, circulating from the ventricles into the subarachnoid space (see **Figure 3-2**). From the subarachnoid space, the CSF flows to the back of the brain, down around the spinal cord, and then back to the brain, where it is reabsorbed into the blood through the arachnoid membrane. The amounts of cerebrospinal fluid produced and absorbed are equally balanced so that under normal conditions, the amount of CSF within the central nervous system remains constant.

Another protective device is the *blood–brain barrier*, a structural arrangement of capillaries that selectively determines which substances can move from the blood into the brain. While substances such as oxygen and glucose are necessary

Figure 3-2   Circulation of Cerebrospinal Fluid

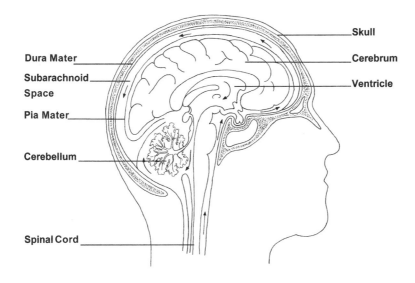

for brain survival and consequently move freely across the blood–brain barrier, other potential harmful substances, such as toxins, are prevented from crossing into the brain.

The central nervous system is composed of white matter and gray matter. **White matter** makes up the inner part of the brain and the outer portion of the spinal cord and consists of myelinated covered axons that conduct nerve impulses. It is called white matter because of its whitish appearance due to the myelin covering. **Gray matter** makes up the thin outer layer of the brain and the inner portion of the spinal cord. Small segments of gray matter are also embedded deep within certain parts of the white matter of the brain. Gray matter consists of groups of neuron cell bodies. It is called gray matter because of its grayish appearance. Gray matter of the brain receives, sorts, and processes nerve messages, while gray matter of the spinal cord serves as a center for reflex action (automatic response to stimuli).

STRUCTURE AND FUNCTION OF THE BRAIN

The brain is directly connected to the spinal cord and serves as the primary center for the integration, coordination, initiation, and interpretation of most nerve messages. It regulates and monitors many unconscious body functions, such as heart and respiratory rate and coordinates most voluntary movements. In addition, it is the site of higher cognitive processes such as learning, generating and relaying thoughts, reasoning, judgment, memory, consciousness, and emotion. The brain also has a sensory function, which is responsible for vision, hearing, touch, taste, and smell. Language function, including the ability to communicate and to comprehend, is also controlled by the brain. Finally, the brain controls basic behavior patterns and the display of general personality traits, which are characteristic of how each individual responds to stimuli.

The brain is protected by the bony covering of the skull (**cranium** or *cranial bones*). The largest part of the brain, the **cerebrum**, is covered with a thin outer layer of gray matter called the **cortex**, which contains billions of nerve cells. The cortex has three specialized areas, which serve three major areas of function:

- The *motor cortex* coordinates voluntary movements of the body.
- The *sensory cortex* is responsible for the recognition or perception of sensory stimuli, such as touch, pain, smell, taste, vision, and hearing.
- The *associational cortex* is involved in cognitive functions such as memory, reasoning, abstract thinking, and consciousness.

The cerebrum is divided into two halves, called the *right hemisphere* and the *left hemisphere*. These two hemispheres communicate with each other. Dividing the hemispheres and connecting specific areas of the two hemispheres are bundles of nerve fibers called the *corpus callosum*. Each hemisphere has centers for receiving information and for initiating responses. The left hemisphere mostly receives information from and sends information to the right side of the body, whereas the right hemisphere mostly receives information from and sends information to the left side of the body.

Deep within the cerebral hemispheres are groups of gray matter called **basal ganglia**, which are part of the *extrapyramidal system*. (*Extrapyramidal* denotes nerve fiber tracts that lie outside the pyramidal tract, a relatively compact group of nerve fibers that originate from cells in the outer layer of the brain.) Extrapyramidal function is concerned with postural adjustment and gross voluntary and automatic muscular movements. The basal ganglia help to maintain tone in muscles in the trunk and extremities, enabling individuals to maintain balance and posture and to engage in movements such as walking. The basal ganglia also play a role in enabling individuals to react swiftly, appropriately, and automatically to stimuli that demand an immediate response, such as after tripping, enabling the individual to adjust his or her movement to avoid a fall.

Each hemisphere of the cerebrum is divided into lobes that contain areas related to specific functions (see **Figure 3-3**). The **frontal lobe** is located in the front of each hemisphere and contains motor areas that initiate voluntary movement and skilled movements, such as those involved in handwriting.

Figure 3-3   **Areas of Brain Function**

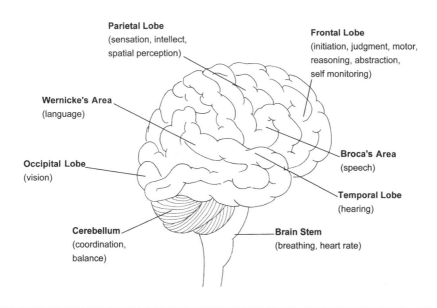

Parietal Lobe
(sensation, intellect, spatial perception)

Frontal Lobe
(initiation, judgment, motor, reasoning, abstraction, self monitoring)

Wernicke's Area
(language)

Occipital Lobe
(vision)

Broca's Area
(speech)

Temporal Lobe
(hearing)

Cerebellum
(coordination, balance)

Brain Stem
(breathing, heart rate)

© Jane Tinkler Lamm.

Other areas in the frontal lobe control higher intellectual functions such as foresight, analytical thinking, and judgment. The **parietal lobe** is located in the middle of each hemisphere and is primarily the sensory area, integrating and interpreting sensation such as touch, pressure, pain, and temperature. Some memory functions are also located in the parietal lobe, especially those responsible for storage of sensory memory. The **temporal lobe** is located under the frontal and parietal lobes and is primarily responsible for the interpretation of and distinction between auditory stimuli. The **occipital lobe** is located at the back or posterior portion of each hemisphere. It is the primary area for reception and interpretation of visual stimuli.

Several parts of the cerebrum are involved in the language function, which consists of the process of receiving, interpreting, and integrating visual and auditory stimuli as well as the ability to express thoughts in a coordinated way so that others can comprehend them. Language function is located in the left hemisphere of the cerebrum in most individuals, whether they are right- or left-handed. An area located over the temporal and parietal lobes, called **Wernicke's area**, is the major area responsible for *receptive function* (speech understanding), or the ability to integrate visual and auditory information so as to understand communication received. An area located in front of the temporal lobe and in the frontal cortex, called **Broca's area**, is responsible for speaking ability and is closely associated with motor areas that control the muscles needed for articulation. This area contributes to *expressive function* (speech formation), or the ability to integrate and coordinate words so that the meaning can be comprehended.

A structure known as the *thalamus* lies within the center of the brain. The thalamus acts as a relay station that sorts, interprets, and directs sensory information. Below the thalamus is the *hypothalamus*, which coordinates neural and endocrine activities. This structure helps regulate the body's internal environment and behaviors that are important to survival, such as eating, drinking, and reproduction. Below the hypothalamus is the *pituitary*, an endocrine gland.

The *limbic system* comprises a group of structures consisting of both gray and white matter that surround the thalamus. The limbic system plays a role in expression of instincts, drives, and emotions as well as the formation of memories. A band of gray matter called the *hippocampus* is involved in learning and long-term memory, helping to determine where important and relevant aspects of facts will be stored.

Beneath the occipital lobe of the cerebrum is a structure called the *cerebellum*. The cerebellum is primarily responsible for the coordination and integration of voluntary movement and for the maintenance of equilibrium, posture, and balance of the body. It also regulates and coordinates fine movements of the extremities, which are initiated by the frontal lobe.

The **brain stem**, which is located beneath the cerebellum at the base of the brain just above the spinal cord, acts as a relay station, transmitting nerve impulses between the spinal cord and the brain. It is the primary center of involuntary functions. Control of vital organ functions, such as regulation of heartbeat or respiration, occurs in the brain stem. Areas in the brain stem also regulate the diameter of blood vessels, contributing to the control of blood pressure. Reflex actions, such as coughing and swallowing, are controlled in the brain stem as well. Finally, the brain stem contains scattered groups of cells, called the **reticular formation**, which are involved in the initiation and maintenance of wakefulness and alertness.

The brain requires both oxygen and nourishment in the form of *glucose* in order to function and to survive. Oxygen and glucose are transported to the brain by blood carried by four major arteries: two *carotid arteries* and two *vertebral arteries*. The vertebral arteries join to form the *basilar artery*. The carotid and basilar arteries then connect at the base of the brain to form the *circle of Willis,* from which *cerebral arteries* branch out to carry blood to the rest of the brain.

STRUCTURE AND FUNCTION OF THE SPINAL CORD AND PERIPHERAL NERVOUS SYSTEM

The Spinal Cord

The spinal cord is part of the central nervous system and extends from the brain stem to the lower part of the back. Bony coverings called *vertebrae*

surround the spinal cord and protect it. This bony covering, as a whole, forms the vertebral column. The *vertebral column* consists of 7 *cervical vertebrae*, located in the neck area; 12 *thoracic vertebrae*, located in the upper and middle back; and 5 *lumbar vertebrae*, located in the lower back. The *sacrum*, located below the lumbar vertebrae, consists of fused (joined) bone. At the tip of the sacrum is the *coccyx*, or tailbone (see **Figure 3-4**).

The spinal cord conducts impulses to and from the brain. The outer white matter of the spinal cord, which consists of bundles or tracts of myelinated fibers of sensory (*afferent*) and motor (*efferent*) neurons, conveys electrical impulses up and down the spinal cord between the **peripheral nervous system** (those nerves lying outside the central nervous system) and the brain. In most instances, sensory information traveling up the right side of the spinal cord

Figure 3-4   The Spine

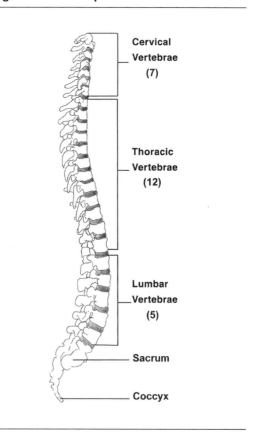

Cervical Vertebrae (7)

Thoracic Vertebrae (12)

Lumbar Vertebrae (5)

Sacrum

Coccyx

© Jane Tinkler Lamm.

crosses over to the left side of the brain, so the left hemisphere of the brain would, for example, interpret pain in the right hand. Conversely, motor impulses originating in the left brain cross to the right side of the spinal cord and initiate a response to the right side of the body. Because of this crossover effect, damage on one side of the brain typically causes manifestations on the opposite side of the body.

The inner gray matter of the spinal cord, which is composed of cell bodies and *unmyelinated* neurons, acts as a coordinating center for reflex and other activities, such as voluntary movements and control of internal functions. A reflex center in the gray matter of the spinal cord is where sensory and motor neurons connect; this part of the spinal cord serves as a center for spinal reflexes. A **reflex** can be defined as an automatic response to a given stimulus. Spinal reflexes control not only muscle reflexes but also the reflexes of internal organs.

The gray matter within the spinal cord resembles the letter "H." The projections of the H are named according to the direction to which they project. The *posterior horns* extend toward the back, and the *anterior horns* project toward the front. Cerebrospinal fluid, which nourishes and protects the spinal cord, fills both the *central canal*, located within the center of the gray matter, and the subarachnoid space surrounding the outer portion of the spinal cord.

Motor (efferent) impulses originate in the motor cortex of the brain, extend down the spinal cord through *descending tracts*, and exit through motor spinal nerve roots that extend through openings between the vertebrae that surround the spinal cord. Sensory (afferent) impulses from the body enter the spinal cord through spinal nerve roots that also extend through openings between vertebrae and then travel up *ascending tracts* in the spinal cord to the brain.

Spinal nerve roots are named for the vertebral level from which they exit. For example, the nerve roots that leave the spinal cord at the *cervical* level are labeled C1 through C8, and the nerve roots that leave at the **thoracic** level are labeled T1 through T12 (see **Figure 3-5**). The sensory (afferent) nerve fibers from outside

the central nervous system carry body sensations into the *sensory nerve roots* (posterior roots) at the back of the spinal cord, where they are then carried up the spinal cord to the brain. Motor (efferent) impulses travel from the brain down the spinal cord and exit from *motor nerve roots* (anterior roots) at the front of the spinal cord. Motor nerve fibers then carry impulses to the voluntary muscles of the body.

Many types of neurons work together to transmit impulses through the spinal cord. Sensory impulses entering the spinal cord at the lumbar region are relayed vertically to the brain through a number of connecting sensory neurons. Motor impulses from the brain to the peripheral nerves, however, are conducted through two separate categories of motor neurons. *Upper motor neurons* originate in the brain and are contained entirely within the central nervous system. *Lower motor neurons*, although originating in the central nervous system, have fibers extending to the peripheral nerves in voluntary muscles. Alteration of function of either upper or lower motor neurons can generally affect the voluntary muscles. The location of the alteration of function determines the nature of the manifestations.

Peripheral Nervous System

A nerve is a bundle of fibers outside the central nervous system that transmits information between the central nervous system and various parts of the body. The peripheral nervous system consists of all nerves that extend from the brain and spinal cord. To function effectively, the peripheral nerves must be connected to the central nervous system. Some peripheral nerves connect directly to the brain (*cranial nerves*); others connect directly to the spinal cord (*spinal nerves*). Cranial and spinal nerves are essential links between the rest of the body and the central nervous system.

The 12 pairs of peripheral nerves that connect and transmit messages directly to the brain are called **cranial nerves**. Some cranial nerves contain only sensory fibers, whereas others contain both sensory and motor fibers. Cranial nerves mediate many aspects of sensation and muscular

Figure 3-5   Spinal Nerves

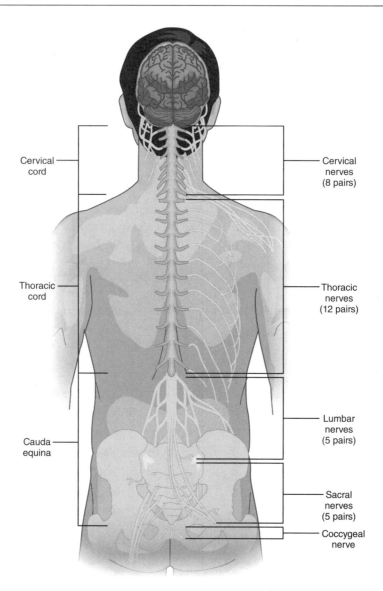

activity in and around the head and neck. Cranial nerves and their related functions are described in **Table 3-2**.

The 31 pairs of peripheral nerves that connect and transmit messages directly to the spinal cord are called **spinal nerves**. Each nerve divides and then subdivides into a number of branches. Nerves at each level travel to specific parts of the body, conveying information between those areas and the central nervous system. Spinal nerves and their related functions are described in Figure 3-5.

Nerves control both voluntary and involuntary functions in the body. Nerves that control voluntary functions (such as movement of the muscles in the extremities) are called **somatic nerves**. Nerves that are concerned with the control of

Table 3-2 Cranial Nerves and Related Functions

Cranial Nerve	Area of Function
I. Olfactory	Smell
II. Optic	Vision
III. Oculomotor	Movement of eye muscles
IV. Trochlear	Eyelids
V. Trigeminal	Sensation in head, face, and teeth, motor activity of chewing
VI. Abducens	Pupil dilation, focusing of lens
VII. Facial	Taste, sensation of external ear, control of salivary glands, tears, muscles in facial expression
VIII. Vestibulocochlear	Sensation of sound, balance, orientation of head
IX. Glossopharyngeal	Swallowing, sensation of pain, taste, touch from tongue and throat
X. Vagus	Heartbeat, digestion, speech, swallowing, respiratory function, gland functions
XI. Accessory	Movement of head and shoulders, muscles of pharynx and larynx in throat, production of voice sounds
XII. Hypoglossal	Tongue movement, speech, swallowing

involuntary functions are part of a subcategory of the peripheral nervous system called the **autonomic nervous system**.

The autonomic nervous system integrates the work of vital organs, such as the heart and lungs. Its primary function is to coordinate the activity of internal organs so that they can make adaptive responses to changing external situations, thereby maintaining internal equilibrium. Nerve fibers monitor the activities of internal organs as well as changes in the external environment. When changes are necessary to maintain internal **homeostasis** (equilibrium) or to protect the body, the autonomic nervous system stimulates an immediate, involuntary response. For example, in response to a speck of dust in the eye, tears are produced; in response to a fearful situation, the heart beats faster.

The autonomic nervous system is divided into two subsystems:

- The sympathetic nervous system
- The parasympathetic nervous system

These two systems work both together and in opposition to control internal organs and regulate their function. Hormones and emotions can affect both systems.

The sympathetic nervous system becomes active during periods of stress and in emergencies. It prepares the body for action, deepening respirations, making the heart beat faster, dilating the pupils, stimulating production of stress hormones, and increasing blood supply to the large muscles of the body.

In contrast, the parasympathetic nervous system dominates when the body is a rest. It activates those mechanisms that focus on body conservation, such as decreasing the heart rate and constricting the pupils of the eye. The parasympathetic nervous system is also an important component of sexual arousal in both males and females.

BIBLIOGRAPHY

Falvo, R. E. (2001). *Human physiology: Physiology 201 core curriculum.* Champaign, IL: Stipes.

Sherwood, L. (2007). *Human physiology: From cells to systems* (6th ed.). Australia, South Melbourne, VIC: Thomson Brooks/Cole

Tortora, G. J., & Derrickson, B. H. (Eds.). (2011). *Principles of anatomy and physiology* (13th ed.). Hoboken, NJ: John Wiley and Sons.

Widmaier, E., Raff, H., & Strang, K. (Eds.). (2010). *Vander's human physiology: The mechanisms of body function.* New York, NY: McGraw-Hill.

CHAPTER 4

Traumatic Brain Injury

OVERVIEW OF TRAUMATIC BRAIN INJURY

Traumatic brain injury (TBI) is an acquired injury to the brain resulting from a bump, blow, or jolt to the head or penetrating head injury. Although once often fatal, improved detection, prompt neurological intervention and interventions to prevent complications have greatly decreased mortality; however TBI is a leading cause of incapacitation (Katzenberger et al., 2013) with at least 1.4 million new cases being reported in the United States annually (Ling, 2016).

Major causes of TBI are falls, motor vehicle accidents, work-related injury, assaults and violence, including gunshots to the head, and blast injuries (Ling, 2016), as well as sports and bicycle-related injuries (DeKosky, Ikonomovic, & Gandy, 2010; Im, Hibbard, Grunwald, Swift, & Salimi, 2011). Blast injuries from explosions have also been a significant cause of TBI in recent years. Although civilians are also susceptible to blast injuries, military personnel are at significant risk for TBI from explosive devices (CDC, NIH, DoD, & VA Leadership Panel, 2013; Yu, Murphy, & Tsao, 2016).

Residual effects of TBI can result in lifelong challenges affecting all areas of function including cognitive, behavioral/emotional and physical effects that impact on interpersonal, social, and occupational function, affecting both the individual and his or her family (Giacino et al., 2012). Changes associated with a TBI can impact an individual's ability to maintain or attain employment, engage in leisure activities, carry on social relationships, or in some instances can affect their ability to live independently (Bowen, Moore, & Okun, 2016).

Any preexisting chronic health conditions at the time of injury as well as other injuries, such as spinal cord injury, which may also have been sustained at the time of brain injury, compound challenges to functional ability. In addition, if alcohol and/or substance abuse was a contributing factor in the cause of the initial injury, it may be an continuing issue after injury adding further complexity to rehabilitation and the individual's ability to reach optimum functional capacity.

Traumatic brain injury can occur at any age. The individual's age and developmental stage of life (see chapter 2) at the time of injury also impacts the physical, social, and emotional implications of TBI. The full effects of TBI in childhood may not be immediately apparent, especially if the injury is mild. Even when residual effects of TBI are recognized in childhood, the different challenges residual effects present at each stage of development may be overlooked. Some cognitive, communication, or behavioral issues may only become apparent after the individual has reached adulthood. Although considerable attention has been given to the functional consequences of TBI that occurs in adulthood, less attention has been paid to the functional consequences adults experience when they were brain injured as a child (Brenner et al., 2007).

In both children and adults, TBI, as a nonreversible injury, has lifetime implications not only for personal, social, and economic areas of life but also has implications for general health (Masel & DeWitt, 2010). Residual effects of TBI can contribute to physical inactivity, weight gain, or other behaviors, all of which can increase chances of developing chronic conditions, such as obesity, heart disease, and diabetes, which in turn compound functional consequences associated with TBI (Reis et al., 2015).

TYPES OF TRAUMATIC BRAIN INJURY

The type of TBI is one determinant of the functional sequelae individuals experience after injury. Due to the nature of the injury, damage to the brain in TBI may be more diffuse and extensive than damage from other nontraumatic conditions, such as stroke or meningitis. The impact on brain function resulting from TBI depends on three factors:

- The cause of the injury
- The area of the brain injured
- The extent of the injury

Traumatic brain injuries are described according to the type of injury (local, diffuse, or fracture of the skull) and mechanism of injury (i.e., the event that caused the injury) and are divided into one of three types:

- Closed head injury
- Open or penetrating head injury
- Blast injury

Closed Head Injury

Closed head injury describes injury to the brain occurring as a result of blunt trauma to the head or rapid motion of the brain within the skull due to violent forces of acceleration. Common causes of closed head injuries are motor vehicle accidents, falls, direct blows to the head, or sports-related injuries. Injury to the brain occurs when the skull strikes an immovable object (such as a car dashboard in an auto accident or the floor in a fall), when acceleration forces from a moving object strikes the skull (such as a baseball bat or a fist) or when external forces cause the brain to move rapidly within the skull (such as in shaken baby syndrome). Damage to the brain can be *focal* (damage occurring in a localized area of the brain) or *diffuse* (damage occurring over a more widespread area of the brain). Functional consequences depend on the location of the damage and the degree to which other structures within the brain were damaged.

Damage to the brain from closed head injury can result from both the initial impact (primary phase) as well as from the brain tissue reaction to the initial injury (secondary phase). The primary phase of brain injury refers to immediate damage to the brain tissue from the initial impact.

The primary phase consists of *coup–contrecoup* and consists of injury to the brain at the site of initial impact and injury to the brain on the opposite side. *Coup injury* refers to damage to the brain at the site of impact due to the skull hitting the brain. Depending on the force, the brain can then be placed in motion from the initial impact so that it moves backward, hitting the opposite side of the skull, sustaining additional damage at that site (*contrecoup*) (see **Figure 4-1**). Because of violent movement of the

Figure 4-1   Coup–Contrecoup Injury

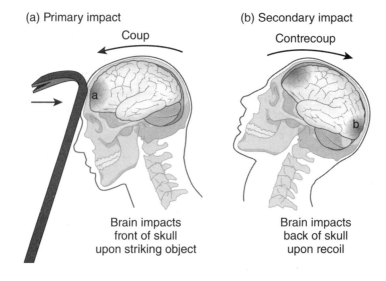

(a) Primary impact
Coup
Brain impacts
front of skull
upon striking object

(b) Secondary impact
Contrecoup
Brain impacts
back of skull
upon recoil

brain within the skull, internal neuronal structures in the brain twist or tear, causing diffuse injury.

The *secondary phase* of TBI begins immediately after the initial brain injury can continue for a prolonged period. The secondary phase refers to brain tissue reaction to the initial injury, such as **edema** (swelling), **intracranial hemorrhage** (bleeding within the cranial vault), or formation of a **hematoma** (sac filled with blood). Because the brain is contained in the skull, and there is no room for expansion, the brain becomes compressed, intracranial pressure increases, and the brain is deprived of blood supply and oxygen, causing additional neurological damage.

Potential threat of damage to the brain in the secondary phase of injury may not be immediately apparent. Unless identified early so that intervention can be instituted promptly, these events can cause additional permanent brain damage or death. Monitoring of intracranial pressure helps to detect rises in pressure, which can indicate cerebral edema or acute bleeding within the skull, so that appropriate interventions can be administered. Hematomas, may form more slowly so that intracranial pressure rise is subtle and gradual, and not initially recognized. Hematomas in the intracranial cavity are classified according to their anatomical location (see **Figure 4-2**). Examples include the following:

- Epidural hematoma
- Subdural hematoma
- Intracerebral hematoma

An *epidural hematoma* occurs in the space between the outer membrane of the brain (the *dura mater*)

and the skull (see chapter 3). Although bleeding generally occurs rapidly, it may not be recognized immediately after an injury. Initially after injury, individuals with epidural hematoma may seem lucid and able carry on a conversation, however as bleeding continues and the hematoma expands, they may gradually slip into unconsciousness hours later. Because epidural hematomas may go unnoticed initially, thus postponing treatment, they carry a high mortality rate (Ling, 2016).

A *subdural hematoma* occurs in the space beneath the dura mater. Although manifestations may be immediately apparent, they may also appear gradually, becoming evident days or even weeks after the injury. In both instances, immediate action is essential in order to stop the bleeding and to relieve the intracranial pressure before permanent damage to the brain occurs.

Intracerebral hematomas may occur in different locations in the brain depending on the site of the blow to the head. They may occur at the point of impact (*coup injury*) in the area opposite the point of impact (*contrecoup injury*) or in other locations. Hematomas can be identified through computerized tomography (CT) or magnetic resonance imaging (MRI). When an intracerebral hematoma is identified, surgery may be indicated in order to drain the blood in the hematoma or, in some instances, to remove the hematoma completely.

Open Head Injury

Open head injury refers to an injury in which the skull is fractured (such as with a blow to the head in which the skull is broken). *Penetrating injury* refers to an open head injury in which the skull has been fractured or penetrated by a foreign object such as a bullet, nail gun, or knife. Fracture or penetration of the skull can force hair, skin, bone, or other fragments into the brain, lacerating and injuring internal structures of the brain as well as increasing the potential for infection.

Functional consequences experienced with open or penetrating injury may be more localized and related to the specific area of the brain affected. If secondary injury occurs from bone or other fragments that have been driven into the brain, functional consequences may be more extensive.

**Figure 4-2   Types and Locations
of Intracranial Hematoma**

TYPES OF INTRACRANIAL HEMATOMAS

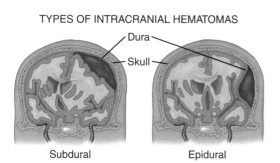

Subdural   Epidural

Blast Injury

Brain injury resulting from blasts is not clearly understood (Wang & Huang, 2013). Brain trauma associated with blasts does not appear to fit completely into either closed or open head injury categories because the primary nature of the injury is unclear. The extent to which brain damage is the direct result of blast-induced pressure waves on the brain and the extent to which damage occurs from secondary effects of the blast has yet to be determined. Likewise, brain trauma experienced from a blast is not always easily identified since manifestations may overlap with manifestations of other conditions such as posttraumatic stress. Consequently, it may be difficult to distinguish between manifestations that are the result of direct injury to the brain from those manifestations associated with emotional trauma (Warren et al., 2015).

Changes in atmospheric pressure following an explosion creates a blast wave. *Primary injury* can occur because blast wave–induced changes in atmospheric pressure cause acceleration of brain tissue resulting in displacement, and shearing forces, which injure internal brain structures, cause diffuse injury (Ropper, 2011). *Secondary injury* may be sustained from flying debris that strike the individual in the blast (MacDonald et al., 2011). *Tertiary injury* can result as, from the blast force, the individual is thrown against solid objects in the environment, causing additional injury. Secondary and/or tertiary blast injuries have been identified in many cases of TBI resulting from explosion, however the degree to which primary blast injury impacts on manifestations experienced with explosions remains unclear (Wang & Huang, 2013).

ASSESSING THE SEVERITY OF TRAUMATIC BRAIN INJURY

Neurological assessment and a number of other evaluation instruments are utilized for classification and to assess degree of injury, as predictors of discharge disposition, and as indicators of the type of rehabilitation services needed in early stages of management of TBI after hospitalization (Ling, 2016).

In the initial stages of brain injury, one tool for determining level of severity is the Glasgow Coma Scale (Jennet, Snoek, Bond, & Brooks, 1981). The Glasgow Coma Scale is a tool for assessing the degree of consciousness. It is typically used in the early postinjury period in the emergency and the critical care unit. The initial assessment provides a baseline from which subsequent changes in neurological status can be measured. The Glasgow Coma Scale is a standardized system by which three areas of function (eye opening, verbal response, and motor response) are assessed. Repeated observations through the Glasgow Coma Scale assists health professionals monitor improvement or deterioration of individuals' level of responsiveness. The scale assesses the level of consciousness along a continuum ranging from alert to coma. Scores are assigned according to the level of response in each of the three areas mentioned above. The range of scores that may be obtained on the scale is from 3 to 15. The lower the score, the deeper the level of unconsciousness and generally the greater the functional consequences.

Another instrument, the Glasgow Outcome Score (GOS), is generally used to assess and summarize functional capacity and outcome after brain injury. The GOS is divided into five categories that range from poor outcome with a range of 1–3 (*death, persistent vegetative state, severe disability*) to good outcome with a range of 4–5 (*moderate disability* or *low disability*) with expectation of return to regular activity.

A third instrument, the Glasgow Outcome Scale Extended (GOSE) is a functional outcome scale and was developed to address the perceived limitations of the Glasgow Outcome Scale so that small, but perhaps meaningful, changes in function could be measured (Scholten et al., 2015). It contains eight categories ranging from *dead* to *good recovery* with the ability to live independently and return to work or school.

The Rancho Los Amigos Cognitive Scale is a scale of cognitive functioning and was originally developed as a behavioral rating scale (Hagan, Malkmus, & Durham, 1972). In the acute stages of brain injury it is used to establish a baseline for comparison later to measure improvement in cognitive function and to give a gross indication of stages of recovery after brain injury. In the later stages of

Table 4-1   Revised Los Amigos Scale of Cognitive Functioning

Level I	No Response = Does not respond to visual, auditory, or tactile stimuli—Total assistance
Level II	Generalized Response = Reflex response to external stimuli. No apparent purposeful movement—Total Assistance
Level III	Localized response = Responds to stimuli, such as turning head in direction of sound or withdrawing from painful stimuli. Able to follow simple commands such as "Squeeze my hand."—Total Assistance
Level IV	Confused and Agitated = Demonstrates restlessness and agitation. Verbalizations may be incoherent and/or inappropriate—Maximal Assistance
Level V	Confused Nonagitated = Maybe able to follow simple instructions. Unable to self-monitor. Not oriented to person, place, or time. May wander randomly—Maximal Assistance
Level VI	Confused/Appropriate = Able to follow simple instructions. Increasing awareness of self and basic needs. Able to engage in self-care with supervision—Moderate Assistance
Level VII	Automatic = Oriented to person and place within environments that are familiar. Overestimates abilities. Difficulty recognizing appropriate social interaction. Able to carry out activities of daily living with some supervision—Minimal Assistance
Level VIII	Purposeful/Appropriate = Oriented to person, place, and time. Initiates and carries out activities of daily living with minimal assistance. Low frustration tolerance—Stand-By Assistance
Level IX	Purposeful, Appropriate = Able to initiate and carry out activity of daily living tasks independently. Acknowledges limitations when they interfere with task—Stand-by Assistance
Level X	Purposeful/Appropriate = Independently able to carry out steps to complete tasks at home, work, or leisure. May require more time to complete tasks. Accurately estimates abilities—Modified Independent

Data from Hagan, C., & Durham, P. (1987). Levels of cognitive functioning. In Rancho Los Amigos Hospital (Ed.) *Rehabilitation of the head injured adult: Comprehensive physical management*. Downey, California: Professional Staff Association of Rancho Los Amigos Hospital.

recovery it can be used as a broad indicator of the extent to which independent functioning is possible and to determine placement as well as the level of care that may be needed. The scale ranges from I (no response) to VIII (Purposeful/Appropriate) and up to X (Postacute/Stable) (see **Table 4-1**). Higher scores indicate higher functional level.

The Disability Rating Scale was developed to quantify functional capacity of individuals with TBI and their progress from the time of injury through rehabilitation to the time they reenter the community (Rappaport, Hall, Hopkins, Belleza, & Cope, 1982). This scale evaluates individuals on eight categories of functional ability. The highest score possible is 30. The lower the individual scores on the Disability Rating Scale, the better. Functional ability is scored on the following areas:

- Level of arousal, awareness, and responsiveness
- Cognitive skills needed for self-care
- Dependence on others

- Psychosocial adaptability, including flexibility and ability to adapt to different people and situations

In the treatment and rehabilitation phase after injury, individuals may remain at one level of unconsciousness or coma for an extended period of time or may move from one level of consciousness to the next. Measurement tools described above help health professionals assess changes in levels of consciousness during the postinjury period and the potential for independent function so that specific interventions can be instituted as the individual moves through different levels of recovery in order to build and restore functional capacity to the degree possible.

CATEGORIZATION OF TRAUMATIC BRAIN INJURY

Determination of severity of brain injury is based on the extent of the injury, the location of the brain damaged, as well as associated manifestations. Brain injuries are classified as *mild, moderate*, or *severe*. The most reliable predictor of functional recovery, especially for severe brain injury is the Glasgow Coma Scale score on initial evaluation (Bernat & Wudicks, 2016). In general, the lower the initial Glasgow Coma Scale score, the less the chances of significant functional recovery (Ling, 2016).

Potential consequences of brain injury vary tremendously depending on the type of injury and the area of brain injured as well as premorbid factors. In general, the more severe the injury, the more permanent functional consequences or deficits are experienced (Im et al., 2011). Although much attention has been devoted to moderate and severe brain injury, there is increasing awareness that mild brain injury, which may go undetected, may also have long-term functional consequences (Ling, 2016).

Mild Brain Injury

Mild brain injuries account for approximately most of all TBIs (Ling, 2016) and are characterized by a traumatically induced disruption of brain function, in which there is at least one of the manifestations listed in **Table 4-2**. Individuals with mild brain injuries have a Glasgow Coma Scale score of 13 or higher and may have few, if any, outer signs of brain injury or no detectable anatomic injury to the brain.

Concussion is a subset of *mild brain injury* and can be defined as a traumatically induced transient disruption of brain function (Hamon et al., 2013). Although concussion, in the past, was thought to have no long-term consequences, studies have now shown that manifestations, such as poor concentration, decreased attention span, and memory difficulties may be experienced hours or days after the injury (Marula et al., 2016), and there is increasing concern that recurrent concussions can contribute to development of long-term manifestations of cognitive dysfunction (Hamon et al., 2013; Ling, 2016).

Individuals with mild brain injury may experience subtle but disruptive manifestations that persist months or even years after the initial injury (Maruta et al., 2016). Manifestations associated with mild brain injury may not only cause individuals considerable distress but can also adversely affect both social and occupational functioning. This group of manifestations, now known as *postconcussion*

Table 4-2   Manifestations of Mild Brain Injury

Individual experiences at least one of the following:

1. Brief loss of consciousness (30 minutes or less)
2. Brief alteration of consciousness (up to 24 hours)
3. Posttraumatic amnesia for 0–1 day
4. Glasgow Coma Scale (best score of 13–15 within 24 hours)
5. Normal appearing brain on CT scan

Data from The Management of Concussion/mTBI Working Group. (2009). VA/DoD Clinical Practice Guidelines for Management of Concussion/Mild Traumatic Injury. *Journal of Rehabilitation Research & Development, 46*(6), CP1–CP68.

syndrome, can include headache, **vertigo** (dizziness), **tinnitus** (ringing in the ears), sleep disturbance, depression, irritability, reduced attention span, or memory impairment. Because there often are few, if any, objective signs of brain injury with mild brain injury, individuals experiencing these manifestations may have their credibility questioned or may be labeled as malingerers.

Moderate Brain Injury

Moderate brain injury is defined by a Glasgow Coma Scale score of 9 to 12. Individuals with moderate brain injury may experience loss of consciousness from a few minutes to several hours. They may develop confusion or disorientation, which may last for a few days or several weeks. Physical, cognitive, or psychosocial deficits from moderate brain injury, may last for weeks to months or, in some cases, may be permanent.

Severe Brain Injury

Individuals with a Glasgow Coma Scale score of 8 or less are considered to have *severe brain injury* (Ling, 2016) characterized by impaired consciousness/coma. **Coma** is defined as prolonged unconsciousness in which there is little, if any, meaningful response and the individual is unable to be awakened even by vigorous stimuli (Bernat & Widicks, 2016). Coma, resulting from severe brain injury may last for an extended period of time, lasting from days to months. Individuals are classified as being in a "*vegetative state*" when there is absence of awareness of the environment with no purposeful voluntary behavior in response to stimuli and no language comprehension or expression, despite giving the appearance at times of wakefulness. There are no interventions currently available to reverse long-standing vegetative state (Bernat & Widicks, 2016).

MANIFESTATIONS OF TRAUMATIC BRAIN INJURY

The brain not only monitors and regulates many unconscious bodily process such as cardiac and respiratory function but it also coordinates most voluntary movements and is the site of consciousness and all intellectual functions. Consequently, brain injury can have a profound impact on all areas of an individual's life and can impact any and all areas of functional ability, including:

- Physical function
- Perceptual function
- Speech and language
- Cognition
- Personality and behavior

Not all individuals with TBI are affected in the same way or to the same extent. Functional effects depend on the area of the brain injured, the extent of the damage, and whether the injury was diffuse or localized. Some individuals may only experience slight functional incapacity in a few areas, while others experience functional disability in a number of areas.

Physical Function

Brain injury can affect a number of motor functions, including ambulation, coordination, balance, strength, endurance, and fine motor skills. Rehabilitation programs evaluate and intervene to help the individual increase mobility, motor dexterity, and stamina in order to achieve greater independence.

Movement and Balance

When injury is more localized, such as with a gunshot wound and confined to one hemisphere of the brain, manifestations are related to the extent of injury and the hemisphere affected. Because each hemisphere of the brain controls the opposite side of the body, injury to one hemisphere affects function of the body on the opposite side. Consequently, injury to the right hemisphere of the brain can cause paralysis or weakness of the left side of the body (*left hemiplegia*), affecting the left arm and leg, while injury to the left hemisphere of the brain can result in paralysis or weakness of the right side of the body (*right hemiplegia*), affecting the right arm and leg. Resulting paralysis or weakness may interfere with the individual's ability to walk, so that assistive such as a cane, a walker, or a brace may be required for ambulation, In some instances, when there is severe weakness or paralysis of the extremities, a wheelchair may be required.

When the injury is diffuse, such as in closed head injury, changes in movement affecting both sides of the body may be present, resulting in problems with muscle coordination (**ataxia**). As a result, balance may be affected so that the individual walks with an unsteady gait or lurches from side to side as they walk. Other motor changes may include **dyskinesia** (abnormal movements) or **dystonia** (abnormal muscle tone). Dystonia can entail either too little tone (**flaccidity** or *hypotonicity*), which decreases the ability to move, or too much muscle tone (**spasticity** or *hypertonicity*), which heightens reflexes or exacerbates abnormal movement.

Individuals can be helped to increase strength and flexibility which subsequently enhance ambulation and balance through a number of interventions including exercises and physical therapy. Orthotic devices may be prescribed for some motor difficulties, such as gait deviation, muscle weakness of an extremity, or to stabilize a joint. In some instances, medications, such as muscle relaxants may be utilized for manifestations such as spasticity.

Coordination

Even when motor function of muscles remains intact and muscle strength and sensation are normal, individuals may experience problems with coordination in which there is loss of ability to organize and sequence specific muscle movements to perform a task (**apraxia**). Although with apraxia individuals are aware of what they want to do and how to do it, they are unable to organize and sequence muscle movements adequately in order to perform the task. Consequently, any number of tasks—from dressing and eating to performing more complex activities such as typing or driving—may be affected. Interventions designed to improve walking and coordination as well as interventions designed to help individuals identify and modify situations that make manifestations worse may also be utilized to improve functional ability.

Fatigue and Endurance

One residual effect after TBI may include extreme fatigue and lack of endurance when completing both mental and physical tasks, especially when tasks are unfamiliar or require significant concentration. Fatigue can also exacerbate other manifestations related to brain injury, compounding detrimental effects on daily functioning and well-being.

Mental fatigue as well as physical fatigue may be more common after TBI. Mental and physical activities that, prior to injury, were once easy for the individual may, postinjury, seem exhausting to complete. Sleep patterns may be also altered after TBI, affecting quality of sleep, which further contributes to fatigue (Viola-Saltzman & Musleh, 2016). Performance levels can deteriorate throughout the day due to fatigue. Consequently individuals may find that it preferable to perform most tasks earlier in the day rather than postponing tasks till later in the day.

Programs that help the individual pace and plan activities, incorporate rest periods throughout the day and learn strategies to maximize quality of sleep at night may help the individual to maximize energy and increase functional capacity.

Eating and Swallowing

Swallowing reflexes may be affected after TBI so that individuals have difficulty with swallowing (**dysphagia**), and, in some instances, individuals may also experience difficulty with chewing. Because of difficulty with swallowing or performing chewing movements, food may be pocketed in one side of the mouth, increasing the risk of gagging or choking. If the gag reflex is also impaired, susceptibility to choking is also increased.

Inability or difficulty related to swallowing can be dangerous because of the risk of *aspiration* (food or liquid entering the lungs rather than the stomach). Interventions to decrease risk of choking or aspiration may include programs that help the individual learn strategies for safe eating and swallowing. In some instances, individuals with swallowing difficulty may require a special diet consisting of soft pureed food that are easier to swallow, or they may need tube feedings in order to prevent aspiration of food into the lungs.

Bowel and Bladder Function

In some instances bladder or bowel function may be affected after brain injury. Individuals may experience **incontinence** (involuntary excretion of urine or solid waste from the body). Incontinence may be due to the individual's inability to recognize the need to urinate or defecate or because of loss of voluntary control of sphincter muscles, which maintain continence. In other instances, other physical impairments, such as difficulty with ambulation, may make it difficult for the individual to reach restroom facilities in time.

Some individuals may, after brain injury, experience inability to urinate at will or to completely empty the bladder when urinating. If bladder and/or bowel function are affected after TBI a bladder and/or bowel retraining program may be instituted. In some cases, if bladder and/or bowel problems persist, adult incontinence protection garments may be needed, or an *indwelling urinary catheter* (a tube inserted into the bladder) in order to drain urine may be utilized.

Perceptual Manifestations

Perceptual ability affects the ability to identify, organize, and interpret information in order to understand the environment and involves vision, hearing, sensation, smell, taste, perception of body balance and position, and perception of the social environment. Although perception is shaped by many factors, it is reliant on the nervous system to receive and process information from the environment. The type of and degree to which perceptional ability is affected after brain injury depends on the area of the brain injured. Although some perceptual changes may improve over time, other perceptual consequences resulting from brain injury may remain permanent.

Recognition

In some instances, individuals lose the ability to recognize familiar things such as words, faces, or objects (**agnosia**). When the brain injury is localized (especially to the right side), individuals may experience a condition called **anosognosia** (one-sided or unilateral neglect) in which body parts or objects on one side of the body are ignored. For example, an individual with anosognosia may shave only one side of the face or put on only one shoe. In some instances, anosognosia is visual, so that there is an inability to perceive objects on either the right or left side of the central field of vision. For example, individuals may only eat food on one side of the plate, leaving the food on the other side untouched, or, when surrounded by people, they may only acknowledge people locate on their unaffected side.

In some cases, anosognosia may affect the ability to recognize auditory stimuli on the affected side so that even though the physical mechanisms involved in hearing are intact on the affected side, auditory stimuli on that side are ignored and only auditory stimuli to the unaffected side evokes a response.

Although there is no direct cure for deficits of perceptual loss, individuals can be helped to learn compensatory modalities with alternative cues and organizational strategies to improve functional ability.

Visual–Spatial Relations

Visual–spatial deficits cause problems with depth perception and judgment of distance, size, position, rate of movement, form, and the relation of parts to wholes. Visual–spatial changes resulting from brain injury interfere with the ability to interpret visual information accurately. Consequently, individuals with visual deficits may have difficulty orienting position and navigating movement within the environment, or they may demonstrate inaccurate judgment of space or distance, under- or overestimating the relationship of distance between two objects. As a result, their movements may seem careless or clumsy, such as frequently bumping into furniture, having difficulty navigating doorways, knocking items off tables or counters, or missing the table when attempting to put a glass down.

Other activities, such as reading, dressing, or driving may also be affected by visual–spatial deficits. For example, when reading, the individual may continually lose their place on the page, or when dressing they may confuse the inside and outside of clothes as well as confusing left and right. Difficulty in judging distances, even if visual–spatial deficits are minimal may make it difficult for individuals to perform tasks such as driving a car.

Programs designed to assist individuals with visual–spatial deficits to learn compensatory strategies can enhance their ability to maneuver in their environment. Retraining skills programs may include repetitive exercise to help individuals compensate for deficits in order to perform a specific task. In some instances individuals may be helped to learn how to modify their environment so that provides more supports and reduces demands.

Vision and Hearing

Visual consequences of TBI may be present even though the eye itself was not injured. Although the eye may still receive light rays, which create an image, in order for a visual image to be perceived, it must be converted into an electrical image that is transmitted to the brain where it is perceived and interpreted. When the neural network of the brain that receives, perceives, or interprets these electrical impulses is damaged, visual deficits may occur.

Visual consequences of TBI can include total blindness, **diplopia** (double vision), blurred vision, cuts in the peripheral field of vision (*blind spots*), **hemianopsia** (loss of vision in half the visual field), or color blindness.

Hearing consequences of TBI may also be present even though the ear itself was not injured. As with vision, in order for hearing to take place the brain must receive, perceive, and interpret auditory signals. When the portion of the brain responsible for transmitting nerve impulses or interpreting auditory signals is injured, hearing deficits (**sensorineural hearing loss**) may result.

Individuals may experience partial or total hearing loss, or they may experience ringing in the ears (**tinnitus**). Injury to areas of the brain that interpret and process auditory signals may result in *central auditory processing disorder,* which affects the efficiency and effectiveness with which the brain recognizes and uses sound. In these cases, even though basic hearing mechanisms are intact, the individual is unable to process information they hear in the same way as others because of decreased coordination between the brain and the ear.

Programs for both vision and hearing deficits experienced after TBI are based on individual need after evaluation of specific strengths and deficits. Visual programs include specific regimes that enhance the individual's visual capability and can help them to improve control of their visual system and increase visual efficiency. Management of hearing deficits are based on the type of hearing loss and can include assistive devices and/or training in the use of compensatory strategies to enhance hearing.

Comprehension of Sensation

Brain injury involving parts of the brain responsible for sensation can lead to a variety of consequences, such as numbness (*anesthesia*), the inability to feel pain (*analgesia*), or the inability to sense movement of body parts. Individuals may also experience abnormal sensations (**paresthesia**) such as pain, tingling, or burning in various locations in the body.

Interventions for problems with sensation depend on individual need. If the individual experiences numbness or lack of sensation in a body part, steps to prevent injury from burns, pressure, or other environmental hazards are important. Interventions, such as stretching exercises, massage, or at times medications, may be used to reduce discomfort experienced with paresthesia.

Taste and Smell

Sense of taste and smell may also be affected by TBI. Individuals may lose total sense of smell (**anosmia**) if the olfactory nerve or corresponding area of the brain has been injured. Although loss of sense of smell may not appear to be a significant consequence of brain injury, it can have important functional implications. Loss of sense of smell can affect the ability to detect hazards such as smoke, gas leaks, or to smell spoiled food. Loss of sense of smell also has social implications, impacting the ability to detect body odor or the overuse of perfumes or after shaves. Lack of sense of smell also affects the ability to taste. Inability to taste may affect the individual's will to eat and, consequently, can also affect nutritional status.

In some cases, improvement in taste and smell may improve over time. When taste and smell are affected, programs that help individuals learn strategies to compensate for losses may be instituted. For example, for safety issues individuals may need to be made aware of the necessity of devices such as smoke alarms or gas detectors in their environment. When taste is affected, a clinical dietitian may be able to offer recommendations for tips, such as making food visually appealing, or using a variety of food textures in meals to increase the individual's willingness to eat.

Speech and Language

Communication is basic to human interaction and has an impact on all areas of activities from social and family interactions, to recreation, to employment. Depending on the area of the brain injured, a number of mechanisms that affect communication may be impacted.

Speech

Speech refers to the physical ability to produce sounds and/or movement of the lips, tongue, or other structures that are used to speak. **Articulation** refers to the position and placement of the tongue and muscles of the palate necessary to enunciate words and sentences. When an area of the brain that controls motor ability of the muscles used in movement of lips, tongue, or other parts of the speech mechanism is injured, individuals may experience weakness or paralysis of the muscles involved in speech. As a result, the ability to move or sequence movements of the tongue or other structures necessary for precise speech is affected—a condition is called **dysarthria**. Dysarthria results in a range of difficulties with pronunciation, varying from slurred speech to speech that is nearly unintelligible.

In some instances, although motor ability of structures involved in speech is not affected, injury to the brain affects the individual's ability to plan, organize, and smoothly execute a learned movement necessary for speech. In this case, even though there is no muscle weakness or paralysis, clarity of speech is affected, a condition called **apraxia of speech**.

Speech difficulties may range from mild to severe. Depending on the degree of speech involvement from brain injury, a number of interventions to assist individuals develop compensatory mechanisms to address specific speech issues may be instituted.

Language

Language refers to how words, gestures, and other symbols are put together to convey and understand concepts. Injury to language-oriented areas of the brain can affect the individual's ability to use words, gestures, or symbols to convey concepts, as well as the ability to understand them. The inability or decreased ability to communicate through speech, writing, or signs is called **aphasia**. There are two types of aphasia: *receptive* and *expressive.*

Receptive aphasia involves injury to the portion of the brain responsible for interpreting auditory or visual stimuli. When the word processing area of the brain is injured, individuals may have difficulty understanding or interpreting the meaning spoken words or meaning of signs or symbols. If the visual center of the brain is affected, individuals may have difficulty distinguishing between and interpreting written words. When both areas are involved, individuals will be unable to understand either spoken or written word, or signs or symbols, although the ability to produce speech may be unimpaired.

Expressive aphasia refers to individuals' inability to communicate what they want to say verbally or in writing, even though they know what they want to say. In other instances, individuals may experience **anomia**, difficulty finding words they want to say, or **paraphrasia**, in which they are unable to use words correctly and coherently. In the latter instance, spoken words or word combinations are so jumbled and misused that speech becomes intelligible.

Speech and language therapies are directed toward improving communication through strategies to enhance listening, speaking, reading, and writing skills or assisting the individual to convey messages through compensatory strategies or alternative means of communication. The success of interventions to assist individuals to gain a functional level of communication skill or to learn compensatory skills is dependent on the extent of damage as well as on the individual's motivation and adjustment to their limitations.

Cognitive Manifestations

Cognition refers to mental processes important to memory and learning, information processing and concept formation, attention, and concentration, as well as executive function, a complex group of skills used to plan, problem solve, and make decisions using sound judgment. The degree of cognitive dysfunction after TBI can range from severe to more subtle impairments that are only noticeable when the individual is fatigued or under stress.

Memory and Learning

Memory encompasses the ability to encode, store, and retrieve information, while learning encompasses the ability to acquire new information or modify existing knowledge, skills, or behavior. After TBI, some individuals may experience difficulty with remembering or learning new information. The type and degree of memory or learning problems occurring after TBI varies from individual to individual.

Memory problems affect the individual's ability to recognize and recall people, places, facts, and concepts as well as to problem solve, form goals, organize, and plan. Memory for both new and old information may be affected.

Several types of memory exist:

- *Immediate memory* lasts only seconds or minutes unless converted into short-term memory. An example of immediate memory is remembering a phone number long enough to dial the number but not committing it to memory for later use.

- *Short-term memory* lasts from minutes to hours, but information is lost if not converted to long-term memory. An example of short-term memory is learning facts for an exam but not committing the facts to long-term memory for future use.
- *Long-term memory* refers to memories that are stored and able to be retrieved in the future, whether weeks or years ahead.

Some individuals may lose the ability to acquire new memories or to recall recent conversations and events. In some instances individuals with brain damage may experience **confabulation**, in which, with no intent to deceive, they fabricate, distort, or present false information about past events that they believe to be true.

Perservation, defined as repetitive speech or thoughts or repetitive and continuous behavior, may also occur after TBI. For example, the individual may become stuck on one theme during conversation, repeating a question, phrase, or concept again and again.

Perseveration can also pertain to tasks, which the individual repeats over and over, such as continuing to wipe the same spot on a counter until someone intervenes. In some instances, preservation may affect adaptive skills affecting the ability to learn from past experience so that the individual continues to use the same strategy to solve a problem even though it is clear the strategy doesn't work.

Some individuals experience *retrograde amnesia,* in which they are unable to remember events that occurred or information learned prior to the injury. Retrograde amnesia does not impair the formation of new memories and often includes loss more recently acquired memories rather than memories formed in the more distant past.

Individuals with brain injury may be unable to remember previously learned skills that were once very familiar, such as dressing, or preparing a sandwich either because they are unable to remember the steps involved or because, after completing the first steps of the task, they forget their original goal.

Memory and learning issues may be one the most limiting of all the potential cognitive consequences of brain injury. Deficits affect the ability to learn, store, and retrieve information. The ability to generalize, or to transfer or apply what has been learned in one setting to another setting, may be lost. For instance, even though an individual has learned and can perform a task in a rehabilitation setting, they may be unable to then perform the same task in his or her own home.

In some instances, over time, memory may gradually improve. Although memory may not be restored to preinjury status, memory specialists can teach individuals memory strategies which help them to compensate for memory loss. Memory specialists can also help individuals identify situations such as fatigue, sleep loss, or emotional stress, which can affect memory so that interventions to minimize these situations can be taken.

Attention and Concentration

After brain injury, individuals may experience disrupted attention and concentration as well as decreased speed and efficiency of information processing (Maruta et al., 2016). Even in mild cases of brain injury, individuals may find that it takes more cognitive effort to pay attention and that they are more easily distracted.

Suffering from difficulty with attention, concentration may make it difficult for the individuals to understand information, follow a train of thought, or accurately interpret information they receive. They may have difficulty focusing on one task or difficulty shifting from one task to another, moving from one task to another without completing any. In other instances they may have difficulty performing multiple tasks at one time, such as writing notes while talking on the telephone or carrying on a conversation while involved in another task, such as polishing furniture. Individuals may also have difficulty retaining directions that include multiple components, such as asking an individual to stand up, turn off the television, close the windows, and lock the door.

Cognitive rehabilitation can assist individuals to gain insight into attention and concentration issues and to learn strategies that help them learn to focus attention as well as to increase ability to concentrate.

Information Processing and Concept Formation

The speed and efficiency of information processing may be disrupted after TBI so that more time to synthesize verbal or visual input is required. As a result, individuals may have delayed responses, making it difficult to maintain the pace in a social setting. Individuals may also have difficulty forming and understanding concepts, or have problems with abstract thinking. As a result, the individual may think only in concrete terms, taking cues and stimuli literally. For instance, in a money exchange in which there is reference to the denomination of currency, the phrase "Do you have anything smaller?" may be taken quite literally to mean the physical size of the currency rather than the monetary value.

Interventions, tailored to the individual and their degree of impairment, that promote self-directed strategies, which can be generalized to tasks of daily living have been found to be helpful in some cases (Cicerone et al., 2012).

Problem Solving and Decision Making

Planning, organizing, and sequencing tasks, may be difficult after brain injury making even apparently simple tasks problematic. For example, when preparing a meal, the individual may not realize that food items that take more time to cook should be prepared first. Consequently, when cooking dinner, they may fully prepare the mashed potatoes before even starting to make the meatloaf. In other instances, there may be difficulty following steps in order. For instance, when dressing, individuals may put on their slacks before they put on underwear or put their socks on over their shoes.

Difficulty with problem solving may consist of the inability to recognize problems as they occur, or, when a problem is identified, the inability to generate alternative solutions or to select a solution when one is presented. Reasoning and decision making may also be affected. The individual may be unable to view the situation as a whole, considering only the portion of the information which is immediately apparent. For example, they may recognize that in order to reach an out-of-town location they can take a train, but they may be unable to recognize the need to have money in order to buy a ticket.

Individuals may also have difficulty thinking of or planning for the future. For instance, they may see no need to have some food supplies to be readily available at home until they are hungry, or they may use all of their money for a taxi ride to a specific destination without thinking about how they will be able to pay for the ride back.

Individuals may also demonstrate the inability to initiate and sustain activity so that tasks are delayed or not completed. For example, when given the task of straightening a room, they may be unable to initiate the task on their own without prompting, or they may be unable to complete the task without continued guidance and direction. Performance may be inconsistent so that even though tasks are performed well on one day, on subsequent days performance may be inadequate.

Breaking tasks into smaller steps, and receiving frequent feedback and guidance can enhance individual's ability to perform tasks.

Judgment

After TBI, individuals may have difficulty accurately analyzing situations and potential consequences of their decisions or they may overestimate their ability and resources. These deficits result in impairment of judgment which can lead to risk taking–behaviors with potential self-endangerment or endangerment to others. For example, the individual may see no harm in leaving a sleeping child in a running car in a closed garage in order to not disturb the child and to keep the child warm.

In other instances, individuals may behave impulsively without anticipating the consequences of their behavior. For example, an unemployed individual may withdraw all money from their checking and savings account to buy a new sports car without thinking about whether they can afford it or if, after buying the car, they will be able to pay other bills.

Support groups for the individual and their family as well as programs for cognitive remediation that provide specific interventions to raise awareness of deficits in judgment, and provide strategies for monitoring situations for potential harm, can be used to enhance function and decrease risk.

Personality and Behavior

Depending on the degree and location of brain damage, TBI may bring about subtle or pronounced changes in personality that can affect family and social relationships and complicate reentry into community, work, and social settings. Family members may express feeling that they are "living with a stranger," or friends and colleagues may describe the individual as being completely different from the person they once knew. For example, an individual who, preinjury, may have been kind, loving, and thoughtful, may after injury exhibit frequent bouts of anger and insensitivity. An individual who was once calm and rational may, postinjury, become unpredictable and volatile, or an individual who was once outgoing and gregarious may, postinjury, become withdrawn and reclusive.

Family, friends, or acquaintances may not recognize personality changes as being related to the brain injury, especially if the changes are subtle. They may, instead, blame the individual, attributing the behavior to willful uncooperativeness, lack of consideration, or laziness. Programs to lend support and help others understand changes and how they related to brain injury as well as teaching target strategies to deal with specific behavioral issues can be helpful.

Disinhibition

Disinhibition in which individuals lose the ability to self censor may also be a consequence of brain injury. Because disinhibition impairs the individual's ability to filter or monitor their behavior, the ability to follow social or cultural rules may be lost. Consequently, they may speak without considering how inappropriate, rude, or insensitive their remarks may be. They also may be unable to self- monitor or control urges so that they eat or drink in access, make inappropriate sexual remarks, touch individuals inappropriately, exhibit inappropriate sexual behavior in public, or become over demanding sexually.

Inadequate and impaired social skills may make it difficult for individuals to function effectively within the environment. Medical, environmental, and psychotherapeutic strategies can be implemented to assist individuals' ability to achieve their optimal level of function within the family, community, and work environment.

Anger

After brain injury, anger or irritability can be a direct physiologic consequence of injury to the brain, but it can also be the result of frustration as the individual attempts to adjust to changes brought about by residuals of brain injury and their long-term implications. They may feel isolated or misunderstood, or they may have difficulty adjusting to functional and role changes. Anger can be expressed actively or passively, verbally or physically.

Support groups and peer mentoring can help individuals to feel less isolated. Learning anger management techniques as well as identifying situations that trigger frustration and anger can also be helpful so those situations can be minimized or avoided.

Depression

Depression has an effect on health, productivity, and quality of life and can exacerbate manifestations of brain injury, slow the pace of cognitive recovery, and impede social functioning and performance of activities of daily living (Garrelfs, Donker-Cools, Wind, & Frings-Dresen, 2015). Although depression can be a physiological result of brain injury, it is also a natural reaction to the loss. Individuals with brain injury can experience a number of losses related to cognitive, motor, sensory, social, and vocational functions.

At times, it may be difficult to discern the extent to which depression is the direct result of physiologic changes in the brain after injury and the extent to which depression is the result of the grieving process as the individual gains awareness of losses, restrictions, and alterations in lifestyle resulting from their injury.

After experiencing brain injury, some individuals have no memory of what they were like prior to the injury. Others may develop an increasing awareness of their condition and its implications, or an awareness that they are unable to perform tasks they performed previously. They may recognize role changes they are experiencing and sense a change of status within family, social, and work settings that diminishes their self-image.

As a result, they may become preoccupied with feelings of worthlessness and grief because of the inability to assume former roles. As a part of grieving, individuals may experience sleep disturbances, become increasingly sad and withdrawn, showing little initiative or motivation.

Neither the individual nor others in the environment may recognize the manifestations as a consequence of depression. As a result, appropriate help may not be sought. Identifying depression is the first step toward finding seeking help to resolve it. Although no single intervention works for everyone, psychotherapeutic and behavioral interventions, peer support, enhancement of positive interactions within the environment, and at times medication are useful tools often used to reduce to manifestations of depression.

Self-Awareness

Self-awareness has practical implications for motivation, involvement, and outcomes. Compensatory strategies designed to assist individuals to regain optimal function after brain injury can only be effective if the individual acknowledges that deficits exist. One of the consequences of TBI, however, may be the individual's limited awareness or acknowledgment of their limitations and the subsequent implications of their injury. They may underestimate the severity of their physical, cognitive, and behavioral limitations and overestimate their ability, setting unrealistic goals.

Individuals may also demonstrate lack of insight into the appropriateness of their behavior, remaining oblivious to subtle reactions or emotional cues from others. They may be unable to monitor and adjust their own actions according to feedback from others, or they may discount feedback because it conflicts with their own views of their behavior or performance.

At times psychological denial of limitations can be a contributing factor to limited self-awareness. In other instances sociocultural or environmental influences may promote or encourage individuals' views, thus contributing to their unrealistic assessment of their ability. Interventions to assist individuals with limited self-awareness consist of identification of the extent to which neurological, psychological, and sociocultural/environmental factors contribute to decreased self-awareness and then planning appropriate psychotherapeutic, behavioral, compensatory or faciliatory strategies.

CONDITIONS ASSOCIATED WITH TRAUMATIC BRAIN INJURY

Posttraumatic Seizures and Posttraumatic Epilepsy

Posttraumatic seizures is a term used to describe seizures occurring within the first 24 hours or first few weeks after TBI. They are related to increased intracranial pressure caused from swelling (**edema**) of the brain or from other direct results of injury and often resolve after swelling in the brain subsides. It is important to distinguish between posttraumatic seizures and a condition called *posttraumatic epilepsy,* a condition in which there are ongoing, recurrent seizures after the immediate postrecovery period. Seizures associated with posttraumatic epilepsy may be mild or severe and may be attributed to the formation of scar tissue in the brain. If they are severe, they can be significantly disabling and are more likely to require management with ongoing antiepileptic medications.

Posttraumatic Hydrocephalus

Individuals with TBI may also develop *posttraumatic hydrocephalus,* a condition characterized by increased volume of circulating cerebrospinal fluid due to blockage of flow, overproduction, or decreased reabsorption of cerebral spinal fluid into the body. The accumulation of cerebrospinal fluid causes increased pressure on the brain *(increased intracranial pressure),* that can result in increasing neurological or functional deterioration. If left untreated, posttraumatic hydrocephalus can cause increased brain damage, increased functional incapacity and in some instances can be fatal.

Posttraumatic hydrocephalus may be treated surgically by implanting a drain or, in more severe cases, a shunt into a ventricle of the brain in order to empty the cerebrospinal fluid to another part of the body, usually the abdominal cavity. Although the drain may be temporary until the problem resolves, the shunt may be permanent. The prognosis for individuals who develop posttraumatic hydrocephalus varies depending on the severity and the presence (or absence) of additional brain damage.

Chronic Traumatic Encephalopathy

Although in the past, damage to the brain was thought to be stable after the initial injury, increasing studies have demonstrated that after TBI in some instances there is continuing deterioration of brain tissue over time (Green, 2015; Maruta et al., 2016). *Chronic traumatic encephalopathy* (CTE) is a term used to describe progressive neurological deterioration associated with repeated brain injury (Bieniek et al., 2015; Stein, Alvarez, & Mckee, 2015). Most often CTE has been associated with sports injuries, but the condition is increasingly now also associated with blast injury (McKee, Stein, Kieman, & Alvarez, 2015).

Manifestations of CTE include behavior and mood changes, impairment of memory and other cognitive functions, and dementia. In addition to management of individual manifestations, current efforts are directed to arriving at clinical diagnosis criteria for early recognition of CTE as well as identifying risk factors and protocols for prevention of injury.

Substance Abuse

Substance abuse has been found to be a contributing factor in a number of accidents that result in TBI (O'Connor, 2016). Individuals with substance abuse issues prior to injury may continue to abuse substances after injury, given the preinjury propensity for abuse paired with stress of adjusting to changes associated with brain injury.

Individuals with no prior history of substance abuse preinjury may also be more vulnerable to substance abuse postinjury. They may use substances as a way of coping with adjustment to changes brought about by brain injury, or substance abuse may be related to manifestations resulting from brain injury such as poor impulse control, impaired judgment, and inability to self-monitor or self-regulate.

Substance abuse after brain injury, whether or not it was present preinjury can contribute to poor rehabilitation outcomes as well as predispose

to further injury. After brain injury, there may be increased sensitivity to effects of alcohol or drug so that deficits in cognitive and/or psychomotor function are intensified. Abuse of drugs or alcohol also affects psychosocial function, making it more difficult for individuals to integrate into the community or the workplace.

If an individual is prone to seizures after TBI, drugs and/or alcohol lower seizure thresholds, increasing seizures risk. In addition, alcohol and drugs can interact with prescribed medications, causing deleterious effects. Assessment of alcohol and drug use should be an ongoing throughout the rehabilitation process and if substance abuse is identified, the individual should be referred to a substance abuse program, and, if possible, one that has been specifically adapted for individuals with TBI.

MANAGEMENT OF TRAUMATIC BRAIN INJURY

Comprehensive, individualized interdisciplinary management and rehabilitation provided by a diverse team of professionals is necessary to achieve both short-term goals and global outcomes for individuals with TBI. Interventions directed toward preventive, restorative, and compensatory strategies are instituted to assist the individual to achieve optimal function in all areas of daily life. The course of recovery and rehabilitation of individuals with TBI varies but is almost always lengthy, ranging from months to years.

Physicians involved in the care of individuals with TBI usually include a primary physician such as an internist or family physician, as well as specialists such as a *neurologist*, a *neurosurgeon*, and a *physiatrist*. Other health professionals involved in the individual's care, treatment, and rehabilitation may include a variety of health professionals such as nurses, respiratory therapists, physical therapists, dietitians or nutrition specialists, speech/language pathologists, audiologists, pharmacists, occupational therapists, recreational therapists, clinical or counseling psychologists, neuropsychologists, cognitive retrainers, social workers, and rehabilitation counselors.

Initial Management of Traumatic Brain Injury

The initial treatment for individuals experiencing TBI is directed toward stabilizing the condition and preventing additional brain injury from secondary causes such as swelling (**edema**) and bleeding. Initial management is also directed toward maintaining nutritional status and preventing other complications that could compromise recovery and/or function.

In the initial stages after brain injury, individuals are immobile, predisposing them to complications such as pneumonia, pressure sores (*decubitus ulcers*), urinary tract infections, and blood clots, any of which can impede recovery. If increased muscle tone or paralysis of extremities is present after brain injury, permanent deformities such as **contractures** (deformity and immobility of a joint due to permanent contraction of a muscle) can occur. If left untreated, contractures can contribute to mobility limitations, reduced functional range of motion, and decreased future functional ability. Interventions to prevent and treat contractures are directed toward improving range of motion by placing joints in a position of function, passive stretching exercises, and in some instances splinting or bracing joints in order to minimize disability from contracture.

Neurosurgical procedures are sometimes indicated in the immediate-treatment phase of brain injury. Careful observation is essential to detect early signs of increased intracranial pressure due to swelling of the brain or intracranial bleeding, which, unless relieved, could cause additional injury or even death. When brain swelling is the cause of increased intracranial pressure, medications may be administered to decrease swelling of the brain, thus decreasing intracranial pressure. As mentioned previously, when increased intracranial pressure is due to the volume of cerebral spinal fluid, surgical placement of a drain or shunt to allow excess cerebrospinal fluid to drain into the general body circulation may be needed.

As discussed earlier in the chapter, increased intracranial pressure can also be caused by accumulation of blood in or around the brain, such as from a blood clot (e.g., a *subdural or epidural hematoma*) or because of hemorrhage. In order to relieve the pressure a surgical procedure in which two small holes are drilled into the skull (*burr holes*) may be necessary to provide entry into the skull so that the blood clot removed or bleeding controlled. In some instances, a **craniotomy** (a surgical procedure in which the skull is surgically opened) may be necessary to remove a clot or foreign object or to control bleeding. If TBI involves an open skull fracture, surgery may be necessary to remove fragments of bone or other foreign materials and to repair the skull.

Other injuries—such as spinal cord injury, musculoskeletal injury, or injury to internal organs—may have also occurred at the time of brain injury. Presence of other associated injuries compound the recovery and rehabilitation process.

Postacute Management and Rehabilitation

After the condition has stabilized, appropriate postacute management requires early and active intervention by the interdisciplinary team. The goal is to help individuals achieve as much independent function as possible in as many areas as possible. In the early phases after brain injury, *physical therapy* may focus on activities to prevent joint and muscular complications. *Physical therapists* work with individuals early after the initial phase of brain injury to provide range-of-motion exercise to extremities, thereby preventing deformity, and later in the recovery period to assist with ambulation. Later physical therapy may be directed toward helping individuals improve balance, muscle control, ambulation, and other physical movements. Individuals who experience **hemiplegia** (paralysis on one side of the body) may need special instruction in ambulation techniques (*gait training*).

Depending on the extent of permanent injury to the brain, individuals may use assistive devices to perform a variety of functions and activities. Braces or splints may be necessary to help individuals increase their functional capacity and become independent. Individuals with paralysis of an arm may be taught to use special tools such as a plate guard to keep food from sliding off the plate, or special eating utensils or other tools designed to help in activities of daily living. If the individual has paralysis of an upper extremity, the weight of the paralyzed arm can cause separation of the arm from the shoulder joint (**subluxation**). To prevent separation from occurring, individuals may wear a sling to support the arm.

Often cognitive changes—rather than physical changes—hamper effective daily functioning for individuals with brain injury. In these instances, *cognitive remediation* strategies designed to ameliorate sensory and perceptual, language-related, and problem-solving deficits may be a major focus of rehabilitation. Cognitive strengths and weaknesses are identified through observation and *neuropsychological assessment*. How cognitive abilities and limitations in areas such as memory, organizational ability, reasoning, or judgment affect the individual's ability to function in the environment is evaluated, and cognitive strategies are devised to help them compensate for or remediate those shortcomings as needed. Individuals are then helped to transfer these strategies from the clinical setting to their own environment. In some instances, depending on the individual's life circumstances and the extent of his or her brain injury, long-term supportive care may be needed.

Most individuals who have experienced brain injury should abstain from alcohol and all drugs that are not part of the management plan. As noted earlier, the use of alcohol and other substances can increase potential for seizures after brain injury. In addition, taking alcohol or drugs in combination with prescribed medications can lead to danger-ous interactions. Furthermore, alcohol and other substances may accentuate any residual deficits from brain injury, increasing the chances of ad-ditional accident or injury as well as impairing individuals' ability to function to their optimal capacity.

Individuals with brain injury may need assis-tance to increase their awareness or orientation to time, place, and person. *Occupational therapy* can help individuals with brain injury integrate avail-able sensory information so that they can use it as a basis for motor activity and increase their ability to perform activities of daily living. Helping indi-viduals learn skills and use assistive devices that would help them with activities of daily living, such

as skills related to personal hygiene, dressing, or eating, may also be a focus of therapy.

Speech and language therapies may focus on the mechanical difficulties of speech, the formation and execution of language, or the development of alternative communication systems. *Speech and language therapists* may help individuals with both verbal and nonverbal communication. Focus may be on speech or language acquisition, or on conversational skills training. The *speech therapist* can also help individuals with brain injury develop social skills that relate to communication so that they learn techniques to enhance communication and ways to structure the environment to maximize their communication effectiveness. In some instances, alternative methods of communication, such as writing or using a picture board, may be used.

If individuals have impaired swallowing capabilities, *speech pathologists* may be involved in helping individuals learn how to swallow again. In some instances, speech pathologists may also be involved in cognitive remediation.

Clinical or counseling psychologists may conduct psychotherapy or counseling with the individual with brain injury and family members to facilitate adjustment. *Neuropsychologists*—psychologists who specialize in neurological testing and assessing brain function—may be involved in neurological assessment, through conducting comprehensive neuropsychological evaluations. Some neuropsychologists may also be involved in cognitive retraining or remediation in which individuals with brain injury learn ways to compensate for areas of cognitive function with which they may have difficulty.

After the individual's condition is stable and they reached optimal functional capacity, they may return home with family support and with appropriate accommodations based on individual need. Several types of focused programs—namely, home-based programs, outpatient rehabilitation programs, community reentry programs, day treat-ment, residential community reentry or transitional living programs, or neurobehavioral programs may be implemented to improve overall function and quality of life while attempting to help indi-viduals gain optimal involvement in family, com-munity, and work settings. These programs offer interventions designed to improve physical and/or cognitive functioning as well as helping individuals adjust and become integrated into the community or work environment. Individuals with significant residual physical, cognitive, or behavioral deficits may require a program that provides continuing supervision and care in meeting basic needs, such as a supported living program or independent living center.

FUNCTIONAL IMPLICATIONS OF TRAUMATIC BRAIN INJURY

Personal and Psychosocial Issues

Aside from psychological manifestations directly related to brain injury itself, individuals with TBI may experience a number of emotional reactions as they cope with the stress and changes their injury has brought about and as they work toward incorporating those changes into their daily lives. Emotional adjustment and adaptation after TBI are unique to the individual and appear to be influenced by a number of factors, including extent and location of injury, social support, educational attainment, and premorbid functioning (Bowen et al., 2016). Consequently, the range of emotional reactions experienced after TBI is vast and individually determined, ranging from depression to mood swings to psychosis (Stéfan, Mathé, & SOFMER Group, 2016).

Just as physical, cognitive, and emotional changes associated with brain injury can cause stress, anxiety, and depression, so can stress, anxiety, and depression influence physical, cognitive, and emotional adaptation (Shields, Ownsworth, O'Donovan, & Fleming, 2016). Adaptation is an individual and dynamic process. Although psychological responses to TBI vary from individual to individual, it is safe to assume that, whether the injury is mild or severe, some psychological, emotional, and behavioral manifestations will be experienced. How individuals view the brain injury in terms of its cause, as well as the extent to which they blame themselves or others for the injury, can influence both their emotional reactions and their subjective well-being.

Emotional manifestations may vary in different phases of adaptation. In the early stages of

adaptation, individuals may deny or not recognize the extent of manifestations of the injury. In later stages of adaptation, as individuals become aware of their limitations, they may experience anger or frustration because of difficulty with various previously mastered tasks, such as dressing or driving, or difficulty with functions, such as memory, speech, or language.

After brain injury, individuals may perceive environmental demands as antagonistic and as greater than their ability to adequately respond. In turn, they may feel vulnerable and unprotected and exhibit anxiety in response to their uncertainty. Feelings of anxiety may be compounded by feelings of worthlessness due to the inability to perform tasks or duties once performed easily prior to the injury. Some individuals may experience feelings of guilt because of inconveniences or problems they believe they are causing their family.

After TBI, individuals' comprehension of the world around them changes. They may experience changes in their thought processes or have difficulty grasping and processing new information. They may have difficulty with perception of events or interactions, or experience difficulty making logical connections or knowing how to respond.

Depression is common after TBI and can have a major impact on overall outcome (Wee et al., 2016), including higher incidence of suicide (Nowranqi, Kortte, & Rao, 2014). Although depression experienced after TBI may, in part, be the direct result of injury to brain tissue, psychosocial factors clearly make significant contributions as well (Wee et al., 2016).

Some manifestations attributed to brain injury itself may actually be associated with *posttraumatic stress disorder* (PTSD) especially with mild TBI (Warren et al., 2015). Posttraumatic stress disorder often occurs after individuals experience extreme stress due to an extremely traumatic event or exposure to threatened death. Development of PTSD is not uncommon after TBI and can hinder individuals from achieving their optimal level of function (Im et al., 2011). This problem, in combination with depression, may have a major impact on outcome.

As mentioned previously, substance abuse may have been a contributing factor to the original accident that caused the TBI. After the injury, individuals may maintain the same pattern of substance abuse behavior they followed prior to the injury. Given this possibility, substance abuse evaluation should be conducted routinely and a management plan instituted as needed. For some individuals, substance abuse may represent a maladaptive means of coping with the stress and depression experienced following brain injury. In either case, after TBI, alcohol or other drugs can exacerbate existing impairments in function, can cause untoward interactions with other prescribed medications, or can precipitate seizures. If substance use was a significant part of the individual's social relationships, prior to injury, they may need to identify and be encouraged to participate in social and recreational activities that do not involve alcohol or other drugs.

Counseling and psychotherapy are important aspects of total rehabilitation for most disabling conditions and can be used to treat depression, reduce denial, increase self-esteem, or help individuals form realistic goals. In the case of individuals with TBI, however, additional challenges may be present if the individual has lost the capacity for insight or is unable to participate in abstract reasoning. In this case, counseling may be directed toward providing emotional support for both the individual and the family, and toward helping all involved adjust and relate to one another in the context of the changes brought about by TBI.

Activities and Participation

After the acute phase of brain injury, individuals—especially those with moderate to severe injury—are often transferred to an inpatient rehabilitation facility where physical, cognitive, and behavioral function are assessed. During the acute phase of rehabilitation, the individual, family members, and interdisciplinary members of a health team assess the individual's level of functioning in each area and implement a plan to assist the individual and optimize his or her level of activity and participation upon return to the home and community.

The complexity of brain injury has far-reaching consequences, including impacts on general activities of daily living. After discharge from acute care facilities, it is important that individuals continue to receive services presumed to be critical to maintain activities of daily living and to prevent secondary complications.

Assistive Devices and Home Modification

The degree to which home modifications or assistance in independent living is needed depends on the individual's level of physical, cognitive, and perceptual function. Although the goal of rehabilitation is to assist the individual to achieve optimal level of independence in as many areas as possible, safety is also an area of concern due to issues related to problem solving, judgment, and impulse control associated with brain injury.

Depending on the specific physical manifestations experienced by the individual as the result of TBI, accommodations, modifications, and assistive devices in the home may be necessary. For example, if the individual experiences paralysis of an upper extremity, items kept in cabinets and cupboards may need to be moved for ease of reach, and special adaptive devices may be needed to assist the individual in dressing or eating. In the case of physical manifestations experienced in lower extremities, bathroom modifications such as a raised toilet seat, grab bars, and bench in the shower or tub may be needed, or doorways may need to be modified to accommodate a wheelchair. In other instances, adaptive devices such as a leg brace may be needed.

Operating a Motor Vehicle

The acquisition of a driver's license and the ability to operate a motor vehicle symbolize independence and contribute to self-esteem. However, the consequences of TBI, whether related to physical or cognitive function, may pose an obstacle to safe driving. The ability to operate a motor vehicle post-TBI depends not only on the individual's physical ability but also on any cognitive and emotional manifestations that could cause harm to either the individual or the general public. Driving is a complex task. Physical manifestations after TBI may necessitate modification of the motor vehicle to facilitate driving; in some instances, severe physical manifestations may preclude driving as an option.

Even when physical manifestations do not pose a barrier to driving, cognitive, emotional, or behavioral manifestations could affect the individual's capacity to drive safely. As a result of their injury, individuals may exhibit poor judgment, impulsivity, outbursts of anger, inability to concentrate, or slower reflexes. Driving requires organizational ability, problem solving, decision-making ability, reflex actions, visual–motor skills, coordination, and physical manipulation. If the individual has difficulty in any of these areas, his or her ability to drive safely may be questioned. In the event that seizures are one of the residual effects experienced after TBI, the ability to drive will be further compromised. Comprehensive assessment of the individual's ability in all areas is needed to assess the ability to drive safely (Liddle, Hayes, Gustafasson, & Fleming, 2014).

Nutrition and Hygiene

Eating behavior may, in some instances, also be affected by brain injury. Some individuals may experience manifestations of TBI that make swallowing difficult. In other instances, individuals may refuse to eat or forget to eat, or they may experience a constant urge to eat, or overeat because they have forgotten that they have just eaten. In these cases, monitoring of eating habits, monitoring of weight gain or loss, and assessment of general nutritional status are needed. Specific strategies to ensure adequate nutrition and stabilization of weight may need to be implemented. For instance, individuals may need to follow a regular schedule so that they take meals at the same time each day. In some instances, when swallowing difficulties are severe, a feeding tube may be necessary to maintain nutrition.

Cognitive Function and Cognitive Remediation

After TBI, individuals may experience a number of cognitive manifestations that affect activities and participation. There may be difficulty with information processing—that is, the process by which information is taken in, and subsequent actions, reactions, and responses to incoming information are made. Individuals may have difficulty with attention and concentration, making it difficult to focus. For example, a family member may ask the individual to watch the pot on the stove, and to turn off the stove when the water boils; the individual

may instead become preoccupied with watching a bird out the window or how the dishes are stacked in the sink, while the pot boils dry. Individuals may also experience perceptual difficulties so that information taken in is misinterpreted or distorted. For example, a stranger's smile may be misinterpreted by the individual with TBI as an invitation to sit next to that person at a restaurant. Individuals may be overwhelmed by information coming in and have difficulty sorting information, prioritizing, and recognizing what is important. As an example, if a sink is filled and running over, the individual may get a mop for the floor rather than turning off the faucet or taking the stopper out of the sink drain. Individuals may experience difficulty with abstraction or conceptualization so that they take analogies literally and need explanations to be given in concrete terms.

Individuals may also have difficulty with memory. Memory problems can interfere with the ability to perform what might seem to be even small tasks of daily living following injury. Encouraging individuals to keep a notepad on which to list scheduled events, appointments, and important information can help them remember specific events. Keeping notes that have been strategically placed in the home or at work can help individuals remember specific tasks that might otherwise be overlooked, such as turning off the lights or closing the door.

Cognitive remediation is used to identify cognitive deficits and to develop interventions that assist individuals with improving cognitive function. Interventions are directed toward cognitive skills such as memory, language, planning, and other cognitive functions which are used in everyday life and which enhance integration into the social and work environment. Interventions involved in cognitive remediation consist of exercises and practice of specific skills in order to restore deficit function as well as assisting individuals to develop compensatory and adaptive strategies to facilitate improvement in processing of information.

Sexuality

Sexuality is more than sexual activity or a sexual act. It is the collection of traits that encompass the whole individual, defining who he or she is in terms of communication and daily interactions.

Traumatic brain injury causes a myriad of cognitive, psychological, and physical changes that in some way affect the sexuality of the individual with the injury (Moreno, Arango Lasprilla, Gan, & McKenal, 2013; Sander & Maestas, 2014).

As a result of TBI, individuals may experience social isolation and loss of social contact through loss of friends, or loss of social role. They may not have had a sexual partner at the time of the injury or may have had limited social or sexual experience prior to the injury so that meeting potential partners and establishing a relationship may be more difficult. When opportunities to increase social interaction do occur, individuals with brain injury may, in their desire to be accepted, be overly anxious, become vulnerable, and be taken advantage of.

Individuals with TBI who do not have a sexual partner may need to learn acceptable outlets through which they can express sexual needs. Cognitive changes that inhibit or regulate emotional responses can result in disinhibition, impaired judgment, or other cognitive factors that regulate impulse control and can have a negative impact on the individual's ability to establish a relationship. In these instances, affected persons may engage in socially uncomfortable behaviors such as making inappropriate sexual advances or responses or engaging in masturbation in public (Turner, Schöttle, Krueger, & Briken, 2015). Individuals may need to be helped to learn appropriate social interaction skills such as how to interpret social and environmental cues, make social contacts, and express sexual needs appropriately.

If individuals were already established in a relationship prior to injury, reactions to sexual issues after the injury may be based on each person's premorbid personality and the dynamics of the relationship. After TBI, sexuality and sexual functioning of both the individual experiencing TBI and his or her partner are affected. Individuals and their partners may benefit from programs directed at addressing expectations and enhancing communication regarding sexuality and sexual function. Psychological factors such as depression or decreased self-esteem can decrease sex drive. Anxiety or emotional reactions of the individual's sexual partner may also adversely affect sexual function and drive.

Physical changes after TBI may also affect sexual function. Sensory–motor changes can cause erectile dysfunction in males or decreased lubrication in females. Motor changes leading to spasticity or ataxia or other issues of mobility may affect sexual performance. Individuals or family members may be reluctant to bring up sexual problems, or in some instances the individual with TBI may be unaware that a problem exists. Talking openly about sexuality and assessing specific sexuality issues in the context of their specific values will enable individuals to discuss specific concerns and to identify ways to adapt to changes in sexuality. In addition, identification of specific sexuality issues can lessen the effects of any problems that do arise.

Social and Family Participation

Social relationships can influence health and well-being, influence overall adjustment to chronic health conditions or incapacitation, and serve as important contributors to rehabilitation. Social relationships and social supports are derived from both the broader social environment and the more intimate environment of the family. The degree to which individuals are incorporated into the larger community and how they are incorporated into their family system after TBI can have significant impact on the extent to which they adjust to and manage manifestations of their injury.

After TBI, social relationships for individuals are often drastically altered. Individuals with TBI undergo changes in temperament, behavior, and skills that may not be clearly understood by the community at large and changes in personality, behaviors, or activity may be misinterpreted and attributed to causes other than the TBI itself (Degeneffe & Lee, 2010). When individuals with TBI attempt to resume relationships, former life activities, and roles within the community, they may experience rejection or failure and social isolation, which in turn may contribute to lowered self-esteem.

Although social roles and social relationships in the broader community are important to function and quality of life, the family is a central aspect in many individuals' environments. No relationship is more significantly modified after TBI than that of the family. Traumatic brain injury dramatically and permanently affects not only the individual experiencing it but also the whole family system. Consequently, maximizing healthy family function and adaptation is crucial to enhancing function and quality of life for the family as well as for the individual family member with TBI.

Traumatic brain injury disrupts the family system, altering family structure, as well as altering roles and responsibilities of individual family members. The individual with TBI may no longer be able to assume the role and responsibilities once integral to the family's function. The individual's condition may necessitate that family members assume new roles and functions, as adjustments are made to compensate and accommodate for the role and responsibilities the individual with TBI may no longer be able to fulfill

Stresses on families inherent in the caregiving responsibilities and adjustment to manifestations of TBI may affect family members' ability to serve as an emotional resource and source of support for the individual with TBI. Often more troublesome for family and friends are not the physical ramifications and residuals of the injury but rather the behavioral and personality changes the individual experiences as a direct result of brain injury. Such personality changes may put additional strain on family relationships.

Not only must the family cope with profound physical, cognitive, and emotional changes in the individual, but the stress of caregiving and the financial burden can also be extreme. Because TBI occurs suddenly, neither the family nor the individual has the opportunity to prepare for its emotional and economic impact. Normal family development is disrupted, and any prior family stress may be exacerbated.

Families can play a pivotal role in facilitating reintegration of the individual with TBI into community life and can significantly influence how the individual reacts to the injury and its residual effects. Depending on the circumstances of the injury, family members may place blame on the individual or on others, may be angry, or may express other negative emotions, which can have a negative impact on the individual and his or her rehabilitation potential. Family members may misinterpret personality changes or specific behaviors of the individual as deliberate or spiteful, coming from deep-seated anger toward the family, or they may assume the individual could control the behavior if he or she wanted to. Individual family members may feel trapped and resent the caregiving roles they must now assume, reminding the individual with brain injury of his or her dependence or belittling the individual. In other instances, the family may seek to foster even more reliance of the individual on the family. Glad to have the individual home again, rather than fostering independence and achievement of fullest functional potential, the family may instead encourage the person's dependence.

Depending on the severity of the brain injury, the personality and coping ability of the caregiver, and the previous relationship between the individual and his or her family, the situation can breed resentment and stress, which in turn can negatively affect rehabilitation potential. Even when caregiving duties are accepted willingly and not considered a burden, adjustment to changes in the individual after injury can precipitate strain and emotional turmoil in family members, and be a source of profound stress. The primary caregiver may neglect his or her own physical and emotional needs, as well as the needs of other family members. In some instances, the behavior of the individual with TBI may make even simple social interactions embarrassing, so that the family eventually feels it is easier to stay within their home environment, becoming increasingly socially isolated.

Marital relationships can also begin to deteriorate. If significant marital strain was present prior to the brain injury, postinjury stress will be increased and consequently exacerbate the strain. Determining premorbid family function can be helpful in identifying problems and working toward solutions.

Support, counseling, and education of the family about the nature of the condition, ways to cope with the individual's behavior, and identification of resources can help to restore family equilibrium. Family members should be given the opportunity to work through their feelings and be assured that their feelings are natural. Emphasis should be placed on maintaining the well-being of self and others in the family unit as well as attending to the needs of the individual with brain injury. Overall, the individual and family should be assisted in attaining realistic expectations and directed to pursuing reasonable goals. Community resources and social support can be helpful in facilitating adaptation of the family.

VOCATIONAL ISSUES AFTER TRAUMATIC BRAIN INJURY

Gainful employment is significantly affected following TBI (Frostad Liaset & Lorás, 2016). Physical, cognitive, or emotional manifestations resulting from TBI may reduce the individual's ability to return to work at the same level as prior to injury, and in some instances may prevent individuals from returning to work at all (Frostad Liaset & Lorás, 2016). Unemployment rates for individuals with brain injury are high and often become higher over time (Cuthbert et al., 2015). Return to work for individuals with TBI has a multifactorial perspective. Because of the wide variation of manifestations related to TBI, no one model can be applied to all individuals. The disparate changes that may occur as a result of TBI present challenges not encountered with many other disabilities. The degree to which individuals with TBI are able to maintain employment depends on the extent of the injury and any associated functional manifestations as well as their prior background, age at the time of brain injury, pre-injury education, occupation, and work history (Frostad Liaset & Lorás, 2016). Personal motivation and support from family are also important factors in determining the individual's rehabilitation potential. Owing to the fact that behavioral and cognitive disabilities in TBI may be less visible and, therefore, less easy to categorize, services to address these needs may not be obtained, further impeding the individual's ability to return to work.

Factors that seem most closely related to the ability to return to work and to maintain employment after brain injury include the severity of injury experienced, the individual's age, pre-injury behavior problems, and work history prior to brain injury (Frostad Liaset & Lorás, 2016). As the severity of brain injury increases, the rate of successful return to work decreases. Persons with greater manifestations and associated impediments may require more extended time and more extensive rehabilitation services before placement. Although the majority of individuals with mild brain injury may be able to return to work, individuals with moderate and severe brain injury have poorer outcomes. Even when job placement is accomplished, for individuals with moderate to severe manifestations, job retention may be difficult.

The type of occupation in which individuals were engaged prior to their injury also appears to influence the return-to-work outcome, with the highest rates of return to work being found among persons with higher decision-making jobs (Frostad Liaset & Lorás, 2016). Likewise, age appears to be a significant determinant of return to work. Generally, the older the individual is at the time of injury, the less likely he or she is to return to work.

Lastly, work history prior to brain injury appears to be related to ability to return to work after injury. Those individuals with a poor work history prior to experiencing brain injury are more likely to have more problems returning to work after brain injury has occurred (Cuthbert et al., 2015)

Cognitive deficits and psychosocial difficulties may have more profound implications for an individual's ability to return to work than do any physical manifestations. Individuals who retain average to above-average intellectual abilities and interpersonal skills after TBI occurs are often better able to compensate for other limitations and maintain or gain employment. For others, however, levels of interpersonal functioning and cognitive self-awareness are often limited. Brain injury may result in drastic changes in personality and personal ability as well as impaired self-awareness, which is also a frequent contributor to employment problems. Individuals who experience emotional liability may experience more difficulty in reentering the workplace and in dealing with coworkers.

Memory impairment may be a debilitating effect of brain injury. Individuals with memory problems may forget what they have learned and may benefit from experience to only a limited extent. Helping individuals find alternative ways to perform tasks and develop strategies to reduce, organize, and retrieve information can reduce the disabling effects of memory impairment. Given that individuals may have difficulty organizing their day, techniques such as implementing structured routines, using written notes or lists, or audiotaped reminders may help improve performance. Generally the use of notes or lists will be most effective if information is kept simple, with no extraneous details. Too much information may cause the individual to become overwhelmed and confused.

Individuals with TBI may be unaware of their deficits and may overestimate their abilities. Judgment may also be affected. Poor self-awareness or inaccurate self-perception can, in turn, contribute to employment problems. Individuals may be unable to recognize job errors and may consistently rate their performance more highly than their employer does. As a result, they may realize only a limited benefit from feedback.

The ability to communicate verbally or in writing or to comprehend words and concepts influences all aspects of job selection, training, and performance (Meulenbroek & Turksta, 2016). Special considerations need to be given when limitations in ability to communicate are present. Visual–perceptual skills are integral to many jobs, both skilled and unskilled. The ability to perceive details, and to scan, match, or accurately perceive patterns may affect a number of daily life activities, including reading, driving, and general ability to navigate the environment.

Motor skills limitations affecting finger dexterity, eye–hand coordination, or eye–foot coordination may also be present in case of brain injury. When these limitations exist, work involving precision or operation of certain tools or equipment may be difficult. Individuals who have experienced paralysis of one of the upper extremities may be limited in their ability to lift, carry, pull, or push. If one of the lower extremities has been affected, individuals may require assistive devices such as a cane, walker, braces, or wheelchair. Consequently, ambulation may be restricted to short distances. Ambulation on uneven surfaces should be avoided and, if a wheelchair is used, environmental modifications may be required. Reduced speed of performance of various tasks, physical stamina, and endurance should also be taken into account. Often individuals may be able to perform a task well if they are allowed to take their time rather than feeling pressured to rush. Competitive environments in which speed is a priority may not be the best choices for individuals with brain injury and may actually contribute to decreased quality of work.

Traumatic brain injury is not a progressive condition, and the individual's overall life expectancy is not affected. Traumatic brain injury is, however, a lifelong condition. Just as rehabilitation needs of individuals vary depending on the age at which the injury occurred, so will rehabilitation needs change over the individual's lifetime. Consequently, ongoing monitoring and contact with individuals may be necessary to help them maintain their maximum potential in the workplace.

In some instances, supported employment or job coaching may be appropriate. In other instances, performance-based feedback or prompts may be sufficient to help the individual maintain employment. Returning to gainful employment represents a series of complex challenges because of the number, complexity, and interaction of problems possible, all of which may contribute to difficulty in maintaining long-term employment. Monitoring performance and maintaining communication with the employer can contribute to job retention. Helping individuals learn compensatory strategies, providing appropriate workplace accommodations, and educating employers about the nature of brain injury and its consequences can greatly increase the chances of successful job placement.

CASE STUDY

John, a 20-year-old student, received a TBI as the result of an auto accident in which he was texting while driving. When he was evaluated at the trauma unit at the hospital, his Glasgow Coma Scale score was 7. After his condition stabilized, John was referred to a rehabilitation center for ongoing management. Residual effects experienced from his injury are information processing difficulty and trouble with short-term memory.

1. Which level of brain injury did John experience based on the Glasgow Coma Scale score?
2. Given the residual manifestations John experienced as a result of his injury, which issues may be important to address as he considers whether he will return to school?
3. Which specific accommodations may John need?

REFERENCES

Bernat, J. L., & Wudicks, E. F. M. (2016). Coma, vegetative state, and brain death. In L. Goldman & A. I. Schafer (Eds.), *Goldman-Cecil medicine* (25th ed.). Philadelphia, PA: Elsevier Saunders.

Bieniek, K. F., Ross, O. A., Cormier, K. A., Walton, R. L., Soto-Ortolaza, A., Johnston, A. D., ... Dickson, W. W. (2015). Chronic traumatic encephalopathy pathology in a neurodegenerative disorders brain bank. *Acta Neuropathologica, 130*(6): 877– 889.

Bowen, L. N., Moore, D. F., & Okun, M. S. (2016). Is blast injury a modern phenomenon? Early historical descriptions of mining and volcanic traumatic brain injury with relevance to modern terrorist attacks and military warfare. *Neurologist 21*(2): 19–22.

Brenner, L. A., Dise-Lewis, J. E., Bartles, S. K., O'Brien, S. E., Godleski, M., & Selinger, M. (2007). The long-term impact and rehabilitation of pediatric traumatic brain injury: A 50 year follow-up case study. *Journal of Head Trauma Rehabilitation, 22*(1), 56–64.

CDC, NIH, DoD, & VA Leadership Panel. (2013). *Report to Congress on traumatic brain injury in the United States: Understanding the public health problem among current and former military personnel*. New York, NY: Author.

Cicerone, K. D., Langenbahn, D. M., Braden, C., Malec, J. F., Kalmar, K., Fraas, M., ... Ashman, T. (2012). Evidence-based cognitive rehabilitation: Updated review of the literature from 2003–2008. *Archives of Physical Medicine Rehabilitation, 92*, 519–530. doi:10.1016/j.apmr.2010.11015.Review

Cuthbert, J. P., Pretz, C. R., Bushnik, T., Fraser, R. T., Hart, T., Kolakowsky-Hayner, S. A., ... Sherer, M. (2015). Ten-year employment patterns of working age individuals after moderate to severe traumatic brain injury: A national institute on disability and rehabilitation research traumatic brain injury model systems study. *Archives of Physical Medicine and Rehabilitation, 96*(12), 2128–2136.

Degeneffe, C. E., & Lee, G. K. (2010). Quality of life after traumatic brain injury: Perspectives of adult siblings. *Journal of Rehabilitation, 76*(4), 27–36.

DeKosky, S. T., Ikonomovic, M. D., & Gandy, S. (2010). Traumatic brain injury: Football, warfare, and long-term effects. *New England Journal of Medicine, 363*(14), 1293–1296.

Frostad Liaset, I., & Lorás, H. (2016, March). Perceived factors in return to work after acquired brain injury: A qualitative meta-synthesis. *Scandinavian Journal of Occupational Therapy, 23*(6), 446–457.

Garrelfs, S. F., Donker-Cools, B. H., Wind, H., & Frings-Dresen, M. H. (2015). Return-to-work in patients with acquired brain injury and psychiatric disorders as a comorbidity: A systematic review. *Brain Injury, 29*(5), 550–557.

Giacino, J. T., Whyte, J., Bagiella, E., Kalmar, K., Childs, N., Khademi, A., ... Sherer, M. (2012). Placebo-controlled trial of amantadine for severe traumatic brain injury. *New England Journal of Medicine, 366*(9), 819–826.

Green, E. A. (2015). Editorial: Brain injury as a neurodegenerative disorder. *Frontiers in Human Neuroscience, 9,* 615. doi:10.3389/fnhum.2015.0061

Hagan, C., Malkmus, D., & Durham, P. (1972). *Rancho Los Amigos scale*. Downey, CA: Rancho Los Amigos Hospital.

Hamon, K. G., Drezner, J. A., Gammons, M., Guskiewicz, K. M., Halstead, M., Herring, S. A., ... Roberts, W. O. (2013). American Medical Society for Sports Medicine position statement: Concussion in sport. *British Journal of Sports Medicine, 47*(1), 15–26.

Im, B., Hibbard, M., Grunwald, I., Swift, P. T., & Salimi, N. (2011). Traumatic brain injury. In S. R. Flanagan, H. Zaretsky, & A. Moroz (Eds.), *Medical aspects of disability*, (4th ed., pp. 65–87). New York, NY: Springer.

Jennet, B., Snoek, J., Bond, M. R., & Brooks, N. (1981). Disability after severe head injury: Observations on the use of the Glasgow Outcome Scale. *Journal of Neurology and Neurosurgical Psychiatry, 44*, 285–293.

Katzenberger, R. J., Loewen, C. A., Wassarman, D. R., Petersen, A. J., Ganetzky, B., & Wassarman, D. A. (2013). A Drosophila model of closed head traumatic brain injury. *Proceedings of the National Academy of Sciences of the United States of America*, 110(44). E4152–E4159.

Liddle, J., Hayes, R., Gustafsson, L., & Fleming, J. (2014). Managing driving issues after an acquired brain injury: Strategies used by health professionals. *Australian Occupational Therapy Journal. 61*(4): 215–23. doi:10.1111/1440-1630.12119

Ling, G. S. F. (2016). Traumatic brain injury and spinal cord injury. In L. Goldman & A. I. Schafer (Eds.), *Goldman-Cecil medicine* (25th ed.). Philadelphia, PA: Elsevier Saunders.

MacDonald, C. L., Johnson, A. M., Cooper, D., Nelson, E. C., Werner, N. J., Shimony, J. S., ... Brody, D. L. (2011). Detection of blast-related traumatic brain injury in U.S. military personnel. *New England Journal of Medicine, 364*(22), 2091–2100.

Maruta, J., Spielman, L. A., Yarusi, B. B., Wang, Y., Silver, J. M., & Ghajar, J. (2016). Chronic post-concussion neurocognitive deficits. II. Relationship with persistent symptoms. *Frontiers in Human Neuroscience, 10*(45). doi:10.3389/fnhum.2016.00045 eCollection 2016

Masel, B. E., & DeWitt, D. S. (2010). TBI: A disease process not an event. *Journal of Neurotrauma 27*(8), 1529–1540.

McKee, A. C., Stein, T. D., Kieman, P. T., & Alvarez, V. E. (2015). The neuropathology of chronic traumatic encephalopathy. *Brain Pathology, 25*(3): 350–364.

Meulenbroek, P., & Turksta, L. (2016). Job stability in skilled work and communication ability after moderate-severe traumatic brain injury. *Disability Rehabilitation, 38*(5), 452–461.

Moreno, J. A., Arango Lasprilla, J. C., Gan., C., & McKenal, M. (2013). Sexuality after traumatic brain injury: A critical review. *NeuroRehabilitation, 32*(1), 69–85.

Nowranqi, M. A., Kortte, K. B., & Rao, V. A. (2014). A perspectives approach to suicide after traumatic brain injury: Case and review. *Psychosomatics, 55*(5):430–437. doi:10.1016/j.psym.2013.11.006

O'Connor, P. G. (2016). Alcohol use disorders. In L. Goldman & A. I. Schafer, (Eds.), *Goldman-Cecil medicine,* (25th ed.). Philadelphia, PA: Elsevier Saunders.

Rappaport, M., Hall, K. M., Hopkins, K., Belleza, T., & Cope, D. N. (1982). Disability rating scale for severe head trauma: Coma to community. *Archives of Physical Medicine and Rehabilitation, 63:* 118–123.

Reis, C., Want, Y., Akyal, O., Ho, W. M., Applegate, R., Stier, G., … Zang, J. H. (2015). What's new in traumatic brain injury: Update on tracking, monitoring and treatment. *International Journal of Molecular Science, 16*(6). 11903–11965.

Ropper, A. (2011). Brain injuries from blasts. *New England Journal of Medicine, 364*(22), 2156–2157.

Sander, A. M., & Maestas, K. (2014). Information/education page. Sexuality after traumatic brain injury. *Archives of Physical Medicine and Rehabilitation, 95*(9), 1801–1802.

Scholten, A. C., Haagsma, J. A., Andriessen, T. M., Vos, P. E., Streyerberg, E. W., Van Beeck, E. F., & Polinder, S. (2015). Health-related quality of life after mild, moderate, and severe traumatic brain injury patterns and predictors of suboptimal functioning during the first year after injury. *Injury, 46*(4), 616–624.

Shields, C., Ownsworth, T., O'Donovan, A., & Fleming J. (2016). A transdiagnostic investigation of emotional distress after traumatic brain injury. *Neuropsychogical Rehabilitation, 26*(3), 410–445. doi:10.1080/09602011.2015.1037772

Stéfan, A., Mathé, J. F., & SOFMER Group. (2016). What are the disruptive symptoms of behavioral disorders after traumatic brain injury? A systematic review leading to recommendations for good practices. *Annals of Physical Rehabilitation Medicine, 59*(1): 5–17. doi:10.1016/j.rehab.2015.11.002

Stein, T. D., Alvarez, V. E., & McKee, A. C. (2015). Concussion in chronic traumatic encephalopathy. *Current Pain and Headache Reports, 19*(10): 47. doi:10.1007/s11916-015-0522-z

The Management of Concussion/mTBI Working Group. (2009). VA/DoD Clinical Practice Guidelines for Management of Concussion/Mild Traumatic Injury. *Journal of Rehabilitation Research & Development, 46*(6): CP1–CP68.

Turner, D., Schöttle, D., Krueger, R., & Briken, P. (2015). Sexual behavior and its correlates after traumatic brain injury. *Current Opinions in Psychiatry, 28*(2), 180–187.

Viola-Saltzman, M., & Musleh, C. (2016). Traumatic brain injury-induced sleep disorders. *Neuropsychiatric Disease and Treatment, 12*:339–348. doi:10.2147/NDT.S69105 eCollection 2016.

Wang, E. W., & Huang, J. H. (2013). Understanding and treating blast traumatic brain injury in the combat theater. *Neurology Research, 35*(3), 285–289.

Warren, A. M., Boals, A., Elliott, T. R., Reynolds, M., Weddle, R. J., Holtz, P., … Foreman, M. L. (2015). Mild traumatic brain injury increases risk for the development of posttraumatic stress disorder. *Journal of Trauma and Acute Care Surgery, 79*(6), 1062–1066.

Wee, H. Y., Ho, C. H., Liang, F. W., Hsieh, K. Y., Wang, C. C., Wang, J. J., … Kuo, J. R. (2016). Increased risk of new-onset depression in patients with traumatic brain injury and hyperlipidemia: The important role of statin medications. *Journal of Clinical Psychiatry, 77*(4), 505–511.

White, R. J., & Likavec, M. J. (1992). The diagnosis and initial management of head injury. *New England Journal of Medicine, 327*(21), 1507–1510.

Yu, K. E., Murphy, J. M., & Tsao, J. W. (2016). Blast from the past: A retrospective analysis of blast-induced head injury. *Neurologist, 21*(2), 17–18.

CHAPTER 5

Stroke

OVERVIEW OF NONTRAUMATIC BRAIN DAMAGE

The brain, like any other tissue, requires oxygen to function. Oxygen is carried in blood by hemoglobin. When there is too little oxygen in the blood supply (**hypoxia**), brain function is altered. When there is no oxygen available (**anoxia**), brain tissue may be permanently damaged resulting in neurological manifestations (Brain Injury Institute, n.d.)

Generally, brain damage is classified as one of two types:

- Traumatic brain injury
- Nontraumatic brain damage

Whereas *traumatic brain injury* refers to injury to the brain from an external force, *nontraumatic brain damage* refers to conditions that restrict or interfere with blood and oxygen reaching parts of the brain, consequently causing damage to brain tissue (The Children's Trust, 2016). Examples of conditions that can cause nontraumatic brain injury are choking, near-drowning, or carbon monoxide poisoning; infections, such as meningitis and encephalitis; occlusion of a blood vessel supplying the brain by a blood clot; rupture of a weakened blood vessel in the brain; and congenital structural aberrations of blood vessels in the brain (Boss & Heuther, 2014).

Although the manifestations of nontraumatic brain damage can be similar to those experienced with traumatic brain injury, often nontraumatic brain damage is associated with other chronic underlying conditions, which, unless adequately managed, can cause additional nontraumatic brain damage. One of the most common causes of non-traumatic brain damage is *stroke*.

OVERVIEW OF STROKE

Stroke (also called *cerebral vascular accident* [*CVA*]) is the fifth leading cause of death and a major cause of incapacitation in the United States (American Stroke Association [ASA], n.d. a). It is caused by decreased blood flow and subsequent inadequate oxygen supply to part of the brain leading to tissue damage, which causes neurological manifestations that can affect a number of body functions. Stroke is related to a number of other chronic conditions, such as cardiac disease, **arteriosclerosis** (*ischemic vascular disease*), **hypertension** (high blood pressure), high cholesterol, and diabetes (ASA, n.d. a; Boss & Huether, 2014).

Other risk factors for stroke include smoking, obesity, physical inactivity, heavy alcohol use, and use of illicit drugs, especially cocaine and amphetamines (Fonseca & Ferro, 2013). Individuals who have a mechanical prosthetic valve in the heart to counteract atrial fibrillation, those who are on dialysis for chronic renal failure, and individuals with *carotid stenosis* (narrowing of the carotid artery due to atherosclerosis) are at higher risk for ischemic stroke (Boss & Huether, 2014).

CLASSIFICATION OF STROKE

Strokes are classified as follows:

- Ischemic stroke (occlusion or blockage of a blood vessel that diminishes blood flow to brain tissue)
- Hemorrhagic stroke (rupture of a blood vessel in the brain)

Ischemic Stroke

About 85% of the strokes are *ischemic strokes,* in which occlusion of a blood vessel reduces or eliminates blood flow to an area of the brain (Mayo Clinic, 2016). If reduction in blood flow is severe, **infarction** (death) of brain tissue in the area supplied by that vessel occurs.

A common cause of ischemic stroke is a blood clot (**thrombus**) formed inside an artery that supplies brain tissue with blood. This condition, called *cerebral thrombosis,* blocks blood flow to an area of the brain, preventing brain tissue from obtaining needed oxygen. In the absence of oxygen, the brain tissue experiences infarction within a short period of time. The amount and severity of damage depend on the degree and duration of decreased blood flow (Boss & Heuther, 2014).

Another cause of ischemic stroke is **embolism**, in which a clot that has formed in another part of the body breaks free and travels through the blood vessels to the brain, lodging in one of the cerebral arteries. In some instances, an *embolus* may be a substance, such as globule of fat, bubble of air, or foreign substance, that has entered the bloodstream and consequently occludes a vessel (Boss & Heuther, 2014; Mayo Clinic, 2016).

At times, temporary blocking of the cerebral arteries causes slight, temporary neurological deficits that lead to "mini-strokes," referred to as **transient ischemic attacks (TIAs)**. An important distinction between TIA and stroke is that the **ischemia** (deficiency of blood supply) associated with TIA is not severe enough to cause an infarction, whereas death to brain tissue occurs with stroke, causing permanent damage. Although the neurological deficits experienced from TIAs are usually temporary, their occurrence forewarns of the possibility of a larger stroke within a year unless the underlying condition that precipitated the TIA is adequately managed (Boss & Heuther, 2014).

Hemorrhagic Stroke

Hemorrhagic stroke occurs because of rupture of a blood vessel, causing *intracranial hemorrhage* (hemorrhage into the brain tissue). In this instance, death of brain tissue occurs not only because a certain area of the brain has been deprived of oxygen but also because the escaped blood causes increased pressure in the brain (*increased intracranial pressure*) that compresses brain tissue against the skull, causing further damage.

A common cause of cerebral hemorrhage is uncontrolled **hypertension** (high blood pressure) (Boss & Heuther, 2014). Other causes of hemorrhagic stroke include **aneurysm**, in which a thin-walled out pouching protrudes from a blood vessel. Aneurysms may be due to either weakness of the wall of the vessel or a congenital aberration. In many instances, aneurysms cause no manifestation until they burst (Boss & Huether, 2014). Aneurysms may rupture directly in the brain (*intracerebral hemorrhage*), often into the **subarachnoid space** (the space that is filled with cerebrospinal fluid). As blood fills the subarachnoid space, *acute hydrocephalus* (sudden buildup of fluid in the brain) may occur, impeding the normal flow and absorption of cerebral spinal fluid), which in turn causes increased *intracranial pressure* and subsequently more damage (Mayo Clinic, 2016; National Institute of Neurological Disorders and Stroke [NINDS], 2016).

Another potential cause of hemorrhagic stroke is *arteriovenous malformation (AVM)*, a congenital aberration characterized by a tangled web of arteries and veins connected by an abnormal passageway. AVMs may also cause hemorrhage into the subarachnoid space. These conditions also often go undetected unless they cause cerebral hemorrhage, although in some instances severe headaches or seizures may be the first manifestation (ASA, n.d. d.).

Cocaine or alcohol abuse can also contribute to the potential for hemorrhagic stroke.

MANIFESTATIONS OF STROKE

Whether a stroke is ischemic or hemorrhagic, the amount, degree, and type of function affected by stroke depend on three factors:

- The side of the brain affected
- The specific area of the brain that has been damaged
- The amount of damage that has occurred

After a stroke produces the initial damage to an area of the brain, surrounding brain tissue becomes **edematous** (swells) and inflamed, which leads to additional damage (Boss & Heuther, 2014). Although death of brain tissue causes permanent damage, areas of the brain that have experienced only swelling may recover, and function in these areas may be restored. Consequently, individuals experiencing stroke may not know the extent of their permanent functional limitations until weeks or even months after the initial event.

After suffering a stroke, a variety of *motor, sensory, cognitive,* and *communication* functions may be affected (Mayo Clinic, 2016), either singularly or in combination. In addition to the area of the brain damaged and the amount of damage that has occurred, the nature of functional manifestations experienced with stroke will, for the most part, be affected by whether the brain has been damaged on the left or right side. Individuals who experience stroke on the left side of the brain will have manifestations that affect the right side of the body and that are consistent with functions controlled by the left side of the brain. Likewise, individuals who experience stroke on the right side of the brain will have manifestations that affect the left side of the body and functions controlled by the right side of the brain (Boss & Heuther, 2014).

Not all individuals with stroke have the same functional manifestations. The type and amount of function that are affected depend on the location and extent of the brain damage. Individuals may experience any or a combination of the general functional difficulties discussed next as a result of stroke.

Motor Manifestations

Individuals may experience weakness or paralysis on the side of the body opposite of the area of the brain that has been damaged by stroke. Consequently, voluntary control of power and strength in the extremities on the affected side of the body may be diminished. Either or both upper or lower extremities on one side of the body may be affected. If an upper extremity is involved, fine hand motions that are needed for writing, buttoning clothes, using eating utensils, or grooming may be affected. If a lower limb is affected, ability for walking or weight bearing may be affected.

Individuals may experience inability to manage the accuracy of muscle movement or limb position (**ataxia**). If an upper extremity is affected, they may have difficulty grasping or handling items. When a lower extremity is affected, they may walk with a wobbly, unsteady, staggering gait. As a result, there may be increased susceptibility to falls (Claflin, Krishnan, & Sandeep, 2015). In some individuals, equilibrium may be affected, making it difficult to maintain balance with resulting postural instability.

Coordination of movement that is unrelated to weakness or paralysis may also be affected. *Apraxia* is a term used to describe a manifestation in which individuals loses the ability to carry out purposeful, coordinated voluntary motor skills movements, despite having the physical ability to do so. The loss of the ability to conduct motor planning and to execute these voluntary movements efficiently is not related to weakness or paralysis but rather to damage to the area of the brain that is responsible for voluntary coordinated movement. When a lower extremity is involved, ambulation may be difficult. When an upper extremity is involved, individuals may have difficulty controlling the accuracy needed for activities so that grasping or reaching for objects is difficult. Apraxia can interfere with the ability to carry out activities of daily living and can impede independent functioning.

Sensation Manifestations

In some instances, individuals have sensation on one side of the body affected as a result of stroke. All sensations, or only one or two, including touch, pain, and sense of position, may be affected. Sensations may be totally lost, lessened, or sometimes misinterpreted (NINDS, 2014). Alteration of sensory function or sensory loss may result in an unawareness of potential dangers to the affected side of the body, such as being too close to a hot stove.

Although loss of feeling or the inability to perceive movement of an extremity is most common in stoke, in some instances rather than feeling numbness, individuals may experience uncomfortable sensations such as tingling, burning, or pain (**paresthesia**).

When the portion of the brain responsible for perceiving visual images is damaged, the ability to perceive objects on one side of the visual field may be diminished. Consequently, individuals may be unable to perceive half of the visual field (**hemianopsia**). As a result, individuals may be able to perceive only half of a visual image. For instance, they may see food on only one half of the table.

Some individuals lose the ability to judge depth and distance, which can affect their ability to navigate within their environment. For example, individuals may stumble over or bump into furniture, run into the side of the door when trying to pass through it, or miss the edge of a table when trying to put down a glass.

The ability to recognize auditory or other sensations may be affected as well. Some individuals may be unable to recognize or identify certain objects, even though they recognize that the object is present and are able to describe its physical properties. Although they know that the object is there, they may be unable to assign any meaning to it or its use. For example, they may see a cup placed in front of them and describe the cup's appearance, but not recognize how the cup is to be used or for what purpose.

Cognitive Manifestations

Cognitive function includes many domains, including memory, language, visual–spatial processes, and executive function, which incorporates decision making, judgment, planning, sequencing, and organizing. A wide variety of cognitive manifestations affecting any of these functions may be present after stroke (Sun, Tan, & Yu, 2014).

Some individuals experience problems with memory. The degree to which memory is affected may be related to the side of the brain that was damaged. In some instances, individuals may have difficulty learning new material or retaining information that is newly learned. In other instances, individuals may have difficulty retaining more complicated information or may have a short retention span. There may also be difficulty with generalizing from one setting to another and with perception of time.

After stroke, individuals may have difficulty reading (**alexia**) or writing (**agraphia**) due to cognitive difficulties rather than motor difficulties. In other instances, individuals may have difficulty recognizing once-familiar images or objects (**agnosia**).

Communication Manifestations

Communication is a multifaceted process that involves both receiving and delivering information, whether through behavior, speaking, writing, reading, or signing. Any difficulty with motor, visual, or cognitive function can affect an individual's ability to communicate.

Speech refers to the physical ability to produce sounds and the movement of the lips, tongue, or other structures that are used to produce language. **Language** refers to how words, as symbols, are put together to convey and understand concepts. Both the ability to use certain muscles to form words and project speech and the ability to use and understand words (language) are controlled by the brain. When the area of the brain that controls either speech or language is damaged, limitations in either area may occur.

Motor difficulty in structures related to speech may affect the individual's ability to speak. Coordination and accuracy of movement of the muscles, lips, tongue, or other parts of the speech mechanism may be impaired secondary to weakness or paralysis of muscles needed to speak, a condition called **dysarthria**. Impairments may range from speech that is slightly slurred to speech that is unintelligible. Paralysis or weakness of muscles may also cause vocal cord dysfunction, which in turn can affect voice quality.

Other motor problems can cause *articulation disorders* in which there is no significant weakness or incoordination for reflexive action but rather the inability to position and sequence muscle movements properly. For example, individuals may be able to scrape a food particle off their teeth with their tongue, yet be unable to coordinate the muscles that move the tongue so as to produce a phonetic sound, a condition known as **apraxia of speech**.

Approximately 20% of individuals have difficulty with expression and comprehension of language after stroke (ASA, 2015a). The ability to transmit/or understand verbal or written language (**aphasia**) may be hampered. Although a number of types of aphasia exist, two categories are commonly distinguished:

- Nonfluent (*expressive or motor*) aphasia
- Fluent (*receptive or sensory*) aphasia

Broca's aphasia is a type of *nonfluent aphasia* characterized by articulation problems, hesitancy, and reduced vocabulary and grammar. When *Broca's area* of the brain is damaged, an individual's speech may be labored, slow, or difficult to understand, and small connecting words, such as prepositions, may be omitted. Individuals may be able to understand and read simple material; however, as the complexity or length of the message increases, difficulty in completing these tasks becomes more apparent. Although individuals are able to comprehend material, they may have difficulty expressing their thoughts in speech and writing because of difficulty putting words and sentences together logically, or they may have word-finding difficulties (**dysnomia**). Reading ability may be better than writing ability.

Wernicke's aphasia is present when Wernicke's area of the brain is damaged. Wernicke's aphasia is a type of *fluent aphasia* in which there is effortless speech, relatively normal grammatical structure, and increased verbal output, but with reduced information content so that what the individual says makes little sense. Auditory and reading comprehension is usually poor. Individuals with Wernicke's aphasia are typically unaware of their communication difficulties.

In some instances, individuals may experience **global aphasia**, in which there is severe difficulty communicating because of both inability to use language (inability to use words and organize them into coherent sentences) and severe difficulty in understanding language, either written or spoken.

Language difficulties may differ depending on the area of the brain damaged. Because the center of language function is located in the left cerebral hemisphere for most individuals, communication problems can occur when damage involves the left side of the brain. By contrast, individuals with right cerebral damage often have intact language function.

Brain damage can affect all forms of communication, including the ability to speak, comprehend, or convey language through either written or verbal means. The type of communication difficulty and the degree of communication difficulty individuals experience after stroke are greatly dependent on the side of the brain that incurred the damage.

MANIFESTATIONS OF LEFT- VERSUS RIGHT-SIDED BRAIN DAMAGE

Although general functional manifestations as outlined previously may be experienced by many people with stroke, certain patterns of functional manifestations appear to be related to whether the damage occurred on the left or right side of the brain, although exceptions can occur (see **Figure 5-1**) (Cleveland Clinic, n.d.). Because the center of language function is located in the left cerebral hemisphere for most individuals, communication deficits can occur when damage involves the left side of the brain. By contrast, individuals with right cerebral damage often have intact language function.

Left-Sided Brain Damage

The most visible sign of left-sided brain damage, regardless of the underlying cause, is *right-sided motor and sensory paralysis* (right-sided **hemiplegia**). The degree of paralysis depends on the extent of the damage. Either or both extremities on the right side may be affected to varying degrees, ranging from total paralysis to limited ability to use a limb. For individuals who are right-handed,

Figure 5-1   Left- vs Right-Sided Brain Damage

Right-Sided Brain Damage

- Spatial-perceptual deficits
- Quick impulsive behavior
- Performance memory deficits
- Left-sided paralysis

Left-Sided Brain Damage

- Speech language deficits
- Slow, cautious behavior
- Language memory deficits
- Problem solving
- Right-sided paralysis

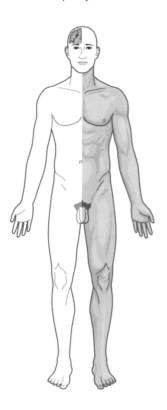
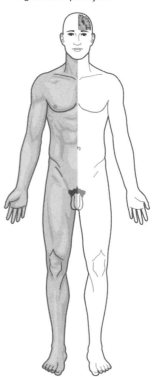

everyday tasks such as feeding oneself, dressing, or a number of other motor activities may be significantly affected.

Most people, regardless of whether they are left-handed or right-handed, have the language center located in the left hemisphere of the brain. The language center, which processes language symbols, affects auditory comprehension, speaking, reading, and writing. Consequently, left-sided stroke may interfere with the individual's ability to comprehend and use language (aphasia). The ability to communicate through speech, writing, or signs in left-sided brain damage are compromised because of damage to the language processing center of the brain rather than because

of impairment of the musculature involved in producing speech.

Although individuals with left-sided brain damage may be able to understand more than they can speak or write, they may have problems with both understanding and speaking. Some people have trouble pronouncing words because of the inability to coordinate muscles used in speech (**dysarthria**), causing their words to be slurred, slow, or difficult to understand, yet their language skills are intact (Cleveland Clinic, n.d.).

Even though individuals may have difficulty with speech and language, their ability to learn and communicate should neither be underestimated nor overestimated. Usually individuals with this type of communication difficulty will be able to understand short, concise statements better than long, complicated sentences. Individuals' ability to understand should not be underestimated even when they are unable to speak. Likewise, in those individuals who are able to speak, their ability to understand should not be overestimated.

Besides difficulty with language, individuals with left-sided brain damage tend to be slow, hesitant, anxious, and disorganized, especially when they are presented with new or unfamiliar situations. Reassurance and frequent reinforcement for tasks performed correctly help reduce anxiety and enhance these individuals' ability to perform.

Right-Sided Brain Damage

The most visible sign of right-sided brain damage is *left-sided motor and sensory paralysis* (ASA, n.d. a). Often right-sided brain damage is accompanied by some degree of visual perception loss or loss of visual motor integration that affects spatial and perceptual function. Functional consequences of spatial and perceptual difficulty can be manifested in several ways. Individuals may experience loss of depth perception or lack of awareness of stimuli on the left side of the body, causing difficulty with navigation within the environment. For instance, individuals may miss the table with a glass when putting it down or bump into a doorway when attempting to go through it. Individuals with right-sided brain damage may also have difficulty processing visual cues. Consequently, an uncluttered, simple, and structured environment can help to prevent distraction and may enhance the individual's ability to perform certain tasks. Spatial/perceptual manifestations of right-sided brain damage may also affect the individual's ability to read. For instance, the person may have an inability to move down the page without skipping lines.

Problems with memory may also be present with right-sided brain damage such that individuals are unable to recognize familiar people or places. In other instances, memory consequence is manifested as disorientation in familiar environments so that individuals may require specific instructions about how to get from place to place. In other instances, memory difficulty may result in individuals forgetting where they have placed personal items and then concluding that someone else must have taken the items.

Because language function is often not affected with right-sided brain damage, the abilities of individuals with right-sided brain damage may be overestimated by others as well as by the individuals themselves. Individuals may be disinhibited and unaware of limitations they may have and consequently overestimate their own abilities to perform tasks, acting quickly and impulsively. As a result of diminished self-awareness, they may tend to set unrealistic goals and appear insensitive to the needs of others. In other instances, individuals may have difficulty decoding nonverbal cues from others and, as a result, be oblivious to others' reactions or feelings.

COMPLICATIONS AND OTHER ISSUES ASSOCIATED WITH STROKE

Medical poststroke complications occur relatively frequently and have been shown to contribute to poor outcomes. The number of complications is extensive; the following complications are some of the most common and some treatment for them (Teasell et al., 2013).

Spasticity and Contractures

When an extremity is paralyzed after stroke, it is initially flaccid; however, due to damage to the part of the brain that moderates muscle function, reflexes to the extremity become overactive, causing spasticity—a condition in which muscles contract and become rigid. Spasticity can cause pain and interfere with positioning of the extremity as well as function. A variety of physical modalities, such as stretching, cooling, or heating of the extremity, as well as medications may be used to manage spasticity.

Owing to flaccidity of an extremity and tightening of supporting tissue around joints of the extremity, a condition known as **contracture**, in which a joint becomes immobilized in a position of nonfunction, may occur. Appropriate positioning of extremities, range-of-motion exercises, stretching, and splinting are all interventions that may be utilized to prevent contractures from occurring (ASA, 2015b).

Poststroke Seizures

Some individuals experience poststroke seizures as a direct result of injury to the brain. Seizures may occur immediately after stroke or may not occur until months afterward (Silverman, Restrepo, & Mathews, 2002). Management of poststroke seizures is individualized and dependent on the functional impact of the seizures as well as on individual preferences (Kilcullen, 2014).

Pain

Individuals may experience pain after stroke as a direct result of brain injury. This condition, called *central pain syndrome*, causes the individual to experience diffuse and intense burning, tingling, or aching pain. Individuals are encouraged to avoid situations that may trigger the pain or may be educated in relaxation techniques that may prove helpful.

A second type of pain experienced may be shoulder pain directly related to paralysis of an upper extremity, such that there is stretching or spasticity of the muscles supporting and around the shoulder joint. Support for the arm through use of a sling as well as other therapeutic exercises to decrease pain and increase function may be utilized (Teasell et al., 2013).

Dysphasia

Some individuals experience difficulty with swallowing (**dysphasia**) after stroke. This condition not only has implications for nutrition but also can lead to pneumonia if individuals aspirate some of the food they are attempting to swallow. Interventions such as modifying a diet to include foods that are more easily swallowed may be utilized to work around dysphasia. In some instances, individuals may work with a swallowing therapist to help restore swallowing function. In other instances, they may have a feeding tube inserted into their

stomach to maintain nutrition and avoid food aspiration (Stroke Association, 2015).

Bowel and Bladder Control

As a result of stroke, some individuals lose the ability to control bowel or bladder function, which can be a source of frustration and social embarrassment. Bowel and or bladder difficulties may be a direct result of damage to neural pathways that control voluntary function. In other instances, it may be the result of difficulty getting to the toilet in time or inability to adequately adjust clothing for toilet use. Sometimes bowel or bladder problems may be attributed to cognitive causes in which the individual does not recognize the need to evacuate bladder or bowel or does not remember how to find bathroom facilities. Interventions for managing bladder and bowel problems depend on the cause but may include regulation of fluid intake, establishing regular scheduled toileting patterns, establishing an effective bowel regime, or utilizing strategies or assistive devices that facilitate toilet use (Teasell et al., 2013).

Emotional Liability

After stroke, some individuals may exhibit a partial loss of emotional control, a condition known as *emotional liability*. Rather than being due to depression or sadness, this condition is a direct result of brain damage. With emotional liability, individuals may engage in prolonged crying or switch from laughing to crying, or from crying to laughing, when there is no apparent relationship between the emotional outburst and what is going on around them. The emotional reaction can often be diverted if the individual's attention can be directed to another activity. The individual's family may need support and guidance in dealing with the individual's outbursts.

Depression

Depression is common after stroke (Salter et al., 2013). Although adaptation to loss of various functions after stroke may involve a period of mourning, ongoing and prolonged depression may become a complication that impedes individuals' functional capacity and participation in the rehabilitation process. In addition, manifestations of depression may be misinterpreted as resulting in cognitive difficulties so that adequate interventions for management of depression are not appropriately instituted.

Underlying Conditions Associated with Stroke

Individuals who have experienced one stroke are at higher risk for a subsequent second stroke (National Stroke Association [NSA], n.d. a). Often stroke is precipitated by an underlying chronic condition such as hypertension, arteriosclerosis, or diabetes. Consequently, ongoing management of underlying conditions is also important to prevent further strokes from occurring and to optimize the individuals' rehabilitation process. Due to physical, cognitive, or emotional manifestations of stroke, however, management of underlying conditions may be more difficult.

MANAGEMENT OF STROKE

Comprehensive rehabilitation and other therapeutic programs are often required for months to years after stroke to help individuals recover ability and adapt to the residual effects of stroke. The overall goal of rehabilitation after stroke is to help the individual reestablish, and optimize, his or her independence and to return to preexisting roles and relationships to the extent possible (NINDS, 2014). Recovery and adaptation after stroke necessitates a multifaceted process that requires attention to the physical, cognitive, and psychosocial aspects of function. A comprehensive approach to rehabilitation entails a multidisciplinary team approach involving a number of professionals, including physiatrists, rehabilitation nurses, physical therapists, occupational therapists, speech therapists, nutritionists, psychologists, social workers, and rehabilitation counselors. Individuals experiencing stroke, along with their family and friends, need support, education, and training to optimize rehabilitation efforts. In addition, the individual's physical environment should be evaluated and modified to compensate for manifestations of stroke that may impede optimal functional capacity.

After stabilization in the early phases of stroke, the major focus of management is restoration of function, reduction of limitations, and prevention of complications. Most natural motor and functional recovery occurs in the first three months after stroke (Claflin et al., 2015), although additional progress can be made through continuing rehabilitation. *Physical therapy* and *occupational therapy* are usually instituted in the early stages of rehabilitation and continue to be provided during the postacute phase. In the early stages of rehabilitation, the focus is on helping individuals increase strength and prevent deformities, such as *contractures*, that might interfere with functional capacity.

Many individuals have some limitations in walking after stroke, which places them at risk for falls and subsequent fractures. Consequently, improving functional walking capacity is a major goal of physical rehabilitation (Teasell & Nussein, 2014). As rehabilitation progresses, goals such as achieving independent walking, helping individuals use assistive devices such as a cane or walker, and performing transfers such as from bed to chair become primary goals.

When the hand and arm are also affected, management is directed toward helping individuals achieve self-care tasks such as feeding, bathing, and toileting and in educating them in the use of assistive devices for carrying out tasks of daily living. *Speech therapy* is instituted for those individuals who experience *aphasia*. Because the types and severity of aphasia vary widely, management is based on individual needs.

After the acute phase of stroke rehabilitation, individuals may move to an extended residential care facility for continued rehabilitation, or they may return home and continue rehabilitation on an outpatient basis. The degree to which individuals are able to achieve optimal function varies and depends on a number of factors, including the location and extent of stroke as well as any preexisting conditions. Other factors of importance are the individual's psychological state, degree of social support, and general environment. For this reason, attention must also be given to the individual's family and social network as well as the physical and social environment in which they function.

FUNCTIONAL IMPLICATIONS OF STROKE

Personal and Psychosocial Issues

The effects of stroke are far-reaching. Not only is stroke associated with many physical and neurobehavioral manifestations, but cognitive, emotional, and social role functioning is affected as well (Teasell & Nussein, 2014). Changes associated with stroke have many long-term psychological and social implications. Adjustment to any change of function due to a chronic condition can be difficult, of course, but manifestations of stroke can offer particular challenges. Stroke can result in loss of functional independence, thereby altering an individual's perception of competency, identity, self-concept, and self-esteem (Brewer, Horgan, Hickey, & Williams, 2013). In some instances, the individual may not accurately perceive the functional implications of the stroke, which may interfere with effective rehabilitation efforts.

The psychosocial, physical, and economic consequences of stroke can pose a major challenge to the family as well as to the individual (ASA, n.d. b). Stroke can create a psychosocial crisis for the family not only because of the functional manifestations the individual experienced due to stroke but also because of the resulting increased caregiving responsibilities that family members must assume, often with little training or support). Although in the past much of this rehabilitation effort took place in the hospital before discharge, individuals who experience stroke may now be discharged much earlier, with much of the rehabilitation that had previously taken place in the hospital being conducted on an outpatient basis. Families may be unprepared for the complexity of interventions needed, the economic consequences, and their own role in contributing to effective rehabilitation outcomes for the individual after stroke (ASA, n.d. b).

Stroke rehabilitation must focus not only on recovery of muscle strength, range of motion, or mobility, but also on rebuilding of individuals' identity, roles, and relationships (Nauert, n.d.). Depending on the extent of brain damage experienced with stroke, individuals may require extensive and ongoing rehabilitation.

Activities and Participation

Physical, cognitive, and emotional residual manifestations of stroke can affect self-care or activities of daily living and community integration. Ongoing rehabilitation efforts involve optimizing functional capacity and societal roles as desired. Continued follow-up with a multidisciplinary team of professionals is necessary to work toward continued optimal capacity, monitor progress, identify barriers, and assess continued needs.

Activities of Daily Living

Because self-care and activities of daily living are often altered by stroke, the individual may need to learn alternative methods of performing routine tasks. Fatigue is often a secondary manifestation after stroke. Thus individuals may need to space out activities or arrange for frequent rest periods during the day. Activities that could once be completed in a short amount of time may need to be divided into a series of smaller tasks carried out over time.

Family Participation

Even when alternative methods are utilized, help from family members or others may be necessary. Family members can become overwhelmed by the responsibility but be reluctant to express their own feelings of frustration or helplessness (ASA, n.d. b). Unless families are helped to cope with their frustration and learn strategies to help them adjust to the situation, increased stress can disrupt family function and interfere with the individual's progress. In some instances, families may become overly protective so that the individual with stroke is hampered from reaching optimal function and independence. Wanting to shield the individual from what is perceived as stressful, family members may exclude the individual from family problems or decision making or limit his or her inclusion in family activities. At times it may be difficult to determine the degree to which the individual's ability or inability to function is due to the stroke itself or the degree to which ability or inability is induced by the situation. It is important for family members to reassure the individual that he or she continues to be a valued and needed member of the family unit, and it is helpful for the family to have the individual participate in as many family and other activities as possible.

Families can help by demonstrating confidence, encouraging the individual, and enabling the family member to do as much for himself or herself as possible. Although the family can be the most effective resource for assisting the individual to reach his or her goals, help and support from other professionals can help to reduce stress and provide assistance to the family in areas where needed. Continued guidance and support from professionals can help families resolve difficulties they may be experiencing in adjusting to role changes and responsibilities that are the result of manifestations of stroke.

Social Participation

Manifestations of stroke can alter social performance and precipitate significant role changes. Members of the larger social environment may lack a thorough understanding of stroke and its implications for physical, and emotional function, or they may misinterpret manifestations of stroke, such as emotional liability and problems with memory, attention, or judgment. Rather than attributing behaviors to results of stroke, poststroke individuals may be perceived to be rude, insensitive, or irresponsible. In other instances, the people in the broader social community may feel uncomfortable due to their own perceived inadequacy in knowing how to respond to individuals with stroke, consequently avoiding interactions altogether.

Rebuffs from people in the social environment can cause the individual with stroke to experience social anxiety and produce low self-esteem. Individuals with stroke may experience frustration and less self-assurance in the struggle to cope with social demands. Promoting greater awareness in the community can help create more openness and acceptance. Nevertheless, after stroke, an individual may need to learn and adopt compensatory mechanisms or strategies to be implemented in a variety of social interactions.

Sexuality

Sexuality involves much more than just sexual intercourse. Regardless of their ability or desire to engage in sexual activity per se, after stroke, individuals continue to need warm, close personal relationships and to feel attractive to others. There are many different ways to fulfill a need for closeness; sexual intercourse is only one way. If individuals were sexually active prior to the stroke, resuming sexual activity would be a natural part of general activity (NSA, n.d. b).

Patience and loving communication are essential to a satisfying relationship. If the individual has a partner, there may be unspoken fears that both are frightened to discuss, which can in turn lead to isolation and stress in the overall relationship. Individuals who have experienced stroke may fear that they will be rejected by or are unattractive to their partner. The partner may fear that engaging in sexual activity will precipitate another stroke. Obtaining assistance from professionals who can help both partners discuss their fears can help to strengthen the relationship.

Environmental Modifications and Assistive Devices

Making home modifications or identifying accessible areas in the community environment help the individual with stroke to achieve increased independence (ASA, 2015b). In addition, a number of assistive devices are available for increased function. Assistive devices need not be costly, and sometimes the most effective device can be devised from simple materials already available in the home.

Many stroke survivors want to resume driving (ASA, 2015c). This is not unusual; driving is a symbol of independence to the individual. Often survivors don't realize the difficulties they may have when driving after a stroke. A good way to determine if the individual is ready to drive safely is to have a driving evaluation by a Driver Rehabilitation Specialist. This specialist tests for visual perception, functional ability, reaction time, judgement and cognitive abilities of the individual behind the wheel. If the stroke survivor is cleared to drive there are many equipment options that can be added to a vehicle for accessibility and driving (hand pedals on the steering column).

VOCATIONAL IMPLICATIONS OF STROKE

The number of individuals who return to work after stroke ranges from 19% to 73% (Treger, Shames, Giaquinto, & Ring, 2007). The extent to which an individual is able to return to work is multifactorial. Age, education, social support, and severity of stroke all contribute to vocational potential. In addition, the type of job, its physical demands and complexity, interpersonal and language requirements, and visual perceptual requirements of the job must be considered. Although there is the common misperception that stroke affects mostly older individuals and, therefore, has less vocational impact, many people at the time of stroke are still active in the workforce. Approximately one-third of individuals who experience stroke are younger than the age of 65 (Centers for Disease Control and Prevention, 2015; National Stroke Association, 2016).

Vocational implications for individuals with stroke vary widely, depending on the specific and individual manifestations exhibited. Specific functions that should be considered are cognitive function, such as memory, problem-solving ability, and spatial and temporal orientation, as well as motor abilities, including coordination, balance, speed of performance, and muscle dexterity.

If communication skills are affected, alternative means of communicating in the workplace or computer-assisted communication may be needed. In many instances, even though individuals' communication may be difficult to understand, patience and practice will enable coworkers to establish basic patterns of communication that make interchange in the workplace possible.

When manifestations of stroke include difficulty with motor skills such as ambulation, manual dexterity, or coordination, demands of the job that include walking, lifting, pulling, or pushing should be evaluated, and workplace modification or specific devices to assist in motor tasks may be needed.

If individuals experience poor motor speed or decreased processing ability as a manifestation of stroke, they may feel rushed or stressed when trying to perform tasks. An environment that has minimal distractions and is free from clutter can be beneficial in such cases. If individuals feel pressure to perform, they may experience stress, and consequently the quality of their work may be affected. Individuals may experience fatigue as a direct consequence of brain damage, or job stress may lead to fatigue. Dividing tasks into smaller steps and taking advantage of frequent rest periods can help to decrease fatigue. Providing an environment in which the individual experiences less pressure and stress can help increase both productivity and quality of work.

Another factor that may either enhance or diminish individuals' ability to reach their full vocational potential may be transportation. Often the individual's ability to drive is affected by stroke owing to motor manifestations such as paralysis, visual spatial manifestations, or cognitive manifestations that include judgment. If the individual is no longer able to drive, finding an alternative way to reach the place of employment is important to facilitate return to work.

Realistic expectations about level of performance are an important component of success. If the individual, his or her family, or the workplace has not adequately and realistically evaluated the employee's capacity to perform, or if they have not provided the modifications or assistive devices that would enable the individual to carry out job tasks, the probability of failure increases. In such circumstances, individuals may become so discouraged that they lose the motivation to try. Ongoing evaluation of progress in the workplace, provision of resources to meet needs as they arise, and continued support all contribute to vocational success (Rehabilitation Institute of Chicago, n.d.).

CASE STUDY

Ms. L., a 49-year-old accountant, had complained of headaches for several days before collapsing in her office. She was immediately taken to the emergency room by ambulance and was found to have experienced a stroke due to cerebral aneurysm on the left side of her brain.

1. Which residual manifestations might Ms. L. experience as a result of left-sided brain damage?
2. How might the manifestations affect her ability to continue her work as an accountant?
3. Depending on the extent and type of residual manifestations, which types of work modification or assistive devices may be beneficial to Ms. L. in continuing her current line of work?

REFERENCES

American Stroke Association. (n.d. a). About Strokes http://www.strokeassociation.org/STROKEORG/AboutStroke/About-Stroke_UCM_308529_SubHomePage.jsp

American Stroke Association. (n.d. b). Caregiver Guide to Stroke. http://strokeassociation.org/STROKEORG/LifeAfterStroke/ForFamilyCaregivers/CaringforYourself/Caregiver-Guide_UCM_457471_Article.jsp#.V0nQcuQ0OgN

American Stroke Association (n.d. d). What is an arteriovenous malformation (AVM)? Received 5/27/16. http://www.strokeassociation.org/STROKEORG/AboutStroke/TypesofStroke/HemorrhagicBleeds/What-Is-an-Arteriovenous-Malformation-AVM_UCM_310099_Article.jsp#.V0icu-Q0OgM

American Stroke Association. (2015a). Aphasia vs. Apraxia. http://www.strokeassociation.org/STROKEORG/LifeAfterStroke/RegainingIndependence/Communication Challenges/Aphasia-vs-Apraxia_UCM_310079_Article.jsp#.V0im5-Q0OgM

American Stroke Association. (2015b). Home modifications for stroke Survivors. http://www.strokeassociation.org/STROKEORG/LifeAfterStroke/RegainingIndependence/HomeModifications/Home-Modifications-for-Stroke-Survivors_UCM_311015_Article.jsp#.V0nZTeQ0OgM

American Stroke Association. (2015c). Driving After Stroke. http://www.strokeassociation.org/STROKEORG/LifeAfterStroke/RegainingIndependence/Driving/Driving-After-Stroke_UCM_311016_Article.jsp#.V0naEeQ0OgM

Boss, B. J., Huether, S. E. (2014). Disorders of the central and peripheral nervous systems and neuromuscular function. In: K. L. McCance, S. E.,Huether, V. L. Brashers, & N. S. Rote, (Eds.). *Pathophysiology: The Biologic Basis for Disease in Adults and Children*. (7th ed.). St. Louis Mo: Elsevier-Mosby; 581–607.

Brain Injury Institute (n.d.) Brain injury types. http://www.braininjuryinstitute.org/Brain-Injury-Types/Hypoxia.html

Brewer, L., Horgan, F., Hickey, A., & Williams, D. (2013). Stroke rehabilitation: Recent advances and future therapies. *QJM: An International Journal of Medicine,106*(1), 11–25.

Caswell, J. (2013). Returning to work. *Stroke Connection,* http://www.strokeassociation.org/idc/groups/stroke-public/@wcm/@hcm/@mag/documents/downloadable/ucm_463026.pdf

Centers for Disease Control and Prevention. (2015). Stroke Facts. http://www.cdc.gov/stroke/facts.htm

Claflin, E. S., Krishnan, C., & Sandeep, P. K., (2015). Emerging Treatments for Motor Rehabilitation after Stroke. *Neurohospitalist.* 5(2): 77–88.

Cleveland Clinic (n.d.). Diseases & Conditions: Stroke and the Brain. http://my.clevelandclinic.org/health/diseases_conditions/stroke/hic_Stroke_and_the_Brain

Fonseca, A. C., Ferro, J. M. (2013). Drug abuse and stroke. *Current Neurology Neuroscience Reports, 13*(2), 325. doi:10.1007/s11910-012-0325-0

Kilcullen, W. (2014). Seizures after a stroke. *Stroke Net.* http://www.strokenetwork.org/newsletter/articles/seizures.htm

Mayo Clinic. (2016). Stroke. http://www.mayoclinic/diseases-conditions/stroke/symptoms-causes/dxc20117265

National Institute of Neurological Disorders and Stroke. Post-Stroke Rehabilitation. Know Stroke. (2014). *NIH Publication. 14,* 1846. https://stroke.nih.gov/materials/rehabilitation.htm

National Institute of Neurological Disorders and Stroke. (2016). Cerebral Aneurysms Fact sheet. http://www.ninds.nih.gov/disorders/cerebral_aneurysm/detail_cerebral_aneurysms.htm

National Stroke Association (n.d. a) Preventing another stroke. http://www.stroke.org/we-can-help/survivors/stroke-recovery/first-steps-recovery/preventing-another-stroke

National Stroke Association. (n.d. b). Sex and sexuality. http://www.stroke.org/we-can-help/stroke-survivors/living-stroke/lifestyle/relationships/sex-and-sexuality

National Stroke Association. (2016). Returning to work after a stroke. http://www.stroke.org/we-can-help/survivors/living-stroke/lifestyle/returning-work-after-stroke

Nauert, R. (n.d.) Psychosocial effects of stroke can be significant. PsychCentral. http://psychcentral.com/news/2009/06/19/psychosocial-effects-of-stroke-can-be-significant/6635.html

Rehabilitation Institute of Chicago. (n.d.). Important issues for stroke survivors to consider when returning to work. National Institute on Disability and Rehabilitation Research, Grant No. H133B080031. https://www.ric.org/app/files/public/3548/Return-to-work-recommendations-for-stroke-survivors.pdf

Salter, K. Mehta, S. Bhogal, S., Teasell, R., Foley, N., & Speechley, M. (2013). Post Stroke Depression. http://www.ebrsr.com/sites/default/files/chapter18_depression_final_16ed.pdf

Silverman, I. E. Restrepo, L., & Mathews, G. C. (2002). Post-stroke seizures. *Archives of Neurology 59*, 195–201.

Stroke Association (2015). Swallowing problems after a stroke. https://www.stroke.org.uk/resources/complete-guide-swallowing-problems-after-stroke.

Sun, J-H., Tan, L., & Yu, J-T. (2014). Post-stroke cognitive impairment: Epidemiology, mechanisms and management. *Annals of Translational Medicine 2*(8), 80. doi:10.3978 /j.issn.2305-5839.2014.08.05

Teasell, R., Foley, N., Salter, K., Hussein, N., Viana, R., & Campbell, N. (2013). Medical Complications Post Stroke. http://www.ebrsr.com/sites/default/files/Chapter17_Medical -Complications_FINAL_16ed.pdf

Teasell, R., & Nussein, N. (2014). Motor Rehabilitation. Stroke Rehabilitation Clinician Handbook. http://www .ebrsr.com/sites/default/files/Chapter%204A_Lower%20 Extremity%20and%20mobility%20post%20stroke_June%20 18%202014.pdf

The Children's Trust. (2016). Non-traumatic brain injury. *Brain Injury Hub*. http://www.braininjuryhub.co.uk /information-library/non-traumatic

Treger, I., Shames, J., Giaquinto, S., & Ring, H. (2007). Return to work in stroke patients. *Disability and Rehabilitation,* 291397–1403.

CHAPTER 6

Epilepsy and Other Conditions of the Nervous System

EPILEPSY

Overview of Epilepsy

The epilepsies are a group of conditions in which there is an underlying neurological condition that causes disruption of electrical activity in the brain, which in turn affects consciousness, movement, or actions through a seizure. *Seizure* is a general term used to describe a state in which there is temporary loss of control over certain body functions.

Approximately 1 in 10 people will experience a seizure during the course of a lifetime. Although the essential feature of epilepsy is recurrent seizures, not all seizures are attributable to epilepsy. Seizures can be the consequences of an acute condition, such as alcohol or drug intoxication or withdrawal, **hypoxia** (diminished oxygen), hypertension, stroke, or trauma. This type of seizure is called *acute symptomatic seizure* (Wiebe, 2016). In these cases, there is temporary disruption of electrical activity in the brain caused by the acute condition, but unless there is damage that causes permanent changes in brain function seizures do not persist after the acute condition is resolved (St. Louis & Granner, 2007).

Epilepsy, in contrast, is a condition in which there are recurrent, seizures due to a permanent, underlying neurological condition in which function of the neurons in the brain is disrupted so that they create atypical electrical discharges resulting in a seizure. Although acute conditions (such as stroke or head injury) can result in permanent damage to the brain resulting in epilepsy, many times, no clear-cut cause for epilepsy can be identified.

Types of Seizures

The type of seizure individuals experience varies and depends on area of the brain affected. The type of seizure experienced determines the type of medication the individual receives to manage seizures. Manifestations of seizures can range from muscle spasms or confusion to total loss of consciousness. Seizures can be mild or severe, can occur frequently or rarely, and can change their pattern of occurrence over time. Depending on the type, seizures usually last from only seconds to minutes. Between seizures, most individuals are able to function without difficulty.

Broadly, seizures in epilepsy may be classified as either focal, in which abnormal nerve cell discharge is limited to *one specific part* of the brain or *generalized*, in which nerve cells discharge abnormally throughout the *whole brain.*

Manifestations of Focal and Generalized Seizures

Focal Seizures

Manifestations of focal seizures vary widely, depending on which part of the brain is affected. Focal seizures types classified according to manifestations during the seizure. For example a focal seizure that involves jerking or movement in one part of the body would be classified as a *motor seizure*. If the seizure involves a manifestation in which the individual experiences an unpleasant smell, the seizure would be classified as an *olfactory seizure*.

Focal seizures are also classified according to the degree of change in consciousness or awareness during the seizure. When consciousness or awareness is impaired during a seizure, the seizure is described as a *dyscognitive seizure*. For example, during a seizure the individual may pace, wander, aimlessly, or utter unintelligible sounds.

Generalized Seizures

Generalized Tonic–Clonic Seizures (Grand Mal)

An abnormal discharge of nerve cells throughout the brain results in a *generalized tonic–clonic seizure*, sometimes called a *grand mal seizure*. Some individuals experience an **aura** (warning sign) immediately before the seizure begins. Auras can consist of things such as seeing a flash of light, having an unusual taste in the mouth, or experiencing other unusual sensations. As the seizure develops, individuals lose consciousness and collapse, entering a **tonic** state characterized by generalized body rigidity. Muscles then enter a **clonic** state, in which the whole body undergoes rapid, jerky movements. The teeth are clenched tightly together, and control of the bladder or the bowel may be lost. The seizure generally lasts less than a few minutes. When it ends, consciousness is gradually regained, but individuals may experience confusion, difficulty in speaking, and headache. Although postseizure manifestations usually disappear within several hours, the fatigue experienced may be overwhelming, often necessitating an extended period of rest or sleep. Although a tonic–clonic seizure may be frightening to those who witness it, individuals experiencing the seizure are usually in no imminent danger unless the immediate environment contains hard, sharp, or hot hazards. No attempt should be made to move individuals experiencing a seizure except as necessary to protect the individual from hazards.

To avoid injury, there should be no attempt to restrain individuals during a tonic–clonic seizure, to pry open clenched teeth, or to place hard objects in the individual's mouth. Individuals should be placed on their side during a seizure so that secretions can drain from the mouth and do not compromise the airway. If the seizure lasts for five minutes or longer, emergency medical care should be sought immediately.

Absence Seizures (Petit Mal)

Like tonic–clonic seizures, *absence seizures* are classified as generalized seizures because nerve cells discharge throughout the entire brain (Wiebe, 2016). Absence seizures are characterized by brief blank spells or staring spells and a loss of awareness of the surroundings. The seizure generally lasts for only seconds. The individual does not fall, and there are usually no outward motor manifestations of absence seizures, although abnormal blinking or slight twitching may occur occasionally. Because of the limited visible manifestations of the seizure, those around the individual may misinterpret an absence seizure as daydreaming or inattentiveness.

When children experience frequent absence seizures, their school performance may be disrupted. Because there may be no significant signs that are easily observed during seizure activity, absence seizures may not be identified and the poor school performance may be erroneously attributed to other causes. Recognition of manifestations and appropriate identification are crucial to enable children to achieve their maximum potential. Absence seizures may disappear spontaneously with age, although some individuals who have experienced absence seizures later go on to develop tonic–clonic seizures.

Status Epilepticus

Status epilepticus is a term used to describe seizures that are prolonged or that come in rapid succession without full recovery of consciousness between seizures. This condition is a medical emergency that can be life threatening. Accordingly, status epilepticus requires immediate healthcare attention and management (Wiebe, 2016).

Identification and Confirmation of Epilepsy

Individuals having a seizure for the first time usually undergo evaluation to determine whether the seizure is a manifestation of an acute health condition or neurological condition that can be treated and resolved, or a manifestation of a chronic neurological problem that will require ongoing management. Extensive physical examination and blood tests are usually part of initial screening, as is a detailed history of precipitating factors that appeared to trigger the seizure.

When individuals have more than one seizure, or when other manifestations or history indicate that epilepsy may be the cause of seizure activity, a more extensive medical evaluation is conducted. A primary diagnostic tool for evaluating individuals after seizures is *electroencephalography (EEG)*, a noninvasive procedure in which the electrical activity of the brain is recorded and the results are printed graphically. *Magnetic resonance imaging (MRI)*, a noninvasive procedure that produces rapid detailed images of body structures, may also be used to identify structural anomalies in the brain that are related to seizures.

Management of Epilepsy

Management of epilepsy depends on the cause and type of seizures experienced, and the probability of recurrence (Davidson & Derry, 2015). Individuals who have had only a single seizure (*acute symptomatic seizure*) are evaluated in order to determine the cause. If the seizure was due to an acute condition, interventions to manage or resolve the condition are warranted. When a cause for the seizure cannot be determined, whether the individual receives further treatment depends on the likelihood of recurrence (Wiebe, 2016).

If seizures are caused by a tumor, scar tissue, or another condition that can be corrected, surgical intervention to remove or repair the tumor or scar tissue may be indicated. In some instances when seizures are not effectively managed by medication and are severely incapacitating, surgery may be directed toward resection of the part of the brain responsible for the seizure activity (St. Louis & Granner, 2007).

Medications are a mainstay of seizure control with the ultimate goal of to obtaining complete freedom from seizures with minimum side effects (Wiebe, 2016). A number of new antiepileptic drugs have been approved for management of epilepsy, enabling the health professionals and the individual to work together to match medications the individual's particular need (Chong & Lerman, 2016).

Although medications do not cure epilepsy, they can effectively manage seizures and enable many individuals to carry on full and productive lives. Successful management of seizures, however, requires the individual's strict, long-term adherence to medication instructions. Medications used to manage epilepsy are also not without side effects. Toxic effects are common during long-term management with anticonvulsant medications. Depending on the medication, side effects may include gum overgrowth, nausea, dizziness, clumsiness, visual difficulty, or fatigue.

Once medication for management of seizures has begun, it is generally maintained for at least two years, regardless of whether the individual has remained seizure free (Browne & Holmes, 2001). If there have been no recurrent seizures after this time, medication may be withdrawn. Individuals who have not experienced any additional seizures since beginning the medication or who have experienced side effects may be tempted to alter or discontinue their medication. The consequences of this course of action could be dangerous or even life threatening. For this reason, individuals should never attempt to alter or discontinue their medication without consulting with a healthcare provider.

Levels of the medication in the blood are periodically monitored. Based on the medication's concentration in the blood and its effectiveness in managing seizure activity, medication dosages may be altered. The levels of the anticonvulsant medication in the blood also serve as an indication of the individual's adherence to the medication plan.

In some cases, even when individuals are compliant with taking anticonvulsant medications, seizures are not effectively managed. Many of these individuals experience several seizures per month or, at times, several seizures per day, despite following a strict management plan. When surgery is indicated for seizures that are severely incapacitating and unable to be effectively managed with medication, a portion of the brain where seizures are triggered may be removed, a portion of the brain may be resected, or the affected portion of the brain may be disconnected from the rest of the brain. The surgery itself may leave residual effects. The amount of incapacity experienced, if any, after this type of surgery depends on the individual circumstances. In fact, some individuals may still need anticonvulsant medications even after surgery.

Alcohol can lower a person's seizure threshold and, therefore, precipitate seizures. Alcohol and anticonvulsant medications may also interact and cause untoward effects. Consequently, individuals with epilepsy should first consult with a healthcare provider about the safety of alcohol use in their specific case.

Individuals with epilepsy should be helped to identify those factors that may trigger a seizure. They should avoid activity that would be hazardous if a seizure should occur, such as swimming alone or operating heavy equipment. A medical identification bracelet should be worn by individuals with epilepsy at all times.

The general prognosis for individuals with epilepsy depends on the type of seizure, the underlying cause, the administration of appropriate management, and the individual's willingness and ability to follow the management plan. If their condition is accurately diagnosed and appropriately managed, most individuals with epilepsy can live active, productive lives. Prompt detection and early medical intervention can greatly improve the ability to manage seizures and enhance the general quality of life for the individual with epilepsy.

Functional Implications of Epilepsy

Personal and Psychosocial Issues

Individuals with epilepsy may face many psychological and psychosocial challenges (Wiebe, 2016). They must learn to deal with uncertainty related to whether and when another seizure will occur. No matter how well seizures are managed, individuals live with the possibility—even if remote—that another seizure will occur. The time, place, and social circumstances under which a seizure may occur are unknown. If individuals experience a seizure in public, they risk feelings of embarrassment and onlookers' potential misperception of the seizure. Individuals may feel they have no control over their lives and behavior. At times, even when seizures are adequately managed, anxiety over the possibility of having a seizure or other psychosocial consequences may be the most incapacitating factor associated with the condition. As a result, individuals may have difficulty establishing interpersonal relationships, building self-esteem, and obtaining or maintaining employment.

Activities and Participation

Social and Family Participation

In the period between seizures, epilepsy is an invisible health condition with no outward signs. Although considerable effort has been devoted to educate the public about the condition, misinformation and lack of acceptance still exist and epilepsy continues to carry a stigma for many individuals. In some cultures, historical misconceptions about epilepsy have linked it to demonic possession and insanity. In other instances, people with epilepsy were not permitted to participate in various events because of their condition. Even when seizures are relatively well managed, individuals may still fear having the occasional seizure and the physical and social consequences that the seizure may bring.

Attitudes have changed for the better in recent years thanks to public education programs, improved placement of individuals with epilepsy into the workforce, and increased ability to manage seizures. Nevertheless, individuals with epilepsy may still experience unjust restrictions, denying them access to participation in routine activities. The stigma and shame associated with epilepsy may cause individuals or their family to deny or minimalize the condition. Individuals may try to pass as someone without a health condition because of anticipated rejection due to real or perceived public attitudes.

Family is crucial to the adjustment of an individual with a condition that has associated incapacitation. Depending on the point at which the epilepsy is identified and the reaction of the family, both adjustment and emotional development of the individual can be affected. When epilepsy is identified in childhood, parental feelings of fear, anxiety, guilt, overprotectiveness, or mourning can influence not only the child's ability to accept his or her condition and associated manifestations but also the child's self-concept and social adjustment. Overly protective parents may foster dependency in their child. Children, in turn, may learn to use their condition as an excuse for inactivity or avoidance of responsibility. As teenagers, concerns related to whether they will drive a car, participate in sports, or engage in dating may cause additional stress and lessening of self-esteem.

Identification of epilepsy in adulthood can also disrupt interpersonal and family relationships. Individuals' social identity may be threatened, such that they go to great lengths to conceal their condition to avoid potential rejection. Partners of individuals with epilepsy may be fearful of observing a seizure or concerned that the disorder is hereditary. Due to anxiety and misinformation, they may be unwilling to learn more about the condition or to provide the support that the individual with epilepsy needs.

Sexuality

Sexual activity, in most cases, need not be affected by epilepsy, although some medications used to manage seizures may have some effect on libido, and issues of low self-esteem may produce greater limitations (Luef & Madersbacher, 2015). Individuals may be reluctant to form intimate relationships because of the fear of having a seizure. Counseling may be necessary to help individuals overcome fear so that appropriate intimate relationships can be established.

Operating a Motor Vehicle

In the past, individuals with epilepsy were restricted from driving motor vehicles because of concerns for both public and personal safety. Today, every state in the United States permits individuals with controlled seizures to drive; however in most states people with uncontrolled seizures are restricted from licensure (Krumholz, Hopp, & Sanchez, 2016)

The ability to operate a motor vehicle has a direct impact on an individual's independence and social well-being. Specifically, inability to drive can limit social interaction, educational experiences, and employment opportunities.

Alcohol Use

Alcohol consumption is frequently a part of social occasions. Individuals with epilepsy should consider the potential hazards of alcohol consumption, especially in regard to taking alcohol when they are also taking anticonvulsant medication, as well as the potential of lowering seizure threshold. However, each individual situation must be considered in terms of the person's specific needs.

Sports and Recreation

Sports activities are another important means of socializing as well as helping individuals build self-confidence and self-esteem. In some situations, restrictions on participation in various activities are placed on individuals with epilepsy even though no basis for limiting activity exists. Although some individuals may have seizures precipitated by fatigue or other sports-related circumstances, others may experience a reduction in the incidence of seizures with exercise. Given this variability, the individual's specific circumstances should be considered rather than issuing blanket restrictions; each case should be considered individually. Restrictions may be necessary for specific activities that present a hazard should a potential seizure, which involves loss of consciousness, take place. For instance, individuals with epilepsy should not swim alone. Likewise, activities such as operating an airplane, rock climbing, or other activities in which a seizure could cause severe and possibly fatal consequences should be avoided. In most instances, applying common sense enables individuals to participate in activities while avoiding potential hazards.

Routine Activities

Between seizures, most individuals with epilepsy are unaffected in their ability to carry on routine activities. However, individuals may be concerned about possible injury while performing routine tasks if a seizure should unexpectedly occur. Concerns about setting clothes on fire from gas stoves, falling in the shower, or a number of other situations that would have potential for injury in the event of a seizure may cause the individual anxiety and interfere with routine activities as a result. Consequently, individuals may need help in establishing common sense safety precautions for activities of daily living. Family, friends, and coworkers should also be informed about appropriate measures to take if a seizure occurs.

Despite effective management of seizures, some individuals may still feel the weight of restrictions of freedoms, activities, and events that others take for granted. For example, individuals may be required to obtain a written statement from a healthcare provider to verify that they can return to regular activities after a seizure occurs. Individuals may need to avoid certain theaters, bars, or other establishments that use strobe lights for decoration or effect if flickering lights precipitate seizures.

Taking medication regularly as recommended, obtaining proper rest, and reducing stress are other self-management issues that individuals with epilepsy must consider. In addition, the social stigma associated with epilepsy—whether real or perceived—can cause stress and influence social function. The uncertainty associated with the condition, as well as restrictions, potential social isolation, and difficulty with employment, may require adjustment and coping skills for the individual to achieve his or her full potential.

Vocational Issues in Epilepsy

Most individuals with epilepsy have the same range of IQ as the general population, unless other conditions that affect intellectual function are involved. Even so, individuals with epilepsy are likely to experience both unemployment and underemployment (Wo, Lim, Choo, & Tan, 2015). Many problems in the workplace related to individuals' ability to obtain or maintain employment continue to be inspired by misperceptions and stigma rather than by actual physical limitations. Although some individuals with epilepsy may have neuropsychological manifestations that can affect employment, most do not. Consequently, special

considerations for individuals in the workplace should reflect their individual situation rather than any generalizations.

Epilepsy is a chronic condition that requires ongoing monitoring and management. Medication is, of course, a major part of management and necessitates close monitoring and diligence in adhering to the medication plan. If individuals do not closely adhere to the medication plan and seizures are not effectively managed as a result, employment can also be affected.

Even when seizures are effectively managed, there remains the chance of unpredictable seizure with loss of consciousness, which may in turn place individuals with epilepsy or others at risk of injury. Consequently, some occupations—such as airplane pilot or interstate truck driver—may be unrealistic for the individual to pursue, however many jobs with reasonable accommodation are suitable (Krumholz et al., 2016). Understanding how seizures affect job function is critical. It is important to assess the types and numbers of seizures individuals have, the degree to which seizures are effectively managed with medication, and the individual's level of adherence in following the management plan. Determination of situational patterns for seizures (such as a regular time when seizures occur) or factors that precipitate seizures (such as fatigue, stress, or flickering lights) is key to helping individuals avoid or alter situations in which seizures may occur. If fatigue tends to precipitate a seizure, care should be taken so that the individual does not become overly tired. Likewise, if seizures are related to the individual's sleep pattern, he or she may be unable to work on a rotating shift. It is also helpful to know whether individuals experience an aura prior to the seizure and, therefore, would be able to remove themselves from dangerous situations prior to the seizure's onset. Individuals who experience seizures should probably not work alone in an isolated environment, especially if the environment imposes some threat of danger if a seizure should occur.

Individuals may question whether they should disclose that they have a seizure condition. Job seekers may choose to disclose their condition to an employer after they have outlined their qualifications and skills for the job, or they may want to establish credibility in the workplace before disclosing that they have a seizure condition (Fraser & Miller, 2005). If, when, and how an individual discloses his or her condition depends on the individual variables and the particular situation.

Employers that fear risk of lawsuits arising from workplace injuries may be overly conservative in applying restrictions on employees with epilepsy. Nevertheless, many jobs once thought to be inappropriate for individuals with epilepsy may not be contraindicated if proper safety equipment is used. In addition, many states have specific regulations protecting employers from excessive liability if injury occurs even though adequate safety precautions were maintained. Work potential can be maximized with continued education of employers, adequate safety precautions, and consideration of individual needs.

OTHER CONDITIONS INVOLVING THE BRAIN

Any infection of the brain or the membranes that surround the brain and spinal cord can cause serious neurological effects, some of which may be permanent. Two examples of infections that can affect the brain are meningitis and encephalitis.

Meningitis

Meningitis refers to an inflammation of the **meninges** (membranes surrounding the brain and spinal cord). It can be caused by bacteria, viruses, or other organisms. Many types of meningitis exist, and the specific name given to the meningitis infection is frequently related to its cause or location.

The hallmark of meningitis is its rapid onset. Confirmation of meningitis is made by a *lumbar puncture* (spinal tap), in which a needle is inserted between the vertebrae and into the subarachnoid space. Cerebrospinal fluid is aspirated and examined microscopically for organisms.

Individuals with meningitis are usually acutely ill, initially with fever and flu-like manifestations. Within a short period of time, they develop severe headache, neck rigidity, and visual discomfort when exposed to bright lights (*photophobia*). If the cause is bacterial in origin, prompt management with antibiotics reduces the chance of progression of the condition. The use of medication and prompt

management intervention have greatly reduced the number of fatalities from meningitis; however, if this infection occurs in individuals whose physical state is weakened or if identification of the condition and medical management are delayed, it can still be fatal. Although most individuals with meningitis recover completely, some may have residual neurological deficits such as deafness, paralysis, or cognitive difficulties (Romero, 2016).

Encephalitis

Encephalitis is an inflammation of the brain due to direct invasion of an organism. It may be caused by an endemic virus, such as the West Nile virus, herpes simplex virus, or varicella-zoster virus (chicken pox), or a number of other viruses (Aksamit, 2016). Some individuals with encephalitis experience severe headache, stiff neck, and coma. There is no adequate intervention to manage encephalitis, except for maintaining comfort and preventing complications. Manifestations can subside in a few weeks, leaving no permanent damage; however, some individuals may develop irreversible neurological changes and the condition can also be life threatening (Romero, 2016).

Although encephalitis (or meningitis) and resulting deficits can occur in any age group, children and older adults are often the most susceptible to more severe manifestations of the condition. Individuals with compromised immune systems, such as those with human immunodeficiency virus (HIV) infection or acquired immunodeficiency syndrome (AIDS), individuals with cancer, or those who have received organ transplants, are also at greater risk (Aksamit, 2016).

Sleep Apnea

Sleep apnea refers to frequent episodes of breathing cessation (**apnea**) during sleep. There are two types of sleep apnea: *obstructive sleep apnea* and *central sleep apnea.*

Obstructive sleep apnea, the most common type of sleep apnea, is a chronic condition characterized by obstruction of the upper airway during sleep, resulting in disturbed sleep with loud snoring and excessive daytime sleepiness. Prevalence is greater in men than in women, and obstructive sleep apnea is associated with excessive weight, poorly controlled hypertension, and heart failure (Basner, 2016). It is also associated with serious health consequences, such as cardiovascular disease, depression, impaired visual/motor skills, and accidents (Pavelec, Rotenberg, Mauer, Gillis, & Verse, 2016).

A second type of sleep apnea, *central sleep apnea,* can occur when the brain fails to send appropriate messages to muscles needed for breathing to initiate respiration. Central sleep apnea can be caused by stroke or by infections affecting the brain stem; it can also be caused by neuromuscular conditions that involve respiratory muscles.

The goal of management of sleep apnea is to decrease sleep fragmentation and reduce resulting **asphyxia** (insufficient intake of oxygen). Management strategies may include treating underlying conditions, weight loss, sleep positioning, oral appliances to maintain an open airway, or the use of mechanical treatment such as *continuous positive airway pressure (CPAP)*. The PAP machine consists of a mask that the individual wears, headgear to hold the mask in place, hosing, and a compact airflow generator which delivers positive airway pressure.

CPAP helps to improve sleep efficiency, quality of life, and mental function and is the first line treatment for obstructive sleep apnea (Basner, 2016).

Narcolepsy

Narcolepsy is a complex neurological sleep disorder involving the central nervous system that is linked to a disruption of the sleep control mechanism and characterized by episodes of excessive sleepiness and uncontrollable sleep that occurs during the day (Vaughn, 2016). The affected individual may fall asleep at any time and during any activity, such as while engaging in conversation, while driving, while eating, or when reading.

Identification of narcolepsy is usually based on a persistent history of excessive daytime sleepiness not due to other causes and confirmed through tests conducted at a sleep disorders clinic. Management usually consists of planned short nap periods during the day and, in some instances, prescription of medications—namely, central nervous system stimulants.

The physical, psychosocial, and vocational implications of narcolepsy can be devastating (Jennum, Ibsen, Petersen, Knudsen, & Kjelberg, 2012). Individuals who are not adequately diagnosed and treated may have difficulty reaching their full potential either in school or in employment. Even with appropriate management, manifestations of narcolepsy may not be adequately managed. Fear of embarrassment, which may result from the unpredictability of narcolepsy attacks, can cause individuals to limit their social interactions. Safety concerns regarding operation of potentially dangerous equipment may be an issue if manifestations are not adequately managed. Employers, teachers, and others coming in contact with the individual should be educated to understand the individual's condition so that if an attack does occur, manifestations will not be misinterpreted.

CASE STUDY

Ms. S. experienced her first generalized tonic seizure at age 18, shortly after she entered college. After several other seizures in the next year, she began taking medication to manage her seizures. She is now beginning her junior year in college and plans to pursue a career as an elementary school teacher but has concerns regarding the appropriateness of her career choice given her history of seizures.

1. Which specific information about Ms. S.'s health condition may be relevant to her career choice?
2. Which aspects of employment as an elementary school teacher may be important to consider?
3. Are there any accommodations that may be needed? If so, which accommodations should be pursued?

REFERENCES

Aksamit, A. J. (2016). Acute viral encephalitis. In L. Goldman & A. I. Schafer (Eds.), *Goldman-Cecil medicine.* (25th ed., pp. 2500–2504). Philadelphia, PA: Elsevier Saunders

Basner, R. C. (2016). Obstructive sleep apnea. In L. Goldman & A. I. Schafer (Eds.). *Goldman-Cecil medicine,* (25th ed., pp. 638–642). Philadelphia, PA: Elsevier Saunders

Browne, T. R., & Holmes, G. L. (2001). Epilepsy. *New England Journal of Medicine, 344*(15), 1145–1151.

Chong, D. J., & Lerman, A. M. (2016). Practice update: Review of anti-convulsant therapy. *Current Neurology and Neuroscience Reports, 16*(4), 39. doi:10.1007/s11910-016-0640-y

Davidson, L., & Derry, C. (2015). Seizure classification: Key to epilepsy management. *Practitioner, 259*(1785), 13–19.

Fraser, R. T., & Miller, J. W. (2005). Epilepsy. In H. H. Zaretsky, E. F. Richter III, & M. Eisenberg (Eds.), *Medical aspects of disability* (pp. 268–288). New York, NY: Springer.

Jennum, P., Ibsen, R., Petersen, E. R., Knudsen, S., & Kjelberg, J. (2012). Health, social, and economic consequences of narcolepsy: A controlled national study evaluating the societal effect on patients and their partners. *Sleep Medicine, 13*(8), 1086–1093.

Krumholz, A., Hopp, J. L., & Sanchez, A. M. (2016). Counseling epilepsy patients on driving and employment. *Neurologic Clinics, 34*(2), 427–442.

Luef, G., & Madersbacher, H. (2015). Sexual dysfunction in patients with epilepsy. *Handbook of Clinical Neurology, 130,* 383–394.

Pavelec, V., Rotenberg, B. W., Mauer, J. T., Gillis, E., & Verse, T. (2016). A novel implantable device for the treatment of obstructive sleep apnea: Clinical safety and feasibility. *Nature and Science of Sleep, 8,* 137–144.

Romero, J. R. (2016). Enterovirusus. In L. Goldman & A. I. Schafer (Eds.), *Goldman-Cecil medicine,* (pp. 2239–2244).

St. Louis, E. K., & Granner, M. A. (2007). Seizures and epilepsy in adolescents and adults. In R. E. Rakel & E. T. Bope (Eds.), *Conn's current therapy,* (pp. 1046–1055). Philadelphia, PA: W. B. Saunders.

Vaughn, B. V. (2016). Disorders of sleep. In L. Goldman & A. I. Schafer (Eds.), *Goldman-Cecil medicine,* (25th ed., pp. 2415–2424). New York, NY: Elsevier Saunders

Wiebe, S. (2016). The epilepsies. In L. Goldman & A. I. Schafer, (Eds.), *Goldman-Cecil medicine.* (25th ed., pp. 2399–2409). Philadelphia, PA: Elsevier Saunders

Wo, M. C., Lim, K. S., Choo, W. Y., & Tan, C. T. (2015). Employability in people with epilepsy: A systematic review. *Epilepsy Research, 116,* 67–68.

CHAPTER 7

Traumatic Spinal Cord Injury

OVERVIEW OF TRAUMATIC SPINAL CORD INJURY

The spinal cord transmits electrical messages to and from the brain that facilitate motor, sensory, and autonomic function. When injury or other conditions interfere with impulse transmission, depending on the location of interference, the motor, sensory, or autonomic functions may be affected.

Although other conditions such as spinal cord tumors, congenital conditions, such as spina bifida, or conditions such as herniated disc can cause a combination of sensory, motor, or autonomic deficits, the most common cause of altered spinal cord function is traumatic spinal cord injury. Common causes of traumatic spinal cord injury are motor vehicle accidents, sports injuries, falls, work-related injuries, or violence such as gunshot wounds (Ling, 2016).

Following traumatic spinal cord injury, transmission of impulses between the brain and other parts of the body below the level of injury is disrupted. Consequently, there is usually irreversible loss of sensory function and voluntary motor control below the level of injury (Guertin, 2016). Individuals may experience numbness, complete paralysis, or exaggerated, absent, or diminished reflexes below the level of the injury. The extent of the functional consequence or loss depends on which part of the spinal cord is injured and whether the cord is bruised, compressed, or severed. For instance, in some cases, swelling, bleeding, or a tumor may compress the cord without severing it. In these instances, removal of the source of compression may restore function if the spinal cord has not been permanently damaged. When the spinal cord is severed, however, transmission of nerve impulses may be permanently lost or disrupted.

TYPES OF SPINAL CORD INJURY

When the spinal cord is completely severed, below the level of injury there is no coordinated neural communication with the brain. Consequently, the individual experiences no voluntary motor or sensory function below the level of injury. When the spinal cord is *not* completely severed, the individual can have some motor or sensory function below the level of the injury. In some instances, one portion of the spinal cord may be nonfunctional, while another portion maintains some function or in some instances some certain nerve tracts may still be functioning, but in an abnormal way.

MANIFESTATIONS RELATED TO LEVEL AND SEVERITY OF INJURY

Manifestations experienced as a result of traumatic spinal cord injury relate not only to whether or not the spinal cord is completely severed but also to the level at which the injury occurred. If spinal nerves are unable to transmit messages between the central nervous system and the peripheral nervous system, function below the level of injury will be disrupted (see **Figure 7-1**).

The degree of functional loss depends on the degree to which the spinal cord is injured and the location of injury. In the case in which the spinal cord is only partially severed the

Figure 7-1   Spinal Nerves

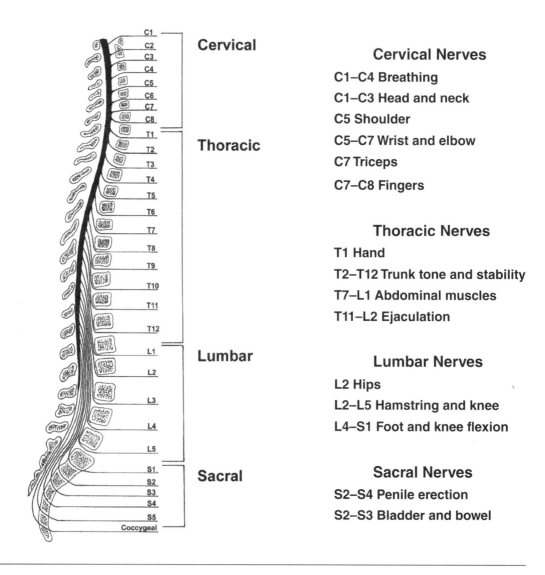

Cervical

Thoracic

Lumbar

Sacral

Cervical Nerves

C1–C4 Breathing

C1–C3 Head and neck

C5 Shoulder

C5–C7 Wrist and elbow

C7 Triceps

C7–C8 Fingers

Thoracic Nerves

T1 Hand

T2–T12 Trunk tone and stability

T7–L1 Abdominal muscles

T11–L2 Ejaculation

Lumbar Nerves

L2 Hips

L2–L5 Hamstring and knee

L4–S1 Foot and knee flexion

Sacral Nerves

S2–S4 Penile erection

S2–S3 Bladder and bowel

© Jane Tinkler Lamm.

individual may experience **paraparesis** meaning that some function exists below the level of injury. For example, if *afferent* nerve roots (*sensory tracts*), which carry messages *to* the brain were injured, some degree of sensory loss *below* the level of injury may exist, or if *efferent* nerve roots (*motor tracts*), which carry messages *from* the brain were injured, some motor loss *below*

the level of injury may be experienced. When both sensory and motor tracts are injured, both motor and sensory loss below the level of injury can be affected

In general, the higher the level of the spinal cord injury, the greater the functional implications. When the individual's injury affects only the lower extremities, they experience **paraplegia** (paralysis of lower extremities). If all four extremities are affected they experience **tetraplegia** (paralysis of all four extremities).

GENERAL PHYSICAL IMPLICATIONS OF TRAUMATIC SPINAL CORD INJURY

A wide range of functional abilities can be affected in spinal cord injury. The degree to which sensory, motor, or reflex function are affected depends on the level and extent of injury (Nas, Yazmalar, Sah, Aydin, & Önes, 2015).

Pulmonary Function

The higher the level of spinal cord injury, the more the pulmonary system is affected due to involvement of muscles used for breathing. When the diaphragm is weakened or paralyzed, as with injuries to the cervical area, assistance with breathing through mechanical ventilation may be necessary.

Even when ventilator support is not required, owing to weakened chest muscles or weakness or paralysis of pulmonary muscles, individuals may be unable to cough effectively to clear their lungs of mucus. This problem can, in turn, predispose to pulmonary infections or pneumonia

Ambulation

Ambulation is affected to some degree regardless of the level of injury, with the exception of injury at the sacral level (S2–S4), in which ambulation may return to near the preinjury state. Individuals with spinal cord injuries above T12 usually require a wheelchair for ambulation. At lower levels of injury (i.e., L1 or lower), ambulation for short distances may be possible with braces or crutches.

Bladder and Bowel Control

Most individuals lose at least some voluntary control of bladder and bowel function after spinal cord injury (Hagan, 2015). Depending on level of injury and degree of functional ability as well as bladder function, a number of urinary collection devices for bladder management may be used (Sorokin & De, 2015). In some instances bladder incontinence pads may be used for urine leakage. In other cases, individuals may be able to perform, intermittent

self-catheterization several times a day in order to empty the bladder. In lower-level injuries, such as at the lumbar level, bladder evacuation may be accomplished by applying external pressure to the lower abdomen.

In spinal cord injuries at the thoracic or cervical level, most individuals experience *neurogenic bladder* (a condition in which bladder muscles are paralyzed and the individual is unable to empty the bladder voluntarily). In these instances, a number of bladder evacuation devices may be used. One type of device, used for males is the condom catheter, or Texas catheter, which is an external collection device consisting of a sheath worn over the penis. The condom catheter has an opening at the end that is connected to a tube attached to a leg bag, worn by the individual. Another device, the indwelling catheter, may be used for drainage of urine. When an indwelling catheter is used, the catheter is inserted into the bladder through the urinary meatus. The catheter is usually attached to a tube, which is then also attached to a leg bag for by the individual, or the catheter may be clamped and then released to empty the bladder periodically. In other instances, individuals may have a suprapubic catheter, in which an indwelling catheter is inserted through a surgical opening on the lower abdomen above the bladder. The suprapubic catheter is also attached to a leg bag. Leg bags for each of these devices is then emptied periodically during the day.

Neurogenic bowel is the term used to describe paralysis of the lower rectal and anal muscles causing inability to control bowel evacuation. Loss of voluntary bowel function is frequently one of the most distressing factors for individuals with spinal cord injury, altering their body image (Coggrave, Burrows, & Durand, 2006). Consequently, an effective bowel management program is important to individuals' overall rehabilitation. Bowel management programs help the individual learn how to empty the lower bowel and to establish a consistent routine so that involuntary bowel evacuation can be avoided (Johnson, Mowrey, & Bergman, 2008). Bowel management may be accomplished through use of suppositories, small-volume enema, digital stimulation or manual evacuation of stool, and by dietary means consisting of consuming foods with high fiber content, avoidance of gas-producing foods, and adequate hydration.

Sexual Function and Fertility

Nerves to the genital region are almost always affected to some degree by spinal cord injury (Hou & Rabchovsky, 2014). This does not mean, however, that other aspects of sexuality—such as sexual attraction to others, sexual desire, and the need to express oneself as a sexual being—are changed. Many men and women remain sexually active after spinal cord injury, although modifications of sexual behavior and function typically need to be made.

Genital function is controlled by the *parasympathetic* and *sympathetic* nervous systems as well as by motor nerves. The amount of function retained after spinal cord injury depends on the level of injury as well as on whether the injury is *complete* or *incomplete*. The higher the level of injury, the more significantly genital function will be affected

Most individuals with a spinal cord injury—both males and females—will have little sensation directly in the genital area (Hou & Rabchovsky, 2014). Because mobility is affected in spinal cord injury, many individuals will also need to use an alternative technique for sexual performance.

Males, regardless of the level of spinal cord injury, may continue to have reflex erections. Also, in many instances, erection can be produced through manual stimulation. The ability to produce an erection through psychological arousal is absent in many men with spinal cord injuries, although individuals with lower spinal cord injuries may demonstrate a weakened sexual response due to psychological stimuli. Some individuals have used techniques such as penile implants to achieve intercourse.

Ejaculation is absent for many men with spinal cord injury; if it does occur, individuals may experience *retrograde ejaculation*, such that semen is deposited into the bladder rather than externally (Ducharme, 2006). As a result, fertility in males is significantly affected, especially in males with complete severance of the spinal cord. Techniques such as *electro-ejaculation*, in which ejaculation is stimulated through electrical means, have been used to obtain sperm for artificial insemination.

Females with spinal cord injuries are still able to engage in sexual intercourse, although the lubrication produced by psychological arousal is usually absent (Forsythe & Horsewell, 2006). Genital sensation may be diminished or absent; however, in some instances, women have reported orgasm after injury (Anderson, Borisoff, Johnson, Stiens, & Elliot, 2007). Menses typically are absent during the first months after injury, with the return of menstruation occurring within 6 months after injury. In most instances, female fertility is unaltered by spinal cord injury (Ahn & Berliner, 2011). Consequently, women who do not wish to become pregnant need to use some form of contraception. When women with spinal cord injuries become pregnant, they are able to carry the pregnancy to term, although because of altered sensation, it may be more difficult for them to determine when labor begins.

PHYSICAL IMPLICATIONS OF SPECIFIC AREAS OF TRAUMATIC SPINAL CORD INJURY

Cervical Level (C1–C8)

An injury to the spinal cord at the cervical level (C1 through C8) results in **quadriplegia** (paralysis of both upper and lower extremities) (see **Figure 7-1**). Injuries at C1 or C2 can be fatal because the functioning of all muscles, including the muscles of respiration, is lost. Due to weakness or paralysis of muscles of respiration with injuries at the cervical level, especially those involving injury at the C1 through C4 level, respiratory assistance with a mechanical respiratory device or ventilator may be necessary. Individuals with higher-level injuries are more susceptible to respiratory infections and pneumonia due to their inability to expectorate mucus effectively owing to paralysis or weakness of respiratory muscles.

Individuals with injuries at the cervical level will likely require assistance from others for self-care. Most individuals with spinal cord injuries at C4 or above use a personal attendant for hygiene care, dressing, and transfers. Wheelchair ambulation may be possible through use of a mouth stick, which individuals can employ to manipulate an electric wheelchair.

With an injury at the C5 level, some gross movement of the upper extremities, such as bending the arm at the elbow, is possible. Individuals may be able to hold a light object between the thumb and finger, or may be able to maneuver small objects with the assistance of hand splints. Assistance will still be required for most activities, but individuals may be capable of transfer on their own with the assistance of special equipment. Although total independent living without some assistance may not be feasible, independent electric wheelchair ambulation is possible.

Individuals with injury at C6 also have gross motor movement of upper extremities and may be able to retain some independence in self-care, such as feeding and dressing with the aid of special orthotic equipment. Propelling a wheelchair manually may be possible, with a modified hand rim, although many individuals continue to operate a motorized chair. With the use of hand splints, individuals may also be able to write. Independent transfer from bed to chair or to a car may also be possible, as is driving with the use of special assistive devices.

Individuals with C7 injuries are capable of straightening their arm and are able to sit up in bed, dress themselves, and transfer. With some adaptations in the environment, almost total independence may be achieved. Fine motor movements of the hands are affected, but writing may be possible with the use of a special device that can be strapped to the hand. Likewise, driving is possible with hand controls.

With C8 injuries, individuals have some sensation in their hands and may become totally independent with a modified environment and some assistive devices.

Thoracic Level (T1–T12)

Spinal cord injuries occurring at T1 or lower result in **paraplegia** (paralysis of the lower extremities). Upper extremities for the most part are unimpaired, with the exception of T1 injuries, in which there may be slight weakness and some loss of flexibility

in the hands. Individuals with an injury between T1 and T3 experience paralysis of the muscles of the trunk even though the upper extremities are functional. Consequently, they may need a brace or other support to maintain posture in an upright position. In most cases, individuals with injuries at T1 through T12 are able to attain total independence in self-care, wheelchair ambulation, and transfer. Although individuals with injuries at T7 to T12 may be able to walk with the use of long leg braces, because of the strenuous nature of the activity, ambulation may be possible for only short distances.

Lumbar Level (L1–L5)

Many of the muscles of mobility are intact with L1 through L5 injuries. All upper body muscles and many of the leg muscles remain functional. Ambulation with braces or use of a cane or crutches may be possible, especially for short distances. Individuals are able to gain total independence in care, although hand controls may be necessary for operating a motor vehicle. Bowel and bladder function are still affected, however, reflex emptying of bowel and bladder may be possible.

Sacral Level (S1–S4)

Ambulation is usually possible with little or no equipment. Bowel and bladder function may still be affected to some degree. In most instances, individuals are able to recover most preinjury function.

INITIAL MANAGEMENT OF TRAUMATIC SPINAL CORD INJURY

The initial management of traumatic spinal cord injuries focuses on preventing further injury, stabilizing individuals' physical condition, and, in some instances, performing surgery to realign the spinal column or achieve decompression of the spinal cord (Ling, 2016). Many individuals with spinal cord injuries—especially those who received the injury as the result of an accident—may have other injuries such as fractures, injuries to internal organs, or traumatic brain injury, further complicating their care and rehabilitation.

Figure 7-2   Halo Brace

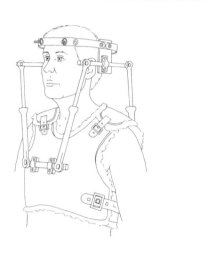

© Jane Tinkler Lamm.

For cervical spine injuries, despite the possibility of surgical intervention, *skeletal skull traction* (placement of a pin or wire into the bony skull structure, which is then attached to traction) is still at times used for immobilization and/or realignment, with the eventual use of *cervical orthosis* such as the *halo vest* for continued stabilization (see **Figure 7-2**) (Kari, Karmali, & Fatoye, 2016). With the halo vest, metal pins are inserted into the skull and attached to a metal "halo" that surrounds the head. The halo is attached with two metal rods to a vest worn on the torso of the individual. The advantage of the halo vest is that it enables individuals to be mobile earlier while still providing stabilization of the cervical spine (Kazi, de Matas, & Pillay, 2013).

POSTACUTE MANAGEMENT AND REHABILITATION AFTER TRAUMATIC SPINAL CORD INJURY

After their physical condition has been stabilized and any acute medical needs are met, individuals are usually transferred to a rehabilitation unit, where they learn skills or how to use assistive devices that will help them to achieve the maximum level of independence. A wide variety of health professionals, such as physiatrists, physical therapists,

rehabilitation nurses, occupational therapists, orthotists, psychologists, social workers, and rehabilitation counselors, are usually involved in this phase of rehabilitation.

Physical therapy begins as soon as possible to prevent complications such as **contractures** (permanent contraction of a muscle such that a joint becomes fixed or immobile), as well as to build strength.

As an individual's condition stabilizes, management is directed toward teaching self-care including dressing, hygiene, grooming, and bladder and bowel care. Most individuals with traumatic spinal cord injury become mobile with the use of a wheelchair. Many types of wheelchairs with a variety of options, including detachable armrests and footrests, removable back panel, lapboard, and carryall bag, are available. Power-operated wheelchairs are available for individuals who have little or no use of their upper extremities. These battery-operated chairs can be controlled with a switch adapted to the particular individual's ability. Power-operated chairs are, however, more difficult to transport due to their size and weight.

POTENTIAL COMPLICATIONS ASSOCIATED WITH TRAUMATIC SPINAL CORD INJURY

In addition to altered functional capacity, individuals with traumatic spinal cord injury are confronted with a number of short-term and long-term issues that require ongoing constant attention (Guertin, 2016). Individuals with traumatic spinal cord injury are at risk of developing additional health problems that could result in a secondary condition and, consequently, more functional implications (Hagan, 2015). Development of complications can hamper individuals' ability to work as well as interfere with their social relationships. Some complications associated with spinal cord injury can also be fatal.

The risk of developing complications is related to the level of injury. In general, the higher the level of injury, the greater the risk of developing secondary incapacitating conditions (Nas et al., 2015). It is, therefore, imperative that individuals with spinal cord injuries, family members, and professionals working with them be aware of this risk and the prevention strategies to lessen the risk. When complications do arise, it is crucial that they be treated immediately.

Pressure Sores (Decubitus Ulcers)

One of the most common complications associated with spinal cord injury is pressure sores, also called **decubitus ulcers** (Joseph & Nilsson-Wikmar, 2015). Pressure sores develop when continuous pressure is exerted to a body part over time (van Weert et al., 2014). These wounds are formed when soft tissue is pressed between bony areas of the body and an external surface. People with spinal cord injuries are at increased risk of developing pressure sores, which result from lack of blood supply (**ischemia**) to a body pressure point. Areas of the body that are particularly vulnerable include the buttocks, sacrum, heel, and back. Pressure on a body part interferes with blood supply, eventually resulting in breakdown and ulceration of the skin. Because individuals with spinal cord injury are often immobile, areas of pressure on certain bony prominences are more likely to develop. As individuals with spinal cord injury usually have no sensation below the level of injury, they are unable to feel pressure; moreover, because of the paralysis, they are unable to easily shift their weight to relieve the pressure. Inadequate skin care, irritation, and nutritional deficiency can further contribute to the development of pressure sores.

Pressure sores are incapacitating, increase medical costs, and contribute to delayed rehabilitation (Cho, Beom, Yuk, & Ahn, 2015). These sores may appear to be small on the surface, but the depth of the ulcer may be more extensive. Pressure sores that are not adequately managed can progress from redness to breakdown of the skin, infection, and eventually skin tissue death (**necrosis**), which could extend through the tissue all the way to the bone. Deep pressure sores may require hospitalization or surgical intervention for their management.

Individuals with spinal cord injury must be aware of the risk of pressure sores and the importance of skin self-monitoring. Education about the importance of decreasing the amount of pressure on bony prominences by regularly changing position, good nutrition, and good skin care is an important part of the rehabilitation process. A number of types of wheelchair cushions are available to help distribute pressure to prevent skin breakdown and extend endurance in a wheelchair. In addition to using the correct cushion, individuals with spinal cord injury should learn how to position the cushion properly.

Spasticity

Spasticity refers to exaggerated involuntary movement of muscles that results in exaggerated muscle jerks, hyperexcitability of reflexes, and muscle spasms. It can restrict activities of daily living, cause pain and fatigue, disturb sleep, contribute to the development of contractures, and affect individuals' self-image (Hagan, 2015). Not everyone with traumatic spinal cord injury develops spasticity. Some persons who do not experience spasticity immediately after injury may nevertheless experience it long after leaving the rehabilitation facility.

Because communication between the *peripheral nervous system* and the brain is interrupted by spinal cord injury, signals received by the *peripheral nerves* are "short-circuited." Rather than traveling to the brain to be interpreted and appropriately adapted, the signal instead returns from the spinal cord directly to the muscle. The resulting muscle contractures can sometimes be violent and can occur with even slight stimulation. Spasticity can be incapacitating, not only because it is disruptive and can potentially cause embarrassment to the individual but also because in some instances it can be so strong that it causes individuals to fall from their wheelchairs. In addition, spasticity can contribute to formation of contractures. Although in some instances spasticity can be useful to help individuals perform certain functions, such as shifting position or standing, more often it is a source of discomfort.

There is no unique way to successfully manage spasticity in all individuals. Instead, how spasticity is managed is based on individual goals. For example, management may be focused mainly on preventing complications such as contractures. In other instances, management may be directed toward increasing individuals' ability to perform various motor tasks.

When spasticity is a cause of concern for an individual, a physical rehabilitation program using a variety of modalities may help diminish its frequency. In other instances, antispasticity medications may be used to reduce spasticity. Botulinum toxin—a neurotoxin—may also be injected into a muscle to temporarily inhibit spasms, increasing range of motion and function as well as helping to reduce pain (Shalkh, Phadke, Ismall, & Boullas, 2016). In other instances, medications that block nerves may be injected so that nerve conduction is disrupted, thereby relaxing muscles (Ling, 2016).

Contractures

Contractures (loss of range of motion, or fixed deformity of a joint) may occur in paralyzed limbs if the joints are not moved through their regular range of motion. Contractures of the upper extremities in individuals with quadriplegia can interfere with the use of assistive devices. If individuals with paraplegia or quadriplegia develop contractures of the hip or knee, it may be difficult to assume adequate positioning in a wheelchair. Regular movement of joints through the full range of motions via passive exercise conducted by another person or through use of special equipment can prevent contractures from occurring. In addition, proper wheelchair seating and correct positioning of joints can help reduce the risk of contractures.

Osteoporosis

Bone is a dynamic substance that is characterized by continual deposition and reabsorption of calcium. The combined stress of weight bearing and muscle pull that occurs with activity helps bones maintain their calcium content. Conversely, inactivity can contribute to softening and weakening of bones (**osteoporosis**). Bone mineral density is lost in paralyzed limbs after spinal cord injury due to mechanical, hormonal, and neural factors (Dudley-Javoroski et al., 2016). Individuals with spinal cord injuries have an increased rate of calcium removal from the bone and, therefore, are more susceptible to fractures, which could be caused by either falls or simple activities such as wheelchair transfer (Frotzier, Cheikh-Sarraf, Pourrtehrani, Krebs, & Lippuner, 2015). Calcium, which is excreted through the urinary system, can also contribute to formation of urinary tract stones. In some instances, calcium is deposited in soft tissues so that the function of a joint or muscle is disrupted.

Adequate diet, passive and strength-building exercises, and electrical stimulation to the muscles are all techniques that can be used to help reduce the risk of developing osteoporosis. In addition, proper training in safety procedures when operating a wheelchair and transferring can help prevent occurrence of falls and potentially broken bones if osteoporosis is present.

Chronic Pain

Chronic pain is a significant issue for individuals with traumatic spinal cord injury (Cardenas et al., 2013). The frequency and severity of pain in those who experience it varies widely. Although the degree to which chronic pain interferes with daily functions inside and outside the home differs from individual to individual, in general pain can contribute to increased distress and decreased social integration.

Pain in spinal cord injury can be incapacitating and persistent and can occur both above and below the level of injury. The most common type of chronic pain experienced in individuals with traumatic spinal cord injury is *neuropathic pain*, which is the result of atypical processing of sensory messages due to the spinal cord injury (Ling, 2016). Individuals may also experience musculoskeletal pain due to poor posture or overuse of musculoskeletal structures during activities such as transfer.

A variety of interventions are utilized for management of chronic pain after traumatic spinal cord injury, including medication and alternative interventions such as massage and acupuncture. Pain relief is often achieved only over short periods of time; in many individuals, pain proves to be refractory to management.

Because pain is an individual phenomenon, in most instances management of pain in individuals with traumatic spinal cord injury is also individualized. It may encompass, in addition to medication, a holist approach that includes exercise, stress reduction, counseling, or alternative interventions such as acupuncture.

Cardiovascular Complications

Cardiovascular complications after spinal cord injury are of major importance since they account for the highest cause of death in this group (Phillips & Krassioukov, 2015). In the acute stage after a spinal cord injury, individuals are susceptible to **thrombophlebitis** (formation of blood clots in the legs) or **pulmonary embolism** (a blood clot that travels to the lungs), a potentially life-threatening disorder (Partida, Mironets, Hou, & Tom, 2016).

Individuals may also experience **orthostatic hypotension**, a condition in which the blood pressure becomes significantly lower when the individual moves from a flat position to an upright position, resulting in manifestations such as dizziness or fainting (**syncope**) (Nas et al., 2015). In some individuals, orthostatic hypotension may persist after the initial rehabilitation period. Orthostatic hypotension or *postural hypotension* can affect activities of daily living and interfere with ability to participate in a variety of other activities (Partida et al., 2016). Management of orthostatic hypotension is directed toward individuals recognizing factors that may precipitate an episode—for example, heat stress or alcohol ingestion. Some individuals may use compression bandages or support stockings on the lower extremities to prevent pooling of blood in the extremities. In other instances, medications may be utilized to ward off this complication.

Individuals with spinal cord injury also have a more sedentary lifestyle, which can affect the cardiovascular system as a whole. Because of increased susceptibility to cardiovascular conditions, individuals with spinal cord injuries should refrain from smoking or use of tobacco products as well as excessive alcohol consumption. Good nutrition, an exercise program, and weight control are other important measures for prevention of cardiovascular disease. Individuals with spinal

cord injuries, because of their increased risk of developing cardiovascular conditions, should undergo regular healthcare examinations and seek out comprehensive healthcare programs that are familiar with and accommodate the needs of individuals with spinal cord injury.

Autonomic Dysreflexia

Autonomic dysreflexia is a complication of spinal cord injury usually above T6. It is caused by loss of coordinated response by the autonomic nervous system, causing an exaggerated response to stimuli below the level of the injury, such as an overextended bladder, pressure sores, or constipation (Fausel & Paski, 2014). This atypical reflex condition is characterized by a sudden rise in blood pressure, profuse sweating (**diaphoresis**), and headache as the result of excessive neural discharge from the autonomic nervous system. Unless immediate management is instituted to decrease the blood pressure, this condition carries a risk of stroke. Identifying and avoiding situations or conditions that trigger autonomic dysreflexia are important in the prevention of this condition.

Difficulty with Thermoregulation and Sweating

Body temperature is under the direct control of the autonomic nervous system. Normally when cold or warm is perceived by peripheral receptors a message is sent to the hypothalamus in the brain. The message is interpreted and an appropriate response stimulated (i.e., shivering in order to maintain heat, or perspiring in order to cool the body). With spinal cord injury, this connection is lost due to autonomic nervous system dysfunction, and individuals are unable to regulate body temperature effectively (Trborich, Ortega, Schroeder, & Fredrickson, 2014). Consequently individuals with spinal cord injury may experience abnormal regulation of body temperature or may be less able to respond to changes in environmental temperatures.

The inability to effective respond to changes in temperature put individuals at risk of developing

hyperthermia (abnormally high body temperature) or **hypothermia** (abnormally low body temperature).

This may place individuals at risk in situations in which there are extreme environmental temperatures, or during some activities, such as exercise.

Although normally sweating can help individuals regulate body temperature, individuals with spinal cord injury, due to autonomic nervous system dysfunction may experience **hyperhidrosis** (excessive sweating) above or below the level of injury (Iwase, Inukai, Nisimura, Sato, & Sugenoya, 2014). The condition can be a source of embarrassment as well as discomfort for the individual.

Pneumonia and Other Pulmonary Problems

Pneumonia and other pulmonary complications are common in individuals with spinal cord injuries, especially those with quadriplegia (Johnson et al., 2008). Although these complications become less likely 1 month after the injury, individuals with spinal cord injuries continue to be more prone to developing pulmonary conditions, such as pneumonia, which can be both incapacitating and life threatening. Individuals with high cervical or high thoracic injuries, because of their weakened chest muscles, have more difficulty in expanding the lungs and clearing secretions. Consequently, they are more susceptible to infection of the lungs. Individuals with higher-level injuries may also have difficulty deep-breathing and removing secretions, contributing to their increased risk of pulmonary complications. Individuals with spinal cord injuries should avoid exposure to persons with pulmonary infections as much as possible, as well as avoid smoking and air pollution.

Urinary Tract and Bowel Complications

Urinary tract infections are the most frequent complication of spinal cord injury (Sekulić et al., 2015). Individuals with spinal cord injuries are especially prone to urinary tract infections because of the inadequate emptying of their bladder. The bladder may not empty often enough or may not empty completely, leaving urine in the bladder

that then acts as a reservoir for infection. Because individuals with spinal cord injury are generally unable to control their bladder, they may need to have a catheter inserted into the bladder to drain urine and prevent incontinence. The bladder and its contents usually contain no pathologic organisms, but there is always the potential for the introduction of infectious organisms when a catheter is inserted into the bladder. For individuals with spinal cord injury, urinary tract infection can be a serious, incapacitating, and, at times, life-threatening problem. Untreated urinary tract infection can lead to **pyelonephritis** (infection of the kidney) and, in severe cases, **septicemia** (infection in the blood).

Due to inactivity because of paralysis, the amount of calcium in the blood increases. As a result, the risk of developing kidney stones (**renal calculi**) is increased. A stone may form in the kidney itself or may lodge in the **ureters** (tubes leading from the kidney to the bladder) so that it obstructs urine flow, causing urine to back up into the kidneys (**urinary reflux**) and eventually damaging the kidney itself.

Education of individuals with spinal cord injuries about the urinary tract, risk of its infection, and ways to decrease the risk of infection or stone formation is crucial in preventing secondary urinary tract complications. In addition, individuals with spinal cord injuries should be made aware of the importance of self-monitoring and promptly reporting manifestations so that immediate identification of infections or other conditions and appropriate management may be instituted.

Secondary conditions related to bowel elimination may also be problematic. Incontinence of fecal material may not only contribute to skin breakdown and urinary tract infection but also result in social isolation if individuals become concerned about the possibility that incontinence might occur. Other problems may relate to **impaction** (fecal matter that becomes hardened and is unable to be evacuated) and **paralytic ileus** (a condition in which the intestine ceases to function). Individuals can decrease their risk for developing these conditions by establishing a pattern of regular elimination, monitoring their diet and fluid intake, and learning specific techniques to enhance optimal bowel function.

Altered Manifestations of Other Health Conditions

Because of the lack of sensation that accompanies most spinal cord injuries as well as the interruption to nerve pathways, manifestations of various conditions unrelated to the spinal cord injury itself may not be recognized and, as a result, may not receive prompt attention and management. For example, because pain is not felt, appendicitis may not be discovered until the appendix ruptures.

In some instances, manifestations of a condition may be expressed differently in individuals with traumatic spinal cord injury than in individuals without spinal cord injury. For example, individuals without spinal cord injury may experience severe flank pain in response to a kidney infection, whereas individuals with spinal cord injury may experience an abrupt increase in spasticity with the same infection. As a result, the manifestation may not be recognized as being related to kidney infection and, consequently, the kidney infection may not be immediately identified and managed. Individuals with traumatic spinal cord injuries, caregivers, and professionals should be made aware of alterations in the presentation of manifestations of infectious or other conditions and should be alerted to report or investigate new manifestations or accentuated old manifestations as soon as they are noted.

FUNCTIONAL IMPLICATIONS OF TRAUMATIC SPINAL CORD INJURY

Personal and Psychosocial Issues

Traumatic spinal cord injury can bring about drastic life changes in terms of both physical and psychosocial functioning. Manifestations of spinal cord injury may necessitate change in employment, bring about changes in social patterns and relationships, and alter general activities of daily living. In addition to experiencing changes in movement and sensation, individuals with traumatic spinal cord injury experience decreased mobility and independence, changes in bowel and bladder functioning, and changes in sexual functioning. These changes can contribute to altered self-concept or loss of self-esteem. How individuals adjust to changes associated with traumatic spinal cord injury will, to some degree, be related to how they conceptualize the losses experienced, their individual coping style, and the amount and type of social support available (Pollard & Kennedy, 2007).

Adaptation to incapacitation varies from individual to individual (Lucas, 2007). Life satisfaction does not appear to be related to the severity of the injury but rather to how individuals perceive alteration in function related to life goals and meaning or purpose in their life (deRoon-Cassini, de St. Aubin, Valvano, Hastings, & Horn, 2009; Park, Edmondson, Fenster, & Blank, 2008). Perception of the degree of loss of physical function, and its relationship to family and social relationships, work, or other life goals, may be more important in predicting any individual's subjective well-being than the manifestations of the injury itself.

Although depression is common after spinal cord injury, this condition is not universal and is not necessary for adjustment to occur. Some individuals are more likely to exhibit depressive manifestations after traumatic spinal cord injury than others. Individuals who had difficulty coping with stress or who had a history of substance abuse or relationship problems prior to the injury may demonstrate difficulty adjusting after injury, consequently psychological manifestations after injury may have greater impact on overall rehabilitation than the physical consequences of the injury (O'Donnel et al., 2013).

After spinal cord injury, changes in function that affect perceived roles in work, social, or family environment can alter personal identity and can trigger loss and stress reactions. Posttraumatic stress disorder (PTSD) has also been linked to traumatic spinal cord injury in some (Otis, Marchand, & Coutois, 2012).

Not all individuals with spinal cord injury experience incapacitating psychological manifestations. In general, individuals who demonstrate greater internal locus of control and a sense that the world is manageable and meaningful also exhibit less psychosocial distress and better adaptation (Schöenberg et al., 2014)

Activities and Participation

Environmental Modifications

Given the physical ramifications of traumatic spinal cord injury and the environmental constraints imposed by such injury, individuals must make modifications not only in their daily routines but also in their personal, social, and occupational spheres. For example, extra time may be needed for daily activities related to personal hygiene. Individuals may need to conform their daily routines to a structured bowel and bladder program. Transportation or moving from one place to another may require extra time and planning. Awareness of environmental constraints, environmental modifications that are needed, and assistive devices that can support functional capacity enables individuals to establish and adjust daily routines and enhance their ability to participate in social and occupational activities. For individuals using wheelchairs, the environment should be conducive to wheelchair use. There needs to be accessible entrance into buildings and interior doors wide enough for wheelchair passage. If the entrance to a building is not level with the ground, a ramp can provide access. For multilevel buildings, elevators are needed in lieu of stairs. Thick carpeting can also impede smooth wheelchair passage.

Furniture of standard height may be uncomfortable or awkward, especially for transfer. Modification of furniture legs to shorten them may be necessary. Counter or desk heights may also need to be modified for the wheelchair to fit under the structure. Bathroom facilities may need to be altered—for example, by lowering the toilet seat or providing hand bars—or devices such as a toilet transfer board may be needed.

Individuals with spinal cord injuries must adopt new behaviors and mobility techniques to function in the environment, but they must also continually adapt to their changing environment. Although spinal cord injury causes radical changes in mobility and independence, most individuals are able to return to their community, and many can return to their own homes with environmental modifications. The degree of successful reentry into the community depends to a great degree on the individual's social support, access to adequate housing and transportation, and availability of quality attendant care if needed.

Operating a Motor Vehicle

Motor vehicles, in addition to being a mode of transportation, serve as a symbol of independence. A wide range of vehicle options and special assistive devices are available for use after spinal cord injury. Hand-operated controls and other modifications enable individuals with paraplegia as well as individuals with quadriplegia who have gross motor movement of the upper extremities to operate motor vehicles and transport wheelchairs. The vehicle should meet the needs of the specific individual (Norweg, Jette, Houlihan, Ni, & Boninger, 2011).

Social and Family Participation

Traumatic spinal cord injury affects the individual who has been injured as well as the network of others around him or her. Societal reactions may vary depending on the degree of experience persons have had with individuals with spinal cord injury. People in the social environment may be uneducated about how to interact with someone in a wheelchair. There may be instances of insensitivity, such as standing in front of the individual in a wheelchair at an art museum, thereby blocking the person's view, or asking insensitive questions. In other instances, individuals in the social environment may attempt to assist without being asked, and without help being needed, such as by grabbing the handles of the wheelchair and pushing the individual in a direction he or she may not wish to go. In still other instances, people in the social environment may avoid the individual with spinal cord injury altogether because they are unsure how they should behave. Although public education programs can be useful, the most beneficial solution may be for the individual with spinal cord injury to be prepared for societal reactions he or she may encounter and to learn to be assertive and how to respond.

Although many families adjust to changes associated with spinal cord injury of the family member, some relationships and roles may need to be reexamined, negotiated, and redefined. In some instances, family members may experience shock, denial, anger, or depression after the injury. Depending on the circumstances surrounding the injury, they may blame the individual or others for the injury, which may in turn contribute to hostility, pessimism, anxiety, and higher levels of social distress. In other instances, families may feel overwhelmed because of financial strains, caregiving responsibilities, or role changes. Family relationships may be further strained if there is stress related to financial strains or if responsibilities related to providing assistance to the individual with spinal cord injury are perceived as overwhelming.

Family members may need education about spinal cord injury as well as encouragement and support so they can cope and, in turn, offer support to the individual. Role obligations may need to be shifted, negotiated, and shared.

A variety of professionals can assist family members in addressing pertinent issues and managing stress. Education and feedback can facilitate communication between the individual and family members, thereby providing a structure for understanding and problem solving.

Recreational Activities

The focus of many rehabilitation programs specializing in spinal cord injury is on helping individuals attain optimal function related to self-care or employment. Typically, only minimal attention is given to recreational activities, which could enable individuals to become active in a larger social sphere. Lack of structured peer recreation activities and peer support can lead to social isolation and impede individuals' feeling of living effectively with their condition.

After spinal cord injury, the level of participation in social and recreational activities will depend on the attitude and interests of the individual, the number of recreational opportunities and resources available, access to appropriate assistive devices, and adequate sources for equipment repair. Assistive devices that enable individuals with spinal cord injuries to participate in many sports and other recreational activities are available, although other considerations—such as adequate transportation, quality attendant care if needed, and other environmental restrictions—must also be considered.

The trend toward increased access to public buildings, businesses, and services is enabling individuals with spinal cord injuries to participate more fully in a broader range of community activities as well as to explore and pursue a number of social roles. Unfortunately, many architectural and attitudinal barriers still exist. Consequently, to live most effectively with their condition, individuals with spinal cord injuries must learn self-efficacy and take on the role of self-advocate (Craig, Nicholson, Guest, Tran, & Middleton, 2015).

Sexuality

Attitudes and beliefs of society often reduce human sexuality to the physical components rather than recognizing that the physical aspects of sexual activity are merely one part of sexuality. Sexuality also relates to feelings of sexual attraction, emotional intimacy, and affection (Sakellariou, 2006). Although physical changes associated with spinal cord injury usually necessitate some modification in sexual behavior, individuals with spinal cord injury continue to be sexual beings. Sexual adjustment is an integral and necessary part of total psychological adjustment.

Individuals with traumatic spinal cord injury should be provided with opportunities to obtain accurate and complete information about sexual activity in conjunction with spinal cord injury, and information should be provided in the context of their personal values. Discussion of sexual needs and reassurance that sexual expression is still possible in their life are important parts of rehabilitation.

Alteration of physical mobility after spinal cord injury may alter certain aspects of sexual relations and will most probably necessitate modification of technique. Elimination of physical barriers and provision of appropriate accommodations are important aspects of enabling individuals with spinal cord injuries to engage in sexual activity. Depending on the extent of immobility associated with the injury regarding use of upper extremities, personal assistance may be required to engage in sexual activities, meaning that more than two people may be involved in the process (Sakellariou, 2006). This type of accommodation, like any other accommodation, should be handled with delicacy and sensitivity.

Bowel and bladder care may need to be performed prior to engaging in sexual activity to prevent incontinence during the activity. Concerns about experiencing bladder or bowel incontinence during sexual activity may be a deterrent to engaging in sexual activity. Learning bladder and bowel management techniques and performing them prior to sexual activity can reduce some of the stress and anxiety associated with concerns about incontinence.

Sexual attraction to others, sexual desire, and the need to express oneself as a sexual being continue after spinal cord injury. Many men and women remain sexually active after spinal cord injury. Modification of sexual techniques, assistive devices, and other accommodations provide the means by which sexual activity can be continued after spinal cord injury.

VOCATIONAL ISSUES AFTER TRAUMATIC SPINAL CORD INJURY

Employment rates for individuals with spinal cord injury vary widely (Cotner et al., 2015). Employment for an individual with spinal cord injury, just as with other health conditions, depends on the person's psychosocial characteristics as well as the physical, social, economic, and political environment (Meade, Reed, Saunders, & Krause, 2015).

A critical factor in employment after spinal cord injury is the extent to which an individual can return to work in the same occupation in the same position as prior to the injury. The level of injury and the individual's previous occupation determine, to a great extent, the amount and type of activity the person will be able to perform and the assistive device or special accommodations needed. For instance, individuals with injuries at the thoracic level will probably require a wheelchair for mobility but will have full use of the upper extremities. Consequently, an individual who is an accountant, for instance, would be able to continue in his or her profession with only some environmental modifications. In contrast, an individual with a high cervical injury with no upper extremity function who had worked as a construction worker may require change of occupation or retraining for another type of position in the field that does not require the same type of physical mobility and stamina. In all instances, the individual's interest and aptitude should be considered.

Environmental barriers such as steps, table heights, and width of doorways will need to be considered in the work environment. Given that many individuals with spinal cord injuries also have difficulty with temperature regulation, the work environment should be climate controlled. Other factors to be considered are the individual's ability to sit for long periods of time, strength, endurance, and transportation available. With a higher level of injury, in which there may be diminished breathing capacity or for which ventilator assistance is required, attention to environmental pollution and cleanliness of the air in the work environment should be considered. Other workplace modifications, such as flexible scheduling including shorter work days or longer rest periods, may also be helpful to attaining or maintaining employment.

Unless individuals have an associated brain injury, there should be no cognitive deficits associated with spinal cord injury. Preinjury education, vocational interests and skills, and congruence with level of functional capacity after injury are important considerations in vocational placement. Age and the presence of financial disincentives are other factors that may influence an individual's employment status (Cotner et al., 2015).

Spinal cord injury is a lifetime condition. As natural physiological changes occur with aging, additional interventions or equipment may be needed. Consequently, periodic checkups should be instituted to identify individuals who are experiencing difficulty in the workplace or who encounter new barriers to access so that appropriate accommodations can be instituted.

CASE STUDY

Sean, an 18-year-old high school senior, experienced a spinal cord injury (C6) during a high school football game. Sean had begun work with his father, the owner of a construction company, during the summer and had hoped to go to a technical school to learn more about construction. After graduating, he had planned to join his father in the construction business.

1. How will Sean's level of injury affect his functional capability?
2. Which types of assistive devices will Sean most likely need to achieve his greatest level of independence?

3. How will Sean's level of injury affect his future plans regarding his interest and career choice?

4. Which specific issues might be important for Sean to address when he considers his vocational plan?

REFERENCES

Ahn, J., & Berliner, J. (2011). Spinal cord injury. In S. R. Flanagan, H. Zaretsky, & A. Moroz, (Eds.), *Medical Aspects of Disability*. (4th ed., pp. 531–547). New York, NY: Springer

Anderson, K. D., Borisoff, J. F., Johnson, R. D., Stiens, S. A., & Elliott, S. L. (2007). Spinal cord injury influences psychogenic as well as physical components of female sexual ability. *Spinal Cord, 45*(5), 349–359.

Cardenas, D., & Jensen, M. P. (2006). Treatments for chronic pain in persons with spinal cord injury: A survey study. *Journal of Spinal Cord Medicine, 29*(2), 109–117.

Cardenas, D. D., Nieshoff, E. C., Suda, K., Goto, S., Sanin, L., Kaneko, T. ... Knapp, L. E. (2013). A randomized trial of pregabalin in patients with neuropathic pain due to spinal cord injury. *Neurology, 80*(6), 533–539.

Chan, S. K. K., & Man, D. W. K. (2005). Barriers to returning to work for people with spinal cord injuries: A focus group study. *Work, 25,* 325–332.

Chen, S. C., Lai, C. H., Chan, W. P., Huang, M. H., Tsai, H. W., & Chen, J. J. J. (2005). Increases in bone mineral density after functional electrical stimulation cycling exercises in spinal cord injured patients. *Disability and Rehabilitation, 27*(22), 1337–1341.

Cho, K. H., Beom, J., Yuk, J. H., & Ahn, S. C. (2015). The effects of body mass composition and cushion type on seat interface pressure in spinal cord injured patients. *Annals of Rehabilitation Medicine, 39*(6), 971–979.

Claydon, V. E., Steeves, J. D., & Krassioukov, A. (2006). Orthostatic hypotension following spinal cord injury: Understanding clinical pathophysiology. *Spinal Cord, 44,* 341–351.

Coggrave, M., Burrows, D., & Durand, M. A. (2006). Progressive protocol in the bowel management of spinal cord injuries. *British Journal of Nursing, 15*(20), 1108–1113.

Cotner, B. A., Njoh, E. N., Trainor, J. K., O'Connor, D. R., Barnett, S. D., & Ottomanell, L. (2015). Facilitators and barriers to employment among veterans with spinal cord injury receiving twelve months of evidence based supported employment services. *Topics in Spinal Cord Injury Rehabilitation, 21*(1), 20–30.

Craig, A., Nicholson, P. K., Guest, R., Tran, Y., & Middleton, J. (2015). Adjustment following chronic spinal cord injury: Determining factors that contribute to social participation. *British Journal of Health Psychology, 20*(4), 807–823.

deRoon-Cassini, T. A., de St. Aubin, E., Valvano, A., Hastings, J., & Horn, P. (2009). Psychological well-being after spinal cord injury: Perception of loss and meaning making. *Rehabilitation Psychology, 54*(3), 306–314.

Ducharme, S. (2006). Medical and psychosocial aspects of infertility for men with spinal cord injury and their partners. *Sex Disability, 24,* 73–75.

Dudley-Javoroski, S., Petrie, M. A., McHenry, C. L., Amelon, R. E., Saha, P. K., & Shields, R. K. (2016). Bone architecture adaptations after spinal cord injury: Impact of long-term vibration of a constrained lower limb. *Osteoporosis International, 27*(3), 1149–1160.

Ehde, D. M., Jensen, M. P., Engel, J. M., Turner, J. A., Hoffman, A. J., & Cardenas, D. D. (2003). Chronic pain secondary to disability: A review. *Clinical Journal of Pain, 19,* 3–17.

Elliot, T. R., & Frank, R. G. (1996). Depression following spinal cord injury. *Archives of Physical Medicine and Rehabilitation, 77,* 816–823.

Fausel, R. A., & Paski, S. C. (2014). Autonomic dysreflexia resulting in seizure after colonoscopy in a patient with spinal cord injury. *ACG Case Reports Journal, 1*(4), 187–188.

Forsythe, E., & Horsewell, J. E. (2006). Sexual rehabilitation of women with a spinal cord injury. *Spinal Cord, 44,* 234–241.

Frotzier, A., Cheikh-Sarraf, B., Pourtehrani, M., Krebs, J., & Lippunder, K. (2015). Long bone fractures in persons with spinal cord injury. *Spinal Cord, 53*(9), 701–704.

Guertin, P. A. (2016). New pharmacological approaches against chronic bowel and bladder problems in paralytics. *World Journal of Critical Care Medicine, 5*(1), 1–6.

Hagan, E. M. (2015). Acute complications of spinal cord injuries. *World Journal of Orthopedics, 6*(1), 17–23.

Hou, S., & Rabchovsky, A. G. (2014). Autonomic consequences of spinal cord injury. *Comprehensive Physiology, 4*(4), 1419–1453. doi:10.1002/cphy.c130045

Iwase, S., Inukai, Y., Nisimura, N., Sato, M., & Sugenoya, J. (2014). Hemifacial hyperhidrosis associated with ipsilateral/contralateral cervical disc herniation myelopathy. Functional consideration on how compression patterns determine the laterality. *Functional Neurology, 29*(1), 67–73.

Jennings, W. (2007). Expert opinion: Frequently asked questions (FAQs): Changing urinary catheters in people with spinal cord injury, residing in the community. *Australian and New Zealand Continence Journal, 13*(2), 46–49.

Johnson, K., Mowrey, K., & Bergman, M. J. (2008). Neurotrauma: Spinal cord injury. In E. Barker, (Ed.), *Neuroscience nursing: A spectrum of care*. (3rd ed., pp. 368–402). St. Louis, MO: Mosby.

Joseph, C., & Nilsson-Wikmar, L. (2015). Prevalence of secondary medical complications and risk factors for pressure ulcers after traumatic spinal cord injury during acute care in South Africa. *Spinal Cord, 54*(7), 535–539. 20. doi:10.1038/sc.2015,189

Kari, M. T., Karmali, M., & Fatoye, F. (2016). Evaluation of the efficiency of cervical orthoses on cervical fracture: A review of the literature. *Journal of Craniovertebral Junction and Spine, 7*(1), 13–19.

Kazi, H. A., de Matas, M., & Pillay, R. (2013). Reduction of halo pin site morbidity with a new pin care regimen. *Asian Spine Journal*, 7(2), 91–95.

Ling, G. S. F. (2016). Traumatic brain injury and spinal cord injury. In L. Goldman & A. I. Schafer, (Eds.). *Goldman-Cecil medicine,* (25th ed., pp. 2364–2382.). Philadelphia, PA: Elsevier Saunders.

Lucas, R. E. (2007). Adaptation and the set-point model of subjective well-being. *Current Directions in Psychological Science, 16,* 75–79.

Meade, M. A., Reed, K. S., Saunders, L. L., & Krause, J. S. (2015). It's all of the above: Benefits of working for individuals with spinal cord injury. *Topics in Spinal Cord Injury Rehabilitation, 21*(1), 1–9.

Nas, K., Yazmalar, L., Sah, V., Aydin, A., & Önes, K. (2015). Rehabilitation of spinal cord injury. *World Journal of Orthopedics, 6*(1), 8–16.

Norweg, A., Jette, A. M., Houlihan, B., Ni, P., & Boninger, M. L. (2011). Patterns, predictors, and associated benefits of driving a modified vehicle after spinal cord injury: Findings from the National Spinal Cord Injury Model Systems. *Archives of Physical Medicine Rehabilitation, 92*(3), 477–483.

O'Donnel, M. L., Varker, T., Holmes, A. C., Ellen, S., Wade, D., Creamer, M. ... Forbes, D. (2013). Disability after injury: The cumulative burden of physical and mental health. *Journal of Clinical Psychiatry, 74*(2), e137–143.

Otis, C., Marchand, A., & Coutois, F. (2012). Risk factors for posttraumatic stress disorder in persons with spinal cord injury. *Topics in Spinal Cord Injury Rehabilitation, 18*(3), 253–263.

Park, C. L., Edmondson, D., Fenster, J. R., & Blank, T. O. (2008). Meaning making and psychological adjustment following cancer: The mediating roles of growth, life meaning, and restored just-world beliefs. *Journal of Consulting and Clinical Psychology, 76,* 863–875.

Partida, E., Miranets, E., Hou, S., & Tom, V. J. (2016). Cardiovascular dysfunction following spinal cord injury. *Neural Regeneration Research, 11*(2), 189–194. doi: 10.4103/1673-5374.177707

Phillips, A. A., & Krassioukov, A. V. (2015). Contemporary cardiovascular concerns after spinal cord injury: Mechanisms, maladaptions, and management, *32*(24), 1927–1942.

Pollard, C., & Kennedy, P. (2007). A longitudinal analysis of emotional impact, coping strategies, and post traumatic psychological growth following spinal cord injury: A 10 year review. *British Journal of Health Psychology, 12*(3), 347–362.

Sakellariou, D. (2006). If not the disability, then what? Barriers to reclaiming sexuality following spinal cord injury. *Sex Disability, 24,* 101–111.

Schöenberg, M., Reimitz, M., Jusyte, A., Maier, D., Badke, A., & Haulzinger, M. (2014). Depression, posttraumatic stress, and risk factors following spinal cord injury. *International Journal of Behavioral Medicine, 21*(1), 169–176.

Sekulić, A, Nikolić, A. K, Bukumirić, Z., Trajković G. (2015). 1074–1079.

Shalkh, A., Phadke, C. P., Ismall, F., & Boullas, C. (2016). Relationship between botulinum toxin, spasticity, and pain: A survey of patient perception. *Canadian Journal of Neurological Science, 43*(2), 311–315.

Sorokin, I., & De, E. (2015). Options for independent bladder management in patients with spinal cord injury and had function prohibiting intermittent catheterization. *Neurourology and Urodynamics*, *34*(2), 167–176.

Trborich, M., Ortega, C., Schroeder, J., & Fredrickson, M. (2014). Effect of cooling vest on core temperature in athletes with and without spinal cord injury. *Topics in Spinal Cord Injury Rehabilita*tion, *20*(1), 70–80.

van Weert, K. C., Schouten, E .J., Hofstede, J., van de Meent, H., Holtstag, H. R., & van den Berg-Emons, P. (2014). Acute phase complications following traumatic spinal cord injury in Dutch level 1 trauma centres. *Journal of Rehabilitation Medicine, 46*(9), 882–885.

CHAPTER 8

Multiple Sclerosis

OVERVIEW OF MULTIPLE SCLEROSIS

Multiple sclerosis (MS) is an inflammatory, *demyelinating* condition of the central nervous system that affects nearly twice as many women as men (Boss & Huether, 2014) and is the second only to trauma as the most incapacitating neurologic condition affecting young adults (Calabresi, 2016). It is a multifaceted and progressive disease with a myriad of physical, psychological, social, vocational, and economic implications. Individuals with Northern European heritage as well as individuals living in more temperate climates appear to be more susceptible (Calabresi, 2016). There is increasing evidence that genetic factors alone do not increase susceptibility but rather the interaction of genetic predisposition with environmental factors, such as cigarette smoking, increased levels of vitamin D, or exposure to the Epstein Barr virus (Ascherio & Munger, 2016).

Some experts believe that multiple sclerosis is an autoimmune condition in which the body's immune system attacks segments of *myelin* (Waid et al., 2014). The triggers of the autoimmune response that causes the body's immune system to attack myelin are unknown.

Multiple sclerosis is a lifelong condition. Because multiple sclerosis is usually not fatal, and many individuals live a normal life span with average life expectancy being only slightly less than those without the condition (Calabresi, 2016). Nevertheless, throughout their life, individuals with MS can expect varying degrees of alteration in functional capacity.

Because the manifestations and course of the condition are so individualized, there is no formula for predicting or estimating the degree or speed at which functional changes may occur.

THE ROLE OF MYELIN

The functional unit of the nervous system is the neuron. Each neuron has a cell body and an axon, a long nerve fiber that transmits electrical messages in a manner similar to an electric wire. **Myelin** is a fatty, protective sheath that surrounds and insulates the axon in the brain and spinal cord and promotes rapid transmission of nerve impulses. When areas of myelin are destroyed and scar tissue *(plaque)* forms (see **Figure 8-1**), transmission of nerve impulses is slowed or blocked by the plaque, altering neurological function in a specific area. How and where manifestations of the blocked nerve transmissions are experienced depend on the extent and precise location of the scarring or plaque formation. The term *multiple sclerosis* comes from the multiple areas of scarring (**sclerosis**) that occur when myelin surrounding nerve fibers in the brain and spinal cord is destroyed.

TYPES OF MULTIPLE SCLEROSIS

There are three major clinical types of multiple sclerosis: *relapsing remitting, secondary progressive*, and *primary progressive* (Calabresi, 2016).

- Relapsing–remitting is characterized by fluctuating course of relapses with associated neurologic deficits, followed by periods of partial or total recovery after relapse

Figure 8-1   Scarring after Loss of Myelin

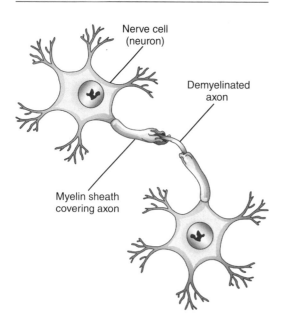

Nerve cell
(neuron)

Demyelinated
axon

Myelin sheath
covering axon

- Secondary progressive is characterized by cessation of fluctuations with slow deterioration and progression
- Primary progressive is characterized by deterioration from beginning.

Approximately 90% of individuals with multiple sclerosis experience the *relapsing–remitting type* of multiple sclerosis (Boss & Huether, 2014), in which there are periods of **exacerbations** (when manifestations become worse), also called *relapses*, alternating with periods of **remission** (when manifestations become better). Most individuals with relapsing–remitting type of multiple sclerosis progress to the *secondary progressive* after 20 years to 40 years (Calabresi, 2016).

INITIAL MANIFESTATIONS OF MULTIPLE SCLEROSIS

The manifestations of multiple sclerosis are diverse and unpredictable, appearing in varying combinations and patterns. Manifestations vary dramatically from individual to individual. They can also vary from time to time in the same person, and depend

on the location and extent of myelin destruction. Consequently, not all persons with multiple sclerosis experience the same manifestations or progression of the condition.

Initial manifestations are often subtle, such that the condition may not be immediately identified. Individuals may first experience fatigue, slight muscle weakness, or difficulty with vision, which then resolves. Due to the vagueness and intermittence of manifestations, the individual may ignore the episode and not seek health care immediately. When health care is sought, manifestations may be so vague or inconsistent that the healthcare provider may attribute them to an acute condition or to stress or malingering; in the latter case, the provider may consequently be reluctant to conduct further tests.

Prior to having multiple sclerosis identified as the cause of manifestations, many individuals have gone from one healthcare provider to another with a host of vague complaints for which no explanation is given. This time lag may induce anxiety, self-doubt, and depression owing to the continuing vague manifestations, which cannot be explained.

Manifestations of multiple sclerosis fluctuate and often involve sensory or visual manifestations, in addition to fatigue, weakness, and impaired balance or coordination, depending on the part of the central nervous system affected (Calabresi, 2016). As manifestations become more pronounced, permanent consequences in a variety of areas become more apparent; these changes are irreversible.

POTENTIAL MANIFESTATIONS OF MULTIPLE SCLEROSIS
Systemic Changes

Fatigue is common in multiple sclerosis (Calabresi, 2016). It may be described as a perception of lack of physical or mental energy that interferes with usual activities and that is experienced as a general and persistent feeling of tiredness with decreased stamina for activities such as walking or standing.

Sensitivity to heat is also experienced in many individuals with multiple sclerosis. For those who do experience heat sensitivity, even minor fluctuations in environmental temperature can cause manifestations to worsen (Campellone, 2015).

Sensory Manifestations

Sensory manifestations in multiple sclerosis can vary from decreased sensation to pain. Some individuals experience a sensation of numbness or tingling in some part of the body (**paresthesia**), or sensations such as insects crawling on the skin, burning, or electrical sensation.

Pain is relatively common in multiple sclerosis (Solaro & Uccelli, 2011). Some people may experience brief and *paroxysmal pain* (sharp, intermittent, sudden, and spontaneous pain). In other instances, individuals with multiple sclerosis experience chronic pain, which can affect psychosocial and vocational function, in turn influencing their emotional state, interpersonal relationships, ability to rest, and capacity to work.

Vision

Any portion of the visual system may be affected by multiple sclerosis. Persons with this disease may experience intermittent episodes of *optic neuritis*, in which there are transient visual manifestations such as dimness or blurring of vision, and often pain over the eye (Baloh & Jen, 2016). Some individuals experience visual disturbances, such as **diplopia** (double vision) due to weakness of ocular muscles. Others experience partial vision loss, which can be acute or chronic if there is damage to the optic nerve. In some instances, individuals experience eye movement manifestations such as **nystagmus**, in which there is a repetitive back-and-forth movement of the eye due to damage to areas of the brain (Shelat, 2015).

Motor Manifestations

Multiple sclerosis may be characterized by muscle weakness, or a partial or complete paralysis of any part of the body. There may be spasm, or involuntary contraction of muscles, with associated cramps, especially in the lower extremities.

Individuals may also experience difficulty with coordination and balance (**ataxia**) or dizziness (**vertigo**). As a result, they may walk with a wide, staggering, unstable gait, which may be misinterpreted by the casual observer as indicative of intoxication.

Individuals may also experience tremor of the head or a particular tremor of the hands called an *intention tremor*. Intention tremor occurs only when the individual tries to engage in a purposeful activity, such as reaching for a glass. When the hand is a rest, no tremor is present.

Many individuals with multiple sclerosis experience **spasticity** (muscle spasm), which may be aggravated by sudden movement or position.

Speech and Swallowing

When there is damage to the nerves that control movement in the mouth or throat, individuals may experience difficulty swallowing (**dysphagia**) or difficulty with speech. Swallowing difficulties may cause affected persons to choke when eating and can contribute to aspiration of food or liquids into the lungs, precipitating lung infections or pneumonia. Swallowing difficulties can also contribute to malnutrition.

Speech difficulties may be manifested as slurred speech, unclear articulation of words (**dysarthria**), or changes in voice quality (**dysphonia**). In other instances, there may be scanning speech, in which the individual enunciates slowly with frequent hesitations at the beginning of a word or syllable.

Cognitive Changes

Cognitive changes are common in individuals with multiple sclerosis, regardless of type (O'Connell, Langdon, Tubridy, Hutchinson, & McGuigan, 2015). When cognitive changes do occur, individuals most frequently experience difficulties with attention, conceptualization, memory, or new learning. Some individuals have difficulty with abstract reasoning and problem solving, as well as difficulty with tasks that require either rapid or precise motor responses. When cognitive manifestations are present, the individual may be seen by a neuropsychologist to determine the extent and type of cognitive function lost. Individuals experiencing difficulties with memory may use compensatory techniques to assist with memory function, such as making lists, keeping a calendar, or minimizing distractions.

Depression

Over 50% of individuals with multiple sclerosis, experience depression (Calabresi, 2016), although the degree to which it is a reaction to the condition and the degree to which it is a manifestation of neurological dysfunction is not known. Some individuals, rather than experiencing depression, experience an inappropriate euphoria (Duncan, Malcom-Smith, Ameen, & Solms, 2015). Feelings of euphoria may interfere with the individual's ability to adapt to manifestations of multiple sclerosis and can affect judgment and decision making.

Bowel or Bladder Control

Multiple sclerosis may also affect bladder and bowel function—which, in turn, can interrupt social and occupational activity. Some individuals experience neurogenic bladder, in which there is sensation of urgency and frequency of urination, sensation of incomplete bladder emptying, or **urinary retention** (the inability to empty the bladder of urine). In some instances, individuals may experience **incontinence** (loss of control of the bladder or bowel). The most frequent bowel manifestation in multiple sclerosis is constipation.

Sexual Function and Fertility

Sexual function is often affected with multiple sclerosis, although this topic is often under-discussed with healthcare providers (Darij et al., 2015). Alteration in sexual function may be a direct result of nerve damage resulting from myelin destruction and associated scarring, but contributing factors may also include psychological issues such as depression, altered self-image, and anxiety (Pintér, Cseh, Sárközl, Illigens, & Siepmann, 2015).

Erectile dysfunction is frequent in men with multiple sclerosis, and both women and men frequently experience loss of libido and or *inorgasmia* (inability to achieve orgasm) (Calabresi, 2016).

Women may also experience a decrease in vaginal lubrication and **dyspareunia** (painful intercourse) (Pintér et al., 2015). Women with multiple sclerosis are, however, able to become pregnant and carry pregnancy to term. There is no evidence that pregnancy causes an increase in manifestations or exacerbations of the condition (Pozzilli, Pugliatti, & ParadigMS Group, 2015).

Fatigue

Although multiple sclerosis entails a number of manifestations that can interfere with function in the long term, regardless of the level of disability, many individuals with multiple sclerosis experience severe fatigue that may be as disabling as the other manifestations experienced (Garg, Bush, & Gappmaier, 2016; Tur, 2016). Although fatigue may at times be related to other secondary conditions, such as urinary tract infection, which can be identified and treated, more often fatigue is directly related to multiple sclerosis itself. Fatigue can be managed through both pharmacological and nonpharmacological means.

IDENTIFICATION AND CONFIRMATION OF MULTIPLE SCLEROSIS

There is no definitive laboratory test for identification of multiple sclerosis. Instead, diagnosis of multiple sclerosis is based on clinical history, manifestations, and the results of a full neurological examination. In addition, tests performed may include *magnetic resonance imaging* (MRI), a scan that can detect plaques that can suggest MS, or *evoked potential*, an electrical test that assesses the time it takes a nerve impulse from an area of the body to reach the brain. Collection and examination of cerebrospinal fluid may be conducted as well, especially to rule out other causes of manifestations, such as infection.

GENERAL MANAGEMENT OF MULTIPLE SCLEROSIS

Multiple sclerosis is a lifelong condition with varying degrees of progression rates of functional change. Consequently throughout life, individuals can expect varying degrees of alteration in functional capacity. Because manifestations and course of the condition are so individualized, there is no formula for predicting or estimating the degree or speed at which functional change may occur. Manifestations of multiple sclerosis often fluctuate between periods of *remission* (when manifestations get better) and periods of *exacerbation* (when manifestations get worse). Although manifestations may partially resolve when the condition is in remission, each exacerbation can bring about additional functional changes that are permanent.

Given the variability in presentation and disease course, interventions are directed toward managing individual manifestations, maintaining function, and modifying the course of the condition so that future exacerbations can be prevented or delayed to the extent possible. Both nonpharmacological and pharmacological approaches may be use for management of manifestations as well as for prevention of exacerbations.

Nonpharmacological approaches, such as maintaining a healthy lifestyle, and identifying potential triggers of exacerbation, such as stress, heat, or fatigue, may decrease chances of exacerbation occurring. Physical therapy, stress reduction, and alternative and complementary therapies may also be used to help manage manifestations (Calabresi, 2016).

Pharmacological approaches may be used to decrease discomfort experienced from manifestations, such as bladder problems, spasticity, or emotional manifestations such as depression. Pharmacological approaches can also be used to modify the course of the condition. Corticosteroids may be used to shorten the duration and severity of manifestations when the individual experiences an acute exacerbation. Immune-mediated therapies, classified according to their immunological mechanism of action, may also be used to decrease relapses, increase time between relapses, and minimize additional damage to the nervous system (Dubey, Sguigna, & Stüve, 2016). The type of medication used varies with the individual.

Managing Systemic Manifestations

Individuals who experience fatigue may find it helpful to determine any coexisting factors that contribute to feelings of fatigue, such as medication side effects, sleep disturbances, or depression, so that they may be managed accordingly. Individuals may also learn activity modification and energy conservation strategies, such as having frequent rest periods, breaking activities into several steps, or otherwise pacing activities. Use of energy-conserving assistive devices, such as motorized scooters, or other assistive devices that can make activities more energy efficient can be useful as well. In addition, other strategies such as stress management and maintaining a cool, climate-controlled environment to avoid elevation in core body temperature may prove beneficial.

Chronic Pain Management

A variety of pharmaceutical interventions may be utilized in management of pain in multiple sclerosis.

Physical therapy and *occupational therapy* may be helpful in assisting individuals to minimize pain due to spasms or postural difficulty. In other instances, cognitive-behavioral therapy has been found to be useful in helping individuals with MS manage pain (Gottberg et al., 2016). Some alternative treatment methods, such as acupuncture, hypnotherapy, and biofeedback, may also be beneficial.

Management of Motor Difficulties

In general, individuals with multiple sclerosis should remain as active as they can without developing excessive fatigue. Physical therapy may be utilized to help individuals with problems of mobility or to train them in the use of assistive devices, such as walkers, if needed. Specific exercises that help to decrease calcium loss from bones, strengthen weak muscles, and maintain muscle strength and joint mobility may be recommended as well. Physical therapy that includes massage and passive range-of-motion exercises may also be beneficial.

Management of Spasticity

Because spasticity varies from person to person, management of spasticity is individually determined. Interventions often include medication as well as nonpharmacologic interventions such as stretching and range-of-motion exercises, strengthening exercises, balance and coordination exercises, or changes in daily activity. Medication and nonpharmacologic approaches may be used individually or in combination. Pharmacologic approaches often include medications such as *muscle relaxants* or *antispasmodics*. Unfortunately, when the individual takes doses of these medications high enough to control spasticity, muscle weakness may be exacerbated.

Management of Speech and Swallowing Difficulties

When speech or swallowing difficulties are an issue, a *speech therapist* may be consulted to help the individual improve function in either swallowing or speech. For swallowing difficulties, the individual may be given exercises to improve swallowing or taught to alter positioning, which can decrease the risk of choking during food ingestion. For speech difficulty, the individual may be taught oral exercises that strengthen muscles used in speech or may use assistive devices, such as a communication board and voice amplifier, to facilitate the ability to communicate.

Management of Cognitive Difficulties

Evaluation by *neuropsychologist* or other health professional can be helpful to determine the extent and type of cognitive difficulty the individual may be experiencing so that a strategy can be designed in accordance with individual need. Because memory deficit is the most frequently encountered cognitive difficulty in multiple sclerosis, strategies such as making lists, keeping notes, and avoiding distractions may enhance function. In addition, cognitive-behavioral therapy may prove useful.

Bladder and Bowel Management

Although some individuals with multiple sclerosis never experience urinary problems, for those who do, *anticholinergic medications*, which inhibit the effects of the parasympathetic nervous system, are sometimes helpful in relieving bladder manifestations such as frequency and urgency. Conversely, *cholinergic medications*, which stimulate the effects of the parasympathetic nervous system, may be helpful in relieving urinary retention. Bladder training may be helpful in reducing and managing bladder control problems. Use of a catheter or sanitary pads may decrease the embarrassment associated with possible leakage of urine. Other

bladder control strategies focus on monitoring the times of day when fluids are ingested and ensuring ready availability of restrooms to minimize the chance of accidents. If the individual has problems with urinary retention, he or she may be taught to insert a catheter into the bladder to drain accumulated urine.

Because a common bowel problem associated with multiple sclerosis is constipation, health providers may assess factors that contribute to constipation, such as medications, decreased fluid intake, or lack of fiber and bulk in the diet. If such factors are identified, strategies such as increasing fluid intake, altering the diet to include more roughage, or developing a regular toileting schedule may be implemented.

Management of Depression

Depression is common in individuals with multiple sclerosis; indeed, suicide rates are higher among persons with MS than in the average population (Strupp et al., 2016). Many individuals with multiple sclerosis indicate that depression, lack of control, social isolation, progressive disease, and high level of disability have led them to have suicidal ideation (Emrich, 2014). *Antidepressant* medications, along with psychological consultation, may be utilized for manifestations of depression (Calabresi, 2016).

FUNCTIONAL IMPLICATIONS OF MULTIPLE SCLEROSIS

Personal and Psychosocial Issues

Most individuals with multiple sclerosis are young adults who have lived through the formative years of childhood and adolescence as relatively healthy individuals and are at a stage of their life in which they are beginning to assume many social and economic responsibilities, such as engaging in a career, establishing intimate personal relationships, and perhaps starting a family. When multiple sclerosis is identified, the first reaction may be one of relief due to the apprehension experienced prior to having an explanation for the manifestations provided. Other individuals, however, may experience new anxiety due to the unpredictability and nature of manifestations.

Restrictions on abilities, activities, and social relationships call for significant initial psychosocial adjustment and alteration of self-concept as well as continual readjustment as exacerbations and remissions occur and as new incapacitating features of the condition emerge. Consequently, the long-term experience of living with multiple sclerosis through young adulthood, middle age, and older adulthood requires not just initial acceptance of the condition, but continued flexibility and adjustment as the condition changes. Individuals may react in a number of ways.

The ambiguity of multiple sclerosis and the erratic nature of the manifestations can produce significant stress. Some persons who have recently been diagnosed with multiple sclerosis may be unwilling to accept the condition and continue to search for someone who will provide an alternative explanation for the manifestations. In other cases, individuals who have searched for years for an explanation for their vague and elusive neurological manifestations may feel a sense of relief at finally being given a definitive cause to explain what they have been experiencing. Others may react with shock and disbelief; still others may demonstrate fear and anxiety. As with other chronic conditions, the individual's reaction to the diagnosis of multiple sclerosis depends on a number of person-specific factors.

As the implications of having multiple sclerosis are accepted, individuals may attempt to gain some control over the condition and its manifestations. Although they may adapt to the realization that multiple sclerosis is a lifelong condition, its unpredictability remains a source of stress. The ability to come to terms with uncertainty may have a salient impact on their adjustment to the condition. Despite planning, unforeseen exacerbations may occur, interfering with plans and activities without warning. Exacerbations can renew a sense of vulnerability, undermining optimism or enthusiasm for long-range planning and causing anxiety about the future.

Mild conditions of MS may produce minimum manifestations that are not easily recognized by the casual observer. This can create a conflict in terms of expectations of others, who may expect more of the individual than he or she is able to do. In other instances, due to vague or subtle manifestations, casual observers may misinterpret manifestations, such as fatigue, as lack of motivation, avoidance of responsibility, or attention seeking. To counteract this perception, individuals with MS may either push themselves beyond their limits or feel isolated and deserted. Consequently, they may not receive the acceptance, encouragement, and social support that can contribute to adjustment.

Learning to live with a lifelong condition such as multiple sclerosis is dependent on individuals' ability to foster a positive attitude and to continue to engage in activities that help them to effectively manage manifestations of MS, adjust to role changes, and maintain a positive self-concept

Activities and Participation

Social and Family Participation

Multiple sclerosis affects not only the individual but also the family; thus it can have a significant impact on family dynamics. With other conditions, such as traumatic spinal cord injury, changes in functional capacity are immediate and permanent, enabling the individual and family to plan accordingly. In multiple sclerosis, alterations in functional capacity are unpredictable, variable, and fluctuating so that the individual and family must make ongoing alterations and adjustments. Uncertainty combined with increasing changes in functional capacity may result in gradual dependence on others for both social and practical support and necessitate additional care-giving roles for family members, placing a strain on family relationships.

Because many individuals experience multiple sclerosis during young adulthood, implications for the family, especially children, can be significant. High levels of social support can assist in the adjustment of individuals with MS, affecting their perception of quality of life, and can be a strong predictor of the family's ability to cope and function effectively (Aghael, Karbandi, Gorji, Golkhatm, & Allzadeh, 2016). Individuals with multiple sclerosis may face a number of qualitative changes in their social networks and personal relationships. Due to declining mobility or function, they may experience a decrease in social interaction or a deterioration in social relationships.

Even when individuals have mild cases of multiple sclerosis, manifestations of the condition can be stressful. In mild cases, individuals may have few visible manifestations or may experience only vague manifestations of weakness or fatigue. Family, friends, and colleagues, who may be unable to observe visible signs of incapacity, may not understand why the individual cannot keep pace with others or why he or she is unable to continue to perform tasks in the same time frame as in the past. The individual may be accused of being lazy or attempting to get out of an activity when, in fact, his or her level of energy is reduced due to the condition. As a result, individuals may attempt to push themselves beyond their capability or beyond what is in their own best interest with regard to management of their condition.

Bladder problems resulting from multiple sclerosis may cause embarrassment, leading an individual to withdraw from social and work activities. A variety of steps can be taken to minimize the social limitations that such problems may present, as described previously.

Although alcohol is not contraindicated for most people with multiple sclerosis, if balance problems are experienced as a result of the condition, alcohol will compound the problem. Likewise, alcohol can be dangerous when taken in combination with some medications. Consequently, individuals with multiple sclerosis should always consult with their healthcare provider before deciding whether alcohol may be consumed on social occasions.

Because of the wide variation in the course of progression of multiple sclerosis and associated functional limitations, a comprehensive evaluation of the individual's environment must be performed to ensure that adequate modifications and compensations are made to allow maximal function. Increasing the individual's functional capabilities has the potential to positively affect social and psychological function.

Sexuality

Although sexual dysfunction may be the direct result of damage to nerves, sexual function may also be altered in persons with MS due to secondary causes such as fatigue, muscle spasm, or paralysis. In other instances, sexual function is altered due to psychosocial issues such as depression, changes in self-image or self-esteem, or strain in interpersonal relationships.

Assistive Devices and Home Modification

As multiple sclerosis progresses, the ability to perform a number of activities of daily living becomes reduced. Alterations in performance of such activities can have a major impact on personal independence, quality of life, social roles, and family relationships. Although individuals may be able to continue to carry on a number of personal activities of daily living, such as toileting, grooming, dressing, and ambulation, there may be increasing need for assistance to carry out more complex tasks such as housekeeping, cooking, shopping, and transportation.

For many individuals with multiple sclerosis, exposure to heat can have a temporary adverse effect on manifestations. Environments in which body temperature is increased, such as during hot or humid weather, fever, or even a hot bath, can make these individuals feel worse, although heat does not necessarily cause a worsening of the condition itself. Individuals should, therefore, avoid hot and humid environments.

VOCATIONAL ISSUES IN MULTIPLE SCLEROSIS

Many individuals with multiple sclerosis experience problems with unemployment and underemployment, especially since it is usually identified during the peak years of employment (Cadden & Amett, 2015). Educational attainment, severity of manifestations, and presence of alteration in cognitive function appear to be significant predictors for employment status for many individuals with multiple sclerosis (Honan, Brown, & Hine, 2014; Li, Fitzgerald, Bishop, Rumril, & Wang, 2015).

The course of multiple sclerosis varies greatly among individuals. Consequently, each individual's vocational potential must be considered separately. Individuals with mild manifestations, those with slowly progressive multiple sclerosis, or those who have extended periods of remission are capable of being gainfully employed for many years. Others who have more serious manifestations of the condition can, with appropriate accommodations and assistive devices, often remain employed despite exacerbations or progression of the condition.

Functional abilities related to mobility, communication, vision, and cognitive function are common areas that need to be addressed. Specific accommodations and needs for each person with multiple sclerosis must be evaluated individually. For example, individuals who experience manifestations such as paralysis of the lower extremities will require wheelchair accommodations. Individuals who experience communication difficulties, such as slurred speech, may need other types of accommodations or considerations regarding job placement. Individuals with balance problems may need to avoid situations in which falling could be hazardous or may need a walking aid, such as a cane or crutches, which could be helpful in preventing a catastrophic fall. If vision is affected, specific accommodations related to visual needs may be warranted. If cognitive function is affected, individuals may benefit from cognitive retraining or memory enhancement programs.

Both emotional stress and physical stress can cause a temporary worsening of manifestations for individuals with multiple sclerosis. The degree of emotional stress that the individual experiences on the job, as well as the level of physical activity required, should be considered. Excessive fatigue, particularly to the point of over exhaustion, should be avoided. Although individuals do not need to curtail their physical activity, they should avoid pushing themselves beyond their limits. Individuals may minimize the effects of fatigue on their job productivity by learning to self-pace so that more strenuous activities are planned when energy levels are higher, such as at the beginning of the day. Individuals should learn to moderate their pace and find activity levels conducive to optimizing their energy. Frequent rest periods may be needed throughout the day. It may be important for individuals to break tasks into smaller steps, resting at intervals in between steps. Adapting work hours to individual needs, involving individuals in more sedentary work, or using energy-saving technology may be advisable to increase work capacity.

Because heat also affects manifestations, individuals with multiple sclerosis should avoid hot and humid environments. They should avoid prolonged exposure to the sun and during hot days stay in an air-conditioned environment as much as possible.

Individuals with multiple sclerosis have increased susceptibility to complications from infectious conditions. For this reason, environments offering significant exposure to people with colds, flu, or other infectious conditions should be avoided.

Although limitations are associated with the condition, many people with multiple sclerosis are able to continue to work with only minor adjustments. Even so, discrimination in the workplace continues to be a barrier for some individuals with multiple sclerosis (Roessler, Rumrill, Hennessey, Nissen, & Neath, 2011). Loss of time at work during exacerbations should be expected, although generally these episodes are not excessive. Provision of assistive devices, new equipment, ready access to restrooms, or job restructuring can enhance the individual's ability to continue work. Specifically, environmental factors, accommodations that allow for more sedentary work, flexibility in schedule, and use of technology can be instrumental in helping individuals with multiple sclerosis maintain employment.

CASE STUDY

Ms. C., a 25-year-old high school teacher, began finding it increasingly difficult to climb the stairs to her classroom on the second floor of the school building. In the following months, she also began to notice blurring of her vision when she was grading students' papers. After several healthcare consultations, she learned that she had multiple sclerosis. In addition to adjusting to differences in functional capacity that she experienced, Ms. C. became concerned about how her health condition might affect her ability to continue as a teacher.

1. Which specific factors of multiple sclerosis should Ms. C. consider with respect to her ability to continue to work as a teacher?
2. Which accommodations may be beneficial to Ms. C. in her current line of work?

REFERENCES

Aghael, N., Karbandi, S., Gorji, M. A., Golkhatmi, M. B. & Allzadeh, B. (2016). Social support in relation to fatigue symptoms among patients with multiple sclerosis. *Indian Journal of Pallative Care, 22*(2), 163–167.

Ascherio, A., & Munger, K. L. (2016). Epidemiology of multiple sclerosis: From risk factors to prevention—An update. *Seminars in Neurology, 36*(2), 103–114.

Baloh, R. W., & Jen, J. (2016). Neuro-ophthalmology. In L. Goldman & A. I. Schafer (Eds.), *Goldman-Cecil medicine.* (25th ed., pp. 2573–2579). Philadelphia, PA: Elsevier Saunders.

Boss, B. J., & Huether, S. E. (2014). Disorder of central and peripheral nervous system and the neuromuscular junction. In K. L. McCance, S. E. Huether, V. L. Brashers, & N. S. Rote (Eds.), *Pathophysiology: The biological basis for disease in Adults and children,* (7th ed., pp. ; 618–621). St. Louis, MO: Elsevier-Mosby.

Cadden, M., & Amett, P. (2015). Factors associated with employment status in individuals with multiple sclerosis. *International Journal of MS Care, 17*(6), 284–291.

Calabresi, P. A. (2016). Multiple sclerosis and demyelinating conditions of the central nervous system. In L. Goldman & A. I. Schafer, (Eds.), *Goldman-Cecil medicine.* (25th ed., pp. 2471–2480). Philadelphia, PA: Elsevier Saunders.

Campellone, J. V. (2015). *Multiple sclerosis.* NIH U.S. National Library of Medicine. Retrieved from https://www.nlm.nih.gov/medlineplus/ency/article/000737.htm

Darij, A., Tatjana, P., Goran, T., Nebojsa, S., Irena, D., Sarlota, M., & Jelena, P. (2015). Sexual dysfunction in multiple sclerosis: A 6 year follow up study. *Journal of Neurological Sciences, 358*(1–2), 317–323.

Dubey, D., Sguigna, P., & Stüve, O. (2016). Managing disability in progressive multiple sclerosis: Current treatment options. *Neurology, 18*(6), 27. doi:10.1007/s11940-016-0412-7

Duncan, A., Malcom-Smith, S., Ameen, O., & Solms, M. (2015). Changing definition of euphoria in multiple sclerosis: A short report. *Multiple Sclerosis, 21*(6), 776–779.

Emrich, L. (2014). Living with MS: Increased risk of depression, anxiety, and suicidal thoughts. *MultipleSclerosis.net.* Retrieved from https://multiplesclerosis.net/living-with-ms/living-ms-increased-risk-depression-sucidal-thoughts

Garg, H., Bush, S., & Gappmaier, E. (2016). Association between fatigue and disability, functional mobility, depression, & quality of life in people with multiple sclerosis. *International Journal of MS Care, 18*(2), 71–77.

Gottberg, K., Chruzandeer, C., Backenroth, G., Johansson, S., Ahlström, G., & Ytterberg, C. (2016). Individual face-to-face cognitive behavioral therapy in multiple sclerosis: A qualitative study. *Journal of Clinical Psychology, 72*(7), 651–662. doi:10:1002/jclp.22288

Honan, C. A., Brown, R. F., & Hine, D. W. (2014). The multiple sclerosis work difficulties questionnaire (MSWDQ). Development of a shortened scale. *Disability Rehabilitation, 36*(8), 635–641. doi:10:3109/09638288.2013.805258

Li, J., Fitzgerald, S. M., Bishop, M., Rumril, P. D., & Wang, F. (2015). Disease related and functional predictors of employment status among adults with multiple sclerosis. *Work, 52*(4), 789–797.

O'Connell, K., Langdon, D., Tubridy, N., Hutchinson, M., & McGuigan, C. (2015). A preliminary validation of the Brief International Cognitive Assessment for Multiple Sclerosis (BICAMS) tool in an Irish population with multiple sclerosis (MS). *Multiple Sclerosis and Related Disorders, 4*(6), 521–525.

Pintér, A., Cseh, D., Sárközl, A., Illigaens, B. M., & Siepmann, T. (2015). Autonomic dysregulation in multiple sclerosis. *International Journal of Molecular Science, 16*(8), 16920–16952.

Pozzilli, C., Pugliatti, M., & ParadigMS Group. (2015). An overview of pregnancy related issues in patients with multiple sclerosis. *European Journal of Neurology, 22* (Suppl 2), 34–39. doi:10.1111/ene.12797

Renoux, C., Vukusic, S., Mikaeloff, Y., Edan, G., Clanet, M., Dubois, B., ... Adult Neurology Departments KIDMUS Study Group. (2007). Natural history of multiple sclerosis with childhood onset. *New England Journal of Medicine, 356*(25), 2603–2613.

Roessler, R., Rumrill, P., Hennessey, M., Nissen, S., & Neath, J. (2011). The employment discrimination experiences of adults with multiple sclerosis. *Journal of Rehabilitation, 77*(1), 20–30.

Shelat, A. M. (2015). *Nystagmus.* Bethesda, MD: U.S. National Library of Medicine, NIH. Retrieved from https://www.nlm.nih.gov/medlineplus/ency/article/003037htm

Shevil, E., & Finlayson, M. (2006). Perceptions of persons with multiple sclerosis on cognitive changes and their impact on daily life. *Disability and Rehabilitation, 28*(12), 779–788.

Solaro, C., & Uccelli, M. M. (2011). Management of pain in multiple sclerosis: A pharmacological approach. *Nature Reviews Neurology, 7*(9), 519–527.

Strupp, J., Ehmann, C., Galushko, M., Bücken, R., Perrar, K. M., Hamacher, S., ... Golla, H. (2016). Risk factors for suicidal ideation in patients feeling severely affected by multiple sclerosis. *Journal of Pallative Medicine, 19*(5), 523–528.

Tur, C. (2016). Fatigue management in multiple sclerosis. *Current Treatment Options in Neurology, 18*(6), 26. doi:10.1007/s11940-016-0411-8

Waid, D. M., Schreiner, T., Vaitaitis, G., Carter, J. R., Corboy, J. R., & Wagner, D. H., Jr. (2014). Defining a new biomarker for the autoimmune component of multiple sclerosis: Th40 cells. *Journal of Neuroimmunology, 270*(1–2), 75–85.

CHAPTER 9

Neurodegenerative and Neuromuscular Conditions

OVERVIEW OF NEURODEGENERATIVE AND NEUROMUSCULAR CONDITIONS

Neurodegenerative Conditions

Neurodegenerative conditions consist of a number of conditions that may either be inherited or acquired and that show progressive deterioration of the *central nervous system* over time. Neurodegenerative conditions may progress slowly or rapidly, and the cause for many is unknown. Both the course and the progression of the neurodegenerative conditions depend on the type and vary from individual to individual. Examples of *neurodegenerative conditions* of the central nervous system include the following:

- Parkinsonism
- Huntington's disease
- Alzheimer's disease

Neuromuscular Conditions

Neuromuscular conditions affect the *nerves* or *muscles,* which results in degeneration of motor neurons in the areas of the *central and peripheral nervous systems,* leading to muscle weakness and **atrophy** (shrinkage) of muscle. In some conditions, involuntary movements are also present. Neuromuscular conditions may be either acquired or inherited, and in some instances the cause is unknown. Examples of *neuromuscular conditions* include the following:

- Amyotrophic lateral sclerosis
- Muscular dystrophy
- Myasthenia gravis

NEURODEGENERATIVE CONDITIONS

Parkinsonism

Parkinsonism is a general term to describe a condition in which four basic manifestations occur:

- Tremor
- Rigidity
- **Akinesia** (absence of movement)
- Postural disturbance (Lang, 2016b)

Parkinson's disease is a common cause of these manifestations, but a number of other conditions can also cause these manifestations. When the manifestations stem from another condition, the individual is said to have *secondary Parkinsonism* rather than Parkinson's disease.

Secondary Parkinsonism

Secondary Parkinsonism can be associated with the ingestion of certain drugs (prescription or illicit) or exposure to toxic substances, such as carbon monoxide or other chemicals. Secondary Parkinsonism gained attention in the early 1980s when the "designer drug" MPTP, which mimicked the action of heroin, entered the street market. A number of young adults, after taking the drug, suddenly developed permanent manifestations of severe Parkinson's disease. Some medications used to manage psychiatric conditions may also produce Parkinsonian-like side effects if not closely monitored.

Examples of other conditions that can cause secondary Parkinsonism include the following:

- Alzheimer's disease
- Encephalitis
- Brain tumor
- Head trauma
- Huntington's disease

Parkinson's Disease

Parkinson's disease is a slowly progressive neurodegenerative condition of the central nervous system that leads to progressive loss of motor function. Although its cause remains unknown, evidence suggests that both genetic and environmental factors may play a role in its etiology (Lang, 2016b). Parkinson's disease involves extensive degenerative changes in the *basal ganglia* (gray matter embedded in the white matter of the brain, which has a role in complex movements) and the loss of or decreases in levels of dopamine (a neurotransmitter) in the basal ganglia.

Most of the incapacitating manifestations associated with Parkinson's disease are due predominantly to drastic reductions of levels of dopamine in the brain.

Manifestations of Parkinson's Disease

Four manifestations of Parkinson's disease are most commonly seen:

- **Bradykinesia** (slowness of movement) or akinesia
- Muscle rigidity
- Postural disturbance
- Tremor

Bradykinesia

In early stages of the condition, individuals may exhibit extreme slowness in initiating or maintaining movements (bradykinesia). Individuals who have Parkinson's disease may walk with small, shuffling steps (*shuffling gait*) and may have difficulty in rising from a chair or bed. They may also find it difficult to initiate or to stop voluntary movements. While walking, for example, they may experience *gait hesitation* when they suddenly "freeze," taking seconds to regain motion; in other instances, they may continue five or six more steps beyond where they want to stop.

Bradykinesia can interfere with activities such as shaving, buttoning clothes, or cutting food—all of which take longer and become more difficult to perform as the condition progresses. Because Parkinson's disease affects both the central and autonomic nervous systems, some individuals may also experience urinary or bowel problems.

Muscle Rigidity

Individuals with Parkinson's disease are sometimes said to have a *poverty of spontaneous movement*. For instance, they may blink less frequently and develop a mask-like, expressionless face. They may develop difficulty swallowing (**dysphagia**), which results in accumulation of saliva in the mouth with subsequent drooling. Because the individual is unable to swallow quickly, the rate of swallowing food decreases and eating becomes slower and more deliberate as the condition progresses. As food collects in the mouth and in the back of the throat, individuals may be prone to coughing and choking episodes, which can cause aspiration of food or liquid into the lung, precipitating lung infection or pneumonia.

Motor changes related to Parkinson's disease may cause speech changes related to incoordination and reduced movement of muscles that control breathing, voice, pronunciation, and rate of speaking. Volume of speech may be decreased (**hypophonia**), and there may be no verbal inflections. Individuals' ability to write may also be affected. For example, reduction in amplitude of movement may affect an individual's ability to write so that handwriting gradually becomes smaller and smaller (**micrographia**) until it is no longer legible.

Postural Disturbance

As the condition progresses, individuals lose postural stability and demonstrate gait irregularities, predisposing them to falls (Li et al., 2012). Posture becomes stooped, and individuals' arms fail to swing with their stride when they are walking. The risk of falls is greater due to loss of postural reflexes, making it difficult to maintain an upright position if the individual is suddenly bumped or jarred. To keep from falling, individuals may inadvertently quicken their steps as if to "catch up" with their own center of gravity (*propulsion*). Muscle tone is increased, creating muscle rigidity, which also interferes with movement and causes severe immobility. Because greater effort is necessary to engage in voluntary movement, fatigue is increased as well.

Tremor

Tremor of an extremity, usually most noticeable in one hand, is the most frequent early manifestation of Parkinson's disease. The tremor intensifies when the hand rests in the lap (*resting tremor*) and diminishes with voluntary movement. The tremor, however, is not present during sleep.

Cognitive and Emotional Changes

Mental and behavioral changes do not always occur as a result of Parkinson's disease, but both cognitive changes and changes in emotions and behavior can be part of the manifestations. Dementia can also occur in some individuals later in the course of the condition. Risk factors for dementia associated with Parkinson's disease include advanced age and longer duration of the condition (Leegwater-Kim & Waters, 2007). Apathy, passivity, depression, and loss of initiative may be noted. Some studies indicate that depression is present in a large number of individuals with Parkinson's disease and can have a more dramatic effect on quality of life than the actual manifestations of the condition or side effects of management. As the individual becomes aware of his or her decreasing cognitive abilities, depression related to losses may result. The degree to which depression reflects physiological changes and the degree to which it represents a reaction to the condition itself, however, are not known.

Identification of Parkinson's Disease

There is no single test that can be used to identify Parkinson's disease. Instead, identification of

Parkinson's disease is usually based on the presence of tremor, stiffness, and slow movement and ruling out other causes of Parkinsonism. Because many other conditions may have similar manifestations in early stages of development, and because initially manifestations may be attributed to aging, appropriate identification of Parkinson's disease as the source of manifestations is often missed. Tests such as *magnetic resonance imaging* (MRI) may be conducted to rule out other causes of manifestations.

Management of Parkinson's Disease

There is no cure for Parkinson's disease. This condition is characterized by progressive debilitation, although the progression occurs slowly over years. Currently, no specific intervention has been proved to modify the progressive course of Parkinson's disease (Lang, 2016b). Consequently, intervention is directed toward reducing the effects of manifestations and preventing complications, thereby enabling the individual to remain active longer. Intervention usually consists of medication, physical therapy, and exercise, along with maintenance of general health.

Pharmacologic Interventions

Some medications are used in the early stages of Parkinson's disease for early treatment of tremor or **dyskinesias** (abnormal involuntary movement). Medication called *levodopa* (L-dopa) is most often used in management of Parkinson's disease as the condition progresses (Lang, 2016b). This drug decreases manifestations of Parkinson's disease by helping to increase the level of the neurotransmitter dopamine in the brain. At first, small amounts are typically utilized; over time, the dosage is gradually increased. Although helpful, levodopa can have serious side effects and demonstrates limited long-term efficacy. Some individuals may experience nausea or abnormal involuntary movements, dyskinesia, or, in some instances, psychiatric disturbances. These effects are generally related to the dosage of the medication, occurring more frequently with higher dosages. In some individuals, levodopa can cause mental confusion or decrease alertness.

Nonpharmacologic Interventions

Nonpharmacologic approaches to treatment of Parkinson's disease include regular exercise, physical therapy, speech therapy, and psychosocial support (Leegwater-Kim & Waters, 2007). Exercise and activity are especially important for individuals with Parkinson's disease because of the tendency of the muscles to be stiff and rigid. Muscles can *atrophy* without the stimulation that exercise provides, decreasing the individual's capacity for self-care. A daily exercise routine, such as walking a specified distance, doing simple calisthenics, or performing active range-of-motion exercises, is encouraged.

Other interventions are directed toward preventing complications. Individualized physical therapy focusing on joint mobility, correction, and prevention of postural abnormalities of the trunk and limbs, and maintenance of regular gait is important to help individuals maintain function as long as possible. Passive stretching of extremities, muscle massage, resistive exercises, and training are techniques used by physical therapists to achieve this goal.

Surgical Interventions

Neurosurgical intervention as a management technique for Parkinson's disease continues to be explored. *Deep brain stimulation (DBS)* has been used with some success (Lang, 2016b). This procedure involves implanting an electrode into a target area of the brain. The electrode is then tunneled under the skin to an external stimulator, which can be switched on or off by the individual with Parkinson's disease.

Surgical procedures appear to be most helpful for those individuals whose manifestations are not satisfactorily controlled with medication.

Assistive Devices and Environmental Modifications

Parkinson's disease is a chronic, lifelong condition characterized by progressive deterioration. Because of its gradual onset and slow progression, most individuals have many years after their diagnosis in which they can remain productive and functional. Assistive devices such as rolling walkers and canes can provide stabilization and assist in mobility. Devices such as wrist weights may be used for hand tremor, and handwriting aids may assist in writing.

Environmental modifications can help to prevent potential falls and enhance mobility. For example, furniture may be rearranged so as to provide a wide path between points as well as to provide something for the individual to hold on to when ambulating. Obstacles such as footstools should be removed to prevent falls. Throw rugs should be removed or tacked down to prevent falls. Smooth floor surfaces are preferable to carpet to enhance mobility.

Functional Implications of Parkinson's Disease

Personal and Psychosocial Issues

Parkinson's disease is a visible neurological condition. Difficulty with movement, stooped posture, and tremor of an extremity are visible signs that may cause the individual with Parkinson's disease to be self-conscious. In addition, lack of facial expression and of spontaneous movements when talking, as well as reduced volume or voice quality, may interfere with verbal and nonverbal communication. Acquaintances or strangers as well as family members may attribute lack of expression to disinterest, dementia, or low-intellectual ability (Lyons, Tickle-Degnen, Henry, & Cohn, 2004), causing the individual to become stressed or frustrated by the attitudes of others. Consequently, the individual with Parkinson's disease may begin to withdraw from or be reluctant to participate in social interactions, which in turn increases stress and creates a sense of social isolation. Stress can make manifestations of Parkinson's disease worse, further contributing to the individual's social isolation.

Anxiety may occur from the time Parkinson's disease is first identified and may continue as manifestations of the condition progress. In addition, many people with Parkinson's disease experience depression, which can have a more significant impact on quality of life and life satisfaction than many of the physical manifestations (Dural, Atay, Akbostanci, & Kucukdeveci, 2003; Gage & Storey, 2004).

For individuals who had prided themselves on their efficiency, communication, or manual skills, deterioration of these skills can be particularly stressful. Because Parkinson's disease is progressively incapacitating, the individual and his or her family must continually readjust to increasing loss of functional capacity, which can in turn contribute to anxiety and depression. If mental deterioration, confusion, or personality changes occur, family members may have increased difficulty coping with these changes. In some instances, individuals with Parkinson's disease may demonstrate decreased initiative and impaired judgment, which can be another source of familial stress.

Activities and Participation

Activities of daily living such as dressing or bathing can be very tiring and time consuming for persons with Parkinson's disease. Individuals should allow enough time so they do not feel rushed. In addition, rigidity and slowness of movement can become worse in crowds or social situations when the individual feels stressed. Family members or others should be helped to understand that attempting to push or pull the individual forward makes matters worse, and that it is most helpful to allow the individual to move at his or her own pace. Given that balance is sometimes a problem, special safety precautions, such as grab bars or a tub bench/shower chair, should be used when bathing. Clearing the environment of potential hazards can prevent accidents and hence further complications resulting from falls. Use of walking aids, such as crutches or a walker, may also help individuals prevent falls.

Sexuality

Information about sexual function in Parkinson's disease is scarce, although sexual problems are frequently present in neurological disorders. Depression is considered a contributor to sexual problems in the general population. Given that individuals with Parkinson's disease frequently experience depression, it stands to reason that some sexual problems may exist. Medications taken for manifestations of Parkinson's disease may also contribute to sexual incapacity. Furthermore, factors common to many types of chronic health conditions can lead to a lack of interest in sexual activities. As time needed for activities of daily living (such as dressing, eating, and personal hygiene) and for management requirements increases, interest in and energy for sexual activity may decline.

Vocational Issues in Parkinson's Disease

Whether persons with Parkinson's disease can continue working is an individual decision that is based on the specific circumstances. In most instances, work that is more sedentary and that does not require significant verbal communication may be continued longer than work that requires more strenuous activity. Because individuals with Parkinson's disease have difficulty with balance and gait, jobs that require considerable walking, stooping, or bending should be avoided. Transportation to and from work may be the largest obstacle to maintaining employment.

Highly stressful occupations should be avoided because increased stress tends to increase the severity of manifestations that the individual experiences. For some individuals, work becomes increasingly difficult and the effort to continue working may produce a tremendous strain. For these individuals, not working may bring a sense of relief from the physical and mental stress of attempting to continue carrying out various tasks and responsibilities. For others, the inability to work may have a detrimental effect. In most cases, individuals will be able to continue working if the work is not extremely demanding physically or does not require manual dexterity. Scheduling frequent rest periods and restructuring the workload may help increase the total amount of work that can be done during the workday. Because stiffness and muscle rigidity are common manifestations of the condition, working in a cold environment should be avoided because of the increase in muscle stiffness that could be experienced.

Huntington's Disease

Huntington's disease is a progressive, genetic condition of the central nervous system in which neurons of the brain degenerate. It is characterized by disorders of movement, cognition, and behavior

(Lang, 2016a). Most individuals develop manifestations between the ages of 30 and 50 years of age, although some individuals may have onset prior to the age of 20, a condition known as juvenile Huntington's disease (Lang, 2016a). The condition advances slowly and progressively. Although the rate of deterioration varies from person to person, as does the rate at which manifestations appear, Huntington's disease has severe functional implications and can result in death after 15 to 20 years (Lang, 2016a).

Manifestations of Huntington's Disease

Huntington's disease is characterized by three types of manifestations:

- Cognitive deficits
- Motor consequences
- Behavioral changes

Cognitive changes usually occur in the early stages, with the individual at first becoming increasingly absent-minded and having difficulty with concentration. As the condition progresses, mental deterioration (**dementia**) occurs.

Early motor manifestations involve movements of the fingers that give the impression that the individual is fidgeting. As the condition progresses, movement and coordination continue to deteriorate, with *bradykinesia* and rigidity interfering with the individual's ability to walk. Jerky, involuntary movements (**chorea**) are present as well. Motor difficulty also affects the individual's ability to speak and to swallow.

Personality and behavioral changes associated with the condition range from delusions to impulse-control problems.

Identification of Huntington's Disease

Identification of Huntington's disease is usually based on the individual's manifestations, family history, and genetic testing (Lang, 2016a).

Management of Huntington's Disease

There is no intervention known to slow the progression of or cure Huntington's disease. Interventions are usually directed toward preventing complications and managing manifestations.

Physical therapy is a major component of the management program for individuals with Huntington's disease. It can assist the individual in improving or stabilizing motor ability, preventing contractures, or adapting the environment to promote safety as well as maximum independence. Occupational therapists may help individuals improve coordination abilities and activities of daily living skills. Speech therapists may help individuals maximize their speech capability and their ability to swallow. In some instances, cognitive retraining and memory training may be useful. Training in ways to avoid exposure to upper respiratory infections as well as other communicable health conditions is also advised.

It is sometimes difficult to distinguish which behavioral manifestations are related to the condition itself and which are related to the individual's anxiety about having the condition. *Psychotropic medications* may be used to help alleviate or control behavioral manifestations regardless of their cause. Medication may be utilized for anxiety or depression, irritability, or mood swings. In some instances, psychotropic medication may be used to control some of the involuntary, jerky movements individuals may be experiencing.

A major portion of management is directed toward assisting individuals and their family in managing self-care as the condition progresses. Individual counseling, family counseling, and genetic counseling of family members may be important interventions.

Functional Implications of Huntington's Disease

Personal and Psychosocial Issues

Individuals and their families must cope with continued losses, both physical and mental, as the condition progresses as well as with the knowledge that Huntington's disease is a progressive condition in which continued deterioration can be expected. For individuals with Huntington's disease, their condition-related cognitive and behavioral changes may make it more difficult for them to cope. Both the individual with Huntington's disease and the family may feel helpless and hopeless. As a result, they may be reluctant to participate in activities designed to maintain or improve their current level of function.

Faulty judgment and impulsivity related to behavioral changes can result in unsafe situations for individuals with Huntington's disease. Individuals who are in denial about their condition and their areas of incapacity may also expose themselves to situations that could result in unsafe practices or injury.

Activities and Participation

As the condition progresses, individuals become less able to care for themselves and, therefore, more dependent on others. As communication becomes more difficult, social interactions become more challenging, often leading to increasing social isolation. Personality changes that may produce violent or hostile behaviors further stress support systems.

Because Huntington's disease has a genetic component, family members may be under additional stress given the possibility that they may themselves be at risk for developing the disease. Counseling, education, and support can help to reduce the stress that family members may be experiencing.

Vocational Issues in Huntington's Disease

Huntington's disease is a progressive, degenerative condition. However, in the early stages before mental deterioration and physical incapacitation are present, short-term training may be appropriate. As the condition progresses and individuals have increasing difficulty with memory, communication skills, and physical ability, sheltered employment may be the most feasible alternative.

Alzheimer's Disease and Other Dementias

Dementia is a broad term characterizing decline from prior levels of cognitive functioning in of reasoning, memory, language, visuospatial ability, or changes in personality or behavior that interferes with daily function (Knopman, 2016). Although the prevalence of dementia increases with advanced age, it may also be secondary to neurological disorders associated with conditions such as stroke or head injury, and can also occur in individuals with long standing intellectual disability. Although Alzheimer's disease is the most prevalent type of dementia, other types of dementia,

including vascular dementia, and dementia associated with conditions such as Parkinson's disease (discussed earlier in the chapter) account for at least 25% (Knopman, 2016). Some dementias are reversible when the cause is removed or corrected. Other dementias, such as Alzheimer's disease are progressive and irreversible.

Alzheimer's Disease

Approximately 200,000 people younger than 65 years of age have Alzheimer's disease (Alzheimer's Association, 2009). No clear cause of Alzheimer's disease has been discovered. Prevalence increases with age; in addition to age, other risk factors associated with developing Alzheimer's disease include family history, diabetes, hypertension, cardiovascular conditions, and head injury (Knopman, 2016).

Manifestations of Alzheimer's Disease

Alzheimer's disease is progressive and initial manifestations may be subtle, insidious, and not easily recognized. Initial subjective reports of memory difficulties may be attributed to normal aging and involve inability to recall names or misplacing items. As the condition progresses, individuals may have difficulty with concentration, memory, orientation, and calculation (Reisberg et al., 2011). Memory lapses gradually become more pervasive, such that individuals have difficulties performing daily tasks such as paying bills, cooking meals, and using transportation. In later stages, assistance may be required for bathing, toileting, and eating. In the terminal stages, individuals may lose the ability to communicate and require total care.

Emotional, behavioral, and psychiatric manifestations may also be noted. Agitation, emotional outburst, and violence may be present. Some individuals demonstrate manifestations of psychosis or delusions. Sleep disturbances are also frequent.

Identification of Alzheimer's Disease

Identification of Alzheimer's disease is primarily based on physical and neurological examination ruling out other conditions that may mimic manifestations (such as medication side effects or interactions, depression, or thyroid dysfunction), clinical history of manifestations, progression of cognitive incapacity, and family and social history. A number of structured neuropsychological and behavioral tests may also be used to evaluate individual's cognitive function. Although these tests are not specific for Alzheimer's disease, they do provide information regarding the extent to which cognitive function is incapacitated. Brief screening tests such as the Mini–Mental State Exam (MMSE) (Folstein, Folstein, & McHugh, 1975) may be used to assess memory, orientation, and concentration. Longer and more detailed tests, such as the Consortium to Establish a Registry for Alzheimer's Disease (CERAD) (Morris et al., 1989), test immediate and delayed recall, language skills of naming and verbal fluency, and drawing ability.

At times, in addition to the original identification of Alzheimer's disease or other dementias, neuropsychological tests such as those mentioned previously may be used to measure change in cognitive function.

Management of Alzheimer's Disease

Several medications are available for management of Alzheimer's disease, even though there is no clear-cut evidence showing that they alter the progression or functional decline of the condition (Knopman, 2016). Other medications are utilized to manage specific manifestations of Alzheimer's disease, such as agitation, depression, sleep disturbance, or psychiatric manifestations.

Nonpharmacologic interventions are useful to improve the individual's ability to function for as long as possible and to improve the family's ability to manage manifestations of the condition. Specific behavioral management techniques to manage disruptive behaviors, interventions to manage incontinence, or other complications such as contractures in later stages can prevent excessive premature incapacity.

Functional Implications of Alzheimer's Disease

Personal and Psychosocial Issues

In the early stages of the condition, as individuals become aware of their incapacities, they may exhibit depression, anger, or grief as they cope with loss of function, changing relationships, and often loss of job. Cognitive therapy in which individuals are seen individually and encouraged to identify positive experiences and pleasant activities may be helpful. Support groups for the individual and his or her family as well as education and training may help in adjustment and decrease the sense of social isolation that may be present.

Activities and Participation

Behavioral management programs may assist the individual's family to learn techniques to reduce or eliminate agitation or other disruptive behaviors. Daycare centers for individuals with later-stage dementia are also useful to provide them with a club-like environment that provides pleasant events and activities.

Vocational Issues in Alzheimer's Disease

The degree to which individuals with Alzheimer's disease are able to continue employment after manifestations appear depends on the type of work in which the individual is engaged and the work environment. In the initial stages of Alzheimer's disease, job restructuring or modification may sometimes enhance the individual's ability to remain in the workplace longer. As the condition progresses, helping individuals maintain a sense of purpose through assisting in tasks appropriate to their level of functioning may be of benefit.

Vascular Dementias

Dementia may also be associated with other conditions such as cerebrovascular disease, cardiovascular disease, atrial fibrillation, or diabetes. Dementia may result if there direct damage to the brain, such as with stroke, or if there is occlusion or narrowing of the major cerebral vessels.

Manifestations of vascular dementia may not follow a particular pattern but rather may be associated with specific events, such as a small stroke that leads to additional decline in cognition and function. Vascular dementia is identified by neurological examination and identification of causative factors. Vascular dementia can be prevented, in some cases, with careful control of the underlying condition that puts the individual at risk.

NEUROMUSCULAR CONDITIONS

Amyotrophic Lateral Sclerosis

Amyotrophic lateral sclerosis (ALS) is also some-times referred to as *Lou Gehrig's disease* in memory of the baseball player who died of ALS in 1941 (Orrell, 2007). ALS belongs to a classification of conditions characterized by gradual degeneration of *motor neurons*, the nerve cells that convey impulses to the voluntary muscles. Motor neurons in the brain (*upper motor neurons*) transmit messages to motor neurons in the spinal cord (*lower motor neurons*), which in turn send messages to muscles in the body. When upper or lower motor neurons are damaged, as in ALS, the muscles are unable to function and control over voluntary motion is lost.

The exact cause of ALS is unknown however risk factors appear to include increasing age, male gender, and genetic susceptibility. Researchers are also investigating physical exercise and environmental factors as potential contributing factors (Shaw, 2016)

Manifestations of ALS

Initial manifestations of ALS may be subtle, including muscle weakness of an extremity, awkwardness or stumbling when walking, difficulty with manual dexterity, or slurring of speech. As muscular weakness gradually progresses, muscle atrophy occurs, and there may be **spasticity** (stiffening of muscles) with exaggerated reflexes (**hyperreflexia**). Other manifestations may include difficulty swallowing (**dysphagia**) and increased difficulty forming words (**dysarthria**). As muscles in the chest and diaphragm are affected, individuals may notice difficulty with breathing (**dyspnea**).

As the condition progresses, individuals become increasingly weak and immobile with progressive paralysis. In later stages of the condition, affected persons may require assistance to breathe. Although voluntary function is gradually lost, cognitive function, sensation, vision, eye movement, and hearing are usually not affected (Shaw, 2016).

The rate of progression of the condition varies. Gradually, however, individuals will lose the ability to stand, walk, or use their arms. Because of decreased ability to swallow, individuals are at risk of aspirating food or liquids, contributing to the possibility of developing *aspiration pneumonia*.

Identification of ALS

There is no specific diagnostic test to detect the presence of ALS. Instead, identification of ALS is usually based on the manifestations that the individual exhibits and their progression, the individual's health history, and the process of ruling out other conditions to which manifestations can be attributed.

Management of ALS

There is no cure for ALS. Management goals are generally directed toward helping individuals and families cope with manifestations of the condition, assisting individuals with ALS to remain independent as long as possible, promoting comfort, and preventing complications. Management of manifestations focuses on maintaining muscle function, relieving discomfort, and forestalling complications such as respiratory infections and **decubitus ulcers** (pressure sores). Medications to reduce spasticity may be utilized, although they can also increase muscle weakness and cause sedation. Physical therapy may be helpful to maintain function and to reduce painful manifestations brought on by muscle spasm. Range-of-motion and stretching exercises can help to reduce spasticity as well as prevent complications such as **contractures** (shortening of a muscle resulting in immobility of a joint).

Occupational therapists can provide support and help individuals to adapt their environments so as to maximize function. Speech pathologists may be required to help individuals who have difficulty with swallowing. If individuals have breathing difficulty, respiratory therapists may be consulted to help individuals learn techniques to assist with respiratory management.

Because most individuals with ALS maintain mental alertness and have the ability to continue meaningful relationships, facilitation of communication is imperative to enhance quality of life as well as productivity. Individuals with speech difficulties may utilize speech therapists to help them learn techniques to communicate. Devices such as voice amplifiers may be helpful for individuals who can speak clearly but not loudly. In other instances, devices that are triggered by eye blinking may be a useful tool to enhance communication.

Functional Implications of ALS

Personal and Psychosocial Issues

Individuals with ALS experience increasing loss of function and increased dependence on others over time. Despite the significant changes that their condition brings about, individuals with ALS retain their cognitive and intellectual ability and still have needs for recreation, entertainment, and companionship. Adjustment and adaptation to the condition and resulting loss of function are individually determined. Whereas some individuals may experience feelings of hopelessness, others have been found to view the future with hope and enthusiasm, and many continue to live productive lives and make significant contributions (Luté et al., 2012).

Factors that appear to be relevant in adjustment to ALS include the degree of social support and the presence or absence of the perception that they are a burden to others (Luté et al., 2012).

Activities and Participation

Friends and acquaintances may withdraw from the individual with ALS because they are unsure of what to expect and are uncomfortable interacting with the individual. Abandonment by social contacts creates social isolation and decreased support. Helping individuals with ALS and their families learn how to talk with friends about ALS as well as community education programs to create ALS awareness can enhance understanding, decrease discomfort, and facilitate social interaction.

Modifications of roles of family members are often required. Because individuals with ALS need substantial help with most activities of daily living, family members most often find themselves in a caregiving role even in the early stages of the condition. Expenditures for health care and equipment can be sizable. If the individual with ALS is also the major financial provider for the family, money issues may become a major concern. Family members may quit work to assume the caregiving role, which further contributes to financial distress. Family members may also have feelings of powerlessness, anger, or anxiety about the future. They may vacillate between resentment and guilt.

Interventions that help families reduce stress and obtain support through community resources and support groups can help to alleviate some of the feelings of anxiety and fear about the future that are commonly experienced by family members as they try to deal with ALS and help them to feel nurtured, emotionally supported, and less isolated.

Vocational Issues in ALS

As ALS progresses, the degree of physical limitation increases, with activity becoming increasingly more difficult. This condition generally progresses fairly rapidly over a course of 3 to 5 years, although some individuals survive for as long as 10 years (Shaw, 2016). Many individuals' live productive lives after ALS has been identified, continuing to work despite advanced manifestations. As new interventions emerge that may slow progression of ALS and prolong survival, the ability to maintain competitive employment may also increase, depending on the requirements of the job and the way in which manifestations affect the individual's ability to perform.

Physical demands of work should be light and sedentary for individuals with ALS. Even if the individual is still ambulatory, a wheelchair-accessible work environment should be considered, as he or she will most likely require a wheelchair for ambulation as the condition progresses. Transfer may become more difficult in later stages of his or her condition. Because communication can be a problem, occupations in which the ability to speak makes up an important part of the job should be avoided.

Muscular Dystrophy

Overview of Muscular Dystrophy

Muscular dystrophy is a group of inherited muscle conditions characterized by weakness and progressive degeneration of skeletal muscle (Hara et al., 2011). It features muscle fiber degeneration with atypical muscle regeneration (**dystrophy**), usually consisting of fat and connective tissue that replaces muscle fibers.

A number of types of muscular dystrophy exist. Some examples are:

- Duchenne's muscular dystrophy
- Becker muscular dystrophy
- Facioscapulohumeral muscular dystrophy
- Limb–girdle muscular dystrophies
- Myotonic muscular dystrophy

The major types of muscular dystrophy are characterized by primary degeneration of muscle fiber with progressive muscle weakness. Muscular dystrophies affect people of different ages, have different patterns of muscle involvement, and demonstrate different rates of progression.

Manifestations of Muscular Dystrophy

Duchenne's muscular dystrophy is the most common inherited muscle disease, typically identified in boys between 2 and 5 years of age (Selcen, 2016). It is characterized by progressive muscle weakness (Mendell et al., 2010) that results in in clumsiness, frequent falls, difficulty running, and difficulty going up stairs. Later, shoulder muscles become weakened, making it difficult to raise the arms or lift objects. Intellectual disability, attention-deficit/hyperactivity disorder, or autism spectrum disorder may also be associated (Selcen, 2016). By late adolescence, as the condition progresses, some individuals may begin using a wheelchair. Some individuals develop **scoliosis** (curvature of the spine) that compromises respiratory function.

Becker muscular dystrophy is a milder form of Duchenne's muscular dystrophy and may be identified in boys after the age of 5 or later as teenagers, and at times even in adulthood (Selcen, 2016). It progresses more slowly, such that individuals often retain the ability to ambulate decades after the condition is identified.

Facioscapulohumeral muscular dystrophy can affect both males and females. It is generally characterized by progressive muscle weakness of the face, shoulders, arms, abdomen, and feet, contributing to foot drop. It may be identified in childhood, but often is not identified until adulthood.

Limb–girdle muscular dystrophy usually affects the hips and shoulders first, then progresses to the arms and legs, although progression is usually slow. This condition may be identified in childhood or not until adulthood.

Myotonic muscular dystrophy can be identified in childhood, but more often is identified in adulthood. It progresses slowly and is characterized by weakening of muscles in the arm and legs, as well as muscles of the head, neck, and facial muscles, causing a characteristic facial droop. Individuals may have a drooping eyelid (**ptosis**) or cataracts. In addition, overall systemic features may affect cardiac function or lead to development of diabetes mellitus.

Identification of Muscular Dystrophy

In addition to health history and family history, blood tests that quantify levels of enzymes indicating muscle damage (*creatine kinase* [*CK*]) or tests that measure electrical activity in the muscle (*electromyography*) may be utilized. In some instances, *muscle biopsy* may be taken to distinguish muscular dystrophy from other possible muscle conditions.

Management of Muscular Dystrophy

There is no cure for muscular dystrophy. Management interventions are directed toward preventing complications and maintaining mobility function as long as possible. Physical therapy is essential to help prevent contractures of the joint and to maintain muscle strength and maximum functional capacity. In some instances, surgical procedures may be indicated, especially if contractures have formed and interfere with function. Occupational therapy may be useful in helping individuals to use assistive devices. Devices such as braces can provide support for weakened muscles of the extremities as well as maintain joints in a position of function. Other devices such as walkers or wheelchairs may be used to assist in mobility.

Individuals who have compromised respiratory function should avoid exposure to others with respiratory infections and keep up-to-date with influenza shots and pneumonia vaccines. In cases of severe respiratory incapacity, a ventilator assist device may be needed. Those individuals who have systemic involvement, such as in myotonic muscular dystrophy, should undergo regular electrocardiogram, measurement of respiratory function, and blood glucose measurements in an effort to detect potential complications so they can be adequately managed (Selcen, 2016).

Functional Implications of Muscular Dystrophy

Personal and Psychosocial Issues

Individuals with muscular dystrophy have unique psychosocial issues related to their condition, and multiple factors influence their ability to cope. Age of onset, family and social resources, specific manifestations, and open communication all contribute to individuals' ability to adjust and meet demands associated with their condition and achieve emotional balance. The degree to which individuals are able to engage in age-appropriate tasks, develop peer relationships, and engage in social patterns in light of the physical manifestations of their condition is an important indicator of the level of adjustment (Hendrickson et al., 2009).

Activities and Participation

Reactions of the family to muscular dystrophy affect individuals' adjustment to their condition. Families may experience a number of stressors, including the need to obtain adequate resources as well as the practical difficulties involved in providing care to the individual. Open, respectful communication between family members and the individual can be an important aspect to decrease stress and anxiety within the family while simultaneously enhancing the well-being of the individual with muscular dystrophy.

Vocational Implications of Muscular Dystrophy

Adequate education and training are essential for occupational success. Individuals who have had muscular dystrophy identified as children and progressed through the school system with appropriate support and guidance for educational planning that takes into account functional capabilities have an excellent chance to achieve their vocational objectives. Consideration of the type of muscular dystrophy and its associated characteristics and course is important so that the individual's capabilities are appropriately matched to the job.

Because most types of muscular dystrophy involve alteration of mobility, and in many instances use of assistive devices, such as braces, walkers, or wheelchairs, work that is more sedentary may be more suitable than work that requires walking or standing. Although cognitive function may be affected in some types of muscular dystrophy, in many instances it is not affected, so that a wide range of work opportunities relying on intellectual capacity may be chosen.

Myasthenia Gravis

Overview of Myasthenia Gravis

Myasthenia gravis is an autoimmune neuromuscular condition in which there is interruption in transmission of nerve impulses to muscle at the point at which nerves initiate contraction of a muscle that can occur at any age (Evoli &Vincent, 2016).

Manifestations of Myasthenia Gravis

The initial manifestation of myasthenia gravis is usually painless muscle weakness that increases with muscle use and decreases after rest of the muscle. Sensation is usually not affected. Although any skeletal muscle can develop symptoms, eye muscles are frequently affected, resulting in double vision (**diplopia**) and/or drooping eyelids (**ptosis**). Muscles of the throat may also be affected, causing slurred speech as well as difficulty with chewing and swallowing. Weakened muscles of the mouth may also result in the appearance of a snarl when the individual attempts to smile. Muscles of upper and lower extremities may be affected, such that individuals may notice difficulty with shaving or brushing their hair without rest periods. Lower extremity involvement may make it difficult for the individual to walk long distances and at times cause the individual to collapse when walking.

Manifestations can vary in severity from time to time, with periods of remissions and exacerbations. Manifestations often become worse with exertion and later in the day. Involvement of muscles of respiration is less common; if respiratory muscles are involved, however, respiratory complications can occur. The condition progresses slowly, and many individuals are able to remain functionally active and live productive lives with no significant incapacities.

Identification of Myasthenia Gravis

Identification of myasthenia gravis is usually based on health history, manifestations, blood test to detect specific antibodies indicative of an autoimmune condition, or *electromyography,* a test that evaluates nerve-to-muscle electrical transmissions.

Management of Myasthenia Gravis

In most instances, medications that prolong and enhance the ability of neurotransmitters to activate muscles are utilized. Immunosuppressive therapy may also utilized both in initial therapy and in long term treatment (Evoli & Vincent, 2016).

Functional Implications of Myasthenia Gravis

Personal and Psychosocial Issues

Changes in both appearance and physical strength may cause anxiety and alter individuals' feelings about their interactions with others. Emotional support and education about the condition can contribute to individuals' and their significant others' ability to adapt to the changes that become manifest.

Activities and Participation

Exertion usually exacerbates weakness associated with myasthenia gravis; given this tendency, individuals may carefully plan activities to conserve energy. Rearrangement of the home can prevent unnecessary energy expenditure. If chewing and swallowing become difficult, individuals may consume small, frequent meals with food that is easily swallowed and allow plenty of time for meals. If respiratory muscles are affected, individuals should attempt to avoid respiratory infections.

Because most regular activity can be continued with myasthenia gravis, social relationships are not severely affected. As speech may become more difficult to discern after prolonged periods of speaking, individuals may avoid situations in which long periods of speaking are required.

Vocational Issues in Myasthenia Gravis

Many individuals with myasthenia gravis are able to continue their ordinary activities with minor modification. Although strenuous or repetitive activities may be more difficult, light activities of short duration are usually not affected. Long periods of walking or standing may also be difficult, so pacing of activities with frequent rest periods may be needed. If individuals' regular occupation is physically demanding or frequent rest periods are not possible, a change of work structure or retooling for a more sedentary line of work may be necessary.

CASE STUDY

Mr. S., a 65-year-old college professor, has over the last few years developed hypophonia, muscle rigidity that has affected his balance, and micrographia— manifestations that have been identified as caused by Parkinson's disease.

1. Which specific issues regarding Mr. S.'s manifestations might affect his potential for continuing teaching as a college professor?
2. Are there accommodations that Mr. S. may use to enhance his functional capacity either at home or at work? If so, which specific accommodations might he find helpful?

REFERENCES

Alzheimer's Association. (2009). Prevalence. In *2009 Alzheimer's disease facts and figures* (pp. 10–19). Chicago, IL: Author.

Dural, A., Atay, M. B., Akbostanci, C., & Kucukdeveci, A. (2003). Impairment, disability, and life satisfaction in Parkinson's disease. *Disability and Rehabilitation, 25*(7), 318–323.

Evoli, A. & Vincent, A. (2016). Disorders of neuromuscular transmission. In L. Goldman & A. I. Schafer (Eds.), *Goldman-Cecil Medicine* (25th ed., pp. 2547–2553). Philadelphia, PA: Elsevier Saunders.

Folstein, J. F., Folstein, S. E., & McHugh, P. R. (1975), Mini-Mental State: A practical method for grading the cognitive state of patients for the clinician. *Journal of Psychiatric Research, 12,* 189.

Gage, H., & Storey, L. (2004). Rehabilitation for Parkinson's disease: A systematic review of available evidence. *Clinical Rehabilitation, 18,* 463–482.

Hara, Y., Balci-Hayta, B., Yoshida-Moriguchi, T., Kanagawa, M., Belltrán-Valero de Bernabé, D., Gündesli, H., ... Campbell, K. P. (2011). A dystroglycan mutation associated with limb–girdle muscular dystrophy. *New England Journal of Medicine, 364*(10), 939–946.

Hendrickson, J. G. M., Poysky, J. T., Schrans, D. G. M., Schonten, E. G. W., Aldenkanp, A. P., & Vles, J. S. H. (2009). Psychosocial adjustment in males with Duchenne muscular dystrophy: Psychometric properties and clinical utility of a parent-report questionnaire. *Journal of Pediatric Psychology, 34*(1), 69–78.

Knopman, D. S. (2016). Alzheimer's disease and other dementias. In L. Goldman & A. I. Schafer (Eds.), *Goldman-Cecil medicine* (25th ed., pp. 2388–2398). Philadelphia, PA: Elsevier Sunders.

Lang, A. E. (2016a). Other movement disorders. In L. Goldman & A. I. Schafer (Eds.), *Goldman-Cecil medicine* (25th ed., pp. 2461–2470). Philadelphia, PA: Elsevier Saunders.

Lang, A. E. (2016b). Parkinsonism. In L. Goldman & A. I. Schafer (Eds.), *Goldman-Cecil medicine* (25th ed., pp. 2454–2461). Philadelphia, PA: Elsevier Saunders.

Li, F., Harmer, P., Fitzgerald, K., Eckstrom, E., Stock, R., Galver, J., ... Batya, S. S. (2012). Tai chi and postural stability in patients with Parkinson's disease. *New England Journal of Medicine, 366*(6), 511–519.

Luté, D., Pauli, S., Altintas, E., Singer, U. Merk, T., Uttner, ... Ludolph, A. C. (2012). Emotional adjustment in amyotrophic lateral sclerosis (ALS). *Journal of Neurology, 259*(2), 334–341.

Lyons, K. D., Tickle-Degnen, L., Henry, A., & Cohn, E. (2004). Impressions of personality in Parkinson's disease: Can rehabilitation practitioners see beyond the symptoms? *Rehabilitation Psychology, 49*(4), 328–333.

Mendell, J. R., Campbell, K., Rodino-Klapac, L., Sahenk, Z., Shilling, C., Lewis, S., ... Walker, C. M. (2010). Dystrophin immunity in Duchenne's muscular dystrophy. *New England Journal of Medicine, 363*(15), 1429–1436.

Morris, J. C., Heyman, A., Mohs, R. C., Hughes, J., van Belle, G., Fillenbaum, G., ... CERAD investigators. (1989). The Consortium to Establish a Registry for Alzheimer's Disease (CERAD). I: Clinical and neuropsychological assessment of patients with Alzheimer's disease. *Neurology, 39,* 1159.

Orrell, R. W. (2007). Understanding the causes of amyotrophic lateral sclerosis. *New England Journal of Medicine, 357*(8), 822–823.

Reisberg, B., Franssen, E. H., Souren, L. E. M., Kenowsky, S., Jamil, I. A., Anwar, S., & Auer, S. (2011). Alzheimer's disease. In S. R. Flanagan, H. Zaretsky, & A. Moroz (Eds.), *Medical aspects of disability* (4th ed., pp. 25–64). New York, NY: Springer.

Selcen, D. (2016). Muscle diseases. In L. Goldman & A. I. Schafer (Eds.), *Goldman-Cecil medicine* (25th ed., pp. 2537–2547). Philadelphia, PA: Elsevier Saunders.

Shaw, P. J. (2016). Amyotrophic lateral sclerosis and other motor neuron diseases. In L. Goldman & A. I. Schafer (Eds.), *Goldman-Cecil medicine* (25th ed., pp. 2522–2526). Philadelphia, PA: Elsevier Saunders.

CHAPTER 10

Post-Polio Syndrome and Other Conditions of the Nervous System

OVERVIEW OF POLIOMYELITIS AND POST-POLIO SYNDROME

Poliomyelitis (or simply *polio*) is an acute infectious viral condition that was prevalent in the United States in the first half of the 20th century. With the advent of the polio vaccine, and widespread immunization, poliomyelitis has mostly been abolished in the United States. Although the condition has been largely eradicated it is still, however, prevalent in some countries (Freedman, 2016).

The virus enters the body when contaminated water or food is ingested or when hands that have been contaminated with the virus touch the mouth. The poliovirus targets the nerve cells that control muscles. The brain stem, spinal cord, and neuromuscular system may all be affected. The nerve cells or motor neurons damaged by the poliovirus are located in the *anterior horn* of the spinal cord and extend to the muscles. As neurons are affected, muscle cells lose the ability to contract, resulting in paralysis. If motor cells are able to overcome the virus, paralysis may be temporary. If, however, motor cells are unable to overcome the virus, they die, resulting in permanent paralysis or, in some instances, ongoing weakness of affected muscles. Poliomyelitis itself is not a progressive condition. Consequently, many individuals who contracted the condition 30 or more years ago adapted to the manifestations or paralysis, muscle weakness, or other residual effects.

In the late 1970s, a number of people who had experienced the initial poliomyelitis infections decades before began reporting unexpected manifestations, which ranged in severity from mild to severely incapacitating (Gordon & Feldman, 2002). At first, these individuals were not taken seriously. Many were classified as having emoional disturbances or new manifestations were merely attributed to aging. In the early 1980s, as more and more individuals who had experienced poliomyelitis decades earlier reported new manifestations, the term *post-polio syndrome* was coined to describe this new phenomenon.

Manifestations of Post-Polio Syndrome

Post-polio syndrome is a noncontiguous neurological disorder that produces a variety of manifestations in individuals who experienced an acute poliomyelitis infection many years earlier. The cause of post-polio syndrome is unknown (McNalley et al., 2015). It appears that most of the motor neurons originally damaged in the initial bout of poliomyelitis are involved in post-polio syndrome.

Common manifestations include the following:

- Slowly progressive muscle weakness
- Generalized and muscular fatigue
- Gradual decrease in muscle size (muscle **atrophy**)

- Muscle pain (**myalgia**) and joint pain
- Increasing skeletal changes such as curvature of the spine (scoliosis)
- Respiratory muscle weakness
- Difficulty swallowing (dysphagia)

Individuals who had previously been able to walk without use of assistive devices may require them because of manifestations of post-polio syndrome. Those who had used assistive devices for ambulation may find it necessary to begin to use a wheelchair.

Post-polio syndrome is progressive, meaning that manifestations will become increasingly worse. Despite increasing incapacitation, however, individuals will not experience the level of functional manifestations that they experienced when polio was in its acute state. With appropriate exercise, strength and function can be improved and incapacitation slowed, if not halted.

Identification Post-Polio Syndrome

Identification of post-polio syndrome involves ruling out or eliminating other conditions that may be responsible for the new manifestations. Manifestations of post-polio syndrome may be difficult to distinguish from those associated with other degenerative conditions of muscles and joints, such as *osteoarthritis* or *osteoporosis.* General health evaluation, routine laboratory tests, *electromyographic* studies (a graphic record of the contraction of a muscle as the result of electrical stimulation), and *nerve conduction* studies may help to identify and exclude other conditions. *Magnetic resonance imaging* may be used to exclude other conditions of the spine that could cause similar manifestations.

Management of Post-Polio Syndrome

No specific intervention is available to alter the course of post-polio syndrome. Individuals with manifestations of increasing muscle weakness, fatigue, and pain should first have a thorough physical examination by a healthcare provider to rule out other potential causes of manifestations. Interventions are largely directed toward managing manifestations experienced with post-polio syndrome and assisting individuals to maintain their functional status and independence as long as possible. Good health practices, including proper nutrition and adequate rest, are important to maintain optimal function.

Generalized fatigue is managed with lifestyle changes consisting of energy conservation measures. Physical activities should be paced to prevent excessive fatigue. Individuals may require frequent rest periods throughout the day. Use of additional assistive devices, such as use of a wheelchair rather than crutches, may help to conserve energy.

Increasing muscle strength through nonfatiguing exercise may be used to treat mild to moderate weakness. Exercises that are tolerable and that do not contribute to more weakness and fatigue may be recommended. Physical therapists generally instruct individuals about proper exercise protocols so that overuse and excessive fatigue can be avoided. Individuals are typically instructed to exercise for short intervals, resting between bouts of exercise, and to exercise only every other day to prevent excessive muscle fatigue.

Individuals with respiratory difficulty may require noninvasive *positive-pressure ventilation* at night. Because individuals with post-polio syndrome are more susceptible to infectious conditions, pneumonia and influenza vaccines are usually recommended.

The use of braces to decrease mechanical stress on the joints may be used to minimize muscle and joint pain. Changes in orthotics or in the mode of ambulation may be required. Moving from braces or crutches for ambulation to a wheelchair can also reduce stress on joints. If the individual with post-polio syndrome is overweight, weight reduction may be recommended to reduce fatigue and stress on the muscles and joints. For individuals whose respiratory muscles were affected by the initial infection, weight control can help to prevent respiratory difficulty as well.

Functional Implications of Post-Polio Syndrome

Personal and Psychosocial Issues

Given that poliomyelitis is not a progressive condition, many individuals believed their recovery to be permanent and adapted and adjusted to the functional incapacity and residual effects associated with the condition. Individuals with residual manifestations from poliomyelitis have likely worked for years to minimize incapacity and maximize their assets. After developing their own self-image and self-esteem based on their abilities, many have gone on to lead full and productive lives. When new, unexpected manifestations associated with post-polio syndrome threaten their self-image, function, and independence, the effect can be stressful and anxiety provoking.

Manifestations of this new "secondary condition" can be both frightening and frustrating for the individual, who again must adjust and adapt to continuing functional implications, to the potential use of new assistive devices, and to alteration of lifestyle. After previously regaining function and establishing a self-identity through much physical and emotional effort, facing new manifestations and changing abilities can be discouraging. Individuals may recall experiences from the initial poliomyelitis infection that can trigger anxiety about the uncertainty of their future. They may reject new assistive devices because they view them as symbols of loss of physical ability that they feel they earned through great effort.

Individual reactions to new manifestations may not be immediately recognized by others, who assume that because they have lived with their change in abilities for years, adjustment and coping are completed. Post-polio support groups can help the individual share experiences of others with similar issues, provide opportunities for brainstorming regarding techniques or devices that have helped others to increase a sense of empowerment, and decrease the sense of isolation that may be experienced. Emphasizing and recognizing assets and identifying ways to continue activities that are most valued can help individuals safeguard their lifestyle rather than eroding it.

Activities and Participation

Many people experiencing post-polio syndrome had their initial experience with acute poliomyelitis at a time when public fears concerning polio and attitudes toward individuals with any form of incapacity set them apart. Consequently, individuals with poliomyelitis may have attempted to minimize their condition so as to blend into general society or sought to cope by hiding manifestations or incapacity. Although public attitudes have changed to a considerable degree, the changing and shifting abilities that accompany post-polio syndrome may cause the individual to experience the same type of anxiety noted with the acute poliomyelitis infection.

Gaining knowledge about post-polio syndrome and its implications can help individuals to be their own best advocate. Unfortunately, not all healthcare providers are well informed about post-polio syndrome. Individuals who have current knowledge about their condition and implications can work in cooperation with health professionals to identify those strategies that best meet their needs. Individuals may need to find ways to reduce their schedules or develop other alterations that can be helpful in maintaining activity. Review of additional adaptive devices that may be needed—whether for ambulation, daily activities, or breathing (if respiration is affected)—is important to optimize function.

Vocational Issues in Post-Polio Syndrome

Most individuals with poliomyelitis have achieved gainful employment and lived productive lives with residuals of polio (Gordon & Feldman, 2002). The onset of manifestations related to post-polio syndrome, however, may make a number of alterations necessary in the work setting. Depending on performance requirements, the individual may be unable to perform all of the job duties. Thus alteration of job duties or retraining for other job duties may be necessary. In some instances, individuals may need to change occupations. In others, early retirement may be necessary.

Even when remaining in the current job is possible, individuals may experience increased fatigue or altered stamina and strength so that frequent rest periods may be needed; some persons may also need a more sedentary job structure. The ability to lift, reach, walk, or climb may be altered owing to increased muscle weakness and fatigue, making such job restructuring necessary.

Manifestations of post-polio syndrome—whether pain, weakness, or fatigue—may necessitate use of additional assistive devices. Individuals who once ambulated without assistive devices may require a cane, crutches, or braces. Individuals who once used crutches or braces may require a wheelchair for ambulation. Adaptation in the workplace for accommodation of assistive devices may be needed. If, owing to increased manifestations, the individual's current mode of transportation is no longer accessible, transportation to and from work may emerge as a barrier to employment. In addition, because of increased manifestations that diminish physical capabilities or stamina, individuals may require extra time to get ready for work.

In some instances, the onset of new manifestations and increasing change in capacity may result in depression, which can interfere with the individual's ability to work effectively. Supportive counseling may be necessary to enable the individual to cope with increasing manifestations of the post-polio syndrome.

GUILLAIN–BARRÉ SYNDROME

Overview of Guillain–Barré Syndrome

Guillain–Barré syndrome is an acquired inflammatory condition of the *peripheral nerves* (nerves lying outside the central nervous system). The exact cause of this syndrome is unknown, but it appears to be an immune-mediated condition, often following infection that appears to sensitize the immune system to antigens that are shared between the infecting organism and the peripheral nerves (Shy, 2016).

Manifestations of Guillain–Barré Syndrome

Weakness is the most common initial manifestation of Guillain–Barre syndrome (Shy, 2016). The severity varies greatly. Muscular weakness that usually begins in the lower extremities and spreads upward (*ascending paralysis*). Paralysis of both upper and lower extremities can occur, and chest and facial muscles can be affected. If breathing is affected, support of ventilation may be needed.

Identification of Guillain–Barré Syndrome

Identification of Guillain–Barré syndrome is usually based on manifestations and physical examination. *Electromyography* may be used to differentiate manifestations from other causes of generalized weakness.

Management of Guillain–Barré Syndrome

Due to the potential for rapid incapacitation, individuals with Guillain–Barré syndrome require hospitalization for observation. Because respiratory muscles can be affected, respiratory failure can be a potentially life-threatening condition that may require assistance for ventilation. Other early interventions may consist of *plasmapheresis* (exchange of the individual's plasma for albumin) or intravenous infusion of *human immunoglobulin,* both of which may shorten the time to recovery (Willison, Jacobs, & van Doom, 2016).

Other interventions are primarily directed toward specific manifestations and used to prevent additional complications. General physical rehabilitation is started early, usually under the guidance of a physiatrist (a physician who specializes in rehabilitation and physical medicine). Physical therapists are usually involved in the early stages of the condition to help individuals prevent muscle atrophy (shrinkage), contractures, or pressure sores. Occupational therapists help individuals learn how to strengthen muscles, use energy conservation techniques, and perform activities of daily living. If speech or swallowing is affected, a speech therapist may be needed to help individuals improve speech patterns or facilitate swallowing.

Most individuals experience a slow spontaneous recovery over a period of weeks or months with only about 20% having long-term disability (Shy, 2016).

Functional Implications of Guillain–Barré Syndrome

Personal and Psychosocial Issues

The initial stages of this syndrome can be extremely frightening. Individuals who were previously healthy may suddenly find themselves paralyzed and unable to care for themselves. If respiration is affected and individuals are placed on mechanical ventilation, the inability to breathe in itself is frightening. In addition, individuals on a respirator are unable to communicate, further adding to their apprehension and feelings of helplessness.

Even though most individuals regain function, the unpredictability of the condition and progression of manifestations lead to fear, frustration, and concern for the future. Depending on the individual's situation and the extent of time needed to recover, financial concerns, fear of permanent incapacity, and loss of dependence can be extremely stressful and can have long-standing psychological effects even after the individual has reached maximum recovery.

Activities and Participation

Although most individuals recover from Guillain–Barré syndrome with no residual effects, some individuals may continue to experience persistent weakness that can interfere with function (Shy, 2016). The psychosocial impact of the acute stages of the condition, along with the long rehabilitative process, may contribute to difficulty in returning to a full level of activity for some individuals.

Vocational Issues in Guillain–Barré Syndrome

Because individuals with Guillain–Barré syndrome have, in many instances, been incapacitated for a lengthy period of time, most will require an extensive period of rehabilitation. This intervention may include driver retraining, learning to pace activities, and, in some instances, reemployment training. Individuals may, after a certain amount of activity, continue to experience muscle aches or other sensations that interfere with everyday activity. Initially, they may consider returning to work on a part-time basis and anticipate the need for periodic rest periods during the day. In the case of individuals who require wheelchair use for a period of time after hospital discharge, architectural barriers at their employment site should be considered.

INFECTIONS OF THE CENTRAL NERVOUS SYSTEM

Any infection of the brain or the membranes that surround the brain and spinal cord can cause serious neurological effects, some of which may be permanent. Two common types of infections of the central nervous system are meningitis and encephalitis.

Both meningitis and encephalitis, along with their resulting residual effects, can occur in any age group. Nevertheless, children and older adults are often the most susceptible to more severe manifestations of both conditions. Individuals with compromised immune systems, such as those with HIV or AIDS, individuals with cancer, or those who have received organ transplants, are also at greater risk.

Meningitis

Meningitis refers to an inflammation of the **meninges** (membranes surrounding the brain and spinal cord and the cerebrospinal fluid). It can be caused by bacteria (*bacterial meningitis*), viruses (*viral meningitis*), or other causes such as drug hypersensitivity or tumors (Nath, 2016). Many types of meningitis exist, and the specific name given to the meningitis infection is frequently related to its cause. For instance, *staphylococcal meningitis* and *pneumococcal meningitis* are named for the organisms responsible for these infections. The nonspecific term *aseptic meningitis* refers to an inflammatory process involving the meninges when there is no evidence of bacteria; it is usually caused by a viral infection. *Mumps meningitis* refers to meningitis caused by the mumps virus.

The meninges of the brain and spinal cord can be infected in several ways. For instance, infection may enter from the upper respiratory tract. Normally, the lining of the throat is sufficient to act as a barrier to the bacteria; however, when the barrier is insufficient, the infecting organisms may invade the bloodstream and reach the meninges, causing them to become inflamed. The organisms gain access to the cerebrospinal fluid and begin to multiply. The infectious organisms may also gain entrance to the blood from another site and then infect the meninges. In addition, infection may occur by direct contamination after skull fracture.

Individuals with meningitis are usually acutely ill, initially with fever. Within a short period of time, they develop severe headache, neck rigidity, and visual discomfort when exposed to bright lights (**photophobia**). As the condition progresses, individuals become confused and often lose consciousness.

Meningitis is identified by a history of manifestations of rapid onset, including fever, stiff neck, and change in mental status. *Lumbar puncture* (spinal tap), in which a needle is inserted between the *vertebrae* and into the *subarachnoid space,* may be performed to aspirate cerebrospinal fluid so it can be examined microscopically for organisms.

If the cause is bacterial in origin, prompt intervention with antibiotics reduces the chance of progression of the condition or the development of complications. The use of prompt intervention with medication has greatly reduced the number of fatalities from meningitis; however, if this disease occurs in individuals whose physical state is weakened or if it is not immediately identified and intervention is delayed, it can still be fatal.

Although many individuals with meningitis recover completely, some may have residual neurological effects, such as deafness, seizures, paralysis, or cognitive difficulties.

Encephalitis

Encephalitis is an inflammation of the brain itself, due to direct invasion of an organism. In the United States, the most common cause of epidemic encephalitis is the West Nile virus, a mosquito-borne virus (Aksamit, 2016). The most nonepidemic cause of encephalitis in the United States is the herpes simplex virus type 1 (Aksamit, 2016; Whitley, 2016).

Individuals with encephalitis initially have nonspecific flu-like manifestations such as fever and muscle pains (myalgia). As the condition progresses, they may experience sore throat, cough, vomiting, and diarrhea. Manifestations usually progress over several days to involve headache, photophobia, and potentially seizures or altered state of consciousness.

Encephalitis is identified through manifestations, computed tomography (CT) scan of the brain, and analysis of the spinal fluid through *lumbar puncture.* Effective management of viral encephalitis is not currently available for most types of viral encephalitis, except for herpes simplex encephalitis (Aksamit, 2016). Consequently, management in the acute phases of the condition consists of monitoring and supportive care. The permanent residual manifestations associated with viral encephalitis are dependent on the cause and may

include sensorineural deafness or hydrocephalus. Approximately 40% of individuals who develop herpes simplex encephalitis experience residuals of seizures, memory problems, or behavioral difficulties (Aksamit, 2016).

OTHER CONDITIONS AFFECTING THE NERVOUS SYSTEM

Lyme Disease

Lyme disease is a multisystem inflammatory condition that affects the nervous system as well as joints and muscles. It is the result of an infection caused by a type of organism called a *spirochete* and is transmitted by the bite of an infected tick. Lyme disease is rarely, if ever, fatal and is not contagious. In its early stages, this condition is characterized by a reddened area around the site of the tick bite. Although most people, if intervention is started early, have no permanent effects from this condition, some may go on to develop a variety of residual effects. Residual effects can include neurological manifestations such as difficulties with gait, sensations of pain, or confusion, **dyspnea** (difficulty breathing), **syncope** (fainting); *Lyme arthritis*, affecting joints, commonly the knee (Wormser, 2016); or in some instances cardiac manifestations consisting of **palpitations** (awareness of heartbeat) (Zimetbaum, 2016).

Identification of Lyme disease is usually based on manifestations and blood tests. Early intervention with antibiotics can significantly improve outcomes and prevent the chronic effects. Some individuals who continue to have feelings of fatigue and joint pain are said to have *post–Lyme disease syndrome.* In other instances, individuals with persistent pain and cognitive difficulties are said to have *chronic Lyme disease* (Wormser, 2016).

Bell's Palsy

Sudden partial or complete paralysis of one side of the face is characteristic of *Bell's palsy* (Shy, 2016). Individuals may experience a sagging eyebrow, inability to close the eye, and drooping of one side of the mouth. Bell's palsy occurs when a nerve running from the brain to the face becomes inflamed. As the inflammation progresses, the nerve swells, becomes compressed, and is no longer able to transmit signals; consequently, paralysis results.

Interventions with steroids is generally instituted (Shy, 2016). Although most individuals recover from Bell's palsy within a month, during the acute phase, if individuals are unable to close the eye, the eye may need to be protected with an eye patch or artificial tears may need to be used. Individuals may also take anti-inflammatory steroids soon after the manifestations appear.

Central Sleep Apnea

There are two types of sleep apnea. The most common type, *obstructive sleep apnea* (Vaughn, 2016) (see chapter 29). The second type of sleep apnea, *central sleep apnea,* occurs when the brain fails to appropriately communicate with muscles needed for breathing to initiate respiration. It can be caused by stroke or by infections affecting the brain stem; it can also be caused by neuromuscular conditions that involve respiratory muscles.

Sleep apnea is characterized by frequent episodes of **apnea** (cessation of breathing) during sleep and daytime sleepiness (Vaughn, 2016). As a result of inadequate breathing during sleep, the individual is aroused from sleep, begins again to breath, and then attempts to resume sleeping. The result is that sleep is fragmented and not restful. Over time, sleep apnea can have both physiological and psychological consequences.

Identification of central sleep apnea usually involves observation and testing at a *sleep clinic,* where brain waves, respiratory effort, heart rate, and levels of oxygen in the blood are monitored overnight. When central sleep apnea is identified, intervention often consists of a *continuous positive airway pressure (CPAP)* machine, which is a mechanical device that the individual wears at night to assist breathing.

Narcolepsy

Narcolepsy is a complex neurological sleep condition causing impairment of the sleep-wake cycle and resulting in excessive daytime sleepiness with sudden involuntary attacks of sleep lasting from a few seconds to several minutes. Manifestations of narcolepsy may also include cataplexy (sudden loss of voluntary muscle control so that the individual is unable to move), dream-like hallucinations while awake, or total paralysis after falling asleep or just after waking (Vaughn, 2016). It can occur at any time and during any activity, such as while engaging in conversation, while driving, while eating, or even while reading. In some instances, individuals may maintain sufficient wakefulness to perform complex behaviors, but not enough for conscious awareness of behavior (Barateau, Lopez, & Dauvilliers, 2016).

Identification of narcolepsy is usually based on a persistent history of excessive daytime sleepiness, not due to other causes and confirmed through tests conducted at a sleep disorders clinic. Intervention usually consists of planned short nap periods during the day and, in some instances, management with medications—namely, central nervous system stimulants.

The physical, psychosocial, and vocational implications of narcolepsy can be devastating. Even with appropriate management, manifestations of narcolepsy may not be adequately managed. Fear of embarrassment, which may result from the unpredictability of narcolepsy manifestations, can cause individuals to limit social interactions. Safety concerns regarding operation of potentially dangerous equipment may be an issue if the individual's manifestations are not adequately managed. Employers, teachers, and others coming in contact with the individual should be educated to understand the individual's condition so that if an attack does occur, manifestations will not be misinterpreted.

GENERAL FUNCTIONAL IMPLICATIONS OF CONDITIONS OF THE NERVOUS SYSTEM

Personal and Psychosocial Issues

While in many instances conditions such as meningitis, Lyme disease, and Bell's palsy resolve with few residual effects, in some instances residual manifestations of some conditions can include neurological effects such as deafness, paralysis, or cognitive deficit. Uncertainty about how functional capacity may be affected can be a source of anxiety during the acute phases of the conditions.

When individuals experience changes in appearance, such as facial paralysis in Bell's palsy, or functional incapacitation, such as gait spasticity in Lyme disease or deafness in meningitis, changes in self-concept and body image may be present as individuals adjust to changes in appearance and new levels of functional ability. Individuals who had been previously active may suddenly face the prospect of adjusting to loss of functional capacity. Depending on the type of residual effect present, individuals may use a variety of assistive devices to achieve increased functional capacity. Although assistive devices can increase sense of independence, some individuals may have a negative emotional reaction to use of assistive devices, viewing the device as a symbol of the inability.

Conditions such as central sleep apnea or narcolepsy may interfere with the individual's ability to effectively engage in activities related to work and daily living. In many instances, manifestations of the condition may be misinterpreted by others as laziness, disinterest, or malingering, in turn altering social relationships.

Just as neurological conditions have a spectrum of functional consequences, so the adjustment and adaptation of people experiencing them are highly individualized. Hence individuals with the same condition will not have similar reactions.

Activities and Participation

The effects of conditions such as encephalitis, Bell's palsy, and Lyme disease depend on the presence of any residuals and, if so, the extent and type of activity affected. Conditions such as central sleep apnea and narcolepsy may require alterations in daily schedules and routines or transportation. When fatigue is one of the manifestations, as in central sleep apnea, it may be necessary to space out activities or to arrange for frequent rest periods during the day. It is sometimes helpful to divide activities that were once completed in a short amount of time into a series of subtasks, allowing rest periods between each step.

Many factors associated with conditions of the nervous system can affect social function.

A supportive environment, including family, plays an instrumental role in individuals' response to their condition. Assistive devices, if needed, present visible cues to others that alert them to levels of physical capacity. In some instances, such as in central sleep apnea or narcolepsy, when there are no readily apparent outward manifestations or assistive devices to provide cues, others in the environment may be unaware that limitations of function or activity exist. Misinterpretation or misperception of the individuals' functional ability can negatively affect social interactions and, in turn, influence personal adjustment.

In some cases, manifestations of the condition may be more troublesome to the individual exhibiting the manifestation than to those persons around the individual. For instance, individuals experiencing facial paralysis with Bell's palsy may fear rejection and consequently withdraw from close personal interactions, while friends and family members, willing and anxious to provide help and support, are hurt by what they view as the individual's rejection. In other instances, individuals may assume that others would not want to interact with them because of their condition, when actually they are greatly admired by others because of their ability to cope.

VOCATIONAL ISSUES IN CONDITIONS OF THE NERVOUS SYSTEM

Unless there are residual effects from conditions, vocational function should not be affected after the acute and rehabilitative phases of conditions such as meningitis, Bell's palsy, and Lyme disease. When residual effects are present, vocational function depends on the type and extent of residual effect experienced. In some instances, extended time away from work may be required for recovery and rehabilitation. Each person and his or her specific needs, abilities, and interests should be considered individually.

Conditions such as central sleep apnea and narcolepsy may require alteration in schedule as well as education of employers and coworkers regarding the nature of the condition and specific accommodations that may be needed.

CASE STUDY

Ms. R. is a 50-year-old woman who experienced polio as a child. Residual consequences of polio consisted of weakness in both lower extremities. Today she ambulates using canes and braces. Ms. R. works as a legal secretary in a small metropolitan city. As part of her job, she frequently accompanies her employer to meetings at different locations in the city as well as to court. Recently she has begun experiencing increasing weakness in her lower legs as well as shoulder pain. After consulting her healthcare provider, Ms. R. was told she is experiencing post-polio syndrome.

1. Which specific issues involving post-polio syndrome should Ms. R. consider with regard to her work?
2. Are there accommodations that Mrs. R. would need in her job to enable her to maintain her optimal level of independence? If so, which accommodations may be needed?

REFERENCES

Aksamit, A. J. (2016). Acute viral encephalitis. In L. Goldman & A. I. Schafer (Eds.), *Goldman-Cecil medicine,* (25th ed., pp. 2500–2504). Philadelphia, PA: Elsevier Saunders.

Barateau, L., Lopez, R., & Dauvilliers, Y. (2016). Treatment options for narcolepsy. *CNS Drugs, 30*(5), 369–379.

Freedman, D. O. (2016). Approach to the patient before and after travel. In L. Goldman & A. I. Schafer (Eds.), *Goldman-Cecil medicine,* (25th ed., pp. 1881–1885). Philadelphia, PA: Elsevier Saunders.

Gordon, P. A., & Feldman, D. (2002). Post-polio syndrome: Issues and strategies for rehabilitation counselors. *Journal of Rehabilitation, 68*(2), 28–32.

McNalley, T. E., Yorkston, K. M., Jensen, M. P., Truitt, A. R., Schomer, K. G., Baylor, C., & Molton, I. R. (2015). Review of secondary health conditions in postpolio syndrome: Prevalence and effects of aging. *American Journal of Physical Rehabilitation, 94*(2), 139–145.

Nath, A. (2016). Meningitis: Bacterial, viral, and other. In L. Goldman & A. I. Schafer (Eds.), *Goldman-Cecil medicine,* (25th ed., pp. 2480–2495). Philadelphia, PA: Elsevier Saunders.

Shy, M. E. (2016). Peripheral neuropathies. In L. Goldman & A. I. Schafer (Eds.), *Goldman-Cecil medicine,* (25th ed., pp. 2527–2537). Philadelphia, PA: Elsevier Saunders.

Vaughn, B. V. (2016). Disorders of sleep. In L. Goldman & A. I. Schafer (Eds.), *Goldman-Cecil medicine,* (25th ed., pp. 2415–2424). Philadelphia, PA: Elsevier Saunders.

Whitley, R. J. (2016). Herpes simplex virus infections. In L. Goldman & A. I. Schafer (Eds.), *Goldman-Cecil medicine,* (25th ed., pp. 2223–2227). Philadelphia, PA: Elsevier Saunders.

Willison, H. J., Jacobs, B. C., & van Doom, P. A. (2016). Guillian-Barré syndrome. *Lancet, 388*(10045), 717–727. doi:10.1016/S0140-6736(16)00339-1

Wormser, G. P. (2016). Lyme disease. In L. Goldman & A. I. Schafer (Eds.), *Goldman-Cecil medicine,* (25th ed., pp. 2021–2026). Philadelphia, PA: Elsevier Saunders.

Zimetbaum, P. (2016). Cardiac arrhythmias with supraventricular origin. In L. Goldman & A. I. Schafer (Eds.), *Goldman-Cecil medicine,* (25th ed., pp. 356–367). Philadelphia, PA: Elsevier Saunders.

CHAPTER 11

Developmental Conditions: Cerebral Palsy and Spina Bifida

Revised by Elizabeth Moran Fitzgerald

OVERVIEW OF DEVELOPMENTAL CONDITIONS

Developmental disabilities are a group of conditions due to an impairment in physical, learning, language, or behavior areas (Centers for Disease Control, n.d.a). According to the Centers for Disease Control (CDC), about one in six children in the United States have one or more developmental disabilities or developmental delays. Developmental conditions are those that are present from birth, or shortly afterward, and that persist throughout life. Special needs of individuals with a developmental condition was first acknowledged through passage of the federal law known as the *Mental Retardation Facilities Construction Act of 1963 (PL 106-442),* which provided for federal support for centers and services for children and adults with mental retardation. Later, other conditions, including cerebral palsy, epilepsy, autism, and other neurological conditions, were added to the scope of coverage.

The term *developmental disability* came into use with passage of the *Developmental Disabilities Act of 1975 (PL 94-103).* This term replaced diagnostic categories (such as mental retardation or cerebral palsy) with a general term that encompassed a wide variety of conditions that occur in childhood, are lifelong, affect intellectual or physical functioning, and require ongoing special services and support.

Although categorizing an individual as having a developmental disability provided guidance for assessment, management of manifestations, or eligibility for services, unfortunately it also created a basis for labeling, stereotyping, discrimination, and segregation. In an attempt to avoid such pitfalls, the *Developmental Disabilities Assistance and Bill of Rights Act of 1990* emphasized functional capacity rather than categorizations and stressed empowerment of individuals with developmental disabilities (McLaughlin & Wehman, 1996). Over the years, there has been a major transformation in how developmental conditions are conceptualized, moving from the *medical model* to conceptualization based on the *social model*, which focuses on enhancing opportunities and providing support for individuals with developmental conditions to help them achieve independence, productivity, and integration and inclusion into the community.

The *Developmental Disabilities Assistance and Bill of Rights Act of 2000* (Public Law 106-402) defines developmental disability as follows:

A severe chronic disability of an individual that:

a) is attributable to mental or physical impairment or combination of mental and physical impairment;

b) is manifested before the individual attains the age of 22;

c) is likely to continue indefinitely;

d) results in substantial functional limitations in three or more of the following areas of major life activity: self-care, receptive and expressive language, learning, mobility, self-direction, capacity for independent living, and economic self-sufficiency;

e) reflects the individual's need for a combination and sequence of special, interdisciplinary, or generic services; individualized support; or other forms of assistance that are of lifelong or extended duration and are individually planned and coordinated.

Although the causes and characteristics of specific developmental disabilities vary, a common feature of developmental disabilities is limitation in one or more areas of function:

• Speech or language
• Attention or affect
• Cognitive or learning ability
• Self-direction or social behavior
• Motor skills and mobility
• Self-care and independence

Of course, many of the needs and concerns of individuals with developmental conditions are the same as those of individuals without specific conditions. The Developmental Disabilities Act, however, is a law that was enacted to provide support and enhance quality of life of those individuals with developmental conditions. A major focus when working with individuals with developmental conditions is identifying specific needs, developing strategies that minimize the degree of incapacitation experienced, and providing necessary supports to enhance functional capacity. Although the family is an important factor when working with individuals with any incapacitating condition, family is especially important in the case of individuals with a developmental condition.

Developmental disability encompasses a wide range of intellectual and physical conditions, such as autism, muscular dystrophy, and sickle cell anemia. This chapter focuses on two of the more common developmental conditions that affect physical function:

• Cerebral palsy
• Spina bifida

CEREBRAL PALSY
Overview of Cerebral Palsy

According to *A report: The definition and classification of cerebral palsy 2006* (2007), the following definition of cerebral palsy was agreed upon: "Cerebral palsy (CP) describes a group of permanent disorders of the development of movement and posture, causing activity limitation, that are attributed to non-progressive disturbances that occurred in the developing fetal or infant brain. The motor disorders of cerebral palsy are often accompanied by disturbances of sensation, perception, cognition, communication, and behavior, by epilepsy, and by secondary musculoskeletal problems." (p. 9). The aforementioned definition emphasizes that CP involves a variety of disorders caused by various factors acting at different points in fetal development. The definition also emphasizes the importance of comorbidities that accompany the orthopedic and neurologic manifestations of CP (Rethlefsen, Ryan, & Kay, 2010). It is the most common major disabling motor disorder of childhood (Rosenblaum et al., 2008). No two individuals with cerebral palsy have exactly the same manifestations. The type of cerebral palsy and the manifestations experienced depend on the location and the extent of the injury to the brain. Whereas some individuals have minor, barely detectable manifestations, others experience significant functional manifestations.

Deaths in children with CP have become very rare in recent years due to advances in neonatal care and increased survival rates for preterm and low birth weight infants. Unless the child with CP has very severe disabilities, he/she will likely survive into adulthood (Haak, Lenski, Hidecker, Li, & Paneth, 2009).

In many instances, the exact cause of cerebral palsy is unknown. Other potential causes of cerebral palsy vary widely and can include the following:

Prenatal (before birth)
  ♦ Exposure of the mother to toxic chemicals or infectious conditions during pregnancy.
  ♦ Rh or ABO blood type incompatibility between mother and fetus, such that the mother's immune system produces antibodies that destroy the fetus's red blood cells.

Usually testing during the prenatal period identifies Rh or blood type incompatibility so that early intervention can be instituted.

♦ Lack of oxygen to the brain of the fetus before birth due to conditions such as umbilical cord strangulation, premature separation of the placenta from the uterus, or prolonged labor (which stresses the fetus).

Perinatal (during and shortly after the birth process)

♦ Birth trauma in which the infant's skull is injured during delivery.
♦ Fetal **anoxia** (lack of oxygen).

Postnatal (after birth)

♦ Traumatic brain injury, such as in infant abuse.
♦ Meningitis, encephalitis, or other infections.
♦ Exposure to toxic chemicals.
♦ Anoxia due to situations such as drowning or carbon monoxide poisoning.

Classification of Cerebral Palsy

In 2001, the World Health Organization (WHO) published the International Classification of Functioning, Disability, and Health (ICF) to standardize health and disability data worldwide (WHO, 2001). The ICF describes disability as dysfunction at one or more of three levels: *impairment* of body structures (for example, organs or limbs) or functions (physiologic or psychological), limitations in *activities*, and restriction of *participation* (involvement in life situations). *A Report: The Definition and Classification of Cerebral Palsy 2006* (p. 12, 2007) stated that a classification system must be reliable in order to be useful. The report outlined the components of CP classification to include the following: (1) Motor abnormalities; (2) accompanying impairments; (3) anatomical and neuro-imaging findings; and (4) causation and timing.

Classification of Impairments

Motor Abnormalities

According to Delgado and Albright (2003), 80% of children with CP have some type of movement disorder. Motor abnormalities should be operationally defined to include the nature and typology of the motor disorder, including tonal abnormalities and movement disorders. The individual's functional motor abilities and limitations in motor function should also be described (*Report*, 2007, p. 12).

Cerebral palsy is most frequently classified as either spastic, dyskinetic, or ataxic (Horstmann & Beck, 2007).

• *Hypertonia*, which is defined as "abnormally increased resistance to externally imposed movement about a joint" (Sanger, Delgado, Gaebler-Spira, Hallet, & Mink, 2003). It can be caused by spasticity, dystonia, or rigidity. Hypertonia in patients with CP is most frequently rated using the Modified Ashworth Scale (MAS) (Bohannon & Smith, 1987) or the Tardieu Scale (Boyd & Graham, 1999).

• *Spasticity* is hypertonia in which resistance to passive movement increases with increasing velocity of movement. Spasticity varies with direction of the movement (Sanger et al., 2003). It is caused by a hyperactive stretch reflex mechanism. Treatments which may reduce spasticity include botulinum toxin, baclofen, selective dorsal rhizotomy, and orthopaedic surgery (Rethlefsen et al., 2010).

• *Dystonia* is defined as "a movement disorder in which involuntary sustained or intermittent muscle contractions cause twisting and repetitive movements, abnormal posture, or both" (Sanger et al., 2003). When dystonic movements are present at rest and do not relax upon attempts at passive movement, they cause hypotonia. Dystonia can also be classified as hyperkinetic.

• *Hyperkinetic movements* are defined as "any unwanted excess movement" (Sanger et al., 2010) performed voluntarily or involuntarily by the patient, and represent what had been referred to as extrapyramidal symptoms. In individuals with CP, the most common hyperkinetic movements include dystonia, chorea, athetosis, and tremors.

Topography or Limb Distribution

The traditional classifications of limb distribution for patients with the hypertonic (primarily spastic) form of CP continue to be used clinically in some countries and include the following:

- hemiplegia (manifestations are found on only one side of the body, such as an arm and a leg on the right side)
- diplegia (all extremities are affected, but lower extremities are more severely affected)
- quadriplegia/tertraplegia (manifestations affect all four extremities)
- triplegia (three limbs are involved)

However, according to data from Surveillance of Cerebral Palsy in Europe (2000), the aforementioned classifications have been shown to have poor interrater reliability (Rethlefsen et al., 2010). The lack of definition of how much upper extremity impairment is needed to classify patients with CP as quadriplegic versus diplegic leads to inconsistencies between raters. Furthermore, according to Rethlefsen et al., children with hemiplegia often have some motor signs on the contralateral side, which could place them in a category of asymmetric, diplegia, quadriplegia, or triplegia. Consequently, some experts recommend abandonment of these labels and advocate for simplified classifications such as unilateral or bilateral, with an indication of upper and lower extremity function (*Report*, 2007; Bax et al., 2005). According to experts (*Report*, 2007), if the traditional terms (e.g., diplegia, quadriplegia, and hemiplegia) continue to be used, then a complete description of the motor impairments in all body regions or a limb-by-limb description of motor impairment and tonal abnormalities seen in each limb are recommended.

Classification of Activity Limitation

Gross Motor Function Classification

In the past, patients' gross motor functional limitations were categorized as mild, moderate, or severe. However, the literature suggests that such terms were not standardized or validated and therefore merely provided information about the patient's ambulatory function. Rosenbaum and colleagues introduced a new classification system for gross motor function in children with CP, the Gross Motor Function Classification System (GMFCS) (Rosenbaum, Palisano, Bartlett, Galuppi, & Russell, 2008).

The GMFCS rated patients' ambulatory function, including use of mobility aids, and performance in sitting, standing, and walking. The limitations of the original GMFCS have been addressed in an updated version of the scale, the GMFCS-Expanded and Revised (GMFCS-ER) (Palisano, Rosembaum, Bartlett, & Livingston, 2008), which has been demonstrated to be valid and reliable in multiple studies (Jahnsen, Aamodt, & Rosembaum, 2006; McCormick et al., 2007; McDowell, Kerr, & Parkes, 2007; Palisano et al., 2008). The GMFCS-ER includes children up to 18 years of age. It also incorporates aspects of the ICH and recognizes that a child's environment may affect gross motor performance. The GMFCS-ER classifies a patient's level of gross motor function based on his/her typical performance rather than best capability. It classifies gross motor function on a 5-point scale with descriptions of skills for various age groups. The levels are:

Level I: Walks without limitations
Level II: Walks with limitations
Level III: Walks using a hand-held mobility device
Level IV: Self-mobility with limitations; may use powered mobility
Level V: Transported in a manual wheelchair

Functional Mobility Scale

Graham, Harvey, Rodda, Nattrass, and Pirpiris (2004) designed the Functional Mobility Scale (FMS) as a measure of ambulatory performance in children with CP. This scale recognizes that children may demonstrate different ambulatory abilities and use different assistive devices to walk varying distances (Rethlefsen et al., 2010). The scale is administered by patient/parent interview. Since this scale focuses on ambulation, it is not intended as a substitute for the GMFCS-ER.

Manual Ability Classification System

The Manual Ability Classification System (MACS) was developed to describe upper extremity performance in activities of daily living for children with CP (Eliasson et al., 2006). Similar to the GMFCS-ER, the MACS acknowledges that upper-limb function is influenced by personal, environmental, and contextual factors. The scale reports on performance of upper-limb tasks in activities of daily living (ADL), regardless of how these activities are accomplished. It is a 5-category scale intended to apply to children of all ages and has been found to be reliable and valid (Eliasson et al., 2006; Morris, Kurinczuk, Fitzpatrick, & Rosenbaum, 2006; Plasschaert, Ketelaar, Ninjnuis, Enkelarr, & Gorter, 2009). The levels of the scale are described at www.macs.nu and are as follows:

> Level I: Handles objects easily and successfully
> Level II: Handles most objects but with somewhat reduced quality or speed of achievement
> Level III: Handles objects with difficulty; needs help to prepare or modify activities
> Level IV: Handles a limited selection of easily managed objects in adapted situations
> Level V: Does not handle objects and has severely limited ability to perform even simple actions

Rethlefsen et al., (2010) note that both the GMFCS-ER and the MACS have improved the description of gross motor and manual abilities in patients with CP. However, these experts note that neither scale identifies the cause of activity limitation. These scales are helpful to categorize the child's ability to function in daily life.

Communication Function Classification

The Communication Function Classification System (CFCS, www.cfcs.us) was initially developed to address the paucity of information in the literature on the communication skills of patients with CP. However, now the CFCS is being used to describe communication performance of individuals with any disability (Hidecker et al., 2011). The intent of the CFCS is to provide a quick and simple instrument to help parents and clinicians understand how different communication environments, tasks, and partners affect communication as well as to help the individual to set goals to enhance communication. The CFCS is designed as a 5-level classification system (CFCS I, II, III, IV, and V) modeled after the GMFCS and MACS. The CFCS provides a valid and reliable classification of communication performance and activity limitations that can be used by researchers and clinicians. Regardless of the type or classification of cerebral palsy experienced, interventions and training programs can help individuals manage manifestations and increase functional capacity. Consequently, management is designed to enhance individuals' abilities and foster independence. The new classification tools will help clinicians to communicate more effectively and enhance their ability to evaluate interventions, thereby improving the quality of life for persons with CP.

Identification of Cerebral Palsy

Manifestations of cerebral palsy may not be immediately recognizable after birth but rather may be identified months or sometimes even years later, when the child's development appears to be delayed. Motor development and language development occur in an orderly series of stages that lead to increased independence. When milestones in these stages of development are not reached, investigation of causes for delay are usually explored. Parents of the child may be the first to seek evaluation because of concerns regarding their child's developmental delays.

There is no definitive test that confirms or rules out cerebral palsy. A thorough health history; evaluation of specific manifestations including reflexes, muscle tone, and posture; a full neurological examination; and ruling out other causes for developmental delay are mainstays in identification of cerebral palsy. Although sometimes the specific cause may be identified, often it is not.

Manifestations of Cerebral Palsy

Depending on the part of the brain affected, cerebral palsy is characterized by *irregularities of movement,* including alterations in the following aspects:

- Muscle tone
- Muscle control
- Posture (Gold & Salsberg, 2011)

Movement Irregularities

Spasticity is one of the most common manifestations and is characterized by exaggerated muscle tone resulting in muscle stiffness and strong muscle contraction. Spasticity interferes with dexterity and the ability to perform various muscle movements. In addition to affecting mobility, spastic contraction of muscle groups can be a source of pain.

Ataxia (inability to control the accuracy of muscle movement) may be experienced by some individuals with cerebral palsy. In walking, ataxia affects balance and coordination, causing inaccurate foot placement and readjustment of position, resulting in a staggering gait. In the upper extremities, ataxia may result in overshooting or uncertain aim when reaching or grasping.

Other irregularity in movements that some individuals may experience affects the ability to conduct purposeful movements or causes movement when none is desired. Individuals may have one or a combination of the following types of movement irregularity:

- **Chorea**: purposeless, jerky, or abrupt movements, especially of the upper extremities
- **Athetosis**: slow, continuous writhing movements
- **Choreoathetosis**: combination of chorea and athetosis

Some individuals may have a combination of spasticity, ataxia, or irregularity of voluntary muscle movement. In rare instances, **atonia**, in which there is lack of muscle tone and muscles are flaccid, may be present.

Other Manifestations

Although cerebral palsy primarily affects muscle control and movement, the brain is responsible for many other activities as well. Consequently, depending on the parts of the brain affected, manifestations of cerebral palsy may include the following issues:

- Alteration of vision
- Alteration in hearing
- Communication difficulties
- Seizures
- Alteration of intellectual ability
- Learning difficulties
- Behavioral difficulties
- Bowel or bladder difficulties (Odding, Roebroeck, & Stam, 2006)

Vision may be affected if there is injury to the part of the brain that interprets visual images or from weakness of muscles responsible for eye movement. Manifestations of visual alterations may include changes in visual acuity, in which there is blurring of vision, **myopia** (nearsightedness), or **hyperopia** (farsightedness). Individuals may also experience visual field difficulty, such **hemianopsia**, in which only half of the visual field is perceived; *peripheral loss,* in which images at the periphery of the visual field are not perceived; or *central loss,* in which objects in the central field of vision are not perceived. Some individuals may demonstrate *oculomotor* difficulties, in which there is difficulty with muscles controlling movement of the eye, resulting in problems with depth perception or manifestations such as **strabismus** (eye misalignment, or "crossed eyes") or **amblyopia** (lazy eye). In some instances, the portion of the brain responsible for interpreting visual images has been injured so that although the eye itself is unaffected, individuals are unable to fully process or interpret visual information.

Likewise, *hearing* may be affected if the portion of the brain responsible for processing sound is injured. In this case, the injury to a portion of the brain blocks auditory pathways, causing severe hearing loss. In other instances, individuals may be able to hear sounds, but may be unable to interpret auditory input. Hearing difficulties may not be immediately identified in persons with cerebral palsy because of the focus on motor difficulties, which are more easily recognizable.

Language development is related to hearing acuity; consequently, any loss in hearing may affect the individual's ability to learn and interpret language. *Speech* may also be affected if injury to the brain affects muscles used for forming words, resulting in **dysarthria** (difficulty with coordination and accuracy of movement of the lips, tongue, or other parts of the speech mechanism).

Seizures are a common manifestation of cerebral palsy and differ depending on the part of the brain involved (Carlsson, Hagberg, & Olsson, 2003). Seizures result from irregular and excessive nerve impulses from certain areas of the brain. When seizures are experienced in cerebral palsy, they may be either generalized or partial.

Intellectual disability is defined as difficulty in both intellectual and adaptive function. Although individuals with cerebral palsy experience a higher incidence of intellectual difficulties than the general population (Taylor & Kopriva, 2002), many have average or above-average cognitive function (Whaley & Wong, 1995). Unfortunately, due to their altered physical appearance and often difficulty with speech and language, individuals with cerebral palsy may be assumed to have less than average intelligence when no cognitive difficulty is present. When intellectual difficulties are present, manifestations range from mild to severe.

Learning difficulties alter the affected individual's ability to acquire or use information through sources such as reading, writing, mathematical calculations, listening, speaking, or reasoning. In cerebral palsy, if present, these issues may be a direct result of intellectual difficulties, or they may be associated with other manifestations such as hearing loss, behavioral problems, or social delay.

Although not all individuals with cerebral palsy experience *behavioral difficulties*, behavioral problems are more prevalent in children with cerebral palsy than in those without chronic health conditions and are more frequent when intellectual disability is also present (McDermott et al., 1996). Behavioral difficulties may result from frustration due to difficulty with completing tasks, inability to communicate effectively, or emotional reactions to external events. Behavioral difficulties can also result from a secondary condition such as *attention-deficit/hyperactivity disorder* or *autism*.

Bowel or bladder problems may be present in some individuals. When present, urinary incontinence may be a direct result of neural damage, or it may result from the inability to attend or respond to sensations indicating the need to urinate or defecate. In other cases, it may be the result of individuals being unable to reach toilet facilities in a timely fashion. Bowel problems more often experienced in the form of constipation, which may be related to insufficient fluid or bulk in the diet.

Although not a manifestation per se, *fatigue* may affect functional capacity. Due to difficulty with motor control and coordination, muscle spasms, and possible involuntary movement, individuals with cerebral palsy may experience greater energy expenditure as they perform everyday tasks, resulting in fatigue. Evaluation of individuals' total energy output and adjustment of tasks and schedule to fit individual needs can help preserve energy and prevent excessive fatigue. Adequate rest at night and establishment of rest periods throughout the day can decrease fatigue.

Complications of Cerebral Palsy

Cerebral palsy is a lifelong condition. Although the condition itself is not progressive, over time its manifestations can precipitate a variety of complications secondary to the cerebral palsy that can alter functional capacity or well-being (Sandstrom, 2007). The best management of complications is through prevention. Specific complications may include the following conditions:

- **Contractures** (loss of range of motion or fixation of a joint) result from the hyperactive stretch reflexes found in spasticity. As a result, muscle shortening occurs that limits the joint's range of motion. Joints of both the lower and upper extremities may be affected. Contractures can seriously affect individuals' functional capacity in terms of walking, siting, and self-care. Contractures can be prevented through regular passive exercise, bracing or splinting, or surgical intervention such as tendon lengthening.
- **Scoliosis** (lateral curvature of the spine) may also be present. It is usually the result of uneven muscle pull on one part of the spine, often due to poorly supported sitting posture. Scoliosis not only affects mobility but can also cause limited respiratory function, which in turn contributes to additional complications. Training that helps individuals increase posture control or use of orthotic devices that help postural alignment can prevent or lessen scoliosis.
- *Dental problems* may be present, such as **dental caries** (tooth decay) or **gingival hyperplasia** (gum overgrowth). Dental problems are sometimes due to prenatal causes or side effects of medications, but more often reflect difficulty with performing adequate oral hygiene. Training on the importance of proper oral hygiene and regular dental care, appropriate brushing techniques, and (perhaps) toothbrush adaptations are important interventions to prevent dental complications.

- **Osteoporosis** (reduction in bone mass) and **osteopenia** (diminished bone tissue) are common in individuals with cerebral palsy (Houlihan & Stevenson, 2009). Decreased bone density can lead to fractures that can limit functional capacity. Factors such as immobilization, side effects of medicine, or inadequate dietary sources of vitamin D and calcium can contribute to lessened bone density. A specific program of weight-bearing and muscle activity as well as consumption of a diet adequate in calcium can help to prevent osteoporosis and osteopenia.
- *Respiratory infections* in individuals with cerebral palsy may be life threatening as well as incapacitating. Scoliosis, which compromises the ability to fully ventilate the lungs and aspiration of food into the lungs due to difficulty with swallowing are both factors that contribute to the potential for respiratory infection. Training that helps individuals improve breathing patterns and lung expansion, education on techniques for coughing to remove mucus, and institution of interventions to prevent scoliosis and facilitate swallowing can all decrease the chances of developing respiratory infection.

Degenerative joint disease may develop in individuals with cerebral palsy. Although cerebral palsy is not a progressive or degenerative condition, increasing functional impairment may be evident throughout life (Ando & Ueda, 2000). In one study, 35% of the adults with cerebral palsy reported reduced walking ability, and 9% had stopped walking completely (Andersson & Mattsson, 2001). Poorly aligned joints may predispose individuals to degenerative joint disease, resulting in pain and increased immobility. Reducing stress on joints, proper alignment, and regular exercise can help to maintain walking ability and decrease chances of developing degenerative joint disease (Andersson, Asztalos, & Mattsson, 2006).

Management of Cerebral Palsy

Interventions begin at an early age in individuals with cerebral palsy and continue throughout life as needs change. Health care transition (HCT) describes the purposeful movement of adolescents from child to adult-oriented care (Carroll, 2015). Nurses and other health care professionals can serve as advocates, mentors, and guides to help the individual with CP and his/her family through the transition process. The type of intervention used at any one time depends on the specific needs and manifestations of the individual at his or her particular life stage. Management is directed toward helping individuals reach their optimal functional capacity by providing functional supports based on specific manifestations and preventing complications that could interfere with functional capacity. All aspects of management plans should be directed toward giving individuals the opportunity to control and manage their own situation as much as possible. Major goals of management often include maintenance of range of motion of joints to prevent contractures and other joint irregularities and increasing muscle control and coordination to counteract irregular postures. In addition, environmental modifications that facilitate the ability to perform activities of self-care, increase mobility, and enhance social function are important to achievement of optimal functioning (Ostensjo, Carlberg, & Vollestad, 2005).

Specific Management Interventions

- Physical therapy is used in cerebral palsy to restore, maintain, or promote optimal movement and to increase and enhance motor skills and balance. Depending on the extent to which mobility is affected, physical therapists may also help individuals to effectively use assistive devices such as a cane, walker, or wheelchair.
- Occupational therapy helps individuals enhance their ability to function at home, school, in public settings, and at work. Through the use of occupational therapy, individuals learn techniques and strategies to manage activities of daily living and other daily functions. An occupational therapist can help to secure items that may be of help in reaching this goal and train individuals in their use. For instance, a number of modifications, such as Velcro-fastened footwear or Velcro fasteners instead of zippers for ease of dressing may

help individuals achieve greater independence. Other assistive technologies such as remote-controlled appliances and devices may also be useful.

- Orthotics, such as braces or splints, may be used to prevent or correct joint irregularities. Braces or splints can accommodate weakness and instability, and can prevent complications such as contractures by maintaining regular positioning of a joint. Hence, they help improve both functional mobility and appearance. The type of brace or splint selected depends on the type of physical manifestation experienced.

- Medications may be used as an intervention for specific manifestations. For instance, *anticonvulsant medications* may be used if seizures are experienced. *Tone-altering medications* may also be used if excessive muscle spasticity or excessive muscle tone is present. Intramuscular injections of *botulinum A toxin* have been used with some success in temporary reduction of spasticity (Gold & Salsberg, 2011). *Muscle relaxants* such as *baclofen* may also be used to reduce spasticity and tremor.

- Surgical interventions are sometimes indicated for specific manifestations. Orthopedic surgery may be indicated for correction of joint irregularities, such as contractures, that interfere with functional ability. Orthopedic surgery may also be indicated to help spasticity by releasing tight muscles or by lengthening muscles or tendons. Orthopedic surgery is not routinely used to manage spasticity unless spasticity adversely affects function or causes pain, and it appears that surgical intervention will bring about improvement. Neurosurgical procedures may also be used in some instances. A procedure called *selective rhizotomy* (cutting of sensory nerves) may be used to reduce spasticity or treat pain, especially in the lower extremities. Another neurosurgical procedure, insertion of an *intrathecal baclofen pump,* may be used to help spasticity. In this procedure, a pump containing the muscle relaxant medication baclofen is placed under the skin of the abdomen. A needle is then inserted into the spinal fluid and a tube attached to the pump, which gradually releases baclofen. This procedure is typically used when oral muscle relaxants have proved ineffective in relieving spasticity.

- Speech or language therapy may be used if individuals have communication difficulties. Alternative and augmentative communication (AAC) devices are important to promote language development and participation in home, school, and community environments. The American Speech-Language Hearing Association defines an AAC aid as either an electronic or nonelectronic device that is used by an individual to send and receive messages (2004). A wide range of device options exist, including pictures in a book, switches with a single message voice output, complex electronic voice output devices, and iPads (Desai, Chow, Mumford, Hotze, & Chau, 2014). The selection of the most appropriate device can be complex and consultation with a speech-language pathologist is important in the selection of a AAC device. Effective training of the AAC user, parents, teachers, and other family members as well as ongoing support from facilitators and communication partners results in more positive outcomes and lessens the risk for abandonment of the AAC device. The incorporation of AAC devices in the individual's classroom also may improve academic activities (Stasolla et al., 2015).

Speech and language pathologists can also assist with difficulty with chewing or swallowing which in turn can affect nutritional status as well as increase the risk of aspiration and subsequent development of complications such as pneumonia. Speech or language therapists can also assist individuals to learn strategies that improve chewing and swallowing. If difficulty with eating is attributable to spasticity or involuntary movement, special adaptive eating utensils may be used.

- *Audiology* may be necessary if hearing is affected, as hearing is important for full development of language skills, and decreased hearing ability can lead to learning difficulties. Hearing loss may be assessed by an audiologist, and in some instances hearing aids may be used to amplify sounds.

- *Ophthalmology* or *optometry* health professionals may be consulted if visual difficulties are present. Vision affects many aspects of function, and reading in particular. For some types of visual difficulties, glasses may be of use. In other instances, modification of reading material through size of print, wider spacing of letters and words, or contrast of background may be useful. In other instances, computer programs for reading that place one word at a time on the screen and reduce need for fast eye movement, thereby reducing tiredness, may be needed. In the case of eye difficulties due to muscle involvement, such as strabismus, surgery may be indicated.

- *Nutritional and dietary counseling* may be recommended if nutrition or gastrointestinal issues are of concern. Nutritional and dietary counseling can help individuals learn how to adjust their diet and intake so that adequate nutrition is maintained and specific dietary problems such as constipation are avoided.

- *Bowel and bladder training* can help individuals learn to manage evacuation difficulties. Training programs help individuals establish dietary control and a regular evacuation schedule. Training programs can also help individuals increase awareness of sensory stimuli that indicate a need for evacuation. In addition, modification of clothing, such as use of Velcro strips in place of zippers, can increase ease of using toilet facilities.

- *Behavioral therapy, recreational therapy, and social skills training* are other interventions that can be used. *Behavioral therapy* identifies triggers of problem behaviors and helps individuals learn techniques and strategies to change them. *Recreational therapy* helps individuals exercise physical and mental skills and provides stimulation and opportunity for socialization. *Social skills training* helps individuals develop and enhance social skills that enable them to respond appropriately to people and situations.

Functional Implications of Cerebral Palsy

Personal and Psychosocial Issues

Individuals' function evolves as they mature. Chronic conditions or incapacity in childhood has implications for the psychosocial well-being of both the individual and his or her family throughout their life (Barlow & Ellard, 2006). Individuals with cerebral palsy go through the same developmental stages and phases as individuals without cerebral palsy. Meeting and accomplishing the tasks of each stage of development is important to maturation.

Although data regarding psychosocial adjustment of adults with cerebral palsy are limited, cerebral palsy as a developmental condition poses many of the same problems as other developmental disabilities. Misunderstanding of the condition by parents, teachers, or others with whom individuals with cerebral palsy come in contact can perpetuate a sick and dependent status rather than a sense of empowerment. How individuals with cerebral palsy were treated in childhood can influence their self-perception and functioning in adulthood. In particular, childhood conditions can influence body image and prevent affected individuals from becoming involved in social relationships (Cho, 2004).

With any type of developmental condition, there is the risk of overprotectiveness from parents and others, which can impede emotional development by restricting access to experiences that are vital to the development of adequate coping strategies. As a result, children may learn, at an early age, to use maladaptive behavior to achieve goals. If this behavior continues into adulthood, it may impede the ability to integrate effectively into the larger social milieu. When children have been kept overly dependent on parents, have been given little responsibility for home chores, have not been confronted with typical consequences of behavior, or have not learned acceptable means of expressing emotions, their lack of experience and mature social development can serve as an incapacitating factor in adulthood.

In other instances, children who have been the focus of a wide variety of services and activities from an early age may continue these expectations into adulthood, demonstrating a sense of egocentricity, which in turn may limit positive social interactions and lead to further social isolation. If these behaviors persist into adulthood, they may become more of an impediment to social integration than any manifestations of the condition itself. In some individuals, brain damage associated with cerebral palsy may create behavior deficits that can interfere with development and maintenance of social relationships. Caron and Light (2016) have noted that adults with cerebral palsy face barriers to social media use yet want to overcome barriers and learn to use social media to enhance their communication competence. They encourage professionals to expand the use of AAC practice to help individuals with cerebral palsy learn to use social media to help them develop interpersonal communication skills.

Activities and Participation

Communication issues for individuals with cerebral palsy may include hearing or auditory comprehension problems, visual incapacity, or speech difficulties. Individuals with communication problems as the result of cerebral palsy may have grown up in an environment in which family, friends, and others became accustomed to their adaptive communication methods. In adulthood, when relationships change and higher standards of performance are expected, communication may then become increasingly difficult. For instance, those persons unfamiliar with the individual or with cerebral palsy itself may misinterpret problems with hearing or unintelligible speech as lack of cognitive ability. In other instances, because the individual may be difficult to understand, acquaintances may avoid interactions with the individual so that he or she becomes socially isolated. Depending on the severity and type of cerebral palsy, decreased mobility, problems with eating, or problems with personal hygiene may further restrict the individual's social interactions.

Although life expectancy for individuals with a variety of health conditions has, in the past, been less than the life expectancy for the general population, awareness of the importance of preventing complications and advances in health care have expanded the number of adults with cerebral palsy living into older age. Older individuals with cerebral palsy experience many of the same issues

as older adults without cerebral palsy, but recent studies have shown that older adults with cerebral palsy experience more loneliness than other adults in the older-age category (Balandin, Berg, & Waller, 2006). In some instances, increasing levels of dependency due to the aging process and possible relocation due to a change in the individual's ability or a caregiver's inability to continue giving care may contribute to loneliness if the separation necessitates separation from family or friends. Encouraging individuals to develop leisure and recreational activities can facilitate social networking and provide opportunities for developing new friendships, although frequent contact alone does not necessarily protect one from loneliness (Balandin et al., 2006). Although there may be a tendency to provide individuals with cerebral palsy the opportunity for social involvement through specialized services or organizations, involvement in community-integrated activities can facilitate social communication as a way to prevent loneliness, provide for development of friendships, and enhance the individual's sense of personal control (Ballin & Balandin, 2005).

Sexuality

Positive peer interactions in childhood are associated with a number of developmental benefits, but individuals with a congenital condition may not have the same opportunities for developing positive relationships and may consequently be at increased risk for social difficulties (Cunningham, Thomas, & Warschausky, 2007). As adolescents, opportunities to participate in social activities, obtain information related to sexuality, and engage in sexual exploration and relationships may have been limited for individuals with cerebral palsy. Although specific physical limitations and barriers may be associated with sexual activity among such persons, the largest barrier to establishing social and sexual relationships may be related to lack of information or resources (Wiegerink, Roebroeck, Donkervoort, Stam, & Cohen-Kettenis, 2006). In addition, adolescents with cerebral palsy may have a distorted body image and lowered self-concept, which may negatively affect their social competence, dating, and sexual behavior. Although individuals with cerebral palsy experience normal desires as both adolescents and adults, they may lack the skills necessary to fulfill those needs. In addition to barriers of inadequate information, skill, or opportunity for appropriate sexual expression, individuals with cerebral palsy may experience physical barriers because of their condition that make sexual expression more difficult.

Vocational Issues in Cerebral Palsy

Cerebral palsy is not a progressive condition, and progressive deterioration does not occur as a direct result of the cerebral palsy itself. Cerebral palsy is, however, a lifelong condition. Consequently, follow-up throughout the individual's life may be necessary. As individuals age with their condition, additional limitations may occur. For instance, fatigue is a consideration for individuals with cerebral palsy regardless of their age. As individuals become older, however, endurance for the same activities over time may be decreased.

Long-term goals for individuals with cerebral palsy are appropriate and desirable. The degree to which individuals are able to achieve their goals in a specified occupation will depend on their physical, psychosocial, and language abilities, as well as their motivation and social support networks. Specific skills and abilities may be enhanced with compensatory measures or practice. Given that functional limitations associated with cerebral palsy are individualized, specific vocational implications will depend on the manifestations that each individual experiences. In some instances, verbal communication is severely impaired; in other cases, it may be totally unaffected. Some individuals may have limited mobility or ambulation problems, whereas others may have significant difficulty with mobility or ambulation. While some individuals will be ambulatory, others may require use of a wheelchair. In some instances, individuals may have difficulty concentrating or remembering; in other instances, individuals' cognitive abilities are unaffected.

Because most jobs require some degree of social skill, when individuals have difficulty in this area, social skills training may be of benefit (Salkever, 2000). Matching the work setting to the individual's specific needs, interests, and abilities

is important in any health condition; however, in the case of cerebral palsy, attention to these factors may be even more important to increase the potential for vocational success. The Vocational Rehabilitation (VR) program http://dds.dc.gov/service/vocational-rehabilitation-services is an excellent resource. Once eligibility has been established, a VR counselor helps individuals prepare for, gain, and retain employment and offers vocational and rehabilitative services through the establishment of an Individualized Plan for Employment (IPE).

SPINA BIFIDA

Spina bifida (SB) is the second most common complex disability of childhood after cerebral palsy (Young, Anselmo, Burke, McCormick, & Mukherjee, 2014). As a result of advances in health care, 90% of children with SB are living into adulthood (Kinsman & Doehring, 1996; Webb, 2009). Spina bifida is one of several congenital conditions, collectively known as *neural tube defects,* which involve incomplete development of the brain, spinal cord, or coverings of these structures. Other neural tube defects include *anencephaly,* in which infants are born with underdeveloped brains and incomplete skulls, and *encephalocele,* in which infants are born with a hole in the skull through which brain tissue protrudes. In most cases, infants with either of the latter conditions do not survive or, if they do, they experience severe intellectual incapacitation.

Spina bifida does not involve the brain but rather the spinal column. In this condition, one or more vertebrae are left open so that the spinal cord is exposed.

Types of Spina Bifida

Three types of spina bifida are distinguished (see **Figure 11-1**):

- **Spina bifida occulta** refers to an opening in one or more vertebrae of the spinal column. The mildest form of spina bifida, it does not involve any damage to the spinal cord. Many individuals with this form of spina bifida may be unaware that their condition even exists.

Figure 11-1 Types of Spina Bifida

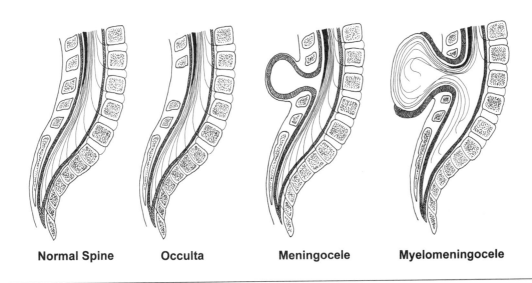

Normal Spine   **Occulta**   **Meningocele**   **Myelomeningocele**

© Jane Tinkler Lamm.

- **Meningocele** refers to a more serious type of spina bifida. In this form of the condition, the **meninges** (the protective covering around the spinal cord) protrude through the opening in the spinal column. The protruding part, called a meningocele, contains only the meninges, not portions of the spinal cord. In some cases, surgery can correct this problem so there is little or no damage to the nerves of the spinal cord. In other instances, individuals with a meningocele may have residual effects resulting from spinal cord damage.

- **Myelomeningocele**, the most common and most severe form of spina bifida, is a condition in which nerves of the spinal cord as well as the meninges protrude through the opening of the vertebrae to the outer part of the body. Because there is no protective covering of the skin, spinal fluid may leak from the protrusion and the risk of infection is great. When this defect occurs, it usually results in **paraplegia** (paralysis of the lower extremities) as well as poor bladder and bowel control. Although surgery is usually

performed immediately to correct the defect, the paralysis of the lower extremities usually persists.

Manifestations of Spina Bifida

Manifestations of spina bifida depend on the type, the part of the spinal cord affected, and the severity of the condition. The severity can range from mild, in which there are few if any manifestations, to severe, which is characterized by muscle paralysis, loss of sensation, and loss of bowel and bladder control. Many children with the severe type of spina bifida also experience **hydrocephalus**, a condition in which fluid builds up in the brain. In these cases, surgical implantation of a *shunt* is necessary so that the fluid can be drained to prevent excessive pressure to the brain. If hydrocephalus is not corrected, cognitive incapacitation can result.

Because spina bifida is congenital, more severe forms of the condition may impinge on motor development. Depending on the social, economic, and psychological circumstances of the individual and the resources available to him or her, cognitive development could also be affected. Although the condition itself is not progressive, problems associated with the condition itself may increase over time. For example, in more severe cases when paralysis is present, uneven posture compounded by vertebral abnormalities may lead to **scoliosis** (lateral S-shaped curvature of the spine). Scoliosis can lead to respiratory problems, impede effective functioning of other internal organs, and decrease endurance. Urinary incontinence is a significant issue in children with spina bifida, affecting 48% to 76% of children often due to the presence of neurogenic bladder (Verhoef et al., 2005). Paralysis and associated bowel and bladder problems can also predispose individuals to develop **decubitus ulcers** (pressure sores). In addition, bowel and bladder problems increase the potential for chronic urinary tract infections.

Management of Spina Bifida

Given that the presence of spina bifida is obvious at birth, and especially with more severe forms, management is usually instigated within 24 hours of birth. Intervention depends on the extent of neurologic problems present, the level of spinal cord affected, and the existence of any complications, such as hydrocephalus or infection. Early surgical interventions have significantly increased the survival rate for people with spina bifida and greatly improved their quality of life. In addition, greater awareness of the potential for complications as a result of spina bifida has led to increased early management of complications as soon as they occur as well as implementation of active measures to prevent complications from occurring.

Functional Implications of Spina Bifida

Personal and Psychosocial Issues

Spina bifida, as a congenital condition, produces important variances in life experiences that have a potential impact on the psychological and social development of the child. The degree to which the child achieves maturity and independence in later life is shaped to a large extent by the biological, psychological, and social experiences of childhood.

Having a new baby is exciting and challenging for all parents. However, in addition to adjusting to life with a new baby, the parents of a child with spina bifida also need to learn as much as possible

about the condition to prepare for the needs of their child. Many excellent resources exist to help parents including the Spina Bifida Association (http://spinabifidaassociation.org) and the National Resource Center (http://spinabifidaassociation.org/resource-directory/).

When a child is born with a congenital condition, parental reactions vary and may include denial, guilt, anxiety, rejection, anger, or overprotectiveness. If, during this vulnerable time, parents are not provided with necessary support, parent–infant attachment and bonding may be altered. Child-rearing style has a profound effect on the child's personality development. Parents who do not establish norms and expectations for a child's behavior may create psychosocial manifestations that have a greater impact than the physical consequences associated with the congenital condition. In addition, a secondary consequence—social isolation—may result from the amount of time needed for health care and hospitalization. Early intervention, active steps to promote socialization and establish friendships, and family support and counseling may help to overcome many of these problems. The Centers for Disease Control and Prevention (2015, December 31) website offers excellent information to help parents understand the needs of their child with spina bifida at each stage of development (http://www.cdc.gov/ncbddd/spinabifida/infant.html).

It is very important for parents to take an active role in managing their child's care. However, as the child enters each stage of development, a normal part of development is gradual separation of parent and child emotionally. When this does not occur because of overprotectiveness or over-involvement of parents, the child may experience prolonged dependence and the inability to take control, which in turn may adversely affect his or her normal development and delays or impede the ability of the child to form his or her own identity. As a result, the individual may develop emotional dependence and remain in the home of the parents past maturity rather than establishing an independent living environment. Parents should talk with their healthcare provider about any questions or concerns. In addition, having support and community resources can help increase parents' confidence in managing their child's needs, enhance quality of life, and assist in meeting the needs of all family members.

Activities and Participation

Social participation is an important determinant of health and has been associated with morbidity, mortality, and quality of life (Levasseur, Richard, Gauvin, & Raymond, 2010). According to Lindstrom (2005), social participation creates opportunities for increased social integration and support, both of which can have a positive impact on health. Unfortunately, children with disabilities are at risk for poor social participation due to a number of complex interactions such as mobility, social competence, incontinence (Fisher, Church, Lyons, & McPherson, 2015), family resources, and other medical issues (Kelly & Altiok, 2011). Children with spina bifida and resulting physical limitations may not be provided with the same opportunities to test their physical and intellectual capabilities as individuals of the same age group without physical difficulties. Doubt about the child's capabilities, or setting expectations that are either too high or too low, can also contribute to low self-esteem and increased dependence. At times, in an attempt to boost the child's self-concept, parents, teachers, and others may shower a child with attention, emphasizing or humoring unrealistic expectations. This approach may, in turn, foster an egocentric personality that may prove to be more of a handicap than any physical limitation the child experiences.

Sexuality

During adolescence, part of development consists of the focus on body image and quest for identity. The child with spina bifida, however, may experience anxiety over appearance, acceptance by peers, and sexuality. Difficulties with interpersonal relationships may arise from having had only limited experience in learning and practicing social skills. Helping individuals with spina bifida to develop appropriate social skills throughout development can foster the ability to form relationships during adolescence and adulthood.

Sexual education is important regardless of the health condition or the age of its occurrence. In the case of congenital conditions, issues of sexuality may be ignored as the individual reaches adolescence. As a result, individuals may have limited opportunities to explore or express their sexual desires. Adult males with more severe forms of spina bifida may have difficulties maintaining an erection and may have difficulties with fertility. Conversely, females may be capable of engaging in sexual relations and have normal fertility, although sensation to the genital area may be absent.

Anticipatory guidance provided to parents from the time they were first told about their child's health condition can be extremely helpful in preventing many of the problems that can negatively affect the child's psychosocial development and can help the child gain full affective and personality growth and maturity. As the child goes through each stage of development, new needs and new demands will inevitably arise. Social encounters outside the home should be encouraged, as well as participation in sports, camping, and other adaptive recreational events designed to promote physical independence and social maturity.

Vocational Issues in Spina Bifida

Unless the individual has associated intellectual difficulties because of other complications associated with spina bifida, his or her intellectual ability should not be altered by this condition. The level of incapacity associated with spina bifida depends on the severity of the condition. Those individuals with paraplegia have the same functional abilities as individuals with paraplegia from other causes. The paucity of literature on work participation among adults with spina bifida in the United States exists. According to Andrén and Grimby (2004), an individual's personal development and social environment may make a significant contribution to the degree to which they achieve their goals. A study by Van Mechelen, Verhoef, Van Asbeck, and Post (2008) on work participation among young adults with spina bifida in the Netherlands revealed that significant determinants of attaining paid work for at least one hour each week were: level of education, level of lesion, hydrocephalus, intelligence quotient, functional independence, and ambulation. The researchers also found that sex, level of education, and self-care independence were significant predictors of full-time employment. The aforementioned study underscores the importance of educational support and self-care independence training for children with spina bifida.

CASE STUDY

Mr. W. is 22 years old. He has ataxic cerebral palsy that has been classified as moderate. Throughout grade school and high school, Mr. W. was included in age-appropriate general education classes with support from special education. His parents have been, and continue to be, supportive of his goals. Mr. W. attended a local university while continuing to live with his parents. He has recently graduated with a bachelor's degree in psychology—a field of study that was of academic interest to him but provided him with few marketable skills that could assure him of a job. Mr. W. is unsure of his career options given his health condition.

1. Which factors regarding Mr. W.'s health condition might be relevant when investigating career options?
2. Which additional information may be helpful to Mr. W. in determining career options?

REFERENCES

A report: The definition and classification of cerebral palsy April 2006. (2007). *Developmental Medicine & Child Neurology, 49,* 8–14. doi:10.1111/j.1469-8749.2007.tb12610.x

American Speech-Language Hearing Association. (2004). Roles and responsibilities of speech-pathologists with respect to augmentative and alternative communication: Technical report. *ASHA Leader, 24*(9), 8.

Andersson, C., Asztalos, L., & Mattsson, E. (2006). Six minute walk test in adults with cerebral palsy: A study of reliability. *Clinical Rehabilitation, 20,* 488–495.

Andersson, C., & Mattsson, E., (2001). Adults with cerebral palsy: A survey describing problems, needs, and resources, with special emphasis on locomotion. *Developmental Medicine and Child Neurology, 43*(2), 76–82.

Ando, N., & Ueda, S. (2000). Functional deterioration in adults with cerebral palsy. *Clinical Rehabilitation, 14,* 3000–3006.

Andrén, E., & Grimby, G. (2004). Dependence in daily activities and life satisfaction in adult subjects with cerebral palsy or spina bifida: A follow-up study. *Disability and Rehabilitation, 26*(9), 528–536.

Balandin, S., Berg, N., & Waller, A. (2006). Assessing the loneliness of older people with cerebral palsy. *Disability and Rehabilitation, 28*(8), 469–479.

Ballin, L., & Balandin, S. (2005). Community participation: Experiences of three older people with cerebral palsy. *AGOSCI News, 15–18.*

Barlow, J. H., & Ellard, D. R. (2006). The psychosocial well-being of children with chronic disease, their parents and siblings: An overview of the research evidence base. *Child Care, Health and Development, 32*(1), 19–31.

Bax, M., Goldstein, M., Rosenbaum, P., Leviton, A., Paneth, N., Dan, B., ... Damiano, D. (2005). Proposed definition and classification of cerebral palsy. *Developmental Medicine and Child Neurology, 47*(8), 571–576.

Bohannon, R. W., & Smith, M. B. (1987). Interrater reliability of modified Ashworth scale of muscle spasticity. *Physical Therapy, 67,* 206.

Boyd, R. N., & Graham, H. K. (1999). Objective measurement of clinical findings in the use of botulinum toxin type A for the management of children with cerebral palsy. *European Journal of Neurology, 6,* S23.

Carlsson, M., Hagberg, G., & Olsson, I. (2003). Clinical and etiological aspects of epilepsy in children with cerebral palsy. *Developmental Medicine and Child Neurology, 50,* 784–789.

Caron, J., & Light, J. (2016). Social media has opened a world of open communication: Experiences of adults with cerebral palsy who use augmentative and alternative communication and social media. *Augmentative and Alternative Communication, 32*(1), 25–40. doi:10.3109/07434618/2015.1052887

Carroll, E. M. (2015). Health care transition experiences of young adults with cerebral palsy. *Journal of Pediatric Nursing, 30,* e157–e164. doi:/10.1016/j.pedn.2015.05.018

Centers for Disease Control and Prevention. (n.d.a). *Developmental disabilities.* Retrieved, from http://www.cdc.gov/ncbddd/developmentaldisabilities/index.html

Centers for Disease Control and Prevention. (n.d.b). *Living with spina bifida: Infants.* Retrieved from http://www.cdc.gov/ncbddd/spinabifida/infant/html

Cho, S. R. (2004). Characteristics of psychosexual functioning in adults with cerebral palsy. *Clinical Rehabilitation, 18,* 423–429.

Cunningham, S. D., Thomas, P. D., & Warschausky, S. (2007). Gender differences in peer relations of children with neurodevelopmental conditions. *Rehabilitation Psychology, 52*(3), 331–337.

Delgado, M. R., & Albright, A. L. (2003). Movement disorders in children: Definitions, classifications, and grading systems. *Journal of Child Neurology, 18* (Suppl 1), S1–S8.

Desai, T., Chow, K., Mumford, L., Hotze, F., & Chu, T. (2014). Implementing an iPad-based alternative communication device for a student with cerebral palsy and autism in the classroom via an access technology delivery protocol. *Computers & Education, 79,* 148–158. Retrieved from doi:10.1016/j.compedu.2014.07.009

Eliasson, A. C., Krumlinde-Sundholm, L., Rosblad, B., Beckung, E., Arner, M., Ohrvall, A. M., & Rosenbaum, P. (2006). The Manual Ability Classification System (MACS) for children with cerebral palsy: Scale development and evidence of validity and reliability. *Devlopmental Medcine and Child Neurology, 48*(7), 549–554.

Fisher, N., Church, P., Lyons, J., & McPherson, A. C. (2015). A qualitative exploration of the experiences of children with spina bifida and their parents around incontinence and social participation. *Child: Care, Health, and Development, 41*(6), 954–962. doi:10.1111/cch.12257

Gold, J. T., & Salsberg, D. (2011). Pediatric disorders: Cerebral palsy and spina bifida. In S. R. Flanagan, H. Zaretsky, & A. Moroz (Eds.), *Medical aspects of disability* (4th ed., pp. 307–347). New York, NY: Springer.

Graham, H. K., Harvey, A., Rodda, J., Nattrass, G. R., & Pirpiris, M. (2004). The functional mobility scale (FMS). *Journal of Pediatric Orthopedics, 24*(5), 514–520.

Haak, P., Lenski, M., Hidecker, M. J., Li, M., & Paneth, N. (2009). Cerebral palsy and aging. *Developmental Medicine and Child Neurology, 51*, 16–23.

Hidecker, M. J. C., Paneth, N., Rosenbaum, P. L., Kent, R. D., Lillie, J., Eulenberg, J. B., ... Taylor, K. (2011). Developing and validating the Communication Function Classification System (CFCS) for individuals with cerebral palsy. *Developmental Medicine and Child Neurology, 53*(8), 704–710. doi:10.1111/j.1469-8749.2011.03996.x, PMC3130799

Horstmann, H., & Beck, F. (Eds.). (2007). *Orthopaedic management in cerebral palsy* (2nd ed.). London, England: Mac Keith Press.

Houlihan, C. M., & Stevenson, R. D. (2009). Bone density in cerebral palsy. *Physical Medicine and Rehabilitation Clinics of North America, 20*(3), 493–508.

Jahnsen, R., Aamodt, G., & Rosenbaum, P. (2006). Gross Motor Function Classification System used in adults with cerebral palsy: Agreement of self-reported versus professional rating. *Developmental Medicine and Child Neurology, 48*: 734–738.

Kelly, E. H., & Altiok, H. (2011). How does participation of youth with spina bifida vary by age? *Clinical Orthopedics and Related Resources, 469*, 1236–1245.

Kinsman, S. L., & Doehring, M. C. (1996). The cost of preventable conditions in adults with spina bifida. *European Journal of Pediatric Surgery, 6,* 17–20.

Levasseur, M., Richard, L., Gauvin, L., & Raymond, E. (2010). Inventory and analysis of definitions of social participation found in the aging literature: Proposed taxonomy of social activities. *Social Science and Medicine, 71*, 2141–2149.

Lindstrom, M. (2005). Ethnic differences in social participation and social capital in Malmo, Sweden: A population based study. *Social Science and Medicine, 60*, 1527–1546.

McCormick, A., Brien, M., Plourde, J., Wood, E., Rosenbaum, P., & McClean, J. (2007). Stability of the gross motor function classification system I adults with cerebral palsy. *Developmental Medicine and Child Neurology, 49*(4): 265–269.

McDermott, S., Coker, A. L., Mani, S., Krishnaswani, S., Nagle, R., Barnett-Queen, L. L., & Wuori, D. F. (1996). A population-based analysis of behavioral problems in children with cerebral palsy. *Journal of Pediatric Psychology, 21*(3), 447–463.

McDowell, B. C., Kerr, C., & Parkes, J. (2007). Interobserver agreement of the Gross Motor Function Classification System in an ambulant population of children with cerebral palsy. *Developmental Medicine and Child Neurology, 49*(7), 528–533.

McLaughlin, P. J., & Wehman, P. (Eds.). (1996). *Mental retardation and developmental disabilities* (2nd ed.). Austin, TX: Pro-ed.

Morris, C., Kurinczuk, J. J., Fitzpatrick, R., & Rosenbloom, P. L. (2006). Reliability of the manual ability classification system for children with cerebral palsy. *Developmental Medicine and Child Neurology, 48*(12): 950–953.

Odding, E., Roebroeck, M. E., & Stam, H. J. (2006). The epidemiology of cerebral palsy: Incidence, impairments and risk factors. *Disability and Rehabilitation, 28*(4), 183–191.

Ostensjo, S., Carlberg, E. B., & Vollestad, N. K. (2005). The use and impact of assistive devices and other environmental modifications on everyday activities and care in young children with cerebral palsy. *Disability and Rehabilitation, 27*(14), 849–861.

Palisano, R., Rosenbaum, P., Bartlett, D., & Livingston, M. H. (2008). Content validity of the expanded and revised Gross Motor Function Classification System. *Developmental Medicine and Child Neurology, 50*, 744–750. doi: 10.1111/j.1469-8749.2008.03089.x

Plasschaert, V. F., Ketelaar, M., Nijnuis, M. G., Enkelarr, L, & Gorter, J. W. (2009). Classification of manual abilities in children with cerebral palsy under 5 years of age: How reliable is the Manual Ability Classification System? *Clinical Rehabilitation, 23*(2), 164–170. doi: 10.1177/0269215508098892

Rethlefsen, S. A., Ryan, D. D., & Kay, R. M. (2010). Classification systems in cerebral palsy. *Orthopedic Clinics of North America, 41*, 457–467. doi:10.1016/j.ocl.2010.06.005

Rosenbaum, P., Palisano, R. J., Bartlett, D. J., Galuppi, B. E., & Russell, D. J. (2008). Development of the Gross Motor Classification System for cerebral palsy. *Developmental Medicine and Child Neurology, 50*, 249–253. doi: 10.1111/j.1469-8749.2008.02045.x

Salkever, D. S. (2000). Activity status, life satisfaction, and perceived productivity for young adults with developmental disabilities. *Journal of Rehabilitation, 66*(3), 4–13.

Sandstrom, K. (2007). The lived body: Experiences from adults with cerebral palsy. *Clinical Rehabilitation, 21,* 432–441.

Sanger, T. D., Chen, D., Fehlings, D. L., Hallett, M., Lang, A. E., Mink, J. W., & Valero-Cuevas, F. (2010). Definition and classification of hyperkinetic movements in childhood. *Movement Disorders, 25*(11), 1538–1549. doi:10.1002/mds.23088

Sanger, T. D., Delgado, M. R., Gaebler-Spira, D., Hallet, M., & Mink, J. W. (2003). Classification and definition of disorders causing hypertonia in childhood. *Pediatrics, 111*(1), e89–e97.

Stasolla, F., Damiani, R., Perilli, V., D'Amico, F., Caffo, A. O., Stella, A., & Leone, A. (2015). Computer and microswitch-based programs to improve academic activities by six children with cerebral palsy. *Research in Developmental*

Disabilities, 45–46, 1–13. Retrieved from doi:10.1016/j .ridd.2015.07.005

Surveillance of Cerebral Palsy in Europe (SCPE). (2000, December). Surveillance of cerebral palsy in Europe: A collaboration of cerebral palsy surveys and registers. *Developmental Medicine and Child Neurology, 42*(12), 816–824.

Taylor, J. R., & Kopriva, P. G. (2002). Cerebral palsy. In M. G. Brodwin, F. Tellez, & S. K. Brodwin, *Medical, psychosocial and vocational aspects of disability* (2nd ed., pp. 387–399). Athens, GA: Elliott & Fitzpatric.

Van Mechelen, M. C., Verhoef, M., Van Asbeck, F. W. A. and Post, M. W. M. (2008). Work participation among young adults with spina bifida in the Netherlands. *Developmental Medicine and Child Neurology, 50,* 772–777. doi:10.1111/j.1469-8749.2008.03020.x

Verhoef, M., Lurvink, M., Barf, H. A., Post, M. W., van Asbeck, F. W. A., Goskens, R. H. J. M., & Prevo, A. J. H. (2005). High prevalence of incontinence among young adults with spina bifida: Description, prediction, and problem perception. *Spinal Cord, 43,* 331–340.

Vocational Rehabilitation Services. (n.d.). Retrieved from http://dds.dc.gov/service/vocational-rehabilitation-services

Webb, T. S., (2009). Medical care of adults with spina bifida. *Journal of Pediatric Rehabilitation Medicine, 2,* 3–11.

Whaley, L. F., & Wong, D. L. (1995). *Nursing care of infants and children* (5th ed.). St. Louis, MO: Mosby.

Wiegerink, D. J., Roebroeck, M. E., Donkervoort, M., Stam, H. J., & Cohen-Kettenis, P. T. (2006). Social and sexual relationships of adolescents and young adults with cerebral palsy: A review. *Clinical Rehabilitation, 20,* 1023–1031.

World Health Organization. (2001). *International Classification of Functioning, Disability and Health.* Geneva, Switzerland: World Health Organization. Retrieved, from: http://www.who.int /classifications/icf/icf_more/en/

Young, N. L., Anselmo, L. A., Burke, T. A, McCormick, A., & Mukherjee, S. (2014). Youth and young adults with spina bifida: Their utilization of physician and hospital services. *Archives of Physical Medicine and Rehabilitation, 95,* 466–471. Retrieved from doi:10.1016/j.apmr.2013.09.0115

CHAPTER 12

Neurodevelopmental Disorders

Revised by Kelly Kazukauskas

[handwritten annotation: Intellectual disability — shift toward more politically correct language.]

The term *developmental disability*, which was instituted by the Developmental Disabilities Act of 1975 (PL 94-102) to describe conditions that are first identified in childhood, are lifelong, and affect intellectual or physical function, continues to be an umbrella term for a wide variety of conditions that affect physical, intellectual, and behavioral functional capacity. Many of these conditions are described in *The Diagnostic and Statistical Manual of Mental Disorders, 5th edition's* (*DSM-V*, American Psychiatric Association [APA], 2013) chapter entitled "Neurodevelopmental Disorders," which includes a variety of disabling conditions that manifest during the developmental period and generate impairments in the major life areas throughout a person's life. These conditions often co-occur and they typically require extensive supports and services (APA, 2013). This chapter focuses on several of the more common conditions affecting intellectual functioning, learning, or behavior that are classified in the *DSM-V* and cross-walked in *The International Classification of Diseases and Related Health Problems* (*ICD-10*) as follows:

- Intellectual Disability (also known as *intellectual developmental disorder*)
- Autism Spectrum Disorder
- Attention Deficit/Hyperactivity Disorder
- Specific Learning Disorder (also known as *learning disability*)

from the term *mental retardation*, a term which has often resulted in social stigma, isolation, and segregation (Matson, Terlonge, & Minshawi, 2008). Social stigma may impact many important life areas, including equality and community inclusion, autonomy and the ability to make choices, disparities in healthcare, and advocacy (Ditchman et al., 2013).

Current research suggests that intellectual disability occurs in approximately 1% of the population, with rates varying based on the income group (high, middle, low) of the country in question (Maulik, Mascarenhas, Mathers, Dua, & Saxena, 2011). Intellectual disability is characterized by impairment in both intellectual and adaptive functioning, featuring significant limitations both in intellectual performance and in adaptive behavior as expressed in conceptual, social, and practical adaptive skills

(Schalock et al., 2010). Additionally, the onset of this disability originates during the developmental period, before age 18 (Schalock et al., 2010).

Many individuals with an intellectual disability also have other health conditions or sensory or motor impairments that further affect their functional capacity. Because both intellectual and adaptive functioning are considered essential features in the diagnosis and treatment of intellectual disability, performance in both areas must be adequately measured during the diagnostic process.

Causes of Intellectual Disability

include brain malformations (such as *neural tube defects*) and chromosomal abnormalities, as discussed previously. *Prenatal* causes of intellectual disability include maternal exposure to infections such as rubella or herpes, maternal abuse of drugs or alcohol, maternal exposure to toxic chemicals or radiation, and exposure to prescription drugs that have *teratogenic* (producing abnormal fetal development) effects. Conditions in utero that cause the fetus to experience **hypoxia** (lack of oxygen supply) can also be prenatal causes of intellectual disability.

Intellectual disability may also occur during the childbirth process (*perinatal*). Pre-term birth, whether spontaneous or medically necessary has been found to be associated with a significantly increased risk for intellectual disability (Langridge

et al., 2013). Complications, such as hypoxia, during the delivery process, which may lead to brain injury, and are associated with an increased risk as well.

Postnatal causes of intellectual disability can be due to brain injury or trauma experienced during childhood as a result of accident or abuse. Childhood infections, such as *meningitis*; exposure to toxic substances, such as lead; metabolic conditions, such as *phenylketonuria* (PKU); and *hypothyroidism* can also be postnatal causes of intellectual disability. Malnutrition, psychological, and social deprivation in childhood are potential causes as well (Handen, 2007; Koger, Schettler, & Weiss, 2005).

Identification of Intellectual Disability

Intelligence refers to individuals' ability to reason, think abstractly, learn, and comprehend complex ideas. Identification of intellectual disability is conducted through measurement of both *intellectual functioning* and *adaptive behavior*, and requires that the individual meet all three of the following criteria:

a) Deficits in intellectual functions, such as reasoning, problem-solving, planning, abstract thinking, judgment, academic learning and learning from experience, and practical understanding confirmed by both clinical assessment and individualized, standardized intelligence testing.

b) Deficits in adaptive functioning that result in failure to meet developmental and sociocultural standards for personal independence and social responsibility. Without ongoing support, the adaptive deficits limit functioning in one or more activities of daily life, such as communication, social participation, and independent living across multiple environments, such as home, school, work, and community.

c) Onset of intellectual and adaptive deficits during the developmental period. (*DSM-V*, APA, 2013)

Handwritten note:

ID

can occur during the prenatal, perinatal, or postnatal period, up until age 18.

Dependent on the type and severity of the disability, it may be identified while the child is in utero or may be identified in the first few months to years of life as developmental milestones are missed. However, intellectual disability is often missed in young children because of misconceptions about the presentation of intellectual disability or the belief that young children cannot be tested. Identifying intellectual disability in young children requires a complete child and family history, including information about the pregnancy. Historically, intellectual ability was primarily determined by use of a single test score on a standardized intelligence test such as the *Wechsler Intelligence Scales for Children* or the *Stanford–Binet Intelligence Scale*, both of which are currently in their fifth revisions and are still widely used. While standardized testing remains an important part of the diagnostic process, the *DSM-V* stresses the importance of evaluating these test scores in conjunction with an individualized cognitive profile based on a thorough neuropsychological assessment. In fact, although the *intelligence quotient* (*IQ*) ranges that have historically been associated with severity of intellectual disability have been included in **Table 12-1**, these ranges have been removed from the level of severity specifiers in the *DSM-V*.

It is important to note that while deficit in intellectual functioning that is confirmed by clinical assessment and standardized intelligence testing is one of the three diagnostic criterion for intellectual disability, determination of the level of severity— *Mild, Moderate, Severe*, or *Profound*—is now based on deficits in adaptive functioning, which must be shown to require ongoing supports in one or more adaptive functioning areas (APA, 2013). Adaptive behavior refers to a person's level of personal independence and social responsibility. Adaptive behavior is a multidimensional concept, and some behaviors are difficult to measure. In particular, adaptive behavior must be considered in the context of the developmental stage of the individual as well as in the context of the individual's specific culture and environment. The severity levels associated with these include three adaptive functioning domains as well: the conceptual domain, the social domain, and the practical domain (Luckasson et al., 2002). Examples of conceptual, social, and practical skills can be found in **Table 12-2**.

Assessment of adaptive function includes a formal clinical assessment as well as a thorough medical, developmental and psychosocial history. Individualized standardized intelligence and adaptive behavior tests used must be psychometrically valid and sound, comprehensive, and culturally appropriate (APA, 2013). Input from individuals

Table 12-1 Historical Ranges of IQ Scores and Corresponding Level of Severity

Classification IQ
Mild 50–55 to 70
Moderate 35–40 to 50–55
Severe 20–25 to 35–40
Profound Below 20–25

Data from American Psychiatric Association. (2000). *Diagnostic and statistical manual of mental disorders* (4th ed., rev.). Washington, DC: Author.

Table 12-2 Examples of Adaptive Skills

Conceptual Skills

Receptive and expressive language
Reading and writing
Money concepts
Self-direction

Social Skills

Interpersonal skills
Gullibility and naiveté
Ability to follow rules and laws
Responsibility

Practical Skills

Activities of daily living

- Eating
- Toileting
- Dressing

Instrumental activities of daily living

- Preparing meals
- Housekeeping
- Telephone use
- Money management
- Job skills
- Maintain safety

closest to the person, such as family members and teachers is also essential in this process.

A number of standardized tests have been developed to measure adaptive functioning, such as the *Vineland Adaptive Behavior Scales* (Carter, Volkmar, & Sparrow, 1998; Conoley & Kramer, 1989; Sparrow, Balla, & Cicchetti, 1984) and the Adaptive Behavior Scale (ABS) (Impara & Plake, 1998; Lambert, Nihira, & Leland, 1993). The ABS consists of two versions: a *School and Community* version (ABS-S: 2) and a *Residential and Community* version (ABS-RC: 2) (Lambert et al., 1993). The School and Community version measures adaptive behavior as it relates to independence and responsibility, whereas the Residential and Community version relates to problem behaviors.

Interpretation of scores from testing, whether intelligence testing or testing of adaptive function, should always be made in the context of the individual, including cultural and environmental variations, language ability, and any sensory, motor, and behavioral factors that may affect testing results. Factors such as the individual's environment and the degree of stimulation and support he or she has received within that environment can also affect the person's abilities. For example, individuals who interpret questions or responses differently owing to their cultural background or who are being given a test not in their native language may have scores that are not reflective of their actual intellectual capacity. Likewise, physical discomfort or other health conditions may affect an individual's ability to perform to maximum capacity during testing. Consequently, test scores alone are not absolute proof of intellectual disability.

Adaptive behavior is also typically assessed through direct observation of the individual as he or she performs various skills used to function in everyday life. Skills assessed usually include communication, calculation, self-direction, social skills, activities of daily living, and job-related skills. When individuals 18 years of age or younger demonstrate a deficient intellectual profile (based on a combination of thorough clinical assessment and standardized testing) and have functional limitations in one or more areas of adaptive functioning, the condition is identified as intellectual disability (APA, 2013).

Classification of Intellectual Disability

Although it might seem that classification of intellectual disability could lead to labeling and stigmatizing, the purpose of classification is to identify specific functional capacities so that supports and services can be tailored to meet each person's individual needs.

There are varying degrees of intellectual disability. In the past, the range of severity of intellectual disability was primarily distinguished based on the classification system outlined in Table 12-1. Classification is, however, multidimensional, and the most recent trends in the field favor the inclusion of not only intellectual ability and adaptive behavior but also health, participation, and context as well.

The American Association on Intellectual and Developmental Disability (Luckasson et al., 2002) developed another system for conceptualizing levels of intellectual disability, which focuses on support needs rather than limitations. This is a strengths-based model, and it defines support needs as intermittent, limited, extensive and pervasive. *Intermittent* indicates a need for support periodically or on a short-term basis during times of transition or crisis. When supports are needed, they may be either high or low intensity (Luckasson et al., 2002). *Limited* is indicative of low-intensity, time-limited supports for specific need areas, such as job training or school transition (Luckasson et al., 2002). *Extensive* refers to a need for ongoing, regular supports on a low-intensity basis to maintain adequate function in the home or work environment (Luckasson et al., 2002). *Pervasive* means that extensive, ongoing, high-intensity support is required for safety and well-being (Luckasson et al., 2002).

Manifestations of Intellectual Disability

Individuals with intellectual disability have a wide range of abilities as well as disabilities. Eighty-five to ninety percent of individuals with intellectual disability are classified in the mild range (Volkmar, Klin, & Paul, 2004). The extent of support needed varies with the individual and with his or her particular circumstances. Some individuals with intellectual disability may also exhibit delays in motor skills development, speech and language problems, or problems with vision or hearing. In addition, emotional challenges and vulnerabilities may be caused by psychosocial or environmental factors. Early intervention, which considers all intellectual, physical, environmental, and social factors, is essential to foster the individual's attainment of his or her full potential.

Individuals with intellectual disability have below-average general intellectual functioning for their stage of development as well as limitations in adaptive functioning or basic skills needed to manage age-appropriate tasks and demands of everyday life, such as communication, conceptualization, self-care, self-direction, self-sufficiency, and safety (APA, 2013). Although actual functional capacity depends on many individual factors, in general, functional disability according to level of intellectual functioning can be classified as mild, moderate, severe, or profound, which can still be found in the *DSM-V* structure of diagnosis (APA, 2013, pp. 34–36).

Mild Intellectual Disability

Generally, individuals with mild intellectual disability are considered capable of attaining a higher level of intellectual functioning. During preschool years, such persons are generally capable of attaining social and communication skills consistent with their peers; consequently, some individuals may not be distinguishable from other children in their age group. As they move into the school-age years supports may be needed in relation to academic skills (reading, writing, and arithmetic) and money or time management. Adults with mild intellectual disability may demonstrate difficulty in executive functioning, including planning, prioritizing, and organizing, and often have limitations with regard to cognitive flexibility.

Socially, individuals with mild intellectual disability may have difficulty accurately perceiving social cues and may be socially immature when compare to age-related peers. Emotional regulation may also be problematic, as well as understanding of risk in potentially dangerous or exploitive social situations.

In relation to the practical domain, individuals with mild intellectual disability are often independent in self-care, although they may need support

with more complex daily living skills. Individuals with mild intellectual disability will likely be able to obtain employment and live independently or with minimal support and supervision, although they may need additional support and guidance when placed in particularly stressful or new situations. Many individuals in this category can live independently in the community.

Moderate Intellectual Disability

Individuals with moderate intellectual disability, in general, may require more supervision in activities of daily living, although they can usually manage self-care. Marked limitations in conceptual skills can be notes throughout development, with achievements progressing slowly in areas such as reading, writing, arithmetic, and management of time and money. Processing abstract information is generally difficult with academic ability remaining in the elementary range. Individuals with moderate intellectual disability are usually capable of learning some vocational skills, although they may function best in a semi-independent or partially supervised work environment, such as supported employment. They may have differing degrees of expressive and receptive language skills.

Individuals with moderate intellectual disability will also require supports in social areas of life, as communication, social understanding, and behavior will typically be less complex than that of peers. In addition, with extended time and support these individuals may be able to perform activities of daily living related to eating, dressing, and hygiene, although supports and reminders may be needed on an ongoing basis in adulthood. They are generally able to live in the community, in a group home, or in a semi-independent setting.

Severe Intellectual Disability

Individuals with severe intellectual disability will generally require extensive support in conceptualization throughout the lifespan. Ability to understand written language, as well as numbers, math, quantity, time, or money will be very limited. While they are school age, they may attain some elementary self-care skills and may learn to read and write on a limited basis; however, for the most part, such persons will require close supervision for most tasks. These individuals generally have limited communication skills and poorly developed motor skills as well. Speech, for example, may be limited to single words or phrases, and they may rely primarily on gestural communication with others. In adulthood, individuals with severe intellectual disability may live in community group homes, in supported apartments or homes, or with their families. Many individuals with severe intellectual disability have an associated health condition that compounds their limitations of function. Most individuals at this level respond best to a consistent caregiver and a low-stimulus environment. Because of the severity of the condition, close supervision and support in most daily activities are usually needed, and they will require supports for responsible decision-making as it relates to the self and to others.

Profound Intellectual Disability

Individuals with profound intellectual disability often have a number of other health conditions that further limit function. For the most part, individuals in this category are dependent on others for all care. Conceptually, individuals with profound intellectual disability have limited understanding beyond the physical world around them. Beyond understanding of simple words and gestures, communication is severely limited. Communication occurs largely through nonverbal means. While they enjoy social interactions, especially with those familiar to them, individual with profound intellectual disability are essentially dependent on others for all areas of life including activities of daily living, self-care, health, and safety.

Interventions in Intellectual Disability

Given that intellectual disability is both a complex and lifelong condition, the overall goal of interventions is to provide opportunities for the individual to enhance development, prevent secondary conditions, and enable the individual to experience age-appropriate activities and conditions as close as possible to those of mainstream society. Individuals with intellectual disability constitute a heterogeneous group with varying needs, skills, backgrounds, and supports. Interventions, therefore,

are individualized based on life stage, current level of functioning, and life goals. Intervention programs or rehabilitation services are crucial to enable individuals to reach their optimal level of functional capacity, to build on strengths, and to identify special talents.

To the extent possible, interventions appropriate to the individual's life stage offer supports and services to the individual and his or her family in the environments in which individuals without disability would participate. Early intervention (birth to 3 years) programs have been found to be significant in enhancing development, decreasing secondary risks, and facilitating independence, inclusion, and productivity, as well as providing family support (McCall & Plemons, 2001). Services may be home-based, school-based, or community-based, depending on individual and family needs and preferences. As individuals move from one life stage to another, they and their families interact with a variety of programs and services to facilitate successful transitions at every important life juncture and to all aspects of life—from going to school, transitioning from school to adulthood, and adjusting to older adulthood. In addition, individuals learn specific functional skills appropriate to their capacity.

Functional Implications of Intellectual Disability

Personal and Psychosocial Issues

Each life stage has its own particular developmental issues that have a relationship to all other stages. As individuals move from infancy, through childhood, to adolescence, into adulthood, and finally into older adulthood, their activities, growth, and behavior change, as do individual needs. Each individual is unique, being associated with a unique set of experiences, environments, and cultural variations. The same is true whether individual has an intellectual disability or not.

Like all individuals, individuals with intellectual disability have a need for family, friends, respect, the right to privacy, and meaningful employment. The concept of *inclusion* refers to the integration and full participation of everyone, regardless of special needs and disabilities or the environment (e.g., school, community), with typical peers, in the least restrictive setting. Although the World Health Organization (WHO, 2001) stresses the importance of full participation and community integration, individuals with intellectual disability, however, may not always enjoy the emotional support needed or may have only limited opportunities for growth. The opinions and expectations most people have about themselves are influenced to a great extent by the behavior of those around them. When minimal expectations or lack of belief in individuals' ability to achieve are communicated, the chance for individuals to progress in attaining goals is diminished. The impact of negative life experiences may reinforce feelings of worthlessness. Because a number of inaccurate and stereotyped ideas about individuals with intellectual disability still exist, barriers to reaching optimal function and independence continue to be present.

Lack of acceptance and devaluation can result in low self-esteem, isolation, or depression. In a study of individuals with intellectual disability by Ailey, Miller, Heller, and Smith (2006), the relationship between depression, perceived social support, loneliness, and life satisfaction was found to be significant. Individuals with intellectual disability may be unable to describe experiences and feelings or may have difficulty communicating needs and wishes, which can cause frustration and acting out. Such behavior may be reinforced by others in the environment and can be instrumental in escaping or avoiding certain tasks.

Providing individuals with support and opportunities that empower them to optimize their functional capacity can contribute to the development of coping skills, which in turn enables them to withstand stress and reach their goals.

Activities and Participation

Intellectual disability, although identified in childhood, is not simply a childhood condition. Individuals with intellectual disability live into adulthood and increasingly are living into older age, which may mean an increasing prevalence of chronic conditions and multiple and complex health problems that change over the life span (Noble, 2001). Individuals with intellectual disability who develop hypertension, diabetes, or other chronic health conditions or psychiatric conditions face additional challenges. The overall goal is for individuals to attain and maintain an optimal level of health and function throughout the life span within the range of their capacity. There are, however, health disparities regarding availability of adequate health care for individuals with intellectual disability as compared to the level of health care available to the general population. *Public stigma* such as healthcare provider attitudes, *structural stigma* such as fee-for-service costs, access to appointments, and time or testing constraints, and *self-stigma,* which may impede self-referral or may preclude personal health and safety care, are all barriers to inclusion in the healthcare system (Ditchman et al., 2013). There continues to be a need for changes in the healthcare system in order to reduce disparities and promote inclusion, as well as a need for provider training and education, to meet the unique needs of persons with intellectual disabilities (Ditchman et al., 2013).

Although societal and employer attitudes are changing slowly, a continued need exists for education and integration of individuals with intellectual disability into society and into the workplace. Although all individuals with intellectual disability can experience stresses resulting from societal stereotypes and attitudes, individuals with mild intellectual disability may confront specific stresses because they may appear "normal" to others, and, consequently, their limitations may not be recognized as a disability. In addition, there continues to be a disproportionate number of persons with intellectual disability in sheltered and supported work environments, who have the capacity to function at a higher level of independence. Myriad reasons for this exist, including attitudes (employer, caregiver, guardian, and self), access (transportation, exposure to opportunities), and support (long-term job coaching options to increase opportunity for successful job tenure). While much progress has been made in this area over the past few decades, there is still a long way to go toward complete inclusion.

Many individuals with intellectual disability are cared for by others in either their own homes or in residential settings, such as assisted-living or group home environments. The level of stress that may be experienced by caregivers and the vulnerability of individuals with intellectual disability raise a concern about the potential for violence, abuse, and neglect toward people with this disability. In 2004, Strand, Benzein, and Saveman reported on the results of a questionnaire that they sent to 164 staff members in 17 different care settings for adults with disabilities in Sweden. In their responses, 74% of the study participants reported being involved in or witnessing violent incidents toward clients, and 14% admitted to being the perpetrator of the violent act. Most of the violence occurred on a daily basis, was both physical and psychological, and tended to occur in close caretaking situations. This study indicates the importance of supportive supervision, education, and outlets for staff and family members, and increased training of individuals with intellectual disability about reporting abusive situations.

Sexuality

Although great strides have been made in terms of the inclusion of individuals with intellectual development into the community, an area that does not receive the same amount of attention, and regarding which there is often a great disparity of views, is that of sexuality (Cuskelly & Bryde, 2004). Individuals with intellectual disability, like all persons, are sexual beings with needs of being liked and accepted, sharing affection, being valued, and sharing thoughts and feelings. Others frequently assume that because of their intellectual disability, such individuals are nonsexual beings, or that they are incapable of controlling sexual urges and, therefore, must be monitored in social settings. Limitations in freedom to express sexuality can come from family members, guardians, care givers, staff, and the general public (Azzopardi-Lane & Callus, 2015). Consequently, these persons may have limited opportunities to develop appropriate social skills. Providing developmentally appropriate sex education can help individuals with intellectual disability to acquire a sense of attractiveness and build a level of social functioning that enables them to develop satisfying relationships with others in adulthood. Because individuals with intellectual disability are vulnerable to sexual exploitation and abuse (Murphy & Elias, 2006), sex education can also provide skills and information that help them learn how to be assertive when uncomfortable situations arise and to report inappropriate behavior of others to individuals whom they trust.

Vocational Issues in Intellectual Disability

The level of occupational functioning for individuals with intellectual disability depends to some extent on the degree of disability. Lack of exposure to or experience in a variety of work settings can be a significant limitation in successful work participation. Because intellectual disability is often accompanied by other health conditions, the physical limitations associated with any other condition must be considered as well. Individuals with intellectual disability usually perform better in a structured environment. Many individuals may need to be taught how to function independently and may need accompanying social skills training.

As with other health conditions, the major barrier to individuals reaching their full potential may be societal stereotypes and prejudice. Although there has been heightened effort toward increasing integrated employment opportunities for individuals with intellectual disability, rehabilitation outcomes—especially for individuals of racial and ethnic underrepresented groups—have been less than ideal. According to Siperstein, Parker, and Drascher (2013), only 34% of persons with intellectual disability are employed while employment rates for the general population far exceed this. Consequently, continued equality in service delivery and assurance and education of potential employers may be crucial factors in successful occupational placement. Limited information is available in the vocational rehabilitation literature on the pattern of work support and employment success of individuals based on the level and degree of intellectual disability they have. However, recent evidence supports the need for early exposure to work and work-related interventions, showing better employment rates long term for individuals with intellectual disability who held jobs prior to leaving secondary education (Siperstein, Heyman, & Stokes, 2014). The authors also found that sheltered workshops, while providing an option to transition *out* of the workforce, rarely act as a pathway into competitive employment if utilized as an employment option early on (Siperstein et al., 2014).

AUTISM SPECTRUM DISORDER

The movement to the *DSM-V* (APA, 2013) brought forth significant changes to the classification and diagnosis of autism-related syndromes, which were previously categorized under the umbrella of *pervasive developmental disorders.* This new unitary diagnostic category includes the previously separate diagnoses of autistic disorder, Asperger's disorder, and pervasive developmental disability not otherwise specified (*DSM-IV-TR*, APA, 2000). The establishment of a single diagnosis, rather than a large category containing five individual diagnoses, was an empirically supported change, although many expressed concern about possible loss of diagnosis and service eligibility (Ozonoff, 2012). According to the *DSM-V*, individuals with a clearly established *DSM-IV* diagnosis of autistic disorder, Asperger's disorder, or pervasive developmental disability not otherwise specified should now be assigned the autism spectrum disorder diagnosis (APA, 2013).

Autism spectrum disorder is an alteration of brain function that has a broad range of behavioral consequences, including impairment in reciprocal social interaction and impairment in verbal and nonverbal communication, play skills, and cognitive and adaptive functioning (APA, 2000; Layne, 2007). Autism spectrum disorder is characterized by two distinguishing features that occur on a continuum based on level of severity: 1) marked deficits in social communication and interactions cross-environmentally, and 2) a pattern of restrictive, repetitive behaviors (APA, 2013). The symptoms of autism spectrum disorder must also present in the early developmental years (although they may not become apparent until later), must cause significant impairment in one of the major life areas (examples: social, educational, or occupational), and must not be better explained by an intellectual disability (APA, 2013).

Autism spectrum disorder is 4.5 times more likely to occur in boys than girls and occurs in all racial, ethnic, and socioeconomic groups (Christensen et al., 2016). Autism spectrum disorder has shown a steady increase in reported prevalence since it was first described in 1943 (Merrick, Kandel, & Morad, 2004). According to the CDC, autism spectrum disorder is identified in approximately 1 in 68 children and affects over 2 million people in the United States alone (Christensen et al., 2016). This is a significant increase from 2002 estimates, which placed the prevalence around 1 in 150 (Christensen et al., 2016). Whether the incidence of autism spectrum disorder is actually increasing, or the reported increase is influenced by heightened awareness by parents and health professionals, or the epidemiological methods used by different groups to arrive at estimates vary, is the source of recent controversy (Baird et al., 2000; Laider, 2005; Williams, Mellis, & Peat, 2005).

Autism spectrum disorder often co-occurs with intellectual disability; however, contrary to popular belief among laypersons it is *not* an intellectual disability in and of itself. Recent data from the CDC Autism and Developmental Disabilities Monitoring Network (ADDM) found that approximately 44% of children with autism spectrum disorder were functioning in the average or above average range intellectually, while approximately 24% were in the borderline range, and approximately 31% had a co-occurring intellectual disability diagnosis (Christensen et al., 2016). Many individuals with autism spectrum disorder also exhibit manifestations of hyperactivity and inattention; as a consequence, this condition is often misidentified as attention-deficit/hyperactivity disorder (APA, 2013).

Manifestations of Autism Spectrum Disorder

Autism spectrum disorder is characterized by behavioral patterns that most commonly include impairments in communication and social interaction. Kanner (1972) was the first to describe children with autism as "having an inability to relate themselves in an ordinary way to people and situations from the beginning of life" (p. 242). Individuals with autism may exhibit manifestations from birth; however, because of the subtlety of early manifestations, the condition may not be identified until manifestations become more noticeable later in development. For example, individuals with autism spectrum disorder who are higher functioning might not be identified until individuals reach school age and difficulties with social interaction become apparent. However, onset typically occurs between 12–24 months of age (APA, 2013).

The range and severity of manifestations vary with each individual. Usually parents report that the child, almost since birth, has been perceived as different. Language delays and inability to relate to social cues are often reported. Parents of children with autism spectrum disorder may report that their child did not enjoy being cuddled, seldom smiled, and did not respond to games such as "peek-a-boo." These children may remain aloof and have problems throughout childhood, with either an improvement in or an exacerbation of behavior in adolescence. They often prefer solitary behavior, preferring to be left alone rather than engaging in explorative behaviors or other social interaction. They may lack the ability to engage in spontaneous or imaginative play and may show strong attachment to inanimate objects rather than people. In particular, abilities related to attention, empathy, communication, and flexibility are affected (Anckarsater et al., 2006).

Activity levels of individuals with autism may range from overactive to very passive. Some children display repetitive or stereotypic body movements or behaviors, such as body rocking, hand flapping, finger flicking, or staring at their hands at close range. In some instances, children may engage in repetitive self-injurious behavior, such as head banging or biting. They may exhibit exaggerated or aggressive responses to people or objects. Rituals and the insistence on sameness or resistance to change are common in individuals with autism. Changes in their environment or routine may be very difficult.

Individuals with autism spectrum disorder often demonstrate hypersensitivity or disproportionate response to sensory stimuli, including touch or sound; however, in some instances they may show a decreased response to pain. Often communication deficits in verbal or nonverbal behavior exist, including the inability to comprehend verbal communication or decipher nonverbal cues. Affected individuals may demonstrate difficulty expressing ideas or needs orally or, conversely,

be highly verbal. *Echolalia,* in which a word or a phrase is repeated numerous times, may be a feature of the condition. Some individuals have difficulty integrating cognitive functions. If autism spectrum disorder accompanies another condition, such as encephalitis, phenylketonuria, or fragile X syndrome, corresponding neurological and other health manifestations will be present. Other medical conditions such as epilepsy are also commonly associated with autism spectrum disorder (APA, 2013).

Causes of Autism Spectrum Disorder

Years ago, autism spectrum disorders were attributed to poor parenting skills, and many people believed that parents who were emotionally unavailable to their children contributed to the development of manifestations of autism. This belief has now been discredited, and parenting skills are no longer thought to be responsible for the development of autism. Although no definitive cause of autism has yet been found, it is most likely that it results from a brain function alteration that is biologically based and arises from a combination of genetic vulnerability and environmental triggers (Blackwell & Niederhauser, 2003).

In 1998 a research study by Andrew Wakefield and colleagues was published in the British medical journal the *Lancet* that claimed to have found a strong connection between the measles, mumps, rubella (MMR) vaccine and the onset of autism spectrum disorder (Ratzan, 2010). Thus began an outbreak of panic over the safety of vaccines. The study was not able to be replicated and an investigation later determined the research to be untruthful and unethical (Ratzan, 2010). The *Lancet* retracted the article in 2004, and it was disclaimed by most of the coauthors who purportedly were involved in the project.

There continues to be considerable concern that a link exists between thimerosal, a mercury-based preservative sometimes used in vaccines, and autism. Until 1999, vaccines against a number of infectious conditions contained thimerosal as a preservative. While the data is mixed and believed by many to be insufficient to support a causal relationship (Tomljenovic, Dórea, & Shaw, 2012), the MMR, varicella (chickenpox), inactivated polio (IPV), and pneumococcal conjugate vaccines have never contained thimerosal. Currently, with the exception of some influenza vaccines, none of the vaccines used in the United States to protect children contains thimerosal as a preservative (Food and Drug Administration, 2012). However, there continues to be a great deal of concern around vaccinations leading many parents to refrain from vaccinating their children.

Identification of Autism Spectrum Disorder

Criteria for identification of autism spectrum disorder, is outlined in *DSM-V* (APA, 2013, pp. 50–51). Diagnostic criteria include deficits in social skills, including communication, social interaction, relationship development and maintenance, as well as restrictive or repetitive behaviors and hyper reactivity to sensory input.

Level of severity is specified individually, based on current symptomatology and level of support needs.

It is possible that the level of severity\may vary based on context. For proper diagnosis, the symptoms identified must be present in the early developmental period, must cause clinically significant impairment in social, occupational, or other important areas of current functioning, and cannot be better explained by intellectual disability (APA, 2013).

Although the *DSM-V* has outlined specific criteria for diagnosing autism spectrum disorder, there continues to be concerns that the new diagnostic criteria are not sensitive enough to identify many of the subtleties that may exist in the milder cases, leading to missed diagnoses and/or loss of service eligibility (Ozonoff, 2012). As a result, the condition may be misidentified or overlooked and, therefore, interventions appropriate to the condition may not be forthcoming. Particularly in the cases of individuals with higher functioning autism spectrum disorder manifestations may not be immediately apparent during assessment conducted in a one-to-one setting. A full history of the individual's behavior and the means by which he or she interacts with others can be an important tool for identification.

There are a number of diagnostic assessments, including the *Childhood Autism Rating Scale* (CARS) (Schopler, Reichler, & Renner, 1988), and screening tools, such as the *Modified Checklist for Autism in Toddlers—Revised with Follow-up* (M-CHAT-R/F) (Robins et al., 2014) which are used to identify autism spectrum disorder. Extensive training and experience are required to administer these tools in a valid and reliable way. Consequently, definitive identification of autism spectrum disorder should be done by clinicians who have extensive experience with the screening instruments and with individuals with autism spectrum disorder.

Management of Autism Spectrum Disorder

Autism spectrum disorder is a lifelong condition. One of the most important aspects of its management is early identification and individualized, intensive behavioral and psychological interventions. In spite of increasing awareness of the prevalence of autism spectrum disorder, delays in identification of the disorder frequently occur due to lack of standardized screening for developmental delays (Filipek et al., 2000). Developmental profiles should focus on speech and language, verbal and nonverbal communication, cognitive function, and motor function. In addition, audiological screening and lead exposure screening should be conducted to rule out other causes of developmental delay.

The hallmark of autism spectrum disorder is social disability. Referrals and resources to help individuals develop social skills, recognize social cues, and learn socially based communication and language skills can help the individual become more socially adept (Giarelli, Souders, Pinto-Martin, Bloch, & Levy, 2005; Landa, 2000). Because coping with change is difficult, maintaining comfortable routines can be helpful to the individual; when change is necessary, it should be introduced gradually.

Individuals on the autism spectrum disorder who have a higher level of functioning (who, for example, may have previously have been diagnosed with Asperger's syndrome) may not adhere to social conventions, such as respecting others' personal space. They may make remarks that are inappropriate in most social environments or talk loudly, relentlessly pursuing a subject of interest to them, even though others show no interest in what they are saying and show little response to the discussion. These individuals may be rigid about adhering to strict routines and become upset or agitated if change is necessary. Some individuals may demonstrate poor gross motor function, appear clumsy, or use repetitive behaviors, such as ritualistic walking patterns and obsessive–compulsive routines.

Higher functioning individuals with autism spectrum disorder often learn to use areas of strength, such as rote verbal skills or savant-like mathematical skills, to compensate for other limitations. Although overall outlook is better for these individuals (APA, 2013), as they reach adulthood they may experience increasing rejection, social isolation, anxiety, and depression.

Communication problems are prevalent in autism spectrum disorder. Consequently, a thorough evaluation of how the individual best communicates, especially in natural settings, is important as it may have meaningful implications for interventions (Kim, Junker, & Lord, 2014). In assessing individuals with autism spectrum disorder, the individual's social, communication, and behavioral strengths and limitations should be incorporated into any rehabilitation plan. As both verbal and nonverbal problems in communication are frequently noted, augmentative systems may be needed (such as signing or use of a communication board) to facilitate communication. Provision of an augmentative communication system that can be successfully used requires careful assessment by skilled professionals. Behavioral protocols—including many employing contingent reinforcement, such as use of tokens—have been used successfully and may facilitate interaction.

Other types of interventions, such as auditory integration training and sensory integration interventions may be helpful to individuals with autism spectrum disorder in some instances. In addition, exercise and physical therapy may be helpful as well. Establishment of any intervention or management plan should always include family members as partners to develop a plan that is best suited for the individual and his or her particular circumstances.

Management planning often involves a multidisciplinary approach including the following elements:

- Audiological exam
- Speech and language evaluation
- Occupational therapy evaluation
- Psychiatric observation and interview
- Neurological exam

Each area of function should be measured against standardized norms and the results used to determine the individual's special needs. As an individual gets older, it will be important to include vocational rehabilitation and therapeutic recreation specialists on the team as well to assist the individual in transitioning into meaningful activity as an adult.

Referral to an early intervention program, which evaluates needs and assists children with neurodevelopmental disorders, is crucial. Early intervention programs involve the whole family and assist in identifying innovative solutions to both behavioral and health problems.

In the management and care of persons with autism spectrum disorder, the main objective is maximization of functional independence and autonomy, and improved quality of life (Hsia et al., 2013). Additional goals include decreasing maladaptive behaviors; reduction of co-occurring mental health concerns, such as mood disorders and anxiety; and mitigation of caregiver stress and burden (Cadman et al., 2012; Carbone, Farley, & Davis, 2010; Myers, Johnson, & American Academy of Pediatrics Council on Children with Disabilities, 2007). While no specific medications are considered standard in management of autism spectrum disorder, a number of pharmacologic agents are prescribed for treatment of related problems, behaviors, and co-occurring disorders. Antipsychotic medications to reduce behavioral symptoms, irritability, and hyperactivity have been used with some success and are beginning to have established evidence for use (Siegel & Beaulieu, 2012). There is insufficient evidence, however, to support the use of mood stabilizers and other medications to treat these and other symptoms such as mood and anxiety (Siegel & Beaulieu, 2012). When medications are employed for management of manifestations, careful monitoring of drug interactions or side effects should be part of the general protocol. In instances where other health conditions coexist with the condition, specific medications for management of those conditions, such as seizures, may be added. When other medications are incorporated within the medication protocol, the potential for drug interactions and subsequent synergistic untoward effects should be considered.

Behavioral and social skills training have been used extensively in the management of specific behaviors in autism spectrum disorder (Blackwell & Niederhauser, 2003). The goal of behavioral training and management is to assist individuals with autism spectrum disorder to approach normal functioning as closely as possible and gain independence. Behavior management helps individuals learn skills to help prevent undesirable behaviors. To be most effective, all individuals involved in a person's care, including caregivers, teachers, and therapists, must apply behavior management consistently over time. Many parents find that this effort requires a significant time commitment, and they may not have the stamina and dedication to maintain the intervention. Although there is no cure or specific intervention for autism spectrum disorder, early intervention and special education programs greatly increase the likelihood of individuals reaching their optimal level of function and independence.

Functional Implications of Autism Spectrum Disorder

Personal and Psychosocial Issues

The goals for individuals with autism spectrum disorder are the same as the goals for most individuals: to live a meaningful, productive adult life, with friends, social outlets, and gainful employment. Individuals' level of achievement often depends not only on which manifestations are associated with the condition but also on how those manifestations have been experienced. Individuals who have been helped to activate their potential and develop skills they are capable of acquiring also experience increased self-worth.

Activities and Participation

Despite level of intellectual and social functioning, many individuals with autism spectrum disorder who are higher functioning continue to live with their parents or with professional support. Nevertheless, the number of higher-functioning individuals with autism spectrum disorder who are gainfully employed is lower than might be expected given their functional abilities (Renty & Roeyers, 2006). As with other health conditions, the extent to which individuals experience limitations because of their condition is often influenced by their environment and social attitudes, as well as by manifestations of the condition itself.

For most families, children leave home to go to college or enter the workforce when they become young adults. In the case of families of individuals with autism spectrum disorder, this transition may be postponed indefinitely.

The educational goals for students with autism spectrum disorder are the same as those for all students: to provide opportunities to acquire the skills and knowledge that will allow them to enter the workforce and lead independent, satisfying lives. However, as these students move closer to exiting the secondary school system, this objective is often not at the forefront of the planning process. Many students with autism spectrum disorder and their parents may experience high levels of stress and anxiety during the transition period from high school into the adult service system. In fact, according to Seltzer, Greenberg, and Orsmond (2010) parents often describe this as "falling off a cliff" due to barriers including lack of continuity, limited access and information, and poor preparation and planning. In other cases parents may be reluctant to allow the individual to achieve greater independence due to feelings of guilt, or they may believe that in allowing their child to leave they are abandoning their own role as parents and providers of care. In some instances, fear of the individual's vulnerability may raise concerns. Either way, expectations for achievement may be set inappropriately low.

Autism spectrum disorder at the higher levels can sometimes be an invisible disability; individuals with this condition are not obviously different to others. Consequently, when they exhibit behaviors associated with the condition, others may not attribute those behaviors to a health condition. For this reason, higher functioning individuals with autism spectrum disorder may not receive the same level of understanding and support experienced by others with a health condition that has more obvious manifestations. These individuals may feel they do not fit into many social and work situations. Inadequate social ability may make it difficult for them to form intimate relationships with others and to find a life partner. They may have difficulty establishing friendships and finding a confidant.

Although parents play a central role in helping their adult child with autism spectrum disorder achieve his or her full life potential, each individual has different strengths, limitations, and life circumstances. As much as possible, individuals should be given opportunities to strengthen their social support network and to receive support that is tailored to their individual needs, thereby enabling them to achieve their greatest level of quality of life.

Sexuality

The skills associated with the core features of autism spectrum disorder, including limitations in communication, social interactional deficits and stereotyped patterns of behavior are important in relation to sexuality, sexual development, and sexual health (Dewinter, Vermeiren, Vanwesenbeeck, & van Nieuwenhuizen, 2013). For individuals with autism spectrum disorder, sexuality is often ignored, although it is of major concern both for the individuals and for their families. Research has shown that individuals with autism spectrum disorder not only engage in sexual behaviors, such as masturbation, but they show interest in romantic and/or sexual relationships with others (Dewinter et al., 2013). Age-appropriate sexual behavior may be present in some individuals with autism, while others may demonstrate inappropriate behavior. Unfortunately, the expression of sexual desires is often disinhibited and/or done inappropriately, which can cause myriad problems. Individuals with autism spectrum disorder, when trying to engage another person in sexual contact, may have difficulty distinguishing between desired and undesired contact, which may be related to their inability to distinguish social and emotional reciprocity (Hellemans, Colson, Verbraeken, Vermeiren, & Deboutte, 2007). Addressing the sexuality-related desires and needs of persons with autism spectrum disorder represents a movement toward normalization and inclusion.

There continues to be a significant need for training and education related to sexuality for persons with autism spectrum disorder, as well as for their families and caregivers.

Vocational Issues in Autism Spectrum Disorder

It has been estimated that from 50%–75% of adults with autism spectrum disorder are unemployed or underemployed, including those with a higher level of functioning (Hendricks, 2010). Historically, only a minority of individuals with autism spectrum disorder have obtained a college or university degree, have lived semi-independently, or have obtained a paid job (Tsatsanis, 2003). Although not all adults with autism are able to work, nearly 35% of adults with autism who are higher functioning, and 10% of adults who are lower functioning work in a supported work environment (Ganz, 2007). Social deficits and the degree of stereotyped and ritualistic behavior can have a detrimental effect on employment regardless of communication skills or intellectual ability (Tsatsanis, 2003).

Individuals with higher functioning autism spectrum disorder usually have typical language and intellectual functioning and may excel in areas not dependent on social interaction. Career choices using computer technology, lab research, or other areas in which there is limited social interaction have been shown to be good options for individuals with this condition.

However, social impairment in autism spectrum disorder can be severely debilitating. Despite the capacity of individuals with autism spectrum disorder to be productive and their ability to make significant intellectual contributions, their apparent social insensitivity and indifference can be severely handicapping. Social skills training can be of help in this regard. Given that change is frequently difficult for individuals with autism spectrum disorder to accept, they may perform better in a structured environment with set routines.

Until recently, few supported employment programs were specifically designed for individuals with autism spectrum disorder, although a growing number of such programs are being developed (Hagner & Cooney, 2005). Some studies indicate that supported employment programs not only increase productivity and satisfaction for individuals with autism spectrum disorder with both higher and lower levels of functioning (Howlin, Alcock, & Burkin, 2005) but can also increase levels of executive functioning in these individuals (Garcia-Villamisar & Hughes, 2007).

Supported employment, in addition to providing individuals with more opportunities to gain employment and increased independence (Hurlbutt & Chalmers, 2004; Tantam, 2003), has also been shown to decrease psychological distress (Tantam, 2000) and to increase quality of life (Beadle-Brown, Murphy, & Wing, 2005).

Each individual with autism spectrum disorder is unique. Consequently, careful appraisal of individual interests, abilities, strengths, and limitations is important to achieve a better vocational outcome.

ATTENTION-DEFICIT/ HYPERACTIVITY DISORDER

Attention deficit/hyperactivity disorder is a neurodevelopmental condition distinguished by persistent patterns of inattention, hyperactivity, and/ or impulsivity that are detrimental to functioning and development (*DSM-V*, APA, 2013). Attention deficit/hyperactivity disorder is associated with higher levels of problems in the home, in social relationships, and at school. One of the most common neurodevelopmental disorders, it is typically first identified in childhood the diagnosis of attention deficit/hyperactivity disorder has recently been extended into adulthood, given findings that upwards of 50% of those diagnosed in childhood continue to demonstrate symptoms into adolescence and adulthood (CDC, 2016; Okie, 2006). Although recently there has been an increasing amount of information about adult attention deficit/hyperactivity disorder, diagnosis requires that symptoms be present before the age of 12 and that they must be present in more than one environmental situation (APA, 2013).

The behavior indicators associated with attention deficit/hyperactivity disorder are common to some degree in children, as all children at one time or another may have difficulty paying attention, sitting still, or may demonstrate impulsive behaviors. There has been a great deal concern about the overdiagnosis of attention deficit/hyperactivity disorder. An important factor in the diagnosis of this disorder is a combination of symptoms that interfere with development and/or the ability to be successful in life arenas, such as school, work, or socialization (APA, 2013).

The percentage of children estimated to have attention deficit/hyperactivity disorder has shown a steady increase over time. While the *DSM-V* reports a rate of 5% in children and 2.5% in adults (APA, 2013), according to the Centers for Disease Control and Prevention (CDC, 2016) US studies have demonstrated rates to be as high as 11% in 4–17 year olds, which represents approximately 4.6 million children. Adult attention deficit/ hyperactivity disorder occurs at a rate of approximately 4.4% in the United States (Kessler et al., 2006). The disorder occurs more frequently in males with ratios at approximately 2:1; although this varies by presentation type (APA, 2013).

Causes of Attention-Deficit/ Hyperactivity Disorder

While one specific cause for the development of attention deficit/hyperactivity disorder is unknown, both environmental and genetically determined biological factors have been found to play a role in its emergence (Vance, Winther, & Rennie, 2012). Factors such as very low birth weight, maternal smoking or alcohol consumption during pregnancy, child abuse or neglect, exposure to teratogens such as lead, and infections have been correlated with attention deficit/hyperactivity disorder (APA, 2013; Taylor & Rogers, 2005). However, these correlations have not been determined to be causal relationships (APA, 2013).

Researchers are paying attention to interplay between environment and genetics during critical developmental periods to identify possible risk and/ or resilience factors that may exist (Vance et al., 2012). As stated by Taylor and Rogers (2005), "A weak risk factor for disorder in the population (e.g., physically harsh treatment) may be stronger on a specific outcome (e.g., aggression) and a very strong influence in a [genetically] vulnerable subgroup" (p. 451). For example, psychosocial factors such as the quality of relationships within the family structure and social interactions with both teachers and peers at school may either create a risk for, or may provide protection against, the development of related symptoms of attention deficit/hyperactivity disorder in someone who may be carrying specific genetic predispositions (Taylor & Rogers, 2005). Conversely, the presence of symptoms of attention deficit/hyperactivity disorder may also influence interactions within the environment; sorting out this relationship may never fully be possible.

While there is emerging evidence that suggests possible gene links, as well as differing brain structure and activity in persons with attention deficit/hyperactivity disorder (Vance et al., 2012), perhaps the strongest evidence for a biological connection can be found by simply looking at family patterns. A significantly high level of heritability exists within this population, which is often observed in first degree relatives (APA, 2013; Vance et al., 2012).

Identification of Attention-Deficit/Hyperactivity Disorder

Attention deficit/hyperactivity disorder typically presents in the early grade school years, although symptoms are sometimes first noticeable when the child is a toddler. It may be challenging to distinguish symptoms of attention deficit/hyperactivity in younger children, as a certain level of rambunctiousness at times is developmentally normal. The presentation of symptoms must be present over the past 6 months, must be developmentally incongruous, must be present in at least two settings, and there must be evidence of adverse impact on academic, vocational, and/or social functioning (APA, 2013). Symptoms of the disorder must also be present before 12 years of age and must not be better explained by another condition or mental disorder.

The assessment and diagnosis of attention deficit/hyperactivity disorder requires a comprehensive, multimodal information gathering process. This should include interviews with parents, teachers, and other individuals who may have relevant insight into the behaviors of the child. Rating scales and checklists are often utilized in this process, which allow parents and teachers to provide observations and information on the presence and prevalence of specific symptoms, as well as

information related to possible coexisting conditions (e.g., the Conners' Rating Scales—Revised; Humphries, 2007). A thorough history of the behavioral problems and related symptoms should be completed by both the parents and teachers, in order to get a complete picture of the presenting problem (Humphries, 2007). Standardized assessment of cognitive and academic ability should also be included in the diagnostic process, as well as actual observations of the child in his or her natural environment, if possible. Given the complexity of attention deficit/hyperactivity disorder and the possible related and/or comorbid conditions that exist, proper diagnosis requires the generation of a comprehensive picture of the child's behaviors, history, environment, and the impact.

Attention deficit/hyperactivity disorder is diagnosed by considering symptoms in a dyadic manner. There are nine symptoms related to inattention and nine symptoms related to hyperactivity and/or impulsivity. In each case, an individual must exhibit a minimum of six symptoms (five if 17 years or older) in order to meet the diagnostic criteria that feature (APA, 2013). A person may meet the criteria for either one or the other, or both.

Attention deficit/hyperactivity disorder expresses itself in three ways: *combined presentation*; *predominantly inattentive presentation*; and *predominantly hyperactive/impulsive presentation* (APA, 2013). Individuals with a combined presentation demonstrate a pattern of inattentive behaviors concurrent with hyperactivity and/or impulsivity. Predominantly inattentive presentation indicates that the criteria for inattention have been met but not those related to hyperactivity/impulsivity. Conversely, the predominantly hyperactive/impulsive presentation is indicative of lower rates of inattention, but diagnostically significant rates of symptoms related to hyperactivity and impulsivity. An overview of the diagnostic criteria can be found in **Table 12-3**.

Once the diagnostic criteria are met, the level of severity (mild, moderate, or severe) should be specified, dependent on the actual number of symptoms present. An individual who meets the minimum number of required criteria, which cause only minor impairments in functioning would be specified as having *mild* attention deficit/hyperactivity

Table 12-3   Symptoms of Attention Deficit/ Hyperactivity Disorder

Symptoms of Inattention (*Must demonstrate a minimum of 6* [*5 if 17 years or older*])

- Often fails to give close attention to details or makes careless mistakes;
- Often has difficulty sustaining attention in tasks or play activities;
- Often does not seem to listen when spoke to directly;
- Often does not follow through on instructions and fails to finish schoolwork, chores, or duties in the workplace;
- Often has difficulty organizing tasks and activities;
- Often avoids, dislikes, or is reluctant to engage in tasks that require sustained mental effort;
- Often loses things necessary for tasks or activities;
- Is often easily distracted by extraneous stimuli;
- Is often forgetful in daily activities.

Symptoms of Hyperactivity/Impulsivity (*Must demonstrate a minimum of 6* [*5 if 17 years or older*])

- Often fidgets with or taps hands or feet or squirms in seat;
- Often leaves seat in situations when remaining seated is expected;
- Often runs about or climbs in situation where it is inappropriate;
- Often unable to play or engage in leisure activities quietly;
- Is often "on the go," acting as if "driven by a motor";
- Often talks excessively;
- Often blurts out an answer before a question has been completed;
- Often has difficulty waiting his or her turn;
- Often interrupts or intrudes on others.

Data from American Psychiatric Association. (2013). *Diagnostic and statistical manual of mental disorders* (5th ed.). Washington, DC: Author.

disorder. The presence of a great number of symptoms causing significant impairment in a number of life areas would yield diagnosis of *severe* attention deficit/hyperactivity disorder.

Research has consistently shown higher rates of co-occurring disorders in persons with attention deficit/hyperactivity disorder. The most common comorbid conditions include mood and anxiety disorders, substance abuse disorders, conduct disorder and oppositional defiant disorder (APA, 2013; Biederman et al., 2006; Vance et al., 2012; Vingilis et al., 2015; Weiss & Weiss, 2004). Specific learning disorders, motor disorders, and autism spectrum disorders have also been found to co-occur with attention deficit/hyperactivity disorder (APA, 2013; Vance et al., 2012). Careful assessment and identification of any co-occurring conditions is extremely important in order to ensure that individuals are receiving the right treatment and the best possible interventions for their specific needs.

Management of Attention-Deficit/ Hyperactivity Disorder

Environmental factors can worsen the severity of symptoms of attention deficit/hyperactivity disorder causing even higher levels of consequence (Miranda, Colomer, Fernandez, Presentacion, & Rosello, 2015). Early identification and management of the disorder can lead to more successful long-term outcomes. The most common approach for the management of symptoms related to attention deficit/hyperactivity disorder continues to be medication, although behavioral therapy approaches are also a viable, evidence-based option. The American Academy of Pediatrics (AAP, 2011) recommends behavior therapy as a first line approach for symptom management in preschool children, followed by the use of appropriate medications if therapy is unsuccessful. For elementary school-aged children and adolescents, a combination of medication and evidence-based behavior therapy is most preferred (AAP, 2011). Adults with attention deficit/hyperactivity disorder are most frequently treated with medications alone.

Central nervous system stimulant medications such as methylphenidate (e.g., Ritalin and Concerta) have been found to be most effective in decreasing symptoms of attention deficit/ hyperactivity disorder with approximately 70%–80% of individuals with having a positive response (AAP, 2011; Humphries, 2006). However, stimulant medications can have a lot of side effects, including loss of appetite, difficulty sleeping, headaches, and irritability (Humphries, 2007). Nonstimulant medications including atomoxetine, guanfacine, and clonidine are an alternative choice when stimulant medications are not preferred or tolerated, although evidence for their success is not as strong (AAP, 2011).

Behavior therapy, which is focused on assisting individuals in changing their behaviors through planning, organization, goal-setting, and rewards, are frequently prescribed for use in both the school and home settings. This requires that parents and/or teachers set clear guidelines for behaviors, structured routines for behavioral control, and positive reinforcements to maximize success (National Institute of Mental Health [NIMH], 2016). Behavioral interventions also often include parental education and/or behavioral parental management training in order to teach parents how to best support their child and to use systems of rewards and consequences to effect behavioral change (NIMH, 2016).

Functional Implications of Attention-Deficit/Hyperactivity Disorder

Personal and Psychosocial Issues

Attention deficit/hyperactivity disorder is associated with myriad psychosocial factors that impact success in different life areas. Problems with family and peers and in school, as well as emotional, behavioral, and conduct problems are all commonly reported (Sarver, McCart, Sheidow, & Letourneau, 2014; Selinus et al., 2015). Research has shown that a diagnosis of attention deficit/hyperactivity disorder is associated with an increased risk for problems in school, including truancy and failure (Norén Selinus et al., 2015). Alcohol and drug abuse is also more prevalent in persons with attention deficit/hyperactivity disorder (Selinus et al., 2015).

Conflicts with siblings and parents may consistently arise, and higher levels of stress and anxiety in the home may cause additional concerns for individuals with this condition (Miranda et al., 2015). Children and adolescents with attention deficit/hyperactivity disorder often struggle in their peer relationships as well, finding it difficult to interact and get along with others.

Some research has also shown higher rates of conduct disorder and antisocial behaviors in individuals with attention deficit/hyperactivity disorder (APA, 2013; Selinus et al., 2015). In a study by Selinus and colleagues (2015), it was found that identification of attention deficit/hyperactivity in early childhood was associated with the highest level of risk among the neurodevelopmental problems for later development of antisocial behavior and impaired daily functioning. Persons with attention deficit/hyperactivity disorder also have a higher number of accidents and injuries, which may also lead to higher rates of related health problems (APA, 2013). These issues speak to the need for early intervention in order to assist individuals in overcoming deficits and learning strategies to promote more successful progress through the developmental stages over time.

Vocational Issues in Attention-Deficit/Hyperactivity Disorder

Psychosocial deficits related to attention deficit/hyperactivity disorder impact the life arenas in adults as well when symptoms of the disorder extend beyond the developmental years. Some suggest that there are cumulative consequences associated with a lifelong diagnosis of the disorder, which subsequently impacts upon quality of life (Brod, Schmitt, Goodwin, Hodgkins, & Niebler, 2011). One important factor that relates to this is employment.

Adults with attention deficit/hyperactivity disorder demonstrate a number of issues in the vocational arena (Das, Cherbuin, Butterworth, Anstey, & Easteal, 2012), including poor occupational performance, work attendance, job attainment and tenure, and interpersonal conflict with supervisors and coworkers (APA, 2013; Stein, 2008). Unemployment and underemployment is a chief concern raised by adults with attention deficit/hyperactivity disorder. A number of factors contribute to these issues. Difficulties in school may lead to underachievement/lower levels of education (Stein, 2008). Symptom management issues, such as difficulty staying on task, self-regulation, and impulsivity may impact upon work performance as well, leading to work performance issues or frequent errors (Painter, Prevatt, & Welles, 2008). Executive/organizational deficits may lead to difficulty with multitasking as well as completion of complex or sequential job tasks (Painter et al., 2008). Related deficits in interpersonal skills may also be problematic during social interactions in the workplace with employers, coworkers and/or customers. Concurrently, because attention deficit/hyperactivity disorder is an invisible disability, workers may be perceived by others as lazy or unreliable. These relationships may be further complicated for individuals who also have issues with conduct or antisocial behavior, which often co-occur with attention deficit/hyperactivity disorder (Stein, 2008). Together, these issues often lead to poor self-concept, decreased self-esteem, and negative beliefs about the world of work among adults with attention deficit/hyperactivity disorder (Painter et al., 2008).

The provision of vocational counseling and support for individuals with attention deficit/hyperactivity disorder can be helpful in navigating these challenges. For example, assessment of vocational interests and abilities in light of a person's specific symptom profile may help identify jobs where those particular symptoms might actual enhance work performance. In addition, assisting a person with attention deficit/hyperactivity disorder in identifying and implementing preferred compensatory strategies in the workplace may assist in managing potential problems. Examples of strategies include recording conversations with supervisors where job instructions are provided, posting written reminders and checklists in strategic places around the workplace, use of a daily calendar system, and reduction of distractions in and around the person's workspace (Painter et al., 2008). An important key to success is individualizing vocational supports and compensatory strategies to the specific needs of the person.

Sexuality

Some findings have shown a connection between attention deficit/hyperactivity disorder and risky sexual behaviors (RSBs; Sarver et al., 2014). This includes earlier start of sexual activity, more casual partners, more lifetime partners, and more sexually transmitted diseases (Barkley, Fischer, Smallish, & Fletcher, 2006; Flory, Molina, Pelham, Gnagy, & Smith, 2006; Ramos Olazagasti et al., 2013; Sarver et al., 2014). However, recent studies have paid particular attention to co-occurring disorders and have found that the relationship between attention deficit/hyperactivity disorder and RSBs appears to

be mediated by co-occurring conduct disorders and/or substance abuse disorders (Ramos Olazagasti et al., 2013; Sarver et al., 2014). This is important as early behavioral interventions for children who may be at-risk for the development of a comorbid conduct or substance abuse problems may subsequently decrease potential for the development of RSBs later in life.

SPECIFIC LEARNING DISORDERS (LEARNING DISABILITIES)

Specific learning disorders (*DSM-V*, APA, 2013; also known as *learning disabilities*) comprise a group of neurologically based processing conditions that affect the individual's ability to acquire or use information through sources, such as reading, writing, mathematical calculations, listening, speaking, or reasoning, in the absence of more global intellectual disability. Specific learning disorders are present in approximately 8%–10% of children under 18 years of age in the United States (National Institute of Neurological Disorders and Stroke [NINDS], 2015). Data is limited related to prevalence in adults but is estimated to be around 4% (APA, 2013). Specific learning disorders are diagnosed in males more frequently than females, at an approximate rate of 2:1 (APA, 2013; Poelmans, Buitelaar, Pauls, & Franke, 2011).

As with other neurodevelopmental disabilities, varying degrees of impairment are associated with specific learning disorders: *mild, moderate,* and *severe*. Severe specific learning disorders affect a large number of academic and functional skills. Although individuals with severe specific learning disorders usually have a lower level of achievement in academic or other areas than would be expected for someone of that age group, it is not indicative of low intellectual ability (APA, 2013; Reschly, 2005). Individuals with severe specific learning disorders may have average or even high levels of intelligence. Nevertheless, the condition can lead to major functional limitation in many areas of daily life (Gillberg & Soderstrom, 2003).

Functional deficits associated with severe specific learning disorders have negative impacts on academic and general life achievements. They can interfere with the individual's ability to read and comprehend information, to carry out mathematical calculations, or to spell or write. Tasks of everyday life, such as using money, paying bills, reading instructions, or completing applications or forms, may be severely compromised (APA, 2013).

Cause of Specific Learning Disorders

Environmental and genetic factors play a role in the development of a specific learning disorder (APA, 2013; Poelmans et al., 2011). Individuals with co-existing neurological conditions, perinatal injury, or genetic predisposition may exhibit specific learning disorders. Environmental factors such as prenatal nicotine exposure and low birth weight increases the risk of development of a specific learning disorder (APA, 2013). However, emerging evidence supports a strong biological component. Specific learning disorders are highly heritable at rates as high as 75% (Poelmans et al., 2011), especially in first-degree relatives (APA, 2013). In addition, imaging studies have shown altered patterns of brain functioning in persons with the specific learning disorder dyslexia (Hoskyn, 2008), which suggests biological indicators. Nevertheless, many individuals with specific learning disorders have no specific identifiable cause to which the condition can be attributed.

Manifestations of Specific Learning Disorders

Specific learning disorders can be manifested in any area of information processing. Individuals generally do not have difficulty with all areas of learning, but may have a disability in just one area. For example, **dyslexia**, an alternative term used to describe difficulties characterized by impairment in reading accuracy, fluency, or comprehension is the most common learning disorder in children (Poelmans et al., 2011). It affects reading in approximately 5%–10% of all school-aged children (Boyd, 2005; Poelmans et al., 2011). Reading disability not only affects academic achievement but also interferes with many other activities that require reading skills, such as reading notices, understanding forms and applications, and reading labels of medicine bottles.

Other types of specific learning disorders may affect writing, including difficulty in handwriting, spelling, or composition. Individuals may have difficulty organizing thoughts in written composition, make numerous punctuation and spelling errors, or have poor handwriting. Academic achievement and other tasks of daily living that require writing are affected with this form of specific learning disorder.

Specific learning disorders may also include difficulty in learning math facts understanding numbers, and difficulty with math reasoning and calculation (**dyscalculia**). Individuals with this type of specific learning disorder have difficulty with simple calculations and following sequences of steps to solve math problems. They may also have difficulty reading numerical symbols or understanding math terms. This type of specific learning disorder, in addition to affecting academic achievement, has implications for other tasks in daily life that rely on mathematical principles and skills, such as counting money, paying bills, and calculating measurements.

Identification of Specific Learning Disorders

Specific learning disorders are often not identified early, and they may not be noticed until the child enters school. When problems are identified, they may be inaccurately interpreted as lack of interest, not trying, or lack of cognitive ability (Dudley-Marling, 2004). Individuals may be labeled as having low intellectual ability and not receive the type of intervention that could accommodate their condition. Although learning disabilities are often identified in school, they may also be first identified in adulthood. In adults, learning disabilities may not be identified unless it becomes obvious that individuals are unable to read signs, written instructions, or complete forms.

There are several key diagnostic features that must be present in order for an individual to meet criteria for a specific learning disorder, which are outlined in **Table 12-4**.

Table 12-4   Diagnostic Features of Specific Learning Disorder

- Persistent difficulties learning keystone academic skills (reading, spelling, writing, calculation and math reasoning), with onset during the formal schooling years.
  - ◆ A lack of progress is made despite the provision of specific interventions at home or in school for six or months.
- Individual performance in the affected academic skill area is well below average for age.
- Learning difficulties are typically readily apparent in the early school years.
- Learning difficulties are specific, meaning:
  - ◆ They are not attributable to intellectual disability;
  - ◆ They cannot be attributed to general external factors (e.g., economic disadvantage);
  - ◆ They cannot be attributed to a neurological, motor, vision, or hearing disorder; and
  - ◆ They may restricted to one academic skill or domain.

Data from American Psychiatric Association. (2013). *Diagnostic and statistical manual of mental disorders* (5th ed.). Washington, DC: Author.

Identification of a specific learning disorder requires a standardized assessment process by a trained clinician and should include a thorough psychosocial evaluation including information about the person's medical, developmental, educational, and family history (APA, 2013). Notably, other factors, such as inadequate educational opportunities (e.g., deficient teaching, high rate of absenteeism) or sensory impairment (e.g., impaired vision or hearing), can also affect ability to learn or ability to gain specific skills, which emphasizes the importance of proper diagnosis and management. Without adequate testing by professionals trained to conduct such tests, identification of a specific learning disorder should not be made. If these other factors are identified, remediation or correction of the underlying problem should be undertaken (if possible).

Management of Specific Learning Disorder

Although a specific learning disorder can be managed, it can be managed successfully only when it is accurately identified. Early intervention

programs such as special educational programs to assist individuals (children and adults) to learn alternative ways of processing information can be beneficial. Provision of special accommodations that enable individuals to adapt to the limitations they are experiencing is also helpful. Those assistive devices or materials that best accommodate the individual's learning needs should be used. Visual aids, materials written in simple phrases, and use of auditory rather than visual learning modes can all help individuals learn material in accordance with their own needs. The underpinning of effective management is tailoring the interventions to best meet each individual's specific needs (Dudley-Marling, 2004).

Functional Implications of Specific Learning Disorder

Personal and Psychosocial Issues

Adults with specific learning disorders face many challenges in employment and daily routines; however, with appropriate interventions and adjustments, educational and employment success and personal satisfaction can be attained. Although early recognition of specific learning disorders and referral to appropriate special education programs can assist many individuals to achieve their full potential, not all individuals are in a situation that affords them this benefit. Individuals who achieve higher levels of success have been found to come from higher socioeconomic backgrounds, have greater social and psychological support systems, and have access to quality special education programs (Greenbaum, Graham, & Scales, 1996).

Individuals with specific learning disorders may experience shame or loss of self-esteem if they are unable to perform learning or other tasks that others take for granted. Self-esteem may be further damaged if individuals are made to feel inadequate or incompetent by others. As adults, these feelings can become internalized and lead to feelings of helplessness. When a specific learning disorder is not identified and individuals do not receive appropriate intervention or have adequate levels of support, the picture can be bleak. Frustrated by school failure, individuals may drop out of high school or obtain entry-level jobs with little hope for advancement. In other instances, individuals may turn to crime or substance abuse.

Activities and Participation

Early identification of learning problems, determination of appropriate expectations, and identification and coordination of specific support systems and educational interventions are critical factors in assisting individuals with a specific learning disorder to achieve their full potential. Individuals who have not had a specific learning disorder identified in childhood but continue to experience the manifestations of their condition in adulthood are frequently ashamed of their limitation and may attempt to hide them and reject services even when they are available. Multi-tiered academic and behavioral interventions may be of benefit in such cases (Reschly, 2005). Providing specific instructional aids, helping individuals identify and acknowledge specific learning needs, and acquiring appropriate supports and resources to meet those needs are examples of interventions that may be instituted.

Vocational Issues in Specific Learning Disorder

Given the wide variety of limitations experienced by individuals with a specific learning disorder, affected persons may need to develop a wide range of compensatory skills and abilities to manage their condition effectively. Individuals should be placed in an environment that suits their specific interests and abilities as well as their particular limitations. Appropriate assessment for identification of the specific type of learning disorder and associated limitations is the first step in successful intervention. When specific limitations are identified, appropriate accommodations can be provided. Individuals should be helped to understand their condition and identify compensatory strategies and techniques that are most helpful for them.

Attention should also be paid to the individual's ability to deal with pressure and criticism. Because individuals may have a history of isolation and negative experiences, they may be more sensitive to pressure to perform or to feedback or criticism about their work or productivity.

Depending on the type of specific learning disorder present, individuals may need accommodations regarding time management, organization, or memory. In other types of learning disabilities, individuals may have difficulty with visual or auditory processing, writing, or reading. Various types of assistive technologies or software, such as personal management software, talking calculators, electronic notebooks, software, display controls, or word processing tools, may also be helpful in enhancing individual performance.

GENERAL ISSUES IN NEURODEVELOPMENTAL DISORDERS

Personal and Psychosocial Issues

Individuals with neurodevelopmental disorders can be found in every age, ethnic, racial, and socioeconomic group. Whether the individual has an intellectual disability, autism spectrum disorder, attention deficit/hyperactivity disorder, a specific learning disorder, or a combination of neurodevelopmental issues, his or her needs and concerns may be as diverse and individualized as those of the general population. This includes mental health needs.

Individuals with neurodevelopmental disorders are generally considered at increased risk for a range of health problems, including mental health concerns (Gustafsson & Sonnander, 2004; Rush, Bowman, Eidman, Toole, & Mortenson, 2004). Unfortunately, the same mental health services available to the general population are often not accessed by persons with neurodevelopmental disorders (Stawski & Merrick, 2006). Often mental health problems go undetected because of communication problems present in many intellectual and other neurodevelopmental disorders, or because manifestations of mental health problems may present differently in this population. At times manifestations are missed because of *diagnostic overshadowing* (the attribution of manifestations to the primary health condition rather than to mental health problems). Even when mental health issues are identified, appropriate interventions may be unavailable due to the misconception that manifestations are not manageable or because mental health professionals have little training or experience working with individuals with neurodevelopmental disorder who also have mental health problems.

The rate of depression in individuals with intellectual or developmental disability is higher than in the general population (Lunsky, 2004). A number of studies have shown that suicidal ideation and attempted suicide occur in individuals with intellectual and neurodevelopmental disorders (APA, 2013; Merrick, Merrick, Lunsky, & Kandel, 2006). However there has been limited research within this population, in particular intellectual disability, on intervention strategies when suicidal behavior is identified (Merrick et al., 2006).

Communication problems are common in individuals with intellectual and neurodevelopmental disorders. For individuals who are unable to communicate adequately, a change in behavior or a demonstration of challenging behaviors may be the first sign of a physical or mental health condition. Assessing the meaning of the behavior as well as the cause, rather than jumping to conclusions about the cause and the appropriate intervention, is an important step in appropriate management. Medications should be used only when needed to manage an underlying health condition—not to control behaviors. Unrecognized health conditions, psychiatric conditions, and environmental changes can all cause changes or exacerbation of behaviors. Family violence and abuse are also associated with individuals with intellectual and neurodevelopmental disorders and should not be discounted as a potential cause for behaviors exhibited by the individual.

Activities and Participation

Individuals with neurodevelopmental disorders have, in the past, been labeled as people incapable of determining their own best interests or negotiating to meet their needs. This myth is slowly being dispelled, as there is increased recognition that each person with a neurodevelopmental disorder has individual strengths that can be utilized to meet life's challenges. Individuals with neurodevelopmental disorders want the same things that most people want in life, including living in a home environment, having the opportunity for friendship and social interaction, and having the opportunity to fulfill educational and vocational goals to the level of their ability. Identifying neurodevelopmental disorders and implementing appropriate interventions as early as possible is important to helping meet these goals (Pinto-Martin, Dunkle, Earls, Fliedner, & Landes, 2005).

Like all people, individuals with neurodevelopmental disorders are sexual persons, and they are entitled to sexual expression, marriage, and children. However, owing to misconceptions, stereotypes, and prejudice, health and rehabilitation professionals, family, and the community may be reluctant to discuss sexuality, to address sexual issues as they arise, or may actively discourage them from sexual practice (Kazukauskas & Lam, 2010). Sexuality is more than anatomical or physical functioning but rather is linked to basic needs of acceptance, affection, value, and self-esteem (Murphy & Elias, 2006). Individuals with neurodevelopmental disorders have the same right to information about sexuality, such as attaining and maintaining intimate relationships and managing complex emotions, as well as information about sexual orientation, sexually transmitted conditions, contraception and abstinence, health implications of pregnancy, and prevention of sexual abuse.

Throughout their life spans, individuals with neurodevelopmental disorders will undoubtedly encounter some of the same challenges that most people encounter. Because of the nature of their mental health needs, however, they are often more vulnerable to a variety of challenges. Individuals with neurodevelopmental disorders should be educated about inappropriate use of illicit drugs and alcohol, development of inappropriate relationships, sexuality, sexual abuse, pregnancy prevention, and prevention of sexually transmitted conditions (AAP, 1996; Kazukauskas & Lam, 2009; Taylor Gomez, 2012). Psychosocial and environmental problems can be a major concern for many individuals with neurodevelopmental disorders. These can be related to the following issues:

- The primary support group (e.g., removal from the home, physical or sexual abuse, parental overprotection)
- The social environment (e.g., difficulty with acculturation, discrimination, death or lossof a friend)
- The educational environment (e.g., conflict with teachers or peers, academic problems,restrictive classroom placement that is inappropriate to meet specific needs)
- Work (e.g., unemployment, difficult work conditions, poor matches between theindividual and the job, underemployment)
- Housing (e.g., inadequate housing, conflict with neighbors or landlords, overlyrestrictive environment)
- Money (e.g., inadequate finances, inadequate public support)
- Health care (e.g., unavailable transportation to facilities, inadequate insurance, inabilityto adequately communicate so as to participate in identification of the condition or inmanagement)
- The legal and justice systems (e.g., victimization, arrest, exploitation, lack ofknowledgeable representation)
- Availability of support services (e.g., conflict with nonfamily caregivers)
- Lack of access to information about assistance available; confusing and uncoordinatedservice systems

Individuals with a neurodevelopmental disorder are likely to experience at least one problem in each of these areas by adulthood (APA, 2013). They and their families should be helped to identify and eliminate barriers and challenges so that they are able to reach the highest quality of life within the range of their ability.

Just as advances in health technology have increased life expectancy for the general population, so have they increased life expectancy for individuals with neurodevelopmental disorders, who are now living longer and confronting the same chronic conditions that others encounter in later life, compounding existing impairments (Heller & Sorenson, 2013). In addition, the prevalence of mental health conditions, including dementia, is increased in a number of intellectual disabilities, such as Down syndrome (Fisher, 2004).

Many individuals with neurodevelopmental disorders continue to live with their families into adulthood. In families without a family member with neurodevelopmental disorder, there is a time when children move out of the parental home to go to school, go to work, or begin their own families. In families in which a family member has a neurodevelopmental disorder, this stage of the family life cycle may be postponed (Krauss, Seltzer, & Jacobson, 2005). In most instances, whether due to incapacitation or death of the primary family caretaker, a decision about moving the individual with a neurodevelopmental disorder to another setting is made. Such decisions affect both the individual and other family members, and they can cause considerable distress and conflict within families. Support for families involved in making this type of alternative residential setting decision should be made available.

Benefits of residential services and supports for individuals with neurodevelopmental disorders are increasingly being realized. Individuals receiving residential services and supports in the community have been found to experience increased personal freedom and opportunities for social activities as well as development of increased level of functional skills, which in turn increases individual independence (Lakin & Stancliffe, 2007).

Vocational Issues

Neurodevelopmental disorders encompass a wide variety of conditions that occur in childhood and are lifelong conditions, affecting intellectual and social function and requiring ongoing special services and support from an interdisciplinary team to meet lifelong opportunities and challenges. Knowledge of the specific condition is important to provide the most effective and least obtrusive support and intervention for individuals with neurodevelopmental disorders as they go about meeting the challenges in their everyday lives. Understanding the characteristics of specific conditions can promote steps toward independence and self-determination.

Although individual needs are often identified though test results and related to the type of health condition and its manifestations, the affirmation that each person is an individual with unique circumstances and goals is essential in the structure of a plan that is most appropriate for that individual. Working with the individual's strengths, interests, and abilities in creative ways produces a better outcome than trying to treat all individuals with the same health condition in the same way (Olney, 2000). Individuals should be assessed in the context of their unique circumstances and preferences. Adequate information should be obtained, which can then be used to make appropriate referrals or to establish plans and interventions to help individuals meet their goals to the best of their ability. Both the strengths and the limitations of the individual serve as a framework for such planning. Services and supports should be identified in conjunction with goals and objectives that have been mutually decided upon by the individual with neurodevelopmental disorder and his or her family.

Employment has the potential for helping individuals with neurodevelopmental disorders achieve independence and social inclusion (Caldwell & Heller, 2007; Cordes & Howard, 2005). Paid and meaningful work can enhance self-image, dignity, and social competence of individuals with neurodevelopmental disorders through social integration and help them gain socially valuable roles. Many individuals with these conditions may not be working because of prejudice and stereotypes that they are unemployable.

In many instances, part-time or supported employment options offer opportunities for individuals for whom work was not previously considered an option. Essential factors that help individuals with neurodevelopmental disorders obtain the best outcome include a job placement that is in accordance with the individual's interests and skills, appropriate transportation arrangements, ongoing monitoring and communication with the employer, adequate training, and advocacy.

Although work remains a primary goal, some concerns regarding work for individuals with neurodevelopmental disorders must also be considered. Individuals with neurodevelopmental disorders may be able to perform a certain set of skills at the job site, but other facets of work, such as time constraints or competition, may produce high levels of stress and make maintaining a satisfactory work environment more difficult. Monitoring anxiety levels and helping individuals improve their ability to cope with stress can increase both job satisfaction and productivity. Most essential are a thorough assessment of the individual, his or her strengths and challenges, and the identification of the job, job setting, and type and degree of support needed to achieve a good match. Individuals with neurodevelopmental disorders should be exposed to a variety of appropriate jobs. As much as possible, the individual's job interest and top job choices should be honored.

CASE STUDY

Mr. C. is a 33-year-old male with attention deficit/ hyperactivity disorder with combined presentation and the specific learning disorder, dyslexia. Mr. C.'s disorders were identified in grade school, and he was placed in special education classes. Although he is functioning in the average range intellectually, he eventually dropped out of school when he was a junior in high school and has had difficulty holding a steady job ever since. Mr. C. currently lives with his parents, but this has become a problematic and highly stressful situation for everyone involved. Mr. C. has a history of impulsive and risky behaviors that have led him to some problems in the home, as well as in his romantic relationships. He has recently had increasingly aggressive and erratic behaviors as well, which led to his parents telling him that he will need to "get help or get out."

1. What are the primary disability-related and psychosocial factors that are impacting upon this case?
2. What types of services do you think would be most helpful in order to assist Mr. C in moving forward?
3. What are some particular issues that you might anticipate in your work with Mr. C.?
4. What else do you need to know?

REFERENCES

Ailey, S. H., Miller, A. M., Heller, T., & Smith, E. V., Jr. (2006). Evaluating an interpersonal model of depression among adults with Down syndrome. *Research and Theory for Nursing Practice, 20*(3), 229–246.

American Academy of Pediatrics. (1996). Sexuality education of children and adolescents with developmental disabilities. *Pediatrics, 97,* 275–278.

American Academy of Pediatrics. (2011). ADHD: Clinical practice guideline for the diagnosis, evaluation, and treatment of attention-deficit/hyperactivity disorder in children and adolescents. *Pediatrics, 128*(5), 1–16. Retrieved from http://www.pediatrics.org/cgi/doi/10.1542 /peds.2011-2654

American Association on Intellectual and Developmental Disabilities. (2013). *Frequently asked questions of intellectual disability.* Retrieved from http://aaidd.org /intellectual-disability/definition/faqs-on-intellectual -disability#.VwnLVI-cHD5

American Psychiatric Association. (2000). *Diagnostic and statistical manual of mental disorders* (4th ed. rev.). Washington, DC: Author.

American Psychiatric Association. (2013). *Diagnostic and statistical manual of mental disorders* (5th ed.). Washington, DC: Author.

Anckarsater, H., Stahlberg, O., Larson, T., Hakanson, C., Jutblad, S. B., Niklasson, L., ... Rastam, M. (2006). The impact of ADHD and autism spectrum disorders on temperament, character, and personality development. *American Journal of Psychiatry, 163,* 1239–1244.

Azzopardi-Lane, C., & Callus, A. (2015). Constructing sexual identities: People with intellectual disability talking about sexuality. *British Journal of Learning Disabilities, 43*(1), 32–37.

Baird, G., Charman, T., Baron-Cohen, S., Cox, A., Swetlenhan, J., Wheelwright, S., & Drew, A. (2000). A screening instrument for autism at 18 months of age: A 6-year follow up study. *Journal of the American Academy of Child and Adolescent Psychiatry, 39,* 694–702.

Barkley, R. A., Fischer, M., Smallish, L., & Fletcher, K. (2006). Young adult outcome of hyperactive children: Adaptive functioning in major life activities. *Journal of the American Academy of Child and Adolescent Psychiatry, 45,* 192–202.

Beadle-Brown, J., Murphy, G., & Wing, L. (2005). Long-term outcome for people with severe intellectual disabilities: Impact of social impairment. *American Journal on Mental Retardation, 110*(1), 1–12.

Biederman, J., Monuteaux, M. C., Mick, E., Spencer, T., Wilens, T. E., Silva, J. M., & ... Faraone, S. V. (2006). Young adult outcome of attention deficit hyperactivity disorder: A controlled 10-year follow-up study. *Psychological Medicine, 36*(2), 167–179. doi:10.1017/S0033291705006410

Blackwell, J., & Niederhauser, C. (2003). Diagnosis and management of autistic children. *Nurse Practitioner, 28*(6), 36–43.

Boyd, M. A. (2005). *Psychiatric nursing: Contemporary practice.* Philadelphia, PA: Lippincott Williams & Wilkins.

Brod, M., Schmitt, E., Goodwin, M., Hodgkins, P., & Niebler, G. (2011). ADHD burden of illness in older adults: A life course perspective. *Quality of Life Research.* doi:10.1007 /s11136-11011-19981-11139

Cadman, T., Eklund, H., Howley, D., Hayward, H., Clarke, H., Findon, J., ... & Glaser, K. (2012). Caregiver burden as people with autism spectrum disorder and attention deficit /hyperactivity disorder transition into adolescence and adulthood in the United Kingdom. *American Academy of Child and Adolescent Psychiatry, 51*(9), 879–888.

Caldwell, J., & Heller, T. (2007). Longitudinal outcomes of a consumer-directed program supporting adults with developmental disabilities and their families. *Intellectual and Developmental Disabilities, 45*(3), 161–173.

Carbone, P. S., Farley, M., & Davis, T. (2010). Primary care for children with autism. *American Family Physician, 81*(4), 453–460.

Carter, A. S., Volkmar, F. R., & Sparrow, S. S. (1998). The Vineland Adaptive Behavior Scales: Supplementary norms for individuals with autism. *Journal of Autism and Developmental Disorders, 28*(4), 287–302.

Center for Disease Control. (2016). *Facts about intellectual disability.* Retrieved from http://www.cdc.gov/ncbddd /actearly/pdf/parents_pdfs/IntellectualDisability.pdf

Centers for Disease Control and Prevention. (2016). *Attention deficit/hyperactivity disorder (AD/HD).* Retrieved from http://www.cdc.gov/ncbddd/adhd/facts.html

Christensen, D. L., Baio, J., Braun, K.V., Bilder, D., Charles, J., Constantino, J. N., ... Yeargin-Allsopp, M. (2016). Prevalence and characteristics of autism spectrum disorder among children aged 8 years—Autism and developmental disabilities monitoring network. In *Morbidity and Mortality Weekly Report Surveill Summ*aries 65(SS-3), 1–23. doi:10.15585 /mmwr.ss6503a

Conoley, J. C., & Kramer, J. J. (Eds.). (1989). *The tenth mental measurements yearbook.* Lincoln, NE: Buros Institute of Mental Measurement.

Cordes, T. L., & Howard, R. W. (2005). Concepts of work, leisure and retirement in adults with an intellectual disability. *Education and Training in Developmental Disabilities, 40*(2), 99–108.

Cuskelly, M., & Bryde, R. (2004). Attitudes towards the sexuality of adults with an intellectual disability: Parents, support staff, and a community sample. *Journal of Intellectual & Developmental Disability, 29*(3), 255–264.

Das, D., Cherbuin, N., Butterworth, P., Anstey, K. J., & Easteal, S. (2012). A population-based study of attention deficit / hyperactivity disorder symptoms and associated impairment in middle-aged adults. *PLoS ONE, 7*(2), 1–9. doi:10.1371 /journal.pone.0031500

Dewinter, J., Vermeiren, R., Vanwesenbeeck, I., & van Nieuwenhuizen, C. (2013). Autism and normative sexual development: A narrative review. *Journal of Clinical Nursing, 22*(23–24), 3467–3483. doi:10.1111/jocn.12397

Ditchman, N., Werner, S., Kosyluk, K., Jones, N., Elg, B., & Corrigan, P. W. (2013). Stigma and intellectual disability: Potential application of mental illness research.

Rehabilitation Psychology, 58(2), 206–216. doi:10.1037/a0032466

Dudley-Marling, C. (2004). The social construction of learning disabilities. *Journal of Learning Disabilities, 37*(6), 482–489.

Filipek, P. A., Accardo, P. J., Ashwal, S., Baranek, G. T., Cook, E. H., Jr., Dawson G., ... Volkmar, F. R. (2000). Practice parameter: Screening and diagnosis of autism. *Neurology, 55*(4), 468–479.

Fisher, K. (2004). Nursing care of special populations: Issues in caring for elderly people with mental retardation. *Nursing Forum, 39*(1), 28–31.

Flory, K., Molina, B. S. G., Pelham, W. E., Gnagy, E., & Smith, B. (2006). Childhood ADHD predicts risky sexual behavior in young adulthood. *Journal of Clinical Child and Adolescent Psychology, 35*, 571–577.

Food and Drug Administration. (2012). *Thimerosal in vaccines.* Retrieved from http://www.fda.gov/BiologicsBloodVaccines/SafetyAvailability/VaccineSafety/UCM096228

Ganz, M. L. (2007). The lifetime distribution of the incremental societal costs of autism. *Archives of Pediatrics and Adolescent Medicine, 161*(4), 343–349.

Garcia-Villamisar, D., & Hughes, C. (2007). Supported employment improves cognitive performance in adults with autism. *Journal of Intellectual Disability Research, 51* (Pt. 2), 142–150.

Giarelli, E., Souders, M., Pinto-Martin, J., Bloch, J., & Levy, S. E. (2005). Intervention pilot for parents of children with autistic spectrum disorder. *Pediatric Nursing, 31*(5), 389–399.

Gillberg, C., & Soderstrom, H. (2003). Learning disability. *Lancet, 362*(9386), 811–821.

Greenbaum, B., Graham, S., & Scales, W. (1996). Adults with learning disabilities: Occupational and social status after college. *Journal of Learning Disabilities, 29*(2), 167–173.

Gustafsson, C., & Sonnander, K. (2004). Occurrence of mental health problems in Swedish samples of adults with intellectual disabilities. *Social Psychiatry and Psychiatric Epidemiology, 39*, 448–456.

Hagner, D., & Cooney, B. F. (2005). "I do that for everybody": Supervising employees with autism. *Focus on Autism and Other Developmental Disabilities, 20*(2), 91–97.

Handen, B. L. (2007). Intellectual disability (mental retardation). In E. J. Mash & R. A. Barkley (Eds.), *Assessment of childhood disorders,* (4th ed., pp. 551–597). New York, NY: Guilford Press.

Hellemans, H., Colson, K., Verbraeken, C., Vermeiren, R., & Deboutte, D. (2007). Sexual behavior in high functioning male adolescents and young adults with autism. *Journal of Autism and Developmental Disorders, 37*, 260–269.

Heller, T., & Sorensen, A. (2013). Promoting healthy aging in adults with developmental disabilities. *Developmental Disabilities Research Reviews, 18*(1), 22–30.

Hendricks, D. (2010). Employment and adults with autism spectrum disorders: Challenges and strategies for success. *Journal of Vocational Rehabilitation, 32*(2), 125–134.

Hoskyn, M. (2008). Neurobiological and experiential origins of dyslexia: An introduction. *Developmental Neuropsychology, 33*, 659–662.

Howlin, P., Alcock, J., & Burkin, C. (2005). An 8 year follow-up of a specialist supported employment service for high-ability adults with autism or Asperger syndrome. *Autism, 9*(5), 533–549.

Hsia, Y., Wong, A. Y. S., Murphy, D. G. M., Simonoff, E., Buitelaar, J. K., & Wong, I. C. K. (2013). Psychopharmacological prescriptions for people with autism spectrum disorder (ASD): A multinational study. *Psychopharmacology, 231*(6), 999–1009. Retrieved from PsycINFO, EBSCOhost.

Humphries, T. (2007). Attention deficit/hyperactivity disorder. In I. Brown & M. Percy (Eds.), *A comprehensive guide to intellectual and developmental disabilities* (pp. 295–307). Baltimore, MD: Paul H. Brookes Publishing Co.

Hurlbutt, K., & Chalmers, L. (2004). Employment of adults with Asperger syndrome. *Focus on Autism and Other Developmental Disabilities, 19*(4), 212–222.

Impara, J. C., & Plake, B. S. (Eds.). (1998). *The thirteenth mental measurements yearbook.* Lincoln, NE: Buros Institute of Mental Measurements.

Kanner, L. (1972). *Child psychiatry* (4th ed.). Springfield, IL: Charles C. Thomas.

Kazukauskas, K. A., & Lam, C. S. (2009). The importance of addressing sexuality in certified rehabilitation counselor practice. *Rehabilitation Education, 23*(2), 127–140.

Kazukauskas, K. A., & Lam, C. S. (2010). Disability and sexuality: Knowledge, attitudes, and level of comfort among certified rehabilitation counselors. *Rehabilitation Counseling Bulletin, 54*(1), 15–25. doi:10.1177/0034355209348239

Kessler, R. C., Adler, L., Barkley, R., Biederman, J., Conners, C. K., Demler, O., ... Zaslavsky, A. M. (2006). The prevalence and correlates of adult ADHD in the United States: Results from the National Comorbidity Survey Replication. *American Journal of Psychiatry, 163*(4), 716–723.

Kim, S. H., Junker, D., & Lord, C. (2014). Observation of Spontaneous Expressive Language (OSEL): A new measure for spontaneous and expressive language of children with autism spectrum disorders and other communication disorders. *Journal of Autism and Developmental Disorders, 44*(12), 3230–3244. doi:10.1007/s10803-014-2180-0

Koger, S. M., Schettler, T., & Weiss, B. (2005). Environmental toxicants and developmental disabilities: A challenge for psychologists. *American Psychologist, 60*(3), 243–255.

Krauss, M. W., Seltzer, M. M., & Jacobson, H. T. (2005). Adults with autism living at home or in non-family settings: Positive and negative aspects of residential status. *Journal of Intellectual Disability Research, 49*(2), 111–124.

Laider, J. R. (2005). U.S. Department of Education data on "autism" are not reliable for tracking autism prevalence. *Pediatrics, 116*(1 Suppl), 120–124.

Lakin, K. C., & Stancliffe, R. J. (2007). Residential supports for persons with intellectual and developmental disabilities. *Mental Retardation and Developmental Disabilities Research Reviews, 13*, 151–159.

Lambert, N., Nihira, K., & Leland, H. (1993). *AAMR Adaptive Behavior Scale—School* (2nd ed.). Austin, TX: Pro-ed.

Landa, R. (2000). Social language use in Asperger syndrome and high functioning autism. In A. Klin, F. R. Volkmar, & S. S. Sparrow (Eds.), *Asperger syndrome* (pp. 125–155). New York, NY: Guilford Press.

Langridge, A. T., Glasson, E. J., Nassar, N., Jacoby, P., Pennell, C., Hagan, R., ... Stanley, F. J. (2013). Maternal conditions and perinatal characteristics associated with autism spectrum disorder and intellectual disability. *PLoS ONE, 8*(1), e50963. doi:10.1371/journal.pone.0050963

Layne, C. M. (2007). Early identification of autism: Implications for counselors. *Journal of Counseling and Development, 85*, 110–114.

Luckasson, R., Borthwick-Duffy, S., Buntinx, W. H. E., Coulter, D. L., Craig, E. M., Reeve, A., ... Tasse, M. J. (2002). *Mental retardation: Definitions, classifications and systems of supports* (10th ed.). Washington, DC: American Association on Mental Retardation.

Lunsky, Y. (2004). Suicidality in a clinical and community sample of adults with mental retardation. *Research on Developmental Disabilities, 25*, 231–243.

Matson, J. L., Terlonge, C., & Minshawi, N. F. (2008). Children with intellectual disabilities. In R. J. Morris & T. R. Kratochwill (Eds.), *The practice of child therapy* (4th ed., pp. 337–361). New York, NY: Lawrence Erlbaum & Associates.

Maulik, P. K., Mascarenhas, M. N., Mathers, C. D., Dua, T., & Saxena, S. (2011). Prevalence of intellectual disability: A meta-analysis of population-based studies. *Research in Developmental Disabilities, 32*, 419–436.

McCall, R. B., & Plemons, B. W. (2001). The concept of critical periods and their implications for early childhood services. In D. B. Bailey, J. T. Bruer, F. J. Symons, & J. W. Lichtman (Eds.), *Critical thinking about critical periods* (pp. 267–288). Baltimore, MD: Brookes.

Merrick, J., Kandel, I., & Morad, M. (2004). Trends in autism. *International Journal of Adolescent Medical Health, 16*(1), 75–78.

Merrick, J., Merrick, E., Lunsky, Y., & Kandel, I. (2006). A review of suicidality in persons with intellectual disability. *Israel Journal of Psychiatry and Related Science, 43*(4), 258–264.

Miranda, A., Colomer, C., Fernández, M. I., Presentación, M. J., & Roselló, B. (2015). Analysis of personal and family factors in the persistence of attention deficit hyperactivity disorder: Results of a prospective follow-up study in childhood. *PLoS ONE, 10*(5).

Murphy, N. A., & Elias, E. R. (2006). Sexuality of children and adolescents with developmental disabilities. *Pediatrics, 118*(1), 398–403.

Myers, S. M., Johnson, C. P., & American Academy of Pediatrics Council on Children with Disabilities. (2007). Management of children with autism spectrum disorders. *Pediatrics, 120*(5), 1162–1182.

National Institute of Mental Health. (2016). *Attention deficit /hyperactivity disorder.* Retrieved from http://www.nimh.nih.gov/health/topics/attention-deficit-hyperactivity-disorder-adhd/index.shtml

National Institute of Neurological Disorders and Stroke. (2015). *NINDS learning disabilities page.* Retrieved from http://www.ninds.nih.gov/disorders/learningdisabilities/learningdisabilities.htm

National Library of Medicine. (2016). *Intellectual disability.* Retrieved from https://www.nlm.nih.gov/medlineplus/ency/article/001523.htm

Noble, J. (2001). *Textbook of primary care medicine* (3rd ed). St. Louis, MO: Mosby.

Norén Selinus, E., Molero, Y., Lichtenstein, P., Larson, T., Lundström, S., Anckarsäter, H., & Gumpert, C. H. (2015). Childhood symptoms of ADHD overrule comorbidity in relation to psychosocial outcome at age 15: A longitudinal study. *PLoS ONE, 10*(9), 1–18. doi:10.1371/journal.pone.0137475

Okie, S. (2006). ADHD in adults. *The New England Journal of Medicine, 354*(25), 2637–2641.

Olney, M. F. (2000). Working with autism and other social communication disorders. *Journal of Applied Rehabilitation Counseling, 66*(4), 51–56.

Ozonoff, S. (2012). Editorial perspective: Autism spectrum disorders in DSM-5—An historical perspective and the need for change. *Journal of Child Psychology And Psychiatry, 53*(10), 1092–1094. doi:10.1111/j.1469-7610.2012.02614.x

Painter, C. A., Prevatt, F., & Welles, T. (2008). Career beliefs and job satisfaction in adults with symptoms of attention-deficit/hyperactivity disorder. *Journal of Employment Counseling, 45*(4), 178–188.

Pinto-Martin, J. A., Dunkle, M., Earls, M., Fliedner, D., & Landes, C. (2005). Developmental stages of developmental screening: Steps to implementation of a successful program. *American Journal of Public Health, 95*(11), 1928–1932.

Poelmans, G., Buitelaar, J. K., Pauls, D. L., & Franke, B. (2011). A theoretical molecular network for dyslexia: Integrating available genetic findings. *Molecular Psychiatry, 16*(4), 365–382. doi:10.1038/mp.2010.105

Ramos Olazagasti, M. A., Klein, R. G., Mannuzza, S., Belsky, E. R., Hutchison, J. A., Lashua-Shriftman, E. C., & Castellanos, F. X. (2013). Does childhood attention-deficit/hyperactivity disorder predict risk-taking and medical illnesses in adulthood? *Journal of the American Academy of Child and Adolescent Psychiatry, 52*, 153–162.

Ratzan, S. C. (2010). Setting the record straight: Vaccines, autism, and the Lancet. *Journal of Health Communication, 15*(3), 237–239. doi:10.1080/10810731003780714

Renty, J., & Roeyers, H. (2006). Quality of life in high-functioning adults with autism spectrum disorder: The predictive value of disability and support characteristics. *Autism, 10*(5), 511–524.

Reschly, D. J. (2005). Learning disabilities identification: Primary intervention, secondary intervention, and then what? *Journal of Learning Disabilities, 38*(6), 510–515.

Robins, D. L., Casagrande, K., Barton, M., Chen, C. A., Dumont-Mathieu, T., & Fein, D. (2014). Validation of the

Modified Checklist for Autism in Toddlers, Revised with Follow-up (M-CHAT-R/F). *Pediatrics, 133*(1), 37–45. doi:10.1542/peds.2013-1813

Rush, K. S., Bowman, L. G., Eidman, S. L., Toole, L. M., & Mortenson, B. P. (2004). Assessing psychopathology in individuals with developmental disabilities. *Behavior Modification, 28*, 621–637.

Sarver, D. E., McCart, M. R., Sheidow, A. J., & Letourneau, E. J. (2014). ADHD and risky sexual behavior in adolescents: Conduct problems and substance use as mediators of risk. *Journal of Child Psychology & Psychiatry, 55*(12), 1345–1353. doi:10.1111/jcpp.12249

Schalock, R. L., Borthwick-Duffy, S. A., Bradley, V. J., Buntinx, W. H. E., Coulter, D. L., Craig, E. M., ... Yeager, M. H. (2010). *Intellectual disability: Definition, classification, and systems of support* (11th ed.). Washington, DC: American Association of Intellectual and Developmental Disabilities.

Schopler, E., Reichler, R. J., & Renner, B. R. (1988). *The childhood autism rating scale.* Austin, TX: Pro-Ed.

Seltzer, M. M., Greenberg, J. S., & Orsmond, G. (2010). *Report #13: The transition out of high school and into adult life for young adults with autism spectrum disorders.* Retrieved from http://www.waisman.wisc.edu/family/reports /autism/report_13.pdf

Siegel, M., & Beaulieu, A. A. (2012). Psychotropic medications in children with autism spectrum disorders: A systematic review and synthesis for evidence-based practice. *Journal of Autism and Developmental Disorders, 42*(8), 1592–1605. doi:10.1007/s10803-011-1399-2

Siperstein, G. N., Heyman, M., & Stokes, J. E. (2014). Pathways to employment: A national survey of adults with intellectual disabilities. *Journal of Vocational Rehabilitation, 41*(3), 165–178.

Siperstein, G. N., Parker, R. C., & Drascher, M. (2013). National snapshot of adults with intellectual disabilities in the labor force. *Journal of Vocational Rehabilitation, 39*(3), 157–165. doi:10.3222/JVR-130658

Sparrow, S., Balla, D., & Cicchetti, D. (1984). *Vineland adaptive behavior scales.* Circle Pines, MN: American Guidance Service.

Stawski, M., & Merrick, J. (2006). Mental health services for people with intellectual disability in Israel: A review of options. *Israel Journal of Psychiatry and Related Science, 43*(4), 237–240.

Stein, M. A. (2008). Impairment associated with adult ADHD. *Primary Psychiatry, 15*(Suppl 4), 9–11.

Strand, M., Benzein, E., & Saveman, B. I. (2004). Violence in the care of adult persons with intellectual disabilities. *Journal of Clinical Nursing, 13*(4), 506–514.

Tantam, D. (2000). Psychological disorder in adolescents and adults with Asperger syndrome. *Autism, 4*(1), 47–62.

Tantam, D. (2003). The challenge of adolescents and adults with Asperger syndrome. *Child and Adolescent Psychiatric Clinics of North America, 12*(1), 142–163.

Taylor, E., & Rogers, J. W. (2005). Practitioner review: Early adversity and developmental disorders. *Journal of Child Psychology & Psychiatry, 46*(5), 451–467. doi:10.1111/j.1469-7610.2004.00402.x

Taylor Gomez, M. (2012). The S words: Sexuality, sensuality, sexual expression and people with intellectual disability. *Sexuality & Disability, 30*(2), 237–245. doi:10.1007 /s11195-011-9250-4

Tomljenovic, L., Dórea, J. G., & Shaw, C. A. (2012). Commentary: A link between mercury exposure, autism spectrum disorder, and other neurodevelopmental disorders? Implications for thimerosal-containing vaccines. *Journal on Developmental Disabilities, 18*(1), 34–42.

Tsatsanis, K. (2003). Outcome research in Asperger syndrome and autism. *Child and Adolescent Psychiatric Clinics of North America, 12*(1), 47–63.

Vance, A., Winther, J., & Rennie, K. (2012). Management of attention-deficit/hyperactivity disorder: The importance of psychosocial and medication treatments. *Journal of Paediatrics & Child Health, 48*(2), E33–E37. doi:10.1111/j.1440-1754.2010.01941.x

Vingilis, E., Erickson, P. G., Toplak, M. E., Kolla, N. J., Mann, R. E., Seeley, J., & ... Daigle, D. S. (2015). Attention deficit hyperactivity disorder symptoms, comorbidities, substance use, and social outcomes among men and women in a Canadian sample. *Biomed Research International,* 1–8. doi:10.1155/2015/982072

Volkmar, F. R., Klin, A., & Paul, R. (2004). *Handbook of autism and pervasive developmental disorders* (3rd ed.). New York, NY: Wiley.

Weiss, M. D., & Weiss, J. R. (2004). A guide to the treatment of adults With ADHD. *Journal of Clinical Psychiatry, 65*(Suppl 3), 27–37.

Williams, K., Mellis, C., & Peat, J. K. (2005). Incidence and prevalence of autism. *Advances in Speech—Language Pathology, 7*(1), 31–40.

World Health Organization. (2001). *International classification of functioning, disability and health.* Geneva, Switzerland: Author.

Yang, Q., Rasmussen, S. A., & Friedman, J. M. (2002). Mortality associated with Down syndrome in the USA from 1983–1997: A population-based study. *Lancet, 359*(9331), 1019–1025.

Diagnosis and Treatment of Psychiatric Conditions: Functional and Vocational Implications

Revised by David B. Peterson

PERSPECTIVES ON PSYCHIATRIC CONDITIONS

A Historical Overview

The diagnosis and treatment of psychiatric conditions has changed dramatically over time as societal views have changed. In the past they have been viewed as manifestations of demonic possession, a sign of moral perversion, or extreme emotion and eccentric behavior (Porter, 2001). Prehistoric cultures viewed psychiatric symptoms as having a magical or religious basis, to be treated with spells or rituals. Ancient Greek and Roman cultures viewed psychiatric conditions as a consequence of immorality, to be exorcized. In the Middle Ages, individuals with psychiatric conditions were hospitalized, but often little more than custodial care was provided and individuals were frequently neglected and mistreated. Regardless of the conceptualization, historically individuals with psychiatric conditions have been confronted not only with manifestations of the condition but also with accompanying negative social attitudes and rejection (Gordon, Tantillo, Feldman, & Perrone, 2004; Kahng & Mowbray, 2004).

In the 1800s, emphasis was on a biological basis of psychiatric manifestations and the development of interventions to cure them (Porter, 2001). When no effective interventions were discovered, psychological rather than biological explanations for the development of and interventions for psychiatric manifestations came into vogue. Nevertheless, strictly psychological approaches also proved to be inadequate to explain the development of psychiatric manifestations as well as inadequate interventions for more serious psychiatric conditions (Porter, 2001).

In the 1950s, the discovery of medications that could manage psychiatric manifestations rekindled the conceptualization of psychiatric conditions as a biological entity. Control of manifestations with medication, along with other social factors, led to deinstitutionalization of large numbers of individuals from state hospitals. Deinstitutionalization shifted the responsibility of care for individuals with psychiatric conditions into community settings, which necessitated the establishment of services in the community to meet their needs (Pollio, North, Reid, Miletic, & McClendon, 2006). Services frequently took the form of community mental health centers designed to address these mental health needs. Although community mental health centers monitored medication effectiveness and addressed many short-term needs of individuals, overall long-term needs—including ongoing support, access to housing, employment, and education—were either unavailable or even ignored. Consequently, individuals with psychiatric conditions often needed to be rehospitalized.

Over the years, in an attempt to simplify psychiatric conditions, clinicians looked for a single factor, such as biological cause, psychological cause, or environmental cause that contributed to development of manifestations; if it could be identified, clinicians thought, it could be corrected. In reality, psychiatric conditions are extremely complex, multidimensional, and individualized so that no single explanation or approach can be adequate for all individuals. Psychiatric conditions incorporate neurobiological and neurophysiological elements as well as psychological, social, and behavioral elements. The effective management of psychiatric conditions requires that all of these elements, in the context of the individual, be considered.

The Recovery Model and Psychiatric Rehabilitation

As with physical conditions, the degree of incapacitation experienced with psychiatric conditions varies. The focus of interventions to manage manifestations of psychiatric conditions began with the medical model, with its tradition in evidence and science, focuses on eliminating or ameliorating psychiatric symptoms with medication and/or psychotherapy. When delivered with humanity and compassion the medical model can make a big difference in people's lives. When integrated with the relatively new *recovery model*, that emphasizes hope, empowerment, peer support, and self-management for individuals with psychiatric conditions, together they prove to be an effective combination in meeting the needs of people living with mental disorders in today's healthcare context. The recovery model seeks to provide accommodations, supports, and services that can enable individuals with psychiatric conditions to live full, productive, and dignified lives within the community, and is now a standard of care in many public mental health service agencies. Many health professionals working with individuals with psychiatric conditions now incorporate a

biopsychosocial model into their practice, integrating concepts from biological and psychological models along with the effects of the social and interpersonal environment surrounding the individual (Peterson & Elliott, 2008).

Psychiatric rehabilitation (also referred to as *psychosocial rehabilitation*) is a multidisciplinary approach to assist individuals with psychiatric conditions in developing skills and supports that will enable them to function at their highest capacity in the residential, educational, or vocational setting of their choice. The definition of psychiatric rehabilitation as approved by the United States Psychiatric Rehabilitation Association (USPRA) is as follows:

> Psychiatric rehabilitation promotes recovery, full community integration and improved quality of life for persons who have been diagnosed with any mental health condition that seriously impairs their ability to lead meaningful lives. Psychiatric rehabilitation services are collaborative, person directed and individualized. These services are an essential element of the health care and human services spectrum, and must be evidence-based. They focus on helping individuals develop skills and access resources needed to increase their capacity to be successful and satisfied in the living, working, learning, and social environments of their choice. (Anthony & Farkas, 2009, p. 9)

One can see considerable overlap between values embraced by the recovery model and psychiatric rehabilitation. Two overreaching goals of psychiatric rehabilitation are work and independence (Peterson & Hong, 2014). Increasingly, emphasis has been placed on treating and managing manifestations through evidence-based interventions that have been shown to be efficacious relative to placebo or no intervention (Duncan, Miller, & Sparks, 2004; Lambert, 2013).

DEFINING PSYCHIATRIC CONDITIONS

Psychiatric conditions, also known as psychiatric diagnoses or mental disorders, have significant societal impact and are leading causes of incapacitation worldwide (Agid et al., 2007; Andersson, Wiles, Lewis, Brage, & Hensing, 2007). In a review of the disability prevalence literature (see Peterson & Hong, 2014), the US Census Bureau's American Community Survey (ACS) estimates that over one-third of those seeking rehabilitation services may have a psychiatric diagnosis affecting cognitive functioning. The National Comorbidity Survey Replication (NCS-R) suggests that over one-quarter of the population presents with psychiatric diagnoses in any given year, and 57.4 percent will have a psychiatric diagnosis within their lifetime; nearly half of those diagnosed will likely have more than one psychiatric diagnosis. It was summarized in the *Monitor on Psychology* that "Mental disorders contribute more to global disability and disease burden than any other category of non-communicable disease" (Martin, 2009, p. 62).

The term *psychiatric disability,* which is used frequently, encompasses a broad range of conditions with a wide variety of manifestations and varying degrees of incapacitation. Although manifestations of psychiatric conditions and the degree of associated incapacitation vary widely, generally psychiatric conditions have been viewed as blocking individuals' goals and interfering with their ability to function effectively within the community. Prejudice and stereotyping of individuals with psychiatric conditions can have more disabling effects than manifestations of the condition itself.

Manifestations of psychiatric conditions can consist of both behavioral actions and subjective feelings. Some psychiatric conditions may be accompanied by limitations in organizational ability, cognitive functions, or social interactions; others are associated with loss of contact with reality (**psychosis**). Still other psychiatric conditions are characterized by significant fluctuations and changes in mood or demonstrations of maladaptive behavior. The extent of incapacitation experienced by individuals as a result of a psychiatric condition depends to a great extent, on the degree to which their manifestations cause subjective distress to the individual, cause distress or disruption perceived by others in the environment, or interfere with their ability to function within their environment.

Unlike many physical conditions, psychiatric conditions can be difficult to define and identify. Moreover, causes of psychiatric conditions cannot always be determined. There are no laboratory tests readily available to confirm the condition. Instead, the primary basis for identifying the condition and predicting functional capacity is the experienced clinical judgment of the professionals who are conducting the evaluation. Moderating variables, such as the ethnic status, education, and socioeconomic status of both the client and the professional, may influence individuals' performance on evaluation as well as professionals' interpretation of the evaluation results.

The American Psychiatric Association in its latest version of its diagnostic taxonomy the DSM-5 (APA, 2013) does not define the term *psychiatric diagnosis* but rather defines a *mental disorder* as:

> a syndrome characterized by clinically significant disturbance in an individual's cognition, emotion regulation, or behavior that reflects a dysfunction in the psychological, biological, or developmental processes underlying mental functioning. Mental disorders are usually associated with significant distress or disability in social, occupational, or other important activities. (p. 20)

It goes on to say that a mental disorder is not. ...

> an expectable or culturally approved response to a common stressor or loss, such as the death of a loved one . . . socially deviant behavior (e.g., political, religious, or sexual) and conflicts that are primarily between the individual and society . . . unless the deviance or conflict results from a dysfunction in the individual as described above. (p. 20)

CLASSIFYING PSYCHIATRIC CONDITIONS

The systems commonly used in the United States to classify psychiatric conditions include the Diagnostic and Statistical Manual of Mental Disorders, Fifth Edition (DSM-5) by the American Psychiatric Association (APA, 2013), and the International

Classification of Diseases, Tenth Revision, Clinical Modification (ICD-10-CM; WHO, 2014). The DSM-5 does not enjoy wide international use, rather, the ICD system has been used by member nations of the World Health Organization (WHO). The following is a review of the historical development of these important classification systems.

Historical Development of the DSM

In 1952 the American Psychiatric Association's Committee on Nomenclature and Statistics published the *Diagnostic and Statistical Manual of Mental Disorders* (DSM-I). This book was the first official manual of mental conditions that had clinical utility. Since its initial publication, the American Psychiatric Association has continued its work to revise and refine the DSM. As more empirical research and field trials were conducted, reliability, descriptive validity, and performance characteristics for diagnostic criteria were improved. Updated versions of the manual bear the number of the edition (e.g., *DSM-II, DSM-III,* and *DSM-IV*). The fourth edition of the manual, DSM-IV, was published in 1994. In 2000, DSM-IV-TR (fourth edition, text revision) was published. The latest effort in empirical documentation on which to base diagnostic decisions is the DSM-5 (APA, 2013). Note the Roman numeral has been changed to conventional numbering that allows subsequent revisions, like that of modern software (e.g., 5.1).

The DSM-5 is the most contemporary effort to establish objective criteria for the identification of psychiatric conditions. In addition to providing specific criteria on which to base identification of a specific condition, it provides consistency among professionals in communicating about psychiatric conditions. The use of the manual for identifying specific conditions requires specialized clinical training and supervision, as the criteria within the manual are complex; they are meant to be guidelines but are not considered absolute and thus require good clinical judgment. In order to understand psychiatric diagnoses, the skilled clinician must be able to distinguish between normal life variations and transient responses to stress, and serious symptomatology manifested as disturbances in behaviors, cognition, personality, physical signs, and

syndrome combinations (APA, 2013). Although all professionals working with individuals with psychiatric conditions should be familiar with the manual, responsibility for definitively identifying a specific condition most frequently lies with psychiatrists, psychologists, social workers, and more recently licensed counseling professionals (e.g., Licensed Mental Health Counselors, Licensed Professional Clinical Counselors).

It should be emphasized that diagnoses should not be used lightly, as they can categorize or label people. It is always best practice to use the least stigmatizing diagnosis possible, and only if it is clinically appropriate. The great value brought about by diagnostic systems is to coordinate the care of similar conditions with the best evidence-based care possible for a given condition (Peterson & Elliott, 2008). Accurate diagnosis of psychiatric conditions leads to appropriate referrals, selection of the most appropriate evidence-based treatments, and ultimately amelioration or elimination of problematic symptoms that negatively impact health and functioning (Peterson, 2011).

DSM-5

Overview of the DSM-5

This overview of the DSM-5 is no substitute for completing appropriate training in psychiatric diagnoses, as well as supervised clinical practice. The DSM-5 was revised to be useful to mental health professionals, consumers of mental health services and their families, and researchers. It aspires to do so by providing clear and concise descriptions of psychiatric diagnoses. As with the DSM-IV-TR, each diagnosis provides explicit diagnostic criteria, dimensional measures that cut across diagnoses, and a concise overview of a given diagnosis, risk factors, associated features, related research, and possible manifestations of the diagnosis (APA, 2013, p. 5).

The DSM-5, and more so its revision process, had its share of critics, as it was revised almost exclusively by psychiatrists, to the exclusion of many other allied health professionals who contributed to previous iterations of the system (Peterson, 2011). Even so, the DSM-5 is an important diagnostic system in the United States.

Research on psychiatric conditions suggests that boundaries between diagnoses are less clear than once thought and that most conditions can be placed on a spectrum with closely related diagnoses that share symptoms, genetic, and environmental risk factors and probable biological bases of behavior (APA, 2013, pp. 5–6). The new organization of the DSM-5 reflects this research. In the last two decades, great advances have been achieved in research regarding psychiatric diagnoses, and information will continue to grow exponentially with advances in science and improve our understanding of psychiatric diagnoses, hopefully reduce social stigma associated with them, and improve treatment outcomes (APA, 2013).

Within the DSM-5 both the ICD-9-CM codes and ICD-10-CM codes are referenced as they relate to the DSM's current diagnoses. Most of the world has been using the ICD-10-CM for some time now, even though the United States only recently updated from the ICD-9-CM in the fall of 2015. Given its 2013 publication date it was necessary to list both versions of the ICD for use in the United States.

The DSM-5 (APA, 2013) is made up of three sections. Section I reviews the history and developmental process of the latest revision of the DSM, and provides a guide to the basics of DSM-5 clinical diagnosis. Section II contains the diagnostic criteria and codes, classifying psychiatric disorders into 22 major categories, an expansion of the DSM-IV-TR's 17 major categories. The primary purpose of Section II is "to assist trained clinicians in the diagnosis of an individual's mental disorders as part of a case formulation assessment that leads to a fully informed treatment plan" (p. 19).

Section III, Emerging Measures and Models, provides new assessment measures, cultural formulations, an alternative model for disorders of personality, as well as conditions for further study. The contents of Section III are suggested to require further study before full implementation with Section II of the manual, but users are encouraged to use them to enhance clinical decision-making (APA, 2013). Included in Section III are 13 symptom domains with dimensional measures of severity proposed for all DSM diagnostic groups. Also included in the Section is the WHODAS 2.0, the

proposed substitute for the GAF system used in the DSM-IV-TR, which will be reviewed further on.

Diagnostic Categories of the DSM-5

The organization of the diagnostic categories in the DSM-5 was changed to harmonize with the most recent version of the Mental and Behavioral Disorders section of the ICD (both versions 10 and 11). This was done in order to minimize the impact of having two different diagnostic systems affecting collection of health statistics and future research replication. Advances in neuroscience are reflected in expanded diagnostic categories and subtypes of neurocognitive disorders (APA, 2013). The 22 new diagnostic categories are listed below. The use of capital letters is as indicated in the DSM-5 (APA, 2013):

1. Neurodevelopmental Disorders
2. Schizophrenia Spectrum and Other Psychotic Disorders.
3. Bipolar and Related Disorders.
4. Depressive Disorders.
5. Anxiety Disorders.
6. Obsessive-Compulsive and Related Disorders
7. Trauma- and Stressor-Related Disorders
8. Dissociative Disorders
9. Somatic-Symptom and Related Disorders
10. Feeding and Eating Disorders.
11. Elimination Disorders
12. Sleep-Wake Disorders.
13. Sexual Dysfunctions
14. Gender Dysphoria
15. Disruptive, Impulse-Control, and Conduct Disorders
16. Substance-Related and Addictive Disorders
17. Neurocognitive Disorders
18. Personality Disorders
19. Paraphilic Disorders
20. Other Mental Disorders
21. Medication-Induced Movement Disorders and Other Adverse Effects of Medication
22. Other Conditions That May Be a Focus of Clinical Attention

Structural Changes

See the DSM-5 pages 809–816 for a thorough discussion of changes from the IV-TR to the fifth revision. The DSM IV-TR had used a multiaxial system which included five axes for describing clinical syndromes (Axes I), personality disorders and mental retardation (Axes II), other health conditions (Axes III), relevant psychosocial or environmental issues (Axes IV) and the clinician's judgement of function (Axes V—Global Assesment of Function or GAF Scale). The DSM-5 has transitioned away from the multiaxial system of diagnosis to a nonaxial system. Axes I and II are combined, and Axis III physical conditions, if they affect psychological functioning, are to be noted along with the psychiatric diagnoses. Axis IV was eliminated, as the DSM-5 task force decided not to further develop its own psychosocial and environmental problems classification schema (APA, 2013, p. 16). This stands to reason given the work of the World Health Organization on the International Classification of Functioning, Disability, and Health (ICF; WHO, 2001), a much more comprehensive classification of psychosocial and environmental functioning (previously reviewed in Chapter 1 of this text). The ICF and its conceptual framework was the basis for the projected substitute for the Axis V GAF, the World Health Organization Disability Assessment Schedule (WHODAS-2; WHO, 2012). The GAF was eliminated due to its inconsistent implementation by clinicians. Finally, with the elimination of the axial system, the order of diagnoses presented in the DSM-5 reflects a developmental and lifespan perspective (APA, 2013).

The frequently used "not otherwise specified" or "NOS" qualifier for DSM-IV-TR, which meant a diagnosis came close to but did not satisfy all of the diagnostic criteria required for the formal diagnosis, has been changed to one of two new options. *Other specified disorder* is used to highlight the specific reason why a set of symptoms does not meet diagnostic criteria. *Unspecified disorder* is the qualifier used if the clinician decides not to highlight the specific reason. Clinical judgment is used in determining whether there is sufficient evidence to use *other specified* versus *unspecified disorder*.

The DSM-5 also has online supplemental information, including more symptom and functional impairment severity measures that cut across diagnostic categories. Additionally, in an effort to enhance cultural sensitivity of DSM diagnoses, the *Cultural Formulation Interview* is provided with supplements (see www.psychiatry.org/dsm5). Pages 14 and 15 of the DSM-5 provide an excellent overview of the myriad cultural, as well as gender issues, that affect the boundary between normality and pathology, as well as the systems in which healthcare is provided.

Diagnostic Changes

Here we review some of the more significant diagnostic changes from moving from the DSM-IV-TR to the DSM-5. There are a number of other detailed changes not covered here; for details the reader is referred to pages 809–816 of the DSM-5.

Some of the diagnostic changes in the DSM-5 include the pervasive developmental disorders combined into an *autism spectrum disorder*, and the term mental retardation has been replaced by *intellectual disability* (or intellectual developmental disorder). Severity of these conditions is estimated using measures of adaptive functioning rather than measures of IQ. The various learning disorders have been combined into one *specific learning disorder* diagnosis. Substance abuse and dependence are now described as *substance use disorders*, and the distinction between tolerance and withdrawal (formerly associated with dependence) and addiction is made clear. The subtypes of schizophrenia have been removed due to their lack of clinical utility. The commonly used cognitive disorder not otherwise specified is now a *neurocognitive disorder*.

ICD-10-CM

The psychiatric diagnostic system most commonly used internationally is the International Statistical Classification of Diseases, 10th Revision (ICD-10; WHO, 1992), recently updated as the International Classification of Diseases, 10th Revision, Clinical Modification (ICD-10-CM; WHO, 2014), which was recently adopted in the United States in the fall of 2015 to replace the well-worn ICD-9-CM. This system was reviewed previously in chapter 1 of this text. The 11th revision of the ICD is scheduled for publication in 2018 (see WHO website on ICD-11 development, http://www.who.int/classifications/icd/revision/en/)

TOOLS FOR IDENTIFYING PSYCHIATRIC CONDITIONS

Identification of psychiatric conditions is as much an art as a science. It requires skill and experience on the part of those evaluating individuals' manifestations and interpreting results of the various tests designed to measure psychological or intellectual function. Many professionals may be involved in testing and evaluation; psychiatrists, clinical psychologists, social workers, and licensed clinical counselors are frequently involved in the identification of psychiatric conditions. Identification of a specific condition is usually based on information gathered from a variety of sources.

Uses of Psychological Testing

Systematic samples of certain types of verbal, perceptual, intellectual, and motor behavior under standardized conditions can be obtained through psychological testing. Psychological tests may be used to evaluate intelligence, personality, or behavior. Results of psychological tests provide partial information needed for the accurate identification of a psychiatric condition. Note, however, that no single test is adequate to offer definitive identification of a specific condition in all situations. Because psychiatric conditions often affect a variety of functions, use of several psychological tests that measure different functions is frequently required.

Intelligence Tests

The term *intelligence* is difficult to define. Theoretically, intelligence consists of a number of skills and abilities, some of which have no means of measurement. Intelligence is a combination of individuals' own unique mental structures and processes plus cultural and educational experiences. Psychological science has developed a number of tests to define intelligence operationally for a variety of capacities. The most commonly used intelligence tests are the *Wechsler Intelligence Scale for Children—Fifth Edition (WISC-V)*, the *Wechsler Preschool and Primary Scale of Intelligence-Fourth Edition*

(WPPSI-IV), the *Stanford–Binet-5 test*, and the *Wechsler Adult Intelligence Scale—IV (WAIS-IV)*.

Limitations of intelligence testing originate from several sources:

- The difficulty of tapping all aspects of intellectual ability
- The effects of individual ability to take the test
- The degree to which the test measures aptitude rather than prior learning and experience
- The effects of cultural variation on test results

One way of classifying levels of intelligence is through a numerical value known as the *intelligence quotient (IQ)*. There is considerable individual variability in abilities, however, and the results of intelligence tests, like the results of other forms of psychological tests, must be evaluated within the context of the individual's cultural and environmental variables. Much intelligence testing involves sampling individuals' intellectual capacity in many different spheres: verbal comprehension, perceptual reasoning, working memory, and processing speed for example. Many tests focus on cognitive processes, including problem solving, adaptive thinking, and other aspects of performance. Tests alone should not be relied upon to determine the level of intellectual functioning.

Mental Status Examination and Assessment through Interview

The structured interview is one way in which the mental functioning of an individual with a suspected condition that affects mental function may be assessed during the initial evaluation. Information obtained in this way may aid both in identifying the condition and in making plans for future interventions. Structured interviews provide information regarding individuals' *orientation, form, and content of thought*, *speech, affect,* and *degree of insight.* Observations made during the interview of the individual's general appearance, behavior, and emotional state are also relevant. The *mental status examination* is a specific type of structured interview used as a screening instrument in assessing intellectual function. Such an examination may be used to detect dementia or impaired intellectual function, as well as to determine the severity of the impairment.

Several mental status examinations of varying lengths have been developed. Although some are part of other instruments that measure functional status, a number of short screening instruments have been devised specifically for the purpose of evaluating mental status. One widely used mental status test is the *Short Portable Mental Status Questionnaire (SPMSQ)*, which is used to assess orientation, personal history, remote memory, and calculation. Another short mental status examination is the *Mini–Mental State Examination (MMSE)*, which is used to assess orientation, memory, and attention, as well as the ability to write, name objects, copy a design, and follow verbal and written commands.

Personality Assessment

Personality may be assessed by either *objective* or *projective* means. Objective personality assessment instruments are structured, standardized tests for which clear and concise criteria have been established. These tests have undergone research and scientific scrutiny to establish their reliability and validity. Although numerous objective personality tests are available, one of the most commonly used is the *Minnesota Multiphasic Personality Inventory-2 (MMPI-2)*. This instrument incorporates validity scales to assess response styles, a variety of clinical scales useful in describing personality function and dysfunction, but not necessarily specific diagnoses. An instrument tied directly to the DSM for diagnostic information in the Million Clinical Multiaxial Inventory-IV (MCMI-IV), recently revised for the DSM-5.

Projective personality tests, such as the *Rorschach inkblot test* and the *Thematic Apperception Test (TAT)*, rely on the test subject to project their unconscious thoughts onto ambiguous stimuli, and the content of their responses is then analyzed to inform personality functioning. The TAT is generally more subjective in nature, and the Rorschach is very time intensive and complex to score and interpret. Projective tests may be more time consuming to administer than are objective tests, and those professionals who administer them require special training. As with all other clinical data, the results of personality assessment tests are merely one part of the total information needed for an accurate identification of a particular mental health condition. No matter which type of test is used, the accuracy of the results depends on the individual's honesty and care in answering test questions. If the individual answers questions in a socially desirable way rather than as an expression of his or her true feelings, test results can be invalid.

Neuropsychological Testing

Standardized neuropsychological test batteries may be used to assess major functional areas of the brain. These tests make it possible to assess a variety of cognitive, perceptual, and motor skills. Traditionally, neuropsychological testing has been used to identify or localize brain damage that has behavioral consequences; however, with newer technological advances such as computed tomography (CT) and magnetic resonance imaging (MRI), this function is now not widely promoted. Neuropsychological tests have become increasingly popular to rule out and monitor the progression of the manifestations of psychiatric conditions that have an identified organic basis. Because individual performance on neuropsychological tests changes with brain function, test results provide a baseline against which future impairment of brain function can be measured; they also provide data that can be incorporated into the process for identifying the condition. Comprehensive standard neuropsychological test batteries are available for adults, but due to the time and expense to administer them their use has fallen out of favor. These include the *Halstead–Reitan Battery* and the *Luria–Nebraska Neuropsychological Battery*. Managed healthcare pressures favor neuropsychological assessment that uses a more modular approach, only administering those tests that are essential, a method that was prescient of the older Benton battery and reflected in the newest comprehensive battery, the Neuropsychological Assessment Battery (NAB).

Behavioral Assessment

Some methods of assessing mental function involve direct, systematic observation of individuals' behavior. Trained observers, family members, or even individuals themselves may monitor and record behavior. Observation and measurement of behavior may take place in individuals' own environment or in a controlled environment. Behavioral assessment methods are being applied to an increasing number of conditions, because they offer not only information that can be used in identification of a condition but also a method of monitoring improvements in behavior once interventions have been initiated.

MANAGEMENT OF PSYCHIATRIC CONDITIONS

No single approach is appropriate for management of all psychiatric conditions. Instead, management of psychiatric conditions is based on a comprehensive assessment of the individual's problems, needs, and strengths. This evaluation usually represents a collaborative effort involving the individual, the family, and professionals from a variety of disciplines, such as psychiatrists, psychologists, social workers, nurses, licensed and rehabilitation counselors. Interventions may be provided in a variety of settings, depending on the individual's particular condition and specific needs. Levels of intervention range from the least restrictive, such as that provided in an outpatient setting, to the most restrictive, such as that provided in an institutional setting. Levels of intervention between these two extremes include intensive outpatient intervention, residential care, and halfway houses.

Intervention in acute episodes of psychiatric conditions may initially focus on alleviating manifestations of the condition, interventions commonly associated with the medical model of care. Ongoing intervention is directed toward preventing recurrence of manifestations and helping individuals attain optimal functional capacity, more consistent with the recovery or psychiatric rehabilitation models of care. Many psychiatric conditions require ongoing intervention or periodic evaluations of the effectiveness of the intervention used. Some psychiatric conditions, like many physical conditions, require daily medication to manage manifestations and are characterized by periods of remission and periods of exacerbation. In many instances, individuals' willingness and ability to adhere to the intervention can determine its success in effectively managing manifestations.

A variety of intervention modalities, including both nonpharmacologic and pharmacologic methods, may be used to reduce, alleviate, and manage the manifestations experienced with psychiatric conditions. More intensive levels of interventions may include, in addition to psychotherapy and pharmacologic intervention, occupational therapy, art and music therapy, and recreational therapy. Often, several different types of interventions are used simultaneously.

Nonpharmacologic Approaches to Management of Psychiatric Conditions

Accurate identification of the condition is considered a cornerstone of management of psychiatric conditions, as it allows for the selection of appropriate interventions designed to eliminate or manage manifestations. Many psychiatric conditions require ongoing medications to manage manifestations. Although medications can reduce manifestations and hospitalizations in individuals with psychiatric conditions, the most effective intervention typically combines psychosocial interventions with medication management. Psychiatric conditions, however, affect multiple areas of function. Consequently, a multitude of personal, environmental, and health factors must be considered in helping individuals function to their optimal capacity (MacDonald-Wilson & Nemec, 2005).

Psychiatric Rehabilitation (Psychosocial Rehabilitation)

Psychiatric rehabilitation (sometimes called *psychosocial rehabilitation*) was described earlier in our review of approaches to care. In summary, it is a multidisciplinary approach that assists individuals with a chronic psychiatric condition to address specific psychosocial issues not addressed by medication alone. Psychiatric rehabilitation has been conceptualized as a process by which individuals are assisted to develop those skills and supports they need to be successful and satisfied in their chosen environment (Anthony, Cohen, Farkas, & Gagne, 2002). Basic goals of psychiatric rehabilitation include *recovery, community integration,* and *improved quality of life.* Psychiatric rehabilitation is *community based, client centered,* and *empowerment oriented* (Leech & Holcomb,

2000), and it helps individuals identify and obtain the resources and support needed to attain their goals (Garske, 1999).

Clubhouse Model

The *clubhouse model* is one of the oldest approaches to psychosocial rehabilitation and provides a wide range of social, health, education, and employment support programs to individuals with psychiatric disability (Coniglio, Hancock, & Ellis, 2012). The model provides recovery focused psychosocial rehabilitation at over 300 sites in over 30 countries around the world (Raeburn, Schmied, Hungerford, & Cleary, 2015).

Clubhouses not only serve as a central meeting place for individuals with psychiatric conditions but also provide informal and experiential strategies to help individuals gain skills that can be integrated into the workplace. Vocational participation may range from clubhouse members performing chores around the clubhouse to members identifying and obtaining employment within the community. In house work contributions are voluntary while community employment involves a tiered employment approach consisting of transitional employment, supported employment, or independent employment. The effectiveness of several of these programs has been evaluated, with mixed results being found (Raeburn, Holcomb, Walter, & Cleary, 2013). Continued research to assess the efficacy of programs in integrating individuals into both society and the workplace is essential to effective rehabilitation of individuals with psychiatric conditions (Raeburn, Schmied, Hungeford, & Cleary, 2014).

Social Skills Training Programs

Social skills training consists of socially focused behavioral interventions directed toward assisting individuals with psychiatric disability to enhance their social performance in conjunction with their specific goals and needs and to improve social functioning within their community. Training programs include a broad range of social skills including verbal and nonverbal behaviors, accurate social perception, ability to process and appropriately respond to social cues and other skills necessary for successful social interaction. Interventions usually begin by targeting small elements of behavior

and then gradually adding elements of behavior, working toward the ideal. Through participation in social skills training groups, individuals learn to make specific responses to specific social situations, to recognize relevant social cues, and to determine appropriate action by using the cues. Such training may involve specific interventions, such as social role modeling, problem solving, positive corrective feedback, behavioral practice, and positive social reinforcement.

Specialized Groups

A variety of specialized groups that focus on meeting a specific need of the individual may be used in conjunction with other programs or services in order to help individuals improve functional ability and overall quality of life.

*Activities of Daily Living Gr*oups may be of help when individuals have difficulty with basic activities of daily living such as bathing or dressing, or difficulty with instrumental activities of daily living such as preparing meals, doing housework, or managing money. Ability to perform these tasks can be an indicator of severity of symptoms as well as an indicator of effectiveness of treatment and can play a key role to independent living and overall well-being. Activities of daily living groups assess the individual's ability to carry out activities of daily living and, when a need is identified, help the individual learn strategies and skills required for day-to-day function.

Isolation and decreased self-esteem may also be experienced by individuals with psychiatric disability. *Self-help groups* provide mutual help, mutual aid, and mutual support and are composed of others with similar conditions. The focus is on helping individuals help themselves while helping others at the same time in a supportive, open environment, with the sharing of common experiences. Self-help groups may exist separately or may be part of services offered by a larger organization. Along the same lines are *drop-in centers* that offer an opportunity for social interaction, recreational activities, and other types of assistance.

A nonprofit grassroots organization offering advocacy and support to individuals with psychiatric disability and their families is the *National Alliance for the Mentally Ill (NAMI).*

NAMI provides education, support, community education and outreach with the goal of eliminating stigma of psychiatric disability and to create positive change within the mental health system and the community.

Some individuals with psychiatric disability require ongoing supervision and may require a period of transition from inpatient to outpatient settings. A number of therapeutic living arrangements may be used to meet their needs, including group homes and day programs. *Group homes* are small, single family homes located with a neighborhood in a community. Individuals with psychiatric disability who reside in group homes are usually unable to live independently. The homes are staffed 24 hours a day. The goal of the staff is to encourage as much independence as possible while providing support and assistance when needed. *Day programs* provide a structured environment in which individuals may participate in the program during the day and return to the community setting at night.

Assertive Community Treatment

Developed in the 1970s, *assertive community treatment* (ACT) is regarded as an organizational framework for delivering services to individuals with psychiatric disability rather than individual services themselves (Test & Stein, 1976). Assertive community treatment programs utilize multidisciplinary teams to provide highly individualized services to individuals with psychiatric conditions in an effort to decrease or eliminate manifestations and to prevent relapse (Dixon, 2000). ACT assists individuals to meet basic needs, improve functioning within the community, and increase their ability to live independently. Rather than using a case management model in which services are distributed among a number of different agencies or services, members of the ACT team work collaboratively to offer direct services to the individual (Weinstein, Henwood, Cody, Jordan, & Lelar, 2011). Members of the ACT team meet the individual in his or her home, providing services and contact based on the individual's unique needs. Team members also monitor management of manifestations and observe for warning signs of potential relapse.

Family Psychoeducation

Family psychoeducation is an intervention in which a professional, an individual with psychiatric condition, and his or her family work in partnership to promote recovery. Through this partnership, current information about the individual's psychiatric condition is communicated to the individual and family, and strategies to help the family develop skills for coping with issues involving manifestations of the individual's condition are developed. Interventions can be used with a single family or conducted with a group of families.

Illness Management and Recovery Programs

Illness management and recovery programs grew out of a recognition that living successfully with any chronic health condition requires collaborative effort between the individual and healthcare provider in order to identify problems, set goals and strategies for self-management, and monitor progress over time (Holman & Lorig, 2000). Although the traditional medical definition of recovery in psychiatric disability focuses on remission of symptoms and return to prior level of functioning, recovery for the individual is more personal in nature, involving individual and subjective aspects of improved function (Mead & Copeland, 2000). Illness management and recovery programs for psychiatric disability emphasize consumer empowerment, establishment of personal goals, acquisition of information and skills to develop mastery over the psychiatric condition by reducing stress, coping with symptoms, and preventing relapse (Mueser et al., 2006).

Integrated Dual Disorders Treatment

Integrated dual disorders treatment (IDDT) was developed for individuals who have both a psychiatric condition and a condition related to substance abuse or dependence. This approach integrates and blends interventions for both psychiatric conditions and substance abuse so that one professional or team provides intervention for both conditions. Techniques used in IDDT programs include individual and group counseling, family psychoeducation, social support, case management, and medication management.

Pharmacologic Approaches to Management of Psychiatric Conditions

Antipsychotic Medications

Management of psychosis may require use of *antipsychotic medications* (see **Table 13-1**). Antipsychotic medications, also known as *major tranquilizers*, and formerly known as *neuroleptics* due to their side effects, can be very effective in managing psychotic symptoms. The first antipsychotic drug, chlorpromazine (Thorazine), was developed in the 1950s, and revolutionized psychiatric care and behavior management in acute care inpatient psychiatric facilities. Since then, numerous other antipsychotic medications have entered the marketplace. Antipsychotic medications are classified into different chemical groups. Medications in each group have varying potency, and individual responses to any of the medications will vary. The medications do not cure psychosis, and those with chronic and severe psychotic conditions may require such medication for a lifetime to effectively manage their symptoms.

Conventional antipsychotic medications were largely replaced by *atypical antipsychotics* (*second-generation antipsychotics*) that were developed after a 1980s study showed that the medication clozapine managed intervention-resistant manifestations in schizophrenia while causing fewer *extrapyramidal side effects* (physical manifestations such as tremor and muscle rigidity) that were common with the older antipsychotic medications

Table 13-1   Common Antipsychotic Agents

Trade Name	Generic Name
Clozaril	clozapine
Haldol	haloperidol
Abilify	aripiprazole
Saphris	asenapine
Latuda	lurasidone
Zyprexa	olanzapine
Invega	paliperidone
Seroquel	quetiapine
Risperdal	risperidone
Geodon	ziprasidone

(Gardner, Baldessarini, & Waraich, 2005). Since then, a number of other atypical antipsychotics have been approved for the management of both manifestations of schizophrenia and acute bipolar episodes and maintenance intervention for bipolar disorders (Masand, 2007), as well as adjunctive therapies for management of treatment resistant depression (Preston, O'Neal, & Talaga, 2013). Although atypical antipsychotics are still widely used, conventional antipsychotic medications have gained increasing favor after recent studies suggested that the atypical antipsychotics are also associated with side effects that can contribute to weight gain and development of conditions such as metabolic syndrome. It has also been found that adherence to the medication plan has not improved with the newer medications (Lieberman et al., 2005).

For over 50 years, manifestations of psychosis have been suggested to be due to disregulation of the neurotransmitter *dopamine,* although other neurotransmitter systems have also been implicated (Tucin, Dolzan, Porcelli, Serretti, & Plesnicar, 2016). As a result, antipsychotic medications have been developed to block the action or transmission of dopamine, with the intent of reducing positive manifestations such as delusions and hallucinations. Blocking of dopamine activity, however, may produce side effects including psychomotor manifestations similar to those seen in Parkinson's disease. These complications are called *extrapyramidal effects*, in recognition of the fact that changes take place in the extrapyramidal tracts of the central nervous system. Extrapyramidal effects are more common with older antipsychotic medications but may include **dystonia** (abnormal muscle tone), **akinesia** (decreased motor activity and apathy), and **akathisia** (extreme restlessness and inability to sit still or remain in one place for any length of time), all of which have acute onset. The most severe extrapyramidal side effect is *tardive dyskinesia*, which comprises abnormal movements of the mouth, such as chewing motions or thrusting movements of the tongue. The side effect of tardive dyskinesia may not be immediately apparent; indeed, it may not develop until years after intervention. Tardive dyskinesia is often related to medication dosage and is irreversible. Frequent monitoring for early manifestations of tardive dyskinesia is important to prevent permanent damage from occurring. *Anti-parkinsonian medications*, such as *benztropine* (*Cogentin*) and *trihexphenidyl* (*Artane*), may be used, especially in conjunction with older antipsychotic medications, to prevent extrapyramidal side effects.

Although atypical or second-generation antipsychotics have been thought to be better tolerated and more efficacious than conventional antipsychotics, they are not without limitations (Masand, 2007). The *Clinical Antipsychotic Trials of Intervention Effectiveness (CATIE)* study compared the effectiveness of several atypical antipsychotics and conventional antipsychotics in the management of schizophrenia (Lieberman et al., 2005). Although rates of discontinuation were slightly lower for individuals taking atypical antipsychotic medications, nearly three-fourths of the individuals discontinued their medications within 18 months, often because of intolerable side effects. Among the side effects associated with antipsychotic medications are weight gain, diabetes, and elevated blood cholesterol, all of which increase the risk of heart disease (Dekker et al., 2005; Sridhar, 2007). In addition, an increased risk of death may be associated with use of antipsychotic medications in older adults (Wang et al., 2005).

In the CATIE Study (Lieberman et al., 2005), sedation was the side effect that accounted for discontinuation of antipsychotic medication in nearly one-third of the participants. Individuals taking antipsychotic medications may also develop photosensitivity, which makes them more sensitive to the effects of the sun and predisposes them to sunburn. Some medications that have potent sedating effects may decrease alertness and produce drowsiness. These manifestations usually subside within 2 weeks after beginning to take the medication. If manifestations persist, alteration in medication may be necessary. Individuals may also experience *orthostatic hypotension*, in which their blood pressure drops when they move from a seated or prone position to a standing position, resulting in dizziness or light-headedness. Individuals may complain of other uncomfortable side effects, such as dry mouth, after beginning antipsychotic medications; these manifestations generally subside within 2 weeks, however. Men on antipsychotic medication may become impotent or

unable to ejaculate; reducing the dosage or changing the medication may alleviate this side effect. Any medication change should always be implemented under the direction of a health professional.

The duration of intervention with antipsychotic medications is determined individually and based on the individual's specific life situation and condition. These medications may be used for up to a year as a prophylactic measure after psychosis is adequately managed. All individuals should have their medications reviewed at least annually by a psychiatrist. There continues to be work on developing better antipsychiatric medications as new hypotheses have been suggested regarding the role in dopamine in producing the manifestations of psychosis in psychiatric disorders. A number of novel medications that impact neurotransmitters are being explored as potential treatment options and may, in the future, change how manifestations of psychosis are treated (Gopalakrishna, Ithman, & Lauriello, 2016).

Antidepressants

Antidepressants may be used as an intervention in conditions in which depression is a manifestation. Although the exact way antidepressants work has not been elucidated, depending upon the class of antidepressant the medications are thought to block the reuptake of the neurotransmitters *norepinephrine* and *serotonin*, thereby increasing their concentration. Levels of both neurotransmitters appear to be reduced in depression. The type of depression and the manifestations experienced, as well as other individual factors, determine the type of antidepressant used. In most cases, medication effects do not occur immediately but rather may take as long as 6 to 8 weeks to show full positive effect.

Tricyclic antidepressants, named for their chemical structure, were once widely used to treat depression. They worked by affecting serotonin and norepinephrine levels in the brain. Today, these medications are not used as frequently as first-line therapy owing to their unpleasant side effects, such as orthostatic hypotension, dry mouth, and urinary retention. More serious issues include potential cardiac arrhythmia, which can result in myocardial infarction, or the ease of overdose and death. They are still employed in some patients with treatment resistant depression. Commonly prescribed cyclic antidepressants include amitriptyline, imipramine, nortriptyline, and trazodone (Preston et al., 2013).

A newer class of antidepressants called *selective serotonin reuptake inhibitors (SSRIs)*, work as effectively as the tricyclics but with fewer side effects and safer with respect to overdosing. They block the reuptake of serotonin in the brain, thought to relieve depression. Popular SSRI's include fluoxetine (or Prozac), citalopram (Celexa), Escitalopram (Lexapro), Paroxetine (Paxil), and sertraline (Zoloft) (Preston et al., 2013).

Newer medications similar to tricyclic antidepressants, which affect both serotonin and norepinephrine, have since been developed, called *serotonin and norepinephrine reuptake inhibitors (SNRIs)*. These dual-action antidepressants include venlafaxine (Effexor), desvenlafaxine (Pristiq), duloxetine (Cymbalta), and mirtazapine (Remeron). One medication worth mentioning, bupropion (Wellbutrin) is a commonly prescribed antidepressant with unique chemical properties not involving reuptake inhibition (Preston et al., 2013).

Monoamine oxidase inhibitors (MAOIs) are older types of antidepressants that are thought to act by blocking the action of the enzyme monoamine oxidase (MAO), which normally helps to break down norepinephrine and serotonin. When the action of MAO is inhibited, the concentration of the neurotransmitters increases. MAO is also responsible for the regulation of metabolism of a substance found in many foods called *tyramine*. When the action of MAO is inhibited and individuals ingest tyramine-containing foods, the accumulation of tyramine in the body can precipitate a severe elevation in blood pressure, causing a *hypertensive crisis* that could result in stroke. To prevent this complication, individuals on MAOIs must adhere to a number of dietary restrictions. Examples of foods to be avoided include aged cheese, wine, beer, chocolate, coffee, raisins, and yogurt. In addition, many other medications, including over-the-counter medications such as sinus medications and cold preparations, can present a hazard. Individuals with chronic alcoholism or liver damage are not good candidates for management of

their condition with MAOIs. Individuals placed on these medications must have the cognitive ability and motivation to precisely follow dietary restrictions so that they can avoid the potentially severe complications with these drugs.

Suicide is always a possibility with individuals who are depressed, and the risk of suicide is influenced by a number of factors (Simon, 2006). The availability of antidepressant medication that could be used in a suicide attempt is a risk that needs to be considered, for example. The risk of attempted suicide may be higher when the antidepressant begins to take effect because suicidal impulses are still present: as individuals' energy returns, so does their motivation to attempt suicide. Suicide is the third leading cause of death among young people (Brent & Mann, 2006). Known risk factors for suicide, especially in young persons with mood disorders, include alcohol abuse, recent loss of a loved one, and a family history of suicidal behavior (Bridge, Goldstein, & Brent, 2006; Friedman, 2006a). Although antidepressants are an important aspect of intervention for depressive disorders, psychotherapeutic modes of intervention should be used in combination with the pharmacologic approach.

Mood Stabilizers

Lithium was one of the first medications effectively prescribed to manage manifestations of bipolar disorder. This element occurs naturally as a salt. Use of lithium for management of psychiatric conditions in the United States began in the 1970s, and this agent has been used in bipolar disorders—both in the management of manifestations and in the prevention of recurring manifestations. In some instances, lithium has been used alone or in combination with antidepressants to treat depressive disorders. Because not all individuals respond to lithium in the same way, the appropriateness of its use is decided on an individual basis. Due to the expensive follow-up work needed to monitor levels of lithium in the blood and potential side effects, lithium is not used as often as it was to treat bipolar disorder.

The way in which lithium works remains unclear. Common side effects include **polyuria** (excessive urination), **polydipsia** (excessive thirst), and, in some individuals, fine hand tremor. Side effects may also include *hypothyroidism* (too little thyroid hormone) or enlargement of the thyroid gland, so individuals should have thyroid function checked regularly. Other potential side effects include fatigue, muscle weakness, and weight gain.

Individuals who use lithium need regular blood tests to measure levels of the medication in the blood and must be regularly monitored by a health professional. If the lithium level is too low, the medication will not be effective. If the level is too high, individuals may experience a variety of side effects. The balance of lithium is easily altered by anything that affects the level of sodium in the body. For instance, a reduction of salt intake, excessive sweating, fear, nausea, and diarrhea can all affect the amount of sodium in the body, thereby causing a buildup of lithium and leading to toxicity. *Diuretics* (substances that cause loss of body fluid), such as some medications, coffee, and tea, also increase lithium levels and can lead to lithium toxicity. Warning signs of toxicity include nausea and vomiting, confusion or disorientation, slurring of speech, irregular heartbeat, and, in severe cases, seizures. Unfortunately the therapeutic level for lithium is also dangerously close to the toxic level of the drug. Overdose of lithium can be fatal.

Anticonvulsant Medications

Now a commonly used first choice in treatment for individuals with bipolar disorders, *anticonvulsant medications* (medications typically used to treat seizures), or mood stabilizers as they have more recently been called, include valproic acid (Valproate), carbamazepine (Tegretol), divalproex (Depakote), and lamotrigine (Lamictal). These medications are especially effective in the acute mania phase. These medications can have long-term side effects, for example, valproic acid may cause liver problems, individuals who are taking this mediation should have liver function tests prior to beginning the intervention and then regularly thereafter.

Antianxiety Medications

Antianxiety medications are generally used for conditions in which anxiety is the predominant manifestation. One popular class of antianxiety medications are the *benzodiazepines* (e.g., diazepam, clonazepam, lorazepam, alprazolam). These medications may have side effects of drowsiness, loss of coordination, or mental slowing, at least initially. Consequently, individuals placed on antianxiety medication should avoid driving or operating certain machinery until they know how they will be affected by the medication. Moreover, individuals taking benzodiazepines should avoid alcohol due to the potential for interaction and possibly life-threatening effects. Important to note that benzodiazepines are not meant for long-term use due to the risk of abuse or physical dependence. Their use should be monitored carefully. Long-term treatment of anxiety disorders is better managed by some classes of antidepressant medications.

Individuals taking benzodiazepines should never suddenly stop the medications because of the severe withdrawal reaction that could potentially occur. Sudden discontinuation effects may include severe manifestations of anxiety and, in some instances, seizures. Before stopping benzodiazepines completely, the dosage should be gradually tapered over time under the supervision of a health professional.

Electroconvulsive Therapy as an Approach for Management of Psychiatric Conditions

Before psychopharmacologic preparations were readily available, electroconvulsive therapy (ECT) was a major mode of treating some psychiatric conditions. Today, psychotherapeutic medications have largely replaced ECT, even though some individuals respond well to ECT. Most large hospitals or academic healthcare centers continue to offer ECT to individuals who are referred for this type of intervention. This therapeutic approach may be especially useful when the long-term administration of medication is contraindicated (Fink, 2000). ECT is often used in the following circumstances:

- Individuals have conditions such as major depression, bipolar depression, or mania and do not respond to medications.
- Individuals' physical health and mental health are threatened without intervention.

- Individuals express a preference for ECT due to its fast-acting nature.
- Individuals have responded favorably to ECT in the past. (Goodman, 2011; Lisanby, 2007)

Although ECT does not cure psychiatric conditions, it can bring about a remission of manifestations. It may be used either alone or in conjunction with psychotherapeutic medications (Lisanby, 2007).

GENERAL FUNCTIONAL IMPLICATIONS OF PSYCHIATRIC CONDITIONS

Personal and Psychosocial Issues

Individuals with psychiatric conditions experience a wide range of manifestations that affect psychological, cognitive, and social functioning. The needs of individuals with psychiatric conditions are multifaceted and complex (Kress-Shull & Leech, 2000). In individuals with a dual diagnosis, problems related to functioning are compounded. Although the benefits of medication as an intervention for psychiatric conditions are substantial, medication usually does not cure the condition but rather merely helps to manage the manifestations. Individuals often have residual manifestations and limitations as a result of their condition, and many are subject to periodic relapses with recurrence of manifestations.

Manifestations experienced vary with the condition, leading to differing degrees of incapacitation. Although fear and anger are normal emotional responses, these responses may be acutely disproportionate to the stimuli in some psychiatric conditions. Some individuals' responses are covert, whereas others' responses are more pronounced. Some individuals manifest their condition through patterns of behavior rather than in emotional forms. Others experience subjective distress, such as an inner sense of weakness, jealousy, or anxiety, although functioning in most of their life is minimally disrupted. Some psychiatric disabilities are characterized by disorganization of mental capacities, which can affect individuals' ability to function in an unstructured environment. Conditions that affect memory and perception can severely limit independent function. Individuals may fail to carry out age-appropriate role functions and have varying degrees of dependence on others.

Individuals may experience stress and anxiety because of manifestations, further compounding the incapacitating component of the condition. The degree to which psychiatric conditions affect individuals' lifestyle depends to a great extent on the nature of the condition. Manifestations of some psychiatric conditions may impair individuals' ability to carry on the activities of daily living to the extent that constant supervision or hospitalization is necessary. In other cases, individuals are able to carry on most activities, albeit in an altered manner. In some instances, individuals may be reluctant to seek appropriate help because of the stigma perceived to be associated with psychiatric conditions. In other instances, individuals may be unaware of the manifestations and their effect on function, and this lack of acknowledgment may further hinder application of the appropriate intervention.

Some individuals with psychiatric conditions may be particularly vulnerable to stress and may lack the ability to withstand pressure or to cope with the normal stresses of everyday life. They may have limited problem-solving ability or find it difficult to engage in self-directed activity. Other individuals may become passive, apathetic, or overly submissive as a direct result of repeated hospitalizations or as a result of the condition itself.

Individuals with psychiatric conditions frequently have comorbid health conditions and associated physical problems that compound manifestations and intervention (O'Day, Killeen, Sutton, & Iezzoni, 2005; Twigger & Houltram, 2006). In addition to the higher incidence of heart disease, diabetes, and obesity that is often associated with medications used to manage psychiatric conditions, tobacco use is higher in individuals with psychiatric conditions than in the general population, further increasing health risk (Osborn, 2001). In addition, the incidence of substance use and abuse is higher in individuals with psychiatric conditions—a comorbidity that further compounds management of the condition (Magruder, Sonne, Brady, Quello, & Martin, 2005).

Activities and Participation

A number of barriers exist for individuals with psychiatric conditions that interfere with their ability to obtain adequate health care to manage health conditions. Individuals may be reluctant to seek health, or they may lack adequate financial resources to do so. In other instances when health care is sought, emphasis may be placed on the psychiatric condition rather than addressing other health issues. Developing strategies to identify empathetic health professionals who are also knowledgeable about issues involved with psychiatric conditions as well as helping individuals learn to be their own advocates in meeting their healthcare needs can help prevent many physical health problems from occurring (O'Day et al., 2005).

At times, appropriate management of psychiatric conditions requires lifestyle changes. For instance, rearrangement of an individual's schedule to make possible attendance at therapy sessions, engaging in a regular exercise program to counter potential weight gain (a side effect of many psychiatric medications), and learning to manage stress can enhance the effectiveness of other interventions. Some medications used in the management of psychiatric conditions may require special lifestyle considerations. For example, the use of MAOIs for depression requires careful monitoring of diet. Other medications have side effects, such as drowsiness and sedation, which affect daily function in a detrimental way.

Either the psychiatric condition or its management may alter sexual function. Individuals with a depressive disorder may lose interest in sexual activity, whereas individuals with a bipolar depression may have excessive sexual interests. Side effects of some medications can alter sexual function as well. In addition, subjective manifestations of lowered self-esteem and self-confidence may make it more difficult for individuals to form intimate relationships.

The impact of a psychiatric condition on social function also depends on the nature of the condition and the individual's reaction to it. Low self-esteem frequently accompanies psychiatric conditions and, in turn, leads to negative self-concept (Knapen et al., 2007). Unfortunately, stigma and myths about psychiatric conditions persist. While society as a whole has become more accepting of individuals with psychiatric conditions, family members may continue to deny the issue, thereby delaying implementation of appropriate

interventions (Hall & Purdy, 2000). If individuals demonstrate bizarre, abusive, or socially offensive behavior, some family members or others within a social group may avoid the individual altogether, resulting in social isolation.

Other psychiatric conditions may lead to social withdrawal. Families of individuals with psychiatric conditions may experience a variety of stresses engendered by the condition. These stresses may be caused by their objective problems in dealing with the individual and his or her condition, as well as by more subjective psychological distress (Hall & Purdy, 2000).

Psychiatric conditions, especially those that require close supervision or long-term care and intervention, may impose financial hardship on the family because of healthcare bills, the individual's economic dependency, and special needs related to household functioning. In some instances, demands of caregiving may require family members to curtail social activities or alter relationships with friends and acquaintances. Time commitments of caregiving may lead to neglect of other family members' needs, further disrupting the family unit. Delivery of family-based services that address ongoing stressors such as financial concerns, housing, and relationship issues promotes development of a stronger family unit and ongoing support (Riebschleger, 2004).

Social barriers are frequently erected against individuals with psychiatric conditions and their families. Social stigma may be the result of either ignorance about psychiatric conditions or feelings of inadequacy in knowing how to interact with individuals with a psychiatric condition. There may be fear of the potential for violence, despite the fact that most people with psychiatric conditions do not commit assaultive acts. Individuals with psychiatric conditions who are free of psychotic manifestations have a drastically reduced risk of violent behavior (Friedman, 2006b). In contrast, substance abuse among individuals with psychiatric conditions can increase the risk for violence (Swanson et al., 2002). Being perceived as dangerous can have a negative impact on relationships, housing, and employment and lead to social distancing, resulting in impairment in social function (Kleinfelder, Telijohann, & Price, 2004). Educating the public that most individuals with psychiatric conditions do not commit violent acts can help to reduce this stigma.

Regardless of the cause of social stigma, it can result in ongoing stress for individuals with psychiatric conditions and their families, as well as pose a barrier to social activity and interaction. Social stigma and stereotypes can also influence the extent of limitations that individuals experience. Limitations sometimes occur not because of the psychiatric condition itself but rather because of the public's reaction to it (Corrigan & Calabrese, 2001). Other issues such as housing instability and, at times, homelessness may further contribute to social stigma, increase stress levels, and negatively influence overall well-being (Tsemberis, Gulcur, & Nakae, 2004).

Increasing emphasis has been placed on social integration of individuals with psychiatric conditions. Nevertheless, although individuals may be living in the community, they frequently may not be an actual part of it (Ware, Hopper, Tugenberg, Dickey, & Fisher, 2007). Full integration includes participation in the community, including maintenance of reciprocal interpersonal relationships, which extends beyond support mechanisms and interaction with other people with psychiatric conditions. It also behooves individuals with psychiatric conditions to accept their responsibility and accountability to the community in which they live.

GENERAL VOCATIONAL ISSUES IN PSYCHIATRIC CONDITIONS

Psychiatric conditions affect a significant portion of the working-age population in the United States (Donnell, Lustig, & Strauser, 2004). The ability of individuals with psychiatric conditions to work depends on the type of condition, the type of work in which they are involved, and the attitudes of those within the work setting. It is important that both professionals and individuals with psychiatric conditions keep in mind that manifestations currently being experienced may not be present in the future and that functional capacity can change (Killeen & O'Day, 2004). Even when individuals experience significant incapacitation as a result of their psychiatric condition, as they learn to

manage manifestations and medications, the level of functional capacity can increase so that return to regular employment in accordance with their interests and talents, and goals can be achieved.

Although work is important to increase self-esteem for individuals both with and without a specific health condition, it can be an especially strong and beneficial tool for those with a psychiatric condition (Tschopp, Bishop, & Mulvihill, 2001). Individuals with a psychiatric condition may lack self-confidence, have a poor perception of their own abilities, and feel a high level of vulnerability and fear of failure (Hoekstra, Sanders, van den Heuvel, Post, & Groothoff, 2004). Although the skills, aptitude, motivation, and objective manifestations of individuals with psychiatric conditions are important, their ability to endure and cope with stress and to engage in active problem solving also determine their ability to work. Job restrictions may be related to job pressure or the ability to work with others, regardless of the individual's particular level of skill or physical and cognitive ability to perform work-related tasks.

As noted earlier, individuals with psychiatric conditions are more vulnerable to stress (Dorio & Marine, 2004). Chronic work stress has been found to amplify the incapacitation associated with psychiatric conditions (Dewa, Lin, Kooehoorn, & Goldner, 2007). To counteract this tendency, individuals should be assisted to develop effective coping mechanisms at work. Discussion with the employer to identify ways to create a less stressful environment may be needed.

Other considerations may relate to individuals' management of their condition. It may be necessary to arrange scheduled absences so that individuals can attend therapy sessions. Some medications used in management of manifestations may produce side effects, such as drowsiness or sedation, that could adversely affect work performance. In addition, individuals' level of adherence to the medication plan is critically important—failure to comply with the medication regimen might potentially lead to relapse and recurrence of manifestations.

Individuals' reactions to the work environment, including noise and distractions, should be taken into account, as should their level of personal responsibility and capacity for self-direction and decision making. Their limited arsenal of interpersonal and coping skills may make it difficult for some individuals to adjust to unforeseen circumstances. Individuals' flexibility to take advantage of chance occurrences and their degree of flexibility in the workplace must be taken into consideration (Szymanski, 2000). Some individuals may require a more structured work environment. In some instances, individuals' expectations of work or assessment of their own capabilities may be unrealistic. Unless these unrealistic notions are identified and dealt with before individuals enter (or reenter) the work setting, discouragement, disappointment, or even relapse may occur.

Supported employment has been found to be an important way to foster empowerment in individuals with a psychiatric condition (Corrigan, 2004) and to help them obtain competitive employment (Bond, 2004). It is a commonly adopted method to help people with a psychiatric condition achieve better and meaningful quality of life through work (Lee, Chronister, Tsang, Ingraham, & Oulvey, 2005; Morris & Lloyd, 2004). In supported employment, individuals work in integrated settings, with monitoring, support, and follow-up being provided on a regular basis. Supported employment provides permanent jobs that are based on individuals' skills and abilities.

Social skills, aptitude, and the ability to work are not necessarily present concurrently in individuals with a psychiatric condition. Employment for each individual must be considered in the context of his or her individual goals, manifestations of the particular condition, and the nature of the work environment. The role that social stigma plays in individuals' perceptions of their own condition and their willingness to accept and follow up with interventions are crucial aspects of the total rehabilitation of individuals with a psychiatric condition.

The unemployment and underemployment rates for individuals with psychiatric conditions remain high (Cook, 2006; Kress-Shull, 2001; Rogers, Anthony, Lyass, & Penk, 2006). Once work is obtained, maintaining employment may also prove to be a challenge for such individuals (Auerbach & Richardson, 2005). Although no one factor accounts for the low employment status of individuals with psychiatric conditions, several

systemic and programmatic barriers exist that may be difficult for them to overcome (Henry & Lucca, 2004). Previous occupational experience appears to be a valid predictor of individuals' ability to return to work (Pluta & Accordino, 2006); specifically, low education and limited work experience predict unfavorable vocational outcomes for individuals with psychiatric conditions (Watzke, Galvao, Gawlik, Huehne, & Brieger, 2006). Given that many individuals have their psychiatric condition identified in adolescence or young adulthood, their lack of opportunities to become established in a career may contribute to their inability to obtain competitive employment. Fewer than 15% of individuals served in the public mental health system are in competitive employment (Gowdy, Carlson, & Rapp, 2004). Low expectations are often embedded in policies and programs, such that individuals are given negative messages regarding their capacity to work (Killeen & O'Day, 2004). Because of concern that stress may cause relapse, individuals with psychiatric conditions may be encouraged to accept unskilled, low-wage positions that are far below their actual skills and capabilities. The amount of stress generated by working for poverty-level wages in a job that does not match the individual's ability is often ignored.

In other instances, financial disincentives may contribute to underemployment or unemployment (Cook et al., 2006; MacDonald-Wilson, Rogers, Ellison, & Lyass, 2003). Often individuals' ability to work is affected by their desire to retain Social Security benefits (Killeen & O'Day, 2004). Individuals may fear that if benefits are relinquished to pursue full-time work, no benefits will be available if they should have a relapse or lose their job. Applying for benefits again after they have been relinquished can be a cumbersome and lengthy process, which individuals with a psychiatric condition may choose to avoid. Consequently, they may remain unemployed or accept low-paying, part-time work rather than lose disability benefits.

Funding of mental health services often exceeds funding for employment services for individuals with psychiatric conditions, with the outcome that employment outcomes may not be the major focus of services provided (O'Brien, Ford, & Malloy, 2005). Continued advocacy, which includes educating not only employers but also policy makers and individuals with psychiatric conditions, is necessary in the ongoing process of reducing unemployment and underemployment among individuals with psychiatric conditions. Although a focus on competitive employment and job development is important, emphasis on job retention through job support is equally important to enhance positive employment and quality-of-life outcomes (Leff et al., 2005).

REFERENCES

Agid, Y., Buzsaki, G., Diamond, D. M., Frackowiak, R., Giedd, J., Girault, J. A., ... Weinberger, D. (2007). How can drug discovery for psychiatric disorders be improved? *Nature Reviews Drug Discovery, 6*(3), 189–201.

American Psychiatric Association. (2000). *Diagnostic and statistical manual of mental disorders* (4th ed., text revision). Washington, DC: Author.

American Psychiatric Association. (2013). *Diagnostic and statistical manual of mental disorders (DSM-5)* (5th ed.). Arlington, VA: Author.

Andersson, L., Wiles, N., Lewis, G., Brage, S., & Hensing, G. (2007). Can access to psychiatric health care explain regional differences in disability pension with psychiatric disorders? *Social Psychiatry and Psychiatric Epidemiology, 42,* 366–371.

Anthony, W. A., Cohen, M. R., Farkas, M., & Gagne, C. (Eds.). (2002). *Psychiatric rehabilitation* (2nd ed.). Boston, MA: Boston University Center for Psychiatric Rehabilitation.

Anthony, W. A., & Farkas, M. D. (2009). *A primer on the psychiatric rehabilitation process.* Boston, MA: Boston University Center for Psychiatric Rehabilitation.

Auerbach, E. S., & Richardson, P. (2005). The long-term work experiences of persons with severe and persistent mental illness. *Psychiatric Rehabilitation Journal, 28*(3), 267–273.

Bond, G. R. (2004). Supported employment: Evidence for an evidence-based practice. *Psychiatric Rehabilitation Journal, 27,* 345–359.

Brent, D. A., & Mann, J. J. (2006). Familial pathways to suicidal behavior: Understanding and preventing suicide among adolescents. *New England Journal of Medicine, 355*(26), 2719–2721.

Bridge, J. A., Goldstein, T. R., & Brent, D. A. (2006). Adolescent suicide and suicidal behavior. *Journal of Child Psychology and Psychiatry, and Allied Disciplines, 47,* 372–394.

Coniglio, F. D., Hancock, N., & Ellis, L. A. (2012). Peer support with in a clubhouse: A grounded theory study. *Community Mental Health Journal, 48*(2), 153–160.

Cook, J. A. (2006). Employment barriers for persons with psychiatric disabilities: Update of a report for the President's Commission. *Psychiatric Services, 57*(10), 1391–1405.

Cook, J. A., Leff, H. S., Blyler, C. R., Gold, P. B., Goldberg, R. W., Clark, R. E., ... Burke-Miller, J. (2006). Estimated payments to employment service providers for persons with mental illness in the Ticket to Work program. *Psychiatric Services, 57*(4), 465–471.

Corrigan, P. W. (2004, Autumn). Enhancing personal empowerment of people with psychiatric disabilities. *American Rehabilitation,* 10–21.

Corrigan, P. W., & Calabrese, J. D. (2001). Practical considerations for cognitive rehabilitation of people with psychiatric disabilities. *Rehabilitation Education, 15*(2), 143–153.

Dekker, J. M., Girman, C., Rhodes, T., Nijpels, G., Stehowwer, C. D., Bouter, L. M., & Heine, R. J. (2005). Metabolic syndrome and 10 year cardiovascular disease risk in the Hoorn study. *Circulation, 112,* 666–673.

Dewa, C. S., Lin, E., Kooehoorn, M., & Goldner, E. (2007). Association of chronic work stress, psychiatric disorders, and chronic physical conditions with disability among workers. *Psychiatric Services, 58,* 652–658.

Dixon, L. (2000). Assertive Community Treatment: Twenty five years of gold. *Psychiatric Services, 51,* 759–765.

Donnell, C. M., Lustig, D., & Strauser, D. R. (2004). The working alliance: Rehabilitation outcomes for persons with severe mental illness. *Journal of Rehabilitation, 70*(2), 12–18.

Dorio, J., & Marine, S. (2004). A comprehensive look at promoting job retention for workers with psychiatric disabilities in a supported employment program. *Psychiatric Rehabilitation Journal, 28*(1), 32–39.

Duncan, B. L., Miller, S. D., & Sparks, J. A. (2004). *The heroic client.* San Francisco, CA: Jossey-Bass.

Fink, M. (2000). Electroshock revisited. *American Scientist, 88,* 162–167.

Friedman, R. A. (2006a). Uncovering an epidemic: Screening for mental illness in teens. *New England Journal of Medicine, 355*(26), 2717–2719.

Friedman, R. A. (2006b). Violence and mental illness: How strong is the link? *New England Journal of Medicine, 355*(20), 2064–2066.

Gardner, D. M., Baldessarini, R. J., & Waraich, P. (2005). Modern antipsychotic drugs: A critical overview. *Canadian Medical Association Journal, 172,* 1703–1711.

Garske, G. G. (1999). The challenge of rehabilitation counselors: Working with people with psychiatric disabilities. *Journal of Rehabilitation, 65,* 21–25.

Goodman, W. K. (2011). Electroconvulsive therapy in the spotlight. *New England Journal of Medicine, 364*(19), 1785–1787.

Gopalakrishna, G., Ithman, M. H., & Lauriello, J. (2016). Update on new and emerging treatments for schizophrenia. *Psychiatric Clinics of North America, 39*(2), 217–238.

Gordon, P. A., Tantillo, J. C., Feldman, D., & Perrone, K. (2004). Attitudes regarding interpersonal relationships with persons with mental illness and mental retardation. *Journal of Rehabilitation, 70*(1), 50–56.

Gowdy, E. A., Carlson, L. S., & Rapp, C. A. (2004). Organizational factors differentiating high performing from low performing supported employment programs. *Psychiatric Rehabilitation Journal, 28*(2), 150–156.

Hall, L. L., & Purdy, R. (2000). Recovery and serious brain disorders: The central role of families in nurturing roots and wings. *Community Mental Health Journal, 36*(4), 427–441.

Henry, A. D., & Lucca, A. M. (2004). Facilitators and barriers to employment: The perspectives of people with psychiatric disabilities and employment service providers. *Work, 22,* 169–182.

Hoekstra, E. J., Sanders, K., van den Heuvel, W. J. A., Post, D., & Groothoff, J. W. (2004). Supported employment in the Netherlands for people with an intellectual disability and a chronic disease: A comparative study. *Journal of Vocational Rehabilitation, 21,* 39–48.

Holman, H., & Lorig, K. (2000). Patients as partners in managing chronic disease. Partnership is a prerequisite for effective and efficient health care. *British Medical Journal, 320*(7234), 526–527.

Kahng, S. K., & Mowbray, C. (2004). Factors influencing self-esteem among individuals with severe mental illness: Implications for social work. *Social Work Research, 28*(4), 225–236.

Killeen, M. B., & O'Day, B. L. (2004). Challenging expectations: How individuals with psychiatric disabilities find and keep work. *Psychiatric Rehabilitation Journal, 28*(2), 157–163.

Kleinfelder, J., Telijohann, S. K., & Price, J. H. (2004). Are university health education programs addressing mental health issues? *American Journal of Health Studies, 19*(4), 226–227.

Knapen, J., Vermeersch, J., Van Coppenolle, H., Cuykx, V., Pieters, G., & Peuskens, J. (2007). The physical self-concept in patients with depressive and anxiety disorders. *International Journal of Therapy and Rehabilitation, 14*(1), 30–35.

Kress-Shull, M. K. (2001). Continuing challenges to the vocational rehabilitation of individuals with severe long-term mental illness. *Journal of Applied Rehabilitation Counseling, 31*(4), 5–10.

Kress-Shull, M. K., & Leech, L. L. (2000). Editorial: Effective psychiatric rehabilitation: A collaborative challenge. *Journal of Applied Rehabilitation Counseling, 31*(4), 3–4.

Lambert, M. J. (Ed.). (2013). *Bergin & Garfield's handbook of psychotherapy and behavior change* (6th ed.). Hoboken, NJ: Wiley.

Lee, G. K., Chronister, J., Tsang, H., Ingraham, K., & Oulvey, E. (2005). Psychiatric rehabilitation training needs of state vocational rehabilitation counselors: A preliminary study. *Journal of Rehabilitation, 71*(3), 11–19.

Leech, L. L., & Holcomb, J. M. (2000). The nature of psychiatric rehabilitation and implications for collaborative efforts. *Journal of Applied Rehabilitation Counseling, 31*(4), 54–60.

Leff, H. S., Cook, J. A., Gold, P. B., Toprac, M., Blyer, C., Goldberg, R. W., ... Raab, B. L. (2005). Effects of job development and job support on competitive employment of persons with severe mental illness. *Psychiatric Services, 56*(10), 1237–1244.

Lieberman, J. A., Stroup, T. S., McEvoy, J. P., Swartz, M. S., Rosenheck, R. A., Perkins, D. O., ... Clinical Antipsychotic Trials of Intervention Effectiveness (CATIE) Investigators. (2005). Effectiveness of antipsychotic drugs in patients with chronic schizophrenia. *New England Journal of Medicine, 353*(12), 1209–1223.

Lisanby, S. H. (2007). Electroconvulsive therapy for depression. *New England Journal of Medicine, 357*(19), 1939–1945.

MacDonald-Wilson, K. L., & Nemec, P. B. (2005). The international classification of functioning, disability and health (ICF) in psychiatric rehabilitation. *Rehabilitation Education, 19*(2 & 3), 159–176.

MacDonald-Wilson, K. L., Rogers, E. S., Ellison, M. L., & Lyass, A. (2003). A study of the Social Security Work Incentives and their relation to perceived barriers to work among persons with psychiatric disability. *Rehabilitation Psychology, 48*(4), 301–309.

Magruder, K. M., Sonne, S. C., Brady, K. T., Quello, S., & Martin, R. H. (2005). Screening for co-occurring mental disorders in drug treatment populations. *Journal of Drug Issues, 35,* 593–605.

Martin, S. (2009, October). Improving diagnosis worldwide. *Monitor on Psychology, 40*(9), 62–65.

Masand, P. S. (2007). Differential pharmacology of atypical anti-psychotics: Clinical implications. *American Journal of Health-System Pharmacy, 64*(2 Suppl 1), S3–S8, quiz S24–S25.

Mead, S., & Copeland, M. D. (2000). What recovery means to us: Consumers perspectives. *Community Mental Health Journal, 36*(3), 315–328.

Morris, P., & Lloyd, C. (2004). Vocational rehabilitation in psychiatry: A re-evaluation. *Australian and New Zealand Journal of Psychiatry, 38*(7), 490–494.

Mueser, K. T., Meyer, P. S., Penn, D. L., Clancy, R., Clancy, D. M., & Salyers, P. (2006). The illness management and recovery program: Rationale, development, and preliminary findings. *Schizophrenia Bulletin, 32*(Suppl 1), S32–S43. doi:10.1093/schbul/sb1022

O'Brien, D., Ford, L., & Malloy, J. M. (2005). Person centered funding: Using vouchers and personal budgets to support recovery and employment for people with psychiatric disabilities. *Journal of Vocational Rehabilitation, 23,* 71–79.

O'Day, B., Killeen, M. B., Sutton, J., & Iezzoni, L. I. (2005). Primary care experiences of people with psychiatric disabilities: Barriers to care and potential solutions. *Psychiatric Rehabilitation Journal, 28*(4), 339–345.

Osborn, D. P. J. (2001). The poor physical health of people with mental illness. *Western Journal of Medicine, 175,* 329–334.

Peterson, D. B. (2011). *Psychological aspects of functioning, disability and health.* New York, NY: Springer Publishing Company.

Peterson, D. B., & Elliott, T. R. (2008). Advances in conceptualizing and studying disability. In S. Brown & R. W. Lent (Eds.), *Handbook of counseling psychology* (4th ed., pp. 212–230). Hoboken, NJ: Wiley & Sons.

Peterson, D. B., & Hong, G. (2014). Psychiatric diagnoses. In M. G. Brodwin, F. W. Sui, J. Howard, E. R. Brodwin, & A. T. Du (Eds.), *Medical, psychosocial, and vocational aspects of disability* (4th ed., pp. 269–284). Athens, GA: Elliott & Fitzpatrick, Inc.

Pluta, D. J., & Accordino, M. P. (2006). Predictors of return to work for people with psychiatric disabilities: A private sector perspective. *Rehabilitation Counseling Bulletin, 49*(2), 102–110.

Pollio, D. E., North, C. S., Reid, D. L., Miletic, M. M., & McClendon, J. R. (2006). Living with severe mental illness: What families and friends must know: Evaluation of a one-day psycho-education workshop. *Social Work, 51*(1), 31–38.

Porter, R. (2001). Mental illness. In R. Porter (Ed.), *The Cambridge illustrated history of medicine* (pp. 278–303). Cambridge, UK: Cambridge University Press.

Preston, J., O'Neal, J. H., & Talaga, M. (2013). *Handbook of clinical psychopharmacology for therapists* (7th ed.). Oakland, CA: New Harbinger Publications.

Raeburn, T., Halcomb, E., Walter, G., & Cleary, M. (2013). An overview of the clubhouse model of psychiatric rehabilitation. *Australasian Psychiatry, 21*(4), 376–378.

Raeburn, T., Schmied, V., Hungerford, C., & Cleary, M. (2014). Clubhouse model of psychiatric rehabilitation: How is recovery reflected in documentation? *International Journal of Mental Health Nursing, 23*(5), 389–397.

Raeburn, T., Schmied, V., Hungerford, C., & Cleary, M. (2015). The contribution of case study design to support research on clubhouse psychosocial rehabilitation. *Bio-Med Central Research Notes, 8*, 521. doi:10.1186/s13104-015-1521-1

Riebschleger, J. (2004). Good days and bad days: The experiences of children of a parent with a psychiatric disability. *Psychiatric Rehabilitation Journal, 28*(1), 25–31.

Rogers, E. S., Anthony, W. A., Lyass, A., & Penk, W. E. (2006). A randomized clinical trial of vocational rehabilitation for people with psychiatric disabilities. *Rehabilitation Counseling Bulletin, 49*(3), 143–156.

Simon, G. E. (2006). The antidepressant quandary: Considering suicide risk when treating adolescent depression. *New England Journal of Medicine, 355*(26), 2722–2723.

Sridhar, G. R. (2007). Psychiatric co-morbidity and diabetes. *Indian Journal of Medical Research, 125*(3), 311–320.

Swanson, J. W., Swartz, M. S., Essock, S. M., Osher, F. C., Wagner, H. R., Goodman, L. A., ... Meador, K. G. (2002). The social–environmental context of violent behavior in persons treated for severe mental illness. *American Journal of Public Health, 92*, 1523–1531.

Szymanski, E. M. (2000). Disability and vocational behavior. In R. Frank & T. Elliot (Eds.), *Handbook of rehabilitation psychology* (pp. 499–517). Washington, DC: American Psychological Association.

Test, M. A., & Stein, L. I. (1976). Practical guidelines for the treatment of markedly impaired patients. *Community Mental Health Journal, 12*, 72–82.

Tschopp, M. K., Bishop, M., & Mulvihill, M. (2001). Career development of individuals with psychiatric disabilities: An ecological perspective of barriers and interventions. *Journal of Applied Rehabilitation Counseling, 32*(2), 25–30.

Tsemberis, S., Gulcur, L., & Nakae, M. (2004). Housing first, consumer choice, and harm reduction for homeless individuals with a dual diagnosis. *American Journal of Public Health, 94*(4), 651–656.

Tucin, A., Dolzan, V., Porcelli, S., Serretti, A., & Plesnicar, B. K. (2016). Adrenosine hypothesis of antipsychotic drugs revisited. Pharmacogenomics variation in nonactue schizophrenia. *OMICS: A Journal of Integrative Biology, 20*(5), 283–289.

Twigger, M., & Houltram, B. (2006). A weighty problem: Monitoring the side effects of medication. *Learning Disability Practice, 9*(10), 28–31.

Wang, P. S., Schneeweiss, S., Avorn, J., Fischer, M. A., Mogun, H., Solomon, D. H., ... Brookhart, M. A. (2005). Risk of death in elderly users of conventional vs. atypical antipsychotic medications. *New England Journal of Medicine, 353*(22), 2335–2341.

Ware, N. C., Hopper, K., Tugenberg, T., Dickey, B., & Fisher, D. (2007). Connectedness and citizenship redefining social integration. *Psychiatric Services, 58*, 469–474.

Watzke, S., Galvao, A., Gawlik, B., Huehne, M., & Brieger, P. (2006). Change in work performance in vocational rehabilitation for people with severe mental illness: Distinct responder groups. *International Journal of Social Psychiatry, 52*(4), 309–323.

Weinstein, L. C., Henwood, B. F., Cody, J. W., Jordan, M., & Lelar, R. (2011). Transforming assertive community treatment into an integrated care system: The role of nursing and primary care partnerships. *Journal of the American Psychiatric Nurses Association, 17*, 64–71.

World Health Organization. (1992). *International statistical classification of diseases and related health problems (ICD-10)* (10th revision). Geneva, Switzerland: Author.

World Health Organization. (2001). *International Classification of Functioning, Disability and Health: ICF.* Geneva, Switzerland: Author.

Word Health Organization. (2011). *International Classification of Diseases Clinical Modification (ICD-9-CM)* (9th Revision). Geneva, Switzerland: Author.

World Health Organization. (2012). *Measuring health and disability: Manual for WHO Disability Assessment Schedule (WHODAS 2.0).* Geneva, Switzerland: Author.

Word Health Organization. (2014). *International Classification of Diseases Clinical Modification (ICD-10-CM)* (10th Revision). Geneva, Switzerland: Author.

CHAPTER 14

Functional Implications of Selected Psychiatric Diagnoses

Revised by David B. Peterson

The National Alliance on Mental Illness (NAMI) publishes national health statistical information on mental illness (see www.nami.org). Estimates derive from various surveys that collected data in 2014 and suggest that one in five adults in the United States, or about 43 million people, experience mental illness in a given year. Of that number about 10 million of them experience severe enough functional impairment to interfere with one or more major life functions. According to the Center for Behavioral Health Statistics and Quality (2015), half of the 20.2 million people estimated to experience substance use issues also have a co-occurring mental illness.

The National Institute of Mental Health (NIMH) within the National Institutes of Health (NIH) on their website (nimh.nih.gov) published more specific prevalence data for the most commonly occurring psychiatric diagnoses in a given year. Based upon 2004 (Kessler et al., 2005) data and the DSM-IV-TR taxonomy in use at the time, the most common psychiatric diagnoses were within the anxiety disorders category, with an 18.1% annual prevalence rate, including such diagnoses as posttraumatic stress disorder, obsessive compulsive disorder, and specific phobias, as well as generalized anxiety disorder. Following substance use disorders (covered in the next chapter) the same data suggest major depression is the third most common with a 6.9% annual prevalence rate, about 16 million people. Bipolar disorder

followed that with a 2.6% annual prevalence rate, or 6.1 million people.

Having explored the functional and vocational implications of psychiatric conditions generally in the previous chapter, here we focus on specific psychiatric diagnoses as currently included in the ICD-10 CM (Word Health Organization [WHO], 2014) and the DSM-5 (American Psychiatric Association [APA], 2013). Diagnoses selected include the most frequently occurring and also some that are the most challenging to manage in treatment.

ANXIETY DISORDERS

Anxiety disorders are the most frequently occurring conditions and share in common some form of excessive anxiety and fear. While fear is an emotional reaction to real or perceived threat, anxiety is the anticipation of such a threat; see pages 189–234 of the DSM-5 (APA, 2013). Common features of these disorders include not only anxiety but also increased arousal and avoidance of situations that the individual perceives as anxiety provoking (Gillock, Zayfert, Hegel, & Ferguson, 2005; Gross et al., 2005; Issakidis, Sanderson, Corry, Andrews, & Lapsley, 2004; Magruder et al., 2005). Individuals with anxiety disorders also frequently have a mood disorder, especially depression (Garakani, Mathew, & Charney, 2006).

Anxiety disorders can be incapacitating and often are not recognized or managed well (Kroenke,

Spitzer, Williams, Monahan, & Lowe, 2007). Approximately one-fourth of the U.S. population experiences some type of anxiety disorder over the course of a lifetime (Kessler et al., 2005; Kessler, Chiu, Demler, Merikangas, & Walters, 2005), and approximately 17% experience severe anxiety (Antai-Otong, 2006a). As mentioned above the annual prevalence rate has been estimated at about 18% for this diagnostic group (Kessler et al., 2005).

Within the DSM-5 the different types of anxiety disorders are dependent upon the types of objects or situation that induce fear and anxiety, and the different types are often co-occurring with one another. These include: separation anxiety disorder, selective mutism, specific phobia, social anxiety disorder (or social phobia), panic disorder, agoraphobia, and generalized anxiety disorder (APA, 2013). No longer included in this category is posttraumatic stress disorder (PTSD), which is now part of a new category of conditions called Trauma- and Stressor-Related Disorders. Also removed from this category and part of its own unique diagnostic group are the obsessive–compulsive and related disorders (e.g., OCD). The prevalence data reported earlier included PTSD and OCD along with the aforementioned anxiety disorders.

A number of psychotherapeutic interventions (e.g., exposure therapy, relaxation techniques) and medications are used to treat anxiety disorders. Although *benzodiazepines* were first-line treatments in the past, due to their addictive potential and the tendency to develop tolerance to this class of medication, SSRIs are now preferred for long-term treatment of anxiety disorders (Preston, O'Neil, & Talaga, 2013; Sheehan & Sheehan, 2007).

Panic Disorder

Panic disorder is an anxiety disorder in which individuals experience feelings of intense fear of discomfort; they are characterized by **panic attacks**, episodes in which the individual has feelings of intense anxiety or terror, accompanied by a sense of impending doom (APA, 2013). During a panic attack, an individual experiences physical manifestations, such as shortness of breath, increased heart rate and palpitations, sweating, and, at times, nausea or other physical discomfort. Panic attacks are not limited to anxiety disorders as they can occur with other psychiatric diagnoses.

Panic attacks that occur spontaneously and do not seem to be triggered by a certain event are called *unexpected* or *uncued* panic attacks. At least initially, they are unpredictable and at times irrational. At other times, panic attacks are directly related to specific situations or stimuli. These episodes are called *situationally bound* or *cued* panic attacks.

Panic attacks can last from a few minutes to a few hours. During attacks, individuals may express fear of losing control, fear of dying, or a feeling that they are detached from reality (Antai-Otong, 2006a). Although the panic attack in and of itself may not be incapacitating, the individual's fears and concerns associated with the attack can cause significant change in behavior, including avoiding certain situations or, in some instances, even giving up a job.

Panic disorder is distinguished from generalized anxiety in that individuals with panic disorders become preoccupied with the physical manifestations associated with the panic attack (Mahoney, 2000). Management focuses on amelioration of manifestations through medication and counseling.

Agoraphobia

Panic disorders are sometimes accompanied by *agoraphobia,* the fear of being in a situation or place from which it might be difficult or embarrassing to escape or in which no help may be available if the individual experiences a panic attack. Although not all individuals who have panic attacks experience agoraphobia, those who do may severely restrict their activity, hampering both social and occupational functioning. They may refuse to venture outside their home alone, or they may be reluctant to travel by car, bus, or other common means of transportation.

Specific Phobia

The term **phobia** refers to fear and anxiety related to specific situations, persons, or objects. Different types of phobias are categorized on the basis of the object feared—for example, *aviophobia* (fear of flying), *gephyrophobia* (fear of bridges), or *xenophobia* (fear of strangers or foreigners).

Incapacitation resulting from phobias may vary from mild to severe. On the one hand, a phobia may be more of a nuisance than a source of incapacitation. On the other hand, it may be so incapacitating that individuals are unable to function effectively in their day-to-day activities if the phobia causes them to avoid particular objects or situations or causes anxiety to the extent that they are unable or unwilling to engage in necessary activities.

Social Phobia (Social Anxiety Disorder)

Social phobia consists of a persistent fear of social situations such as parties or other social gatherings. Individuals with social phobia avoid these situations because of the distress they experience and fear of embarrassment. Social phobia can severely affect individuals, jobs, relationships, and social functioning.

Other conditions within this DSM-5 category but not covered here include separation anxiety disorder, selective mutism, and generalized anxiety disorder; for details, see pages 189–234 of the DSM-5 (APA, 2013).

OBSESSIVE–COMPULSIVE AND RELATED DISORDERS

This is a category new to the DSM-5, separating this group of disorders from anxiety disorders due to emerging research supporting their distinctive nature. See pages 235–264 of the DSM-5 (APA, 2013). *Obsessive–compulsive disorder (OCD)* is a chronic condition that, if not managed, can cause significant incapacitation, with manifestations following a waxing and waning course (Maj, Sartorius, Okasha, & Zohar, 2002). Although OCD usually occurs in late adolescence or early adulthood, its onset can occur anytime throughout the life span, from preschool age to older adults (Zohar, Fostick, Black, & Lopez-Ibor, 2007).

Individuals with OCD have recurrent **obsessions** (persistent thoughts) or **compulsions** (persistent actions) that they are unable to control. For instance, individuals may have recurrent thoughts of the death of a loved one, or they may have an irresistible urge to perform repetitively some behavior that seems purposeless, such as turning a light on and off three times before retiring for the night. Attempts by individuals to ignore the compulsions merely increase anxiety, discomfort, and distress. Individuals with OCD may experience shame regarding manifestations of the condition; in an attempt to keep manifestations secret, they may not seek help. OCD can cause significant distress and social incapacitation. Individuals may become increasingly reluctant to interact socially and may, in some instances, become housebound.

Cognitive-behavioral therapy is a major intervention for OCD (Foa, Franklin, & Moser, 2002). Medication is often used in combination with such therapy, especially for individuals who are unable to function in their jobs or socially owing to manifestations of the condition (Jenike, 2004).

Other conditions within this DSM-5 category but not covered here include body dysmorphic disorder, hoarding disorder, trichotillomania, and excoriation disorder; for complete details, see pages 235–264 of the DSM-5 (APA, 2013)

TRAUMA AND STRESS RELATED DISORDERS

Another diagnostic category new to the DSM-5, this group of disorders was removed form anxiety disorders due to their unique characteristics and the related research. See pages 265–290 of the DSM-5 (APA, 2013).

Posttraumatic Stress Disorder

Posttraumatic stress disorder (PTSD) was formerly included among the anxiety disorders within the DSM-IV-TR, but research supported its inclusion in a new category established in the DSM-5, Trauma and Stress Related Disorders. PTSD continues to be a condition in which manifestations occur after the experience of a traumatic event, such as an automobile accident, plane crash, natural disaster, or act of violence (Hough & Ursano, 2006). War, especially, produces increased risk due to stress, adversity, and physical and psychological experiences in combat (Garske, 2011). Individuals may develop manifestations of the condition after either experiencing a traumatic event themselves or observing a traumatic event. Reactions to a traumatic event may vary with the individual, although manifestations of PTSD generally fall into three broad categories (Strauser, Lustig, & Uruk, 2006):

- Persistent recollection of the event; sleep difficulties; difficulty concentrating; hypervigilance or hyperarousal; exaggerated startle responses when exposed to stimuli related to the traumatic event
- Persistent experience of the event; recall of distressing images; nightmares or flashbacks
- Emotional numbing; avoidance of individuals or situations reminiscent of the event; detachment; loss of interest in previously enjoyed activities or important close relationships

PTSD, which may occur at any age, causes varying degrees of impairment. Individuals with a previous history of mental health problems, or with depression or an anxiety disorder at the time of the traumatic event, are at higher risk for development of this condition (Freedy & Simpson, 2007; Stevenson, 2005). Distress experienced with PTSD can affect mental function, including memory. Individuals with PTSD may have difficulty concentrating. Short-term memory has also been found to be significantly affected in this disorder, which can affect intellectual function (Emdad & Sondergaard, 2006).

Posttraumatic stress disorder is an incapacitating condition that is often accompanied by depression (Ipser, Seedat, & Stein, 2006). When depression is present, the functional status of the person with PTSD is negatively affected (Stapleton, Asmundson, Woods, Taylor, & Stein, 2006).

Physical manifestations of PTSD may also be present. Individuals may experience vague or severe physical manifestations, such as headache, gastrointestinal upset, fatigue, or muscle tension, which do not have an easily identifiable physical cause (Lincoln et al., 2006). Chest pain related to anxiety may also be present and at times may be misinterpreted so that interventions for what could be a cardiac condition are delayed (Alcaras & Roper, 2006). Emotional manifestations of PTSD such as emotional withdrawal, irritability, and distrust of others are frequently experienced as well (Freedy & Simpson, 2007).

When PTSD is identified and appropriately managed, the prognosis is frequently positive (Stevenson, 2005). Conversely, if PTSD is not identified and manifestations persist, it can be debilitating and require ongoing psychological and pharmacological intervention (Ursano, 2002).

Education and counseling can help individuals understand the nature of their condition and facilitate their recovery. Psychodynamic therapies may be used to help individuals explore their feelings and behavior. Cognitive therapy and anxiety management therapies can also be helpful. Group therapy and peer counseling groups reduce isolation and stigma and provide individuals with PTSD the opportunity to discuss and share their experiences with others (Foa, Keane, & Friedman, 2000; Stevenson, 2005). Because manifestations of PTSD also affect other family members, family therapy is helpful to encourage family members to discuss specific issues. Medications such as SSRIs are often used in the management of PTSD to reduce manifestations, including associated depression (Ipser et al., 2006). The alpha blocker Prozasin has proven useful in reducing night terrors associated with PTSD (Preston et al., 2013).

Other conditions within this diagnostic group of the DSM-5 but not reviewed here include reactive attachment disorder, disinhibited social engagement disorder, acute stress disorder, and adjustment disorders. See pages 265–290 of the DSM-5 for details (APA, 2013).

DEPRESSIVE DISORDERS

Depressive disorders were formally combined with bipolar disorders to form the category of mood disorders in the DSM-IV-TR. However, emerging research and contemporary thinking have associated bipolar disorder with aspects of schizophrenia spectrum disorders, viewing them on a continuum of sorts, and so bipolar disorders have their own category within the DSM-5 (APA, 2013), and will be described later.

Depressive disorders have in common sad, empty, irritable mood. The duration, timing, and presumed etiology of symptoms determine what specific depressive diagnosis is appropriate; See pages 155–188 of the DSM-5 for specific diagnostic details (APA, 2013). As mentioned above,

depression is the second most frequently occurring psychiatric diagnosis apart from substance
use disorders (covered in the next chapter). Major
depression has a 6.9% annual prevalence rate, or
an estimated 16 million people in any given year
deal with major depression.

Depressive conditions have been identified
in children in early childhood (Krishnakumar &
Geeta, 2006) and across the lifespan. Hospitalization may be necessary for severe depression due
to disturbance in interpersonal or occupational
functioning. In addition, a strong association
between substance use disorders and depression
has been noted, which contributes further to disability (Compton, Thomas, Stinson, & Grant, 2007).

Major Depressive Disorder

Major depressive disorder represents one of the
leading causes of functional incapacity, second
only to heart disease as a major cause of functional disability (Rytsala et al., 2007). Depression
affects both the individual and the larger society
through factors such as economic cost, time lost
at work, disability days, and pervasive effects on
physical, mental, and social well-being (Lerner
et al., 2004). Not only does it exist as a primary
health condition, but it also has the potential to
coexist with any other health condition (Bishop &
Sweet, 2000). Depression is frequently underi-
dentified, largely because its manifestations can
be confused with manifestations of other health
conditions (Whooley & Simon, 2000).

Manifestations of Major Depression

Major depressive disorder is defined by depressed
mood or loss of interest in nearly all activities (or
both) for at least two weeks, which is accompanied
by three or more of the following manifestations:

- Insomnia or *hypersomnia* (excessive sleeping)
- Feelings of worthlessness or excessive guilt
- Fatigue or loss of energy
- Diminished ability to concentrate
- Substantial change in appetite or weight
- Psychomotor agitation or retardation
- Recurrent thoughts of death or suicide
  (APA, 2000)

Persistent Depressive Disorder (Dysthymia)

*The DSM-5 refers to dysthymia as persistent
depressive disorder,* characterized by manifestations
similar to those experienced in major depression,
albeit to a lesser degree. Although its manifestations are not as severe as those seen major
depression, the chronic nature of this condition
may impair social and occupational functioning.
The essential distinction between major depressive
disorder and dysthymia is the severity and duration of the manifestations. While major depression generally has a more acute onset, individuals
with dysthymia may be chronically depressed for
months or years.

Functional Implications of Major Depression

Personal and Psychosocial Issues

Individuals in the midst of a major depressive
episode experience feelings of hopelessness and
discouragement, loss of interest in activities previously found pleasurable, decreased energy levels,
and difficulty with memory. They may also express feelings of worthlessness or guilt and have
impaired cognitive functions, evident as the inability to concentrate or to make decisions. Other
manifestations, such as insomnia, hypersomnia,
and appetite disturbances resulting in weight gain
or weight loss, are called *vegetative signs.*

Activities and Participation

The degree of incapacitation produced by major
depression varies, although social and occupational
activities are usually affected to some degree.
Chronic depression causes marked impairment
in psychosocial function and work performance
(Keller et al., 2000). With severe depression,
incapacitation can be so great that individuals are
unable to attend to their own daily needs, such as
basic hygiene and nutrition. Prominent factors that
have been found to be predictive of overall degree
of disability are the severity, duration, and number of depressive episodes (Rytsala et al., 2005).
In addition, older age appears to be a major factor
predicting the degree of work disability (Rytsala
et al., 2007).

Diagnoses included in the Depressive Disorders category but not covered here include a new diagnosis, disruptive mood dysregulation disorder, and emerging from proposed diagnosis status in the DSM-IV-TR to actual diagnosis in the DSM-5, premenstrual dysphoric disorder. See pages 155–188 of the DSM-5 for specific diagnostic details (APA, 2013).

BIPOLAR AND RELATED DISORDERS

Bipolar and related disorders is a new category in the DSM-5, placed between schizophrenia spectrum and other psychotic disorders and depressive disorders due to the overlap in presentation across these categories. As mentioned above, bipolar disorders have been estimated to be present in 2.6% of the U.S. population in a given year, or 6.1 million people. Bipolar disorders are conditions characterized by extremes in mood or *mood instability,* associated with three possible types of episodes (Frye, 2011):

- *Mania*
- *Hypomania*
- *Depression*

Manic Episode

A manic episode is a phase of the condition in which the mood becomes distinctly and unrealistically euphoric, behavior becomes hyperactive, and the individual may appear flamboyant and overly enthusiastic. During this episode, individuals may engage in excessive activity, need little sleep, and show little interest in food. Speech becomes rapid, nonstop (*pressured speech),* loud, and difficult to follow because of rapid changes from one unrelated topic to another (*flight of ideas).* Individuals in a manic episode of bipolar disorder may be impulsive and exercise poor judgment, such as engaging in indiscriminate sexual activity or going on extravagant spending binges. They may become involved in grandiose, unrealistic projects or imagine they have superior talents in a specified area. Heightened energy can also turn into severe anxiety, or individuals may demonstrate extremes of anger, aggressiveness, or rage. Mania may also be accompanied by psychotic manifestations such as

psychosis, delusions, and hallucinations, and may result in the need for hospitalization (APA, 2013; McColm, Brown, & Anderson, 2006).

Hypomanic Episode

A hypomanic episode is a milder form of a manic episode associated with the specific diagnosis bipolar II disorder. The DSM-5 makes the distinction between a manic and a hypomanic episode in that the former is "goal directed" and causes "marked impairment in social or occupational functioning," while the latter is just "present to a significant degree" and associated with a clear change in character (APA, 2013, pp. 124–125). Otherwise they share a similar list of seven features with differing criteria and duration.

Major Depressive Episode

In a major depressive episode, individuals become lethargic and sad, and experience feelings of hopelessness and despair. They have difficulty with concentration, decision making, or taking initiative and may experience insomnia and loss of appetite. The DSM-5 notes nine specific characteristics with specific criteria to satisfy the diagnosis (see page 125 of the DSM-5). Although both mania and depression can be debilitating, a major portion of the disability occurring with bipolar II disorder in particular results from depressive episodes occurring in the condition (Howland, 2006a; Mitchell & Malhi, 2004; Post, 2005; Preston et al., 2013).

Course

Individuals may have one or more episodes of mania or hypomania (not necessarily including a major depressive episode), or episodes that alternate between mania/hypomania and depression. When the alterations between mania and depression occur frequently, the episodes are called *rapid cycling.* Episodes of rapid cycling can take place in any combination or sequence, but usually occur 4 or more times in 12 months (Antai-Otong, 2006b). Some individuals experience an episode that contains both manic and depressive features— a so-called *mixed episode.*

Bipolar disorders are commonly associated with severe disability (Huxley & Baldessarini, 2007). Each person with a bipolar disorder is affected differently. A range of personal, social, and environmental factors influence how manifestations of bipolar disorder are evident in each individual (Russell & Browne, 2005).

Onset of bipolar disorder usually occurs in adolescence or young adulthood, although this condition has also been identified as late as in the early 40s (Kennedy et al., 2005; Meyer & Quenzer, 2005) and in children younger than the age of 13 (Perlis, Miyahara, & Marangell, 2004; Spearing, 2002). Individuals often experience a *prodrome,* or period prior to the development of major manifestations during which there is deviation from previous levels of function but manifestations are not recognized as indicative of bipolar disorder (Conus, Berk, & McGorry, 2006).

A high correlation between substance abuse and bipolar disorder has been noted, although the extent to which substance abuse represents an attempt at self-medication or precipitates manifestations is unknown (Salloum & Thase, 2000; Strakowski & DelBello, 2000). Anxiety-related disorders, including social phobias, panic disorder, and obsessive–compulsive disorders, have also been found to co-occur with bipolar disorder (Freeman, Freeman, & McElroy, 2002). Individuals with bipolar disorder are at higher risk for suicide, especially when emerging from major depressive episodes, and for committing violence against others if experiencing anger and aggressiveness during manic episodes (Murphy, 2006).

Classification of Bipolar Disorders

There are three major classifications of bipolar disorder:

- Bipolar I disorder
- Bipolar II disorder
- Cyclothymia (APA, 2013)

Bipolar I Disorder

Bipolar I disorder is the most common of the three major classifications and is characterized by the occurrence of at least one manic episode, which lasts more than one week and interferes with social, interpersonal, or vocational functioning, or by one mixed episode (APA, 2000; Montejano, Goetzel, & Ozminkowski, 2005). Individuals with bipolar I disorder also frequently have one or more major depressive episodes, but they are not required for the bipolar I diagnosis (APA, 2013).

Bipolar II Disorder

Bipolar II disorder is similar to bipolar I disorder, but is characterized by at least one major depressive episode and a hypomanic episode. The presence of the hypomanic episode distinguishes bipolar II disorders from major depressive disorders (APA, 2013). In review, a major depressive episode is characterized by loss of interest in activities, sadness, and depressed mood. In contrast, a hypomanic episode is characterized by elevated or irritable mood over a period of time.

While hypomania is a milder form of mania, Bipolar II disorder is associated with significant impairment in functioning with patients experiencing longer periods of major depression along with mood instability, and a high rate of suicidality (APA, 2013; Preston et al., 2013). If individuals experience a manic or mixed episode, they are then categorized as having bipolar I disorder rather than bipolar II disorder.

Cyclothymia

Cyclothymia is a mood disorder characterized by manifestations similar to those of bipolar disorders, with hypomanic and depressive periods occurring over a 2 year period without ever satisfying the specific criteria for mania, hypomania, or major depression (APA, 2013; Montejano et al., 2005). Owing to the chronic nature of the condition, individuals with cyclothymia experience manifestations of symptoms for years.

Identification of Bipolar Disorders

As with other psychiatric conditions, there is no definitive test for identifying bipolar disorder. Rather, identification is based on history and manifestations, as well as by ruling out other causes.

Bipolar disorders are not always immediately identified even after manifestations are present. Manifestations may be disguised by alcohol or substance abuse or, if manifestations are mild, as in hypomania, they may be denied or ignored. Individuals who experience psychotic manifestations may be identified as having schizophrenia rather than bipolar disorder. If depressive manifestations are present, individuals may be identified as having major depression rather than bipolar disorder. Accurate identification of bipolar disorders is crucial, because it has important implications for management and prognosis (Bowden, 2005).

Management of Bipolar Disorders

Although bipolar disorder is a lifelong condition, appropriate management can have a significant impact on affected individuals' quality of life and ability to function (Montejano et al., 2005). Acute manifestations are usually managed with medication. Once manifestations are stabilized, maintenance management—which may include both medication and psychosocial interventions—is instituted to improve function and to prevent further occurrence of manic or depressive episodes.

In the past, *lithium* was the main drug used in management of bipolar disorders. While still used today, the potential for overdose and the need to monitor lithium levels in the blood have made other medications more appealing to prescribers (Preston et al., 2013). Many different medications may be used depending on the stage and phase of the condition. While in the manic phase, individuals may receive lithium as well as several other medications such as *anticonvulsant medications,* which have mood-stabilizing effects. Likewise, atypical *antipsychotic medications* may be used for management of acute manic episodes.

Individuals who experience anxiety may also be given *antianxiety medications.* If individuals have a major depressive episode, an *antidepressant* may be prescribed as part of the pharmacologic regimen, in addition to lithium, anticonvulsant, or atypical antipsychotic (Preston et al., 2013). Antidepressants for any major depressive episode needs to include careful monitoring when beginning medication, as a person with an as yet undiagnosed bipolar disorder could have a manic episode in response to antidepressant medication (Howland, 2006b; Montejano et al., 2005; Preston et al., 2013). When medication does not adequately control depressive manifestations, *electroconvulsive therapy (ECT)* may be indicated (Tess & Smetana, 2009).

Although management with medication is essential for controlling manifestations in bipolar disorders, nonadherence to medication regimens is high (Conus et al., 2006; Huxley & Baldessarini, 2007). Consequently, effective management of bipolar disorders includes a combination of medication and psychosocial interventions. Strategies that help individuals manage manifestations include psychosocial education in which individuals and their family members receive general information regarding the condition, learn to manage manifestations, and identify potential triggers of mood change. Other strategies, such as cognitive-behavioral therapy, may be used to help individuals learn to monitor their behavior and thoughts and develop a plan for handling stress and crisis. Interpersonal and group therapies as well as participation in self-help groups are other interventions that are used to help individuals gain insight into their management, establish healthy thinking styles, maintain interpersonal relationships, and explore the effects of the condition on self-esteem (Frank et al., 2005).

FUNCTIONAL IMPLICATIONS OF BIPOLAR DISORDER

Personal and Psychosocial Issues

Individuals with bipolar disorders may be concerned about disclosure regarding their condition, stigma, unpredictability of mood, unstable interpersonal relationships, and potential financial and career loss. Accepting and learning about the condition are major steps toward managing it. Strategies to maintain function and prevent relapses can be developed to help individuals learn to observe small changes in their physical, mental, or emotional status that may represent early warning signs of relapse. In this way, individuals become able to implement interventions that can prevent relapse from occurring.

The response to his or her condition differs for each individual. Identification of specific factors, such as fatigue, seasonal changes, or hormonal changes, that serve as triggers for episodes of mania or depression can help each person institute interventions specific to his or her unique response.

Making changes such as maintaining a healthy diet, exercising, getting adequate sleep, taking medication regularly, avoiding alcohol and drug abuse, and adopting a less hectic lifestyle may help individuals to avoid relapse. Maintaining a range of social support networks, such as family and friends, community groups or organizations, religious affiliations, or support groups, can also help individuals better manage their condition.

Activities and Participation

Social adjustment, interpersonal relationships, leisure activities, and vocational function may all be impaired in individuals with bipolar disorders (Huxley & Baldessarini, 2007). In particular, manic episodes impair social and occupational functioning to a considerable extent. During these episodes, individuals may be easily distracted, and attention may shift rapidly from one activity to another with little provocation. Grandiose delusions, in which they believe that they have special skills, knowledge, or relationships, and poor judgment during the manic phase can lead to catastrophic financial losses or illegal activities. A highly structured, calm environment can help to decrease anxiety or hyperactivity. Psychosocial interventions that focus on interpersonal relationships, stress management, and the importance of stability in daily routines can address the interplay between the individual and his or her environment. Psychoeducational approaches employed with individuals and their families can facilitate a supportive environment as well as provide information that promotes healthy thinking styles, corrects distorted thinking, and encourages maintenance of appropriately paced daily activities and management of the condition.

Vocational Issues in Bipolar Disorder

The rates of unemployment and underemployment for individuals with bipolar disorders far exceed the corresponding rates for the general population, despite the former's relatively high premorbid academic and vocational functioning (Hergenrather, Gitlin, & Rhodes, 2011; Huxley & Baldessarini, 2007). Lack of understanding of bipolar disorder and its manifestations may contribute to these low employment rates, as does the stigma associated with psychiatric conditions. Individual and group psychotherapy can have a positive influence on vocational status by helping individuals gain insight into and a sense of control over management of their condition (Lam, Hayward, Watkins, Wright, & Sham, 2005). Early onset of manifestations and a more severe and longer course of manifestations have both been associated with some cognitive impairments, such as impairments in executive function, attention, and verbal and working memory, which may influence functional ability in individuals with bipolar disorders (Smith, Muir, & Blackwood, 2006). In these instances, cognitive remediation may be helpful in improving functional capacity.

Workplace accommodations may assist individuals with bipolar disorders to continue or obtain employment. The extent of accommodations needed depends on the individual's unique circumstances. Examples of specific workplace accommodations that may be needed include flexible scheduling and minimization of distractions in the immediate work environment.

SCHIZOPHRENIA SPECTRUM AND OTHER PSYCHOTIC DISORDERS

The DSM-5 changed this diagnostic category significantly from the DSM-IV-TR. Gone are the subtypes of schizophrenia (e.g., paranoid, disorganized types). Now, as with the bipolar disorders, schizophrenia and other psychotic disorders are described as occurring along a spectrum of psychotic symptoms, including delusions, hallucinations, disorganized thinking and motor behavior, and negative symptoms, described below.

Schizophrenia spectrum and other psychotic disorders can be complex, chronic, lifelong conditions involving a range of emotional, cognitive, and behavioral manifestations. Diagnoses in this category of the DSM-5 include schizotypal personality disorder, delusional disorder, brief psychotic disorder, schizophreniform disorder, schizophrenia, and schizoaffective disorder (see pages 87–122 of the DSM-5, APA, 2013). We will focus here on the diagnosis of schizophrenia, the reader is referred to the DSM-5 regarding the other disorders in this spectrum.

Schizophrenia

The prevalence of schizophrenia in the general population is lower than the 1% previously thought (APA, 2000), now estimated to range somewhere between 0.3% and 0.7% (APA, 2013). An estimated 70% of affected individuals experience their first manifestations in late adolescence to young adulthood (Lyness, 2016). The individual with schizophrenia may be unaware of manifestations and as a result demonstrate unwillingness to seek help for management of manifestations.

Causes of Schizophrenia

There are is number of theories regarding the cause of schizophrenia including structural abnormalities of the brain, brain chemistry, genetic or environmental factors, endocrine or viral disorders, or exposure to toxins, however no single cause has been found for the development of schizophrenia. Neuroimaging studies have identified some variation in structure of the brain of individuals with schizophrenia (Freedman, 2003) and some chemical changes have also been identified (O'Brien, Kennedy, & Ballard, 2008), however, the role these factors play in development of schizophrenia continue to be speculative. The origin of the condition is likely to be multifactorial, most probably stemming from interactions of a number of variables including genetic and environmental factors (Jarskog, Miyamoto, & Lieberman, 2007). It appears that repeated psychotic episodes left untreated may be associated with the enlargement of vesicles in the brain and reduced brain mass (Preston et al., 2013).

Manifestations of Schizophrenia

Manifestations may develop slowly and insidiously. Individuals may show increasing lack of interest in their surroundings and gradually withdraw from family and friends. Personal appearance and hygiene may deteriorate over time. Previous level of function may gradually diminish, and the person may begin to demonstrate inappropriate behavior or responses. Although often development of manifestations proceeds over time, in many cases manifestations have sudden onset, possibly related to a specific precipitating stress. Characteristic manifestations of schizophrenia can include delusions, hallucinations, disorganized speech or behavior or negative manifestations as discussed below.

Delusions

Individuals with *delusions* may experience beliefs that have no grounding in reality. Prominent delusions involve the false belief that their thoughts, feelings, or actions are being controlled by external forces, that their private thoughts are being transmitted to others (*thought broadcasting*), and that thoughts are being inserted into their mind by others (*thought insertion*). Individuals may assign personal significance to events that are unrelated to them, such as the belief that a radio announcer is delivering a special message to them personally (*ideas of reference*). In addition, individuals may exhibit an exaggerated sense of self, such as holding a belief that they alone are able to save the world from disaster (*delusions of grandeur*). In other instances, they may experience *paranoid delusions*, in which they perceive a threat from others or are convinced of conspiracy against them or others.

Hallucinations

Auditory–verbal hallucinations are a common positive symptom of schizophrenia spectrum, however, hallucinations may involve any of the senses (visual, tactile, olfactory) (Thomas et al., 2016). Individuals with auditory hallucinations may, for example, hear voices that direct them to perform a specific task. Individuals with visual hallucinations may see persons or objects that are not present. Tactile hallucinations may be experienced as, for example, insects crawling over the *body*, or olfactory hallucinations as an odor that is not actually present. A challenge in evaluating auditory or visual hallucinations is ruling out natural occurring phenomena that appear to be such, like hearing one's name called in a noisy room, or seeing shadows that may be normal changes in vision due to age.

Disorganized Thinking (Speech)

Individuals may have *disorganized* thinking typically evidenced by the content of their *speech*, in which there is failure to conform to semantic or syntactic rules governing communication. Ideas and topics are fragmented and unrelated with no logical progression of thought (*derailment* or *loose association*) and answers to questions may be obliquely related or unrelated (*tangential speech*). There may also be *poverty of speech*, in which words spoken convey little meaning (*incoherence* or word salad; APA, 2013).

Disorganized Behavior

Behavior may be unpredictable, or inappropriate for the situation. Individuals may exhibit odd mannerisms or movements or may engage in inappropriate sexual behavior. They may demonstrate childlike behavior, engage in inappropriate laughing, or unpredictable agitation. They may have difficulty performing regular activities of daily living, such as attending to personal hygiene so that they appear disheveled. Dress may be inappropriate—for example, wearing multiple layers of clothing in the middle of summer. An extreme manifestation of behavior disorganization in this category is catatonia, or a marked decrease in reactivity to one's environment. See page 88 of the DSM-5 for specific examples (APA, 2013).

Negative Symptoms

Diminished emotional expression and *avolition* are two negative symptoms particularly prominent in schizophrenia versus any other disorder from this spectrum (APA, 2013). *Diminished emotional expression* refers to diminished emotional response exhibiting little facial expression of emotion, often demonstrating a blank look, and almost mask-like appearance. Emotional expression may be limited regardless of the situation. *Avolition* refers to the inability to initiate and pursue goal related activities. There is little motivation, one may appear withdrawn or aloof, showing little interest in surroundings or activities.

Three other negative symptoms include *alogia*, *anhedonia*, and *asociality*. *Alogia* refers to diminished fluency and use of language so that there is reduced spontaneous speech. *Anhedonia* refers to the inability to experience pleasure. Individuals may lose interest or withdraw from activities that they once found pleasurable. They may report not enjoying anything of life or feeling emotionally empty. Anhedonia can be experienced on a physical level, such as no longer enjoying food or being unable to find pleasure in sexual activity, or in a social context, such as no longer enjoying hobbies they once found pleasurable or being unable to enjoy social activities they once liked. Finally *asociality* refers to a lack of desire or motivation to engage in social interactions. Individuals with asociality may be viewed as a loner or as being aloof.

Identification of Schizophrenia

There are no laboratory tools or tests that definitively identify schizophrenia as the cause of observed manifestations, although some neuroimaging and neuropsychological measures have demonstrated some differences between individuals with schizophrenia and those without the disease (APA, 2013). Schizophrenia is identified through personal history and observations of manifestations, as well as by ruling out other potential causes of observed manifestations. Sensitivity to cultural differences and cultural meanings of behaviors that may be misinterpreted as out of the ordinary by individuals not familiar with the individual's culture should also be taken into consideration before attributing observed behaviors to schizophrenia.

Management of Schizophrenia

Although there is currently no cure for schizophrenia, it is a condition from which individuals can ameliorate symptoms and improve their function (Gillam, 2006). Management is directed toward reducing and managing manifestations, assisting individuals to focus on their strengths, and helping them manage difficulties so that they can function more effectively and appropriately within the community.

Pharmacologic and psychosocial interventions are used together to help individuals achieve optimal benefit. Medications for psychotic manifestations (*antipsychotics*) are usually needed throughout life (Leucht et al., 2012). The type of medication and the dose are individually determined. Individuals taking antipsychotic medications should be carefully monitored to determine the effectiveness of the medication in managing manifestations and to identify any side effects or medication-related problems they may be experiencing.

Although antipsychotic medications help reduce the risk of future psychotic episodes and assist individuals to resume independent function, they are not a guarantee against relapse. Likewise, medications used to manage manifestations of schizophrenia are not without side effects, including discomfort (e.g., restlessness, decreased energy, weight gain, muscle spasms, tremors, dry mouth, difficulty with urination, or constipation). Second generation or *atypical antipsychotics* while having fewer and less intense side effects have been shown to increase the risk of developing conditions such as diabetes and cardiovascular disease (Law, 2007; Lieberman et al., 2005; Preston et al., 2013).

Adherence to medication protocols has been shown to be a major problem for individuals with schizophrenia (Rosenheck et al., 2011). In particular, those individuals who experience side effects, who fear that side effects may occur, or who may deny their need for medication may discontinue taking their medication (Gillam, 2006; Stroup et al., 2006). Abrupt discontinuation of antipsychotic medication can be potentially dangerous as well as have profound implications for long-term outcomes (Hui et al., 2006). Individuals expressing concerns about their medication should be referred to the appropriate health professional for advice and monitoring.

In addition to medication, a variety of psychosocial interventions to improve functioning are often part of the management protocol. Psychosocial interventions are directed toward helping individuals improve their coping resources and support systems, thereby minimizing stress from life events and enhancing coping efforts (Beebe, 2007). Counseling and individual or group therapy can assist individuals to understand and accept their condition as well as build self-esteem. Case management, behavioral interventions, social skills training, family groups, and support groups are other interventions that have been used successfully with schizophrenia patients (Revheim & Marcopulos, 2006).

Functional Implications of Schizophrenia

The acute or active phase of schizophrenia severely interferes with personal and social functioning. During this phase, individuals require supervision and direction to meet basic needs and to prevent self-injury. Depending on their particular circumstances and the degree of available support, many individuals are able to function independently and obtain employment after psychosis has been resolved. The degree of independent function that is possible depends on the success of the medication management of the condition, the extent of the individual's insight into the condition, and the extent to which he or she continues to adhere to the management protocol. Some individuals need continued assistance because of repeated exacerbations of residual manifestations or incapacitation.

Personal and Psychosocial Issues

The severity of manifestations and chronicity of schizophrenia have profound effects both on individuals and their families (Rhoades, 2000). The course and outcome for individuals with schizophrenia vary dramatically (Gillam, 2006). Individuals and families can experience social stigma and isolation, disruption of activities of daily life, interruption of future goals, financial burden, and other stressors that have adverse effects on health and well-being.

Individual and family therapy can assist individuals and their families to develop the resources necessary to cope with this chronic, lifelong condition as well as facilitate communication and enhance problem solving, which in turn increases the chance of a positive outcome. Although medication management remains key in helping individuals with schizophrenia achieve their optimal functional capacity (Lyness, 2016), psychosocial interventions are essential in helping individuals and families achieve acceptance and ultimately successful outcomes.

Activity and Participation

Individuals with schizophrenia tend to have a number of health issues, in addition to the manifestations experienced as a result of their condition, which can affect function. They have a 20% shorter life expectancy relative to the general population. People with schizophrenia have a high risk of obesity, twice the risk of developing diabetes, and twice the risk of dying from cardiovascular disease as compared to the general population (Klam, McLay, & Grabke, 2006). Although such risks are increased to some degree because of medication side effects, some of these excess risks are related to lifestyle, such as unhealthy diet, inactivity, and smoking. Smoking, for example, is twice as frequent in individuals with schizophrenia as in the general population (Klam et al., 2006).

Substance dependence or abuse is also a risk for individuals with schizophrenia and is associated with poorer outcomes (Swofford, Scheller-Gilkey, Miller, Woolwine, & Mance, 2000). Other risks include suicide attempts and homelessness.

Appropriate community support and rehabilitation are important to help individuals achieve their optimal level of functioning. Psychoeducational programs, which help individuals and their families with early recognition of relapse and assist them in learning how to cope with the stresses associated with managing this condition, provide additional empowerment and support.

Vocational Issues in Schizophrenia

Employment has numerous potential benefits for individuals with schizophrenia, including structure, socialization, increased income, and increased self-esteem (Twamley et al., 2005). Because individuals with schizophrenia generally experience their first manifestations in adolescence or young adulthood, when job and career choices and skill building are major developmental tasks, they may have limited work skills. Likewise, they may have difficulty with social skills. There may be a need for education focusing on extensive job training, problem-solving skills, money management skills, use of public transportation, and social skills training. Individuals with schizophrenia may have difficulty coping with stress. Consequently, the amount of physical and emotional stress in the workplace and the individuals' ability to cope with stress should be considered.

SOMATIC SYMPTOM AND RELATED DISORDERS

Somatic symptom and related disorders are a new category within the DSM-5 that all share in common somatic symptoms associated with significant distress and impairment. This new category steers away from the DSM-IV-TR emphasis on physical symptoms for which no organic cause can be found. The new focus is on the manifestations of symptoms that, because of how the person presents and interprets these symptoms, cause significant distress and impairment in social, occupational, and interpersonal functioning (APA, 2013). In the DSM-5 there was an effort to reduce the number of overlapping diagnoses within this category in the DSM-IV-TR, making this diagnostic set easier to use by the full spectrum of allied health professionals. See pages 309–328 of the DSM-5 for complete diagnostic details.

Somatic Symptom Disorder

Somatic symptom disorder is characterized by multiple specific or vague somatic symptoms that cause distress or disrupt social or occupational functioning. Because physical manifestations are often similar to manifestations of a variety of health conditions, individuals may receive healthcare interventions for the manifestations even though no organic cause may be found. Individuals with somatic symptom disorder do not consciously produce their symptoms but truly experience them; their suffering is genuine whether or not there is a medical explanation for their condition. Most of those patients who in the past were diagnosed with the now antiquated *hypochondriasis* from previous versions of the DSM are diagnosed with *somatic symptom disorder*. In the special case of someone preoccupied with acquiring an illness but are as yet undiagnosed or have mild symptoms, they are given a new DSM-5 diagnosis of ***illness anxiety disorder*** (see pages 315–318 of the DSM-5).

Conversion Disorder (Functional Neurological Symptom Disorder)

Conversion disorder manifests as individuals losing voluntary motor or sensory function (e.g., paralysis, blindness, or numbness of a body part), for which there is no clinical correlation with recognized neurological or medical conditions; they do not follow a pattern that would correspond to a specific health condition or injury. The individual does not intentionally produce the manifestations. The diagnosis is generally identified in late childhood or early adulthood. Its onset is often sudden and frequently associated with stress. In many instances, manifestations are of short duration.

Factitious Disorder

Factitious disorder is a condition in which individuals *voluntarily* produce psychological or physical symptoms, feigning illness because of a seemingly compulsive need to assume the sick role in the absence of obvious external reward (APA, 2013). A factitious disorder differs from *malingering* (in which individuals also produce symptoms intentionally) in that the goal of malingering is usually obvious, such as a desire to receive an insurance settlement or to collect disability payments; in contrast, in factitious disorders, there is no external incentive for the behavior. In the DSM-5 factitious disorder is either imposed on self as just described, or imposed on other, previously known as *factitious disorder by proxy*.

DISSOCIATIVE DISORDERS

According to the DSM-5 (APA, 2013, pp. 291–308) dissociative disorders "are characterized by a disruption of and/or discontinuity in the normal integration of consciousness, memory, identity, emotion, perception, bodily representation, motor control, and behavior" (p. 291). *Dissociative identity disorder* (remotely known as multiple personality disorder) is a condition with the presence of two or more distinct personality states or an experience of possession accompanied by recurrent episodes of amnesia. *Dissociative amnesia* is the inability to recall events that occurred within a certain period of time or the inability to recall information regarding one's own identity. *Depersonalization/derealization disorder* is a condition with two main characteristics: depersonalization, or experiences of unreality or detachment from one's mind, self, or body, and/or; derealization, or experiences of unreality or detachment from one's surroundings.

PERSONALITY DISORDERS

The APA in the DSM-5 define the 10 specific personality disorders generally as "an enduring pattern of inner experience and behavior that deviates markedly from the expectations of the individual's culture, is pervasive and inflexible, has an onset in adolescence or early adulthood, is stable over time, and leads to distress or impairment" (2012, p. 645). During the revision process for the DSM-5, there was much press surrounding the update of this diagnostic group, with predictions of the entire taxonomy changing dramatically. What actually happened is the same criteria from the DSM-IV-TR were included in the DSM-5 update, and the much touted new model for personality disorders was included in the Emerging Measures and Models section (Part III) of the DSM-5. Readers are referred to pages 761–782 of the DSM to see the proposed alternative model for personality disorders. Here we will focus on the disorders as presented on pages 645–684 of the DSM-5.

Individuals with personality disorders may have no insight into the role that their own behavior plays in creating problems within their environment. They may rationalize their actions, blaming others for their situation or misfortune without examining their own responsibility for the situation at hand.

Ten types of personality disorders are described within the DSM-5 that cause varying degrees of impairment: Paranoid, schizoid, schizotypal, antisocial, borderline, histrionic, narcissistic, avoidant, dependent, and obsessive–compulsive personality disorder (APA, 2013). When a personality disorder exists in combination with other mental conditions, the prognosis is more guarded, and interventions for and management of the personality disorder are more difficult (Gunderson, 2011; Preston et al., 2013). At times, affected individuals may not have a personality disorder that precisely meets diagnostic criteria, but their maladaptive personality traits may still interfere with the management or identification of co-occurring conditions.

NEUROCOGNITIVE DISORDERS

Formerly titled *Delirium, Dementia, Amnestic and Other Cognitive Disorders* in the DSM-IV-TR, in the DSM-5 this category is called

Neurocogitive Disorders (NCDs). The NCD group of diagnoses have in common cognitive deficits that are acquired and represent a decline in functioning, and are not developmental as in the Neurodevelopmental Disorders category of the DSM-5 (see pages 31–86; APA, 2013). This diagnostic group is divided into major and mild categories depending upon symptom presentation and severity (see table on pages 593–595 for these determinants). Subtypes for NCDs include: Alzheimer's disease, vascular, with Lewy bodies, Parkinson's disease, fronto-temporal, traumatic brain injury, HIV infection, substance/medication-induced, Huntingtons' disease, prion disease, another medical condition or multiple etiologies.

Identification of conditions in this category is usually based on a detailed history of manifestations, findings on physical and neurological evaluation, clinical and laboratory studies, and neuropsychological assessments. These conditions affect a variety of cognitive abilities:

- Memory
- Judgment orientation
- Attention
- Computational and organizational skills

Individuals may also experience associated psychomotor or language impairments, sleep disturbances, and other behavioral manifestations. Although some of these conditions remain stable, others have been linked to progressive deterioration and decline of function.

Conditions classified in this DSM category can be acute or chronic. Manifestations of acute conditions are sudden in onset, such as signs and symptoms caused by generalized infection or intoxication. By comparison, manifestations of chronic conditions generally appear more slowly and are characterized by the deterioration of cognitive processes over time, such as manifestations occurring with arteriosclerosis or Alzheimer's disease.

Delirium and Dementia

Delirium and dementia may be either reversible or irreversible. If the underlying cause of the manifestations can be corrected and the brain has not been permanently damaged, the condition is said to be *reversible*. If the underlying cause cannot be corrected or managed, or if the damage to the brain is permanent, the condition is referred to as *irreversible*.

Both delirium and dementia are characterized by alteration of brain function and are often caused by an identifiable organic factor. Both also share manifestations marked by a decrease in cognitive ability or memory from a prior level of functioning. Both conditions can occur secondary to another health condition, such as heart disease in which circulation and consequently oxygen supply to the brain are diminished. Likewise, they can be caused by other factors, including a systemic health condition (e.g., thyroid disease), injury to the brain itself (e.g., ministrokes), or toxic substances (e.g., poisons, alcohol, or other drugs). Manifestations of delirium and dementia may affect psychological, cognitive, or behavior function.

Delirium

Delirium is characterized by an acute disorder of attention and cognitive function, such as difficulty inattention, disorganized thinking, and altered level of consciousness (Inouye, 2016).

Delirium has multiple causes and usually involves a combination of factors, including individual vulnerability because of a preexisting health condition. It can be the initial manifestation of a more serious underlying condition that has gone unrecognized, such as pneumonia. Examples of predisposing factors that may precipitate delirium follow:

- Infection
- Organ system failure
- Inadequate oxygen supply
- Metabolic condition
- Dehydration
- Side effects of medication
- Drug interactions
- Intoxication
- Drug or alcohol withdrawal
- A combination of causes

Manifestations of delirium characteristically develop over a short period of time and include clouded state of consciousness, confusion, or disorientation. Individuals have difficulty with focusing attention, may be easily distracted, and demonstrate disorganized thought processes. In some instances, they may experience delusions or hallucinations.

Delirium may not be immediately recognized if the individual has another health condition that affects cognitive function. When the individual's baseline of cognitive function or behavior is not familiar, manifestations of delirium may be attributed to the original health condition rather than a secondary cause. Identification of delirium relies on recognizing a sudden change in cognitive function or behavior, plus a physical examination and a thorough medical health history including medication or substance use. In some instances, laboratory testing may be used to identify potential underlying causes of delirium.

The cornerstone of management of delirium is recognizing the manifestations, identifying the cause, and correcting it. Consequently, management depends on the cause of the manifestations. If the cause of delirium can be identified and interventions are employed appropriately, and if no permanent brain damage has resulted, the condition is reversible.

Dementia

Dementia is a global deterioration of multiple intellectual abilities, including memory. In addition to memory impairment, impairments may occur in other higher intellectual functions, such as judgment, the ability to abstract, and personality variables. Many causes of dementia exist, some of which are outlined in **Table 14-1**.

Some types of dementia are reversible, such as dementia resulting from a thyroid condition. In this case, when the thyroid condition is resolved, manifestations of dementia are reversed. Some potentially reversible dementias are listed in **Table 14-2**.

Dementia caused by other conditions is not reversible. Some conditions responsible for *nonreversible dementia* are described next.

Table 14-1   Potential Causes of Dementia

Alzheimer's disease
Anemia
Anoxia
Binswanger's disease
Brain tumor
Chronic alcohol/drug use/abuse
Chronic liver disease
Chronic lung disease
Communicating hydrocephalus
Creutzfeldt-Jakob disease
Depression
HIV infection
Huntington's disease
Infections of the central nervous system
Metabolic disorders
Multicerebral infarcts
Multiple demyelinating lesions
Parkinson's disease
Pick's disease
Subdural hematoma
Syphilis
Systemic lupus erythematosus
Thyroid disorders
Uremia
Vitamin B12 deficiency

Table 14-2   Potential Reversible Causes of Dementia

Thyroid disorder
Anemia
Nutritional deficiencies
Depression

Types of Nonreversible Dementia

Alzheimer's Disease

Alzheimer's disease accounts for 60% to 80% of all conditions that are characterized by dementia (Knopman, 2016). It is a progressive, degenerative type of dementia featuring an insidious onset and gradual deterioration of cognitive function, eventually resulting in death. Although Alzheimer's disease has commonly been thought of as a condition that occurs in older age groups, it may occur as early as middle life.

Initial manifestations of Alzheimer's disease may include forgetting of recent events, misplacing items, and becoming lost in familiar surroundings. Memory lapses progress from periodic to consistent. In the early stages of the disease, individuals may be able to continue to perform routine tasks and function in familiar environments. As the condition progresses, performing necessary tasks becomes more difficult. Personality changes may also be present. In some instances, manifestations of aggression, agitation, delusions, and hallucinations may be apparent (Karlawish, 2006). Behavioral and psychiatric symptoms may increase as the condition progresses (Mayeux, 2010).

Although identifiable structural changes occur in the brain that are characteristic of Alzheimer's disease (Goedert & Spillantini, 2006), there is currently no definitive way to identify this disease as the cause of dementia except by direct examination of the brain at autopsy. Tentative identification of Alzheimer's disease is based on detailed personal and social history, progression of manifestations, mental status examination to rule out delirium and determine specific areas of cognitive incapacitation, drug evaluation, and ruling out of other causes through laboratory tests and physical and neurological examinations.

Progression of Alzheimer's disease and the severity of manifestations at different stages vary from individual to individual. Some studies suggest that physical and mental exercise can slow progression of the condition (Marx, 2005), although there is no definitive evidence to prove this hypothesis. Although several medications that mitigate manifestations are currently on the market, there is no cure for Alzheimer's disease. Management is directed toward helping individuals maintain general health, well-being, and functional capacity for as long as possible, as well as supporting the family members responsible for their care.

Vascular Dementia

Vascular dementia, sometimes called *multi-infarct dementia,* occurs when small strokes cause **infarctions** (death of tissues) in areas of the brain that are responsible for cognitive function. The underlying cause of vascular dementia is arteriosclerosis. Arteriosclerosis can contribute to dementia when vessels supplying blood to the brain become narrowed or occluded, diminishing blood flow and hence delivery of oxygen to the brain. Larger vessels, such as the carotid arteries in the neck, are often affected by this condition. Arteriosclerosis is a chronic condition. Risk factors for vascular dementia include cardiovascular disease, diabetes mellitus, and hypertension (Knopman, 2016).

Areas of damage can be identified through use of CT scan or MRI. Once permanent damage to the brain occurs, functional loss owing to affected areas of the brain is not reversible. Management is directed toward controlling the underlying condition responsible for the small strokes so as to prevent further damage from occurring.

Other Causes of Dementia

Dementia may also be experienced as a result of *HIV infection.* In this type of dementia, destruction of brain tissue results in symptoms of forgetfulness, difficulty with concentration and problem solving, and general slowness. Behavioral manifestations of apathy and social withdrawal may also be evident, as well as motor manifestations such as tremor or difficulty walking.

Dementia due to *brain trauma* from a single injury is not progressive, but damage to the brain and its consequent associated manifestations are permanent. Individuals who are exposed to repeated head trauma may have increased manifestations as additional trauma occurs. The degree and severity of manifestations will depend on the extent and location of injury in the brain. Manifestations may range from severe cognitive, motor, and sensory limitations to mild concentration and memory difficulties.

Creutzfeldt-Jakob disease (CJD) is a form of *prion disease*, and a rare type of dementia. It is caused by an accumulation of prion proteins in the central nervous system. In humans, prion disease is thought to result from dietary exposure to meat from animals that have been infected with the prion disease known as bovine spongiform encephalopathy (BSE) (Bosque, 2016). Manifestations frequently include motor disturbances such as ataxia (stumbling gate) or spasticity. There is no cure for CJD; management of this disease consists of support.

Functional Implications of Dementia

Personal and Psychosocial Issues

Dementia affects all areas of function, regardless of its cause, and impacts both the individual and his or her family. In the early stages of dementia, individuals are generally aware that they are unable to function as they had in the past, and they experience compromised self-image as loss of abilities ensues and dependency increases. Depression and anxiety are common in the early stages of dementia (Mayeux, 2010). However, individuals can still maintain enjoyment and participate in a socially supportive environment throughout the stages of the condition. Acceptance and positive affirmations from others can help provide this supportive and positive environment. Individuals with dementia have the same emotional needs as others to feel they are accepted and belong. Self-esteem can be validated by emphasizing individuals' past roles and incorporating their former lifestyle into their current setting as much as possible.

Although aggression and combativeness that can lead to apathy, withdrawal, and depression can be experienced as dementia progresses, these emotions may often result from individuals' feelings of loss of control and limited ability to feel safe. Feelings of security fostered by a supportive environment can reduce agitation.

Activities and Participation

Individuals with dementia strive for continuation of a purposeful life and a sense of well-being within their ability. Activity modification and breaking activities down into manageable "failure-free" tasks can contribute to this goal. Expectations of individuals should be realistic so they are not placed in situations that are beyond their ability to cope. Family members or other caregivers are key

components in quality of life for the individual. Education and training for caregivers throughout progression of the condition can reduce stress and enhance quality of life for all. Support groups for individuals and their families can provide an opportunity for social interaction and promotion of psychological well-being.

Environmental restructuring may be helpful to facilitate movement within the environment. Simplifying the environment and providing visual cues such as pictures of toilets on doors of bathrooms can be of assistance as dementia progresses.

Vocational Implications of Dementia

Many individuals in the early stages of dementia have functional incapacities that force them to quit their jobs, even though they are not incapacitated enough to need full-time care and would prefer to continue working. Ensuring that individuals have the opportunity to engage in some type of productive work can improve morale by providing a sense of usefulness.

CASE STUDY

Mr. B. is a 56-year-old male with schizophrenia. The condition was first identified when he was 17. Since that time, he has had a number of relapses. For the last 10 years, however, he has been able to manage the manifestations well and has not experienced any recent relapses. Mr. B. has been successfully employed as a certified nursing assistant in a nursing home for the last 5 years, and has recently decided that he would like to go to a community college and work on an associate degree in nursing. Mr. B. has used medications as well as a number of other psychosocial interventions to manage his condition. He has become increasingly concerned, however, about the potential long-term effects of the medications and is considering discontinuing them.

1. Are Mr. B.'s career plans feasible given his health condition? Why or why not?
2. Which specific issues might Mr. B. face in working toward his career goals?
3. Which issues should Mr. B. consider regarding his medication?

REFERENCES

Alcaras, N. M., & Roper, J. M. (2006). Chest pain among combat veterans: A conceptual framework. *Military Medicine, 717*(6), 478–483.

American Psychiatric Association. (2000). *Diagnostic and statistical manual of mental disorders,* (4th ed., text revision). Washington, DC: Author.

American Psychiatric Association. (2013). *Diagnostic and statistical manual of mental disorders, (DSM-5)* (5th ed.). Arlington, VA: Author.

Antai-Otong, D. (2006a). Anxiety disorders. *Nursing, 36*(3), 48–49.

Antai-Otong, D. (2006b). The art of prescribing: Treatment considerations for patients experiencing rapid-cycling bipolar disorder. *Perspectives in Psychiatric Care, 42*(1), 55–58.

Beebe, L. H. (2007). Beyond the prescription pad: Psychosocial treatments for individuals with schizophrenia. *Journal of Psychosocial Nursing, 45*(3), 35–43.

Bishop, M., & Sweet, E. A. (2000). Depression: A primer for rehabilitation counselors. *Journal of Applied Rehabilitation Counseling, 31*(3), 38–45.

Bosque, P. J. (2016). Prion diseases. In L. Goldman & A. I. Schafer (Eds.), *Goldman-Cecil medicine,* (25th ed., pp. 2504–2506). Philadelphia, PA: Elsevier Saunders.

Bowden, C. L. (2005). A different depression: Clinical distinctions between bipolar and unipolar depression. *Journal of Affective Disorders, 84*(2), 117–125.

Center for Behavioral Health Statistics and Quality. (2015). *Behavioral health trends in the United States: Results from the 2014 National Survey on Drug Use and Health* (HHS Publication No. SMA 15-4927, NSDUH Series H-50). Retrieved from http://www.samhsa.gov/data/

Compton, W. M., Thomas, Y. F., Stinson, F. S., & Grant, B. (2007). Prevalence, correlates, disability, and comorbidity of DSM-IV drug abuse and dependence in the United States. *Archives of General Psychiatry, 64*(5), 566–576.

Conus, P., Berk, M., & McGorry, P. D. (2006). Pharmacological treatment in the early phase of bipolar disorders: What stage are we at? *Australian and New Zealand Journal of Psychiatry, 40,* 199–207.

Emdad, R., & Sondergaard, H. P. (2006). General intelligence and short-term memory impairments in post traumatic stress disorder patients. *Journal of Mental Health, 15*(2), 205–216.

Foa, E. B., Franklin, M. E., & Moser, J. (2002). Context in the clinic: How well do cognitive-behavioral therapies and medications work in combination? *Biological Psychiatry, 52,* 987–997.

Foa, E. B., Keane, T. M., & Friedman, M. J. (Eds.). (2000). *Effective treatments for PTSD: Practice guidelines from the International Society for Traumatic Stress Studies.* New York, NY: Guilford Press.

Frank, E., Kupfer, D. J., Thase, M. E., Mallinges, A. G., Swartz, H. A., Fagiolini, A. M., ... Monk, T. (2005). Two year outcomes for interpersonal and social rhythm therapy for individuals with bipolar I disorder. *Archives of General Psychiatry, 62,* 996–1004.

Freedman, R. (2003). Schizophrenia. *New England Journal of Medicine, 349*(18), 1738–1749.

Freedy, J. R., & Simpson, W. M. (2007). Disaster-related physical and mental health: A role for the family physician. *American Family Physician, 75*(6), 841–846.

Freeman, M. P., Freeman, S. A., & McElroy, S. L. (2002). The co-morbidity of bipolar and anxiety disorders: Prevalence, psychobiology, and treatment issues. *Journal of Affective Disorders, 68*(1), 1–23.

Frye, M. A. (2011). Bipolar disorder: A focus on depression. *New England Journal of Medicine, 364*(1), 51–59.

Garakani, A., Mathew, S. J., & Charney, D. S. (2006). Neurobiology of anxiety disorders and implications for treatment. *Mount Sinai Journal of Medicine, 73*(7), 941–949.

Garske, G. G. (2011). Military related PTSD: A focus on the symptomatology and treatment approaches. *Journal of Rehabilitation, 77*(4), 31–36.

Gillam, T. (2006). Positive approaches to schizophrenia. *Mental Health Practice, 10*(4), 30–33.

Gillock, K. L., Zayfert, C., Hegel, M. T., & Ferguson, R. J. (2005). Posttraumatic stress disorder in primary care: Prevalence and relationships with physical symptoms and medical utilization. *General Hospital Psychiatry, 27,* 392–399.

Goedert, M., & Spillantini, M. G. (2006). A century of Alzheimer's disease. *Science, 314*(3), 777–784.

Gross, R., Olfson, M., Gameroff, J. J., Shea, S., Feder, A., Lantingua, R., ... Weissman, M. M. (2005). Social anxiety disorder in primary care. *General Hospital Psychiatry, 27,* 161–168.

Gunderson, J. G. (2011). Borderline personality disorder. *New England Journal of Medicine, 364*(21), 2037–2042.

Hergenrather, K. C., Gitlin, D. J., & Rhodes, S. D. (2011). Consumers with bipolar disorder: A theory based approach to explore beliefs impacting job placement. *Journal of Rehabilitation, 77*(3), 14–24.

Hough, C. J., & Ursano, R. J. (2006). A guide to the genetics of psychiatric disease. *Psychiatry, 69*(1), 1–20.

Howland, R. H. (2006a). Challenges in the diagnosis and treatment of bipolar depression—Part 1: Assessment. *Journal of Psychosocial Nursing, 44*(4), 9–12.

Howland, R. H. (2006b). Challenges in the diagnosis and treatment of bipolar depression—Part 2: Treatment options. *Journal of Psychosocial Nursing, 44*(5), 9–12.

Hui, C. L. M., Chen, E. Y. H., Kan, C. S., Yip, K. C., Law, C. W., & Chiu, C. P. Y. (2006). Detection of non-adherent behavior in early psychosis. *Australian and New Zealand Journal of Psychiatry, 40,* 446–451.

Huxley, N., & Baldessarini, R. J. (2007). Disability and its treatment in bipolar disorder patients. *Bipolar Disorders, 9,* 183–196.

Inouye, S. K. (2016). Delirium or acute mental status change in the older patient. In L. Goldman & A. I. Schafer (Eds.), *Goldman-Cecil medicine,* (25th ed. pp. 117–121). Philadelphia, PA: Elsevier Saunders.

Ipser, J., Seedat, S., & Stein, D. J. (2006). Pharmacotherapy for post-traumatic stress disorder: A systematic review and meta-analysis. *South African Medical Journal, 96*(10), 1088–1096.

Issakidis, C., Sanderson, K., Corry, J., Andrews, G., & Lapsley, H. (2004). Modeling the population cost-effectiveness of current and evidence-based optimal treatment for anxiety disorders. *Psychological Medicine, 34,* 19–35.

Jarskog, L. F., Miyamoto, S., & Lieberman, J. A. (2007). Schizophrenia: New pathological insights and therapies. *Annual Review of Medicine, 58,* 59–71.

Jenike, M. A. (2004). Obsessive–compulsive disorder. *New England Journal of Medicine, 350*(3), 259–265.

Karlawish, J. (2006). Alzheimer's disease: Clinical trials and the logic of clinical purpose. *New England Journal of Medicine, 355*(15), 1604–1606.

Keller, M. B., McCullough, J. P., Klein, D. N., Arnow, B., Dunner, D. L., Gelenberg, A. J., ... Zajecka, J. (2000). A comparison of nefazodone, the cognitive behavioral analysis system of psychotherapy, and their combination for the treatment of chronic depression. *New England Journal of Medicine, 342*(20), 1462–1470.

Kennedy, N., Boydell, J., Kalidindi, S., Fearson, P., Jones, P. B., Van Os, J., ... Murray, R. M. (2005). Gender differences in incidence and age at onset of mania and bipolar disorder over a 35-year period in Camberwell, England. *American Journal of Psychiatry, 162*(2), 257–262.

Kessler, R. C., Berglund, P., Demler, O., Jin, R., Merikangas, K. R., & Walter, E. E. (2005). Lifetime prevalence and age-of-onset distributions of DSM-IV disorders in the National Co-morbidity Survey Replication. *Archives of General Psychiatry, 62*(6), 593–602.

Kessler, R. C., Chiu, W. T., Demler, O., Merikangas, K. R., & Walters, E. E. (2005). Prevalence, severity, and comorbidity of 12-month DSM-IV disorders in the National Comorbidity Survey Replication. *Archives of General Psychiatry, 62*(6), 617–627.

Klam, J., McLay, M., & Grabke, D. (2006). Personal empowerment program: Addressing health concerns in people with schizophrenia. *Journal of Psychosocial Nursing, 44*(8), 20–28.

Knopman, D. S. (2016). Alzheimer's disease and other dementias. In L. Goldman & A. I. Schafer (Eds.), *Goldman-Cecil medicine* (25th ed., pp. 2388–2398). Philadelphia, PA: Elsevier Saunders.

Krishnakumar, P., & Geeta, M. G. (2006). Clinical profile of depressive disorder in children. *Indian Pediatrics, 43,* 521–526.

Kroenke, K., Spitzer, R. L., Williams, J. B. W., Monahan, P. O., & Lowe, B. (2007). Anxiety disorders in primary care: Prevalence, impairment, co-morbidity, and detection. *Annals of Internal Medicine, 146*(5), 317–325.

Lam, D. H., Hayward, P., Watkins, E. R., Wright, K., & Sham, P. (2005). Relapse prevention in patients with bipolar disorder: Cognitive therapy outcome after 2 years. *American Journal of Psychiatry, 162,* 324–329.

Law, D. (2007). Physical health: How to minimize the risks faced by patients with schizophrenia. *Mental Health Practice, 10*(6), 26–28.

Lerner, D., Adler, D. A., Cang, H., Lapitsky, L., Hood, M. K., Perissinotto, C., ... Rogers, W. H. (2004). Unemployment, job retention, and productivity loss among employees with depression. *Psychiatric Services, 55*(12), 1371–1378.

Leucht, S., Tardy, M., Komossa, K., Heres, S., Kissling, W., Salanti, G., & Davis, J. M. (2012). Antipsychotic drugs vs placebo for relapse prevention in schizophrenia: A systematic review and meta analysis. *Lancet, 379*(9831), 2063–2071.

Lieberman, J. A., Stroup, T. S., McEvoy, J. P., Swartz, M. S., Rosenheck, R. A., Perkins, D. O., ... Clinical Antipsychotic Trials of Intervention Effectiveness (CATIE) Investigators. (2005). Effectiveness of antipsychotic drugs in patients with chronic schizophrenia. *New England Journal of Medicine, 353*(12), 1209–1223.

Lincoln, A. E., Helmer, D. A., Schneiderman, A. I., Li, M., Copeland, H. L., Prisco, M. K., ... Natelson, B. H. (2006). The war-related illness and injury study centers: A resource for deployment-related health concerns. *Military Medicine, 171*(7), 577–585.

Lyness, J. M. (2016). Psychiatric disorders in medical practice. In L. Goldman & A. I. Schafer (Eds.), *Goldman-Cecil medicine,* (25th ed., pp. 2346–2356). Philadelphia, PA; Elsevier Saunders.

Magruder, K. M., Frueh, B. C., Knapp, R. G., Davis, L., Hamner, M. B., Martin, R. H., ... Arana, G. W. (2005). Prevalence of posttraumatic stress disorder in Veterans Affairs primary care clinics. *General Hospital Psychiatry, 27*(3), 169–179.

Mahoney, D. M. (2000). Panic disorder and self states: Clinical and research illustrations. *Clinical Social Work Journal, 28*(2), 197–212.

Maj, M., Sartorius, N., Okasha, A., & Zohar, J. (Eds.). (2002). *Obsessive–compulsive disorder,* (2nd ed.). Chichester, UK: John Wiley.

Marx, J. (2005). Preventing Alzheimer's: A lifelong commitment? *Science, 309*(5), 864–866.

Mayeux, R. (2010). Early Alzheimer's disease. *New England Journal of Medicine, 362*(23), 2194–2201.

McColm, R., Brown, J., & Anderson, J. (2006). Nursing interventions for the management of patients with mania. *Nursing Standard, 20*(17), 46–49.

Meyer, J. S., & Quenzer, L. F. (2005). *Psychopharmacology: Drugs, the brain and behaviour.* Sunderland, MA: Sinauer Associates.

Mitchell, P. B., & Malhi, G. S. (2004). Bipolar depression: Phenomenological overview and clinical characteristics. *Bipolar Disorders, 6,* 530–539.

Montejano, L. B., Goetzel, R. Z., & Ozminkowski, R. J. (2005). Impact of bipolar disorder on employers: Rationale for workplace interventions. *Disability Management Health Outcomes, 13*(4), 267–280.

Murphy, K. (2006). Managing the ups and downs of bipolar disorders. *Nursing, 36*(10), 58–63.

Perlis, R. H., Miyahara, S., & Marangell, L. B. (2004). Long-term implications of early onset in bipolar disorder: Data from the first 1000 participants in the Systematic Treatment Enhancement Program for Bipolar Disorder (STEP-BD). *Biological Psychiatry, 55*(9), 875–881.

Post, R. M. (2005). The impact of bipolar depression. *Journal of Clinical Psychiatry, 66*(Suppl 5), 5–10.

Preston, J., O'Neal, J. H., & Talaga, M. (2013). *Handbook of clinical psychopharmacology for therapists* (7th ed.). Oakland, CA: New Harbinger Publications.

Revheim, N., & Marcopulos, B. A. (2006). Group treatment approaches to address cognitive deficits. *Psychiatric Rehabilitation Journal, 30*(1), 38–45.

Rhoades, D. R. (2000). Schizophrenia: A review for family counselors. *Family Journal, 8*(3), 258–266.

Rosenheck, R. A., Krystal, J. H., Lew, R., Barnett, P. G., Fiore, L., Valley, D., ... CSP555 Research Group. (2011). Long-acting risperidone and oral antipsychotics in unstable schizophrenia. *New England Journal of Medicine, 364*(9), 842–851.

Russell, S. J., & Browne, J. L. (2005). Staying well with bipolar disorder. *Australian and New Zealand Journal of Psychiatry, 39,* 187–193.

Rytsala, H. J., Melartin, T. K., Leskela, U. S., Sokero, T. P., Lestela-Mielonen, P. S., & Isometsa, E. T. (2005). Functional and work disability in major depressive disorder. *Journal of Nervous and Mental Disease, 193,* 189–195.

Rytsala, H. J., Melartin, T. K., Leskela, U. S., Sokero, T. P., Lestela-Mielonen, P. S., & Isometsa, E. T. (2007). Predictors of long-term work disability in major depressive disorder: A prospective study. *Acta Psychiatrica Scandinavia, 11,* 206–213.

Salloum, I. M., & Thase, M. E. (2000). Impact of substance abuse on the course and treatment of bipolar disorder. *Bipolar Disorders, 2*(3 Pt 2), 269–280.

Sheehan, D. V., & Sheehan, K. H. (2007). Current approaches to the pharmacologic treatment of anxiety disorders. *Psychopharmacology Bulletin, 40*(1), 98–109.

Smith, D. J., Muir, W. J., & Blackwood, D. H. R. (2006). Neurocognitive impairment in euthymic young adults with bipolar spectrum disorder and recurrent major depressive disorder. *Bipolar Disorders, 8,* 40–46.

Spearing, M. (2002, September). *Bipolar disorder* (NIH Publication No. 02–3679). Bethesda, MD: National Institutes of Health, National Institute of Mental Health.

Stapleton, J. A., Asmundson, G. J. G., Woods, M., Taylor, S., & Stein, M. B. (2006). Health care utilization by United Nations peacekeeping veterans with co-occurring, self-reported, post-traumatic stress disorder and depression symptoms versus those without. *Military Medicine, 171*(1), 562–566.

Stevenson, B. (2005). Post-traumatic stress disorder. *Alberta RN, 61*(10), 10–12.

Strakowski, S. M., & DelBello, M. P. (2000). The co-occurrence of bipolar and substance use disorders. *Clinical Psychology Review, 20*(2), 191–206.

Strauser, D. R., Lustig, D. C., & Uruk, A. C. (2006). Examining the moderating effect of disability status on the relationship between trauma symptomatology and select career variables. *Rehabilitation Counseling Bulletin, 49*(2), 90–101.

Stroup, T. S., Lieberman, J. A., McEvoy, J. P., Swartz, M. S., Davis, S. M., Rosenheck, R. A., ... CATIE Investigators. (2006). Effectiveness of olanzapine, quetiapine, risperidone, and ziprasidone in patients with chronic schizophrenia following discontinuation of a previous atypical antipsychotic. *American Journal of Psychiatry, 163,* 611–622.

Swofford, C. D., Scheller-Gilkey, G., Miller, A. H., Woolwine, B., & Mance, R. (2000). Double jeopardy: Schizophrenia and substance use. *American Journal of Drug and Alcohol Abuse, 26*(13), 343–358.

Tess, A. V., & Smetana, G. W. (2009). Medical evaluation of patients undergoing electroconvulsive therapy. *New England Journal of Medicine, 360*(14), 1437–1444.

Thomas, R. J., Chaze, C., Lewin, D., Calhoun, V. D., Clark, V. P., Bustillo, J., ... Turner, J. A. (2016). Functional MRI evaluation of neural networks underlying auditory verbal hallucinations in schizophrenia spectrum disorders. *Frontiers in Psychiatry, 7*(39). Retrieved March 29, 2016, from doi:10.3389/fpsyt.2016.00039

Twamley, E. W., Padin, D. S., Bayne, K. S., Narvaez, J. M., Williams, R. E., & Jeste, D. V. (2005). Work rehabilitation for middle-aged and older people with schizophrenia: A comparison of three approaches. *Journal of Nervous and Mental Disease, 193*(9), 596–601.

Ursano, R. J. (2002). Post-traumatic stress disorder. *New England Journal of Medicine, 346*(2), 130–132.

Whooley, M. A., & Simon, G. E. (2000). Managing depression in medical outpatients. *New England Journal of Medicine, 343*(26), 1942–1950.

Word Health Organization. (2014). *International Classification of Diseases, Clinical Modification (ICD-10-CM)* (10th Revision). Geneva, Switzerland: Author.

Zohar, J., Fostick, L., Black, D. W., & Lopez-Ibor, J. J. (2007). Special populations. *CNS Spectrums, 12*(2 Suppl 3), 36–42.

CHAPTER 15

Substance-Related and Addictive Disorders

Revised by David B. Peterson

HISTORY OF SUBSTANCE USE

Substance use for medicinal, social, psychological, and religious purposes has been part of most cultures and civilizations since the beginning of recorded time. Many major population groups have developed their own knowledge of substances that alter states of consciousness (Weatherall, 2001) and have condoned the use of a wide array of substances, including plants and plant derivatives, alcohol, nicotine, caffeine, inhalants, and tonics, for therapeutic, ritualistic, religious, or recreational purposes (Fabricant & Farnsworth, 2001).

Examples of substance use throughout the ages abound. In ancient civilizations, alcohol—and wine in particular—was considered a gift from the gods. Opium, which has been cultivated for more than 6,000 years, was used both for medicinal purposes, such as pain relief, and for psychological effects, such as sedation and euphoria. Marijuana use has been reported as early as 2000 B.C. for a variety of health problems as well as for its hallucinogenic properties. In some cultures, marijuana use was believed to assist religious men to have visions of the gods and reveal future events. Psychedelic plants were also used in ancient religious ceremonies.

In the Middle Ages, various psychoactive substances were used widely by medieval witches and medicine men as a poison for adversaries, as an analgesic for pain, and as a hallucinogen to generate prophesies (Fabricant & Farnsworth, 2001). Stimulants were often used in the Middle Ages,

when resources were scarce, to combat fatigue and hunger in soldiers (Inaba & Cohen, 1993).

Tobacco, which was largely unknown in Europe, was introduced by Columbus in 1492 after he noted Native Americans smoking. The practice of smoking the dried leaves of the tobacco plant, *Nicotiana*, was brought to England by Sir Walter Raleigh in the 16th century primarily for medicinal use; however, its use as a social drug quickly spread (Weatherall, 2001).

During the 1800s, inhaled nitrous oxide, also called *laughing gas*, was discovered and used for medicinal purposes as well as for recreation. It was frequently used both as anesthetic and as an intoxicant (Fairley, 1978). The hypodermic needle was developed in the 1860s, but its use was later expanded from healthcare purposes to injecting heroin after it was produced commercially in the late 1800s. The availability of heroin created an ever-growing population of individuals who used the drug compulsively and became addicted to it (Inaba & Cohen, 1993). The 20th century saw the introduction of a number of patented medications that could be purchased over the counter and that were used for medicinal purposes as well as becoming sources of abuse (Abbott & Fraser, 1998).

As use and abuse of various substances became viewed as problematic, regulation or prohibition of a number of substances was attempted in an effort to control or prevent their use. When society becomes ambivalent toward use of a substance, when it determines such use to be inappropriate, or when substance use becomes uncontrolled, hazardous, or disruptive to individuals or to others, then substance use is considered to be problematic and in some instances is made illegal.

PREVALENCE OF SUBSTANCE USE

According to the Center for Behavioral Health Statistics and Quality (2015), in 2014 27 million people aged 12 or older used an illicit drug in the past 30 days, which corresponds to about 1 in 10 Americans (10.2%, an increase from 2004, see below). Estimates suggest such use is primarily marijuana (22.2 million), an increase over previous years, and the nonmedical use of prescription pain relievers (4.3 million people). While the use of many types of illicit drugs has not increased in recent years, the percentage of people aged 12 or older in 2014 who were current heroin users was higher than the percentages in most years from 2002 to 2013 (CBHSQ, 2015).

In 2004, approximately 22.5 million people in the United States (9.4% of the population) were classified as either engaging in substance abuse or experiencing substance dependence. Some 3.4 million members of this group were classified as being dependent on or abusing both alcohol and illicit drugs (Substance Abuse and Mental Health Services Administration, 2005).

In many current cultures, the use of a number of substances is condoned, and use of these socially sanctioned substances may have no harmful effects when they are used appropriately and in moderation. Misuse or overuse of substances or use of illegal substances, however, can have severe physical, psychological, or social consequences (Feinstein, Richter, & Foster, 2012).

SUBSTANCE-RELATED AND ADDICTIVE DISORDERS

Collectively, the use of substances so that they become problematic was formerly referred to in DSM-IV-TR as *substance-related disorders; now in the DSM-5 this diagnostic group is called substance-related and addictive disorders* (American Psychiatric Association [APA], 2000; 2013).

Ten classes of drugs are associated with this diagnostic group: Alcohol, caffeine, cannabis, hallucinogens, inhalants, opioids, sedatives/hypnotics/anxiolytics, stimulants, tobacco, and other or unknown substances (APA, 2013, p. 481). One new category was added to this group of diagnoses in the DSM-5, gambling disorder, included due to research suggesting that gambling behaviors affect reward systems similar to those activated by drugs use (APA, 2013).

The remaining substance-related and addictive disorders in the DSM-5 are divided into two broad groups: substance use disorders and substance-induced disorders. The essence of all substance use disorders is the use of drugs despite significant substance-related problems. The use of the terms *addiction* and *dependence* have been left out of the specific diagnoses in this iteration of the DSM due to the continuum of presentations across substances and the lack of diagnostic precision for these terms, as well as the stigma associated with these terms (APA, 2013, p. 485). Substance-induced disorders involve intoxication, withdrawal, and substance-induced mental disorders (e.g., psychotic, bipolar, depressive, anxiety, OCD, sleep, and neurocognitive disorders; APA, 2013).

Etiology

Advancements in research indicate that drugs used to excess are associated with direct activation of a common area of the brain, the limbic system associated with the brain's reward system. The National Institute on Drug Abuse (2014) of the National institute on Health explains that this pleasure center encourages us to repeat behaviors that are important for life. Drugs also can activate this important system and affect the regulation of emotional perception, in part explaining the mood-altering property of drugs.

Most drugs of abuse affect the brain's reward system by flooding it with dopamine, a neurotransmitter that regulates movement, emotion, motivation, and feelings of pleasure. Excessive dopamine levels produce euphoric effects that reinforce ongoing use of a drug. Unfortunately these effects can linger long after the actual effects of the drug wear off (detoxification), due to underlying changes in brain circuitry that persist due to ongoing exposure to the effects of a drug, which may result in intense drug cravings and repeated relapses (APA, 2013).

Beyond the very powerful physical effects of substances on brain functioning, *substance-related disorders* reflect a complex interaction of biological, psychological, social, cultural, and environmental factors. People with lower levels of self-control may be more vulnerable to developing a substance-related diagnosis or addiction (APA, 2013). Substance-related disorders may involve substances that are *licit, illicit, prescribed*, or *not prescribed*. The etiology and management of substance-related disorders entail a complex interface of numerous factors; no one factor alone explains the development of substance-related and addictive disorders.

Just as all chronic and incapacitating health conditions affect physical, social, psychological, and vocational aspects of individuals' lives, so too do conditions related to substance use. Like other chronic, relapsing conditions, substance-related conditions produce a variety of impairments. Implications of these conditions must be evaluated in the context of the individual's specific situation. Conditions related to substance use can occur alone or in combination with one or more other physical or psychiatric conditions. The effects of substance use combined with manifestation of another health condition can cause additional physical, psychological, and social complications, exacerbating the incapacitating effects of both.

SUBSTANCE USE DISORDER

The DSM-5 diagnostic criteria for substance use disorder across the ten listed substances are complex, and the reader is referred to pages 483–485 for details. Pages 585–589 deal with gambling disorder specifically. Substance use disorder as a diagnosis applies to all of the substances listed except for caffeine.

The pathological patterns of behavior associated with substance use disorders criteria addressed in the DSM-5 include impaired control, social impairment, risky use, and pharmacological criteria (drug tolerance and withdrawal) for each substance (p. 483). The level of severity assigned from mild to severe depends on the number of symptoms

present. Course specifiers in the DSM-5 are more straightforward than they were in the DSM-IV-TR, they include in early remission, in sustained remission, on maintenance therapy, and in a controlled environment; the definitions of each are included within each of the criteria sets (APA, 2013). These consequences of substance use may include any of the following:

- Disruption of work or school, such as repeated absences or declining performance
- Neglect of family obligations
- Repeated hazardous behavior, such as driving a motor vehicle or operating machinery while under the influence of the substance
- Recurrent disorderly conduct or problems with interpersonal relationships owing to substance use
- Recurrent legal problems related to use of the substance
- Continued use of the substance despite the negative consequences related to that use

SUBSTANCE-INDUCED DISORDERS

Substance-induced disorders category of the DSM-5 includes *intoxication, withdrawal,* and *other substance/medication-induced mental disorders.*

Intoxication

Intoxication is a term that describes reversible behavioral or psychological changes related to the effect of a substance on the nervous system (APA, 2013). The level of intoxication from a substance is determined by the concentration of the substance in the blood. The concentration, in turn, is determined by the amount of the substance taken into the body as well as the rate at which the substance is absorbed into the bloodstream. The rate at which a substance is absorbed into the bloodstream depends on the route of administration. For instance, substances that are injected directly into a vein (*intravenous [IV] injection*) have an immediate effect, whereas substances that are ingested orally take longer to be absorbed into the bloodstream and, consequently, exert their effects more slowly. The rate of absorption of substances taken orally is also affected by the presence or absence of food in the stomach and the rate of gastric emptying. Body size also affects concentration of substances in the blood. For instance, blood alcohol levels are proportionately lower in large individuals than in small individuals, even though both might consume equal amounts of alcohol under similar conditions. In addition, gender affects risk for specific health problems related to levels of alcohol consumption. Women, with generally lower body weights and lower rates of metabolism of alcohol than men may be at higher risk for developing specific health problems with higher alcohol consumption (O'Connor, 2016).

Withdrawal

Consumption of large amounts of alcohol or other substances at frequent intervals for prolonged periods creates a state of physical dependence such that cessation or reduction in the amount consumed produces distressful and incapacitating physical manifestations known as *substance withdrawal*. Physical manifestations experienced during withdrawal vary in severity, and do not apply to all of the substances listed in the DSM-5 (e.g., hallucinogens).

There are substantial differences in complications as well as management of withdrawal from specific substances. Individuals with mild to moderate withdrawal manifestations who have no preexisting conditions and who have adequate social support may have withdrawal managed at a community-based facility. In contrast, individuals who develop more serious withdrawal manifestations or those who have coexisting psychiatric or physical conditions usually require residential management or hospitalization to manage symptoms of withdrawal and detoxification (Kosten & O'Connor, 2003).

ADDICTION

As noted earlier, the concepts of *addiction* and *dependence* are not employed in the DSM-5 due to varied presentations across substances, the lack of diagnostic precision associated with these concepts, and the historical stigma associated with their use. However, when someone develops a dependence upon a substance it refers to substance use that results in physical or psychological distress related to substance tolerance, withdrawal, or a pattern of compulsive behaviors related to substance use. The DSM-5 diagnostic criteria address conditions from mild to the most severe that would include dependence or addiction, but the entire spectrum is included under the diagnosis substance use disorder.

Developing dependence on a substance may also be marked by compulsive substance use or substance-seeking behavior, in which individuals become so preoccupied with the substance that much of their daily activity revolves around using and obtaining it. Despite the negative consequences of substance use that individuals with substance dependence may have experienced, such as loss of a job or family, they may persist in using the substance.

Addiction as written about in the associated literature emphasizes the *behavioral component* of a substance-related condition rather than physical dependence (Maddux & Desmond, 2000). Addiction comprises a chronic, neurobiological condition that is influenced by psychosocial, genetic, and environmental factors and that is characterized by compulsive substance-seeking behaviors, impaired control over drug use, and continued use of the substance despite negative consequences (Adinoff, 2004; Ruiz, Strain, & Langrod, 2007). The physical and psychological craving for the substance becomes so all-consuming that individuals expend tremendous effort, energy, and financial resources to obtain it, often at the expense of the safety and well-being of themselves and others.

In addiction, substance use evolves into more than merely "wanting" or "liking" the substance. According to Robinson and Berridge, the nervous systems of individuals who are addicted become hypersensitized, which causes pathological craving for the substance, independent of physical signs of withdrawal (Robinson & Berridge, 2001). Compulsive substance-seeking and substance-taking behavior is facilitated by difficulties in decision making and the ability to judge consequences of drug-seeking and drug-taking actions (Robinson & Berridge, 2003).

Predisposition to Addiction

Although only a small number of individuals who use substances become addicted, several factors appear to predispose certain individuals to addiction (Nestler & Hyman, 2016). For instance, a growing body of evidence indicates a *genetic predisposition* in some individuals for development of alcohol-related conditions as well as dependence on other substances such as nicotine, cocaine, and opioids (Ruiz et al., 2007). *Personality traits* such as risk-taking or novelty-seeking traits have also been found to be more prevalent in individuals who abuse or become dependent on drugs (Helmus, Downey, Arfken, Henderson, & Schuster, 2001). Individuals with *psychiatric conditions*—especially schizophrenia, bipolar disorder, and depression—have an increased risk of substance abuse (Leikin, 2007). Individuals with a *dual diagnosis* (experiencing both a psychiatric condition and a substance use disorder) have also been shown to have a more unfavorable prognosis in terms of management and outcome (Kavanagh, McGrath, Saunders, Dore, & Clark, 2002).

Tolerance

When individuals continue to use a substance over time, they may begin to experience diminished effects with the use of the same amount of the substance. Consequently, the amount of the substance taken to achieve the same effects must be increased. This phenomenon is called *tolerance*. The degree of tolerance experienced varies from individual to individual and with the specific substance being used.

Individuals using substances chronically may adapt their behavior so that they are able to continue functioning at work, at home, or in social situations, even though they are under the influence of a substance. Although tolerance is not always an indication of dependence, it is commonly observed in individuals with substance-related conditions. Furthermore, individuals who develop a tolerance for one substance may also develop higher tolerance for related substances, a condition known as *cross-tolerance*.

Detoxification

Detoxification may be a first step in management of severe substance use disorders. The goal of detoxification is to initiate abstinence, reduce manifestations of withdrawal, prevent complications, and retain individuals' participation in recovery interventions (Kosten & O'Connor, 2003). During the detoxification process and when undergoing withdrawal, individuals may experience *nausea and vomiting, tachycardia, hypertension fever*, and *diaphoresis* (profuse sweating). In more severe withdrawal, individuals may experience *disorientation, hallucinations, delirium tremens,* and, in some instances, *seizures*. Withdrawal from some substances, such as alcohol and other sedatives, can be fatal if not managed medically.

Risk factors for more severe withdrawal are older age (40 years or older), high tolerance, other health problems (such as diabetes or cardiovascular disease), and poor nutrition. Individuals who are in lower-risk groups may undergo detoxification at community health settings; by contrast, individuals at higher risk usually require hospitalization.

During the detoxification process, healthcare management may consist of providing adequate hydration, restoring electrolyte balance, providing thiamine and other vitamins, administering sedatives, and monitoring for possible complications. After detoxification, management may include administration of medications that act as substitutes for the abused substances. The goal in providing these medications is to gradually reduce their dosage, thereby eventually eliminating dependency.

SUBSTANCE USE AND CHRONIC HEALTH CONDITIONS

Individuals with a primary chronic health conditions can also have a secondary condition related to substance use. In some instances, substance use may have been a factor in the acquisition of a chronic health condition—for example, traumatic brain injury sustained in a motor vehicle accident while driving under the influence or HIV infection acquired by sharing contaminated needles. Substance use may also be a maladaptive coping mechanism for an individual who is trying to adjust to a chronic health condition. In other instances, individuals may become dependent on substances that were originally used to manage other conditions, such as pain or anxiety. Whether substance use was a precursor of an acquired health condition or a mechanism for coping with a health condition, having two health conditions makes management of both conditions more complex.

A number of factors may place individuals with a chronic health condition at higher risk for substance-related conditions:

- Health factors such as easy access to medication used to alleviate manifestations, such as chronic pain, making it easier to use the medication excessively; or unnecessary or unwarranted use of medication for manifestations that could have been managed by alternative means
- Psychological factors such as depression, boredom, and frustration, in which substances are used as a means of escape from reality
- Social factors such as oppression or alienation, in which substances are used recreationally in an attempt to gain acceptance and normalization (Greer, Roberts, & Jenkins, 1990; Watson, Franklin, Ingram, & Eilenberg, 1998).

The coexistence of a substance-related and addictive disorder with other chronic health conditions can exacerbate and accentuate manifestations of the health condition as well as increase individuals' vulnerability to complications, leading to acquisition of additional health problems. Although substance use can coexist with any health condition, comorbidity between substance use and psychiatric conditions (dual diagnosis) is very common (Allen Doyle-Pita, 2001; Volkow, 2001). Whether a substance-induced condition is the primary or secondary health condition, appropriate intervention and management of substance use are necessary if individuals are to reach their full rehabilitation potential.

PHYSICAL EFFECTS OF ALCOHOL USE

Alcohol is the most widely used and abused substance in the United States (O'Brien, 2013). A wide range of physical and psychiatric complications are associated with alcohol dependence (O'Connor, 2016; Ruiz et al., 2007). Physical complications resulting from alcohol use result both from the direct effects of alcohol on body tissues and from the body's adaptive responses to excessive exposure to alcohol. The effect of alcohol on the body, like the effect of any drug, depends on the interaction

between properties of the specific pharmacologic agent and characteristics of a specific individual. For example, evidence suggests that women tend to be more sensitive to the effects of alcohol and more susceptible to adverse effects of excessive alcohol consumption than are men (Blume, Counts, & Turnbull, 1992; Harley, 1995; Kandall, 1996; Scott-Lennox, Rose, Bohlig, & Lennox, 2000; Urbano-Marquez et al., 1995). Likewise, older adults may be at greater health risk with alcohol consumption due to changes in alcohol metabolism in older individuals (O'Connor, 2016).

The intoxicating effects of alcohol correlate roughly with the alcohol concentration in the blood. Alcohol is quickly absorbed into the bloodstream from the stomach and intestines and rapidly metabolized, making it a fast-acting drug. Because it diffuses quickly into the water contained in all body tissues, blood concentration of alcohol is an accurate reflection of the concentration of alcohol in other body tissues.

Some alcohol is eliminated through the kidneys and lungs, but the liver metabolizes most of this substance. Although a moderate dose of alcohol is normally cleared from the blood in approximately 1 hour, only a fixed amount of alcohol can be metabolized at a time. When the rate of alcohol consumption exceeds the body's ability to metabolize it, alcohol accumulates in the bloodstream, elevating the blood alcohol concentration.

Physical Effects of Alcohol on the Nervous System

The brain is the primary target of alcohol's pharmacologic effect (O'Connor, 2016). The alcohol concentration in the blood reflects the alcohol concentration in the brain. At low levels of intoxication (0.05%), alcohol may produce a sense of relaxation and well-being, feelings of euphoria, and possibly mild muscle incoordination and mild cognitive impairment. As the concentration of alcohol increases (0.11% to 0.20%), neurological signs such as slurred speech, **ataxia** (more severe muscle incoordination), impaired mental impairment, and prolonged reaction time may become apparent. Continued elevation of blood alcohol concentration (0.31% to 0.41%) can produce confusion, mild stupor, and, ultimately, coma. A blood alcohol level of 0.51% or higher usually leads to death from depression of the respiratory center located in the brain.

Another effect in the spectrum of neurological disturbances associated with intensive alcohol intoxication is the occurrence of *blackouts*. These periods of amnesia are characterized by an inability to remember events during the time of the blackout.

Alcohol Withdrawal Syndrome

Individuals who have used alcohol heavily but then decrease their intake or stop using alcohol altogether may experience manifestations related to *alcohol withdrawal*. In withdrawal, individuals may experience a hyperactivity, manifested by insomnia, anxiety, agitation, or tremors, as well as *tachycardia* (fast heartbeat) or diaphoresis (sweating). In severe cases, individuals may also experience nausea, vomiting, and visual and auditory hallucinations.

Alcohol withdrawal can be complicated by seizures and delirium. The most severe form of alcohol withdrawal is delirium tremens. Individuals with delirium tremens experience significant restlessness, gross disorientation, cognitive disruption, elevation of temperature and pulse rate, and, in some instances, psychosis. Although delirium tremens can be fatal, its course is often self-limiting. The acute period of delirium tremens usually lasts from 2 to 10 days, but can be more prolonged in case of severe withdrawal.

To manage withdrawal syndrome, individuals may receive a cross-tolerant drug, such as a sedative. Initially, sedatives are provided in large doses to suppress manifestations of withdrawal. The dose is then reduced or the interval between doses is increased, or both, so that the dosage progressively tapers off to zero. Because of wide variations in drug tolerance, management of withdrawal syndrome is individualized.

ALCOHOL-RELATED HEALTH CONDITIONS

Health conditions directly related to physical effects of chronic alcohol use on body organs are generally caused by dietary insufficiency, the direct toxic effects of alcohol on body tissue, or both. All organ systems may be involved. The outcome of alcohol-related health conditions depends on the nature of the condition and its severity. Although some alcohol-related health conditions are reversible, almost no such condition can be cured if the individual continues to use alcohol to excess.

Nervous System Conditions

Wernicke Encephalopathy (Wernicke's Disease)

Wernicke encephalopathy is a condition occurring most frequently in situations when individuals have engaged in chronic alcohol use combined with poor nutrition and prolonged vomiting (Koppel, 2016). This potentially life-threatening condition is characterized by the sudden onset of confusion, **nystagmus** (involuntary eye movements), and ataxia. Management of Wernicke encephalopathy consists of the replacement of thiamine. Early intervention is mandatory to prevent permanent deficits. Prompt intervention resolves many of the manifestations.

KORSAKOFF SYNDROME

Korsakoff syndrome occurs in about 80% of individuals who survive Wernicke encephalopathy and is characterized by consistent learning and memory impairment, although other aspects of cognitive function, such as alertness, attention, and social interactions and procedural memory may remain intact (Koppel, 2016). Individuals may have mild disorientation to time and place and may engage in *confabulation* in which they fabricate information without the intent to deceive. Korsakoff syndrome does not respond to treatment with thiamine. Consequently, it is important that Wernicke's encephalopathy is recognized and treated early in order to prevent Korsakoff syndrome from occurring.

Peripheral Neuropathy

Although many causes of *peripheral neuropathy* exist, a number of individuals who chronically use alcohol to excess develop disorders of the *peripheral nerves* (nerves outside the central nervous system). Peripheral neuropathy associated with chronic alcohol use is thought to be the result of both the toxicity of alcohol and nutritional deficiencies—specifically, inadequate amounts of thiamine and the other B vitamins. This condition affects the extremities and includes manifestations such as numbness, painful sensations, weakness, and muscle cramps. Burning pain of the feet may also occur. Good nutrition and the administration of supplemental B vitamins can bring about improvement, albeit slowly.

Cardiovascular System Conditions

Cardiomyopathy

Cardiomyopathy (functional and structural changes in the heart muscle) associated with chronic, long-term alcohol consumption results from the direct toxic effects of alcohol on the heart muscle itself. The heart may become enlarged (**cardiomegaly**), and the heart muscle may become more fibrous. The heart's ability to pump effectively may be compromised, with manifestations of congestive heart failure, such as difficulty in breathing and swelling, becoming evident as the cardiac damage progresses. Abstinence from alcohol can improve cardiomyopathy in some individuals (McKenna & Elliott, 2016).

Beriberi Heart Disease

A deficiency in thiamine is thought to contribute to the development of beriberi heart disease. Individuals with this condition have a high cardiac output, even at rest, because of the dilation of the peripheral small blood vessels. Beriberi heart disease responds well to the administration of supplemental thiamine.

Alterations in Heart Rate and Rhythm

Alcohol can affect both the speed at which the heart beats and the rhythm that it maintains. The most common type of arrhythmia associated with alcohol abuse is *atrial fibrillation* (irregular rapid beating of the upper chambers of the heart), followed by *supraventricular tachycardia* (fast heartbeat of lower chambers of the heart). Withdrawal from alcohol dependence can put a heavy load on the heart, sometimes compromising cardiac function so severely during detoxification that death

can result. Given this risk, detoxification should be conducted under careful supervision of health professionals.

Hypertension

Individuals who drink excessively may develop **hypertension** (high blood pressure) (O'Connor, 2016). Hypertension can bring about serious consequences such as *stroke* or *myocardial infarction* (heart attack).

Alterations in Blood

Excessive consumption of alcohol can alter the body's ability to absorb and utilize *folate* (a nutritional substance required to manufacture healthy blood cells). As a result of folate deficiency, formation of *red blood cells*, *white blood cells*, and *platelets* can be affected contributing to *megaloblastic anemia* (the presence of large abnormal red blood cells), *leukopenia* (abnormal decrease in the number of white blood cells), and *thrombocytopenia* (abnormal decrease in the number of platelets). Consequently, individuals may experience anemia, lower resistance to infection, and interference with blood clotting. Administration of supplemental folate, proper nutrition, and abstinence from alcohol can generally reverse these manifestations.

Musculoskeletal System Conditions

Regardless of the person's nutritional status, alcohol has a direct toxic effect on skeletal muscle by destroying muscle fibers, leading to weakness, pain, tenderness, and swelling of affected muscles. **Myopathy** (alteration of structure or function of muscle) related to alcohol use may be either acute or chronic. The more common form is *chronic alcoholic myopathy,* which evolves over a period of months to years. Pain may be less severe in chronic myopathy, although muscle cramps can occur. In addition, muscles may **atrophy** (shrink or become smaller) and weaken. Most manifestations of myopathy improve with the cessation of alcohol use, whereas continued alcohol use leads to continued deterioration in muscles. Excessive alcohol consumption can also contribute to **osteoporosis** (a reduction in bone mass), causing bones to become weakened, fragile, and easily broken. Osteoporosis occurs not only because calcium intake is insufficient, but also because alcohol interferes with the absorption of calcium from the intestines.

In addition to having a direct effect on the musculoskeletal system, alcohol can contribute to major injury. Individuals under the influence of alcohol may have decreased balance and coordination as well as demonstrate impaired judgment. As a result, they may experience injuries from falls, fires, or motor vehicle or pedestrian accidents.

Gastrointestinal System Conditions

Alcohol may affect almost every organ of the gastrointestinal tract. Individuals who consume alcohol excessively have an increased incidence of cancer of the throat and esophagus as well as colorectal cancer (Cho et al., 2004). Whether the increased incidence of cancer is attributable to direct contact of alcohol with the tissues, to the presence of carcinogenic substances in some alcoholic beverages, or to a combination of the two is unknown. Despite the fact that alcohol is considered a **hepatotoxin** (a substance that is harmful to the liver), individuals who chronically use alcohol differ widely in their susceptibility to liver conditions.

Esophagitis and Gastritis

Esophagitis and **gastritis** are inflammations of the esophagus and of the stomach, respectively. Both can occur with acute or chronic abuse of alcohol. The severity of these conditions depends on the individual. In some instances, these conditions produce only mild discomfort; in other cases, the irritation and inflammation lead to ulceration and bleeding. Intervention is directed toward reducing the inflammation. Obviously, abstinence from alcohol is a major management objective.

Alcoholic Hepatitis

Alcoholic hepatitis is an inflammation of the liver brought about by alcohol; it is *not* a contagious form of hepatitis. During the process of alcohol metabolism, fat is deposited in the liver. When individuals consume excessive amounts of alcohol, the ongoing accumulation of fat enlarges the liver, a condition called *fatty liver*. If individuals continue to consume alcohol, liver cells may die, causing

the liver to become inflamed. This inflammatory condition, in which the liver is usually enlarged and painful, constitutes alcoholic hepatitis.

Alcoholic hepatitis can be fatal (Nguyen-Khac et al., 2011). Abstinence from alcohol can reverse the effects of both fatty liver and alcoholic hepatitis. Conversely, individuals who continue to use alcohol have a high chance of developing *cirrhosis* (Garcia-Tsao, 2016). Although liver transplantation has a favorable outcome in many individuals with cirrhosis, healthcare professionals are at times reluctant to perform such transplants based on the view that individuals who use alcohol are responsible for their condition and are likely to resume drinking even after transplant (Brown, 2011; Shawcross & O'Grady, 2010). In many instances, individuals are required to demonstrate a 6-month abstinence period before they can be considered for transplantation (Mathurin et al., 2011).

Cirrhosis

Cirrhosis is a condition that involves **fibrosis** (formation of fibrous tissue) of the liver. It can be caused by a variety of conditions, but is most frequently attributable to either *hepatitis C* or alcoholism (Garcia-Tsao, 2016). When alcohol injures the liver repeatedly over an extended period of time, fibrous tissue replaces liver cells. Circulation within the liver then becomes less efficient, resulting in obstructions and ultimately increasing pressure in the blood vessels.

All blood from the gastrointestinal tract, spleen, pancreas, and gallbladder is carried to the heart through the liver by the *portal system*. As a result of the fibrous changes that occur in the liver with cirrhosis, pressure increases in the portal vein, a condition known as *portal hypertension*. The backflow of blood results in the enlargement of the spleen (**splenomegaly**), accumulation of fluid in the abdominal cavity (**ascites**), and development of esophageal varices (discussed in the next section).

Some individuals with cirrhosis experience no manifestations, especially in the condition's early stages. As the condition progresses, however, they may experience weakness, nausea, loss of appetite (**anorexia**), and **jaundice** (yellow discoloration of the skin and whites of the eyes from the accumulation of bile pigments in the blood).

Identification of cirrhosis is based on the condition's manifestations; results of blood tests; imaging via ultrasound, CT, or MRI; and liver biopsy. When standard health interventions have failed to control the complications of cirrhosis, individuals may be referred for *liver transplantation.*

Management of cirrhosis is largely directed toward mitigating manifestations, but abstinence from alcohol is a necessity for survival. Individuals with cirrhotic changes in the liver have an increased risk of liver cancer as well as a higher risk of a number of other complications. Those persons who continue to abuse alcohol despite cirrhotic changes in the liver or other complications have a significantly decreased survival rate.

Esophageal Varices

Esophageal varices is a condition in which veins in the esophagus become dilated and tortuous as a result of *portal hypertension,* a complication of cirrhosis of the liver. Approximately 60% to 80% of individuals with cirrhosis develop esophageal varices (Garcia-Tsao & Bosch, 2010). Varices may bleed periodically, with bleeding then stopping spontaneously. Individuals with esophageal varices may experience **hematemesis** (vomiting of blood) and **melena** (dark, tarry bowel movements caused by digestion of swallowed blood). Bleeding esophageal varices can be life threatening. High portal pressure may cause them to burst, resulting in hemorrhage and requiring emergency attention to stop the bleeding.

Management is directed toward controlling hemorrhage. The two major interventions for esophageal varices involve *endoscopy,* in which a tube is inserted into the esophagus. The most common of the two procedures, *endoscopic band ligation,* involves placing elastic bands around the esophageal varices, *endoscopic sclerotherapy*, involves injection of a substance into the varices that *scleroses* (hardens) and stops the bleeding (Garbuzenko, 2016). In instances in which endoscopic procedures do not stop the bleeding, more invasive surgical intervention may be needed (Afdhal & Curry, 2010). In some instances, a temporary measure to control acute bleeding may involve insertion of a special tube (*Sengstaken–Blakemore tube*) into the esophagus; a balloon on this tube is then inflated to exert pressure against the bleeding vein.

Pancreatitis

A variety of conditions other than alcohol abuse may cause **pancreatitis** (inflammation of the pancreas). *Alcoholic pancreatitis*, however, is a form of pancreatitis that develops in susceptible individuals after chronic alcohol abuse. In this condition, the pancreatic ducts become obstructed. Normally, the pancreas secretes enzymes into the small intestine to aid in digestion. In contrast, in alcoholic pancreatitis, the enzymes become active while they are still in the pancreas, so that the pancreas essentially begins to digest itself, causing progressive degeneration with scarring and calcification of pancreatic tissues. Pancreatic function is often severely curtailed. Chronic pancreatitis can lead to severe incapacitation from pain, malabsorption of nutrients resulting in weight loss, and diabetes mellitus secondary to the destruction of cells in the pancreas that secrete insulin (*islets of Langerhans*).

Management of pancreatitis is directed toward halting destruction of tissue and alleviating the manifestations. As with other conditions affecting the gastrointestinal tract, effective management requires that individuals abstain from alcohol. If they no longer consume alcohol, many will recover from alcoholic pancreatitis to live a normal life. If they continue to drink, however, the prognosis is generally poor.

MANAGEMENT OF ALCOHOL USE DISORDER

Alcohol use disorder can be a chronic, lifelong condition. It may require long-term management that extends beyond the initial period of detoxification and may involve a wide variety of services, including individual, group, and family therapy. In addition, self-help groups, such as *Alcoholics Anonymous (AA)* for alcohol-dependent individuals and *Alanon* and *Alateen* for their families, are widely recommended.

Typically, the goal of management is abstinence from alcohol and other mood-altering substances. In some circumstances, medications are used to discourage and inhibit the use of alcohol. One such medication, an aversive substance called *disulfiram* (Antabuse), interferes with the normal metabolism of alcohol; as a consequence, individuals who ingest alcohol after taking Antabuse experience severe gastrointestinal distress. Although it has not been shown to have a lasting long-term benefit, this agent may facilitate abstinence in the early recovery phase for individuals prone to impulsive drinking (O'Connor, 2016). Other medications, such as *naltrexone* (ReVia) and *acamprosate* (Campral), help to reduce cravings for alcohol.

Effective management of alcohol dependence includes both pharmacologic and psychosocial interventions. Psychosocial interventions in the form of counseling, psychoeducation, negotiation of behavior change, and specific behavioral agreements are frequently used. Most successful interventions have been demonstrated to combine healthcare interventions, psychosocial counseling, and support networks.

OTHER SUBSTANCE USE DISORDERS

Caffeine Use Disorder

Although *caffeine* is not commonly thought of as a substance of abuse or dependence, individuals who consume large amounts may exhibit signs of withdrawal after abrupt cessation or reduction in caffeine use (APA, 2013). Caffeine is commonly obtained from coffee or tea, but it may also be consumed in soft drinks, chocolate, and over-the-counter drugs, such as weight loss aids and antidrowsiness medications.

Caffeine acts primarily as a stimulant. While moderate caffeine use appears to pose few health risks for most healthy individuals, overuse can produce caffeine intoxication, which can lead to manifestations of anxiety, insomnia, **tachycardia** (rapid heartbeat), **hypertension** (elevated blood pressure), and gastric distress (APA, 2013). Its use can be associated with several psychiatric syndromes, such as caffeine-induced sleep disorder, caffeine-induced anxiety disorder, and caffeine dependence (APA, 2013; Ruiz et al., 2007).

In addition, caffeine interacts with a number of medications and can interfere with their effectiveness. For example, caffeine and sedative drugs such as benzodiazepines have antagonistic effects, so that the sedative effect of a drug, such as Valium, may be blocked when it is taken with caffeine. Caffeine has also been shown to interfere with metabolism of some antipsychotic drugs and

bronchodilating drugs, thereby diminishing their effectiveness (Ruiz et al., 2007).

If caffeine use is found to cause or exacerbate physical or psychiatric problems or interfere with medication efficiency, individuals may need to reduce or eliminate their use of this stimulant. Individuals with caffeine dependence may experience manifestations of withdrawal, such as fatigue, difficulty concentrating, and headache. Gradual reduction of caffeine consumption along with social support can be helpful in this regard. The availability of a large number of decaffeinated products makes it possible to decrease caffeine consumption, if necessary.

Tobacco Use Disorder

Although cigarette smoking is the most common method of tobacco use, other methods of tobacco use include cigars, pipe smoking, and smokeless tobacco with nicotine in all forms of tobacco acting as the major reinforce for repeated use (George, 2016). Nicotine consumed through smoking, chewing, or snuffing tobacco is absorbed through the mucous membranes or surfaces of the lung, producing an immediate reward effect (Maseeh & Kwatra, 2005). Tobacco use is a major contributor to development of cancer, cardiovascular conditions, and pulmonary conditions (Benowitz, 2010). Although tobacco use in the United States has decreased in recent years, many individuals in the general population continue to use it on a regular basis.

Tobacco use disorder, like other conditions characterized by problematic pattern of use leading to deleterious effects, is viewed as a chronic condition that requires ongoing attention (Schroeder & Warner, 2010). Individuals with tobacco use disorder can experience both physiological and psychological withdrawal manifestations within hours after they are deprived of tobacco (Brown, Lejuez, Kahler, Strong, & Zvolensky, 2005). These withdrawal manifestations can include insomnia, irritability, anxiety, depressed mood, increased appetite, and weight gain (APA, 2013). Although most manifestations associated with withdrawal are related to deprivation of nicotine, a number of social factors, such as conditioning and expectancy, also contribute to perception of manifestations and craving for nicotine (Ruiz et al., 2007).

Interventions for Tobacco Use Disorder

Interventions for tobacco use disorder vary widely and consist of pharmacologic and psychosocial approaches. Overall, the success rates for such approaches to cessation of tobacco use appears to be directly related to the smoker's motivation to stop. Nevertheless, emerging evidence suggests that a key factor affecting an individual's ability to stop smoking is how he or she responds to the discomfort and distress related to withdrawal rather than the physical withdrawal manifestations alone (Brown et al., 2005).

Pharmacologic Approaches

Pharmacologic approaches to smoking cessation include a number of methods including nicotine replacement therapies, antidepressant agents, and other medications for smoking cessation.

The goal of nicotine replacement therapy (NRT) is to alleviate withdrawal manifestations. *Nicotine gum* and *nicotine lozenges* contain small amounts of nicotine which is absorbed from the gum. *Nicotine patches* are transdermal patches that are placed on the skin and are designed to release nicotine slowly where it is absorbed through the skin. *Nicotine nasal sprays* is a nicotine solution in a nasal spray bottle. Individuals administer the spray to each nostril every 4–6 hours. *Nicotine inhalers* (e-cigarettes) produce a nicotine vapor, which is inhaled.

Antidepressant agents, *nonnicotine drugs,* such as *Bupropion,* are also used to treat tobacco use disorder. The goal of use of these agents is smoking cessation and the reduction of nicotine craving and manifestations of withdrawal (George, 2016). Other smoking cessation medications such as Varenicline are also used alone or in combination with other medications to treat tobacco use disorder.

Psychosocial Approaches

Counseling to help individuals reduce the stress associated with smoking cessation and a number of behavioral approaches has been used in smoking-cessation programs. *Cognitive-behavioral therapies, motivational interventions, and mindfulness meditation, community support groups*, and *self-help programs* have been employed to augment smoking cessation efforts (George, 2016). Overall, the success rates for pharmacologic and psychosocial approaches to cessation of tobacco use appear to be directly related to the smoker's motivation to stop.

Sedative, Hypnotic, or Anxiolytic Use Disorder

Sedatives, hypnotic, anxiolytic medications are medications that work on the central nervous system to treat anxiety and depression. Whether they are used as an intervention for management of a specific condition or manifestation, or whether they have been obtained illegally, sedatives, hypnotics, or anxiolytic medications may be associated with substance use disorder, including tolerance and dependence (Weaver, 2015).

Medications in this category which are frequently associated with substance use disorder include *benzodiazepines* and *barbiturates.* Benzodiazepines (i.e., Xanax, Klonopin, Valium), the most frequently prescribed anxiolytic, are consequently the most widely associated with substance use disorder (Weiss, 2016). Individuals may also combine sedative-hypnotics with other drugs, such as opioids or stimulants in order to enhance the opioid effect or buffer the effects of withdrawal.

Withdrawal from sedatives–hypnotics is similar to withdrawal from alcohol. Therapeutic withdrawal from a sedative–hypnotic, like therapeutic withdrawal from alcohol, usually involves administration of a cross-tolerant drug to suppress withdrawal manifestations with gradual tapering of the dosage. The drug being withdrawn determines the length of time required for tapering. For some sedatives, 7 to 10 days is sufficient for detoxification. Longer-acting drugs that have been used at high dosages may require 14 or more days for detoxification.

Opioid Use Disorder

Although addiction is often assumed to be associated with illicit or illegal drugs, a growing number of people have become addicted to legal or prescription drugs (Weaver, 2015). Because *opioids* (narcotic drugs such as morphine, meperidine [Demerol], hydromorphone [Dilaudid], oxycodone [OxyContin], and codeine) are frequently used for pain, addiction can occur through regular prescription use (Okie, 2010). In other instances, these medications are obtained illegally. One commonly used illegal opioid is heroin.

In addition to delivering pain relief, narcotics produce euphoria, sedation, and a feeling of tranquility. At first, individuals may take illegal narcotics primarily for the feeling of euphoria. Repeated administration rapidly produces tolerance and intense physical dependence. Eventually, as the dosage or frequency of drug administration increases, individuals need to continue to take the drug regularly to avoid manifestations of withdrawal.

OxyContin (oxycodone) is a medication that is prescribed for pain control but has become increasingly popular as a drug of abuse and addiction. Its popularity is, in part, due to its availability; it also provides an instant euphoria and is less expensive than drugs such as heroin. This medication is taken orally for management of pain, but those individuals using OxyContin for illicit reasons tend to crush it and then swallow or snort the powder or inject the drug after it has been dissolved in water. Numerous negative health consequences are related to opiate use, and especially long-term use of heroin. Drugs that are injected increase individuals' risk of contracting HIV infection or hepatitis C, if needles are shared (Weiss, 2016). Addition of adulterants to substances or use of nonsterile techniques of injection may also produce health complications. Skin abscesses, **cellulitis** (inflammation of tissues), **thrombophlebitis** (inflammation of a vein with associated clot formation), **septicemia** (presence of toxins in the blood), and bacterial **endocarditis** (inflammation of the inner lining of the heart) are all potential complications.

Withdrawal manifestations vary in severity and duration, depending on the particular drug abused. Withdrawal from narcotics is generally not life threatening. Many manifestations of withdrawal are flu-like but may also include anxiety, irritability, and restlessness.

One of three medications are usually used in treatment of opiate use disorder:

- methadone
- buprenorphine
- naltrexone

(Weiss, 2016)

Methadone can be used for purposes of detoxification as well as maintenance. It is provided only in a strictly regulated environment in which the medication is taken under clinical observation and supervision. It reduces opiate craving and blocks effects of other opioid use, and has been found to be effective in decreasing risk of HIV and hepatitis acquired through needle sharing, reducing criminal activity associated with drug-seeking behavior, and helping individuals to reach a socially rehabilitated state so that they can gain employment (Weiss, 2016).

Buprenorphine is a medication that has been found to be helpful both for detoxification and for maintenance in the management of opiate addiction. One potential advantage of buprenorphine is that it can be prescribed by office-based clinicians rather than only in specialized opiate management programs (Donaher & Welsh, 2006; Mintzer et al., 2007; Moore et al., 2007). Another drug, Naltrexone, blocks the euphoric effects of opiates, creating less desire for opiate use. The disadvantage of Naltrexone is the reluctance of individuals to take this medication (Weiss, 2016).

Regardless of the medication used to manage opiate addiction, management with medication is most effective when combined with counseling.

Stimulant Use Disorder

Acting directly on the central nervous system, *stimulants* create an increased state of arousal and concentration and speed up mental and motor activity. Individuals may take stimulants for such effects as increased alertness, increased sense of well-being, increased confidence, reduction of fatigue, or decrease in appetite. *Amphetamines* (e.g., Benzedrine or Dexedrine) and methamphetamine, methylphenidate (Ritalin), cocaine, and caffeine are all stimulants. In addition to exerting effects on the central nervous system, stimulants have generalized systemic effects, including an increase in heart rate, an increase in blood pressure, a rise in body temperature, and the constriction of peripheral blood vessels.

Cocaine is a highly addictive neurostimulant (Pilon & Scheiffle, 2006). Although it has been used by healthcare providers as a local anesthetic (especially for ear, nose, and throat procedures), cocaine remains a drug of wide abuse and an important public health hazard (Leikin, 2007). As with other stimulants, its physical effects may include elevated heart rate, elevated blood pressure, and increased respiratory rate. The immediate effects of cocaine produce subjective feelings of increased alertness and energy, enhanced confidence, and enhanced physical and mental ability (Ruiz et al., 2007).

In recent years, cocaine has become one of the most widely abused stimulants in the United States (Weiss, 2016). It may be taken orally, used intranasally (snorted), smoked, or injected intravenously. The technique of *free-basing* cocaine, which gained popularity in the 1980s, involves heating a flammable solvent such as petroleum or ether, and then using it to heat the cocaine. This process "frees" cocaine hydrochloride from its salts and adulterants, converting it to a form of cocaine that will vaporize. The free-base cocaine can then be inhaled or smoked, usually with a water pipe, for direct absorption through the alveoli in the lungs. The technique rapidly delivers high concentrations of cocaine to the brain and results in blood levels as high as those achieved with injection.

The free-basing technique can cause additional incapacitation due to burns from fires started during the free-basing process. Because of the concerns regarding the dangers of combustion and injury in free-basing, *crack cocaine* has become increasingly popular.

Crack, a solid form of free-base cocaine, is an alkaloid form of cocaine obtained by "cooking" cocaine hydrochloride with bicarbonate of soda (Baldwin et al., 2002). Dependence occurs very rapidly with this form of the drug. Crack is smoked rather than sniffed. Its concentrated form and its route of administration make its potency many times greater than that of cocaine alone. The euphoric effect produced by crack lasts only a matter of minutes, however. To achieve the same euphoria, users may engage in repeated use or binge on large quantities followed by periods of nonuse (Henskens, Mulder, Garretsen, Bongers, & Sturmans, 2005; Hope, Hickman, & Tilling, 2005). Crack cocaine can also be injected, and it is frequently injected in combination with other drugs such as heroin. Crack cocaine is associated with a number of criminal and health-related problems (Holloway, Bennett, & Lower, 2004), and injections of this drug are associated with increased risk of transmitting HIV and hepatitis C (Judd et al., 2005).

Individuals using cocaine, especially at higher dosages, may use depressant drugs in an attempt to counterbalance the former substance's stimulant effects. For example, alcohol and cocaine are commonly combined for this purpose. The simultaneous injection of cocaine and heroin (*speed-balling*) is another combination used by some individuals.

Aside from its psychological, social, and vocational consequences, cocaine use can have serious health consequences. Free-basing or smoking crack cocaine can lead to pulmonary complications, including hemorrhage in the lungs (Baldwin et al., 2002). Chronic use of intranasal cocaine may cause ulceration or perforation of the nasal septum. Cocaine intoxication can produce neurological effects, such as confusion, anxiety, hyperexcitability, agitation, and violence.

More serious effects are the result of acute *cocaine toxicity*, which is dose related, in which individuals can experience stroke or seizures, severe **hyperthermia** (increased body temperature), **arrhythmia** (irregular heartbeat) (Hsue et al., 2007), **myocardial infarction** (heart attack), and, in some instances, sudden death. Another side effect of excessive cocaine use, *cocaine psychosis*, is manifested as paranoia, panic, hallucinations, insomnia, and picking at the skin. The psychotic episode can last from 24 to 36 hours. Individuals with this condition are usually hospitalized and treated with antipsychotic medication.

The substances sometimes added to adulterate cocaine to increase its weight, thereby increasing profit from its sale, may cause other health complications. Problems can result from the nature of the substance used to mix with the cocaine or from the dosage taken. Adulterants such as talc or cornstarch can cause complications ranging from inflammation to **embolus** (matter traveling in the blood) (Low, Jenkins, & Prendergast, 2006).

Adverse behavioral effects are also common with cocaine use. For example, a high prevalence of anger, impulsivity, and violence is associated with cocaine addiction (Goldstein et al., 2005), and chronic use can result in paranoid psychosis (Floyd, Boutros, Struve, Wolf, & Oliwa, 2006).

Phencyclindine (PCP, also known as *angel dust*), procaine, or heroin, may be added to cocaine to potentiate the drug's effects. Because the user can never be certain of the cocaine's potency, however, the effects are not always predictable. The withdrawal syndrome from cocaine consists of a craving for more cocaine, depression, irritability, sleep disturbances, gastrointestinal disturbances, headaches, and, possibly, suicidal ideation. Because it is not unusual for individuals who are cocaine dependent to be dependent on other drugs as well, a withdrawal reaction from those other substances may be experienced, too.

Amphetamines are used in healthcare settings to treat conditions such as attention-deficit disorders. The potential for abuse of these medications is continually present. A newer street drug classified as an amphetamine is *crystalline methamphetamine* (*crystal meth* or *ice*), which is highly addictive, both physically and psychologically (Lukas, 1997). Like crack, crystal meth can be heated and inhaled in a technique similar to that used when smoking free-base cocaine. Crystal meth has greater strength and longer duration of effects, lasting from 8 to 24 hours. Methamphetamine increases energy and alertness and decreases appetite. Its greater stimulation of the brain makes it more dangerous mentally, creating cravings that can continue for years after cessation of use (Wermuth, 2000). Toxic levels can produce severe paranoid thinking with hallucinations. There is also greater risk of suicidal depression. Chronic use of methamphetamine in any form can result in serious psychiatric, cardiovascular, metabolic, and neuromuscular changes. Side effects include shaking, seizures, *cardiac arrhythmias* (irregular heartbeat), and hyperthermia (elevated body temperature). Long-term use can lead to a feeling that the skin is "crawling," anxiety, and insomnia, as well as addiction (Leikin, 2007).

Management of stimulant abuse, and crack/cocaine abuse in particular, involves management of the manifestations rather than alternative intervention options such as those available for opiate abuse. Antidepressants are sometimes used as an intervention if the person has manifestations of

depression, and sedatives such as benzodiazepines may be prescribed for manifestations of agitation and insomnia. Because of their potential for addiction, these medications are used sparingly and for only short periods of time (Harniman, 2006).

Psychosocial interventions include counseling such as motivational interviewing, cognitive-behavioral therapy, and group and family counseling. Other psychosocial interventions such as stress management skills training and support groups are beneficial as well.

Cannabis Use Disorder

When *cannabis* (*marijuana*) is smoked, the psychoactive compound (THC) that it contains produces euphoria, relaxation, dream-like states, and sleepiness. Some individuals report enhanced perceptions of colors, tastes, and textures when under the influence of marijuana.

The use of marijuana for medicinal purposes remains controversial, although it has been reported to reduce pain, spasms, nausea, and a variety of other manifestations in a number of health conditions, including multiple sclerosis, cancer, HIV/AIDS, and glaucoma (Hoffmann & Weber, 2010; Kramer, 2015; Page & Verhoef, 2006). A recent news development regarding Colorado's legalization of cannabis use suggests the beginning of a new era in which the effects of legal recreational use of cannabis may be explored as well.

The psychoactive response to the drug depends to a great extent on the dose, the personality and experience of the user, and the environment in which the drug is used. Often, users report a sense of the slowing of time and impairment in their ability to learn new facts while they are under the influence of cannabis.

Overdose, or for some simply the use of cannabis, can produce anxiety, panic states, and psychosis (Weiss, 2016). Meta-analytic data suggest that marijuana can induce psychosis, especially in those already dealing with a psychiatric diagnosis (Large, Sharma, Compton, Slade, & Nielssen, 2011). On a systemic level, cannabis produces an increase in heart rate, dilation of the bronchioles, and dilation of the peripheral blood vessels.

Chronic smoking of cannabis has been shown to produce inflammatory changes in the lungs that can contribute to the development of chronic conditions such as emphysema, however the degree to which changes are due to marijuana use alone, or in combination with other substances has not been determined. Use of other drugs, including alcohol and tobacco, may compound the adverse effects of cannabis (Hall & Degenhardt, 2009).

Although cannabis is usually smoked, it may be ingested orally. Oral consumption can delay its effects for as long as an hour, and the effects are less potent. *Hashish*, the concentrated form of THC, is also smoked and has considerably higher potency than cannabis.

There is no specific intervention for cannabis abuse. When cannabis use severely hampers individuals' functioning, interventions most often involves psychotherapeutic techniques directed at underlying problems. Because cannabis may be abused in combination with other drugs, management may be multifocal in nature.

Hallucinogen-Related Disorders

Sometimes called *psychedelics, hallucinogens* are drugs that, at some dosage, produce hallucinations or distortions in perceptions or thinking. Individuals under the influence of hallucinogens report increased awareness of sensory input and a subjective feeling of enhanced mental activity. Common hallucinogens include *LSD (lysergic acid diethylamide), psilocybin, PCP* (angel dust), and *mescaline.*

There has been a dramatic increase in synthetic drugs used recreationally such as cathinones (hs), and MDMA (Albertson, Chenoweth, Colby, & Sutter, 2016). Substance analogues, or *designer drugs,* can have dangerous, permanent effects. Users of one class of these drugs, the *methamphetamines*, which include *MDMA* (ecstasy) and *MDEA* (Eve), may be especially susceptible to permanent brain damage because the amount that produces psychological effects is not vastly different from the dosage that produces neural damage (Liechti, Kuntz, & Kupferschmidt, 2005). The designer drug *MPPP* is associated with a Parkinsonian syndrome in some individuals. Designer derivatives of amphetamines produce euphoria but can also have hallucinogenic effects and may cause cardiac arrhythmias (irregular heartbeat), *cerebral hemorrhage* (stroke), hyperthermia (elevated body temperature), altered mental status, panic, and psychosis. Individuals with PCP intoxication are especially prone to agitation and violence (Leikin, 2007).

Hallucinogens are usually taken orally and may be used concurrently with other drugs. One of the most powerful hallucinogens is LSD. Its effects vary with the individual, the dose, and the environment in which the drug is used. Generally, the effects develop within several hours and last as long as 12 hours. Individuals may report heightened sensitivity and clarity, increased insights, a sense of time moving more slowly, and distortions of visual images. Some individuals experience adverse effects from LSD, such as a panic state with severe anxiety.

The physical consequences of abuse of most hallucinogens in and of themselves are not significant. The psychological consequences, however, can be severe. Adverse effects of hallucinogens vary from acute psychosis to self-mutilation or suicide. Accidents can result from misjudgment or impairment. Some individuals experience "flashbacks" in which hallucinations reappear briefly even months after the last drug dose. An overdose of hallucinogens can result in exceedingly high body temperature, seizures, and shock.

Because hallucinogens produce no physical dependence, no specific intervention for management exists. Adverse effects such as panic episodes are usually managed with a supportive environment and observation (Kramer, 2015).

Inhalant Use Disorder

Substances that cause perceptible changes in brain function when they are administered through inhalation are called *inhalants*. Inhalants are generally classified into four categories:

- Aerosols
- Gases
- Solvents
- Nitrites

(Nguyen, O'Brien, & Schapp, 2016)

A wide variety of substances are abused in this way, often because they are readily accessible and inexpensive. For example, commonly used inhalants include airplane glue, typewriter correction fluid, marking pencils, industrial and household chemicals, paint thinners, gasoline, nitrites (poppers, snappers, or rush), and nitrous oxide. Although individuals of all age groups practice inhalant abuse (commonly called "huffing"), it is especially prevalent among adolescents and pre-adolescents (Leikin, 2007).

Although the effects of inhalants are brief, they can be serious, especially with prolonged or long-term use. The adverse effects of inhalants vary according to the type of substance inhaled. Organic solvents such as airplane glue can produce cardiac arrhythmia, bone marrow depression, damage to the kidney and liver, and, in some instances, death.

Prolonged use of *nitrites* is thought to suppress the immune system, thereby increasing the individual's susceptibility to infection. These substances are frequently used to enhance sexual pleasure; consequently, individuals who use nitrites in this way and engage in unsafe sex practices may be at greater risk for developing HIV infection owing to the suppression of the immune system and subsequent increased vulnerability to infection.

Chronic abuse of *nitrous oxide* can result in nerve damage, seizures, bone marrow changes, respiratory depression, or death. Because nitrous oxide distorts the senses, driving during intoxication with this substance is hazardous. Even though the effects of inhalants are brief, their use can result in dependence. No specific intervention is usually indicated for inhalant abuse, although specific psychotherapeutic measures may be implemented to prevent relapse and to help individuals discontinue inhalant use.

HEALTH IMPLICATIONS OF USE AND ABUSE OF OTHER SUBSTANCES

Not only does substance abuse cause psychological, social, and vocational impairments, but it can also lead to criminal activity as users try to obtain drugs or get money to buy drugs. Substance abuse also has serious health consequences.

Dermatologic Complications

Many of the health complications related to drug abuse result from nonsterile injections or from adulterants rather than from the drug itself.

Abscess

Bacterial infection may cause pus to collect in the tissues, forming an abscess. In association with drug use, improper cleansing of the skin before injection or the use of a nonsterile needle may lead to an abscess. In this situation, skin at the site becomes warm, red, swollen, and painful with a **purulent** (pus) discharge. Skin around the area frequently becomes **necrotic** (dies). If the abscess goes untreated, individuals may develop systemic manifestations of fever, loss of appetite, and fatigue. Infection may spread to the bloodstream, creating a generalized systemic infection (**bacteremia**).

Management of an abscess consists of draining the purulent material and **debriding** (removing) the area of dead tissue. Antibiotics are usually recommended, especially if individuals demonstrate systemic manifestations.

Cellulitis

An acute inflammation of the tissues without **necrosis** (tissue death) is called *cellulitis*. When associated with intravenous drug abuse, cellulitis is caused by the invasion of a variety of organisms or by irritation of the tissues from the drug itself. The tissue becomes red and tender, and **adenopathy** (swelling of lymph nodes) may occur. Management of cellulitis depends on the cause. Occasionally, cellulitis progresses to abscess formation.

Other Dermatologic Complications

Injections with nonsterile needles or injections of drugs that have been contaminated by adulterants may leave *needle track scars*. Injections cause a mild inflammatory reaction and, with subsequent injections, produce scarring at the injection site. Injection of a drug into an artery instead of a vein can cause an extreme reaction of intense pain, swelling, and coldness of an extremity. If this condition is not managed properly, *gangrene* may develop, necessitating amputation of the limb.

Cardiovascular Complications

Other than direct effects on the heart from the drug itself, most cardiovascular complications that result from drug use are related to the use of nonsterile injection techniques or to contamination of the drug with adulterants. One potential complication is **endocarditis** (inflammation of the inner lining of the heart), which affects the valves of the heart and can have potentially serious consequences.

Some drugs have a direct toxic effect on the heart muscle or directly affect heart rhythm. In some instances, inflammation of the veins with clot formation (**thrombophlebitis**) may occur because of the toxic effects of the drug.

Pulmonary Complications

The intravenous injection of drugs to which an adulterant such as talc, starch, or baking soda has been added may result in pulmonary complications. Because these "filler" substances do not dissolve, they circulate in the blood and may become lodged in lung tissue. The lodged particles cause an inflammatory reaction in the lungs, resulting in *fibrosis* of the lung tissue. If the fibrous changes are extensive, they may affect the oxygen-exchanging ability of the lungs. Manifestations similar to those of emphysema may then develop. Changes in lung elasticity can eventually result in *pulmonary hypertension* and subsequent *heart failure*.

Lung infections or lung abscesses may occur if infectious organisms become localized in the lungs after the nonsterile injection of a substance. *Aspiration pneumonia,* an inflammation of the lungs, may result from the inhalation of foreign substances or chemical irritants. Aspiration of gastric contents is also a common cause of aspiration pneumonia. Individuals who become unconscious because of a drug overdose may, in their unconscious state, vomit and subsequently inhale the vomitus. If they inhale a large quantity, the results can be fatal.

Individuals who use drugs, including alcohol, to excess may also develop *tuberculosis.* Rather than being a direct result of drug use, this infection is likely to be the consequence of the general lifestyle and living conditions of individuals who abuse drugs. Malnourishment, poor hygiene, and overcrowding all contribute to development of tuberculosis. In addition, because some drugs have an immunosuppressant effect, substance-abusing individuals may be more susceptible to the infection.

An overdose of narcotics or sedative/hypnotics can severely depress the respiratory center, causing cessation of breathing and consequent death. Overdoses of narcotics have also been associated with development of severe *pulmonary edema* (collection of fluid in the lungs), which, without intervention, can result in death.

Gastrointestinal Complications

Because the liver acts as the detoxification center for the body, individuals who chronically use drugs may damage this organ. Some substances appear to be more directly harmful to the liver than others. Chronic, excessive use of solvents, for example, can cause liver necrosis (tissue death). Other substances may cause liver abnormalities such as inflammation or fibrosis.

Hepatitis is a common complication of drug abuse. The *hepatitis A virus (HAV)* is transmitted through the oral–fecal route; thus HAV infection is related to poor hygiene, poor sanitation, and poor environmental conditions. Individuals who abuse drugs may contact hepatitis A through poor living conditions rather than from direct drug use. Infection with the *hepatitis B virus (HBV)* occurs through sexual transmission, mother-to-infant transmission, person-to-person contact, or transmission from blood, blood products, or contaminated needles.

Hepatitis C virus (HCV) is transmitted almost exclusively by contact with blood infected with the virus. Screening of blood transfusions has almost eliminated transmission of hepatitis C through transfusion. Consequently, most HCV transmission in industrialized countries now takes place via intravenous drug use (Wedemeyer & Pawlotsky, 2012). Individuals who use intravenous drugs and share needles are at high risk for developing this condition. Hepatitis C generally becomes a chronic condition and can predispose the individual to development of cirrhosis (Garcia-Tsao, 2016). The only intervention currently used for hepatitis C consists of injections of *interferon* and *ribavirin*; even with treatment, however, approximately half of all individuals with hepatitis C will experience a relapse.

Neurological Complications

Seizures may result from an overdose of drugs or a hypersensitivity to adulterants. They are especially prevalent after an overdose of amphetamines or cocaine. In some instances, stroke may also accompany an overdose. Toxic effects of adulterants on the nervous system can lead to blindness and peripheral nerve damage as well.

Other Health Risks

Individuals who use drugs have a higher incidence of sexually transmitted disease, such as *gonorrhea, syphilis*, and *chlamydia*, related to their general lifestyle and sexual practices. One of the most serious and hazardous complications of drug use is infection with HIV—a risk that is related to both intravenous drug use and unsafe sexual practices. Heavy use of some drugs, such as *ecstasy*, has been shown to induce vulnerability for cognitive disorders, and in some cases affective and anxiety disorders that may persist for more than 5 months after cessation of the drug's use (Thomasius et al., 2005).

Drug abuse during pregnancy has serious implications for the offspring. Some fetal hazards are related to lifestyle of the mother who abuses drugs during pregnancy; these risks, in addition to reflecting effects of the drug itself, may be related to poor prenatal care, poor nutrition, and a generally poor health status. The direct toxic effects of drugs on the developing fetus (**teratogenic** effects) can include neurological or physical irregularities, as well as pose dangers related to withdrawal syndrome in the infant after birth.

IDENTIFICATION OF SUBSTANCE–RELATED AND ADDICTIVE DISORDERS

Identification of a substance use disorders or substance-induced disorders is often delayed or manifestations overlooked, contributing to the condition's continued incapacitating effects, development of health complications, and progression of addiction. Denial and resistance to acknowledging the problem are universal manifestations of substance-related and addictive disorders. Consequently, even if family members or associates have identified a substance use problem, the individual who abuses substances may not acknowledge the condition and may refuse to seek help.

Conditions related to substance use are frequently associated with health and personal concerns. Consequently, many individuals presenting at health or counseling facilities may have coexisting or secondary substance use problems that have not been identified. Some health professionals may feel uncomfortable questioning or confronting individuals about substance use problems so that identification or management of the problem is further delayed. Undetected substance use problems have significant effects on the health and well-being of individuals as well as the health and well-being of their family and others.

Screening Instruments

Routine screening of individuals presenting for health care or counseling can help health professionals determine whether a problem exists and whether a more in-depth assessment is needed. Several hundred screening instruments are available for this purpose. One of the best-known and widely used instruments for alcohol screening is *CAGE,* which is an acronym for italicized letters in each of the four questions in the instrument (Ewing, 1984). Other widely used tests for alcohol screening include *MAST (Michigan Alcoholism Screening Test*; Seizer, 1971) and AUDIT (Alcohol Use Disorders Identification Test; Saunders, Aasland, Babor, De La Fuente, & Grant, 1993). The Drug Abuse Screening Test (DAST) parallels MAST but is designed to screen for drugs other than alcohol (Gavin, Ross, & Skinner, 1989; Skinner, 1982). Each of these screening tests has its own benefits and limitations. The type of screening test used for identifying a substance use problem is based on the circumstances under which the test is used as well as on specific factors related to the individual. The clandestine nature of substance use and the tendency to underreport or withhold information affect the reliability of these instruments.

Direct Drug Screening

Direct testing for the presence of the substance of abuse in the body may involve *breath analyzers* and *blood alcohol tests*. Both tests measure intoxication; neither reveals the extent of abuse or dependence. Screening of blood or urine samples is also used to verify suspected substance use. As with any laboratory test, there is a possibility of false-negative or false-positive results. Newer screening methods are designed to be more sensitive and produce more accurate results.

Drug testing results are valid only if the testing is accomplished under strictly controlled conditions. Many individuals who use drugs are aware of a variety of methods to invalidate test results, such as substituting a specimen from a drug-free individual for their own specimen. The appropriate methods and times of drug screening are highly controversial. Routine screening for drugs without the individual's knowledge and consent evokes a variety of legal and ethical concerns.

Health Evaluation

Identification of substance use during the course of a healthcare examination may rely on information obtained from several sources. Physical manifestations of substance abuse/dependence may include a variety of conditions. Questions about substance use practices should be routinely asked in the examination of individuals with gastrointestinal disturbances, hypertension or heart disease, liver disease, neurological changes, or history of traumatic injuries. Blood cell irregularities, such as a decreased number of platelets or signs of bone marrow depression, or other indirect clinical laboratory signs, such as elevated levels of *gamma-glutamyltransferase (GGT)* or *gamma-glutamyltranspeptidase (GGTP)*, and elevated *red blood cell mean corpuscular volume (MCV)*, may suggest problems with substance abuse. Elevated levels of enzymes such as *serum glutamic oxaloacetic transaminase (SGOT)* and *serum glutamic pyruvic transaminase (SGPT)* may also be associated with substance use, although increased concentrations of SGOT and SGPT can be associated with other conditions (e.g., myocardial infarction) as well.

Behavioral and Psychological Screening

Investigation of subtle psychological or behavioral manifestations is also important in identification of a substance use problem. Depression, hyperactivity, sleep disturbances, anxiety, sexual problems, and personality changes are common manifestations of substance abuse or dependence. In addition, the incidence of accidents and injury is often increased in persons using substances of abuse.

MANAGEMENT OF SUBSTANCE USE CONDITIONS

The first step in the management of a substance-related condition is the identification and acknowledgment of the problem. Screening may be hampered by several barriers:

- Denial of the problem by the individual or family members
- Reluctance of healthcare and mental health personnel to confront or discuss the problem

Once the problem is identified and confronted, assessment for the health and psychosocial problems that typically accompany substance use problems and assessment of the level of the individual's motivation for change are important for effective intervention (O'Connor, 2000). Successful management for substance use conditions generally requires more than one level of intervention during the long recovery process. Specifically, intervention may involve community-based or residential intervention along with continued intervention at a community-based facility. Most individuals receiving intervention for substance use consider themselves "recovering," denoting the long-term, chronic nature of the recovery process. Relapse is a common part of recovery. Rather than being thought of as failure, it can be viewed as an opportunity for learning and growth (American Academy of Pediatrics, 2000).

Many individuals with substance-related conditions eventually experience physical, social, or psychological crises that require residential intervention. The precise intervention varies greatly from facility to facility and depends on the particular type of crisis experienced. Some facilities provide management for substance use conditions solely on a community basis. Others provide a combination of residential and community-based interventions.

Management sometimes begins with detoxification, which may or may not involve residential intervention, depending on the individual, the specific substance of abuse, and the presence of additional complications. Ongoing intervention, which includes a variety of rehabilitation strategies, such as psychotherapy, family therapy, and self-help programs (e.g., *Alcoholics Anonymous* or *Narcotics Anonymous*), is often necessary to prevent relapse. Several psychotherapeutic approaches to the management of substance abuse exist. The specific type of intervention used often depends on the facility and the overall philosophy of the healthcare professionals conducting the intervention. In almost all instances, however, abstinence is a management goal.

In some instances, medications are used in the ongoing management of substance dependence. For example, Antabuse and methadone (or another opiate substitute), as discussed earlier, are commonly used in the management of alcohol dependence and opiate dependence, respectively.

Individuals with a substance use condition may also require ongoing healthcare intervention for any health complications that have resulted from the substance use. Because nutritional deficiencies frequently accompany substance use condition, most detoxification centers and residential facilities provide nutrition therapy as a part of the management plan. Educational programs that stress the importance of nutrition and other aspects of a healthy lifestyle are often incorporated into the general management program.

FUNCTIONAL IMPLICATIONS OF SUBSTANCE ABUSE AND DEPENDENCE

Personal and Psychosocial Issues

The extent to which psychological incapacitation is the direct *result* of a substance-related condition versus the *cause* of the condition is not easily determined. Individuals with substance use conditions frequently have low self-esteem and experience depression. They may have feelings of inadequacy, loneliness, and isolation that lead to increased substance use. Individuals, when influenced and controlled by the substance used, may rely on it rather than on their own resources and may doubt that they have the ability to cope without the substance. Consequently, their self-confidence and self-esteem may be eroded even more.

Individuals who are psychologically dependent on a substance feel a need and longing for the substance; in turn, they become irritable, depressed, anxious, and resentful when the substance is not available. Individuals with a psychological craving for a substance may attribute their need to a personal flaw in their character or may consider their need to be a negative reflection on themselves. Either interpretation further contributes to lowered self-esteem and self-deprecation.

Individuals may use denial or rationalization as a form of self-protection and as a way to minimize their substance use problems. They may deny that a substance use problem exists, or may rationalize their behavior by redefining their substance use so that it appears to be acceptable. Some individuals become aggressive or perform violent acts when they are under the influence of certain substances. Those who are predisposed to this type of reaction may become involved in criminal acts, such as brawls, homicide, rape, or child abuse.

As individuals become increasingly dependent on a substance, the concept of living without it produces fear and dread. Individuals interpret removal of the substance as removal of all joy and excitement from life. As with all types of perceived loss, individuals may experience grief and bereavement.

Recovery from a substance use condition involves restoration of self-esteem and confidence, and it requires a willingness to accept responsibility for one's personal behavior. Individuals need assistance to accept losses that they have experienced and to develop skills for coping in the future. Recovery is a continuing process that incorporates long-term vigilance and a continuing commitment to remain drug free.

Activities and Participation

A substance-related condition affects every aspect of an individual's daily life. As dependence on the substance becomes more pronounced, individuals may lose interest in self-care, show a decreased desire for food, and experience a variety of sleep disturbances, resulting in sleep deprivation. Daily activities may become focused on obtaining more of the substance. Activities once enjoyed may offer little joy or inspire little interest. Individuals recovering from a substance use condition may need to learn or relearn components of a healthy lifestyle such as self-care, including hygiene and grooming, proper diet, and the importance of exercise. These aspects of daily living may be a vital part of an individual's rehabilitation.

Substance use can also affect individuals' ability to drive a motor vehicle. Poor driving performance can result in accidents or arrests, which can in turn lead to the loss of the person's driver's license. Therefore, transportation may become a problem if individuals must depend on others for their transportation needs.

Sexuality

Sexual dysfunction is common in individuals with substance use conditions. Women may experience decreased libido or become promiscuous. Men may experience not only decreased libido but also adverse effects on sexual performance, including impotence—a common side effect of chronic alcohol abuse.

Social Relationships

Social effects of substance-related conditions are widespread, touching family relationships, relationships with friends and associates, and general functioning as a member of society. Individuals' ability to function as a member of a social group may gradually deteriorate as substance use increases. To some extent, social factors may determine the social implications of substance use. For example, the availability of substances within a group or as part of a social event may determine whether individuals with a condition related to substance use participate in the activity.

The extent of social tolerance of individuals' behavior while intoxicated may either curtail or enhance substance use at first. As individuals become increasingly dependent on the substance, however, the substance takes on an increasing importance. Conversely, the importance assigned to individuals' social contacts and activities declines.

Individuals with a substance-related condition may be unable to function within their social networks. Repeated, heavy use of the substance often leads to upheavals in relationships. Social and family relationships are strained and often destroyed if individuals become abusive or violent, or if they engage in socially unacceptable behavior while under the influence of the substance. Individuals' behavior often alienates others, leading to social isolation. Decreasing reliability in performance of social roles and inability to maintain commitments cause those affected by the individual's deterioration in behavior to feel disappointed and angry. Others in the social environment may have to alter their own roles to assume duties that the individual once fulfilled. This shifting of responsibilities places additional burdens on all concerned and may eventually lead to resentment or even banishment of the individual from the group. Family members and associates may begin to withdraw from the individual emotionally. As individuals become increasingly more isolated, feelings of self-loathing, guilt, and shame may develop. Feeling rejected by family and associates, individuals may limit their social contacts to relationships with others who also engage in substance use.

The broader social consequences of substance-related conditions may include legal and even criminal implications. As mentioned earlier, there is a strong correlation between substance use conditions and a variety of accident rates. Motor vehicle accidents, for example, can lead to physical incapacitation not only for the individual with the substance use condition but also for others. Thus the loss of a driver's license and the threat of more serious criminal charges are potential outcomes of substance use conditions. Furthermore, individuals who become dependent on illegal substances may engage in illegal activities to obtain money with which to purchase drugs. Even if individuals do not face criminal charges as a result of their drug-seeking behavior, they can become overly focused on obtaining the drug rather than on functioning in a productive social role.

In some cases, family and social relationships can be salvaged in the recovery process. In other instances, loss of these relationships is permanent.

Depending on individual circumstances, therapeutic recovery may involve the development of new social roles and relationships or the reestablishment of old ones.

VOCATIONAL IMPLICATIONS OF SUBSTANCE ABUSE AND DEPENDENCE

In the early stages of a substance-related condition, individuals may be concerned that the use of the substance will interfere with their work. If substance use progresses to abuse or dependence, however, this focus may be reversed; that is, individuals may become more concerned that their work will interfere with their use of the substance. The substance assumes a penultimate role in the person's life, drastically affecting his or her work performance.

Although early identification of and intervention with workers with a substance use condition are most desirable, the problem may not be recognized until a progressive deterioration of work performance, increased absenteeism, or an increase in job-related accidents occurs. Fear that they will lose their jobs if their employers become aware of these indicators may motivate individuals with a substance use condition to seek assistance in managing their condition.

The ability of individuals to return to their former employment after intervention for a substance use disorder depends on the circumstances. In some instances, the stress and tension associated with the job may be beyond individuals' stress tolerance and coping ability. It may be beneficial to find a less stressful work setting, especially in the early stages of recovery, until the individual's tolerance for stress gradually increases. Physical incapacitation resulting from a substance use condition must also be considered when evaluating vocational potential.

It is essential to identify past work problems, which may extend beyond issues of substance use. Some individuals may need to learn social skills, work-appropriate behaviors, or good hygiene or grooming practices; some need to improve their work skills. Individuals who began using substances at an early age may not have developed sufficient work skills or work history to obtain employment. These individuals, in particular, may require additional education or job training. If individuals return to the same work setting that originally precipitated feelings of inadequacy, which in turn contributed to development of substance use disorders, the return to work may increase the risk of relapse. In some cases, learning new skills or coping strategies may enable individuals to return successfully to the same work setting. In other instances, a new work environment may be necessary.

Loss of a driver's license because of a substance-related condition may make transportation to and from work more difficult. In addition, if driving a motor vehicle had been part of the former employment, job restructuring or job change may be necessary. Some occupations require professional licensure; in such circumstances, revocation of an individual's license as a result of a substance use condition may limit his or her ability to work in that occupation. Many professional licensing boards have provisions for the reinstatement of licensure after documented rehabilitation. If the professional license is reinstated, a probationary period, in which the individual's work performance is closely observed and monitored, may be required to maintain licensure.

Conviction on criminal charges—especially felony charges—may disqualify individuals from employment in some occupations. Although decisions may be made on a case-by-case basis, such charges and their impact on employment in different fields and in different locations must be considered. As with most incapacitating conditions, the attitudes and concerns of employers must be addressed, especially given the social stigma that is often attached to substance use conditions. Employers may require particular encouragement to reinstate or hire individuals who have been convicted of criminal charges. Recognizing the potential for rejection by employers based on these attitudes, recovering individuals may be reluctant to share their complete history with employers or may become defensive when asked questions about substance use. Fear of rejection because of prejudice may be part of the equation when the individual returns to work. With increasing awareness of substance use conditions and with educational efforts directed toward employers, however, individuals may encounter decreasing levels of prejudice.

Many individuals who are recovering from substance use conditions return to their original employment and lead full, productive lives. In all instances, however, abstinence is a prerequisite for continuing productivity. Ongoing long-term management or involvement with self-help groups may also be necessary to prevent relapse.

CASE STUDY

Mr. K. is a 42-year-old male with a high school education. He is an auto mechanic who has been a social drinker since his early 20s. His drinking has gradually intensified over the years, and family and friends have repeatedly confronted Mr. K. about his drinking. On several occasions, Mr. K. was inebriated on the job, and his employer asked him not to return to work. He is divorced from his first wife, with whom he has two children, and is responsible for child support. His second wife of 5 years recently left him and is seeking a divorce. After being convicted on a DUI charge and being arrested for disorderly conduct, Mr. K. was referred to a residential facility. He is now at a community-based facility.

1. When working with Mr. K. to develop a rehabilitation plan, which significant factors would you consider about his situation?
2. How might social factors influence Mr. K.'s rehabilitation?
3. Which additional information would you want to know about Mr. K. to work with him on his rehabilitation plan?
4. Which types of services might be useful for Mr. K.?

REFERENCES

Abbott, F. V., & Fraser, M. I. (1998). Use and abuse of over-the-counter analgesic agents. *Journal of Psychiatry and Neuroscience, 23*(1), 13–34.

Adinoff, B. (2004). Neurobiologic processes in drug reward and addiction. *Harvard Review of Psychiatry, 12*(6), 305–320.

Afdhal, N. H., & Curry, M. P. (2010). Early TIPS to improve survival in acute variceal bleeding. *New England Journal of Medicine, 362*(25), 2421–2422.

Albertson, T. E., Chenoweth, J. A., Colby, D. K., & Sutter, M. E. (2016). The changing drug culture: Emerging drugs of abuse and legal highs. *FP Essentials, 441*, 18–124.

Allen Doyle-Pita, D. (2001). Dual disorders in psychiatric rehabilitation: Teaching considerations. *Rehabilitation Education, 15*(2), 155–165.

American Academy of Pediatrics. (2000). Indications for management and referral of patients involved in substance abuse. *Pediatrics, 106*(1), 143.

American Psychiatric Association. (2000). *Diagnostic and statistical manual of mental disorders* (4th ed., text revision). Washington, DC: Author.

American Psychiatric Association. (2013). *Diagnostic and statistical manual of mental disorders* (5th ed.). Washington, DC: Author.

Andrabi, S., Greene, S., Moukaddam, N., & Li, R. (2015). New drugs of abuse with withdrawal syndromes. *Emergency Medical Clinics of North America, 33*(4), 779–795.

Baldwin, G. C., Choi, R., Roth, M. D., Shay, A. H., Kleerup, E. C., Simmons, M. S., & Tashkin, D. P. (2002). Evidence of chronic damage to pulmonary microcirculation in habitual users of alkaloidal ("crack") cocaine. *Chest, 121*(4), 1231–1238.

Benowitz, N. L. (2010). Nicotine addiction. *New England Journal of Medicine, 362*(24), 2295–2303.

Blume, S. B., Counts, S. J., & Turnbull, J. M. (1992, July 15). Women and substance abuse. *Patient Care, 141*–145, 148–151, 154–156.

Brown, R. A., Lejuez, C. W., Kahler, C. W., Strong, D. R., & Zvolensky, M. J. (2005). Distress tolerance and early smoking lapse. *Clinical Psychology Review, 25*(6), 713–733.

Brown, R. S. (2011). Transplantation for alcoholic hepatitis: Time to rethink the 6 month "rule." *New England Journal of Medicine, 365*(19), 1836–1838.

Center for Behavioral Health Statistics and Quality. (2015). *Behavioral health trends in the United States: Results from the 2014 National Survey on Drug Use and Health* (HHS Publication No. SMA 15-4927, NSDUH Series H-50). Retrieved from http://www.samhsa.gov/data/

Cho, E., Smith-Warner, S. A., Ritz, J., van den Brandt, P. A., Colditz, G. A., Folsom, A. R., ... Hunter, D. (2004). Alcohol intake and colorectal cancer: A pooled analysis of 8 cohort studies. *Annals of Internal Medicine, 140*(8), 603–613.

Christen, A. G., & Christen, J. A. (1994). Why is cigarette smoking so addicting? An overview of smoking as a chemical and process addiction. *Health Values, 18*(1), 17–24.

Donaher, P. A., & Welsh, C. (2006). Managing opioid addiction with buprenorphine. *American Family Physician, 73*(9), 1572–1580.

Ewing, J. A. (1984). Detecting alcoholism: The CAGE questionnaire. *Journal of the American Medical Association, 252,* 1905–1907.

Fabricant, D. S., & Farnsworth, N. R. (2001). The value of plants used in traditional medicine for drug discovery: Environmental health perspectives. *Reviews in Environmental Health, 109*(1), 69–75.

Fairley, P. (1978). *The conquest of pain.* London, England: Michael Joseph.

Feinstein, E. C., Richter, L., & Foster, S. E. (2012). Addressing the critical health problems of adolescent substance use through health care, research and public policy. *Journal of Adolescent Health, 50*(5), 431–436.

Floyd, A. G., Boutros, N. N., Struve, F. A., Wolf, E., & Oliwa, G. M. (2006). Risk factors for experiencing psychosis during cocaine use: A preliminary report. *Journal of Psychiatric Research, 40*(2), 178–182.

Garbuzenko, D. V. (2016). Current approaches to the management of patients with cirrhosis who have acute esophageal variceal bleeding. *Current Medical Research and Opinion, 32*(3), 467–475.

Garcia-Tsao, G. (2016). Cirrhosis and its sequelae. In L. Goldman & A. I. Schafer (Eds.), *Goldman-Cecil medicine,* (25th ed., pp. 1023–1031). Philadelphia, PA: Elsevier Saunders.

Garcia-Tsao, G., & Bosch, J. (2010). Management of varices and variceal hemorrhage in cirrhosis. *New England Journal of Medicine, 362*(9), 823–832.

Gavin, D. R., Ross, H. E., & Skinner, H. A. (1989). Diagnostic validity of the Drug Abuse Screening Test in assessment of DSM-III drug disorders. *British Journal of Addiction, 84*(3), 301–307.

George, T. P. (2016). Nicotine and tobacco. In L. Goldman & A. I. Schafer (Eds.), *Goldman-Cecil medicine,* (25th ed., pp. 145–149). Philadelphia, PA: Elsevier Saunders.

Goldstein, R. Z., Alia-Klein, N., Leskovjan, A. C., Fowler, J. S., Wang, G. J., Gur, R. C., & Volkow, N. D. (2005). Anger and depression in cocaine addiction: Association with the orbitofrontal cortex. *Psychiatry Research, 138*(1), 13–22.

Greer, B. G., Roberts, R., & Jenkins, W. M. (1990). Substance abuse among clients with other primary disabilities: Curricular implications for rehabilitation education. *Rehabilitation Education, 4*(1), 33–44.

Hall, W., & Degenhardt, L. (2009). Adverse health effects of non-medical cannabis use. *Lancet, 374,* 1383–1391.

Harley, D. A. (1995). Alcohol and other drug use among women: Implications for rehabilitation counseling. *Journal of Applied Rehabilitation Counseling, 26*(4), 38–41.

Harniman, B. (2006). Substance misuse: An overview of assessment and treatment options. *Nurse Prescribing, 7*(5), 180–183.

Helmus, T. C., Downey, K. K., Arfken, C. L., Henderson, M. J., & Schuster, C. R. (2001). Novelty seeking as a predictor of treatment retention for heroin dependent cocaine users. *Drug and Alcohol Dependence, 61,* 287–295.

Henskens, R., Mulder, C. L., Garretsen, H., Bongers, I., & Sturmans, F. (2005). Gender differences in problems and needs among chronic, high-risk crack abusers: Results of a randomized controlled trial. *Journal of Substance Use, 10*(2–3), 128–140.

Hoffmann, D. E., & Weber, E. (2010). Medical marijuana and the law. *New England Journal of Medicine, 362*(16), 1453–1456.

Holloway, K., Bennett, T., & Lower, C. (2004). *Trends in drug use and offending: Results of the NEW-ADAM Programme 1999–2002. Finds 219.* London, England: Home Office.

Hope, V. D., Hickman, M., & Tilling, K. (2005). Capturing crack cocaine use: Estimating the prevalence of crack cocaine use in London using capture–recapture with covariates. *Addiction, 100,* 1701–1708.

Hsue, P. Y., McManus, D., Selby, V., Ren, X., Pillutia, P., Younes, N., ... Waters, D. D. (2007). Cardiac arrest in patients who smoke crack cocaine. *American Journal of Cardiology, 99*(6), 822–824.

Inaba, D. S., & Cohen, W. E. (1993). *Uppers, downers, all arounders: Physical and mental effects of psychoactive drugs.* Ashland, OR: CNS Productions.

Judd, A., Hickman, M., Jones, S., McDonald, T., Parry, J. V., & Stimson, G. V. (2005). Incidence of hepatitis C virus and HIV among new injecting drug users in London: Prospective cohort study. *British Medical Journal, 330,* 24–25.

Kandall, S. R. (1996). *Substance and shadow: Women and addiction in the United States.* Cambridge, MA: Harvard University Press.

Kavanagh, D. J., McGrath, J., Saunders, J. B., Dore, G., & Clark, D. (2002). Substance misuse in patients with schizophrenia: Epidemiology and management. *Drugs, 62,* 743–755.

Koppel, B. S. (2016). Nutritional and alcohol-related neurologic disorders. In L. Goldman & A. I. Schafer (Eds.), *Goldman-Cecil medicine,* (25th ed., pp. 2506–2512). Philadelphia, PA:Elsevier Saunders.

Kosten, T. R., & O'Connor, P. G. (2003). Management of drug and alcohol withdrawal. *New England Journal of Medicine, 348*(18), 1786–1795.

Kramer, J. L. (2015). Medical marijuana for cancer. *CA: A Cancer Journal for Clinicians, 65*(2), 109–122.

Large, M., Sharma, S., Compton, M. T., Slade, T., & Nielssen, O. (2011). Cannabis use and earlier onset of psychosis: A systematic meta-analysis. *Archives of General Psychiatry, 68*(6), 555–561.

Leikin, J. B. (2007). Substance-related disorders in adults. *Disease-a-Month, 53,* 313–335.

Liechti, M. E., Kuntz, I., & Kupferschmidt, H. (2005). Acute medical problems due to ecstasy use: Case-series of emergency department visits. *Swiss Medical Weekly, 135*(43–44), 652–657.

Low, G. S., Jenkins, N. P., & Prendergast, B. D. (2006). Needle embolism in an intravenous drug user. *Heart, 92,* 315.

Lucey, M. R., Mathurin, P., & Morgan, T. R. (2009). Alcoholic hepatitis. *New England Journal of Medicine, 360*(26), 2758–2768.

Lukas, S. E. (1997). *Proceedings of the National Consensus Meeting on the Use, Abuse, and Sequelae of Abuse of Methamphetamine with Implications for Prevention, Treatment, and Research.* DHHS Pub. No. (SMA) 96-8013. Substance Abuse and Mental Health Services Administration and Center for Substance Abuse Treatment.

Maddux, J. F., & Desmond, D. P. (2000). Addiction or dependence. *Addiction, 95,* 661–665.

Maseeh, A., & Kwatra, G. (2005). A review of smoking cessation interventions. *Medscape General Medicine, 7*(2), 24–39.

Mathurin, P., Moreno, C., Samuel, D., Dumortier, J., Salleron, J., Durland, F., ... Ducios-Vallée, J. C. (2011). Early liver transplantation for severe alcoholic hepatitis. *New England Journal of Medicine, 365*(19), 1790–1800.

McKenna, W. J., & Elliott, P. (2016). Diseases of the myocardium and endocardium. In L. Goldman & A. I. Schafer (Eds.), *Goldman-Cecil medicine,* (25th ed., pp. 320–339). Philadelphia, PA: Elsevier Saunders

Mintzer, I. L., Eisenberg, M., Terra, M., MacVane, C., Himmelstein, D. U., & Woolhandler, S. (2007). Treating opioid addiction with buprenorphine–naloxone in community-based primary care settings. *Annals of Family Medicine, 5*(2), 146–150.

Moore, B. A., Fiellin, D. A., Barry, D. T, Sullivan, L. E., Chawarski, M. C., O'Connor, P. G., & Schottenfeld, R. S. (2007). Primary care office-based buprenorphine treatment: Comparison of heroin and prescription opioid dependent patients. *Journal of General Internal Medicine, 22*(4), 527–530.

National Institute on Drug Abuse. (2014). *Drugs, brains, and behavior: The science of addiction.* Retrieved from https://www .drugabuse.gov/publications/drugs-brains-behavior-science -addiction/drugs-brain

Nestler, E. J., & Hyman, S. E. (2016). Biology of addiction. In L. Goldman & A. I. Schafer (Eds.), *Goldman-Cecil medicine,* (25th ed., pp. 143–145). Philadelphia, PA: Elsevier Saunders.

Nguyen, J., O'Brien, C., & Schapp, S. (2016). Adolescent inhalant use, prevention, assessment and treatment: A literature synthesis. *International Journal of Drug Policy, 31*, 15–24.

Nguyen-Khac, E., Thevenot, T., Piquet, M. A., Benferhat, S., Goria, O., Chatelain, D., ... AAH-NAC Study Group. (2011). Glucocorticoids plus *N*-acetylcysteine in severe alcoholic hepatitis. *New England Journal of Medicine, 365*(19), 1781–1789.

O'Brien, P. G. (2013). Substance-related disorders. In P. G. O'Brien, W. Z. Kennedy, & K. A. Ballard (Eds.), *Psychiatric mental health nursing,* (2nd ed., pp. 342–369). Burlington, MA: Jones & Bartlett Learning.

O'Connor, P. G. (2000). Treating opioid dependence: New data and new opportunities. *New England Journal of Medicine, 243*(18), 1332–1334.

O'Connor, P. G. (2016). Alcohol use disorders. In L. Goldman & A. I. Schafer (Eds.), *Goldman-Cecil medicine,* (25th ed., pp. 149–162). Philadelphia, PA: Elsevier Saunders.

Okie, S. (2010). A flood of opioids, a rising tide of deaths. *New England Journal of Medicine, 363*(21), 1981–1985.

Page, S. A., & Verhoef, M. J. (2006). Medicinal marijuana use: Experiences of people with multiple sclerosis. *Canadian Family Physician, 52,* 64–65.

Pilon, A. F., & Scheiffle, J. (2006). Ulcerative keratitis associated with crack-cocaine abuse. *Contact Lens and Anterior Eye, 29*(5), 263–267.

Robinson, T. E., & Berridge, K. C. (2001). Incentive-sensitization and addiction. *Addiction, 96,* 103–114.

Robinson, T. E., & Berridge, K. C. (2003). Addiction. *Annual Review of Psychology, 54,* 25–53.

Ruiz, P., Strain, E. C., & Langrod, J. G. (2007). *The substance abuse handbook.* Philadelphia, PA: Lippincott Williams & Wilkins.

Saunders, J. B., Aasland, O. G., Babor, T. F., De La Fuente, J. R., & Grant, M. (1993). Development of the Alcohol Use Disorders Identification Test (AUDIT): WHO collaborative project on early detection of persons with harmful alcohol consumption—II. *Addiction, 88*(6), 791–804.

Schroeder, S. A., & Warner, K. E. (2010). Don't forget tobacco. *New England Journal of Medicine, 363*(3), 201–204.

Scott-Lennox, J. S., Rose, R., Bohlig, A., & Lennox, R. (2000). The impact of women's family status on completion of substance abuse treatment. *Journal of Behavioral Health Services and Research, 27*(4), 366–379.

Seizer, M. L. (1971). The Michigan Alcoholism Screening Test: The quest or a new diagnostic instrument. *American Journal of Psychiatry, 127*(12), 1653–1658.

Shawcross, D. L., & O'Grady, J. G. (2010). The 6-month abstinence rule in liver transplantation. *Lancet, 376,* 216–217.

Skinner, H. A. (1982). The Drug Abuse Screening Test. *Addictive Behavior, 7*(4), 363–371.

Substance Abuse and Mental Health Services Administration. (2005). *National survey on drug use and health.* Retrieved from http:\\www.oas.samhsa.gov/nhsda.htm

Thomasius, R., Petersen, K. U., Zapletalova, P., Wartberg, L., Zeichner, D., & Schmoldt, A. (2005). Mental disorders in current and former heavy ecstasy (MDMA) users. *Addictions, 100,* 1310–1319.

Urbano-Marquez, A., Estruch, R., Fernández-Solá, J., Nicolás, J. M., Paré, J. C., & Rubin, E. (1995). The greater risk of alcoholic cardiomyopathy and myopathy in women compared with men. *Journal of the American Medical Association, 274*(2), 149–154.

Volkow, N. D. (2001). Drug abuse and mental illness: Progress in understanding co-morbidity. *American Journal of Psychiatry, 158*(8), 1181–1183.

Watson, A. L., Franklin, M. E., Ingram, M. A., & Eilenberg, L. B. (1998). Alcohol and other drug abuse among persons with disabilities. *Journal of Applied Rehabilitation Counseling, 29*(2), 22–29.

Weatherall, M. (2001). Drug treatment and the rise of pharmacology. In R. Porter (Ed.), *Cambridge illustrated history of medicine,* (pp. 246–277). Cambridge, UK: Cambridge University Press.

Weaver, M. F. (2015). Prescription sedative misue and abuse. *Yale Journal of Biology and Medicine, 88*(3), 247–256.

Wedemeyer, H., & Pawlotsky, J. M. (2012). Acute viral hepatitis. In L. Goldman & A. I. Schafer (Eds.), *Goldman-Cecil medicine,* (24th ed., pp. 966–973). Philadelphia, PA: Elsevier Saunders.

Weiss, R. D. (2016). Drugs of abuse. In L. Goldman & A. I. Schafer (Eds.), *Goldman-Cecil medicine,* (25th ed., pp. 156–162). Philadelphia, PA: Elsevier Saunders.

Wermuth, L. (2000). Methamphetamine use: Hazards and social influences. *Journal of Drug Education, 30*(4), 423–433.

CHAPTER 16

Conditions of the Eye and Blindness

STRUCTURE AND FUNCTION OF THE EYE

The eyeballs are spherical organs encased in the orbital cavities of the skull (see **Figure 16-1**). Muscles located on the top, bottom, and side of each eye enable the eye to rotate in different directions. The eyelid serves a protective function. Through frequent blinking, it helps to keep the eye moist, preventing irritation. The *lacrimal glands*, which lie in the upper, outer side of the eye behind the eyelid, secrete tears to keep the eyeball moist and help rid the eye of foreign material.

In front of the eye is a transparent curved structure called the *cornea,* which admits light and protects the inner eye from foreign particles and organisms. Although the cornea contains no blood vessels, it is richly supplied with nerve cells. The *sclera* (the white part of the eye) forms the globe of the eye. It is continuous with the cornea. It has the primary function of supporting and protecting the eye and maintaining eye shape. Lining the exposed area of the sclera and inner eyelid is a sensitive membrane called the *conjunctiva*. Lying underneath the sclera and also surrounding the eyeball is the *choroid coat*, which contains most of the blood vessels that nourish the eye.

The colored part of the eye is called the *iris*. At the center of the iris is a round opening called the *pupil*, which admits light to the inner part of the eye. The cornea covers both the iris and the pupil. The iris contracts and relaxes, changing the size of the pupil, thus automatically regulating the amount of light that enters the eye. In bright light, the action of the pupil causes it to become smaller to reduce the amount of light admitted. In the dark, the action of the iris causes the pupil to become larger in order to admit as much light as possible.

Directly behind the iris is a space called the *posterior chamber*. Contained in the posterior chamber are structures called the *ciliary processes,* which produce a transparent fluid called the *aqueous humor.* The aqueous humor escapes from the posterior chamber through the pupil into a space lying between the iris and cornea called the *anterior chamber*. The aqueous humor then drains from the eye into lymph channels and into the venous system through a sieve-like structure called the *canal of Schlemm* (*trabecular network*), which is located at the junction of the iris and the sclera. The balance between the amount of aqueous humor produced and the amount drained helps to maintain normal *intraocular pressure* (pressure within the eyeball).

The aqueous humor nourishes both the cornea and a structure located directly behind the iris called the *lens*. The lens is a small transparent disk enclosed in a transparent capsule. Attachments around the circumference of the lens, called *ciliary muscles,* automatically contract or expand, changing the shape of the lens from fat to thin (or vice versa) in response to the proximity or distance of an object being visualized. These changes in the shape of the lens permit the eye to focus for near or far vision, a process called **accommodation**. To focus on objects in the distance, the ciliary muscles relax, thereby thinning and flattening the lens. To focus on objects close by, the ciliary muscles contract so that the lens becomes more rounded.

Figure 16-1   The Eye

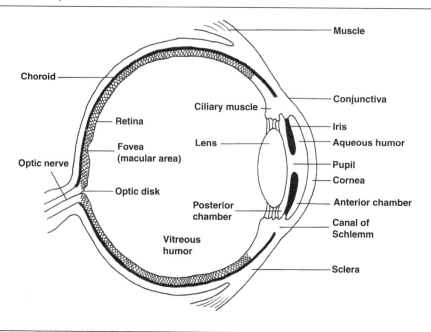

© Jane Tinkler Lamm.

Behind the lens is a larger cavity known as the *vitreous space*. This space is filled with a jelly-like, translucent substance called the *vitreous humor*, which helps to maintain the form and shape of the eyeball.

At the very back of the eye is the innermost coat of the eye, the *retina*. The retina contains two layers: (1) a pigmented layer that is fixed to the *choroid* and (2) an inner layer that contains special light-sensitive cells called rods and cones.

Rods are involved with detecting light and dark as well as shape and movement; they are primarily necessary for night vision and peripheral vision. Rods contain a derivative of vitamin A, called *rhodopsin*; this highly light-sensitive substance breaks down rapidly when exposed to light. The chemical process causes a reaction that activates the rods so that the eye adjusts to varying amounts of light, enabling individuals see in the dark—a process called **adaptation**.

Cones are involved primarily in daylight and color vision as well as in the perception of sharp visual detail. Most of the cones are located in a spot on the retina called the *macula*. The macula is the area of clearest *central vision*. The center of the macula, the fovea, contains no rods and is the area where vision is clearest in good light.

The *optic nerve* enters the back of the eye through an area called the *optic disk*. This area is sometimes called the *blind spot* because it does not contain light-sensitive cells. Light rays pass through the cornea, enter the pupil, pass through the lens, and register on the retina. Sensory cells of the retina receive light stimuli and convert them into electrical impulses. These electrical impulses are then transmitted to the optic nerve, which transmits them to fibers in the brain, which then carries the impulses to the *occipital lobe* of the brain, where they are interpreted.

After exiting the optic disk, the optic nerves from both eyes join together at the base of the brain just in front of the brain stem to form the *optic chiasm*. At this point, half of the nerve tracts from each eye cross over to the opposite side of the brain. Both eyes receive information from a combination of both visual fields. *Depth perception* requires that the brain receive input from both eyes. The portion of the visual field detected by both eyes, which is called the *binocular visual field*, is necessary for depth perception.

MEASURING VISION

The two most common types of testing for vision are *visual acuity testing* and *visual field testing* (Baloh & Jen, 2016). **Visual acuity** is defined as the sharpness of the visual image perceived. Visual acuity tests are used to measure the level of best vision and to measure the need for corrective lenses.

One standard test of visual acuity is the *Snellen test*. The chart used for this test contains a series of letters on nine lines of decreasing size. Lines are identified according to the distance from which they can be read by individuals with unimpaired vision. For example, individuals with normal visual acuity can read the top line of the chart at 200 feet and the last line at 20 feet. When taking the Snellen test, individuals view the chart at the equivalent of 20 feet and read the lines on the chart from the largest to the smallest. The results of the test are expressed as a fraction, with the numerator denoting the equivalent distance from the chart at which the individual being tested views the chart (20 feet) and the denominator denoting the distance from the chart at which a person with normal vision would be able to read the same line. Consequently, a visual acuity of 20/100 means that the individual being tested can see at 20 feet what a person with normal visual acuity could see at 100 feet; thus it indicates that the individual has a visual loss. A result of 20/10 means that the individual being tested has better than normal visual acuity, as he or she can see at 20 feet what individuals with normal visual acuity could see at 10 feet.

Visual field is defined as the size of the area that individuals can see without turning the head or moving the eyes. *Peripheral vision* (side vision) is measured by a curved device called a perimeter. Individuals look into the perimeter, and a test object is systematically moved from outside the peripheral field of vision toward the center until the individual indicates visualization of the object. *Central vision* (vision in the center of the visual field) is tested with the individual looking at a tangent screen, on which a test object is systematically moved across the screen. The individual's ability to see the object at certain points is then mapped, outlining his or her central field of vision.

TYPES OF VISUAL CONDITIONS

When any deviation of normal vision exists, individuals are considered to have a *visual impairment* or *loss*. Visual impairments or visual loss range from *mild visual loss* to *total loss of vision*. In general, conditions involving the eye that result in some type of visual loss can be categorized as follows:

- Refractory errors
- Difficulty with coordination of the eyes
- Opacities of the eye
- Damage to the eye due to injury
- Damage to the eye secondary to other conditions
- Degenerative changes of the eye

Visual loss may be temporary, reversible, progressive, or permanent. Such a loss may involve any of the following components of vision:

- *Central field of vision.* Individuals are able to see images in the periphery of the visual field but not images in the center.
- *Peripheral field of vision.* Individuals are able to see images in the center of the field of vision but not in the periphery *(tunnel vision).*
- *Night vision.* Individuals have difficulty seeing at night *(night blindness).*
- *Color vision.* Individuals have difficulty distinguishing colors, especially red and green. Rarely, individuals have complete lack of color vision with associated low visual acuity *(achromatopsia).*
- *Binocular vision.* Individuals have difficulty with the coordinated use of both eyes to produce a single image. As a result, they may have double vision (**diplopia**).

Severe visual loss can be defined as the inability to read ordinary newsprint even with the aid of glasses. When deviations of vision are great enough to cause *total loss of light perception,* the term **blindness** is used. Many individuals, however, have some usable vision; in such cases, special aids or devices can enable them to perform most tasks. When ordinary glasses, contact lenses, healthcare interventions, or surgery is unable to correct sight to the normal range, individuals are said to have *low vision* or to *be partially sighted*. The term **legal blindness** is used to describe both those who have total loss of vision and those who have some remaining visual function but who are significantly incapacitated by visual loss. In the United States, legal blindness has been defined as follows:

- Visual acuity not exceeding 20/200 or worse in the better eye with correcting lenses
- Central field of vision limited to an angle of 20 degrees or less

CONDITIONS OF THE EYE AND BLINDNESS

Refractive Errors

The most frequent cause for diminished visual acuity is refractive error (Yanoff & Cameron, 2016). *Refractive errors* occur when changes in the cornea, aqueous humor, lens, or vitreous humor prevent proper bending of light rays to converge on the retina. One type of refractive error, **myopia** (nearsightedness), results from elongation of the eyeball so that light rays focus on a point in front of the retina. Individuals with this condition have good visual acuity for close objects but difficulty seeing objects in the distance. The opposite type of refractive error is **hyperopia** (farsightedness), in which the eyeball is shorter than normal so that light rays focus on a point beyond the retina. Individuals with hyperopia have good visual acuity for objects in the distance but have difficulty focusing on things at close range. Another type of refractive error, **astigmatism**, results from irregularity of the shape of the cornea or (at times) the lens so that vision is distorted. Myopia, hyperopia, and astigmatism can occur at any age.

Presbyopia is a condition usually associated with aging in which gradual loss of accommodation occurs due to loss of elasticity of the lens and weakening of the ciliary muscle. Individuals with presbyopia must hold small objects and printed material farther and farther away to see clearly

because the eye can no longer adjust the shape of the lens to allow clear vision of close objects.

Refractory errors are usually remedied with corrective lenses or Lasik surgery (discussed later in the chapter). This procedure attempts to correct nearsightedness by altering the shape of the cornea, causing it to flatten.

Incoordination of the Eyes

To achieve good vision, both eyes must work together so that images from each eye can fuse into a single image. When this does not occur, vision may be impeded to some degree. Incoordination of the eyes can be the result of heredity, disease, or damage to the brain.

Nystagmus is a condition in which the eyes move involuntarily even though the gaze is fixed in one direction. The movement may occur in any direction but most often is horizontal. Nystagmus may be congenital, or it may develop later in life as a result of a neurological or other type of condition. Although this condition may cause little visual disturbance and be unapparent to the individual, it may be distracting and noticeable to others who are interacting with the person.

Strabismus is a condition in which there is misalignment of the two eyes so that the two eyes are not simultaneously oriented. The eyes may be crossed, both turning inward (*esotropia*), or there may be deviation of one or both eyes outward (*exotropia*). Strabismus is classified according to the type and magnitude of misalignment. When the eyes aren't simultaneously stimulated with the same visual image, only one eye will develop normally so that the other eye will not develop the ability to process visual images clearly and vision in that eye will be blurred (**amblyopia**) and binocular vision will be impaired (Yanoff & Cameron, 2016). Strabismus may result from unequal ocular muscle tone or from a neurological condition. It can often be corrected by surgery, by corrective lenses, by medications, or by a combination of the three interventions.

Suppression amblyopia (lazy eye) is a condition in which one eye does not develop good vision, usually because of strabismus. It is usually treated at an early age by placing a patch over the

eye. The eye usually responds to early intervention and the condition is corrected. If the condition is not managed early, however, it can persist for life.

Opacities of the Eye

Opacities of the Cornea

Any condition—including injuries, inflammation, or infection—that causes scarring or clouding of the cornea can cause permanent partial or total loss of vision. Because of its rich nerve supply, inflammation or injury to the cornea can cause severe pain. Prompt intervention for corneal inflammation can prevent subsequent formation of scar tissue that can interfere with vision. When clouding or scarring of the cornea causes permanent visual loss, *corneal transplant* (discussed later in this chapter) may be performed. When corneal transplant is successful, vision may be restored with few, if any, restrictions.

Cataracts

A **cataract** is a clouding or opacity of the lens of the eye. Although cataracts are a common cause of visual loss in older adults, they may also be congenital, inherited, the result of ocular trauma or inflammation, or associated with a variety of other conditions, such as diabetes. They can also be drug induced, such as occurs with use of high levels of certain types of steroids. Individuals with cataracts often describe their vision as looking through a cloudy pane of glass or through a fog.

Although cataracts are generally bilateral, they may form at different rates in each eye. As the lenses become more opaque, vision gradually diminishes. If cataracts are the result of injury, such as from radiation or a foreign object striking the lens, loss of vision occurs more rapidly. Cataracts associated with the aging process progress more slowly over time.

Because there is no way to return the lens to its normal transparency, management of cataracts involves removal of the lens and its replacement with an implant, with glasses, or with both. An intraocular prosthetic lens is typically inserted into the eye at the time of surgery; surgery is usually performed on an outpatient basis. Any implanted lens has a fixed focal length so that vision is clear at only one distance. Thus individuals who have undergone cataract surgery may continue to need corrective lenses, such as bifocals.

Injuries to the Eyes

Eye injuries are common and, in many cases, preventable. The most common type of eye injury is an injury to the cornea caused by a foreign body. Although often considered minor, these injuries can become serious if a scratch or abrasion to the cornea becomes infected or causes scarring, which can in turn impede vision. When the cornea becomes so scarred that vision is severely compromised, a surgical procedure—*corneal transplant* (**keratoplasty**)—may be performed (Gain et al., 2016). Corneal transplantation may also be performed when the shape of the cornea is distorted. Donor eyes for such procedures come from individuals who have recently died. During the surgical procedure, the opaque area of the cornea of the recipient's eye is replaced with the clear donor cornea, which is sutured into place. Because the cornea has no blood vessels, the healing process is slow. Although a corneal transplant can restore vision, graft rejection or need for a second operation may also occur.

More serious injuries to the eye include chemical burns, corneal laceration, and bleeding into the anterior chamber (*hyphema*), all of which can threaten vision. Chemical agents with an alkaline base (such as cleansing agents, fertilizers, plaster, and refrigerants) can penetrate the eye rapidly, leading to cell disruption and tissue death. Chemical agents with an acidic base cause protein coagulation in the eye so that penetration is not as rapid, but scarring of tissue can still result in visual loss. In both instances, immediate irrigation of the eye can decrease the amount of damage to the eye; nevertheless, emergency healthcare intervention should be sought immediately.

Some injuries involve puncture or laceration of the eye. Common causes of such trauma are work-related injuries, such as those associated with chopping or sawing wood, or chiseling or hammering metal on metal, such that a stray fragment of material causes the laceration. In some instances,

the puncture is so small that it may not be detected immediately. Puncture or laceration of the eye warrants immediate healthcare attention.

Deep penetration or laceration of the eye can cause bleeding into the anterior chamber. Blows to the head or the eye can also damage the internal structures of the eye, leading to hemorrhage, retinal damage, or other injury. When bleeding causes increased intraocular pressure, surgical intervention may be needed to relieve the pressure and prevent further damage from occurring.

Any injury to the eye necessitates a consultation with a healthcare provider. The degree of visual loss that results from an eye injury is not only a function of the extent and type of injury, but also, frequently, the consequence of the delay or promptness of emergency intervention.

Most eye injuries are preventable. Using appropriate eye protection for work, home, and sports activities that carry a risk of eye injury is one of the major forms of prevention.

Inflammation and Infections of the Eye

Conjunctivitis is an inflammation of the membrane that lines the eye, the conjunctiva. It may be caused by infectious organisms, such as viruses or bacteria, by allergy, or by chemicals. In most instances, conjunctivitis is easily managed, is self-limiting, and has no permanent effects. Conjunctivitis caused by virus is particularly contagious, however (Kuo, Espinosa, Forman, & Valsamakis, 2016). Some types of infectious conjunctivitis, such as *gonococcal conjunctivitis* and *trachoma,* can cause ulceration of the cornea and subsequent blindness (Yanoff & Cameron, 2016).

Uveitis is an inflammation of the *uveal tract* (iris, ciliary body, choroid). It may be associated with an autoimmune condition such as ankylosing spondylitis or *inflammatory bowel disease* or with either local or systemic infection, such as HIV. Manifestations may include decreased vision and sensitivity to light (**photophobia**). Uveitis is usually treated with topical medication.

Keratitis is an inflammation of the cornea that can be associated with a number of infectious conditions, including herpes simplex (*herpetic keratitis*), or can be a complication of HIV infection. Another common cause of keratitis is use of contacts. Microbial keratitis is associated with the use of contact lenses and is usually caused by improper handling of contact-lens equipment and solutions (Cheung, Nagra, & Hammersmith, 2016). The risk of infection decreases with proper hand washing and with use of the appropriate technique for cleaning and applying contact lenses.

Glaucoma

Glaucoma comprises a group of conditions that result in visual field loss; it is the leading cause of irreversible blindness (Yanoff & Cameron, 2016). Although glaucoma was once linked only to increased intraocular pressure, it is now recognized that, while increased intraocular pressure is a risk factor, this condition can be caused by a variety of conditions (Yanoff & Cameron, 2016). If glaucoma is left unmanaged, permanent damage to the optic nerve can result, causing blindness.

Glaucoma can occur either as a primary condition or secondary to other conditions such as diabetes, trauma, infection, prolonged use of medications such as steroids, and developmental ocular irregularities occurring in childhood. It develops when the amount of aqueous humor produced exceeds the amount being drained from the eye, much like a sink into which water continues to flow even though the drainage pipe is blocked, resulting in overaccumulation of water in the sink.

Several types of glaucoma are distinguished, with the broad categories being based on the reason for the problem with the aqueous flow.

Types of Glaucoma

Primary Open-Angle Glaucoma

The most common type of glaucoma, *primary open-angle glaucoma,* occurs when the outflow of aqueous humor from the eye is reduced. Because the outflow no longer equals the inflow, the amount of aqueous humor builds up, and pressure in the eye increases. Open-angle glaucoma generally progresses slowly over many years, producing no manifestations until the optic nerve is sufficiently damaged to reduce visual acuity and

visual field. At this point, the damage is irreversible. Vision loss generally begins with the loss of peripheral (*side*) vision so that individuals can see only straight ahead, as if looking through a tunnel (*tunnel vision*). Because loss of peripheral vision is often gradual, individuals may be unaware of the problem until the condition has reached an advanced stage. If left untreated, the field of vision continues to narrow until all vision is lost. There is no cure for chronic open-angle glaucoma. If the condition is detected early, however, appropriate healthcare intervention can control it for many years. Consequently, early detection is important.

Secondary Open-Angle Glaucoma

Secondary open-angle glaucoma is also due to reduced outflow of aqueous humor. In this case, however, it is caused by a preexisting or underlying condition such as trauma or steroid use.

Primary Angle-Closure Glaucoma

Primary angle-closure glaucoma develops much more rapidly than primary open-angle glaucoma and is a healthcare emergency. Manifestations include sudden severe pain, sharply decreased vision, nausea and vomiting, and rapid damage to the optic nerve with associated vision loss. Acute angle-closure glaucoma results from an abrupt blockage and obstruction of the canal of Schlemm so that aqueous humor rapidly accumulates in the anterior chamber of the eye. Although acute closed-angle glaucoma is much less common than chronic open-angle glaucoma, it must be managed immediately to prevent blindness. Initially it may be managed with medications, but laser surgery may also be necessary (Yanoff & Cameron, 2016).

Secondary Angle-Closure Glaucoma

Secondary angle-closure glaucoma can result from scarring that blocks the flow of the aqueous humor. Conditions such as diabetes, uncontrolled hypertension, and inflammation of the uveal tract because of other conditions can cause blockage of aqueous humor flow. Intervention usually involves surgery (Yanoff & Cameron, 2016).

Management of Glaucoma

Management of glaucoma is directed toward reducing the intraocular pressure either by decreasing the amount of aqueous humor produced or by increasing its outflow. This goal can be accomplished with medication or through surgical creation of a new pathway for drainage.

Medication for the management of glaucoma, whether eye drops or oral medication, must be used daily on a lifelong basis to control eye pressure and prevent further damage to vision. In any type of glaucoma, early detection and management are critical to prevent irreversible damage to the optic nerve and subsequent blindness. Regardless of the type of glaucoma, lifetime healthcare supervision is required. Most people with glaucoma can lead unrestricted lives without blindness if the condition is identified early and the intervention is followed as recommended.

Management of Primary Open-Angle Glaucoma

Primary open-angle glaucoma may be managed with medication in the form of eye drops alone to decrease production of aqueous humor, or eye drops in combination with oral medication that reduces pressure in the eye, thereby halting progression of the condition. Because eye drops are absorbed into the bloodstream, they may affect other body functions and cause systemic side effects ranging from generalized weakness to central nervous system, cardiovascular, and gastrointestinal manifestations.

Oral medications for the management of glaucoma work by decreasing production of aqueous humor. Like eye drops, these medications can affect other body functions and cause systemic side effects. Consequently, individuals who use eye drops or oral medication for management of glaucoma should be under continuing healthcare supervision—not only to monitor the condition itself but also to identify any side effects of the intervention.

When intraocular pressure cannot be successfully managed with medication, individuals with chronic open-angle glaucoma may have surgery, called *trabeculectomy,* to relieve pressure by creating

a passageway through which the aqueous humor can drain. Individuals may also need to continue using eye drops or oral medication after surgery to manage pressure; however, in some instances, surgery may eliminate the need for medication.

Management of Angle-Closure Glaucoma

Angle-closure glaucoma results from the forward displacement of the iris, which in turn narrows or obstructs the path for aqueous humor outflow. Eye drops called *miotics* constrict the pupil, thereby enlarging the drainage passageway and facilitating the outflow of aqueous humor. Because of the emergency nature of angle-closure glaucoma, oral or intravenous medication is given immediately to relieve pressure on the optic nerve temporarily. Once the pressure level has dropped to a safe level, a surgical procedure called *iridotomy* may be performed. Iridotomy removes a small section of the iris so that the aqueous humor can flow freely from the posterior chamber to the anterior chamber of the eye, preventing further eye damage by relieving built-up pressure. This procedure is often performed with a laser. Iridotomy may sometimes be performed prophylactically in the unaffected eye after an acute attack of glaucoma in the opposite eye.

Surgical procedures also include *trabeculectomy*, in which an alternative filtration path is created for aqueous drainage (Yanoff & Cameron, 2016).

Retinopathy

Any condition that affects the retina is termed a **retinopathy**. Retinopathies are often named for their cause. For example, *arteriosclerotic retinopathy* results from changes that occur in blood vessels in the retina because of arteriosclerosis. *Hypertensive retinopathy* results from changes that occur in these blood vessels because of high blood pressure. In both instances, management of the primary underlying condition can impede the progress of retinopathy.

The most common type of retinopathy, and the most common cause of blindness, is *diabetic retinopathy* (Crandall & Shamoon, 2016). Diabetic retinopathy is the result of damage to the retina and is a complication of diabetes mellitus. It is an important cause of visual loss that can have significant health, social, and financial consequences. Usually there are no manifestations in early stages of diabetic retinopathy. Given this fact, regular comprehensive eye examinations by a healthcare provider are important in helping to prevent visual loss.

Diabetic retinopathy causes visual loss in several ways. There are two categories of diabetic retinopathy:

- Nonproliferative diabetic retinopathy
- Proliferative diabetic retinopathy

Nonproliferative diabetic retinopathy is caused by changes in blood vessel walls, which allow fluids to leak into retinal tissue. At the same time, small blood vessels in the retina may become occluded, disturbing circulation in the retina so that some retinal tissue receives too little oxygen and dies (**necrosis**).

Proliferative diabetic retinopathy results from extensive areas of closure of the small blood vessels in the retina. As a result, retinal tissues receive too little oxygen (**ischemia**), a state to which the body responds by stimulating growth of new vessels. These new blood vessels are abnormally fragile and prone to bleeding, causing hemorrhage into the vitreous humor. The degree of vision loss depends on the amount of hemorrhage. Vessels may burst, filling the back of the eye with blood and resulting in significant visual loss. In some instances, scar tissue associated with new vessels can pull on the retina so that it detaches from underlying tissue.

Surgery may be performed to remove hemorrhage (**vitrectomy**), or laser intervention may be performed to stop the bleeding (Crandall & Shamoon, 2016). *Laser photocoagulation* is a procedure in which an intense beam of light from a laser is used to seal leaking blood vessels of the retina. The laser beam passes through the lens of the eye and vitreous fluid without harming the structures. It is then directed to a very precisely defined area to destroy fragile vessels prone to hemorrhage, or to affected areas of the retina characterized by additional proliferative vessel changes. Laser photocoagulation may help reduce the risk of visual loss, but it does not stop the progression of diabetic retinopathy. Such intervention is usually performed on an outpatient basis.

Retinal Detachment

With a detached retina, the sensory layer of the retina becomes separated from the pigmented (*choroid*) layer, depriving the sensory layer of its blood supply. A detached retina may result from a sudden blow to the head, a tumor in the choroid layer, retinal degeneration caused by other medical conditions, or hemorrhage associated with conditions such as diabetic retinopathy.

Manifestations may develop suddenly or slowly over time. Individuals may notice flashes of light or a loss of vision in different areas of the visual field, or they may experience a complete loss of vision in the affected eye. Usually there is no pain. Retinal detachment in one eye may indicate an increased risk of detachment in the other eye. Prompt identification of the condition and surgical intervention are essential to prevent permanent vision loss.

A surgical procedure called *scleral buckling* is sometimes used to treat retinal detachment. Scleral buckling mechanically restores contact of the retina with the choroid. The area of the sclera that lies over the retinal defect is depressed with an implant so that the choroid and the retina are pressed together. Another surgical procedure, *pars plana vitrectomy (PPV)* is also gaining popularity in the treatment of retinal detachment because it enhances the ability to view the retinal periphery so that additional breaks can be more easily identified (Lai et al., 2016).

Retinitis Pigmentosa

Retinitis pigmentosa is a hereditary, degenerative condition of the retina that causes slowly progressive loss of peripheral vision and, in many cases, blindness (Jones et al., 2016). Although progressive restriction of the visual field occurs as a result of the loss of peripheral vision, the remaining central visual acuity often remains good. Frequently the first manifestation of retinitis pigmentosa is difficulty with night vision (*night blindness*), which usually begins in late youth or early adulthood (Yanoff & Cameron, 2016). Although there is no cure for this condition, a number of assistive devices (as discussed later in the chapter) are available to enhance function.

Macular Degeneration

Degenerative changes in the macula—the part of the eye needed for seeing fine detail and central vision—results in a condition known as *macular degeneration.* Macular degeneration usually occurs after the age of 50, with no apparent cause, although some research has suggested genetic influence may play a role (Yanoff & Cameron, 2016). Painless loss of central visual acuity is usually slow, with visual distortion or blurring of vision being the first manifestation. Eventually individuals may develop a blind spot in the center of their field of vision, which gradually increases in size as the condition progresses. Given that warning signs of macular degeneration are absent until central vision is affected, the importance of regular eye examinations cannot be overemphasized.

Macular degeneration does not result in complete blindness, but it does destroy some or all of the sight in the center of the field of vision. Two types of macular degeneration are distinguished: dry form and wet form. Most cases of macular degeneration are *dry form,* which is characterized by **atrophy** (shrinkage) and thinning of the macula, causing mild to moderate vision loss. The type of macular degeneration called *wet form* is characterized by significant loss of vision due to abnormal blood vessel formation and hemorrhage.

Both types of macular degeneration demonstrate loss of central vision while peripheral vision remains intact. There is no cure for macular degeneration, although the use of assistive devices (as discussed later in the chapter) can help increase visual function. Activities such as reading may become difficult because of distortion of letters or because of parts of words or sentences in the center of the reading material that appear to be missing. Large print with black type and a white background may make reading easier, as may use of assistive devices such as a magnifying glass.

IDENTIFYING FUNCTIONAL CAPACITY OF THE EYE AND EYE CONDITIONS

Comprehensive Eye Examination

Comprehensive eye examinations usually include an external eye exam, which measures eye movements, size of the pupils, and pupils' ability to

react to light. The exam also includes testing of *visual acuity* and *visual field* as described earlier in this chapter. This part of the exam may be performed by an *optometrist* (a nonphysician who specializes in correcting refractive errors). An **ophthalmologist** (a physician who specializes in evaluation and management of conditions of the eye) may conduct tests of visual acuity as well, but also checks ocular movement, function of the optic nerve, and light reflexes of the pupils, and identifies any optic nerve pathology.

As part of the exam, individuals may be asked to view a chart through an instrument called a *refractor*. A light is then shined through the refractor onto the retina to estimate the eye's ability to focus on distant objects. Also included in a comprehensive eye exam is *tonometry* (described in the next subsection) and evaluation of the eyes' structures, including the cornea and iris, retina, and lens.

Tonometry

Tonometry is used to measure pressure in the eye in an effort to detect glaucoma. An instrument called a *tonometer* is placed directly on the cornea after the cornea has been anesthetized with drops of a local anesthetic. The tonometer measures the amount of pressure within the eye, making it possible to detect glaucoma.

Gonioscopy

For *gonioscopy*, a special contact lens that contains a mirror is gently placed on the eye. The ophthalmologist uses the lens like the periscope of a submarine to examine structures inside the eye. This test is especially helpful in detecting glaucoma.

Ophthalmoscopic Examination

A direct *ophthalmoscopic examination* is used to visualize the internal structures of the eye. It is performed with an instrument called an *ophthalmoscope* placed close to the eye. The ophthalmoscope contains a light that shines into the eye and magnifies internal structures so that any changes can be noted.

The internal structures of the eye may also be observed with a *slit lamp,* a type of microscope that is placed in front of the eye of the individual being tested. A finely focused slit of brilliant light is shined onto the eye to magnify details of the cornea, iris, and lens. A slit lamp is especially useful in identifying foreign bodies in the eye, evaluating corneal ulcers, and identifying cataracts.

Fluorescein Angiography

The purpose of *fluorescein angiography* is to detect changes in the blood vessels of the retina. A fluorescein dye is either taken orally or injected into the bloodstream. When the dye reaches the blood vessels of the eye, use of special ultraviolet light enables photography of the vessels for later study. Any swelling or leakage of the vessels of the retina is apparent on the photograph.

MANAGEMENT OF CONDITIONS OF THE EYE AND BLINDNESS

Eyeglasses and Contact Lenses

Corrective lenses may take the form of either eyeglasses or contact lenses. Because so many different types of eye conditions interfere with visual acuity, the type of corrective lenses needed is individually determined. The various types of lenses are recommended by an ophthalmologist or an optometrist. Unlike ophthalmologists, optometrists do not prescribe medications or perform surgery. Lenses for glasses are made by *opticians*, technicians who have been trained to fill optical recommendations. They grind and construct the lens according to the recommended specifications.

When visual acuity at several different distances must be corrected, *bifocal* or *trifocal* lenses may be used. Individuals with *bifocal lenses* use the lower portion of the lens for near vision and the upper portion for far vision. *Trifocal lenses* have three different divisions: one for *near vision*, one for *intermediate vision*, and one for *far vision*.

Although several types of contact lenses are available, the most commonly used are hard and soft corneal lenses. Hard lenses cover the central area of the cornea and are generally more durable. Soft lenses cover the entire cornea and are generally more fragile. Regardless of the type, contact lenses must be individually recommended and

constructed. They are helpful for counteracting a variety of visual conditions, but they do not correct astigmatism.

Generally, there are no complications associated with wearing eyeglasses. Contact lenses, however, can damage the eye if they are not worn and cared for properly. Not all people can or should wear contact lenses. Overwearing of hard lenses can cause corneal abrasions and associated complications. Individuals who do not use good hygienic practices when inserting the contact lens may develop an infection of the eye, in which case contact lenses should not be worn.

Refractive Surgery

Refractive surgery is an alternative to wearing glasses or contact lenses. Growing numbers of individuals are choosing to have this kind of surgery to correct their vision. Myopia (nearsightedness), hyperopia (farsightedness), and astigmatism (irregularity in the shape of the cornea or lens resulting in distortion of the visual image) are the conditions most commonly corrected with refractive surgery.

A number of surgical techniques have been developed for refractory conditions since the first surgery, *radial keratotomy (RK)*, was introduced in the late 1970s. Today, RK has largely been replaced with surgeries that are performed by *laser:*

- Photorefractive keratectomy (PRK)
- Laser-assisted *in situ* keratomileusis (LASIK)
- Laser epithelial keratomileusis (LASEK)

Before individuals have surgery, they are required to have a complete eye examination and must be free of cataracts, glaucoma, macular degeneration, or other eye conditions that would require healthcare intervention. In addition, surgery is contraindicated in the presence of certain health conditions, such as diabetes, pregnancy, autoimmune conditions, and conditions of the immune system. Although refractive surgery is effective in correcting myopia and hyperopia, there is always the potential for complications (Bitz, Hunt, & Cost, 2016). Consequently, individuals should be aware of both the risks and the benefits before undergoing the procedure, since the changes resulting from refractive surgery are generally permanent and irreversible.

Prosthetic Devices and Eye Replacement

When injury or other conditions necessitate removal of the eyeball, or when there is a congenital absence of the eye (**anophthalmia**), a prosthetic eye may be constructed and worn by the individual. The prosthetic eye, while not contributing to vision, serves a cosmetic purpose and can enhance the individual's body image and self-concept.

Assistive Devices and Low-Vision Aids

Assistive devices and low-vision aids should be part of an overall program to enhance the entire life of the individual, not just the individual's visual system. Types of devices used should be based on individual needs as well as willingness and ability to use them. The overall goal with utilization of low-vision aids is to recapture, strengthen, and maintain individuals' self-confidence in their ability to realize safe, independent functioning. These devices enhance remaining visual abilities through use of individually recommended adaptive equipment appropriate to the specific person's lifestyle.

Adaptive equipment for activities of daily living may include both *optical devices,* such as high-powered lenses and telescopic spectacles, and *nonoptical devices,* which are readily available and require no special training, such as large-print reading material or large-button telephones. *Low-technology devices* such as talking watches, raised-dot markings for oven dials, and templates for check signing require little training and may require only simple adaptations. Other devices, such as talking clocks and timers, writing guides, talking books, and audiocassettes, may similarly help to meet the communication needs of individuals with visual loss.

High-technology devices are more sophisticated electronically and may require specialized training. Examples of these devices include video magnifiers and computer systems. Video magnifiers use closed-circuit television and can magnify a printed page on a television screen for reading. Numerous computer software programs and adaptive devices can be used to enlarge printed materials or to convert print into synthetic speech output. These devices include large-print computer monitors, programs that enlarge print size on the screen,

printers that modify font size, synthetic speech software programs with external audio units, and typewriters equipped with synthetic speech output that interface with personal computer units. Speech packages allow for adjustments in the rate of speech and the tone of voice to meet the needs of the individual user.

One of the best-known tactile aids is *Braille.* Hard-copy Braille uses the familiar raised-dot method, whereas soft-copy Braille is stored on electromagnetic tape and presented as patterns by a set of pins that represent a Braille dot. Individuals place their fingers on display units through which the pins protrude. Another type of product is *refreshable Braille displays*—electronic devices that are used to read information sent from a computer to a monitor. This kind of device produces Braille output on a Braille display.

Another type of tactile aid is an electromechanical vibratory system. With this system, a small camera is passed over a line of print, and each printed letter is then displayed as a pattern of vibrations that the individual can feel with the finger.

A number of professionals recommend and provide training in the use of optical, nonoptical, low-technology, and high-technology aids. They include occupational therapists, low-vision specialists, orientation and mobility (O&M) instructors, rehabilitation teachers, and adaptive technology specialists.

The key to successful use of any assistive or adaptive device is involvement of the individual who will ultimately use the device in selecting it, to ensure that the device meets user requirements, capabilities, and needs. Customization of devices to accommodate special needs of individuals ensures that the device can be integrated into the daily routine, helps individuals view the device positively, and helps them use the device to best enhance their own functional capacity.

Orientation and Mobility Training

The goal of orientation and mobility training is to enable individuals with a visual loss to achieve as much mobility as possible according to their capabilities and desires and to recapture, strengthen, and maintain self-reliance for safe and independent function. Orientation and mobility specialists provide training that helps individuals know where they are in relation to their surroundings and learn how to safely navigate within their environment. In particular, O&M specialists help individuals to move independently indoors and outdoors, and in familiar or in unfamiliar environments; they also provide training in the use of public transportation, use of canes, and use of mobility lights or electronic travel aids. Through individualized training, persons with visual loss learn to orient themselves to their environment by using compensatory strategies including illumination techniques and use of contrast, magnification, memorization of location, and auditory and tactile feedback. Compensatory strategies may involve such things as listening for the direction of traffic, arm and hand positioning for guidance along walls and railings, and systematic search techniques for dropped or lost objects.

Mobility Aids

Various types of *mobility aids*, such as sighted guides, guide dogs, canes, and electronic devices, are available to help individuals with visual loss move about the environment more freely. Orientation and mobility specialists can help determine the preferred system for individuals.

Guide dogs not only increase the mobility of the individual with a visual loss but can also provide protection and companionship. These dogs undergo intensive training before being matched with the individual to whom they are assigned. They are taught how to respond to various commands as well as how to deal with curbs, traffic, and other potential hazards in the environment. The individual and the dog train together for a number of weeks to become an effective team. Not all individuals are able to use a guide dog, and some individuals prefer to use other forms of mobility aids, such as a long cane. In most instances, individuals should be cane proficient before using a guide dog.

The most common mobility aid is the *prescription* or *long cane*, which is usually made of aluminum or fiberglass. An O&M specialist recommends the cane according to the individual's height, length of stride, and comfort. The cane is used in a systematic way. The person moves the cane rhythmically in an arc in front of the body to ensure a safe space for the next step. Although

this strategy provides some protection, it does not account for objects above the waist that are in the individual's path. In an attempt to compensate for this type of obstacle, some canes have tone-emitting radar units that make a sound with a differential pitch for the direction and height of obstacles in front of the individual. Some individuals prefer collapsible, folding, or telescopic canes, which are less obtrusive and can be collapsed and slipped into a purse or under a chair when not in use.

Electronic travel aids may also be used. These devices emit light beams or ultrasound waves. When the light beam or ultrasound waves hit an object in the individual's path, the device vibrates or emits a sound.

FUNCTIONAL IMPLICATIONS IN CONDITIONS OF THE EYE AND BLINDNESS

Functional Implications for Individuals Who Are Partially Sighted

Personal and Psychosocial Issues

Individuals who have low vision or who are partially sighted do not quite fit into the category of either the blind or the sighted population. Consequently, they often have special needs that are overlooked. Adjustment to vision loss is not necessarily correlated with the degree of vision remaining. Individuals with partial sight do not have fewer adjustment issues than individuals who are totally blind and, in fact, may have more adaptation difficulties because their partial sight presents an ambiguous situation for others. In addition, individuals with partial sight may exhibit high levels of anxiety because they may be unsure about whether or when they will lose more of their residual vision.

Because partially sighted individuals have some remaining sight, they may attempt to "pass" as a sighted person to avoid potential rejection or avoidance by others. They may deny their condition altogether and associate only with sighted persons in an attempt to be accepted by mainstream society. Some may make excuses for awkward behavior or attempt in other ways to conceal the fact that they have low vision. They may refuse to use low-vision aids, such as a cane, for mobility or reject suitable orientation and mobility training.

In extreme cases, they may engage in dangerous activities such as operating a motor vehicle even though legally, due to their degree of vision loss, they are not eligible to do so.

Activities and Participation

The social community often lacks understanding of the true nature and extent of vision loss so that individuals with low vision are ridiculed in public for appearing to see more than would be expected by a person with vision loss (Vance, 2000). Individuals with partial sight may be viewed as malingerers by family and acquaintances because they can see some things but not others. Even when individuals attempt to function with appropriate assistive devices, they may be suspected of denying their condition by those who expect individuals with visual loss to be dependent and isolated.

Although individuals with moderate to mild visual loss may carry on much of their personal business with low-vision aids, some activities are more restricted. For instance, people often view the ability to drive as very important in the maintenance of independence. This perception makes it extremely difficult for individuals who are losing their vision to give up this activity. Furthermore, by its very nature, the gradual loss of vision creates a time period in which the decision to stop driving is particularly difficult. The emphasis on self-care and independence for individuals with partial vision must be tempered with judgment and concern for the welfare of the individual as well as the welfare of others.

Functional Implications for Individuals with Severe Vision Loss or Blindness

Personal and Psychosocial Issues

Severe vision loss often precipitates a sense of fear and reduced personal competence, which may result in isolation and social withdrawal. Visual loss may be present at birth, or it may develop suddenly or slowly at any time in an individual's life. Often vision loss follows an unpredictable and uncontrollable progression. Adjustment to loss of vision can depend on many factors, including the degree of loss and the age at which the individual experiences that loss.

Persons who have been blind since birth have not, for example, had the opportunity to learn concepts such as distance, depth, proportion, and color. Because of their lack of visual experiences in their environment, such as the observation of tasks or behaviors of others, concepts that sighted individuals often take for granted must be learned by other means. This adaptive learning of tasks then becomes a natural part of their development so that adjustment to visual limitations is incorporated into their self-perception and daily activities as a normal part of growing up.

In contrast, individuals who develop loss of vision later in life are able to draw on visual experiences in the environment as a frame of reference for physical concepts, but may find it more difficult to accept blindness than those who have never had vision. Individuals who lose vision later in life are required to make certain modifications of self-perception as a result of their physical changes and subsequent need for restructuring of daily activities. Persons who are newly blind may experience grief and despair over the loss of visual function. They may become dependent, feel insecure in new situations, and perceive a marked loss of autonomy. Some may become reluctant to interact in social situations because they want to avoid the awkwardness of initial attempts at social interactions. Loss of control over standard methods of initiating conversations (e.g., eye contact and other nonverbal cues), noticeable discomfort or overhelpfulness of sighted persons, and prolonged gaps in conversations may lead newly blind individuals to believe that they are being watched or ignored.

Accommodation to visual loss or blindness is multifaceted. Individuals with a visual loss must adjust their self-concept and personal goals to take into account the realistic limits imposed by vision loss. They must develop adaptive skills and new abilities, and they must draw on personal resources to adjust to their new situation. Individuals who experience traumatic blindness (i.e., a sudden loss of partial or total vision because of an internal or external event, such as a head injury, direct injury to the eye, or chemical burn) may have to cope not only with the sudden loss of vision, but also with insurance company representatives, attorneys, and other legal and bureaucratic aspects surrounding the circumstance of their condition. In these situations, family members may also react to the situation with responses ranging from anger to revenge to overprotectiveness.

Even when individuals with severe visual loss function independently for the most part, they may be dependent on assistance from others in some activities. The greater dependence associated with a severe visual loss or blindness may be a source of conflict and may negatively affect formerly close relationships, especially if others have misperceptions or misunderstanding about the nature of the visual loss. In other instances, individuals, in an attempt to demonstrate self-reliance and independence, may reject help from family and friends, causing alienation and social isolation. Counseling individuals to understand sighted people's reactions may facilitate social interactions and enhance development of constructive and realistic interactions.

Activities and Participation

Vision is important for many activities of daily living. Individuals with little or no vision must learn new techniques for carrying out routine activities of self-care and mobility. They must orient themselves to the home environment so that they may move freely from room to room without risk of injury. Family members can contribute to the individual's mobility within the home by never moving furniture within a room without informing the individual and leaving doors either completely open or completely closed after informing the individual of the plan so that he or she does not bump into a partially open door.

At first, tasks such as pouring water into a glass without spilling it, buttering bread, and cutting meat may seem insurmountable for the individual with severe visual loss. Over time, however, most people with visual loss learn to prepare their meals and dine independently once they have been oriented to the location of food, tableware, and cooking utensils. Cooking can be learned through techniques such as the systematic placement of cooking equipment and utensils and special labeling on cans, frozen foods, oven dials, and other items.

Through training, individuals with severe vision loss or blindness are gradually able to assume

personal responsibility for self-care. Rehabilitation teachers provide in-home training in skills of daily living. Activities such as bathing, combing the hair, shaving, applying make-up, and dressing in a coordinated fashion can all be performed independently through skills training and systematic organization and labeling of personal items.

Although individuals with severe visual conditions or blindness may need someone else's help to read a bill, a check, an invoice, or a personal letter, in some instances documents or forms can be translated into Braille, thereby enabling the individual to have more independence and privacy.

Outside the home, individuals with severe visual loss or blindness can learn techniques of mobility in new environments with the use of a cane or guide dog. Through these techniques, individuals are able to travel to work or to other destinations of their choice. They can also learn methods of carrying money so as to discriminate between bills as well as ways to discriminate between different coins. Individuals can continue to enjoy leisure activities including many outdoor activities, such as swimming, hiking, and fishing. With special adaptive procedures, even bicycling is possible. A number of sports organizations, such as American Blind Bowlers Association, United States Blind Golfers Association, and Beep Ball Teams have also been formed for individuals who are blind.

Social Interaction

Much social interaction and communication are mediated by watching nonverbal actions and reactions of others, such as posture, facial expression, or movement. The absence of these visual cues can place individuals with visual loss at a disadvantage in a social setting, unless all concerned have developed increased awareness and sensitivity to the individual's inability to observe nonverbal cues.

Major obstacles to the effective functioning of individuals with visual loss in social environments include social stereotyping and attitudes of sighted individuals toward individuals with severe visual loss or blindness. Many sighted individuals view individuals who have severe visual loss or who are blind as helpless and dependent. Others believe the myth that people

who have severe visual loss or who are blind develop extraordinary powers of hearing and touch to compensate for the loss of vision rather than recognizing that these individuals have merely learned skills that enable them to be more effective in interpreting their environment. Negative attitudes or stereotypical views held by friends, employers, and casual acquaintances may be based on discomfort with blindness or lack of experience with individuals who have severe vision loss or are blind. Regardless of the cause, these negative attitudes can have a major impact on individuals with severe visual loss or blindness, and can limit their potential especially if they conform to social expectations. Developing an understanding of sighted persons' discomfort, misperceptions, and misinformation can provide the individual with severe vision loss or blindness with a basis for formulating proactive strategies for problem solving, perspective taking, and social inferences, which can ultimately result in fuller social integration.

Sexuality

Although visual loss does not affect sexual activity directly, loss of vision may impinge on self-esteem and self-confidence, which in turn can affect sexual relationships. In addition, loss of visual information significantly affects interpersonal communication, such picking up visual cues from a partner that indicate receptiveness to sexual activity, or seeing the facial expressions or other nonverbal communication that is an integral part of sexual relationships.

Establishing relationships in the sighted world also depends to a great extent on determination of physical attractiveness and on nonverbal cues, such as body language, eye contact, or facial expression. Individuals with severe vision loss or blindness require more direct contact or interaction to assess the initial attractiveness of an individual to them, relying on features of personality or verbal interaction rather than physical cues observed visually. In some instances, due to misperceptions and stereotyping, individuals with severe vision loss or blindness are not permitted the same types of information or education about sexual issues as are

sighted persons. Information about relationships normally developed through visual modeling and observation may not be experienced by individuals with severe visual loss or blindness, especially those who have lacked sight since an early age. Under these circumstances, it may be necessary to teach appropriate skills and social behaviors that are generally learned by observation by sighted individuals.

Family Interaction

Although attitudes of family members are important factors in adjustment to most health conditions, these attitudes appear to exert an especially powerful influence on the adjustment of individuals with severe vision loss or blindness. How families react to individuals with visual loss depends on the particular family's patterns of belief, feelings, and resources. When family members believe that the demands being placed on them exceed their available resources so that their resources are overtaxed, stress and strain may develop. Conversely, if families are able to meet the major needs of their members so that they can pursue realistic goals, they will be better able to cope successfully.

Family attitudes during rehabilitation may determine individuals' motivation to learn and accept major changes in lifestyle. During this time, overprotective or overly anxious families who encourage dependency may prevent or impede rehabilitation. In contrast, families who foster positive attitudes and demonstrate respect and recognition of the individual with severe vision loss or blindness are a major asset to rehabilitation.

GENERAL VOCATIONAL ISSUES IN VISION LOSS AND BLINDNESS

Persons who are blind or who have low vision are underrepresented in the competitive labor market (Eckert et al., 2015). The degree of the vocational impact of a condition that affects vision depends on the nature of the employment, the type and extent of visual loss, and the life stage at which the visual loss occurs. Many individuals with partial vision are able to continue in their field of employment with special adaptive or low-vision aids; others must learn new job skills. When visual loss is progressive, ongoing evaluation and planning for decreasing visual acuity should be part of the rehabilitation plan.

In addition to the manifestations of a specific eye condition, barriers to employment may include deficits in skills or education, lack of work experience, lack of job preparation skills, and lack of motivation or information. Paid reader support may be necessary to gather information about job openings or training opportunities. In other instances, lack of direction or low expectations of family and friends may make it more difficult to continue looking for work or preparing for employment.

In addition to the challenges posed by on-the-job activity, the ability to get to and from work may be a barrier to employment. If individuals are no longer able to drive and no public transportation is available, suitable alternatives for transportation to and from work must be devised. Unreliable transportation can be a major barrier to obtaining and maintaining employment.

For individuals with low vision, level of visual acuity—and, therefore, the individual's ability to resolve visual detail—must be considered in employment in which reading or seeing fine visual detail is required. Accommodations may involve making the image larger through some form of magnification or using an optical device to make the object appear larger. Individuals with low vision may need additional lighting to enhance vision; however, lighting that produces glare can be detrimental to individuals' visual efficiency and comfort. Individuals with visual field deficits may have difficulty with peripheral or central vision. Those with peripheral vision problems may have difficulty detecting objects around them. In addition, peripheral field deficiency can interfere with mobility, and with performing near-vision tasks such as reading or writing. Central vision loss affects individuals' straight-ahead vision, with probably concurrent reduction in visual acuity. Consequently, reading and tasks requiring visualization of detail will be affected. The degree of

functional consequence depends on the size and location of the loss of vision.

CASE STUDY

Ms. L. is a 42-year-old computer programmer who lost her vision as a result of diabetic retinopathy. Ms. L. lives with her husband and teenage son in a small Midwestern community. There is no public transportation available. Ms. L. had been commuting by car 25 miles to her place of employment. You have been asked to begin working with Ms. L. on her rehabilitation plan.

1. Which factors and issues would you consider regarding Ms. L.'s loss of vision and her employment?
2. Which specific assistive devices or other accommodations might Ms. L. require?
3. Which types of services might be helpful to Ms. L. to assist her in reaching her optimal level of independence?

REFERENCES

Baloh, R. W., & Jen, J. (2016). Neuro-opthalmology. In L. Goldman & A. I. Schafer (Eds.), *Goldman-Cecil medicine,* (25th ed., pp. 2571–2579). Philadelphia, PA: Elsevier Saunders.

Bitz, J. B., Hunt, D. J., & Cost, A. A. (2016). Post-refractive surgery complications and eye disease, active component, U.S. Armed forces 2005–2014. *Monthly Surveillance Monthly Report, 23*(5), 2–11.

Cheung, N., Nagra, P., & Hammersmith, K. (2016). Emerging trends in contact lens-related infections. *Current Opinions in Opthalmology, 27*(4), 327–332.

Crandall, J., & Shamoon, H. (2016). Diabetes mellitus. In L. Goldman & A. I. Schafer (Eds.), *Goldman-Cecil medicine,* (25th ed., pp. 1527–1548). Philadelphia, PA: Elsevier Saunders.

Eckert, K. A., Carter, M. J., Lansingh, V. C., Wilson, D. A., Furtado, J. M., Frick, K. D., & Resnikoff, S. (2015). A simple method for estimating the economic cost of productivity loss due to blindness and moderate to severe visual impairment. *Opthalmic Epidemiology, 22*(5), 349–355.

Gain, P., Julliene, R., He, Z., Aldossary, M., Acquarti, S., Cognasse, F., & Thuret, G. (2016). Global survey of corneal transplantation and eye banking. *Journal of the American Medical Association Opthalmology, 134*(2), 167–173.

Jones, B. W., Pfeiffer, R. L., Ferrell, W. D., Watt, C. B., Marmor, M., & Marc, R. E. (2016). Retinal remodeling in human retinitis pigmentosa. *Experimental Eye Research, 150,* 149–165. doi:10.1016/j.exer.2016.03.018

Kuo, I. C., Espinosa, C., Forman, M., & Valsamakis, A. (2016). A polymerase chain reaction-based algorithm to detect and prevent transmission of adenoviral conjunctivitis in hospital employees. *American Journal of Ophthamology, 163,* 38–44.

Lai, F. H., Lo, E. C., Chan, V. C., Breien, M., Lo, W. L., & Young, A. L. (2016). Combined pars plana vitrectomy-scleralbuckle versus pars plana vitrectomy for proliferative vitreoretinopathy. *International Ophthalmology, 36*(2), 217–224.

Yanoff, M., & Cameron, J. D. (2016). Diseases of the visual system. In L. Goldman & A. I. Schafer (Eds.), *Goldman-Cecil medicine,* (25th ed., pp. 2556–2573). Philadelphia, PA: Elsevier Saunders.

Hearing Loss and Deafness

STRUCTURE AND FUNCTION OF THE AUDITORY AND VESTIBULAR SYSTEMS

The system related to hearing and the system related to equilibrium and spatial orientation are closely linked; thus both must be taken into account when considering conditions that affect hearing. Conditions that affect hearing often also affect equilibrium; likewise, conditions that affect equilibrium often affect hearing (Baloh & Jen, 2016).

- The *auditory system* is involved with the detection of sound waves and, consequently, with hearing.
- The *vestibular system* is involved with body equilibrium, orientation, and balance.

THE AUDITORY SYSTEM

The Ear

The ear consists of three divisions: the outer, middle, and inner ear (see **Figure 17-1**). Its components are part of both the auditory and vestibular systems.

The Outer Ear

The *outer ear* includes the *pinna* (auricle) and the *external ear canal* (external auditory meatus). The pinna—the visible portion of the ear—is made up of elastic cartilage covered with skin. Its function is to collect sound waves and conduct them to the *eardrum* (tympanic membrane). The external ear canal is approximately 1 inch long and extends from the opening of the ear to the eardrum. It contains special glands that produce **cerumen** (earwax), which protects the ear against the entry of foreign material.

The Middle Ear

The *tympanic membrane* separates the outer ear from the middle ear. The *middle ear*, also called the *tympanic cavity,* is an air-filled cavity connected to the throat by the *eustachian tube,* which helps equalize air pressure on both sides of the tympanic membrane. Changes of atmospheric pressure, such as occur with change in altitude, necessitate equalization of air pressure in the middle ear. When the ears "pop" during altitude changes, it indicates that the eustachian tube has allowed air in the middle ear to equalize with the pressure outside the head. When this does not occur, discomfort can result. The eustachian tube, which is normally collapsed in adults, opens with yawning or swallowing, allowing air pressure on both sides of the tympanic membrane to equalize. Another pathway connects the tympanic cavity to the *mastoid air cells* within the *mastoid process* of the temporal bone.

The middle ear lies between the eardrum and the inner ear. It contains three small movable bones called *ossicles*, which transfer sound vibrations from the eardrum to the inner ear. These small bones—the *malleus,* the *incus*, and the *stapes*—are connected by small ligaments and are attached to the tympanic membrane by the handle of the

Figure 17-1   The Ear

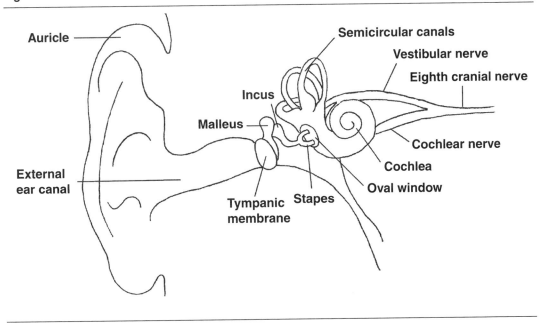

© Jane Tinkler Lamm.

malleus with the footplate of the stapes connected to a thin membrane called the *oval window*, which connects to the inner ear. Also connecting the middle ear with the inner ear is an opening called the *round window.*

The Inner Ear

The *inner ear (labyrinth)* is a fluid-filled cavity that lies deep within the temporal bone of the skull. It is important not only for hearing (as part of the *auditory system*), but also for maintaining body balance and equilibrium (as part of the *vestibular system*). Contained within the inner ear is the *cochlea*, which is part of the *auditory system*, and the *semicircular canals*, which are part of the *vestibular system*. The cochlea has a snail-like appearance and contains tiny hair cells within the *organ of Corti*, the structure responsible for hearing. Movement of fluid within the inner ear stimulates nerve endings in both the auditory and vestibular systems. Impulses from both systems are converted into nerve impulses and transmitted from the inner ear to the brain by the *eighth cranial nerve,* sometimes called the *acoustic* or

auditory nerve. This nerve contains two branches: the *cochlear nerve branch,* which conducts sensory information about sound, and the *vestibular nerve branch,* which conducts impulses regarding body balance and movement.

Mechanism of Hearing

Sound waves enter the external ear and move through the external ear canal, striking the eardrum and causing it to vibrate. The vibration of the eardrum first moves the malleus, which transmits the vibration to the incus; in turn, the incus transmits the vibration to the stapes. The chained movement of the malleus, incus, and stapes conducts sound waves from the eardrum to the oval window, which connects to the inner ear. The stapes' vibration in the oval window activates the fluid in the inner ear, stimulating the tiny hair cells in the organ of Corti. The movement of these hair cells stimulates the nerve endings located around their bases to transmit impulses to the *cochlear nerve*, which carries the impulses to the *auditory center of the brain,* where they are perceived and interpreted as sound.

Sense of Hearing

The sense of hearing comprises the neural perception of *sound energy* and is based on transmission of external sound to the structures of the outer, middle, and inner ear; the nerves to the brain; and portions of the brain involved in processing acoustic information. Vibrations known as *sound waves* produce sound. Sound is characterized by both *pitch* (tone) and *intensity* (loudness). Individuals with hearing loss can have diminished hearing with regard to pitch, intensity, or both.

Pitch

Pitch, or tone, is determined by the frequency of vibrations of sound waves. The faster the vibrations (*frequency*), the higher the pitch. Frequencies are measured in *hertz (Hz)*, or cycles per second. Hearing loss related to frequency results in a distortion of sound so that individuals may be unable to differentiate between many of the sounds of speech. For example, words with similar sounds, such as *cat* and *rat,* may be easily confused. Increasing the volume does not improve the quality of sound or make words clearer if this type of hearing loss exists.

Intensity

Intensity, or loudness of sounds, depends on the *amplitude* of sound waves. The greater the amplitude, the louder the sound. Loudness is measured in *decibels (db)*. Hearing loss related to intensity involves more difficulty in hearing because of reduction in sound volume. With this type of hearing loss, *amplification* of sound may improve hearing. In instances where individuals have hearing loss related to both frequency and intensity, increasing volume alone will not improve overall hearing.

THE VESTIBULAR SYSTEM AND EQUILIBRIUM

The vestibular structures in the ear, which are concerned with maintaining equilibrium, include the *semicircular canals* and a small rounded chamber at their base called the *vestibule.* The semicircular canals contain nerve endings through which balance is controlled. Like the organ of Corti, they contain numerous hair cells that project into the fluid of the inner ear. The movement of the head sets this fluid in motion and moves the hair cells, stimulating the nerve endings, which then transmit the impulses to the vestibular nerve. These impulses are carried to the portion of the brain involved with maintaining equilibrium and coordinating movement.

The *vestibular system* contributes to the sense of balance and equilibrium. Although conditions of the vestibular system can be associated with conditions that affect hearing, such as Meniere's disease (discussed later in the chapter), manifestations related to the vestibular system can also exist with other conditions, as described in this section. No matter what the cause, disturbances of the vestibular system can cause manifestations that interfere with individuals' daily function and can be severely incapacitating.

One of the classic manifestations associated with vestibular dysfunction is vertigo. **Vertigo** is an illusory sense of motion, usually described as a spinning sensation, and often thought of in terms of dizziness. Although vertigo can be associated with many conditions, it is always related to the body's vestibular system. Episodes of vertigo can last from a few seconds to days.

Conditions of the Vestibular System—Vertigo

Physiologic Vertigo

Physiologic vertigo is a term used to describe conditions such as *motion sickness, space sickness,* or *height vertigo* in which there are no other health conditions causing manifestations. Motion-induced vertigo may also be experienced when an individual returns to stationary ground after prolonged exposure to motion, such as on a ship. This condition, called *mal de débarquement syndrome,* is usually temporary but can also last for months, and sometimes years (Baloh & Jen, 2016).

Benign Paroxysmal Positional Vertigo

Benign paroxysmal positional vertigo (BPPV) is the most common cause of vertigo and results from degenerative debris in the form of free-floating calcium carbonate crystals that enter the semicircular canal (Baloh & Jen, 2016). Floating debris in the

fluid causes an illusion of motion, with subsequent vertigo and nausea. Vertigo in BPPV is brought on by head movements or changing of position. Consequently, individuals with BPPV may be at increased risk for falls.

Intervention consists of *particle-repositioning procedures,* in which the individual's head is rotated in sequence into different positions, or habituation exercises that reteach the brain so that vertigo does not occur when the brain is exposed to stimuli from the debris (Kinne & Leafman, 2015).

Vestibular Neuritis

Vestibular neuritis (inflammation of the vestibular nerve), a condition of the inner ear, can cause vertigo that lasts for days or weeks and is extremely incapacitating. During the episode, individuals become nauseous with vomiting and feel a violent spinning of their surroundings. The cause of vestibular neuronitis is unknown. Vertigo can also be associated with head injury or other neurological conditions such as brain tumor or multiple sclerosis.

Meniere's Disease

In addition to affecting hearing, Meniere's disease (discussed later in the chapter) is also responsible for causing vertigo.

Other Conditions Causing Vertigo

Vertigo can also be caused by *infection* in the inner ear, *vascular insufficiency* (lack of blood supply to parts of the vestibular system usually related to conditions such as arteriosclerosis), tumors (such as *acoustic neuroma* or *meningioma),* and conditions affecting the central nervous system such as *multiple sclerosis* or brain injury.

Identification of Conditions of the Vestibular System

Because vertigo often follows an episodic course, its cause may be difficult to identify. Individuals who experience vertigo or who have problems with balance are frequently tested for inner ear and *sensorineural* conditions related to vestibular function. These tests are usually performed either by an audiologist or by another health professional.

In one test of vestibular nerve function, known as the *caloric test,* either cold or hot water is introduced into the external auditory canal. The water stimulates fluids within the inner ear, which in turn stimulate the vestibular nerve. The introduction of the water into the ear creates a reflex response of the eye called *nystagmus* (involuntary horizontal eye movement). By monitoring the direction of eye movements, the audiologist or health professional can determine the origin of the dizziness and identify nerve damage if present.

A test called *nystagmography* may be used to test oculomotor control by inducing and recording eye movements. This test is helpful in identifying the location of the source of vertigo in the vestibular system.

Management of Conditions of the Vestibular System

Management of vertigo—the main manifestation of conditions of the vestibular system—consists of managing the underlying cause when possible. Medications may be used for acute episodes of vertigo, but are not appropriate for chronic use. Individuals with chronic vertigo may be given vestibular rehabilitation exercises to help them compensate for loss of vestibular function (Baloh & Jen, 2016).

HEARING LOSS AND DEAFNESS

Disruption of any part of the hearing system can result in hearing loss. Hearing loss can affect both the *volume* and the *clarity* of sound. Some individuals have hearing loss that results in reduced *hearing sensitivity;* they may be unable to hear soft speech or may have difficulty hearing speech when background noise is present. Other individuals have difficulty with *speech discrimination;* even though volume is adequate, they may be unable to clearly hear certain phonetic elements of speech (for example, consonants such as "x" and "s") because they occur at frequencies where hearing loss is present. Individuals can have both sensitivity loss and discrimination deficit at different degrees.

Any degree of hearing loss is considered a *hearing impairment. Hard of hearing* refers to hearing loss in which individuals have mild to

moderate hearing loss and usually have difficulty understanding conversational speech through the ear with or without a hearing aid. *Deafness* refers to severe to profound hearing loss in which there is the inability to understand conversational speech through the ear, even with amplification. The degree of hearing loss is commonly defined on the basis of the audiogram described later in this chapter and may be classified as:

- Partial
- Total
- Temporary
- Permanent
- Mild
- Profound

Classification of Hearing Loss

In addition to the degree, as described above, hearing loss is classified based on the *type and location* responsible for hearing loss and the *age of onset*.

Type and Location of Hearing Loss

Type and location of the loss are classified as one of four types:

- Conductive
- Sensorineural
- Mixed
- Central

Conductive Hearing Loss

Conductive hearing loss occurs when there is damage, obstruction, or malformation in the external or middle ear, which prevents sound waves from reaching the cochlea in the inner ear. In many cases, correction of the underlying problem can restore diminished hearing. Conductive loss may result from the following causes:

- Buildup of earwax in the ear canal
- A foreign object in the ear
- Infection of the middle ear (**otitis media**)
- Hardening of the small bones in the ear that are important for conducting sound (**otosclerosis**)
- Trauma to the outer or middle ear
- Congenital malformations of the middle or outer ear
- Tumors of the outer or middle ear

Conductive hearing loss is a mechanical problem that alters the loudness of sound but does not reduce its clarity because the inner ear, where sound is "processed," is not compromised. Sometimes conductive hearing loss cannot be corrected, so hearing aids may be used to amplify sound and restore normal loudness. These types of hearing losses are generally of mild to moderate degree. Individuals with mild to moderate conductive hearing loss usually have good success with hearing aids if use of such devices is necessary.

Sensorineural Hearing Loss

Sensorineural hearing loss results from damage or irregularities of the inner ear or the auditory nerve and can lead to total deafness. This type of loss involves damage to the hair cells of the inner ear, which in turn interferes with the reception of nerve impulses. In some cases, the hair cell function of the cochlea is unaffected; rather, the cause of hearing loss is related to the nerve transmission pathway to the brain. With sensorineural loss, hearing is affected not only in terms of loudness but also in terms of pitch or clarity. Individuals may perceive no sound; if sound is perceived, it may be distorted. Sensorineural hearing loss can be caused by a number of factors:

- Hereditary factors
- Genetic (syndrome-related) factors
- Acute infection, such as meningitis or mumps
- *Ototoxic drugs* (drugs that damage nerves of the central nervous system that are associated with hearing)
- Tumors
- Exposure to loud noise
- Trauma to the cochlea
- Disease (discussed later in the chapter)
- Aging (presbycusis)

Sensorineural hearing loss may also be due to an irregularity of or injury to the auditory centers of the brain, such as from head injury or stroke. When this type of hearing loss occurs, the individual is said to have *central deafness*. In this type of deafness, either the ability of the sound stimulus to reach the hearing centers of the brain

is disrupted or the hearing center in the brain receives and processes signals incorrectly.

Sensorineural hearing loss is almost exclusively irreversible. Because it involves damage to the hair cells of the cochlea or nerve cell damage, and because the nerve function cannot be restored, associated hearing loss is usually permanent. Although the cause of sensorineural loss should be evaluated by healthcare professionals, individuals with sensorineural hearing loss should also consult with a licensed audiologist for evaluation and potential fitting of hearing aids as well as communication strategies training.

Mixed Hearing Loss

When individuals have *mixed hearing loss,* they experience a combination of conductive hearing loss and sensorineural hearing loss. The conductive component may lend itself to healthcare intervention, while the sensorineural component remains impervious to intervention. In some instances, individuals may benefit from amplification of sounds. The extent of the hearing loss experienced with mixed hearing loss and the success of intervention depend on the degree and type of sensorineural damage.

Central Hearing Loss

Central loss refers to hearing loss experienced because of impairment in the central nervous system rather than because of impairment or damage of the ear itself or the auditory nerve. For example, damage to the part of the brain that receives, perceives, and interpret sounds, such as with traumatic brain injury, or stroke, or neurological conditions that interfere with the transmission of impulses to the brain.

Age of Onset

Another classification of hearing loss is based on when the hearing loss occurred:

- **Prelingual hearing loss** occurs before the individual acquires language, usually before the age of 3 years.
- **Postlingual hearing loss** occurs after verbal language is obtained.

- **Prevocational hearing loss** occurs after an individual acquires language but before entering the workforce, usually before the age of 19.
- **Postvocational hearing loss** refers to hearing loss that occurs after the individual has started to work.

CONGENITAL VERSUS ACQUIRED HEARING LOSS

Hearing loss may be *congenital* (present at birth) or *acquired* (occurring after birth or later in life). In many instances, hearing loss is multifactorial, caused by both genetic and environmental factors (Williams, 2000).

Congenital Hearing Loss

There are three major causes of congenital hearing loss:

- Genetic (syndrome related)
- Prenatal exposure to drugs or toxins
- Prenatal exposure to infections, such as measles (rubella)

Genetic Hearing Loss

Genetic hearing loss may be part of specific genetically linked conditions that involve a variety of other abnormalities, or it may be an isolated case. Genetically determined deafness may either be present at birth or appear later in adulthood. The degree, progression, and age of onset of genetically based hearing loss vary widely, depending on the specific condition or syndrome. In some instances, genetics may not cause deafness per se but rather predispose individuals to hearing loss induced by noise, drugs, or infection (Steel, 2000).

Prenatal Exposure to Drugs or Toxins or Infection

Maternal exposure to drugs or other substances, or maternal infection such as rubella (measles) during the first trimester of pregnancy, can damage the auditory system of the developing fetus, resulting in congenital hearing loss (Acar, Ocak, Acar, & Kocaöz, 2015).

Acquired Hearing Loss

A number of causes of acquired hearing loss are possible:

- Recurrent ear infections (e.g., otitis media)
- Noise
- Injury
- Viruses
- Degenerative conditions
- Aging
- Ototoxic drugs (drugs that damage the inner ear)
- Tumors (acoustic neuroma)

Recurrent infections of the middle ear, such as otitis media, in early childhood can lead to complications causing conductive hearing loss in young children. Prompt identification and management of infections can decrease the risk of hearing loss (Sharma, Pannu, Arora, & Sharma, 2016). In addition, early intervention when hearing loss is identified in young children can lead to better long-term outcomes, including speech, language, and educational outcomes (Shafer, 2006).

Noise-induced hearing loss is more common among individuals with exposure to loud explosive or industrial noises or to continued exposure to loud noise over time. With brief exposure to loud noise, individuals may experience only temporary hearing loss; however with continued exposure, permanent injury can begin. The degree of permanent injury appears to be related to the duration and intensity of exposure (Baloh & Jen, 2016). Avoiding loud noises and wearing ear protectors during exposure to loud noise can drastically reduce the incidence of noise-induced hearing loss. Many industrial sites in which occupational noise presents a hazard now make a concerted effort to inform employees of the necessity of wearing hearing protectors, although compliance with hearing protection policy may be low (Robertson, Kerr, Garcia, & Halterman, 2007). Acquired hearing loss can also result from injuries, such as traumatic brain injury,

Viruses, such as those associated with measles, mumps, and meningitis, can produce sensorineural hearing loss (Lerner & Eng, 2005) or other conditions that affect the auditory pathway, such as acoustic neuroma.

Stroke or traumatic brain injury that damages part of central nervous system or the area of the brain necessary for interpreting stimuli as sound may also be responsible for hearing loss. Some degenerative conditions, such as multiple sclerosis, can be accompanied by loss of hearing. Tumors, such as *acoustic neuroma,* can also compress a portion of the auditory system, causing hearing loss.

Hearing sensitivity declines gradually and progressively with aging (Baloh & Jen, 2016), although the extent to which degeneration of portions of the auditory system is due to the aging process or to cumulative noise trauma throughout life may be difficult to determine. Hearing loss associated with aging is known as *presbycusis*. The most important consequence of this aging-related decline in hearing sensitivity is difficulty in understanding speech. Hearing loss, coupled with other perceptual and processing effects of aging, may result in confusion, withdrawal, disorientation, and inappropriate responses, which can lead others to assume erroneously that individuals are cognitively incapacitated (Nichols, 2006).

Drugs or other substances that are harmful to the auditory pathway are described as **ototoxic**. Salicylates or certain blood pressure medications taken in high doses can produce transient hearing loss; by contrast, some antibiotics, such as streptomycin and neomycin, can be severely ototoxic, destroying the hair cells of the cochlea (Baloh & Jen, 2016).

Manifestations of Hearing Loss

Hearing loss can lead to depression, social isolation, stress, and functional problems such as impaired balance (Nichols, 2006). The type and degree of hearing loss experienced by individuals, regardless of the cause, are varied. Hearing loss usually involves more than a reduction in the loudness of sound. Some hearing losses, for example, result in a distortion of sound so that words may be heard but are difficult to understand or are garbled. In this case, increasing the loudness is unlikely to enhance the individual's ability to understand what is being said.

Some individuals with hearing loss may develop **recruitment**, a manifestation characterized

by an abnormally rapid increase in the perception of loudness with small changes in signal energy. Individuals with recruitment have a narrow range between a level of sound loud enough to be understood and a level of sound that causes discomfort or pain. Unexpected sounds may startle individuals with recruitment and distract them from interpretation of the sound's meaning. Therefore, increasing loudness of sound does not correct the hearing problem and can actually cause increased discomfort.

CONDITIONS OF THE AUDITORY SYSTEM

Conditions of the Outer Ear

Conditions of the outer ear can contribute to hearing loss when an obstruction disrupts the mechanical transmission of auditory stimuli, thereby decreasing acuity of hearing. Although conditions of the outer ear may not have a major impact on hearing or may be correctable, they may also be disfiguring, leading to cosmetic concerns. Deformities or abnormalities of the outer ear can result from congenital conditions or from trauma. Other conditions of the outer ear that may impede hearing include buildup of earwax, foreign bodies in the ears, and growths (e.g., polyps) that cause obstruction.

For the most part, partial occlusion of the external ear canal has no influence on the efficiency of sound transmission and causes no significant hearing loss. Complete occlusion, however, generally results in a moderate conductive loss. Conditions of the outer ear that cause temporary conductive hearing loss can usually be corrected or alleviated by surgical or mechanical intervention.

Conditions of the Middle Ear

Several conditions of the middle ear may cause temporary or permanent hearing loss.

Perforated Tympanic Membrane

A thickened or perforated tympanic membrane (ruptured eardrum) may or may not impair hearing. Rupture of the eardrum may result from an injury (e.g., a blow to the ear or head or an explosion), infection, or inflammation.

Otitis Media

Otitis media includes two types of conditions:

- *Acute otitis media*—inflammation of the middle ear space
- *Otitis media with effusion*—fluid in the middle ear

Acute otitis media occurs suddenly and often results when an upper respiratory infection or allergy causes swelling of the eustachian tube, interfering with regular drainage, and enabling spread of microorganisms through the eustachian tube in the middle ear. The resulting infection and inflammation cause increased pressure, which in turn leads to bulging of the eardrum, pain, and some diminished hearing. When the infection is managed properly, and if the eardrum has not been ruptured, hearing is usually restored.

Otitis media with effusion refers to a condition in which fluid continues to accumulate after infection of the middle ear has subsided. Otis media with effusion can cause conductive hearing losses due to the collection of fluid in the middle ear or due to rupture or scarring of the tympanic membrane. For the past four decades, concerns about the effects of otitis media with effusion on speech, language, and learning development in young children have led to use of aggressive interventions such as placement of *tympanostomy tubes* to prevent permanent damage. The degree to which prompt insertion of tympanostomy tubes improves developmental outcomes in children who have no other conditions confounding development have been called into question (Berman, 2007; Paradise et al., 2007).

Mastoiditis

Mastoiditis is an infection of the mastoid cells within the mastoid process located in the temporal bone of the skull. Because of the proximity of the mastoid cells to other important structures in the head, this condition may lead to a number of complications, including paralysis of the facial muscles and infection or abscess of the brain. Mastoiditis is not as prevalent as it once was, thanks to the earlier detection of otitis media and intervention with antibiotics. Nevertheless, chronic mastoiditis and associated complications can arise if previous ear infections are not managed.

Otosclerosis

Otosclerosis is a hardening of the ossicles (incus, stapes, and malleus of the middle ear), which transmit sound impulses to the inner ear. Early manifestations may include trouble hearing on the telephone but not in crowds. This condition appears in part to be hereditary. It causes conductive hearing loss because hardening of the ossicles reduces the efficiency of the transfer of sound impulses to the inner ear. Otosclerosis produces progressive hearing loss accompanied by **tinnitus** (ringing or noise in the ear). Some individuals may also have vestibular manifestations such as vertigo (illusion of spinning movement) or problems with equilibrium.

Individuals with otosclerosis often hear amplified speech well and without distortions; consequently, they are usually good candidates for hearing aids. Hearing can also often be restored or improved with surgical intervention, although surgery does not fully remedy the loss. When determining if surgery is appropriate, individuals' lifestyle and occupation are considered. Because surgery may affect vestibular function, individuals who require fine balance for employment may find amplification through hearing aids a better choice than surgery. If individuals' hobbies or occupations expose them to large and rapid changes in barometric pressure, or if heavy lifting is required, hearing aids may also be a better choice because of the chance of postoperative complications or vestibular disturbances.

Conditions of the Inner Ear

Many conditions of the inner ear cause permanent hearing loss; many also affect the vestibular system.

Tinnitus

Tinnitus (ringing or noise in the ears) may or may not be accompanied by hearing loss. It can result from overexposure to loud noise or can be a manifestation of a more serious condition, such as tumor, high blood pressure, or head injury. It can also result from side effects or toxic effects of some medications. In some instances, tinnitus may be a separate entity, not associated with a specific condition and with no identifiable cause. The management of tinnitus depends on the cause. In some cases, if the cause can be identified and managed,

the ringing can be eliminated. In other instances, even though the cause is identified, damage may be permanent and tinnitus cannot be cured.

Most people with tinnitus adjust to its presence and experience no severe residual effects; however, some individuals have difficulty adjusting and experience incapacitating effects of tinnitus, including sleep disturbances and severe emotional distress (Baloh & Jen, 2016). Some individuals complain of problems sleeping because of the constant noise and may need background noise, as from a radio, to mask the sound. A number of interventions, including group cognitive therapy, have been used to help people cope with tinnitus. Adjustment to tinnitus does not appear to be related to the severity of the condition but rather to the coping styles of those affected.

Acute Peripheral Vestibulopathy (Labyrinthitis)

Labyrinthitis (inflammation of the labyrinth of the inner ear) may be acute without resulting in permanent hearing loss. This condition may occur as a complication of otitis media, influenza, or upper respiratory infections. Because the inner ear is involved, manifestations of vertigo, nausea, and vomiting frequently accompany labyrinthitis. Most people gradually improve in one or two weeks, although in some instances manifestations can persist for months (Baloh & Jen, 2016).

Meniere's Disease

Meniere's disease is a chronic condition of the inner ear that encompasses the triad of recurrent severe vertigo, sensorineural hearing loss, and tinnitus. The cause of Meniere's disease is unknown, but it is believed that the condition results from overabundance of fluid (*endolymph*) in the inner ear, because of either overproduction or underabsorption of fluid (Baloh & Jen, 2016). It is also thought that disturbances in the fluid dynamics of the endolymph are involved in associated hearing loss. One or both ears may be affected. Exacerbations are episodic, such that the condition is characterized by remissions and relapses. When episodes do occur, they are dramatic, often incapacitating individuals during the episode.

During an episode of exacerbation, vertigo usually appears suddenly and is often accompanied by

nausea and vomiting. Vertigo associated with Meniere's disease can be severely incapacitating, lasting from a few minutes to hours (Baloh & Jen, 2016). Tinnitus may be either intermittent or constant between exacerbations, becoming worse during an exacerbation. Hearing loss associated with Meniere's disease is variable. Lower tones may be affected first, but all tones are affected as the condition progresses.

Intervention consists of dietary and lifestyle modifications, including management of dietary sodium to help reduce fluid pressure in the inner ear, and use of diuretic medications to decrease fluid volume by increasing urine production (Baloh & Jen, 2016).

Trauma or Other Health Conditions

As discussed earlier in the chapter, sensorineural hearing loss may result from damage to the inner ear or to the acoustic nerve. Among the causes of sensorineural deafness are the following:

- Traumatic head injury
- Exposure to high levels of noise, which can damage the hair cells in the innerear
- Ingestion of ototoxic agents (drugs or other chemicals that destroy the hair cellsof the inner ear or damage the eighth cranial nerve)
- Stroke
- Hypertension and arteriosclerosis, which produce vascular changes in the central-nervous system
- Infections, such as meningitis
- Growths (such as *meningioma* or *acoustic neuroma*) or malignant tumors insidethe head, which may cause hearing loss by mechanically impinging on theacoustic nerve or by involving it directly
- Other neurological conditions, such as multiple sclerosis, that produce changesin the auditory pathway that contribute to hearing loss

Presbycusis

Presbycusis, as discussed earlier in the chapter, is caused by degenerative changes in the inner ear, neural pathways, or both. The reason that presbycusis occurs is unknown. This diagnosis has become a catchall term that encompasses many types of auditory deteriorations, but is commonly thought to accompany aging-related structural changes in the ear. Most often presbycusis occurs in both ears equally. Onset is slow, and hearing loss can vary in degree from mild to severe. Ability to hear higher tonal frequencies is usually affected first, but the ability to hear lower frequencies is gradually affected as well. Hearing loss experienced as a result of presbycusis most often is accompanied by word discrimination difficulties, especially if the hearing loss has greatly affected the individuals' perception of the higher-pitched consonants.

IDENTIFICATION OF HEARING LOSS

Before hearing loss can be evaluated or managed, it must be identified. Individuals with hearing losses may not be aware of the degree of loss, or they may deny that hearing loss exists. An important tool in identification may be simple observation of behaviors that are indicative of a hearing loss.

Indications of possible hearing loss in infants and small children include unresponsiveness to sound, delayed development of speech, and behavior problems (e.g., tantrums, inattention, and hyperactivity). School-aged children with unidentified hearing loss may have speech impairments, demonstrate attention disorders, or demonstrate below-average ability in school.

Adults with unidentified hearing loss may be irritable, hostile, or hypersensitive. They may deny their inability to understand or respond appropriately by blaming others for not enunciating distinctly. They often avoid situations in which hearing is more difficult, such as those where large crowds or large groups are present. Individuals with unidentified hearing loss may speak excessively loud and may require increased volume to hear the television and radio.

Heightened sensitivity and patience are often necessary when encouraging individuals with suspected hearing loss to obtain evaluation and seek intervention. Initial resistance to these recommendations is not unusual.

Health Examination

Healthcare professionals may be the first to recognize or be consulted about a potential hearing loss. Although it is often omitted, screening for hearing loss should be part of every health exam. Various checklists and questionnaires may be used initially

to elicit manifestations associated with hearing loss. The ear canal may also be examined for obstruction and the tympanic membrane visualized with an instrument called an *otoscope*. Likewise, rudimentary auditory screening may be performed.

Tuning forks are sometimes used in routine health examinations as an initial screening method for hearing loss. This method can help differentiate between conductive or sensorineural hearing loss, and problems with both air conduction and bone conduction of sound. It does not quantify the degree of loss, if any exists.

A rudimentary test of the ability to hear by air conduction can be carried out by placing a vibrating tuning fork in the air near the ear, but out of the individual's sight. Hearing by bone conduction is evaluated by placing a vibrating tuning fork in different positions on the individual's skull, which causes vibration throughout the skull, including the inner ear. The inability to hear the sound in either instance is an indication of hearing loss. Irregular test results warrant further testing and evaluation. Because of the gross nature of this screening method, it has been largely replaced by other methods.

When problems with hearing are identified, referral for additional testing may be made. Further testing and evaluation may be conducted by an *audiologist,* a person with a master's or doctoral degree in audiology who specializes in evaluating hearing conditions and providing rehabilitation interventions for individuals with hearing conditions. If testing by the audiologist reveals that additional intervention is necessary, referral is made to an *otolaryngologist* (a physician who specializes in identification and management of conditions of the ear and related structures).

Audiometric Testing

Audiometric testing measures the degree of hearing loss with an electronic device called an *audiometer.* An audiologist usually performs the test.

Tests routinely used by audiologists attempt to define three major aspects of hearing:

- Degree of hearing
- Type of hearing loss
- Ability to understand speech under various conditions

A complete audiometric evaluation usually includes pure-tone air and bone conduction testing, speech audiometry, and acoustic immittance measurement. From audiometric results, the type and degree of hearing loss can be determined as well as the degree of speech understanding.

Pure-Tone Audiometry

The accurate measurement of sound is an important component of a hearing test. Changes in sound intensity are measured in decibels and heard as changes in loudness. Changes in sound frequency are measured in hertz and heard as changes in pitch. The *audiogram* is a method of recording the softest sounds that individuals can hear. A general guide for describing functional implications of degrees of hearing loss associated with decibel losses is found in **Table 17-1**.

Table 17-1	Functional Implications of Degrees of Decibel Loss
26–40 dB	Mild hearing loss. In ideal listening conditions, hearing is minimally affected; there may be difficulty hearing faint, distant speech even in ideal conditions; background noise may interfere with hearing.
41–55 dB	Moderate hearing loss. Hears conversational speech but only at close distances; understanding speech is more difficult with background noses.
56–70 dB	Moderately severe hearing loss. Hears loud conversational speech that is close by. Has difficulty hearing in group situations.
71–90 dB	Severe hearing loss. Conversational speech severely affected. Perception of sound is usually distorted.
Greater than 90 dB	Profound hearing loss. May hear (or feel from vibrations) only very loud sounds. Hearing is not the primary communication channel.

Reproduced from Moore, C. L. (2001b). Racial and ethnic members of under-represented groups with hearing loss and VR services: Explaining the disparity in closure success rates. *Journal of Applied Rehabilitation Counseling, 33*(1), 15–20.

Figure 17-2   Audiogram

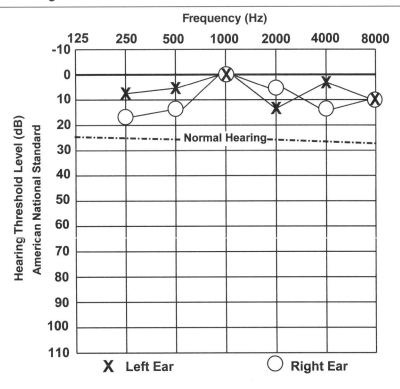

© Jane Tinkler Lamm.

The Audiogram

The individual's ability to detect sound and pitch in each ear is plotted on the audiogram (**Figure 17-2**). A *pure-tone audiogram* is a graph on which an individual's responses to calibrated tones are plotted as *thresholds*. Numbers across the top of the audiogram represent pure-tone frequencies ranging from 125 to 8,000 Hz. Along the side of the audiogram are numbers ranging from –10 to 110 that represent measurement of decibels.

The audiogram illustrates the degree of hearing loss. The *audiometric exam* takes place in a sound chamber to eliminate distracting sounds. An *audiometer* emits sounds (*pure tones*) or words through earphones worn by the individual being tested (*air conduction audiometry*). As the tones are transmitted through the earphones, the individual indicates when sound is first heard. The results of

this test are then plotted on the audiogram. The hearing-level scale is constructed so that average unimpaired hearing equals 0 decibels; unimpaired hearing sensitivity ranges from –10 to 25 decibels. The higher the number on the decibel scale, the greater the degree of hearing loss. The audiogram tests speech frequencies, which range from 250 to 8,000 Hz. The inability to discriminate frequencies within this range may interfere with everyday communication.

Bone Conduction Audiometry

When audiometric testing reveals a hearing loss, the audiologist conducts further testing to determine whether hearing loss is sensorineural, conductive, or mixed in nature. Tests used for this purpose include *bone conduction tests*. The procedure for *bone conduction audiometry* consists of placing a

vibrator on the individual's mastoid process or on the forehead. Calibrated tones are then transmitted through the vibrator directly into the inner ear, bypassing the external and middle ear systems. The individual's responses to the thresholds are plotted on the audiogram and contrasted with the air conduction test results.

To determine the type of hearing loss, thresholds for air and bone conduction are compared. Depending on the differences between the two thresholds, hearing loss is classified as sensorineural, conductive, or mixed.

Speech Audiometry

Although pure-tone audiometry is used to determine individuals' ability to hear specific tones, speech audiometry provides measurements that may indicate more appropriately individuals' ability to understand speech in everyday situations. Two types of speech audiometry measured are the *speech reception threshold (SRT)* and the *speech discrimination threshold (SDT)*. In both tests, individuals wear headphones and listen to words being transmitted through the headphones without any visual cues.

Tests of the speech reception threshold help to identify the lowest intensity, or softest sound level in decibels, at which an individual first understands speech. Words with two syllables (such as *baseball, ice cream,* or *cowboy)*, taken from a standardized list, are presented to the individual through earphones. The individual then repeats the word, thereby demonstrating acuity for hearing the spoken word. The speech reception threshold should correspond closely to the average pure-tone air conduction threshold and provides a check of the accuracy of the pure-tone measurements. The higher the decibel level required for either threshold, the greater the hearing loss. A speech reception threshold or average pure-tone threshold of 25 decibels, for instance, is considered borderline normal hearing for adults. (Limits for children are reduced to 15 to 20 decibels.) A threshold of 26 to 40 decibels is considered a mild hearing loss.

In addition to measuring how loud speech must be to be heard, testing involves determining how well individuals understand speech once it is loud enough to hear. *Speech discrimination tests* (sometimes called *word recognition tests*) help provide this information. During the test, words from standardized lists of phonetically balanced one-syllable words are presented to the individual through earphones without visual cues. The individual must identify and repeat words back to the examiner. The test is scored as the percentage of correctly repeated words. The lower the percentage, the greater the problem in understanding. Individuals with speech discrimination hearing loss may be able to recognize speech but unable to understand it. The speech discrimination score provides a measure of the ability to understand words at a comfortable volume. It assesses the ability to judge acoustic information and distinguish between similar speech sounds, such as the letters "p" and "b" or the letters "t" and "d."

Acoustic Immittance or Impedance Audiometry

Acoustic immittance measurement includes a battery of tests that evaluate middle ear status. *Tympanometry* is a test of acoustic immittance in which the mobility or flexibility of the tympanic membrane is assessed by measuring how much sound energy is admitted into the ear as air pressure is varied in the external auditory canal. The status of the eardrum is assessed by altering the air pressure in the ear canal and measuring the eardrum's response to sound transmissions under these varying conditions and different stimuli. As sound energy strikes the eardrum, some is transmitted to the middle and inner ear, but some is reflected back into the ear canal. If the tympanic membrane is stiff, much of the sound energy is reflected back into the external ear canal. The less impedance, the more sound energy admitted to the middle and inner ear. An increased level of resistance is indicative of a middle ear condition.

The results of this type of testing are plotted on a graph called a *tympanogram*. The ear's response is plotted on the vertical dimension of the graph, and air pressures are plotted on the horizontal dimension.

Acoustic immittance testing may also be used to measure the *acoustic reflex*—that is, movement

of the muscles attached to the malleus and stapes as a response to intense sound. It should occur in both ears in response to a loud sound, even if only one ear is stimulated. Acoustic reflex testing may be helpful in identifying conditions or problems that involve the cochlea or auditory nervous system.

Acoustic immittance testing requires no voluntary responses from the individual. Consequently, tympanometry is frequently used to detect or rule out conductive hearing loss in children or in adults who are unable to cooperate fully during pure-tone testing.

Electrocochleography

Electrocochleography is a procedure in which stimulus-related electrical activity generated in the cochlea and auditory nerve is recorded. For the test, the individual reclines, with electrodes being placed in the external auditory canal. The sound stimulus is then delivered through earphones. This test is useful in evaluation of inner ear fluid disorders such as Meniere's disease.

Auditory Brain Stem Response

The auditory brain stem response (ABR) records electrical activity generated as sound travels from the auditory nerve through the auditory brain stem pathway. During this test, the individual reclines, with electrodes being placed on the mastoid or on the earlobe. A stimulus is then presented through earphones, and electroencephalogram activity is evaluated and the ABR assessed. The ABR is useful in ruling out auditory conditions such as conditions related to the cochlea; degenerative or demyelinating conditions of the auditory system, such as multiple sclerosis; and tumors of the auditory system.

Otoacoustic Emissions

Otoacoustic emissions are measured reflections in the outer ear of mechanical activity in the cochlea. Otoacoustic emissions testing enables measurement of hearing in infants, young children, and difficult-to-test persons such as those with dementia or diminished intellectual function. The technology has enhanced the ability to detect hearing loss early in life.

MANAGEMENT OF HEARING LOSS AND DEAFNESS

Both healthcare and other interventions may be used in the management of hearing loss. Healthcare interventions may involve surgery or medications, whereas other interventions may include use of hearing aids or other assistive listening devices and special training programs.

Management of hearing loss or deafness in most cases involves a variety of professionals. An *otolaryngologist* may provide evaluation and management of hearing loss. Audiologists, in addition to conducting evaluations of hearing function, manage other interventions for hearing loss, including selecting and fitting amplification devices. The audiologist reviews the hearing test results and consults with the individual about his or her listening needs before recommending which style or type of hearing aid would be most beneficial.

Children with hearing loss may also have speech production difficulties because of lack of auditory feedback. *Speech and language pathologists* often work with individuals to help them with particular aspects of speech, language, or both to increase intelligibility.

Auditory training is often helpful for individuals with special problems in communication. Such training may be included in hearing aid orientation or special programs on listening for the sounds of speech and other environmental sounds. Various interventions that are used in the management of hearing loss are discussed in the following sections.

Hearing Aids

A hearing aid is any mechanical or electronic device that improves hearing. The type of hearing aid recommended is highly individualized and fitted according to individual need. The advent of digital technology has advanced the quality of hearing aids significantly over the past decades. In the past, hearing aids were mainly designed to amplify sound; today, these devices are much more complex and combine sound amplification with signal processing for speech, noise reduction, and a number of other functions, including a wireless

link with other communication systems. Several types are available:

- Behind-the-ear style, which curves around the back side of the ear
- In-the-ear style, which fits in the ear canal and outer ear bowl
- Canal style, which fits entirely within the ear canal so it is barely visible

All hearing aids, regardless of type or shape, magnify sound and include the following components:

- Microphone to pick up sound
- Amplifier, which makes sound louder
- Receiver, which conveys sound to the ear
- Battery, which provides power for the hearing aid

Digital Versus Analog Hearing Aids

Prior to 2000, most hearing aids were analog (Fransman & Walker, 2007). *Analog hearing aids* work by increasing volume, but they have little capacity to distinguish pitch (bass sounds versus high-pitched sounds). Because the primary function is to amplify sound, all sounds are amplified indiscriminately. Consequently, although the ability to hear another person talk in a quiet environment is improved, attempting to hear a conversation in a noisy environment is more difficult because all sounds are amplified. Individuals using analog types of aids can control volume; changing volume repeatedly is cumbersome, however, and not helpful for understanding conversations in noisy environments.

Tone control is a feature on conventional analog hearing aids that allows the audiologist to modify frequency sensitivity of the hearing aid amplifier to best respond to the individual's hearing loss. For instance, individuals with hearing loss at higher frequencies have difficulty hearing some higher-pitched tones of speech. Tone control is an attempt to amplify the high frequencies without amplifying the lower frequencies.

Digital hearing aids change acoustic signals into a discrete series of digital signals so that the audiologist can appropriately shape the hearing aid response to the individual's hearing loss. As a result, digital hearing aids can theoretically be programmed for each individual's hearing loss and provide more precision and clarity of sound. Many contain special "noise-reduction circuits" that aid in reducing background noise distraction. Digital hearing aids have become much more affordable in recent years, with technology options ranging from basic digital to premium digital with directional microphones.

Implantable Hearing Aids

Implantable hearing aids are an option for individuals who cannot use cochlear implants or who cannot or prefer not to use external hearing aid devices. Implantable hearing aids facilitate hearing through air or through bone conduction and help transmission of sound vibrations entering the middle ear. Implantable hearing aids may be implanted surgically in which a small device is attached to one of the bones of the middle ear (bone anchored hearing aids [BAHA]) or through a nonsurgical procedure in which a tube is placed into the ear with hearing aid portion inserted directly into the tube (Shin et al., 2016). Although BAHA are mostly used with individuals with conductive loss whose hearing loss is not profound (Edmiston, Aggarwal, & Green, 2015), middle ear implants (MEI), which consist of surgical implants into the middle ear to vibrate bones of the middle ear, may be used for more severe hearing loss or for individuals with sensorineural hearing loss (Koci et al., 2016).

Effective Hearing Aid Use

Hearing aid units are dispensed and fitted by audiologists or hearing aid dispensers. These devices may be fitted to one or both ears. *Monaural* refers to fitting of a single hearing aid; *binaural* refers to fitting of two hearing aids. Recent trends show binaural fittings are becoming the norm for a variety of reasons, including improved localization skills, safety, and ease of hearing in noisy environments.

Most individuals are given a written contract that provides them with a 30-day trial evaluation period, after which, if they are not satisfied, they can receive a refund for the cost of the hearing aid, less any service charges. Although the hearing aid

industry has become more regulated, it is highly recommended that individuals seeking a hearing aid consult with a licensed audiologist who specializes in dispensing of hearing aids. As always, a referral from a friend, family member, or trusted health professional is the best way to assure the individual is working with a skilled and reputable professional.

Although hearing aids may improve hearing and may be beneficial for many individuals, they do not correct hearing in the same way that glasses can improve vision to the 20/20 level (Desselle & Proctor, 2000). Hearing aids can improve volume but not always clarity of speech. Because analog hearing aids work as amplifiers, they make speech louder but not always clearer. In addition, these devices amplify not only speech but other sounds in the environment as well, which can interfere with the individual's ability to decipher speech. Individuals with hearing aids may need speech reading to help them fill in gaps in comprehension of speech that persist despite use of the hearing aid. Digital hearing aids have a unique advantage over analog devices in that they can provide more volume to the soft sounds of speech and less volume to the louder background sounds that can interfere with understanding.

Hearing aids should be carefully recommended in accordance with individual needs. For best practice, they should be dispensed with appropriate verification and orientation regarding proper care and use. Orientation plays a vital role in the success of hearing aid use by helping to establish realistic expectations. Additional audiological rehabilitation training or counseling helps individuals learn ways to enhance communication and minimize communication obstacles.

One potential barrier to effective hearing aid use is the attitude of the individual. Some individuals may resist using hearing aids because they believe society will view them as less capable. Although smaller, less conspicuous hearing aids have improved acceptance, negative attitudes toward hearing aids are one factor that may impede their use among many persons who might otherwise benefit from these devices.

Hearing aids are delicate devices that need routine care and maintenance to ensure maximum function. Batteries must be replaced regularly.

Individuals using hearing aids must be careful to protect hearing aids from damage to the internal components. Specifically, users should refrain from dropping these devices or subjecting them to extremes in temperatures, excess moisture, or exposure to other substances, such as hair spray, that could damage the microphone or receiver.

Assistive Listening Devices and Systems

Assistive listening devices (ALDs) include a wide variety of equipment other than hearing aids that can be used by persons with hearing loss. Some devices may be used independently; others supplement hearing aids. As individuals with hearing loss may have more difficulty perceiving high-pitched sounds common in speech or hearing in background noise, assistive listening devices help to improve the signal-to-noise ratio by facilitating listening and reducing background noise and reverberation.

Telecoil Circuitry

Some hearing aids have special features called *telecoil circuitry or tone control*. Hearing aids with telecoil circuitry feature have a special switch or push button (*T switch*) located on the hearing aid case that activates the telecoil. A telecoil is a very small coil of wire that acts as an antenna, picking up electromagnetic energy that is then delivered to the receiver of the hearing aid and converted into sound. Also available is a plug called a boot or shoe, which is designed to fit over the end of a behind-the-ear hearing aid equipped with *direct auditory input (DAI)*. This device enables individuals to be connected to an external sound source, such as a radio signal or microphone. It improves the signal-to-noise ratio, thereby enhancing sound quality. Telecoil circuitry enables individuals to use other assistive listening devices discussed later in this chapter.

Telephone Devices

Many different types of telephone devices are available to assist with telephone communication. Some of these devices are hearing aid compatible and work in conjunction with the hearing aid telecoil. Such telephones enable the hearing aid user to utilize the telecoil circuitry and thereby receive a clearer signal, without annoying acoustic feedback

a microphone or a direct plug-in wire, to convey the amplified speech signal directly to the receiver (a hearing aid, earphone headset, or neck loop) worn by the individual. When a microphone is used, the speaker talks into the microphone; the sound travels through a cord and then directly reaches the receiver worn by the listener. When a plug-in is used, a wire is plugged into the sound source (such as a television or a radio), and the sound travels through the wire directly to the individual's personal receiver. Using hard-wired systems with television or radio enables individuals with hearing loss to increase the volume on their personal receiver without altering the volume for others in the room.

Hard-wired systems are considered personal listening systems and are more useful in one-to-one communication as opposed to group settings. The systems are small, with the amplifier being contained in a pocket.

Large-Area Systems

Background noise often competes with speech sounds, creating a more challenging listening environment for individuals with hearing loss. Additional reverberation affects sound quality in large groups and brings a more distorted signal to hard-of-hearing individuals. Distance is another factor that has a negative effect for those with hearing loss. A number of devices to enhance hearing in group settings are available. Examples of these *large-area devices* include audio loop systems, FM systems, and infrared systems.

Audio Loop Systems

Audio loop systems are made up of a microphone, an amplifier, and a coil of wire (also called an induction coil) that loops around the seating area. Electricity flows through the coil, creating an electromagnetic field that can be picked up by the telecoil of a hearing aid, which is itself activated through a T switch or push button. The telecoil acts as an antenna and picks up the electromagnetic energy, delivering it to the user's hearing aid. Individuals using the audio loop must sit within or near the loop for it to operate effectively. Audio loop systems can be permanently installed in public meeting rooms, churches, or theaters, or they can be set up on an as-needed basis.

or squeal. Telecoil circuitry allows the hearing aid user to tap into the electromagnetic signal from the telephone; electromagnetic energy is then transferred to the receiver of the hearing aid and converted into sound. Not all phones in use today are compatible with telecoil technology, although the Federal Communication Commission (FCC) has made changes in statutes that require all new phones, including cell phones, to be hearing aid compatible.

Some other telephone devices may be used without a hearing aid. Portable telephone amplifiers can be slipped over a telephone receiver and may be useful for hard-of-hearing individuals who travel and need a louder signal. Other telephone amplification devices may be wired to the telephone handset so that volume is increased, allowing the user to control the amplification level. Public telephones equipped with amplifier handsets, although not always readily available, are becoming more common. These telephones are usually identified with an access sign.

Telecommunication Display Devices

Telecommunication display devices (TDD), also called *teletypewriters (TTY)*, are used to transmit conversations in printed format over regular telephone lines. Individuals on both ends of the line must have compatible devices with which to type their messages and visualize the printed message on a screen or paper. If one individual does not have a TDD, a third-party system may be used or a relay operator may transmit the message to the other individual. Telecommunication relay services allow a person using TDD to communicate with another person using a voice telephone, with the relay operator acting as an interpreter. Special software is also available that allows a personal computer to interact with TDD and provide a synthesized speech signal. In addition, computers are allowing greater access for deaf and hard-of-hearing individuals with email.

Hard-Wired Systems (Personal Listening Systems)

Hard-wired systems are individual devices that amplify speech and minimize outside noise so that speech can be more easily understood. The systems must have a direct connection to the sound source, using either

cues, such as flashing lights; auditory cues, such as increased amplification of sound; or *tactile cues*, such as a vibrator. *Certified Hearing Guide Dogs* (International Dogs, Inc.), for example, are trained to react to certain environmental sounds (e.g., a telephone ringing). The dog does not bark but rather makes physical contact with the individual and then runs to the source of the sound.

Surgical Interventions

Surgical interventions may be performed in some conditions to restore or improve hearing.

Myringotomy

When the middle ear is infected, as in otitis media, or when fluid builds up in the middle ear, surgical intervention may be necessary to drain pus or fluid, thereby relieving pressure and preventing rupture of the eardrum (tympanic membrane). A *myringotomy* is a procedure in which an incision is made into the eardrum for this purpose. Because the procedure is performed under controlled conditions, it seldom leaves enough scar tissue to have a negative effect on hearing.

If fluid has accumulated in the middle ear, a needle may be inserted so the fluid can be removed (*needle aspiration*). A common procedure performed during myringotomy is the placement of *ventilation or pressure-equalizing tubes* in the tympanic membrane to equalize middle ear pressure. When the ventilation tube is in place and operating properly, conductive hearing loss due to middle ear condition is usually completely eliminated.

Mastoidectomy

Since the advent of antibiotics for management of mastoiditis (inflammation of the mastoid bone), *mastoidectomy* is performed less frequently. Mastoidectomy is a surgical procedure to remove infected mastoid air cells, located in the mastoid process. Because the mastoid is a portion of the acoustic system of the middle ear, hearing loss could still be present after surgery, depending on the nature of the surgery.

Tympanoplasty

Surgical procedures involving the middle ear are referred to generally as *tympanoplasty* (repair of

FM Systems

FM systems are wireless devices that work much the same way as FM radios. Sound is picked up and transmitted through a frequency-modulated band directly to a receiver worn by the individual with hearing loss. Wireless FM systems have greatly reduced the hardware needed by persons with hearing loss, especially with regard to hearing aid compatibility. Such systems enhance listening in noisy environments by improving the signal-to-noise ratio.

Infrared Systems

Infrared systems require installation of an infrared light emitter, which is usually piggybacked onto an existing public address system. Sound is transmitted by invisible, harmless infrared light waves and picked up by a receiver, which can take the form of either a headset for use without a hearing aid or a device intended for use with a hearing aid equipped with a T switch. These systems are best suited for use in rooms or meeting areas without windows, as sunlight affects the signal.

Captioning Services and Telecaption Adapters

Closed captioning, in which printed dialog appears on a corner or at the bottom of the screen, may be used for television or movies. Real-time captioning services display the text on a video monitor immediately. All televisions manufactured after July 1993 that are 13 inches or larger must be equipped with closed captioning option. Older models can utilize a decoder that is connected to the television. Captioned feature and educational films are available through a variety of distribution services as well.

Alerting Devices

Hearing enables individuals to respond to sounds such as sirens, the horn of an approaching car, the doorbell, or a baby's cry. Hearing loss can, therefore, hamper individuals' ability to respond to everyday environmental sounds, potentially increasing the risk of accidents and possibly increasing feelings of insecurity. A variety of devices and systems are available commercially to alert individuals with hearing loss to these cues. They may use visual

the tympanic membrane). *Myringoplasty* is a specific type of tympanoplasty in which the damaged eardrum is repaired. Other types of tympanoplasties may be performed for the surgical repair or reconstruction of the ossicles of the middle ear. Repairing or reconstructing the conductive mechanisms of the middle ear may improve or restore the conductive component of individuals' hearing.

Stapedectomy

The most common surgical intervention for otosclerosis is *stapedectomy*, a surgical replacement of an immobile or fixed stapes with a prosthesis. The surgery reestablishes a sound pathway between the middle and inner ear. It usually improves hearing but does not totally restore it.

Cochlear Implant

In hearing individuals, sound travels from the outer ear to the middle ear, and then to the cochlea, where it is converted into electrical impulses that are transmitted through the auditory nerve to the brain for interpretation. When the hair cells within the cochlea become damaged, however, this conversion process cannot take place. Cochlear implants bypass the hair cells of the inner ear, stimulating the auditory nerve directly.

A cochlear implant is a surgically implanted electronic device that transduces sound signals into electrical signals that stimulate the auditory nerve. It consists of the following components:

- A microphone that picks up sound.
- A speech processor (typically worn behind the ear or, in older models, on a belt) that converts sound into digital impulses according to the individual's degree of hearing loss.
- A headpiece held in place by a magnet attached to the implant that has been surgically placed on the other side of the skin behind the ear.
- The implant, which converts signals into electric currents, sends them through a wire surgically placed into the cochlea, and transmits the impulse to the auditory nerve through electrodes at the end of the wire. The auditory nerve then carries these impulses to the brain, where they are interpreted as sound.

Cochlear implants, which were once used mainly for bilateral deafness and severe hearing loss, are now also used by individuals who are unable to have effective oral communication even with the benefit of a hearing aid (Gates & Miyamoto, 2003). Although cochlear implants cannot restore total hearing, this intervention can be life-changing for many individuals, enabling them to hear environmental sounds and improve communication (Sherwood, 2007). Although the sound heard with cochlear implants is not like an acoustic signal, individuals with implants become accustomed to hearing via this electrical stimulation.

Cochlear implants can help *speech reading* by enabling individuals to distinguish beginnings and endings of words, as well as intonation and rhythm patterns being used. Individuals typically hear moderate sounds, although they may have difficulty perceiving speech clearly in noisy environments and hearing music clearly. Implants can also have a positive impact in work environments. In addition to experiencing an improvement in verbal communication, individuals with cochlear implants are better able to hear and identify warning signals (Saxon, Holmes, & Spitznagel, 2001).

Not all individuals who are deaf are candidates for cochlear implants. For adults, in most instances the following criteria need to be met before receiving a cochlear implant:

- Severe to profound sensorineural deafness
- Speech recognition at less than 50% with appropriate hearing aid
- Motivated and psychologically suitable for the implant (Zeng, 2004)

The success rate with cochlear implants varies (Olson, 2006). Individuals who have shorter-term deafness appear to have greater success with implants than those with long-term hearing loss (Gates & Miyamoto, 2003). In children, particularly before the age of two, there has been considerable interest in the impact of cochlear implants on speech and language development. To learn words and acquire language, children must be able to accurately perceive and discriminate distinct sounds in language. Recent research suggests that earlier implant may not have as large an effect on speech perception as

it does on other language skills (Phan, Houston, Ruffin, Ting, & Holt, 2016).

Individuals who receive a cochlear implant should have realistic expectations for their hearing ability after the procedure. Optimal use of the implants requires a commitment to rehabilitation, training, and daily practice. Although the cost of cochlear implants is covered by many insurers, reimbursement for auditory rehabilitation—a key to successful use of implants—may be minimal or nonexistent.

Before receiving a cochlear implant, individuals should be well informed about the issues involved and the facts related to implantation (Chute, 2004). They must be carefully screened with an audiological assessment, thorough hearing history and health examination, and psychosocial assessment. Individuals with prelingual deafness, who often have strong ties to the Deaf community, may be unprepared for the social ramifications of their cochlear implant. Some members of this group (as discussed later in the chapter) are strongly opposed to cochlear implants for cultural reasons. Consequently, in some instances, cochlear implants may socially isolate individuals from friends in the Deaf community who reject the idea of implants (Tucker, 1998).

The use of cochlear implants for young children has also raised a number of issues that are still under debate. Improved technological means to test hearing in infants and young children has made early detection of hearing loss or deafness and early intervention possible. Although studies have demonstrated improved cognitive and speech perception outcomes with cochlear implants at a young age (Roman, Rochette, Triglia, Schön, & Bigand, 2016), others question the ethical implications of cochlear implant in children, prior to their ability to give informed consent (Lantos, 2012; Pass & Graber, 2015).

Other Assistive Interventions Speech Reading (Lip Reading)

Speech reading is a communication skill in which individuals with hearing loss watch for clues from the lips, tongue, and facial expression of the speaker. Only one-third of the English language is visible on the lips, so individuals who speech read often supplement meaning by observing facial expressions of the speaker and gathering conceptual cues (Myers & Thyer, 1997). Speech reading may also be supplemented with a manual communication system such as *cued speech*.

Speech reading requires good lighting. The speaker must face the individual who is speech reading and must be close enough to enable the individual to see the speaker's lip formation. The speaker should use a natural speaking voice and expression, avoiding distortions of the mouth through movements such as grimacing. Speech reading is more difficult when the speaker speaks very rapidly or enunciates poorly, uses distracting hand movements, or has a beard or a mustache that obstructs view of the lips. Speakers should avoid chewing, turning away from the listener, or moving about while talking. The speaker should get the listener's attention before beginning to speak and clarify statements as necessary.

Considerable concentration is required for most people with hearing loss to grasp the spoken word. It is a complex process that can be very tiring when conversation is extended.

Sign Language

Language is a set of symbols combined in a certain way to convey concepts, ideas, and emotions. There are many ways of transmitting language. *Speech* is the verbal expression of language concepts. *Sign language* is a means of communication in which specific hand configurations symbolize language concepts. Several types of sign language exist, with the two most common being *American Sign Language (ASL)* and *Signed English*.

American Sign Language is a distinct and complete language that contains linguistic components constituting a sophisticated, independent language. It is the native language of Deaf culture. ASL has its own grammar and syntax, idioms, and metaphors. It has no written form. Moreover, it is conceptual in nature rather than word oriented. Signs of ASL are abstract symbols that are capable of expressing multiple elements simultaneously.

In contrast, Signed English follows the syntax and linguistic structure of English. Often, people who use Signed English also mouth the words that they sign, a process called *simultaneous communication*.

Cued speech is another system of visual communication. It is phonetically based, using hand shapes to represent speech sounds.

Interpreters

Certified interpreters can provide an important communication link between the deaf or hard-of-hearing individual and the hearing world. Used in both group settings and one-to-one interactions, interpreters are able to translate information so that accurate communication can take place. In situations where it is important for the translation to be precise and accurate, such as healthcare and counseling situations, it is crucial that the interpreter be properly trained and be certified by the *Registry of Interpreters for the Deaf*. In some situations, such as healthcare or counseling interactions, it is beneficial to use a professional interpreter with experience in mental health or healthcare paradigms who can properly assist with complex communication needs. Although family members sometimes serve as interpreters for deaf or hard-of-hearing individuals in more informal situations, in professional situations their use may obscure objective information, so it should be avoided if possible.

The presence of an interpreter can be intrusive and alter the dynamics of the healthcare or counseling interaction. Use of interpreters means that a third party will be present, reducing the sense of privacy that is normally expected in a number of professional situations. Certified interpreters, however, practice under a stringent code of ethics, which requires that all transactions be strictly confidential. It takes some adjustment for the employer, counselor, healthcare professional, or other person working with the deaf or hard-of-hearing individual to become accustomed to having a third party present in situations that normally take place on a one-to-one basis.

FUNCTIONAL IMPLICATIONS OF HEARING LOSS AND DEAFNESS

Personal and Psychosocial Issues

Communication and Development

The needs of people who are deaf or hard of hearing are different from those of individuals with other health conditions. Hearing is vital to verbal communication and to perception of environmental cues; thus any degree of hearing loss interferes with daily function to some extent. It alters speech intelligibility and other basic aspects of hearing such as localization, recognition, or identification of sound. The ability of individuals to adjust to hearing loss depends on the type and degree of loss, the age of onset, and the extent to which the loss interferes with daily communication and activity.

Severe hearing loss or deafness experienced congenitally or in early childhood also has developmental implications (Kral & O'Donoghue, 2010). Hearing loss occurring prior to language development influences individuals' experience and opportunity to gain concepts generally taken for granted in the hearing world. Children who do not have hearing loss learn many concepts from overheard conversations, background information from radio or television, and a multiplicity of other sources. Through this peripheral, daily communication, children learn cultural norms and expectations, generate and shape ideas, and form and enhance values and beliefs. Children who have severe hearing loss or are deaf are not exposed to many elements of communication that would otherwise enrich their language base, help them to formulate concepts, and impart social norms.

Individuals with congenital deafness or with hearing loss acquired before speech development require special programs to help them learn to communicate. Unfortunately, hearing loss in the very young is not always recognized immediately and may be misinterpreted as intellectual deficits, intellectual incapacity, or behavior disorders. Regular development and healthy adjustment of children with hearing loss depend to a large degree on early identification of hearing loss, appropriate management of hearing loss, early social and cultural influences, and parental attitudes and acceptance. Identification of profound hearing loss or deafness in a child can result in parental guilt, overprotection, or rejection. Professional assistance for the family when deafness in an infant is identified may be critical to their acceptance of the child's needs and to their ability to provide a nurturing environment for the child's emotional development. Individuals who have acquired a hearing loss during adulthood have memories of sound,

language, and previous function. Speech patterns have already been learned and can be maintained through special speech and conversation intervention. Individuals who have acquired hearing loss in adulthood may, however, feel uncomfortable and fear that others will reject them if they admit their hearing loss. They may deny that hearing loss exists or develop strategies to hide hearing loss, such as dominating the conversation to minimize the necessity of understanding anyone else or accusing others of not speaking clearly or mumbling. Some individuals exhibit aggressive behavior as a reaction to their hearing loss; others may withdraw completely from situations in which they have difficulty in hearing. Being unable to understand what is being said, individuals with hearing loss may believe that laughter and conversations of others are being directed toward them.

Hearing loss can lead to isolation, loneliness, and frustration, as well as to sensory deprivation. Hearing helps individuals communicate on a daily basis with family and friends and in social and work settings. At the most basic level, it helps individuals keep in touch with the environment. Background sounds, such as the wind in the trees, children playing down the street, and a train whistle in the distance, keep individuals aware of what is happening in the outside world. Hearing also acts as a signal to action. A telephone ringing, a baby crying, the horn of an approaching car, and the sound of footsteps from behind, for example, are all cues for some type of action. Thus, not only must individuals with a loss of hearing alter activities for which hearing is vital, but they also experience a sense of vulnerability because of the inability to hear sounds that once served as cues to action or danger.

Because hearing loss is an invisible form of incapacitation, denial is common, especially for those persons who acquire a hearing loss later in life. They may react with increased sensitivity or irritability when they do not understand words. Increased social pressure to understand may cause anxiety and frustration, and activities and interactions that they once enjoyed may be avoided. Unwillingness to acknowledge hearing loss may result in individuals' refusal to participate in hearing evaluations or reluctance to wear hearing aids.

If the onset of hearing loss is sudden, individuals will not have had the opportunity to adapt gradually as hearing diminishes, nor will they have had the opportunity to develop signing skills. Thus sudden hearing loss may be accompanied by depression, which can in turn interfere with learning and using new communication skills. The effects are circular, intensifying feelings of isolation and making the individual more depressed. Counselors trained in sign language may not be readily available, and the use of an interpreter for counseling sessions may increase individuals' reluctance to participate or to disclose feelings openly.

Any and all of the emotional states experienced by the adult with hearing loss may be experienced by the parents of children who have been identified as hard of hearing or deaf. Just as adults with hearing loss must work through their feelings to achieve a healthy adjustment, so must parents before they can be of optimal assistance to their child. Individuals who have hearing loss depend heavily on visual channels and on manual means of communication. The development of additional health conditions that threaten these resources for communication is of increased concern. A visual impairment or a condition that affects the hands, such as rheumatoid arthritis, can seriously hamper an individual's accustomed means of communication if using ASL or Signed English, necessitating additional training in new ways of communicating.

Deafness and Deaf Culture

A distinction should be made between members of Deaf culture and those who are deaf. Using a capital "D," indicates those individuals who describe themselves as a linguistic minority sharing a culture, not a health condition (Phillips, 1996; Porter, 1999). From the vantage point of Deaf culture, deafness is not a disability, a deficiency, or a handicap but rather a culture unto itself (Lane, 1995). Culture influences knowledge, attitudes, beliefs, values, and perceptions. It underlies the meaning given to action and the means by which experiences in the world are organized and understood. One of the key components of culture is language, which is necessary for communication. Language is an important part of every cultural identity and determines to a great extent who talks with whom

and what is discussed (Rendon, 1992). For those with hearing loss, there is no common language. Indeed, not all individuals with severe or profound hearing loss use the same language to communicate. Some individuals use Signed English; some use ASL; some rely to a large extent on speech reading to communicate. Especially for individuals who are prelingually deaf who use ASL as their primary language, English may viewed as a foreign language.

American Sign Language is a source of pride for the Deaf community. It is a true language, with its own structure and a syntax that has developed over time and that has no written form. Consequently, individuals who use ASL and especially those who are prelingually deaf frequently become part of the larger Deaf culture.

The Deaf community has its own theater, literature, and schools, along with social rules that are different from those of the hearing community (Barnett, 1999). Differences, especially in social norms, patterns, and traditions, can cause misunderstandings and misperceptions by those in the hearing world. Members of the Deaf culture have their own rules for behaviors, such as for getting the attention of individuals with whom they would like to communicate. Stomping a foot or tapping the hand of the individual to get his or her attention may be perfectly acceptable social behavior in the Deaf community, but may be viewed as rude by those in the hearing world. Consequently, individuals in the Deaf community may tend to associate with others in the Deaf community rather than those in the hearing world, may prefer state residential schools for educating the deaf rather than mainstreaming, and may reject efforts to incorporate them into the hearing world. In some instances, pride in the Deaf culture may even preclude procedures such as cochlear implants that could improve ability to hear (Olson, 2006). Individuals in the Deaf community may believe that attempts to correct their hearing imply that they have a health condition that needs a cure, perpetuating the view of the Deaf as disabled. Some may go as far as viewing efforts to cure deafness as an attempt to obliterate Deaf culture (Tucker, 1998). The Deaf culture does not exist in a vacuum. Individuals may be embedded in the Deaf culture,

but they are also imbued with values, attitudes, and behaviors that are part of a larger national culture as well as often part of ethnic minority cultures (Moore, 2001a; Moore, 2001b). This fact creates another layer of diversity.

Activities and Participation

Issues in the Environment

Many daily activities involve the sense of hearing. For individuals with hearing loss, even simple transactions—such as purchasing items from a local store, communicating with a repair person, or obtaining directions—require additional means of communication. In some instances, use of a third party as an interpreter may be a solution; however, individuals who are hard of hearing or deaf may resent the loss of privacy or loss of the sense of independence associated with the use of an interpreter.

Environmental sounds such as a knock on the door and the ringing of an alarm clock are not easily detected by individuals with hearing loss or deafness. Numerous technological devices and special aids are available to alert individuals to environmental sounds. In addition, signal dogs trained to alert their deaf owners to environmental sounds or signals are increasing in popularity. Depending on the degree of hearing loss, special activities—such attending movies, plays, and concerts—may be affected as well. The special devices mentioned previously help individuals participate more fully in such activities. In addition, decoders that provide captioned programming are available to enable individuals with hearing loss to enjoy television.

Issues in Childhood

For children, language plays an important role in regulating social play interactions and is paramount for framing and setting up play activities. Children who are deaf or hard of hearing may have difficulty developing cooperative play with hearing playmates. Promoting socialization between children with hearing loss and their hearing peers includes building on the strengths of the children and fostering a shared communication system that encourages social integration. Hearing loss

at an early age also has implications for literacy (Moreland, Atcherson, Zazove, & McKee, 2015). Low literacy rates may be attributed to lack of consensus on educational methods. Emphasis is often placed on techniques of communication, with less emphasis on content matter. In addition, because English is often a second language to individuals who are deaf, children who are deaf may face the same educational barriers as those experienced by other minority groups whose primary language is not English.

Issues in the Social Environment

The social environment of individuals with hearing loss can be altered due to the need for alternative means of communication. Individuals who have been deaf since birth or early childhood may integrate well with the Deaf community, where a common language is shared. Those who acquire hearing loss later in life, however, frequently do not join the Deaf community and may feel more isolated, feeling that they fit into neither the Deaf community nor the hearing world.

People with acquired hearing loss in adulthood are more likely to maintain social and cultural contacts with the hearing world because they have grown up with the language and culture of the hearing world. Many people who were deaf from an early age and use ASL as their primary language, however, feel that they are part of the Deaf community, with a different culture, as discussed previously.

Individuals with hearing loss may limit social contacts to family members and a few close friends, or they may avoid social contacts altogether because of their inability to understand what is being said. Difficulty in understanding verbal communication can cause withdrawal from social situations in an effort to avoid the embarrassment of giving inappropriate responses to questions or statements. Lack of understanding by others can exacerbate this sense of social isolation. New acquaintances who are unfamiliar with hearing loss or unaware of individuals' inability to hear may perceive them as aloof or even rude because of their failure to respond to a friendly statement that they did not hear. Individuals with hearing loss may have more difficulty keeping up with conversations in group settings, especially if others in the group are unaware of or insensitive to their needs. Group settings with poor lighting make lip reading more difficult, and competing sounds, such as the clattering of dishes in a restaurant, may make communication difficult even for individuals with milder hearing loss.

Engaging in conversation requires cooperation from others. Some people may feel uncomfortable or impatient while attempting to communicate with individuals with hearing loss and, consequently, may avoid contact with them. Some may consider deafness to carry a social stigma because of myths and misconceptions about hearing loss. Such attitudes build a barrier to acceptance by others and inclusion in the larger social community. Societal responses can create difficult and stressful situations for individuals with hearing loss, discouraging their further participation in social functions.

Family Interactions

Although family members serve as a support group for individuals with hearing loss, their attitudes may also impede individuals' acceptance of their condition and subsequent rehabilitation. Family members may perceive a hearing loss as feigned or may attribute the difficulty to inattention. As a result, they may become angry, ignore the individual, or exclude him or her from conversation rather than learning techniques to enhance the individual's ability to maintain an active role in conversation. In many cases, family members who serve as interpreters for those with hearing loss may begin to resent their role, feeling stifled in social interactions.

Sensitivity of family members and others in the social environment to the needs of individuals with hearing loss or deafness is important to enable full participation in social interactions. Without awareness and sensitivity of others, individuals with hearing loss may be unable to actively participate in family discussion, decision making, or conversations at mealtime, or engage in small talk while performing various tasks.

Sexuality

Hearing loss can have an impact on state of mind and can affect behavior. When one of the individuals in a relationship experiences hearing loss, the

communication aspect of the relationship is affected and can become a source of anxiety and misunderstanding. Individuals who are single may have more difficulty meeting potential partners and establishing communication that could lead to a more intimate relationship.

Individuals who have been deaf from childhood may not have received adequate sex education, either due to misperceptions about sex education needs of children who have hearing loss or are deaf, or because of the unavailability of individuals competent or comfortable in communicating information about sexual issues in sign language. Lack of sex education in childhood, in addition to affecting normal developmental issues, can place children at risk of potential sexual abuse.

When hearing loss is acquired, discussion of the impact of hearing loss and alternative means of communication to retain intimacy can be helpful in maintaining a strong relationship. For instance, individuals with hearing loss may no longer be able to recognize romantic cues that were once a part of the relationship. Darkened environments, which may have once been conducive to intimate moments, may further preclude communication, making it difficult for individuals with hearing loss to lip read or pick up facial cues that might enhance understanding and communication.

Support Groups

A number of support groups directed toward individuals with adult- or late-onset hearing loss are available, including Self-Help for Hard of Hearing People (SHHH) and the Association of Late Deafened Adults (ALDA). In addition to offering support to individuals who are hard of hearing or deaf, SHHH and ALDA strive to increase community understanding about the rights and needs of individuals with hearing loss as well as to make social environments more accessible. Many communities also have other types of support groups for people with hearing loss.

VOCATIONAL ISSUES IN HEARING LOSS AND DEAFNESS

Individuals with hearing loss face the same issues with regard to employment as others with health

conditions; however, additional special vocational issues must be considered in the former case. Many jobs require individuals to be alert to auditory cues to perform or to maintain safety. Most jobs also require communication with coworkers or customers. People who are deaf or hard of hearing may have difficulty receiving instructions or supervision, or participating in staff meetings or in-service training. In addition, they may have difficulty interacting as part of work-related social functioning. Assistive devices may be needed to help them with basic communication, or there may be a need for job restructuring, redesigning procedures, or redelegation of assignments to accommodate communication needs.

Just as there are myths and stereotypes about hearing loss in the social world, so there are myths and stereotypes in the world of work. Employers and fellow workers may not understand hearing loss and may be unaware of the special needs of individuals who are deaf or hard of hearing, or the special techniques available to enhance communication. Because hearing loss is an invisible health condition, coworkers or supervisors may not recognize the need for special accommodations or may believe that individuals with hearing loss are feigning the degree of incapacitation. In some instances, individuals' lack of ability to hear may be interpreted as lack of intellectual ability, such that individuals with hearing loss may be relegated to jobs requiring less cognitive ability.

In the work setting, individuals with hearing loss may need special assistive devices, communication aids, and signaling devices. The use of such devices is often dependent on the availability and expense of the purchase and installation of the special items. Equipment may be prioritized according to need if funds are limited. For example, a signaling device that is crucial for safety may be considered vital, whereas equipment that would enhance individuals' performance may not receive as high a priority.

Because visual cues are so important to communication for individuals with hearing loss, good lighting in the workplace is a necessity. Many individuals with hearing loss experience discomfort with loud noises; therefore, noise levels in

the environment should be evaluated. In some instances, it may be necessary for individuals to wear ear protectors to prevent further hearing loss. Room acoustics must also be considered, as the reverberation of sound in an environment can interfere with the effectiveness of a hearing aid. Hearing aids can greatly enhance the performance of some individuals in the work setting. Although technological advances have made hearing aids more durable, these intricate devices remain susceptible to damage from environmental factors. Hearing aids are sensitive to extremes of temperature—especially extreme cold—and they require protection from perspiration in hot and humid environments.

Individuals with hearing loss are a heterogeneous group and should be considered as such. Although special needs associated with hearing loss should be considered, individuals' unique talents and interests should also be taken into account in helping persons with hearing loss adjust to the work environment. With the use of assistive devices, many job opportunities not previously open to individuals with hearing loss are now well within the range of possibilities. However, attitudinal barriers still exist and may preclude the individual with hearing loss from obtaining satisfactory employment.

CASE STUDY

Ms. N. is a 42-year-old attorney who has developed hearing loss as a result of Meniere's disease. On audiological evaluation, she was found to have hearing loss in both ears at the 45-decibel range.

1. To what extent will Ms. N.'s degree of hearing loss interfere with her ability to continue to function in her current occupation? Which specific factors may be important to consider?

2. Given Ms. N.'s type and extent of hearing loss, which adaptive devices or accommodations may be used in her current occupation?

REFERENCES

Acar, B., Ocak, E., Acar, M., & Kocaöz, D. (2015). Comparison of risk factors in newborn hearing screening in a developing country. The Turkish Journal of Pediatrics, 57(4), 334–338.

Baloh, R. W., & Jen, J. (2016). Hearing and equilibrium. In L. Goldman & A. I. Schafer (Eds.), Goldman-Cecil textbook of medicine. (25th ed., pp. 2593–2601). Philadelphia, PA: Elsevier Saunders.

Barnett, S. (1999). Clinical and cultural issues in caring for deaf people. Family Medicine, 31(1), 17–22.

Berman, S. (2007). The end of an era in otitis research. New England Journal of Medicine, 356(3), 300–302.

Chute, P. A. (2004). Cochlear implants: An evolving journey. ASHA Leader 9(3), 7–8.

Desselle, D. D., & Proctor, T. K. (2000). Advocating for the elderly hard-of-hearing population: The deaf people we ignore. Social Work, 45(3), 277–281.

Edmiston, R. C., Aggarwal, R., & Green, K. M. (2015). Bone conduction implants—A rapidly developing field. Journal of Laryngology and Otology, 129(10), 936–940.

Fransman, D., & Walker, S. (2007). Digital hearing aids: A life transformed. Learning Disability Practice, 10(3), 16–19.

Gates, G. A., & Miyamoto, R. T. (2003). Cochlear implants. New England Journal of Medicine, 349(5), 421–423.

Kinne, B. L., & Leafman, J. S. (2015). Effectiveness of the Parnes particle repositioning manoeuvre for posterior canal benign paroxysmal positional vertigo. Journal of Laryngology and Otology, 129(12), 1188–1193.

Koci, V., Seebacher, J., Weichbold, V., Zorowka, P., Wolf-Magele, A., Sprinzl, G., & Stephan, K. (2016). Improvement of sound source localization abilities in patients bilaterally supplied with active middle ear implants. Acta Oto-Laryngologica, 136(7), 692–698.

Kral, A., & O'Donoghue, G. M. (2010). Profound deafness in childhood. New England Journal of Medicine, 363(15), 1438–1450.

Lane, H. (1995). Constructions of deafness. Disability and Society, 10(2), 171–189.

Lantos, J. D. (2012). Ethics for the pediatrician: The evolving ethics of cochlear implants in children. Pediatrics in Review, 33(7), 323–326.

Lerner, P. K., & Eng, N. (2005). Speech, language, hearing, and swallowing disorders. In H. H. Zaretsky, E. F. Richter III, & M. G. Eisenberg (Eds.), Medical aspects of disability (3rd ed., pp. 289–324). New York, NY: Springer.

Moore, C. L. (2001a). Educating the deaf: Psychology, principles, and practices (5th ed.). Boston, MA: Houghton Mifflin.

Moore, C. L. (2001b). Racial and ethnic members of under-represented groups with hearing loss and VR services: Explaining the disparity in closure success rates. Journal of Applied Rehabilitation Counseling, 33(1), 15–20.

Moreland, C., Aicherson, S. R., Zazove, P., & McKee, M. (2015). Hearing loss: Issues in the deaf and hard of hearing communities. FP Essentials, 434, 29–40.

Myers, L., & Thyer, A. (1997). Social work practice with deaf clients: Issues in culturally competent assessment. Social Work in Health Care, 26(1), 61–74.

Nichols, A. D. (2006, October). Hearing loss: Perceptions and solutions. Nursing Homes Magazine, 66–69.

Olson, A. D. (2006). Counseling adults prior to a cochlear implant. *ASHA Leader, 11*(13), 5, 18–19.

Paradise, J. L., Feldman, H. M., Campbell, T. F., Dollaghan, C. A., Rockette, H. E., Pitcairn, D. L., ... Pelham, W. E. Jr. (2007). Tympanostomy tubes and developmental outcomes at 9 to 11 years of age. *New England Journal of Medicine, 356*(3), 248–261.

Pass, L., & Graber, A. D. (2015). Informed consent, deaf culture, and cochlear implants. *Journal of Clinical Ethics, 26*(3), 219–230.

Phan, J., Houston, D. M., Ruffin, C., Ting, J., & Holt, R. F. (2016). Factors affecting speech discrimination in children with cochlear implant: Evidence from early-implanted infants. *Journal of the American Academy of Audiology, 27*(6), 480–488.

Phillips, B. A. (1996). Bringing culture to the forefront: Formulating diagnostic impressions of deaf and hard-of-hearing people at times of medical crisis. *Professional Psychology: Research and Practice, 27*(2), 137–144.

Porter, A. (1999). Sign-language interpretation in psychotherapy with deaf patients. *American Journal of Psychotherapy, 53*(2), 163–176.

Rendon, M. E. (1992). Deaf culture and alcohol and substance abuse. *Journal of Substance Abuse Treatment, 9*, 103–110.

Robertson, C., Kerr, M., Garcia, C., & Halterman, E. (2007). Noise and hearing protection: Latino construction workers' experiences. *American Association of Occupational Health Nurses Journal, 55*(4), 153–160.

Roman, S., Rochette, F., Triglia, J. M., Schön, D., & Bigand, E. (2016). Auditory training improves auditory performance in cochlear implanted children. *Hearing Research, 337*, 89–95.

Saxon, J. P., Holmes, A. E., & Spitznagel, R. J. (2001). Impact of a cochlear implant on job functioning. *Journal of Rehabilitation, 67*(3), 49–54.

Shafer, D. N. (2006). Early hearing diagnosis key to language skills. *ASHA Leader, 11*(14), 5, 53.

Sharma, K., Pannu, M. S., Arora, A., & Sharma, V. (2016). Preventive audiology: Screening for hearing impairment in children having recurrent URII. *Indian Journal of Otolaryngology and Head and Neck Surgery, 68*(2), 163–166.

Sherwood, L. (2007). Ear: Hearing and equilibrium. In L. Sherwood (Ed.), *Human physiology: From cells to systems* (6th ed., pp. 208–220). Belmont, CA: Thompson/Brooks-Cole.

Shin, J. W., Kim, S. H., Choi, J., Park, H. J., Lee, S. C., Choi, J. S., ... Lee, H. K. (2016). Surgical and audiologic comparison between Sophono and bone-anchored hearing aid implantation. *Clinical and Experimental Otorhinolaryngology, 9*(17), 21–26.

Steel, K. P. (2000). New interventions in hearing impairment. *British Medical Journal, 320*(7235), 622–629.

Tucker, B. P. (1998). Deaf culture, cochlear implants, and elective disability. *Hastings Center Report, 28*(4), 6–14.

Williams, P. J. (2000). Genetic causes of hearing loss. *New England Journal of Medicine, 342*(15), 1101–1109.

Zeng, F. G. (2004). Trends in cochlear implants. *Trends in Amplification, 8*(1), 1–34.

Sickle Cell Disease, Hemophilia, and Conditions of the Blood

STRUCTURE AND FUNCTION OF THE BLOOD

Blood circulates continuously through the body and is essential for life. Blood is composed of a liquid and a combination of several types of specialized cells:

- Red blood cells (RBCs), also called *erythrocytes*
- White blood cells (WBCs), also called *leukocytes*
- Platelets, also called *thrombocytes*

The liquid portion of the blood is a watery, colorless fluid called *plasma*. It contains no blood cells but rather is essential for carrying blood cells and nutrients through the circulation, as well as for transporting wastes from the tissues. Plasma also contains vital *plasma proteins* and other important substances.

The total blood volume accounts for approximately 7% of human body weight. Under usual conditions, the quantity of blood in the adult body remains constant. The RBCs, WBCs, and platelets account for approximately 45% of the total blood volume, while plasma accounts for the other 55%. More than 99% of the cells in the blood are red blood cells.

Blood has many functions:

- It carries oxygen and nutrients to the body tissues.
- It facilitates communication between the endocrine glands and other body organs by transporting hormones.
- It carries waste products from the tissues to the organs of excretion, such as the lungs and the kidneys.
- It protects the body from foreign organisms.
- It promotes clotting to minimize excessive bleeding.
- It helps regulate body temperature.

Blood cells are formed by a process called *hemopoiesis* or *hematopoiesis*. Tissues that produce blood cells are said to be *hematopoietic*. Blood cells are produced in the bone marrow as well as in lymphoid tissue and organs. Special cells called *stem cells* are the sources from which all blood cells are formed. Bone marrow is especially rich in stem cells.

Structure and Function of Red Blood Cells (Erythrocytes)

Red blood cells carry oxygen to the tissues. When mature, they are devoid of a nucleus. These cells are usually disk shaped, with a thin center and thicker edges. They are flexible, which allows the cells to adapt their shape to fit through blood vessels of differing sizes. *Hemoglobin* is the red pigmented protein contained within the erythrocytes and is the specific part of the red blood cell that carries oxygen. In addition, hemoglobin contains iron.

Structure and Function of White Blood Cells (Leukocytes)

White blood cells are important to the body's ability to resist or destroy foreign materials and organisms; that is, they are an important component of immune system function. The five types of leukocytes play different roles in defending the body from infection (see **Table 18-1**).

Under normal circumstances, blood contains a fairly consistent number of circulating WBCs. When an infection occurs or when some other foreign stimuli are in the body, WBCs proliferate so that large numbers of them circulate in the bloodstream; this condition is called **leukocytosis**. White blood cells are formed in the bone marrow and play the predominant role in the body's defense system. These leukocytes take action when body tissues have been damaged or invaded by organisms or other foreign materials. Any infection or invasion by foreign substances causes a dramatic increase in the number of WBCs in the blood. Some leukocytes—called *phagocytes*—are scavengers and have the ability to destroy and ingest bacteria or foreign particles; the process of ingesting cells and foreign objects is called **phagocytosis**. The role of WBCs in immunity is discussed in the Introduction to the Immune System chapter.

Structure and Function of Platelets (Thrombocytes) and Coagulation

Platelets are disk-shaped cells that are formed by special cells in the bone marrow. The smallest

Special cells in the bone marrow produce erythrocytes. Several vitamins, such as *vitamin B_{12}* and *folic acid* (which is part of the vitamin B complex), are necessary for the formation of erythrocytes. These vitamins are obtained from the diet. Iron, which is also obtained from the diet, is important for the formation of hemoglobin. Excess amounts of iron and vitamin B_{12} are stored in the liver.

New RBCs are constantly being formed. Although most erythrocytes are released into the blood, some are taken up by the spleen to be stored for emergency use when the RBC count drops significantly below regular levels, such as during excessive bleeding (*hemorrhage*). Newly formed RBCs enter the bloodstream before they are totally mature. At this stage, they are called *reticulocytes*. Within several days, these reticulocytes mature to become erythrocytes. The life cycle of erythrocytes is approximately 120 days. As the erythrocytes reach the end of their lives, they become more fragile and rupture. In addition, some of the old erythrocytes are destroyed in the *spleen*. Special cells within the spleen and liver absorb the old erythrocytes, making room for more new cells.

When the quantity of oxygen supplied to body tissues decreases, the body increases the number of RBCs produced. For example, at higher altitudes, where less oxygen is available in the air, the bone marrow reacts by producing more RBCs, even if an adequate number of RBCs are present in the circulation.

Table 18-1 Types of Leukocytes

Type	Function
Neutrophils	Engulf and destroy foreign substances
Eosinophils	Are involved in allergic reactions
Basophils	Secrete histamine and are involved in allergic reactions
Monocytes	Become macrophages, which destroy foreign substances
Lymphocytes	
B lymphocytes (B cells)	Become cells that secrete antibodies to destroy foreign substances
T lymphocytes (T cells)	Release chemicals that destroy cells invaded by viruses

cells in the blood, they contain no hemoglobin.

The number of platelets circulating in the blood usually does not change. If the number of platelets should decrease, however, the condition is called **thrombocytopenia**; conversely, an increase in the number of platelets is called **thrombocytosis**. Platelets play a crucial role in blood clotting and are involved in an important first step in preventing excessive bleeding after an injury. Approximately one-third of platelets are stored in the spleen for emergency use.

The term **hemostasis** refers to the series of events that stop bleeding from damaged vessels. When bleeding occurs, the damaged blood vessel immediately constricts, going into spasm in an effort to minimize blood loss. The walls of the vessels become sticky, causing the walls to adhere to each other and further restrict blood flow. This sticky surface of the vessels activates platelets so that they group together and adhere to the wall, forming a plug. The plug, in addition to stopping the bleeding momentarily, releases other chemicals that in turn enhance blood coagulation.

Platelets alone cannot stop bleeding indefinitely. Instead, the formation of the plug activates *clotting factors* (coagulation factors from the liver, plasma, and other sources) so that a clot forms to control the bleeding. Clotting involves turning blood from a liquid into a more solid form. The platelet plug acts as a base, allowing the clot to attach and seal the break. For a clot to form, *fibrinogen*—a substance that is formed in the liver and present in the plasma—is converted into *fibrin*. Fibrin forms a matrix at the site that collects blood cells and platelets, resulting in clot formation.

The conversion of fibrinogen to fibrin takes place because of an enzyme called *thrombin*. Thrombin is formed only when needed from a precursor called *prothrombin*, which is found in the plasma. This conversion is made possible by a plasma clotting factor—*factor X*—that becomes activated because of another plasma clotting factor.

Different sets of substances play major roles in both intrinsic and extrinsic blood clotting factors, most of which are named by Roman numerals designated from I to XIII. *Intrinsic clotting factors* precipitate clotting by making contact with substances contained in the blood. *Extrinsic clotting*
factors precipitate clotting by interacting with substances in the tissues outside the blood. For instance, thrombin activates factor XIII, thereby stabilizing the fibrin matrix, whereas other substances in the clotting mechanism may be activated because of substances that have leaked from tissues outside the vessel. *Vitamin K* is necessary for the formation of some clotting factors and is essential to clot formation. To prevent excessive clotting, other body mechanisms are activated as well.

SICKLE CELL DISEASE

Overview of Sickle Cell Disease

Sickle cell disease is a genetic condition are caused by a mutation in the hemoglobin molecule (Steinberg, 2016). Individuals with sickle cell disease have a mutation on a part of hemoglobin that results in the development of *sickle cell hemoglobin*, also known as *hemoglobin S*.

This mutation is passed on by an autosomal recessive gene and occurs most often in individuals of African descent, although it can also occur in individuals of Hispanic, Mediterranean, Middle Eastern, and Near Eastern ancestry (Steinberg, 2016).

Identification of Sickle Cell Disease

In the United States, routine screening of infants for sickle cell disease is required to promote early management of the condition if present (Bonham, George, Dover, & Brody, 2010). Identification of irregular hemoglobin can be done through microscopic examination of blood cells (*sickle cell prep*), although this test cannot distinguish between sickle cell disease and sickle cell trait. Another test, *hemoglobin electrophoresis*, may also be done to identify and measure different types of hemoglobin. In addition, prenatal testing through *amniocentesis* may be conducted in some instances.

Sickle Cell Crisis

The course of sickle cell disease includes periods of painful and incapacitating *vaso-occlusive* events (*sickle cell crisis*) in which the blood supply, and consequently oxygen, is cut off to various body tissues. Sickle cell crisis is marked by rigidity of the sickled red blood cells, increased adhesiveness

on these cells' surface, and decreased red blood cell survival. When the oxygen concentration in the blood is low, the red blood cells' surfaces become sticky and the cells become deformed so that, instead of being disk shaped, they assume the shape of a crescent or sickle. Because of this distortion, the red blood cells become rigid and are unable to adapt their shape to fit through tiny blood vessels. These misshaped red blood cells become entangled with one another and begin to pile up. Eventually, the sickle-shaped red blood cells obstruct vessels and prevent blood flow to surrounding tissue (vaso-occlusive events). A sickled cell is very fragile and is easily destroyed, which severely curtails its average life span. As a result, the bone marrow dramatically increases production of RBCs in an effort to keep pace with the accelerated rate of destruction. Because the rate of production cannot keep pace with the rate of destruction, individuals with sickle cell disease can become severely anemic (*hemolytic anemia*).

The specific causes of sickle cell crisis are unknown; however, certain factors—such as heavy exertional stress, mental stress, infection, dehydration, high altitudes, and extremes in temperature—may be precipitating factors (Steinberg, 2016).

Manifestations of Sickle Cell Disease

Due to the destruction of RBCs (**hemolysis**), many individuals with sickle cell disease experience chronic anemia (hemolytic anemia) with associated fatigue. Because fatigue is not a life-threatening manifestation, it often does not receive the same attention as other manifestations related to sickle cell disease. It can, however, affect individuals' functional capacity and interfere with both daily activities and work-related functioning. In addition to generalized fatigue, some individuals experience difficulty breathing on exertion (**exertional dyspnea**).

Pain, due to lack of oxygen to a body part, is the hallmark of vaso-occlusive events. Although all body parts, including internal organs, may be affected, the hands and feet, back, legs, knees, and chest are especially common sites of pain. If blood flow, and consequently oxygen supply, is severely diminished, the affected tissue may undergo **necrosis** (tissue death). The amount of damage experienced during sickle cell crisis may range from mild to severe, depending on the degree of blockage and the length of time the blockage exists.

Although the degree and frequency of painful episodes vary greatly in different individuals, many persons with sickle cell disease experience pain nearly half the time. Sometimes this pain can be managed with oral analgesics; in other cases, it is severe enough to warrant hospitalization and administration of narcotics and intravenous hydration therapy.

Complications of Sickle Cell Disease

A number of complications are possible with sickle cell anemia. Some individuals have none, while others experience complications that are severe (Steinberg, 2016). This section describes a number of common complications of sickle cell disease.

Immune Function

Chronic anemia associated with sickle cell disease lowers resistance and increases individuals' susceptibility to infection. In addition, the spleen is frequently affected during sickle cell crisis and may be permanently damaged over time due to vaso-occlusive events. Because the spleen is important in immune function, damage to or removal of this organ can cause increased risk of infection.

In some instances, *splenic sequestration crisis* may occur, characterized by acute, painful enlargement of the spleen such that the individual's abdomen becomes very bloated and hard. Splenic sequestration is an acute complication of sickle cell disease and can result in death if it is not recognized immediately and managed appropriately. Individuals with severe spleen involvement may have a **splenectomy** (removal of the spleen) or may require chronic transfusion support.

Individuals with sickle cell disease may be placed on prophylactic antibiotics to decrease their risk of developing an infection that could precipitate sickle cell crisis. Immunizations, avoidance of contact with individuals with infectious conditions, good nutrition, and general health maintenance are extremely important to prevent infections from occurring.

Aplastic Crisis

Aplastic crisis in sickle cell disease, which can be triggered by an infection, refers to an acute and temporary worsening of anemia caused by an abrupt decrease of RBC production by the bone marrow. Because individuals with sickle cell disease already have decreased numbers of RBCs by virtue of their condition, decreased production of RBCs in aplastic anemia can be a life-threatening event. Recovery from aplastic crisis may be spontaneous or, in some instances, transfusion of RBCs may be needed to counteract the shortage of these cells.

Neurological Complications

Occlusion of vessels in the brain can result in a stroke and resulting manifestations, which can be permanent and life threatening and can include cognitive impairment as well as other neurological consequences (see Chapter 5) (Goldstein, 2016).

Ocular Complications

Increased blood **viscosity** (thickness) may cause sickle cell **retinopathy** (damage to the retina of the eye), resulting in vitreal hemorrhage and possibly retinal detachment. Although complications can cause visual loss, many times changes in the eye regress spontaneously with little permanent damage (Steinberg, 2016).

Pulmonary Complications

Acute chest syndrome is a condition characterized by fever, chest pain, and **dyspnea** (difficulty breathing) that affects nearly half of all individuals with sickle cell anemia (Steinberg, 2016). Its consequences may include pulmonary infection and vaso-occlusive events that involve the lungs. If the lungs are the site of repeated vaso-occlusive events or recurrent lung infections, pulmonary function may be compromised, with resulting incapacitation related to limited lung function.

Cardiac Complications

Chronic anemia associated with sickle cell disease causes the heart to pump faster in an attempt to supply additional oxygen to the tissues (Steinberg, 2016). This increased work by the heart can contribute to enlargement of the heart (**cardiomegaly**) and decreased cardiac efficiency.

Renal Complications

Sickle cell disease can cause kidney damage resulting in **hematuria** (blood in the urine) and **proteinuria** (protein in the urine) and eventual *renal failure.*

Skeletal Complications

Occlusion of blood flow during a sickle cell crisis can result in **osteonecrosis** (bone death) and consequent damage to the bones and joints, especially the hip and shoulder joints, leading to pain, swelling, and limited mobility of joints and resulting in decreased mobility. Nearly half of all individuals with sickle cell anemia develop osteonecrosis (Steinberg, 2016). *Avascular necrosis* (tissue death due to lack of blood supply) of *the head of the femur* (thigh bone) may occur with sickle cell disease and may require surgical intervention.

Genital Complications

A condition called **priapism** (sustained, painful erection in the absence of sexual stimulation) may occur in males with sickle cell disease. The condition requires immediate healthcare attention to prevent permanent nerve damage and consequent impotence.

Dermatologic Complications

Some individuals develop painful and nonhealing *leg ulcers* because of the interruption in circulation that occurs during sickle cell crisis. Ulcers are incapacitating and disfiguring, and they may become infected, leading to systemic infection. Because leg ulcers are frequently resistant to healing, individuals may need to be placed on bed rest to facilitate healing of the ulcers. In some instances, skin grafting may be necessary.

Complications Related to Growth and Development

The growth and development of individuals with sickle cell anemia can be affected, although the exact way the condition contributes to delayed growth is still unclear. Although some delay in

physical and sexual maturation occurs, individuals do eventually reach full physical maturity

Management of Sickle Cell Disease

Sickle cell disease is a chronic, lifelong condition. Thus management of this disease is directed toward controlling manifestations and preventing complications. Due to advances in management of sickle cell disease, better supportive care, and early detection and management of complications, the life expectancy of individuals with sickle cell anemia has increased dramatically (Steinberg, 2016). Education of individuals with sickle cell disease and their families regarding sickle cell disease and its genetic basis, as well as about the importance of regular health maintenance, and prompt seeking of health care for any infection or other acute health condition are crucial to ensuring good outcomes. Understanding the triggers of sickle cell crisis can help to prevent incapacitating complications. Individuals should have regular, scheduled health evaluations to monitor the course of their condition and to evaluate the effectiveness of the management plan.

Good nutrition is essential to combat anemia and to maintain the body's resistance to infection. Because of the propensity of those who have sickle cell disease to develop infections, routine immunizations, including administration of pneumonia vaccines, are crucial. Prophylactic antibiotics are often used as well.

Likewise, maintaining adequate fluid intake is important for individuals with sickle cell disease. Adequate hydration minimizes the sickling of red blood cells and decreases blood viscosity. Adequate fluid intake is especially important in situations in which individuals may be exposed to high environmental temperatures.

Anemia associated with sickle cell disease may necessitate transfusion therapy. Repeated transfusions can result in iron overload, which in turn can cause heart and liver failure (Steinberg, 2016). Iron chelation therapy may be used to decrease the risk of this complication. Although stem cell transplantation has been used with success in some individuals with sickle cell anemia, only approximately 10% of individuals are able to find suitable donors (Steinberg, 2016).

Individuals who experience sickle cell crisis usually require hospitalization. During the crisis, management focuses on restoring fluids if dehydration has occurred and on relieving pain associated with the crisis, usually through administration of narcotics. Adequate pain management is a crucial part of management of sickle cell crisis. Pain in individuals with sickle cell disease is often undertreated owing to concerns about narcotic addiction or suspicion of drug-seeking behavior.

Organ damage as a result of sickle cell disease is managed in a similar fashion to organ damage that may be present in other chronic conditions, such as chronic kidney disease and chronic lung disease. If significant organ or bone damage has occurred as a result of sickle cell crisis, individuals may be referred to a pain clinic to help them learn how to manage chronic pain. If infection or another condition precipitated the crisis, interventions directed toward treating the underlying condition are instituted.

Functional Implications of Sickle Cell Disease

Personal and Psychosocial Issues

Sickle cell disease usually manifests itself in childhood, necessitating healthcare attention and, possibly, frequent hospitalizations. Although many individuals with sickle cell disease adjust and learn to cope with their condition, factors related to this condition may disrupt social development and educational progress in other individuals. Psychological coping patterns are relevant both to the experience of pain and to broader adjustment issues.

Because sickle cell disease is hereditary, parents of children with sickle cell disease may experience guilt or fear the loss of their child. As a result, they may become overly protective, promoting dependence in the child. At the same time, the child may learn manipulative behaviors to gain attention. These maladaptive means of coping may persist throughout life, creating a greater barrier to social relationships and work than does the condition itself.

The transition to adulthood for any adolescent may be challenging due to disruption of previously established relationships or other life changes as

youth move from a more protected environment into the adult world. For adolescents with sickle cell disease, prolonged health conditions and multiple hospitalizations may disrupt the formation of sense of self and contribute to difficulty in developing substantive peer relationships. Adherence to a management plan to prevent crisis or complications, such as drinking recommended daily quantities of water or taking prophylactic penicillin, may be especially difficult for members of this age group and require significant support. Adolescents may be reluctant to disclose their condition to avoid the marginalization they may associate with their condition or to avoid being seen as "different" by their peers.

Many adults with sickle cell disease have learned to manage their condition and cope with factors related to it.

Individuals with sickle cell disease have lived with their chronic condition throughout life and, therefore, are frequently familiar with the types and dosages of medication required to relieve pain. Because pain intensity is difficult to assess by the outside observer, health professionals may interpret requests for specific pain medications and dosages as drug-seeking behavior, however there is no evidence to suggest that the rate of addiction in sickle cell disease is different than the rate for the general population (Kotila, Busari, Makanjuola, & Eyelade, 2015)

Sickle cell disease carries the additional stress of unpredictability. Although some factors that provoke a sickle cell crisis may be identifiable, crises are often unpredictable and beyond the individual's control. Not only are these crises painful and incapacitating, but there is also the potential for organ damage each time such an incident occurs. Lack of control over the frequency or severity of sickle cell crises and not knowing the extent of damage that each crisis may inflict can lead to stress.

Activities and Participation

Individuals with sickle cell disease can usually maintain regular schedules and do not need to alter their activities, unless specific activities are found to precipitate a sickle cell crisis. Most activities, if performed in moderation, can be tolerated. Even so, owing to the unpredictability of sickle cell crisis,

sometimes a crisis may necessitate unplanned hospitalization, disrupting work schedules and interfering with participation in social events. The role of stress as a precipitating factor in sickle cell crisis must also be considered. Although stress is frequently associated with negative events, it can also be linked to positive events, such as a graduation celebration or a wedding.

Sickle cell disease affects the entire family. Individuals with sickle cell disease may require significant attention, which may create tension and anxiety. How the family members react to the individual and the degree of support they provide will greatly influence the individual's self-concept and development of social skills.

Vocational Issues in Sickle Cell Disease

Individuals with sickle cell disease often have a lifelong pattern of disruption caused by repeated hospitalizations, which may in turn have affected their academic achievement, job training opportunities, and acquisition of job skills. The degree of physical consequences that individuals experience as a result of sickle cell disease depends on whether organ damage has been experienced. If specific organ or joint damage has been inflicted as a result of repeated sickle cell crises, the individual will have many of the same limitations as individuals who have similar conditions for other reasons. Problems with ambulation, vision, or neurological function can arise if damage to specific areas of the body has occurred, for example. Without organ damage, the physical consequences of the condition will affect the individual's capacity for exertion and strenuous activity. Individuals with sickle cell disease must consider not only the physical demands of a job as related to stamina but also the role that strenuous exertion has in precipitating sickle cell crisis. Because sickle cell disease is a lifelong condition, over the years most individuals learn which types of activities and how much activity they can usually tolerate.

Despite the potential relationship between overexertion and sickle cell crisis, most individuals with sickle cell disease are able to perform moderate work. In instances where individuals with sickle cell disease experience fatigue and chronic pain, a realistic vocational goal may be part-time employment or a more sedentary type of work. Environmental factors such as extremes of temperature, high altitudes, and potential for exposure to infection should be avoided. Because dehydration can precipitate a crisis, individuals should have ready access to water or other fluids in their work environment. Likewise, because of their increased fluid intake and consequently high urine output, ready access to restrooms is required.

Stress in the work environment, including its contribution to the development of sickle cell crisis, is another factor that individuals with sickle cell disease must consider. Not all individuals react to stress in the same way, nor are perceptions of stress always the same. For this reason, the importance of stress must be determined on an individual basis. The degree to which absences due to sickle cell crises become a hindrance to work performance depends on the individual, the frequency of such crises, and the seriousness of the crises when they occur.

The potential for sickle cell crisis and subsequent absences from work should be considered and discussed with employers in advance. Individuals may be reluctant to reveal their condition to the employer because of fear that repeated absences may jeopardize employment. Nevertheless, adequate preparation of employers in advance for potential absences can alleviate problems if absences do occur.

Psychosocial factors and their impact on vocational function cannot be dismissed. The unpredictability of the condition and the continued potential for sudden death as the result of sickle cell crisis may precipitate depression and affect motivation to seek work. If the individual has not developed adequate social skills, social skills training may be needed.

HEMOPHILIA

Overview of Hemophilia

Hemophilia is one of several inherited, chronic bleeding conditions characterized by a deficiency or absence of one of the clotting factors (Ragni, 2016). With this X-linked recessive condition,

males inherit the condition and females have no manifestations but are carriers of the affected chromosome.

In most instances, hemophilia is transmitted when a mother who carries a hemophilia gene and an unaffected father have a son. Under these circumstances, there is a 50% chance that their sons will have hemophilia and a 50% chance that their daughters will be carriers. If the father has hemophilia but the mother is unaffected, none of the sons will be affected, but all daughters will be carriers (Ragni, 2016). Although hemophilia can occur in women, it is extremely rare. If the mother is a carrier and the father has hemophilia, each of their daughters will either have hemophilia or be a carrier, while sons will have a 50% chance of having hemophilia or being unaffected (Ragni, 2016). In some instances, individuals are born with hemophilia despite the lack of a family history. In these instances, the condition is thought to have been caused by a spontaneous mutation rather than heredity (Ragni, 2016).

The degree of severity varies for hemophilia. With new prophylactic infusion therapy, and without complications, individuals with hemophilia now have a life expectancy matching that of the regular population (Ragni, 2016).

Types of Hemophilia

Several types of hemophilia exist, including hemophilia A and hemophilia B, both of which are caused by a defect in a clotting factor. They are differentiated by the specific clotting factor that is deficient. The most common type of hemophilia is *hemophilia A,* caused by a deficiency in blood coagulation factor VIII. The next most common type is *hemophilia B,* in which *clotting factor IX* (also called *Christmas factor*—named after an individual with the condition) is defective (Ragni, 2016).

Manifestations of hemophilia A and hemophilia B are indistinguishable. Both are characterized by the development of excessive bleeding precipitated by even minor incidents. In most instances, the condition is recognized in infancy or childhood when, for example, excessive bleeding occurs after circumcision or spontaneous or easy bruising is identified. In mild cases, individuals may not have hemophilia identified until they reach adulthood.

Identification of Hemophilia

Severe cases of hemophilia are usually identified in infancy after prolonged bleeding following a procedure, such as circumcision. In less severe cases, hemophilia is often suspected on the basis of family history, incidents of prolonged bleeding, and laboratory studies.

Manifestations of Hemophilia

Although individuals with hemophilia do not initially bleed faster, the clotting mechanism is disturbed so that bleeding is prolonged or the oozing of blood may persist after injury. Because the platelet count is decreased in hemophilia, bleeding from a small cut or scratch does not pose a severe problem. In contrast, deficiency in clotting factors can pose danger of internal bleeding into the internal organs, joints, or brain with trauma or surgery.

The severity of hemophilia varies along a continuum from a tendency toward slow, prolonged, persistent bleeding to a tendency toward severe hemorrhage, and is categorized as mild, moderate, or severe depending on level of clotting factor present. Individuals with the *mild form* of hemophilia usually do not experience spontaneous bleeding or excessive bleeding after minor injury, but can develop prolonged bleeding after injury or surgery. Individuals with the *moderate form* of the condition experience spontaneous bleeding and may also have prolonged bleeding after even minor injury. In the most *severe form* of the condition, individuals may experience spontaneous bleeding into the joints (**hemarthrosis**) or brain (**intracranial hemorrhage**), severe nosebleed (**epistaxis**), severe bruising (**ecchymosis**), or **hematoma** (development of a sac filled with an accumulated mass of blood).

Bleeding into the joints is extremely painful and can cause significant joint destruction. Knees and ankles are affected most frequently, although elbows may eventually become involved. Joint irregularity and incapacity of movement may result from damage to the joint structure and from **atrophy** (wasting) of surrounding muscles. Bleeding into the muscles, if severe, may exert pressure on nerves and cause a temporary sensory loss. If the hemorrhage damages muscle tissue, fibrous tissue may form, causing varying degrees of functional loss.

Management of Hemophilia

Hemophilia is not curable and requires management of bleeding throughout the individual's life. With proper care, individuals with hemophilia can manage their condition successfully, such that their life expectancy approaches that of individuals without hemophilia (Acharya, 2016).

The cornerstone to management of hemophilia is prophylaxis and prompt intervention when bleeding occurs. To prevent damage from bleeding, significant blood loss, and joint damage, all bleeding must be detected early and managed promptly. More than 100 comprehensive hemophilia centers are available throughout the United States, all of which help individuals with hemophilia manage their conditions physically and psychologically (Lane et al., 2016).

Management is directed toward preventing any injury that could precipitate bleeding, and toward managing bleeding episodes when they do occur. The mainstay of management of hemophilia is *replacement therapy* with plasma or plasma concentrates that contain the clotting factors that are deficient in the individual's blood. Infusions may be administered during bleeding episodes (*episodic therapy*), or periodically to prevent bleeding (*prophylactic therapy*) (Acharya, 2016). Management of hemophilia with factor concentrates must be individualized for each person (Lane et al., 2016). Because of the higher concentrations of clotting factors, plasma concentrates are given more frequently than is fresh plasma. Clotting factors are usually replaced through *intravenous infusion* (infusing a substance directly into a vein). The amount, type, and duration of the infusion depend on the individual's clotting deficiency, his or her size, and the severity of the bleeding problem. Infusions may be instituted prior to surgery to prevent excessive bleeding.

Early management of bleeding helps to prevent complications. Consequently, learning to administer clotting factor concentrates at home is of major benefit. To do so, individuals must be able to calculate the appropriate dose and mix and administer the concentrate intravenously. Home therapy is appropriate for mild bleeding but is not sufficient when major bleeding occurs. Major bleeding requires healthcare attention.

Complications of Hemophilia

Potential for Infection

Although replacement therapy through infusion is a cornerstone of hemophilia management, prior to development of purification methods of infusion products, testing and other procedures, individuals receiving intravenous transfusions had a chance of contracting blood-borne viruses such as *hepatitis B virus* (HBV), *hepatitis C virus* (HCV), and *human immunodeficiency virus* (HIV). With new technologies, individuals born after 1990 have less chance of being exposed to these viruses through infusion intervention (Ragni, 2016). Although these technologies have virtually eliminated the risk of transmitted viral infections from infusion in developed countries, other countries do not always have access to these resources. Likewise, individuals receiving infusion interventions prior to the 1990s may also have been exposed to viruses during transfusion. In these situations, individuals may have developed complications related to hepatitis B or C infection or HIV.

Joint Complications

Individuals with hemarthrosis may experience severe pain that requires analgesic intervention and joint immobilization for several days. Aspirin should be avoided because it interferes with platelet function and can increase susceptibility to bleeding. Physical therapy or recommended exercise carried out at home may be necessary to maintain the range of motion of the affected joints. If the joints demonstrate severe degeneration, reconstructive orthopedic surgery, such as *joint replacement,* may also be necessary. Individuals with hemophilia should always wear a *MedicAlert identification* bracelet or necklace to alert others to their condition in case of an emergency.

Functional Implications of Hemophilia

Personal and Psychosocial Issues

How individuals respond to having hemophilia as adults depends to a great extent on their experiences with the condition during childhood. Because hemophilia is present from birth, attitudes displayed by parents and significant others during individuals' development may significantly affect both their self-view and their view of their condition. If parents were overprotective, individuals' social and psychological development may have been stunted so that they lack self-confidence and remain overly dependent. If many hospitalizations were required due to the condition, individuals may have experienced multiple school absences, and consequently their educational achievement may be lower than that of other members of their peer group.

Activities and Participation

Physical activity has benefit for everyone, including individuals with hemophilia. Because of a fear of injury, however, such individuals may have not have participated in sports or other activities in which physical and motor skills are learned and mastered. Primary considerations in determining the extent of participation are the severity of the hemophilia, the type of sport in which the individual wishes to participate, and the person's level of awareness of his or her condition. Noncontact sports, such as track and field and tennis, and contact sports, such as basketball and soccer, are less likely to pose a threat of injury than collision sports, such as football, hockey, and rugby, although this point may not be important for individuals with hemophilia.

In some instances, and especially for those individuals with the severe form of hemophilia, inability to predict when bleeding may occur or fear of being unable to manage bleeding may result in passivity and inactivity. At other times, if individuals have had difficulty adjusting to the condition, uncertainty about the future, or denial of either the seriousness of hemophilia or the precautions that need to be taken to manage it, excessive risk taking may result.

Although replacement therapy and home infusions have done much to improve the lives of individuals with hemophilia and to mitigate the consequences resulting from the condition, these therapies are very expensive. The expense of managing this condition may be an additional source of stress. Individuals with inadequate resources to pay for infusions may neglect them altogether or undermanage their condition in an attempt to decrease its cost. Over the long term, inadequate management of hemophilia can cause complications and, in turn, increased functional incapacitation.

Individuals with hemophilia may experience both acute and chronic pain if bleeding into the joints occurs. Consequently, pain medications are frequently used. If medications are not carefully used and monitored, there is the potential for the development of drug dependence, sometimes to the extent that drug rehabilitation is required. Individuals who have not adjusted well to their condition and self-medicate to alleviate their emotional discomfort may be at particular risk.

Although exposure to HIV or HCV as a result of infusion therapy is rare today, individuals who were exposed to and contracted HIV or HCV infection as a result of infusion therapy prior to 1985 may now be living with two chronic, lifelong conditions. As a result, they may experience not only stress and anxiety but also anger, resentment, and depression. Some individuals may feel stigmatized by their condition, and especially by the public's awareness of the link between hemophilia and HIV, and attempt to hide their condition.

Long-term survivors of HIV infection associated with hemophilia are a small group within the HIV-positive community and may not feel the same sense of support from that community as do other members of this group. Those individuals who contracted hepatitis C as a result of transfusion may have increased anxiety because of the knowledge that HCV infection may progress to cirrhosis or liver cancer (Pawlotsky, 2016). Whether individuals have HIV or HCV infection, they may face issues of disclosure, stigma, and uncertain prognosis.

Sexuality

Sexual issues may be of concern for individuals with hemophilia even in the absence of concomitant HIV or HCV infection. Complications, such as joint damage, or the side effects of medications may also interfere with sexual function. Because hemophilia is a hereditary condition, individuals may experience guilt or fear, and may grapple with the decision of whether to have children. The potential impact on long-term relationships and the decision whether to have children may be troublesome. In some instances, there may be avoidance of developing close, meaningful relationships because of the individual's discomfort with having a hereditary condition.

Vocational Issues in Hemophilia

Improved healthcare technology and the availability of self-infused coagulation factors have greatly increased the ability of individuals with hemophilia to decrease manifestations of their condition and maintain employment in a variety of settings (Acharya, 2016). Individuals with severe hemophilia may also be able to perform a variety of job tasks without limitations; however, in severe manifestations of the condition, individuals face increased unpredictability in terms of when the bleeding will occur.

When bleeding does occur, individuals should be able to self-infuse the concentrates in 15 to 30 minutes; however, they will need to take a break from work to perform the replacement therapy. A semiprivate place to perform the infusion, as well as a place to store the equipment and concentrate, will be needed.

Usually, individuals with hemophilia have little functional incapacitation in the vocational setting, unless they experience joint complications. Joint damage and subsequent joint replacement owing to complications of hemophilia may impose the same limitations as does joint damage from other causes. In some instances, surgical correction of damaged joints may be indicated.

Obviously, individuals with hemophilia—especially those with moderate to severe manifestations of the condition—should avoid employment in which there is a direct threat of physical injury. Injuries that may be minimal by most standards can have serious implications for individuals with more severe forms of hemophilia. For the most part, however, primarily abilities and interests determine the vocational functioning of individuals with hemophilia.

One barrier to employment may be lack of understanding on the part of the employer about the relatively few limitations that are actually associated with hemophilia. Because the public has now connected hemophilia and the potential for HIV infection, coworkers may demonstrate fear and anxiety when working with individuals with hemophilia, especially if a bleeding episode occurs. Likewise, coworkers who observe individuals administering self-infusing concentrates, and who do not understand the concepts underlying replacement therapy, may draw false conclusions about the activity, causing further discrimination. Educating employers and coworkers about hemophilia and its management may be one of the most crucial links to vocational success for the individual with hemophilia.

OTHER CONDITIONS AFFECTING THE BLOOD (HEMATOLOGICAL CONDITIONS)

Other hematological conditions (conditions affecting the blood) may be caused by a number of factors, may arise from many different sources, and may be manifested in many different ways. Causes may include all of the following:

- Irregularities of blood cells
- Overproduction or underproduction of blood cells
- Destruction of blood cells
- Irregularities of clotting mechanisms

Anemia

Overview of Anemia

Anemia is general term used to describe conditions characterized by a reduction in the number of red blood cells circulating in the blood. The degree of anemia reflects the ability of the bone marrow to produce red blood cells or to increase the production of red blood cells enough to keep up with their loss or destruction.

Alterations in the plasma or fluid volume in the blood can give a false view of the actual level of red blood cells in the blood. For instance, fluid loss—such as in dehydration, vomiting, or diarrhea—can reduce the fluid volume of the blood, thereby increasing the relative concentration of red blood cells in the blood. Conversely, overhydration or

other conditions in which fluid volume in the blood is increased may present a picture characterized by a relatively low level of red blood cells even though the actual levels remain the same.

Actual reduction in red blood cells can be due to any of the following causes:

- Excessive loss of red blood cells
- Underproduction of red blood cells
- Destruction of red blood cells
- Deficiency in the components of red blood cells that affects their ability to bind to oxygen

Because one of the components of red blood cells is *hemoglobin* (the molecule in the blood that carries oxygen), a reduction in red blood cells also results in a reduction in hemoglobin, with concurrent loss of oxygen to tissues.

Any of the following situations may precipitate anemia:

- Nutritional anemia, in which there is a dietary deficiency in nutrients that contribute to the production of red blood cells, such as *iron-deficiency anemia*
- Inability of the body to absorb certain vitamins that are essential for production of red blood cells
- Failure of the bone marrow to produce enough red blood cells
- Hemorrhage
- Destruction of red blood cells due to toxic organisms, or specific conditions such as sickle cell anemia
- Other chronic conditions

(Bunn, 2016)

Classifications of Anemia

Anemias are sometimes classified by the size and color of the red blood cells. For example, healthy, uniform-sized cells are called *normocytic.* Thus anemias in which the red blood cells are larger than usual are called *macrocytic anemias,* while those in which cells are smaller than usual are called *microcytic anemias.* Uniform-sized cells that are of characteristic color are called *normochromic.* In turn, anemias in which the color of the red blood cells is paler than usual are called *hypochromic anemias.*

Pernicious anemia is an example of anemia caused by the body's inability to absorb certain vitamins needed for red blood cell production. This chronic condition is caused by the inadequate secretion by the stomach of a substance (*intrinsic factor*) that is necessary for the intestines to absorb vitamin B_{12}. It may also be caused by dietary deficiency of vitamin B_{12}. Deficiency of vitamin B_{12} impairs production and maturation of blood cells. Consequently, the body is unable to produce adequate numbers of red blood cells, resulting in anemia.

Aplastic anemia (sometimes called *pancytopenia*) is an example of the body's inability to manufacture enough red blood cells and is caused by inadequate functioning of the bone marrow. Aplastic anemia can occur spontaneously, or it can be the result of damage to the bone marrow produced by drugs, toxic chemicals, or ionizing radiation. It may also be caused by invasion of the bone marrow by cancer or by the chemotherapy used to treat cancer.

Hemorrhagic anemia refers to anemia resulting from significant blood loss and subsequent diminished volume of circulating blood (*hypovolemia*). When significant blood loss occurs, there are not enough red blood cells (and consequently not enough hemoglobin) to carry adequate amounts of oxygen to body tissues. Blood loss resulting in hemorrhagic anemia can be acute (such as from an injury) or chronic (such as from slow, chronic bleeding from the intestines).

Hemolytic anemia is a type of anemia caused by excessive or premature destruction of red blood cells (hemolysis). Hemolytic anemia may occur in association with some infectious conditions (such as *malaria*) or with certain inherited red blood cell conditions (such as sickle cell disease, discussed earlier in this chapter). It may also develop as a response to drugs or other foreign or toxic agents. The spleen usually becomes enlarged (**splenomegaly**) in chronic hemolytic conditions because of the need to remove an excessive number of damaged red blood cells.

Manifestations of Anemia

Regardless of the cause, anemia disrupts the transport of oxygen to tissues throughout the body, resulting in a number of systemic manifestations. For instance, severe anemia increases the workload of the heart. To compensate for decreased oxygen in the tissue, the heart pumps at a more rapid pace (**tachycardia**) in an attempt to increase the oxygen supply to body tissues. Due to an inadequate number of red blood cells circulating throughout the body, individuals with anemia may have pale skin (**pallor**), weakness, or difficulty in breathing (dyspnea). Inadequate oxygen supply to the brain in anemia may cause the individual to be unable to concentrate or to experience irritability.

Fatigue is a major manifestation of anemia. It can reduce the individual's ability to work by decreasing physical and emotional well-being, as well as interfere with cognitive ability. Individuals with anemia may also be more susceptible to infection, a vulnerability that merely adds to the incapacitating effects the initial anemia may have caused.

Identification of Anemia

A thorough health examination and health history are important first steps in identifying possible causes for manifestations. Individuals usually also undergo laboratory testing, including a complete blood count (CBC), reticulocyte count, and microscopic examination of blood cells. In some instances, a microscopic examination of bone marrow may be conducted as well.

Management of Anemia

The first step in managing anemia is to identify the cause and correct it if possible. When the cause is identified, management is specific to the cause. If anemia is the result of blood loss, blood replacement through transfusion may be necessary. In other instances, only dietary, vitamin, or iron supplements may be necessary. Management of anemia associated with chronic conditions such as sickle cell disease was discussed earlier in the chapter.

Thalassemias

Overview of the Thalassemias

The *thalassemias,* or *thalassemia syndromes,* are a group of inherited hemolytic conditions that represent the most common single-gene condition in the world (Benz, 2011; Cappellini, 2016). These conditions are common in individuals with heritage from the Mediterranean region, Africa, the Middle East, India, Southeast Asia, and Indonesia (Cappellini, 2016).

Thalassemias range from mild to severe and are characterized by the production of thin, fragile, red blood cells and defective hemoglobin synthesis. As a result, the hemoglobin content of the red blood cells is inadequate. In addition, some interference with erythrocyte metabolism may occur, which causes the red blood cells to be irregularly formed and consequently decreases their survival time. Thus anemia associated with thalassemia can result both from the increased destruction of red blood cells and from the impaired production of hemoglobin.

Manifestations of Thalassemia

Manifestations experienced with thalassemia are mainly due to the lack of oxygen in the blood as a result of faulty hemoglobin production. Because the thalassemias are genetically based, the condition is lifelong. The type and severity of manifestations experienced depend on the type of thalassemia. Individuals with alpha-thalassemia may have mild anemia or may experience no manifestations at all, although they may be carriers of the faulty gene. Individuals with betathalassemia may experience anemia, fatigue, and enlarged spleen. The more severe forms of betathalassemia, also called Cooley's anemia, may have more severe manifestations. Children may have decreased growth and delayed puberty with underdevelopment or decreased function of testes or ovaries.

Individuals with Cooley's anemia may appear pale and listless, or have jaundice (yellowing of the skin), enlarged spleen, and severe anemia. They may also experience conditions such as **osteopenia** (decreased bone density) or **osteoporosis** (increase in the porous nature of bone), which may make them more susceptible to fractures and subsequent pain. In addition, Cooley's anemia is associated with increased susceptibility to infection.

Identification of Thalassemia

Because the thalassemias are genetically based, a detailed family history as well as genetic studies may be conducted to diagnose these anemias.

In addition, blood tests, such as CBC and hemoglobin studies, are carried out.

Management of Thalassemia

Transfusion is the mainstay of management in more severe cases of thalassemia (Cappellini, 2016). Iron overload is a frequent problem among individuals with thalassemia because of the breakdown of red blood cells and increased absorption of iron from the gastrointestinal tract. The accumulated iron forms deposits in various organs of the body, including the heart, liver, and endocrine glands, which damages the affected organs. Consequently, in addition to transfusion therapy, iron chelation therapy may be necessary to prevent iron overload (Holstein & Hohl, 2012).

Individuals with thalassemia must also make lifestyle adjustments, including increasing calcium intake, participating in regular physical activity, and quitting smoking. Bone marrow transplantation and gene therapy have been used in the management of thalassemia as well (Cappellini, 2016).

Functional Implications of Thalassemia

Personal and Psychosocial Issues

The thalassemias are lifelong conditions. Consequently, reactions to the condition and adjustment in adulthood are often determined by individuals' experiences with the condition during childhood. Individuals who grow up with the condition in a supportive, compassionate atmosphere where they are given increased responsibility for management of their condition in accordance with their level of maturity may have less difficulty transitioning from adolescence to adulthood than do those individuals who experienced an overly protective home environment and uncompassionate peers. In some instances, manifestations of thalassemia such as lack of energy or repeated absences from school due to healthcare appointments or interventions can affect individuals' academic performance.

Prior to the development of management options such as transfusion and iron chelation, many individuals with thalassemia did not survive into adulthood. For this reason, health professionals working with adults with thalassemia are often unfamiliar with the particular needs and challenges of these individuals. Lack of understanding on the part of healthcare professionals can contribute to frustration and discouragement for individuals with thalassemia and lead to decreased adherence with management interventions.

Concerns about the genetic component of thalassemia, the cost of interventions needed to manage the condition, and the time-consuming nature of management can influence relationships and decisions about the future. Counseling and support can help individuals and partners have open and frank discussions, which can assist in relationship stability.

Activities and Participation

Many people are unfamiliar with thalassemia and may hold numerous misperceptions about the manifestations and consequences of the condition, making it difficult for individuals with thalassemia to become full participants in a social group. The degree to which individuals learned to become independent and assertive in discussing their condition with peers when they were children can affect success in social situations in the future. Other factors related to this condition, such as pain, fatigue, associated secondary conditions, time spent in managing the condition, and cost involved in management, can also influence individuals' ability to fully participate. Learning how to plan and manage interventions necessary for management of their condition, as well as developing realistic expectations regarding stamina, can promote involvement in activities and social interaction.

Vocational Implications of Thalassemia

As with many chronic health conditions, the key to creating a successful work environment for persons with thalassemia is open discussion with employers about the nature of the condition and associated special needs. Workplace modification may be needed to enable individuals to conserve energy. Mechanical aids that reduce strain, flexible work hours to accommodate fatigue, or time off for interventions or healthcare appointments necessary for management of the condition can be useful in contributing to effective job function.

In some instances, if possible, home-based workstations can be used to help the individual have access to work while at the same time providing opportunities for rest as needed.

Polycythemia (Erythrocytosis)

Polycythemia (also called *erythrocytosis*) is a condition characterized by an increase in the number of red blood cells, as well as in the concentration of hemoglobin, within the blood. Several types of polycythemia are distinguished. For example, *polycythemia vera* is associated with an *overproduction* of both red and white blood cells. The cause of polycythemia vera is unknown. Because of the increased number of cells in the blood, individuals with this condition may experience hypertension, congestive heart failure, heart attack, or stroke. They may also experience hemorrhage if congestion in the blood vessels causes the vessels to rupture.

When the body's demand for oxygen increases, the bone marrow produces additional red blood cells to meet the increased demand. *Secondary polycythemia* results from increased production of red blood cells and occurs in conjunction with other conditions such as chronic obstructive lung disease or, sometimes, as a result of living at high altitudes. Management focuses on the underlying condition.

In some conditions, such as severe burns, a loss of plasma occurs without a loss of red blood cells, creating a condition similar to polycythemia. Although there is no actual increase in the number of red blood cells, the loss of fluid increases the proportion of red blood cells in the blood. In these cases, management involves fluid replacement to decrease the viscosity of the blood.

Agranulocytosis (Neutropenia)

Agranulocytosis is a marked reduction in the level of a specific type of leukocyte. This reduction in leukocytes is called **leukopenia**. A common cause of agranulocytosis is toxic reaction to certain medications used in the management of chronic conditions, such as medications used to treat epilepsy or medications used to treat certain psychiatric conditions. Agranulocytosis may also result from exposure to certain chemicals or ionizing radiation.

Because white blood cells are important to fight infection, a reduction in the number of these cells increases an individual's susceptibility to infection. Agranulocytosis is a potentially serious condition and, without prompt intervention, can result in death. Management is directed toward removing the toxic agent responsible and providing medications (e.g., antibiotics) to treat the resulting infections.

Purpura

Purpura is a condition characterized by hemorrhage of small blood vessels, forming small purplish spots on the skin (**petechiae**). It can be caused by a drug reaction or clotting factor abnormalities, or it may be associated with other conditions, such as kidney or liver failure, systemic infection, or underlying malignancies (Korman, 2016).

Leukemia

The leukemias are caused by overproduction of various types of white blood cells. They are discussed in greater detail elsewhere in the text.

GENERAL MANAGEMENT OF CONDITIONS AFFECTING THE BLOOD

For many conditions of the blood, management is directed toward alleviating manifestations or eliminating the underlying cause. If a blood condition is caused by a toxic substance, the first line of management is to remove the offending agent. Anemia that is caused by a deficiency may be managed by supplementation or replacement therapy. For instance, iron-deficiency anemia may be treated by the administration of oral or injectable iron preparations. Pernicious anemia may be managed with injections of vitamin B_{12}. When an overproduction of red blood cells occurs, as in polycythemia, management may involve the removal of blood; **venesection** or **phlebotomy** is a procedure in which quantities of blood are removed to reduce the overall volume in the body.

Transfusion

Although transfusion is part of the management for a number of blood conditions and is beneficial in their management, this therapy is not without risk or potential adverse effects. Risks can include transfusion reactions that occur immediately as well as reactions and complications that occur years after the transfusion, including infections, transfusion-related acute lung injury (TRALI), and other transfusion-related complications (Sheppard & Hillyer, 2012). In addition to the risk of such a reaction, there is a risk that a blood transfusion will transmit an infectious condition such as hepatitis or HIV, although careful screening of blood by blood banks has significantly reduced this risk.

Bone Marrow Transplant

Bone marrow transplant is a procedure in which individuals' bone marrow is eradicated and healthy bone marrow is inserted to replace it. Bone marrow transplants are used when the immune system is severely deficient or for conditions such cancers, sickle cell anemia, or thalassemia. Bone marrow cells are obtained from a donor who is carefully matched with the recipient to decrease the chances of rejection of the transplant, as well as to prevent a reaction in which the transplanted cells attack the cells of the individual who has received the transplant.

GENERAL FUNCTIONAL IMPLICATIONS OF BLOOD CONDITIONS

Personal and Psychosocial Issues

Personal and psychosocial implications for a particular individual with a blood condition depend on the condition itself. Some conditions may be managed relatively easily, whereas others may require constant vigilance. Although some conditions may be managed and, in some instances, cured, others require lifelong management and carry a potentially more ominous outcome.

Individuals with conditions affecting the blood generally have no visible reminders of their condition. Without external adaptive devices, such as wheelchairs, crutches, or canes, or any other signs of incapacitation, individuals may react by denying the seriousness of their condition and resist healthcare advice. For example, individuals with hemophilia may engage in risk-taking behaviors, even though injury and subsequent bleeding could occur. Individuals with sickle cell anemia may engage in a flurry of activity, even though associated stress and fatigue may precipitate a sickle cell crisis.

Some blood-related conditions occur later in life, necessitating adjustment at the time that the condition and any associated limitation occur. Conditions such as sickle cell anemia and hemophilia are lifelong, however. Consequently, individuals with these conditions will have coped with their condition in one way or another from childhood into adulthood. Many individuals with either sickle cell anemia or hemophilia experience periodic health needs throughout their childhood and adolescence as a direct result of their condition. Although these experiences can build confidence in the ability to cope, they may also have a negative impact on development. Individuals may carry the coping behaviors and attitudes learned in childhood into the adult years, where they continue to affect the individuals' perceptions of themselves, their condition, and their abilities. Depending on the constructiveness of the coping strategy used, such behaviors may be either an asset or a hindrance.

Although many individuals with sickle cell disease or hemophilia effectively manage their condition and live full and productive lives, the possibility of early death or potential for development of complications of their condition may be a source of anxiety and depression. For example, even though hemophilia can be effectively managed, there may be an underlying fear that an accident or traumatic event may occur in which bleeding cannot be stopped. Individuals with sickle cell disease may fear the possibility of stroke or other life-threatening complication in the event of sickle cell crisis. The ways in which individuals cope with such potential threats to their well-being may range from the adoption of a philosophical view toward life to passivity and withdrawal.

Activities and Participation

The degree to which individuals with conditions affecting the blood can maintain routine daily schedules depends on the specific condition. Different conditions affecting the blood affect activities of daily living in varying degrees, depending on the associated manifestations. Manifestations of fatigue or difficulty in breathing with exertion may require individuals to pace their activities throughout the day to conserve energy. Individuals may need more frequent rest periods, or they may need to divide activities into smaller steps, which they perform throughout the day rather than completing a task all at once.

Good health practices are important to everyone. However, due to the increased susceptibility to infection that is part of many conditions affecting the blood, individuals with these conditions must take extra care to consume well-balanced diets and maintain well-balanced programs of rest and activity. Exercise is especially important to individuals with hemophilia. Regular, moderate exercise can build muscles that protect joints and decrease the incidence of bleeding into the joints. Activities that carry a higher probability of injury, such as contact sports, should be avoided.

GENERAL VOCATIONAL ISSUES IN CONDITIONS OF THE BLOOD

The cause and manifestations of a condition affecting the blood determine its vocational impact. If, for example, the condition has been caused in part by exposure to toxic substances within the environment, hazards should be removed before individuals return to the workplace. If fatigue or dyspnea is a manifestation of the condition, as occurs with anemia, it may be necessary to consider the physical demands of the job and the need for more frequent rest periods. When infection is a potential complication of the condition, individuals should avoid exposure to factors and environments that may precipitate infection.

In all instances, to prevent misunderstanding, if work alterations such as more frequent rest breaks or the need for privacy to perform infusions, such as in hemophilia, are needed, employers should be made aware and fellow workers educated as much as possible about the nature of the condition and the reason for the special work modifications.

CASE STUDY

Ms. B. is a 19-year-old African American female with sickle cell disease. She is a high school graduate and is currently enrolled in a junior college, where she is studying to be an X-ray technician.

Since entering school at the junior college, she has had a number of sickle cell crises that have necessitated her hospitalization. Ms. B. has developed severe damage to joints in her lower extremities as a result of her condition. Although her healthcare provider has recommended that Ms. B. reconsider her occupational goal given her series of sickle cell crises since being in school, she is determined to pursue her education and to become an X-ray technician. She continues to push herself even when she does not feel well.

1. How would you approach Ms. B. about her vocational plans given the healthcare provider's recommendation?
2. How realistic is Ms. B.'s vocational choice?
3. Which health issues as well as other physical and psychological issues would you consider when working with Ms. B. to develop her rehabilitation plan?
4. Which general lifestyle issues might you address with Ms. B. that could contribute to her rehabilitation potential?

REFERENCES

Acharya, S. S. (2016). Advances in hemophilia and the role of current emerging prophylaxis. *American Journal of Managed Care, 22*(5), 116–125.

Benz, E. J. (2011). Newborn screening for a-thalassemia: Keeping up with globalization. *New England Journal of Medicine, 364*(8), 770–771.

Bonham, V. L., George, J., Dover, M. D., & Brody, L. C. (2010). Screening student athletes for sickle cell trait: A social and clinical experiment. *New England Journal of Medicine, 363*(11), 997–999.

Bunn, H. F. (2016). Approach to the anemias. In L. Goldman & A. I. Schafer (Eds.), *Goldman-Cecil medicine,* (25th ed., pp. 1059–1068). Philadelphia, PA: Elsevier Saunders.

Cappellini, M. D. (2016). The thalassemias. In L. Goldman & A. I. Schafer (Eds.), *Goldman-Cecil medicine,* (25th ed., pp. 1089–1095). Philadelphia, PA: Elsevier Saunders.

Goldstein, L. B. (2016). Ischemic cerebrovascular disease. In L. Goldman & A. I. Schafer (Eds.), *Goldman-Cecil medicine,* (25th ed., pp. 2434–2445). Philadelphia, PA: Elsevier Saunders.

Holstein, S. A., & Hohl, R. J. (2012). Thalassemia. In E. T. Bope & R. D. Kellerman (Eds.), *Conn's current therapy 2012,* (pp. 861–865). Philadelphia, PA: Elsevier Saunders.

Korman, N. J. (2016). Macular, popular, and vesiculobullous, and pustular diseases. In L. Goldman & A. I. Schafer (Eds.), *Goldman-Cecil medicine,* (25th ed., pp. 2671–2682). Philadelphia, PA: Elsevier Saunders.

Kotila, T. R., Busari, O. E., Makanjuola, V., & Eyelade, O. R. (2015). Addiction or pseudoaddiction in sickle cell disease patients: Time to decide—A case series. *Annals of Ibaden Postgraduate Medicine, 13*(1), 44–47.

Lane, S. J., Sholapur, N. S., Yeung, C. H., Iorio, A., Heddle, N. M., Sholzberg, M., & Pai, M. (2016). Understanding stakeholders important outcomes and perceptions of equity, acceptability, and feasibility of a care model for haemophilia management in the US: A qualitative study. *Haemophilia, 22(Suppl 3),* 23–30. doi:10.1111/hae.13009

Pawlotsky, J. M. (2016). Chronic viral and autoimmune hepatitis. In L. Goldman & A. I. Schafer (Eds.), *Goldman-Cecil medicine,* (25th ed., pp. 1000–1006). Philadelphia, PA: Elsevier Saunders.

Ragni, M. V. (2016). Hemorrhagic disorders: Coagulation factor deficiencies. In L. Goldman & A. I. Schafer (Eds.), *Goldman-Cecil medicine,* (25th ed., pp. 1172–1181). Philadelphia, PA: Elsevier Saunders.

Sheppard, C. A., & Hillyer, C. D. (2012). Adverse effects of blood transfusion. In E. T. Bope & R. D. Kellerman (Eds.), *Conn's current therapy 2012,* (pp. 777–785). Philadelphia, PA: Elsevier Saunders.

Steinberg, M. H. (2016). Sickle cell anemia and other hemoglobinopathies. In L. Goldman & A. I. Schafer (Eds.), *Goldman-Cecil medicine,* (25th ed., pp. 1095–1104). Philadelphia, PA: Elsevier Saunders.

CHAPTER 19

Introduction to the Immune System

STRUCTURE AND FUNCTION OF THE IMMUNE SYSTEM

The immune system is a complex organization of specialized cells and structures that has specific defenses to protect the body against foreign substances known as *antigens*, including bacteria, viruses, parasites, toxins, allergens, and tumors. The immune system also promotes the inflammatory process (such as the red and swollen tissue that surrounds a splinter or as in response to a cut) so as to initiate healing. When an antigen is present, the body produces substances called *antibodies* to help fight off invasion by the "foreign" substance. This *antigen–antibody reaction* forms the basis for immunity.

The basic principle behind immune system function is the ability to distinguish *self* from *nonself*. A special molecule, *major histocompatibility complex (MHC)*, also known as *human leukocyte antigen (HLA)*, marks cells in the body as self. Anything that lacks this biological marker is considered nonself. When the immune system recognizes a substance as nonself—that is, as foreign (an antigen)—it activates a number of mechanisms to eliminate the foreign substance.

The immune system also includes a number of barriers that protect against foreign substances entering the system. For instance, the skin and organisms on it provide a first-line protective barrier against invasion by harmful organisms. In addition, saliva, tears, and gastric juices contain substances that kill organisms before they can become harmful. Should foreign substances enter the body, the immune system has many mechanisms available to fight the invasion on an internal level. The reactions of the immune system to antigens are collectively called the *immune response*.

Sometimes, despite the many mechanisms in place, the immune system does not work properly, and the line between self and nonself becomes blurred. For instance, the immune system may fail to recognize cells in the individual's own body (self) and attack them, causing an *autoimmune* condition, such as *rheumatoid arthritis* or *type 1 diabetes*. At other times, the immune system overreacts to a foreign substance, causing an *allergic reaction*. In still other instances, the immune system may compromise the health status of individuals who have undergone procedures such as organ transplantation, because the new organ is perceived by the immune system as a foreign substance, and not as self. Consequently, an immune response is triggered and the transplanted organ destroyed, unless health interventions are implemented to suppress the immune system.

Although the immune system works effectively most of the time, when the concentration of a foreign substance or its virulence is too great for immune defenses, individuals become ill, such as when individuals succumb to the flu, or when they develop more serious infectious health conditions, such as tuberculosis.

TYPES OF IMMUNITY

The immune system can be divided into two components:

- Innate (nonspecific; natural) immunity
- Adaptive (specific; acquired) immunity

Innate Immunity

Innate immunity is the body's first line of defense. It provides a nonselective response and requires no previous exposure to an antigen. This type of immunity includes several mechanisms of protection:

- Physical barriers such as the skin, mucus that traps organisms, and the flushing action of saliva and tears.
- Antimicrobial substances contained in tears and saliva, and other body fluids that break down organisms, making them more vulnerable.
- Substances in the gastrointestinal tract that contain chemicals that are toxic to many organisms and, therefore, prevent their growth and proliferation.
- Inflammation, which is a response to tissue damage. The inflammatory process brings cells to the injured area that destroy and ingest foreign material so that tissue repair can begin. As a result of the inflammatory process, the affected area becomes red, warm, and swollen, and the inflamed area becomes walled off to prevent or delay bacteria from spreading.

Adaptive Immunity

Adaptive immunity involves specific types of cells (T cells and B cells, as discussed later in this chapter) and their derivatives. It requires prior exposure to an antigen to be activated. When the cell recognizes an antigen, this type of immunity ensures that mechanisms are activated to neutralize or destroy the antigen.

Adaptive immunity is further subdivided into *cellular immunity (cell-mediated immunity)* and *humoral immunity.* Each component has a different role and function.

- Cellular immunity is characterized by the role of T lymphocytes. It fights viruses and bacteria, cancer, and some allergens, and plays a role in the autoimmune response.
- Humoral immunity is characterized by the transformation of B cells into cells that produce and secrete antibodies to specific antigens.

ORGANS OF THE IMMUNE SYSTEM

The immune system has numerous other structures that contain components to fight foreign substance or antigens (**Figure 19-1**). These internal lines of defense include the following elements:

- Tonsils and adenoids
- Thymus
- Spleen
- Bone marrow
- Gut-associated lymphoid tissue (Peyer's patches)
- Lymphatic system
- Antibodies
- Complementary system
- White blood cells

Tonsils and Adenoids

The *tonsils* are lymphoid tissue found at the back of the throat that are part of the lymphatic system (discussed later in this chapter). They help protect the body against harmful organisms that are ingested. The *adenoids,* which also consist of lymphoid tissue, are located at the back of the throat and protect against organisms that are breathed in. Although both the tonsils and the adenoids are part of the body's line of defense against antigens, neither is considered crucial because the immune system has so many other components. Consequently, if the tonsils and adenoids become infected, especially repeatedly, they are often removed.

Thymus

The *thymus* is located toward the upper center portion of the chest behind the sternum (breast bone). It produces T cells. Although the thymus is more active in children and adolescents, production of T cells from this source continues throughout adulthood.

Spleen

The *spleen* is located in the upper left quadrant of the abdomen. It filters blood and helps to destroy microorganisms. It also disposes of aged blood cells and stores white blood cells and platelets.

Figure 19-1   The Immune System

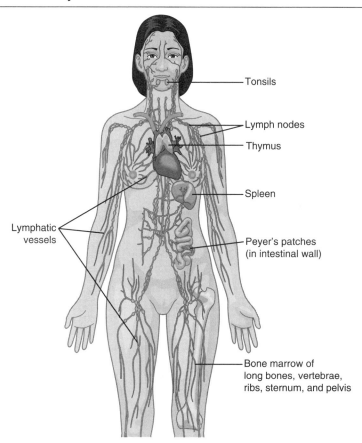

- Tonsils
- Lymph nodes
- Thymus
- Spleen
- Lymphatic vessels
- Peyer's patches (in intestinal wall)
- Bone marrow of long bones, vertebrae, ribs, sternum, and pelvis

Bone Marrow

The *bone marrow* manufactures *red blood cells, white blood cells,* and *stem cells*. White blood cells, which are discussed in more detail later in this chapter, are important components of immune function.

Gut-Associated Lymphoid Tissue (Peyer's Patches)

Peyer's patches are lymphoid tissue located in the lining of the small intestine. They destroy harmful organisms before they enter the bloodstream.

Lymphatic System

The lymphatic system plays a major role in defense against invading organisms and other foreign substances. This special circulatory system is distinct from the general blood circulation, but intermingles with it. Lymphatic circulation, rather than having a pump like the heart in the general circulatory system, depends on muscle movement to circulate the fluid within it. The lymphatic system consists of *lymph vessels, circulating lymph fluid* (clear fluid that bathes the body's tissue), and *lymph nodes* (small structures of the immune system that are located throughout the body and act as filters). Lymph nodes also serve as temporary storage reservoirs for *lymphocytes* (white blood cells that fight infection).

Antibodies

Antibodies are substances that respond to antigens, binding to the antigens to disable them or stop their action. In addition, antibodies signal the complement system (discussed next).

Complement System

The *complement system* consists of proteins that are found in the blood and manufactured by the liver. As part of immune function, they enhance the ability of antibodies and other cells to remove harmful organisms for the body. These proteins rupture membranes of the antigen and stimulate the inflammatory process.

White Blood Cells

White blood cells (also called *leukocytes*) start as stem cells and are mostly produced in the bone marrow to fight harmful substances in the body. White blood cells are classified into two general categories based on their appearance under the microscope: *granulocytes* and *agranulocytes* (see **Table 19-1**). The types of white blood cells in each category work together to destroy bacteria and viruses.

Granulocytes

- *Neutrophils* are the first line of defense when there is a cut or injury. They go to the site of inflammation, engulf foreign organisms, and destroy them by a process called *phagocytosis.*
- *Eosinophils* focus on parasites, especially on the skin and lungs, and release toxins to kill them.
- *Basophils* carry histamine to the site of injury, facilitating the inflammatory process by causing blood vessels to dilate so that additional body resources can move to the site to assist in defense and healing.

Agranulocytes

- *Monocytes* are the largest white blood cells. When they leave the blood, they are called

macrophages. Macrophages perform phagocytosis as well as clean up dead neutrophils and other debris from the inflammatory process.
- *Lymphocytes* are formed in the lymphatic tissue. Although found in the blood, they tend to congregate in lymph tissue such as lymph nodes, the spleen, and the thymus. Lymphocytes are discussed in more detail later in the chapter.

DEFENSE AGAINST MICROORGANISMS

The primary microorganisms that the immune system defends against are *bacteria* and *viruses.* Bacteria are organisms that are capable of living and reproducing on their own. Some bacteria are harmless and beneficial, such as those found in the healthy intestines of humans. Bacteria that cause disease are called *pathogens.* They cause harm by attacking tissues directly, or by producing poisonous substances called *toxins.* As noted earlier, the human body's natural defense against foreign substances, including bacteria, is the creation of *antibodies* to fight the foreign substance.

In contrast to bacteria, viruses are unable to survive or reproduce without invading another cell, called a *host cell.* To survive, a virus enters a living host cell and uses the reproductive capacity of that cell for its own replication. Consequently, when a virus enters a cell, it instructs the cell to reproduce the virus.

Not all viruses are harmful to humans, although some can cause health conditions ranging from mild conditions, such as the common cold, and to more serious conditions, such *as poliomyelitis* or HIV infection. Usually, the body recognizes viruses as foreign and activates the immune system to attack and destroy the offending agent. Some types of viruses that are not destroyed by this process can remain inactive *(dormant)* in the body for long periods without causing problems; however, they remain integrated within the genetic material of the cell and are capable of replicating when triggered to do so. For example, the *varicella zoster virus* initially causes chickenpox, but years later can cause herpes zoster *(shingles).*

Table 19-1   Types of White Blood Cells

Granulocytes	Agranulocytes
Neutrophils	Monocytes
Eosinophils	Lymphocytes
Basophils	B lymphocytes
	T lymphocytes

AUTOIMMUNE RESPONSES

Cells carry specific protein markers to ensure that the body recognizes its own tissue as self and not foreign. Sometimes, however, the immune system becomes unable to recognize the body's own tissues and begins to produce antibodies and T cells that attack the body's own cells. When the immune system directs a response to attack the body's own cells as if they were foreign substances, individuals are said to have an *autoimmune condition*. Examples of autoimmune conditions include *systemic lupus erythematosus* and *rheumatoid arthritis*.

OTHER CONDITIONS ALTERING IMMUNE RESPONSES

A variety of other conditions can alter the body's immune response. For instance, individuals receiving an organ transplant must have their immune system suppressed to prevent rejection of the donor tissue. As a result, they are more prone to infections. Individuals with certain types of cancers, such as *lymphoma* and *leukemia*, may become *immunodeficient* and develop serious infections. In addition, management of cancer with chemotherapy or radiation therapy may weaken the immune system.

Individuals who overuse or abuse narcotics or steroid drugs can also alter the immune response, leaving them more prone to infections. Although immunodeficiency is the key characteristic in a number of other conditions, the most widely known condition affecting immunity is HIV infection.

LYMPHOCYTE FUNCTION

The two major types of lymphocytes are *B lymphocytes* and *T lymphocytes*. B lymphocytes mature in the bone marrow and migrate to lymphoid tissue, such as the lymph nodes and spleen. These lymphocytes have the capability of recognizing and selectively responding to antigens. In response to recognition of an antigen, antibodies (*immunoglobulins*) are produced. Antibodies, in turn, enter the bloodstream, recognize and bind to the antigen, and destroy it (humoral immunity). Thus antibodies do not penetrate cells but rather interact with circulating antigens.

When antibodies are produced because of exposure to an antigen, resulting in the body's generation of its own antibodies, the process is described as *active immunity*. If antibodies from another person or animal are introduced into an individual, the process is called *passive immunity*.

T lymphocytes mature in the thymus and are regulators and controllers of the immune system. When these lymphocytes are exposed to an antigen, rather than producing antibodies, they react to the antigen directly, attacking body cells that have been invaded by the foreign substance or malignancy (cellular immunity).

T cells comprise several different subsets of cells that behave differently. *Killer T cells* (*CD8* or *cytotoxic* T cells) release chemicals that destroy the targeted cell. *Helper T cells* (*CD4*) do not kill cells but rather help coordinate the immune response, activating B cells to make antibodies against antigens, as well as activating and enhancing the activity of cytotoxic cells and macrophages. Helper T cells are activated by a substance called *interleukin-1*, which is produced by macrophages. Helper T cells then produce *interleukin-2, interferon*, and other chemicals that stimulate B cells to make antibodies. A subset of helper cells, called *regulatory T cells* or *suppressor T cells*, inhibit both the innate and the adaptive immune responses as a way of minimizing harmful effects of the immune response.

Usually, helper cells outnumber killer cells by a 2:1 ratio. After the initial invasion by a foreign substance, T cells form a "memory." If a "remembered" organism invades the body again, the immune response is more intense. Killer T cells, in addition to working to rid the body of infected cells, attack cancer cells and are responsible for the rejection of grafts or transplants.

BIBLIOGRAPHY

Falvo, R. E. (2001). *Human physiology: Physiology 201 core curriculum*. Champaign, IL: Stipes.

Sherwood, L. (2007). *Human physiology: From cells to systems* (6th ed.). Australia: Thomson Brooks/Cole.

Tortora, G. J., & Derrickson, B. H. (Eds.). (2011). *Principles of anatomy and physiology* (13th ed.). Hoboken, NJ: John Wiley and Sons.

Widmaier, E., Raff, H., & Strang, K. (Eds.). (2010). *Vander's human physiology: The mechanism of body function*. New York, NY: McGraw-Hill.

CHAPTER 20

Human Immunodeficiency Virus (HIV) Infection

OVERVIEW OF HIV INFECTION

Human immunodeficiency virus (HIV) infection is a health condition that was once considered fatal; now, however, with appropriate management, many individuals with HIV infection continue to live full, productive lives (Centers for Disease Control and Prevention [CDC], 2016). HIV infection consists of a spectrum of conditions ranging from nonexistent manifestations to manifestations associated with severe depletion of the immune system and associated complications.

Two distinct viruses cause HIV infection:

- HIV-1 is the most prominent form worldwide and is responsible for most cases of HIV infection (Avert, 2015).
- HIV-2 is more uncommon and initially concentrated in West Africa; it is now found in the United States, Europe, South America, and India as well. HIV-2 can also cause immunodeficiency, although this infection is thought to be less virulent than HIV-1 (Maldarelli, 2016).

MECHANISM OF HIV INFECTION

HIV infection is caused by a *retrovirus* called human immunodeficiency virus. A retrovirus uses a complicated process called *reverse transcription* (RT) to reproduce itself. In this process, a viral enzyme called *reverse transcriptase* is used to integrate the virus's genetic material into the genetic material of other cells. In so doing, HIV essentially takes over these cells—primarily the *CD4 cells* (often called helper T cells because they help the body fight off infection)—to produce more HIV. The virus multiplies extremely rapidly, and errors that are caused by this rapid generation of cells are not corrected so that the virus mutates constantly. Some of the cells containing the virus burst, releasing HIV directly into the blood. Consequently, both infected cells and virus may be found in the blood and, therefore, travel to other sites. This characteristic of the virus—that is, its rapid generation and the constant mutations—makes it very difficult for the body to destroy HIV. It also explains why the virus rapidly becomes resistant to medications that are used to kill it (Rote & Huether, 2014).

HIV destroys a subset of helper T cells (CD4+) and impairs the cells' ability to recognize antigens. As a result, profound deterioration of the immune system occurs, such that the body has no defense against even the least aggressive organisms. The virus reproduces within the CD4 cell itself, producing additional HIV, which in turn invades other T cells. The number of CD4 cells decrease and the body cannot respond to new antigens. In this way, the immune response becomes dysfunctional and is overwhelmed with the HIV virus and the individual moves into the last stage of HIV, which is called AIDS (CDC, 2015).

PHASES OF HIV INFECTION AND MANIFESTATIONS

HIV-1 begins to replicate in the mucosa almost immediately after exposure, although the virus, at this point, cannot be detected in the blood. This phase, called the *eclipse phase,* generally lasts 7 to 21 days (Carter & Hughson, 2013). The term *sero-conversion* refers to the phase in which the body begins producing HIV antibodies and cytotoxic lymphocytes in response to the infection. Even though antibodies are present in the blood during this stage, manifestations may be vague or flu-like. Thus, unless the individual has a high degree of suspicion that he or she has been exposed to HIV, testing may not be sought. The virus can still be transmitted to others, however. Some individuals may experience **lymphadenonopathy** (swelling of lymph nodes) during this stage of infection, but in many cases they remain free of manifestations for months, or sometimes years.

If individuals with HIV do not receive interventions to fight the infection, or if their body has become resistant to interventions, immune function continues to deteriorate until it is unable to fight off infections. In the initial stages of immune system deterioration, individuals may experience weight loss, diarrhea, and some opportunistic infections such as **candidiasis** (yeast infection). As the immune system continues to decline, more severe opportunistic infections such as Kaposi's sarcoma or tuberculosis may begin to emerge. Opportunistic infections and complications of HIV are discussed later in the chapter.

TRANSMISSION OF HIV

When an individual is infected with HIV, the virus is found in the blood as well as in body secretions. Transmission can occur in a variety of ways:

- Infusion of infected blood or blood products
- Accidental stick with an infected needle
- Intravenous drug use and sharing of equipment
- Anal, oral, or genital intercourse
- Contact with a cut or open wound on the skin
- Fetal transmission from a woman with HIV infection to her unborn child
- Transmission of HIV from mother to infant through breastmilk

There is no evidence that transmission can occur in any way other than direct blood-to-blood or sexual contact with an infected individual. For example, the virus does not appear to be transmitted through coughing, sneezing, or casual contact. Moreover, because all viruses require living tissue to survive and multiply, the virus dies quickly once outside the body (AIDS.gov, 2015).

PREVENTION OF HIV INFECTION

Although advancements in management of HIV infection have greatly extended the life span of individuals infected, the most promising advance in management of HIV consists of combination prevention programs (Avert, 2015). Education is an important component of preventing HIV transmission. A large percentage of individuals are unaware of their HIV infection until manifestations appear in the later stages of the condition (Avert, 2015). Early identification and behavioral interventions such as counseling, needle exchange, and use of condoms can help reduce transmission of HIV through reducing risk behavior as well as by providing an opportunity for early intervention, which can help delay progression of the condition (Avert, 2015). In the United States, HIV infection is often not identified until it is at the advanced stage, so many individuals affected may not take precautions to prevent transmission.

Scientists continue to work on developing an effective vaccine against HIV. Although enormous progress has been made in understanding of HIV, the unique characteristics of this virus continue to pose challenges and obstacles to vaccine development (Rote & Huether, 2014). In addition, a number of studies have been undertaken to investigate whether antiretroviral therapy could reduce sexual transmission of HIV, thereby reducing the incidence of HIV infection (Del Rio & Cohen, 2016).

IDENTIFYING HIV INFECTION

Identification of HIV is important to facilitate implementation of appropriate interventions, including management, notification and testing of partners, and education of individuals and family members about methods of preventing transmission of HIV.

The procedures most commonly used to identify HIV infection consist of blood tests that identify not the virus itself but rather the presence of antibodies that the body has produced against the virus. *Enzyme immunoassay (EIA)*, which is a blood test, is usually performed first. If the EIA test is positive for HIV antigens, a more specific test, the *Western blot*, is then conducted. A positive Western blot confirms the HIV infection. In an attempt to minimize barriers to testing for HIV, rapid screening tests that use a finger stick or salivary testing, with results becoming available in 20 to 40 minutes, have been approved by the FDA. If these tests are positive, the results still need to be confirmed by the EIA and Western blot tests (U.S. Preventive Services Task Force, 2016).

Because many individuals with HIV in the United States do not receive testing until they experience manifestations, the Centers for Disease Control and Prevention (CDC) and U.S. Preventive Services Task Force (USPSTF) issued new recommendations in 2013 that would integrate screening into routine healthcare services (USPSTF, 2015). Voluntary screening for HIV is now recommended for all individuals from ages 13 to 64 regardless of their specific risk and pregnant women and those who present in labor whose status is unknown (CDC, 2015; Westergaard & Gupta, 2012).

MANIFESTATIONS AND COMPLICATIONS OF ADVANCED HIV INFECTION

Infection with HIV affects all body systems. If individuals do not receive interventions to manage HIV, or if for various reasons interventions are ineffective, all body systems can be affected both in terms of function and susceptibility to opportunistic infection and malignancy.

An *opportunistic infection* is one that would not occur in individuals with sufficient immune system function. Many organisms commonly found in the environment pose no threat when there is an adequately functioning immune system. However, individuals with advanced HIV infection have an immune system that is no longer able to defend against or resist these organisms. Without protection from the immune system, these individuals are susceptible to opportunistic conditions and infections that under usual circumstances would not become full-blown diseases. Common manifestations and complications associated with advanced HIV are described later in the chapter.

MANAGEMENT OF HIV INFECTION

Medication

Development of antiretroviral therapy (ART) and advances in the management of HIV infection have improved the quality of life and life expectancy of individuals living with HIV significantly (Rote & Huether, 2014). Since 1995, deaths from HIV infection in the United States have declined to the extent that HIV is now considered a chronic condition to be managed, rather than a terminal disease (Deeks, Lewin, & Havlir, 2013).

New medications used in the management of HIV are being introduced and guidelines for *antiretroviral therapy* (ART) updated as new studies of their effectiveness evolve (Westergaard & Gupta, 2012). ART involves taking a combination of HIV medications to prevent the virus from multiplying. There are currently a total of 28 antiretroviral drugs approved by the FDA in the treatment of HIV infection (Gulick, 2016). In the past, medication regimes consisted of taking up to 20 pills a day divided into doses every 8 hours. As new drugs have been developed and approved, coformulations with more than one medicine in a single pill have become available, making the medication regime much more manageable. Currently there are four one-pill, once daily pills that have been approved by the FDA for HIV treatment (Gulick, 2016).

Selected combinations of antiretroviral drugs, known as highly active antiretroviral therapy (HAART) act on different parts of the virus replication preventing viral replication. *HAART* therapy, has produced a remarkable effect in controlling progression of HIV and prolonging the life expectancy of those persons infected with the virus (Rathbun & Butler, 2016).

Prevention of Opportunistic Infections

In addition to medication, much of the management of HIV infection is geared toward supportive care and prevention of opportunistic infections. Individuals should have adequate rest, should engage in a program of moderate exercise, and should maintain adequate nutrition. As the condition progresses, individuals may need to modify their exercise program and allow for more frequent rest periods to conserve energy. As much as possible, they should attempt to prevent opportunistic infection. For example, in addition to maintaining good health practices, they should avoid crowds and people with known infections such as colds and flu. If they develop manifestations of infection, they should consult a healthcare provider immediately.

Many individuals with HIV and other chronic diseases are interested in other modalities that they have heard that others have taken or seen on the Internet that will "cure" their disease. The Center for Complementary and Alternative Medicine is a part of the National Institutes of Health. Many individuals are interested in adding complementary therapies (therapy works with current treatment) such as massage, meditation, acupuncture, dietary supplements, and herbals. Complementary treatments should be discussed with the healthcare provider to make sure that the complementary and traditional treatments don't conflict. Alternative therapy (therapy used instead of ordered medications and treatments) such as garlic, St. John's Wort, and cleansing fasts are often substituted for their traditional treatments and often the individual with HIV will not discuss it with their healthcare provider. This can compromise or negate the effectiveness of their treatment. It is important that any supplements, herbal or other treatments that are taken, are discussed with the healthcare provider (National Center for Complementary and Alternative Therapy, 2016).

Some medication are single drug and some are combination drugs. The efficacy of the drug may decrease with time so that the medications may need to be changed in order to enhance effectiveness (Gulick, 2016). The U.S. Department of Health and Human Services (USDHH, 2016) provides guidelines for the medications.

Opportunistic Infections

In the later stages of HIV infection, if opportunistic or neurologic manifestations occur, management is directed toward the specific infection or manifestation. It is not unusual for individuals with later-stage HIV infection to experience a number of hospitalizations for acute opportunistic infections.

Individuals with HIV infection should take precautions not to transmit the virus. They should fully understand the importance of practicing safe sex, of informing sexual partners of their condition prior to sexual activity, and of not sharing needles, razors, toothbrushes, or any other items that could be contaminated with blood. Education and support are crucial interventions to reduce the risk of HIV transmission, as well as to increase individuals' willingness and ability to adhere to medication management guidelines (CDC, 2015).

Adherence

To realize the maximum effectiveness of the medications and protect against organism resistance, individuals must take medications correctly and consistently as inconsistent or inaccurate use of antiretroviral drugs can be harmful (AIDSinfo, 2016a).

Early antiretroviral protocols were complicated and difficult for many individuals to follow. In addition, many of the medications used to treat HIV had serious and uncomfortable side effects and dangerous medication toxicities (AIDSinfo, 2016b).

When ART protocols are instituted, it is of paramount importance that individuals adhere to the management plan. If the medications are not taken correctly, they may lose their effectiveness. Because of the importance of adherence to the medication protocol, in the last decade concerted effort has been put forth to develop potent, yet well-tolerated, and convenient medication protocols that would enhance adherence and long-term use (Gulick, 2016). As a result, medications have been developed that include more than one medicine in a single pill, making one pill once daily treatment possible and consequently increasing adherence rates (Gulick, 2016).

Although antiretroviral drugs have been improved, like all medications, the possibility of side effects and toxicity still exist. Some side effects, such as nausea, vomiting, diarrhea, cannot only be uncomfortable for the individual but can contribute to nonadherence. More serious side effects/toxicity such as kidney or liver problems may also be experienced. Consequently, it is important for the individual and their healthcare provider to have regular close communication and monitoring regarding any side effects or signs of toxicity so that the drug protocol can be altered appropriately.

COMPLICATIONS OF HIV INFECTION

Neurologic Manifestations and Complications

HIV causes inflammation in the central nervous system early and may cause a variety of neurological conditions over the course of the disease (Berger & Nath, 2016). Individuals with HIV infection may develop complications related to the nervous system that are the result of HIV itself, the result of an opportunistic infection, or due to medication side effects.

HIV dementia (also called *HIV-associated neurocognitive disorders [HAND]*) may occur in mild form or may be severe enough to interfere with daily function. Individuals in older age groups and those who have history of substance abuse or addiction are at higher risk for development of HIV dementia (Berger & Nath, 2016). Initial manifestations may include cognitive decline, such as poor memory, poor concentration, or forgetfulness.

Peripheral neuropathy (a condition involving the peripheral nerves) may also be associated with HIV infection, medication side effects, or opportunistic infection. Individuals with peripheral neuropathy may experience manifestations ranging from numbness of the extremities to burning of the feet and legs, progressing to severe pain, which can be incapacitating.

Dermatologic Complications

Skin manifestations are frequently the initial feature of HIV infection. Although the incidence of skin complications associated with HIV infection has decreased with the advent of antiretroviral medications, a number of skin complications may still occur (Maurer, 2016).

Skin complications may include infections such as *herpes zoster*, *herpes simplex*, or *human papillomavirus*; inflammatory conditions such as *psoriasis*; or a rare form of cancer called *Kaposi's sarcoma*. Kaposi's sarcoma—a rare form of cancer that is not usually seen in individuals with healthy immune systems—is characterized by pink, brown, or purplish blotches on the skin (Rose & Harris, 2015).

Pulmonary Complications

Pulmonary complications are common in individuals with HIV infection and can result from both infectious and noninfectious causes related to the HIV infection itself, medications used in treatment, or unrelated to HIV (Crothers & Morris, 2016). Complications, such as acquired bacterial pneumonia, or opportunistic infections, such as *pneumocystis pneumonia*, can present considerable risk. Lung cancer is a leading cause of mortality in individuals with HIV (Crothers & Morris, 2016). Other pulmonary conditions, including *latent tuberculosis*, can become active with decreasing CD4 and declining immune system effectiveness (Colebunders & French, 2016).

Chronic obstructive pulmonary disease, including emphysema and chronic bronchitis (see Chapter 29) is also increasingly associated with HIV infection, as is higher rate of lung cancer. The increased incidence of both conditions is possibly due to the confounder of greater rate of tobacco use in individuals with HIV (Crothers & Morris, 2016).

Cardiac Complications

Individuals with HIV infection are at increased risk of developing coronary artery disease (Pham & Tores, 2015). The cardiac complications associated with HIV are caused by the HV infection itself as well as side effects of antiretroviral therapy. Although some increased risk is attributable to traditional risk factors for coronary heart disease such as tobacco use, diabetes, or hypertension, some risks are directly related to the chronic inflammation associated with HIV and ART associated elevation of blood lipids (Masur, Healey, & Hadigan, 2016). Due to the increased risk, individuals with HIV should be assessed for cardiac complications regularly and interventions to prevent or modify cardiovascular risk instituted.

Gastrointestinal Complications

The opportunistic infection *oral candidiasis* (yeast infection–oral thrush) is commonly seen in individuals with compromised immune systems, including those with HIV (Maurer, 2016). The fungus *Candida* frequently invades the oral cavity and causes a superficial infection in the mouth and throat, which is manifested by pain and white plaques. It also commonly infects the esophagus (*candida esophagitis*), causing difficulty swallowing (**dysphagia**) and severe pain.

Acute or chronic diarrhea occurs frequently in individuals with HIV infection and may be caused by medications or by an opportunistic infection (Knox & Wanke, 2016). Kaposi's sarcoma, as well as appearing on the skin as noted earlier, may also develop in any location in the gastrointestinal (GI) tract, causing bleeding. Damage to the liver after ART is initiated may occur and is more common when hepatitis C and hepatitis B are also present (Colebunders & French, 2016)

Weight loss can be the result of additional caloric requirements brought about by the metabolic demands associated with condition, but can also be due to difficulty eating or swallowing because of oral thrush or other gastrointestinal infection, side effects of medications used for treating HIV, or depression. As individuals lose weight and become increasingly malnourished, susceptibility to opportunistic infection increases.

Ophthalmologic Complications

Individuals with HIV, especially if advanced, can develop opportunistic infection of the eye such as *cytomegalovirus (CMV) retinitis,* which can result in loss of vision in both eyes (Nishijima et al., 2015).

Metabolic Complications

Individuals with HIV infection experience an increased incidence of a number of metabolic disorders including diabetes mellitus (see Chapter 23), chronic

kidney disease (see Chapter 30) and liver disease. The causes of metabolic complications with HIV are multifactorial, including ART toxicity, chronic inflammation, and dysfunction of the immune system.

Musculoskeletal Complications

Manifestations related to the musculoskeletal system may be present in individuals with HIV either because of the infection itself or due to medication side effects. Individuals may experience weakness, numbness, or discomfort in the extremities (Berger & Nath, 2016). Some medications have been associated with loss of bone mineral density during initial treatment, however, bone mineral density loss appears to stabilize after (Gulick, 2016).

Malignancies

A number of malignancies have higher incidence in individuals with HIV, including lung cancer, Hodgkin lymphoma, oropharyngeal cancers and liver cancers. These cancers, are categorized as non-AIDS-defining malignancies (NADM), because they are not considered as AIDS-defining by the Centers for Disease Control (Uldrick & Yarchoan, 2016).

Immune Reconstitution Inflammatory Syndrome (IRIS)

Individuals who have begun ART may develop a condition known as *immune reconstitution inflammatory syndrome (IRIS)* (Colebunders & French, 2016). IRIS develops as immunity is restored relative to certain infections and noninfectious antigens. As a result, individuals may experience paradoxical worsening of manifestations of an opportunistic infection that is already established or may develop a new opportunistic infection, which previously had shown no manifestations, although the organism was present.

MANAGEMENT OF COMPLICATIONS OF HIV INFECTION

Management of HIV-related complications depends on the organ or body system affected. Many of the interventions for a specific condition occurring as a complication of HIV infection are the same interventions that would be instituted for the specific condition if HIV were not present.

FUNCTIONAL IMPLICATIONS OF HIV INFECTION

Personal and Psychosocial Issues

The personal and psychological challenges faced by individuals with HIV infection are diverse (Davis, Mbuqua, Koch, & Johnson, 2011). Each experience is unique to the individual and his or her particular circumstances.

After first learning that HIV infection is present, individuals may experience shock and denial. As the reality of being HIV positive is gradually realized, individuals are confronted with the knowledge that they have a lifelong condition that requires constant vigilance and management, and one that can be incapacitating and life threatening. Although the advent of HAART interventions have made it possible for many people with HIV to live full and productive lives, the interventions do not work for everyone, and in some instances may not be available to everyone. Realizing the maximum effectiveness of antiretroviral intervention also requires commitment to adherence and perhaps significant lifestyle changes, which can also be anxiety provoking, as can the knowledge that interventions do not eradicate the virus. Consequently, there is always the threat that the condition could progress.

In some instances, individuals may not have disclosed activities related to sexual preference, drug use, or unsafe sexual practices prior to discovering they are HIV positive. The potential need to disclose to family or friends such activities or practice that had previously been hidden can cause additional stress, which combines with the stress arising from the knowledge that they are HIV positive. Individuals may also fear actual or potential transmission of HIV to intimate partners, possible rejection by family or friends, potential loss of employment, and economic stress due to HIV-related healthcare costs.

Stress may also be experienced because of the complexity of and potential risks associated with interventions for management of HIV infection. Not only can medication protocols be complex and expensive, additional concerns regarding potential toxic effects of medications or side effects that may be incapacitating may be another source of stress and anxiety.

Although many individuals with HIV show resilience to stress associated with HIV and adapt well, others experience severe emotional distress. Studies indicate that almost 48% of individuals with HIV infection report manifestations of depression, generalized anxiety, or panic disorder. Other studies report that the incidence of substance abuse and mental health conditions in individuals with HIV infection is higher than that in the general population (Westergaard & Gupta, 2012). While depression, anxiety, or substance use may be the direct result of reaction to the stress associated with having HIV infection, mental health conditions or substance abuse or dependence may have been preexisting conditions and may have contributed to the individual's exposure to HIV owing to increased vulnerability or lifestyle practices. Regardless of the nature of these comorbid conditions, mental health or substance-related conditions have implications not only for quality of life but also for effective management of HIV. Because major focus is often on management of HIV itself, mental health conditions or substance abuse/dependence issues may not be appropriately addressed or managed.

Uncertainty can be another source of distress during the course of HIV infection. It is impossible to predict when, how rapidly, or if the infection will progress to a later phase. Following periods of being very unwell, individuals with HIV infection may then recover and experience periods of well-being, followed by development of another infection that can again be incapacitating. Given this type of unpredictability, individuals may find it difficult to set goals for the future, or they may abandon personal aspirations. Psychological and social support are crucial throughout the course of the disease to help individuals cope with possible changes in self-image and self-esteem that may be experienced as a result of the challenges experienced with HIV infection. Hope can be fostered through inclusion and active participation in decision making regarding management of the condition as well as goal development for the future.

Activities and Participation

All chronic health conditions have an impact not only on the individual with the condition but also on those persons around that individual. In the instance of HIV infection, associated social stigma may be a strong contributor to stress experienced by the individual and his or her family and friends. This stigma may be based on misinformation about how HIV is transmitted, prejudicial attitudes about groups perceived to be linked to HIV transmission, or generalized fear or avoidance of individuals with this chronic or perceived terminal health condition. Misinformation and social prejudice can affect social interactions at school, at work, or in the general community. People may avoid individuals with HIV infection due to fear of exposure through even casual contact or they may devalue individuals due to their condition. As a result, individuals with HIV may find themselves increasingly socially isolated, which in turn can contribute to depression or maladaptive behavior.

Social prejudice may be related to perceptions of the individual's group affiliation. When HIV infection first emerged more than a quarter of a century ago, those affected were frequently among already stigmatized populations such as homosexual men, injection-drug users, and immigrants from developing countries. Although HIV infection exists in every segment of society, affected individuals may still be socially marginalized owing to preexisting prejudicial attitudes against some groups. These social judgments, which stem from preconceived ideas about HIV, including factors assumed to be associated with development of the condition that are viewed as "morally unacceptable," may contribute to discriminatory behaviors toward and social ostracism of individuals with HIV infection. Although public education about HIV and its modes of transmission has helped to change some attitudes among the general population, some individuals with HIV infection may continue to experience rejection and abandonment.

In turn, these experiences may contribute to their feelings of depression and despair.

Individuals with HIV infection may also experience anger and resentment toward the society-imposed isolation that hampers HIV-infected individuals in their efforts to obtain social support and, at times, even the health care afforded to individuals with other chronic or life-threatening conditions. Individuals who have become infected with HIV through healthcare interventions such as blood transfusions may experience additional anger at contracting the condition as "innocent victims."

Although physical function can decline if interventions to manage HIV infection are unavailable, if such interventions are ineffective, if drug resistance occurs, or if there is nonadherence to the management plan, in many instances individuals living with HIV infection are able to continue most activities of daily living and live full and productive lives. Individuals with HIV infection require a balance of periods of activity and rest to prevent overfatigue, as well as development of a healthy lifestyle, including nutrition and exercise. A moderate, regular program of exercise can help individuals maintain optimal emotional and physical health.

Sexuality

Having HIV infection may require that individuals reexamine and redefine their current relationships. There is no direct effect on sexual function associated with HIV infection; however, because of the possibility of transmission of the virus to others via sexual contact, individuals with HIV infection may be fearful of engaging in sexual activity. Individuals with HIV infection should inform their sexual partners about their condition prior to sexual contact and should engage in only safe sexual practices. Partners of individuals with HIV infection may react to knowledge of the partner's HIV-positive status in a variety of ways, ranging from loving support to total abandonment.

Women with HIV infection who become pregnant can transmit their HIV infection to their children. Although antiretroviral therapy during pregnancy can minimize the chances of transmission (Gulick, 2016), knowledge of HIV infection may alter decisions to become pregnant, may cause additional stress during pregnancy and may be a source of stress in intimate relationships.

VOCATIONAL IMPLICATIONS OF HIV INFECTION

Since the advent of antiretroviral therapy with expanded treatment access, employment prospects have sharply increased among individuals with HIV infection who are receiving antiretroviral treatment (Quinn, 2016). Maintaining vocational roles despite significant health issues is important in meeting individuals' emotional and economic needs. Work, in addition to meeting financial needs, is a source of social contact and offers a sense of belonging. The advent of new interventions to manage the condition and the associated increase in life expectancy has provided a more positive outlook for individuals with HIV infection.

Many factors—including psychosocial, financial, health, and legal factors—may affect individuals' ability and willingness to maintain employment. Individuals may be confronted with conflicting pressures about whether they should continue to work. Contextual factors, such as disability benefits and health insurance or drug plans, may also influence their decisions.

For individuals with HIV infection, the most serious impediments to successful functioning in the workplace may be overt or covert discrimination, and prejudice. Although protected under the Americans with Disabilities Act (ADA), HIV-positive individuals may worry that they will lose their jobs as a result of their condition, regardless of their continued mental and physical ability to work. In other instances, if the condition progresses, lack of physical stamina or other complications associated with the condition may necessitate work modification.

When individuals with HIV infection do maintain employment, there are usually no special restrictions, unless complications occur. Because of the mode of transmission of the virus, such individuals should avoid occupations in which their blood may contaminate the blood of others. Because infection can have such serious consequences for HIV-positive individuals, they should also avoid job situations in which they are likely to be exposed to infection. If individuals experience increasing fatigue, they may need to undertake less strenuous work or arrange for shorter work schedules or more frequent rest periods. Complications such as cognitive changes, motor incoordination, or other conditions associated with HIV may also affect an individual's capacity to function in the work setting.

CASE STUDY

Mr. G. is a 26-year-old male who is HIV positive. He contracted HIV from his partner, who died of the infection last year. Mr. G. has a high school education and is a certified nursing assistant working in a nursing home, where he performs routine care for nursing home residents, such as bathing, lifting, turning, and feeding. He has been employed at the nursing home for the past 10 years. Mr. G. tells you he loves his work and very much wants to continue it as long as possible, both for financial reasons and because his health insurance is tied to his employment. He also tells you that work has been therapeutic for him after the loss of his partner. Mr. G. states that his employer is unaware of his condition because it has not interfered with his job performance. Lately, however, Mr. G. has had more difficulty keeping up with the physical demands at work because of fatigue, and in the past few weeks he has developed lymphadenopathy. He has begun a new experimental medication that he also believes might have some side effects that could interfere with his ability to work. Mr. G. has a strong support group of friends; however, his family has severed all ties to him.

1. Is it appropriate for Mr. G. to withhold information about his condition from his employer and to continue to work in the current setting? Why or why not?
2. What is Mr. G.'s rehabilitation potential?
3. Which factors will influence Mr. G.'s rehabilitation potential?
4. Which health and healthcare factors related to Mr. G.'s condition would you consider when helping him develop a rehabilitation plan?

REFERENCES

AIDS.gov. (2015a). *Stages of HIV infection.* Retrieved from https://www.aids.gov/hiv-aids-basics/just-diagnosed-with-hiv-aids/hiv-in-your-body/stages-of-hiv/

AIDS.gov. (2015b). *Overview of HIV treatment.* Retrieved from https://www.aids.gov/hiv-aids-basics/just-diagnosed-with-hiv-aids/treatment-options/overview-of-hiv-treatments/

AIDS.gov. (2016). *Drug resistance.* Retrieved from https://www.aids.gov/hiv-aids-basics/just-diagnosed-with-hiv-aids/treatment-options/drug-resistance/index.html

AIDSinfo. (2015). *The stages of HIV.* Retrieved from https://aidsinfo.nih.gov/education-materials/fact-sheets/19/46/the-stages-of-hiv-infection

AIDSinfo. (2016a). *HIV treatment: Following an HIV regimen: Steps to take before and after starting HIV medicines.* Retrieved from https://aidsinfo.nih.gov/education-materials/fact-sheets/21/55/following-an-hiv- regimen---steps-to-take-before-and-after-starting-hiv-medicines

AIDSinfo. (2016b). *Side effects of HIV medications.* Retrieved from https://aidsinfo.nih.gov/education-materials/fact-sheets/22/63/hiv-medicines-and-side-effects

Avert. (2015a). *HIV Strains and types.* Retrieved from http://www.avert.org/professionals/hiv-science/types-strains

Avert. (2015b). *HIV and AIDS HIV prevention programmes overview.* Retrieved from http://www.avert.org/professionals/hiv-programming/prevention/overview

Berger, J. R., & Nath, A. (2016). Neurologic complications of human immunodeficiency virus infection. In L. Goldman & A. I. Schafer (Eds.), *Goldman-Cecil medicine,* (25th ed., pp. 2328–2332). Philadelphia, PA: Elsevier Saunders.

Carter, M., & Hughson, G., (2013). Primary infection. *Nam AIDS Map.* Retrieved from http://www.aidsmap.com/Primary-infection/page/1044761/

Centers for Disease Control and Prevention. (2015a). *Guidelines for HIV.* Retrieved from http://www.cdc.gov/hiv/guidelines/index.html

Centers for Disease Control and Prevention. (2015b). *HIV transmission.* Retrieved from http://www.cdc.gov/hiv/basics/transmission.html

Centers for Disease Control and Prevention. (2015c). *HIV/AIDS: HIV testing.* Retrieved from http://www.cdc.gov/hiv/testing/

Centers for Disease Control and Prevention. (2015d). *What is HIV?* Retrieved from http://www.cdc.gov/hiv/basics/whatishiv.html

Centers for Disease Control and Prevention. (2016). *Living with HIV.* Retrieved from http://www.cdc.gov/hiv/basics/livingwithhiv/index.html

Chou, R., Selph, S., Dana, T., Bougatsos, C., Zakher, B., Blazina, I., & Korthuis, P. T. (2012). *Screening for HIV: Systematic Review to Update the U.S. Preventive Services Task Force Recommendation.* Evidence Synthesis No. 95. AHRQ Publication No. 12-05173-EF-1. Rockville, MD: Agency for Healthcare Research and Quality.

Colebunders, R., & French, M. A. (2016). Immune reconstitution inflammatory syndrome in HIV/AIDS. In L. Goldman & A. I. Schafer (Eds.), *Goldman-Cecil medicine,* (25th ed., pp. 2332–2335). Philadelphia, PA: Elsevier Saunders.

Crothers, K., & Morris, A. (2016). Pulmonary manifestations of human immunodeficiency virus and the acquired immunodeficiency syndrome. In L. Goldman & A. I. Schafer (Eds.), *Goldman-Cecil medicine,* (25th ed., pp. 2305–2318). Philadelphia, PA: Elsevier Saunders.

Davis, S. J., Mbuqua, A., Koch, D. S., & Johnson, A. (2011). Recognizing suicide risk in consumers with HIV/AIDS. *Journal of Rehabilitation, 77*(1), 14–19.

Deeks, S. G., Lewin, S. R., & Havlir, D. V. (2013). The end of AIDS: HIV infection is a chronic disease. *The Lancet, 382*(99030), 1525–1533. Retrieved from http://www.thelancet.com/journals/lancet/article/PIIS0140-6736%2813%2961809-7/abstract

Del Rio, C., & Cohen, M. S. (2016). Prevention of human immunodeficiency virus infection. In L. Goldman & A. I. Schafer (Eds.), *Goldman-Cecil medicine,* (25th ed., pp. 2285–2287). Philadelphia, PA: Elsevier Saunders.

Department of Health and Human Services. (2016). *Antiretroviral Guidelines for Adults and Adolescents. Guidelines for the use of antiretroviral agents in HIV-1-infected adults and adolescents.* Retrieved from http://aidsinfo.nih.gov/contentfiles/lvguidelines/AdultandAdolescentGL.pdf

Gulick, R. M. (2016). Antiretroviral therapy of human immunodeficiency virus and acquired immunodeficiency syndrome. In L. Goldman & A. I. Schafer (Eds.), *Goldman-Cecil medicine,* (25th ed., pp. 2287–2292). Philadelphia, PA: Elsevier Saunders.

Knox, T. A., & Wanke, C. (2016). Gastrointestinal manifestations of HIV and AIDS. In L. Goldman & A. I. Schafer (Eds.), *Goldman-Cecil medicine,* (25th ed., pp. 2302–2305). Philadelphia, PA: Elsevier Saunders.

Maldarelli, F. (2016). Biology of human immunodeficiency viruses. In L. Goldman & A. I. Schafer (Eds.), *Goldman-Cecil medicine,* (25th ed., pp. 2280–2285). Philadelphia, PA: Elsevier Saunders.

Masur, H., Healey, L., & Hadigan, C. (2016). Infectious and metabolic complications of human immunodeficiency virus and acquired immunodeficiency syndrome. In L. Goldman & A. I. Schafer (Eds.), *Goldman-Cecil medicine,* (25th ed., pp. 2292–2302). Philadelphia, PA: Elsevier Saunders.

Maurer, T. (2016). Skin manifestations in patients with human immunodeficiency virus infection. In L. Goldman & A. I. Schafer (Eds.), *Goldman-Cecil medicine* (25th ed., pp. 2318–2322). Philadelphia, PA: Elsevier Saunders.

National Center for Complementary and Alternate Medicine: NIH. (2016, February 16). *HIV.* Retrieved from https://nccih.nih.gov/health/hiv

Nishijima, T., Yashiro, S., Teruya, K., Kikuchi, Y., Katai, N., Oka, S., & Gatanaga, H. (2015). Routine eye screening by an ophthalmologist is clinically useful for HIV-1-infected patients with CD4 count less that 200/uL. *PLoS ONE 10*(9), e0136747. doi:10.1371/journal.pone.0136747

Pham, T. V., & Tores, M. (2015). Human immunodeficiency virus infection-related heart disease. *Emergency Medicine Clinics of North America*, *33*(3), 613–622.

Quinn, T. C. (2016). Epidemiology and diagnosis of human immunodeficiency virus infection and acquired immunodeficiency syndrome. In L. Goldman & A. I. Schafer (Eds.), *Goldman-Cecil medicine,* (25th ed., pp. 2272–2278). Philadelphia, PA: Elsevier Saunders.

Rathbun, R. C., & Butler, J. (2016). Antiviral therapy for HIV infection. *Medscape.* Retrieved from http://emedicine.medscape.com/article/1533218-overview

Rose, L., & Harris, K. E. (2015, April 15). *Kaposi Sarcoma.* Retrieved from http://emedicine.medscape.com/article/279734-overview#a4

Rote, N. S., & Huether, S. E. (2014). Infection. In K. L. McCance, S. E. Huether, V. L. Brashers, & N. S. Rote (Eds.), *Pathophysiology: The biologic basis for disease in adults and children* (7th ed., pp. 322–327). St. Louis MO: Elsevier-Mosby.

Uldrick, T. S., & Yarchoan, R. (2016). Hematology and oncology in patients with human immunodeficiency virus infection. In L. Goldman & A. I. Schafer (Eds.), *Goldman-Cecil medicine,* (25th ed., pp. 2322–2328). Philadelphia, PA: Elsevier Saunders.

U.S. Preventive Services Task Force. (2015). *Final update summary: Human immunodeficiency virus (HIV) infection: Screening.* U.S. Preventive Services Task Force. Retrieved from http://www.uspreventiveservicestaskforce.org/Page/Document/UpdateSummaryFinal/human-immunodeficiency-virus-hiv-infection-screening

U.S. Preventive Services Task Force. (2016). *Screening for HIV clinical summary of U.S. preventive services task force recommendation.* Retrieved from http://www.uspreventiveservicestaskforce.org

Westergaard, R., & Gupta, A. (2012). The patient with HIV disease. In E. T. Bope & R. D. Kellerman (Eds.), *Conn's current therapy 2012,* (pp. 86–104). Philadelphia, PA: Elsevier Saunders.

CHAPTER 21

Introduction to Cancers: General Methods of Identification and Management

STRUCTURE AND FUNCTION OF THE CELL

The basic unit of all living things is the *cell*. The human body contains approximately 75 trillion cells. Although different types of cells perform different functions, all cells have certain basic characteristics in common:

- All cells require nutrition and oxygen to live.
- Almost all cells have the ability to replicate.

Replication of cells is a controlled process in which cells die and form at an approximately equal rate in adults, maintaining a balance in the number of cells present at any time. The precise way in which cell growth and reproduction are regulated within the human body is unknown. Similarly, little is known about the mechanism that controls the number of each specific cell type that is produced. Some cells, such as those that make up the layers of the skin and the lining of the intestine, grow and replicate frequently. Other cells, such as those that make up the musculature of the gastrointestinal tract, may not replicate for years. Although it was once thought that cells that make up neurons, the functional units of the nervous system, do not replicate at all, evidence is now available that shows in some instances nerve cells can replicate (Mu & Gage, 2011).

Different body tissues are made up of different types of cells. These different types of cells are named for their specific characteristics. For example, *epithelial cells* are found in the skin, the lining of body organs (e.g., the lining of the intestine), and glandular tissue (e.g., the breast or prostate). Blood vessels, lymph vessels, and other lymph tissue are composed of *endothelial cells*. Different types of cells are also found in muscle, nerve, bone, and other tissues in the body.

Every cell contains *DNA*—the genetic material that serves as the blueprint for all the body's structures. *Genes*, which are composed of DNA, carry hereditary information about all characteristics of the organism. Although each cell contains all the genes for a particular organism, it expresses only particular genes. This discrimination in the use of genes is the basis for different cell types. Genes determine how cells grow, as well as when or whether the cells divide to form new cells. Before cells can replicate, however, genes must replicate themselves. After its genes replicate, the cell divides, forming another cell identical to itself. It is through this systematic, organized replication of cells that continuity of life is maintained.

DEVELOPMENT OF CANCER

Cancer is not a single condition but rather many different conditions grouped under a single heading. More than 100 types of cancers have been identified. Cancers can arise from any type of cell and are classified according to the cell of origin. Frequently, the term *tumor* is assumed to be synonymous with *cancer*; however, not all tumors are cancerous. A **tumor**, also called a *neoplasm*, is a new and irregular growth of cells that serves no useful function and may interfere with healthy tissue function (Rote & Virshup, 2014). The reason for the proliferation of cells is often unknown.

Tumors may be **benign** (noncancerous) or **malignant** (cancerous). Although benign tumors may disturb body function by exerting pressure on surrounding tissues, thereby preventing surrounding organs from obtaining a sufficient blood supply, they usually grow slowly, do not invade surrounding tissue, remain localized, and generally do not recur once removed. Cells in benign tumors usually closely resemble regular cells in the tissue of their origin.

Malignant tumors, by contrast, consist of irregular cells that exhibit uncontrolled and destructive growth as well as the ability to invade surrounding tissues and move to other parts of the body. Some of the more virulent cancer cells are described as *anaplastic*, meaning that their appearance takes on irregular characteristics so that they are less differentiated than are the regular cells from which they are derived.

Cancer develops when an alteration (*mutation*) in the DNA within a regular cell occurs. As a result, the control mechanism that regulates cell replication is lost. Because their replication is uncontrolled, cancer cells replicate more rapidly—at a rate exceeding the rate at which the regular cells in the tissue die.

The original site of cancer cell reproduction is called the *primary site*, sometimes referred to as the *primary tumor*. Cancer cells do not remain confined to the original site but rather extend into and invade surrounding tissues as they replicate.

In addition, cancer cells are less adhesive than are regular cells. Selected cancer cells may break off from the original cluster, enter the bloodstream or the lymph system, and travel to other parts of the body, where they begin another irregular pattern of reproduction. The movement of cancer cells from the original site to another part of the body is called **metastasis**. Cancer cell reproduction at this additional site is called a *secondary tumor*, meaning that metastasis has occurred and that the secondary tumor is not the original site of cancer growth.

Cancer cells compete with regular cells for nutrients. Reproduction of cancer cells is not well regulated, and some cancer cells replicate at a more rapid rate than do regular cells. Eventually, available nutrients are taken from the regular cells to nourish the cancer cells.

CAUSES OF CANCER

The exact cause of cancer is unknown. Many causes probably exist, and it may be necessary for a variety of factors to be present for cancer to develop. Although specific causes are unknown, several factors are known to increase the risk of cancer:

- Ionizing radiation
- Some chemicals and pollutants
- Alcohol
- Diet, obesity, and physical inactivity
- Tobacco exposure
- Some infectious agents (viruses and some bacteria)
- Chronic physical irritation to a body part
- Ultraviolet rays (sun)
- Hereditary predisposition
- Suppressed immune response (McCance, 2014; Hunter, 2016)

Chemicals or other substances that are thought to cause cancer are called **carcinogens**. Some carcinogens may be present in the environment, but are not readily evident. Individuals may be exposed to carcinogens within the environment or workplace for a number of years before cancer develops. Some substances may not be carcinogenic per se, but may serve as cocarcinogens, promoting tumor growth. Other factors, such as hormonal secretion, diet, and stress, have been implicated as potential factors in the development of or propensity for cancer, but the specific mechanisms that contribute to this relationship are unknown.

TYPES OF CANCERS

There are more than 100 types of cancer (National Institute of Health [NIH], 2015). Any type of cell in the body may be the source of cancer. Cancers are named for the type of tissue from which they originated. Examples of some common types of cancers and the corresponding tissue from which they arise are described here:

- **Carcinoma**: cancer of the epithelial cells
- **Sarcoma**: cancer of the bone, muscle, or other connective tissue
- **Lymphoma**: cancer of the lymphatic system
- **Leukemia**: cancer of blood cells or blood precursor cells
- **Melanoma**: cancer of pigment-producing cells, usually of the skin

Because the specific behavior of cancer cells depends on the type of cell from which they originated, no generalizations can be made about cancer. Each type of cancer may progress at a different rate and may respond to different types of intervention in different ways. Consequently, classification of cancer is important in determining both management and outcome.

STAGING AND GRADING OF CANCER

When cancer is identified, it is important to determine not only the cancer type but also the extent to which cancer cells have spread. This process is called **staging**. Staging of cancers not only helps healthcare providers determine an individual's **prognosis** (prediction of the course and outcome of the condition), but also helps to determine the type of intervention that is most appropriate.

Many types of staging systems are used. Indeed, staging systems continue to change as more research is conducted and more is learned about cancer. The following factors are usually considered in staging systems:

- Site of the primary tumor
- Size and number of tumors
- Lymph node involvement
- Cell type and grade
- Presence or absence of metastasis

Summary Staging

Cancer registries sometimes use summary staging, a system that groups cancer cases into categories. Example categories include the following (SEER Training Module, n.d.):

- In situ: Cancer cells remain superficial in tissue in which they originated.
- Localized: Cancer cells are limited to the organ in which they originated with no evidence of spread.
- Regional: Cancer cells have spread to nearby organs or lymph nodes.
- Distant: Cancer cells have spread to distant organs or lymph nodes.
- Unknown: Stage cannot be determined due to inadequate information.

TNM Staging

The most common system for staging is the *TNM system,* which classifies cancer according to tumor size, node involvement, and metastasis. The letter "T" stands for *tumor;* "N" for *node;* and "M" for *metastasis.*

When there is no evidence of a primary tumor, the stage is defined as *T0.* If cancer cells are present but have not invaded surrounding lymph nodes or organs, the stage is defined as *Tis* (previously called *in situ*). As the tumor increases in size, it may be staged from *T1* to *T4,* depending on the tumor size and involvement. *TX* means the tumor cannot be measured.

When there is no lymph node involvement, the *N* staging is *N0.* If cancer cells extend beyond he initial tissue site and involve lymph nodes in the surrounding area, however, the stage is either *N1, N2,* or *N3* (previously called regional involvement), depending on the degree of involvement and irregularity of nodes. *NX* means the nodes cannot be evaluated.

If cancer cells remain at the original site, even though surrounding tissues and lymph nodes are involved, the *M* staging is *M0.* When cancer cells have metastasized to another area of the body, staging is either *M1, M2,* or *M3,* depending on the extent of metastasis. *MX* means that metastasis cannot be evaluated.

Generalized Staging

Often the TNM system is assumed to correspond to the following *generalized stages:*

- Stage 0: cancer in situ
- Stage I, II, or III: the higher the number, the more extensive the cancer
- Stage IV: metastasis

Histologic Studies and Grading

Histologic studies and *grading* are laboratory procedures in which the type and structure of cancer cells are determined microscopically. Cells are examined to determine their type and the extent to which they differ from their regular precursors. Histologic grading is based on the appearance of cells and the degree of differentiation. Cells are graded as follows:

- Grade I: *mild dysplasia* (cells are slightly different from regular cells)
- Grade II: *moderate dysplasia* (cells are more irregular)
- Grade III: *severe dysplasia* (cells are very irregular and poorly differentiated)
- Grade IV: *anaplasia* (cells are immature and undifferentiated; cells of origin are difficult to determine)

The histologic type of cell and the grading of the cell are important in the determination of the interventions instituted *and* the prognosis. Individuals with tumor cells that are *well differentiated* (more similar to the cell of origin, with a more organized structure) may have a better prognosis, for example, than do individuals with tumor cells that are considered *anaplastic* (containing more irregularities in structure).

GENERAL PROCEDURES FOR IDENTIFICATION OF CANCER

In general, the earlier cancer is identified, the better the outcome. Some cancers grow and invade surrounding tissue without causing physical manifestations;

these cancers are called *occult malignancies.* Tests and procedures used to detect irregularities before manifestations develop are called *cancer screening procedures.* When manifestations occur or when screening procedures have positive or suspicious results, additional testing is necessary.

Radiographic Procedures (X-Ray)

In addition to conventional X-rays, *computed axial tomography (CAT scan), magnetic resonance imaging (MRI), ultrasound,* and, occasionally, *arteriography* may be helpful in identifying an irregularity in anatomic structure or the presence of a tumor. *Mammography* is a soft-tissue radiographic examination of the breast that is frequently used as a screening procedure even though there are no manifestations; this modality can reveal cancerous lesions before they can be detected by direct examination of the breast. Although radiographic tests are important in identifying irregularities, they are rarely used alone for the identification of cancer. Instead, confirmation of the presence of cancer requires histologic testing.

Surgery for Identification of Cancer

In some instances, surgical procedures may be performed to confirm or rule out the presence of cancer. Depending on the size and location of the tumor, the surgical procedure may be relatively minor, such as the removal of an external wart or polyp, or it may be a major intervention, such as *exploratory laparotomy* (the surgical opening of the abdomen for the purpose of investigation).

Regardless of the type of surgical procedure performed, an accurate identification of cancer as well as cancer type can be made only after a microscopic examination of the tissue removed. For such an examination, a **biopsy** is performed to remove a small portion of tissue from the body. Biopsy may be done by inserting a needle into the tumor and removing some cells through the needle (*needle biopsy*). It may also be done by making an incision and removing a portion of the tumor (*incisional biopsy*). The type of biopsy depends on the size and location of the tumor.

Cytology

The study of cells that have been scraped from tissue surrounding the area of interest is called *cytology*. Perhaps the best-known example of cytology used for this purpose is the *Papanicolaou smear (Pap smear)*. Cells from sputum specimens that have been expectorated from the lungs as well as other types of fluids may also be examined through cytology for identification of cancer.

Endoscopy

An *endoscopic examination* involves the insertion of a tubular device into a hollow organ or cavity to visualize the inside of the structure directly. This procedure may be performed through a natural body opening or through a small incision. Examples of endoscopic examinations include bronchoscopy, sigmoidoscopy, gastroscopy and esophagoscopy, and laryngoscopy (examination of the larynx or vocal cords). Endoscopy can also be used to obtain a tissue sample from an internal structure for a histologic examination.

Nuclear Medicine Procedures

Nuclear medicine procedures can be used in the identification of cancer as well as its management if cancer is present (Schlumberger et al., 2012). For identification of cancer, nuclear medicine procedures utilize small amounts of radioactive materials (*radiopharmaceuticals*) that are injected intravenously, swallowed, or inhaled, depending on the body part to be examined. The radioactive material gradually accumulates in the area of the body being examined. Radioactive emissions from the materials may then be detected by special cameras that provide precise pictures of the body part being investigated.

Nuclear medicine procedures may be used with CT or MRI to correlate and interpret information from both procedures into a special view (*image fusion* or *coregistration*). In some facilities, special imaging modalities such as *single photon emission computed tomography (SPECT/CT)* and *positron emission tomography/computed tomography (PET/CT)* are available. These special devices are able to perform both exams at the same time.

Laboratory Tests

Although laboratory tests per se may not be a definitive tool for identifying cancer, the results of such tests may provide information that indicates impaired physiologic function, which could be an indication of cancer, such as the anemia or altered white blood cell count associated with leukemia. In some instances, laboratory tests are used for screening purposes. For example, substances such as *alpha-fetoprotein* and *carcinoembryonic antigens* are usually found in embryonic and fetal tissues, but disappear after birth. In later life, however, tumors may produce these substances. Consequently, elevated levels of either substance in adults may be an indication of certain types of cancers or other conditions.

GENERAL MANAGEMENT OF CANCER

Many modalities are available to prevent, control, or cure cancer. Management modalities can be classified as follows:

- Surgery
- Chemotherapy
- Radiation (external or internal)
- Biological (immunotherapy, hormone therapy, gene therapy)
- Bone marrow transplantation

These interventions may be used alone or in combination. Indeed, many management approaches involve multiple types of interventions rather than one. When interventions consist of several different types of interventions, management is said to be *multimodal.*

A number of factors are considered when deciding which approaches are the best choices for the management of a particular cancer. A major consideration is the *type of cancer* itself. Because different cancers grow at different rates, metastasize to different parts of the body, and react differently to various forms of intervention, the histologic type of cancer is a major determinant in management decisions. The *stage of cancer* is also considered. The extent to which cancer has invaded surrounding tissues and the presence of any metastases determine how aggressive and which type of intervention should be instituted. Tumor location and its relationship to other vital organs determine the accessibility of the tumor for removal.

The goal of cancer management also influences the type of intervention used. Goals for management of cancer can include any of these:

- Cure
- Extension of life
- Prevention of metastasis
- Palliation

In terms of cancer management, *cure* is usually defined as no evidence of cancer for 5 years after intervention, indicating a regular life expectancy for the individual. Management for the prevention of metastasis, also called *adjuvant therapy,* is directed toward eliminating cancer that, although not detectable and having no manifestations, may be present and may cause a recurrence of cancer. *Palliative therapy* is directed toward the relief of manifestations or complications of cancer, such as obstruction or severe pain, rather than toward cure.

Factors related to the specific individual must also be taken into consideration. Other coexisting chronic conditions unrelated to the cancer, the cancer itself, or the age of the individual may compromise the ability to withstand certain interventions. In some cases, individuals may choose to forgo some types of interventions due to the risks and side effects involved, which they may feel outweigh the benefit of the intervention.

Cancer may be managed with either systemic or local interventions. Often, such management consists of a combination of the two. Cancer may be managed surgically, chemically *(chemotherapy)*, with radiation, or with other means—separately or in combination.

Surgical Procedures

Surgical procedures are usually directed toward the local management of cancer and may be preventive, curative, palliative, or reconstructive (Rote & Virshup, 2014). *Preventive surgery* may be performed when precancerous or suspicious lesions are discovered. For example, a mole or polyp that, although not malignant, has a high probability of

becoming malignant in the future may be removed. *Curative surgery* is generally more extensive. It may involve not only the tumor but also an organ or surrounding tissue. Depending on the size and location of the tumor, curative surgery can affect subsequent function only minimally, can impair function severely, or can cause permanent disfigurement. *Palliative surgery* is directed toward reducing the size or retarding the growth of the tumor, or relieving severe discomfort associated with the presence of the tumor. In all instances, the goal of palliative surgery is to prolong or increase quality of life rather than to cure the cancer. *Reconstructive surgery* is directed toward restoring maximal function or correcting disfigurement.

Surgical procedures used in management of cancer may be considered either simple or radical. *Simple surgical procedures* usually involve removal of the tumor, while surrounding structures and organs remain intact. *Radical surgical procedures* are more extensive. In radical surgery, not only is the tumor removed but some underlying tissue (e.g., muscle or organ) is removed as well. Radical surgery often results in alteration in function or appearance to some degree. With advances of healthcare techniques, fewer radical procedures are now being performed.

Chemotherapy

Chemotherapy is an intervention that uses *antineoplastic medications* (chemical agents that destroy cancer cells) for the management of cancer. It can be curative in many cancers, but can also be used for prevention or palliation (Doroshow, 2016). In some cancers, chemotherapy *(adjuvant chemotherapy)* may be used in conjunction with other interventions, such as surgery or radiation, to augment the effectiveness of those interventions and eliminate micrometastises (Rote & Virshup, 2014). The newest agents to treat cancer are called targeted therapy. They work with other chemotherapy drugs but are targeted for specific cancer cells. They show promise and studies of their use are continuing (NIH, 2014).

Chemotherapy can be administered at home, in health facilities on an outpatient basis, or in an inpatient setting. Administration of a chemotherapeutic agent can be oral, by injection, by catheter or port, or topical. Some individuals may use a portable device (*infusion pump*) that pumps small amounts of the chemotherapeutic agent constantly into a vein (*infusion therapy*). In other instances, high concentrations of chemotherapeutic agents may be injected directly into a body cavity, such as the bladder or the peritoneal cavity, to manage localized tumors.

Administration of the chemotherapeutic agent can take anywhere from a few minutes to a few hours. The agent can be administered daily, weekly, or monthly. The type of chemotherapeutic agent used and the duration of the intervention depends on the cancer type, the individual's response to the medication, his or her general health, and the type of chemotherapeutic medication used. If more than one chemotherapeutic agent is used (as in combination therapy), medications can be given either together or alternately, depending on the medications involved.

Single chemotherapy drugs, given alone, rarely provide a cure; it generally takes a combination of two or three antineoplastic medications together in the management of cancer (Rote & Virshup, 2014). Chemotherapeutic agents may be classified according to their mechanism of action, their chemical structure, their relationship to another medication, and sometimes their origin (i.e., because they are derived from the same plant). Because some chemotherapeutic agents act in more than one way, certain medications may be included in more than one category. Although most chemotherapeutic agents affect growth and reproduction of cancer cells in some way, different medications work by affecting different phases of the cell cycle. Some examples of general types of chemotherapeutic agents follow:

- Alkylating agents: prevent cancer cells from reproducing
- Antimetabolites: prevent cancer cells' division in part of their reproductive phase and interfere with cell growth
- Antitumor antibiotics: interfere with cancer cell replication

Unfortunately, chemotherapeutic agents can damage healthy structures as well. For instance, alkylating agents can damage bone marrow over time, whereas antitumor antibiotics can cause damage to the heart over time. In addition to destroying and damaging cancer cells, these chemotherapeutic agents can damage regular cells that grow rapidly, such as the cells of the hair follicles, skin, and lining of the gastrointestinal tract, and cells in the bone marrow. As a result, toxic side effects of chemotherapy may include hair loss (**alopecia**), loss of appetite, nausea, vomiting, diarrhea, and fatigue. Suppression of bone marrow function may interfere with the production of various components of blood, contributing to manifestations such as anemia, bruising due to decreased blood clotting ability, and increased susceptibility to infection because of decreased production of white blood cells (American Cancer Society, 2015).

In some instances, if the chemotherapeutic agent is administered in small doses over time, toxic side effects may be reduced. This type of intervention delivers the maximal dosage of the medication to the tumor site and may result in fewer systemic side effects. Newer medications to offset side effects of chemotherapy may help to ameliorate the toxic effects of medications used at higher doses in chemotherapy.

Not all individuals who receive chemotherapy experience all possible side effects. Those who do not have severe side effects can, for the most part, continue their daily activities. No special precautions are necessary, with the exception of avoiding exposure to individuals with colds or flu because resistance to infection may be lowered during chemotherapy.

Radiation Therapy

Radiation therapy can be used to cure cancer, to relieve manifestations, or to keep cancer under control; radiation can be given alone or as part of the treatment management after chemotherapy (NIH, 2015). It may be conducted *externally* or *internally*. Such therapy can be used as the primary intervention or in combination with other interventions. Ionizing radiation can be delivered through high-energy rays (*teletherapy*); through radioactive implants, seeds, or wires; or intravenously with radioisotopes (Doroshow, 2016). Radiation therapy damages cancer cells and causes cancer cell death.

External radiation therapy is performed through a machine that beams high-energy rays directly to the cancer cells so that the maximum effect of the radiation occurs within the tumor itself. Even though radiation penetrates the skin and underlying tissue, there is minimal damage to these structures. This is especially true of newer techniques such as intensity-modulated radiation therapy that allow more exact focus of high-energy beams to the specific cancer site, thereby reducing damage to healthy tissue.

Internal radiation therapy involves inserting small amounts of radioactive material into the body, a procedure called *brachytherapy*. A radioactive substance is delivered to the tumor site through implants, needles, beads, or seeds. The interstitial implant may be removed after a specific period of time, or it may be left in place permanently, depending on the half-life of the radioactive source.

Although newer techniques offer more protection to healthy cells, like chemotherapy, radiation therapy can affect growth and reproduction of regular cells, resulting in potentially toxic side effects. The number of regular cells exposed to the radiation, the dosage of radiation, the part of the body receiving radiation therapy, and unique characteristics of the individual determine the side effects experienced. These side effects may appear either immediately or some weeks or months after the radiation therapy was administered. Some individuals experience generalized manifestations similar to those of radiation sickness: nausea, vomiting, loss of appetite, fatigue, and headache. Other individuals experience side effects specific to the area irradiated, such as sore throat if the head or neck has been irradiated, or localized skin reactions, such as radiation burn. Like chemotherapy, radiation therapy may cause bone marrow depression, resulting in anemia, lowered resistance to infection, and possibly hemorrhage.

Biological Therapies

Immunotherapy

Another approach to the management of cancer is *immunotherapy*. Because human cancer cells express cancer-associated antigens, the goal of immunotherapy is to stimulate and strengthen the individual's own immune system so that it recognizes cancer cells as foreign objects and destroys them (*active immunotherapy*). *Passive immunotherapy* uses antibodies created outside the body to help fight cancer cells. With this approach, the ability of the body's own immune system to fight cancer cells is strengthened.

Immunotherapeutic agents can also help to increase the susceptibility of cancer cells to the *cytotoxic agents* (chemicals that are detrimental to or destroy cells). Many immunologic approaches to cancer management are already being used, including *interferon* and *interleukin-2*. Interferon is thought to enhance the actions of cell-killing cells that attack and destroy cancer cells. It also slows cell division and suppresses tumor growth. Another example of immunotherapy involves administration of bacille Calmette–Guérin (BCG), which is used in the management of superficial bladder cancer (Bajorin, 2016; Clark, 2012).

Hormone Therapy

Hormone therapy can be used to increase the benefits of chemotherapy in cancers that are hormone dependent (such as certain breast cancers that are estrogen dependent and prostate cancers that are androgen dependent). Hormones are not used to kill cancer cells but rather to keep the cancer cells from growing, which means that individuals remain in remission for extended periods of time. Hormone preparations work either by blocking hormone receptors so that the cancer cells cannot use estrogen or androgen, or by preventing the individual's body from making hormones.

Monoclonal Antibodies

Monoclonal antibodies are specific antibodies made in the laboratory that are designed to attack a specific antigen. Although monoclonal antibodies are used for a number of health conditions, they are also used as an intervention for cancer, although they may be more effective in some cancers than in others. When used in the management of cancer, they may be used alone or used in combination with other interventions. Monoclonal antibodies are usually given intravenously and can generate some short-term side effects with their initial administration, such as fever, chills, nausea, and vomiting.

Gene Therapy

Gene therapy as an intervention for management of a number of health conditions, including cancer, is currently in its infancy. This type of therapy works by modifying the genetic structure of the cells to suppress or inhibit growth.

Bone Marrow and Hematopoietic Stem Cell Transplantation

Hematopoietic stem cells are immature cells that can develop into red blood cells, white blood cells, or platelets. *Bone marrow* or *stem cell transplantation* is an intervention used for a number of different conditions, malignant as well as nonmalignant. In cancers, stem cell transplant replaces bone marrow cells that have been destroyed or damaged by chemotherapy or radiation with healthy bone marrow stem cells.

Bone marrow stem cells can be obtained from several sources. Cells can be removed either from a donor (*allogenic transplant*) or from the individual's own body (*autologous transplant*).

For allogenic transplants, the donor and the recipient must be closely matched in terms of *human leukocyte antigens (HLAs)*, which are proteins or markers used by the immune system to recognize foreign substances. The closer the HLA match between donor and recipient, the greater the chance of transplant success and the lower the risk of *graft-versus-host disease (GVHD)*, in which the transplanted cells attack cells of the individuals who receive them (Keating & Bishop, 2016). In addition, in some instances transplanted cells appear to generate an immune reaction that enhances destruction of malignant cells.

With autologous transplants, cells are removed from the individual's own body prior to irradiation or chemotherapy, and then later reinfused. The advantage of autologous infusions is that they eliminate the risk of rejection and GVHD (Keating & Bishop, 2016). The disadvantage is that there is risk of contamination with tumor cells from the individual's body. Also, autologous transplants lack the extra antitumor effect that may be found with allogenic transplants.

Obtaining Bone Marrow Stem Cells

The process of obtaining bone marrow stem cells is called *harvesting*. Bone marrow stem cells may be harvested through extraction of bone marrow directly or from a vein. Extraction of bone marrow stem cells requires that the individual undergo a minor surgical procedure under general anesthesia. Bone marrow is extracted from a large bone in the body (usually the pelvic area) via needle biopsy.

Stem cells also circulate in the peripheral blood in small quantities. Peripheral stem cell harvesting removes cells from the peripheral blood, thereby avoiding a surgical procedure. In this procedure, blood is removed through a catheter in one arm and circulated through a special machine that isolates stem cells. The blood that has had the stem cells removed is then returned through a catheter into a vein in the other arm.

An alternative source of stem cells is from umbilical cord blood previously stored in cord blood banks. Consequently, no additional harvest procedures are required with this approach. Although stem cells from umbilical cord blood represent an allogenic source, because of the immature nature of the cells, the chances of the recipient developing GVHD are less; however, the donor still must be matched somewhat with the recipient of the cells (Keating & Bishop, 2016). In addition, because there is generally only a small volume of stem cells in umbilical cord blood, obtaining stem cells from this source is not always feasible for adults.

Transplantation

Prior to bone marrow transplantation, individuals receive large doses of radiation (often total body irradiation) or chemotherapy to eradicate any viable marrow, kill tumor cells, and suppress the immune system so as to reduce the chance of rejection of the transplant. As a result of the immune system suppression, however, individuals receiving a transplant are highly susceptible to infection. After the individual receives an infusion of cells from the donor, the person's bone marrow regenerates using the new cells.

Because of the immunosuppression that occurs prior to surgery, individuals may have an increased susceptibility to infections. In addition, with allogenic stem cell transplant, a number of immunosuppressive medications may be used to prevent GVHD. As immunologic tolerance becomes more firmly established, these medications are usually gradually discontinued (Keating & Bishop, 2016).

BIBLIOGRAPHY

Falvo, R. E. (2001). *Human physiology: Physiology 201 core curriculum.* Champaign, IL: Stipes.

Sherwood, L. (2007). *Human physiology: From cells to systems* (6th ed.). Australia: Thomson Brooks/Cole.

Tortora, G. J., & Derrickson, B. H. (Eds.). (2011). *Principles of anatomy and physiology* (13th ed.). Hoboken, NJ: John Wiley and Sons.

Widmaier, E., Raff, H., & Strang, K. (Eds.). (2010). *Vander's human physiology: The mechanism of body function.* New York, NY: McGraw-Hill.

REFERENCES

American Cancer Society (2015). *Chemotherapy drugs: How they work.* Retrieved from http://www.cancer.org/acs/groups /cid/documents/webcontent/002995-pdf.pdf

Bajorin, D. F. (2016). Tumors of the kidney, bladder, ureters, and renal pelvis. In L. Goldman & A. I. Schafer (Eds.), *Goldman-Cecil medicine,* (25th ed. pp. 1345–1351). Philadelphia, PA: Elsevier Saunders.

Clark, P. E. (2012). Malignant tumors of the urogenital tract. In E. T. Bope & R. D. Kellerman (Eds.), *Conn's current therapy 2012,* (pp. 889–897). Philadelphia, PA: Elsevier Saunders.

Doroshow, J. H. (2016). Approach to the patient with cancer. In L. Goldman & A. I. Schafer (Eds.), *Goldman-Cecil medicine,* (25th ed., pp. 1206–1222). Philadelphia, PA: Elsevier Saunders.

Hunter, D. J. (2016). Epidemiology of cancer. In L. Goldman & A. I. Schafer (Eds.), *Goldman-Cecil medicine,* (25th ed., pp.1222–1225). Philadelphia, PA: Elsevier Saunders.

Keating, A. & Bishop, M. R. (2016). Hematopoietic stem cell transplantation. In L. Goldman & A. I. Schafer (Eds.), *Goldman-Cecil medicine,* (25th ed., pp. 1198–1204). Philadelphia, PA: Elsevier Saunders.

McCance, K. L. (2014). Cancer epidemiology. In K. L. McCance, S. E. Huether, V. L. Brashers, & N. S. Rote (editors). *Pathophysiology: The biologic basis for disease in adults and children,* (7th ed., pp. 402–437). St. Louis MO: Elsevier-Mosby.

Mu, Y., & Gage, F. H. (2011). Adult hippocampal neurogenesis and its role in Alzheimer's disease. *Molecular Neurogeneration, 6,* 85–92.

National Institute of Health: National Cancer Institute (2014). *Targeted therapies.* Retrieved from http://www.cancer.gov /about-cancer/treatment/types/targeted-therapies

National Institute of Health: National Cancer Institute (2015). *What is cancer?* Retrieved from http://www.cancer.gov /about-cancer/understanding/what-is-cancer

Rote, N. S., & Virshup, D. M. (2014). Cancer biology. In K. L. McCance, S. E. Huether, V. L. Brashers, & N.S. Rote (Eds.), *Pathophysiology: The biologic basis for disease in adults and children* (7th ed., pp. 363–401). St. Louis MO: Elsevier-Mosby.

SEER Training Modules. National Institute of Health: National Cancer Institute (n.d.). Reviewed at http://training .seer.cancer.gov/citation.html

Schlumberger, M., Catargi, B., Borget, I., Deandreis, D., Zerdoud, S., Bridji, B., ... Tumeurs de la Thyroide Refractaires Network for the Essai Stimulation Ablation Equivalence Trial. (2012). Strategies of radioiodine ablation in patients with low-risk thyroid cancer. *New England Journal of Medicine, 366*(18), 1663–1672.

CHAPTER 22

Specific Cancers and Their Management

Cancer is not one condition, but rather a number of different conditions of varied types that can occur in any region of the body. Most cancers are named for where they begin (e.g., lung cancer begins in the lung but may spread to other parts [metastases] of the body) (National Institute of Health [NIH], 2016a). The procedures used to identify cancer, the interventions used in cancer management, and the functional limitations associated with cancer differ depending on the type of cancer, advanced stage of cancer, and the anatomic site involved. In many instances, a combination of interventions—including surgery, chemotherapy, and irradiation—is used. In the management of cancer in its very early stages, surgery alone may be sufficient.

CANCER OF THE GASTROINTESTINAL TRACT

Cancer may involve any part of the gastrointestinal (GI) tract or accessory organs. Management of such cancer often involves the removal or major resection of the organs involved. Because manifestations of cancers of some organs such as the liver and the pancreas frequently become evident only late in the course of the condition, interventions may be directed toward palliation rather than cure (Doig & Heuther, 2014).

Cancer of the Mouth

Oral cancer can form in any part of the mouth or throat. Risk factors smoker or history of head or neck cancer (NIH, 2016b). Surgical management for cancer of the mouth may include removal of the tumor as well as removal of the nearby lymph glands to determine whether the cancer has spread. If cancer has spread to the neck or other tissues, more radical surgery may be indicated, resulting in facial deformity or disfigurement due to the amount of tissue removed. If the tongue has been partially removed, speech may be affected. Reconstructive surgery may be required to minimize these effects.

Cancer of the Esophagus

Cancer of the esophagus has been linked to smoking and alcohol use, especially when individuals engage in both behaviors (Brashers & Heuthers, 2014). Other risks include gastroesophageal reflux disease, obesity, and Barrett's esophagus (Doig & Heuther, 2014), in which irregular tissue extends from the opening of the stomach into the esophagus. Management of cancer of the esophagus may consist of radiation therapy with or without chemotherapy or surgery.

When esophageal cancer is localized, the affected part of the esophagus may be removed and reattached to the remaining part of the esophagus (NIH, 2016c). When the cancer is more severe, **esophagectomy** (removal of some or all of the esophagus) may be necessary. Depending upon the extent of the surgery the individual may have voice changes (NIH, 2016c). If the individual has the esophagus removed, an artificial opening must be made into the stomach, with a feeding tube inserted through which liquid feedings can be introduced. Following feeding, the opening is then "plugged" to prevent leakage. As a consequence of esophageal removal, individuals lose the ability to eat or drink through the mouth. Obviously, the ramifications of this type of surgery may influence individuals' willingness to have surgical versus other forms of interventions for their cancer.

Cancer of the Stomach

Cancer of the stomach varies with the geographic location of the individuals affected, with the incidence of stomach cancer being higher in some countries than in others. Risk factors for developing cancer of the stomach include environmental factors (including dietary intake and cigarette smoking), genetic factors, and predisposing conditions (e.g., *Helicobacter pylori* infection, chronic gastritis) (Doig & Heuther, 2014). Management of stomach cancer may consist of partial or total removal of the stomach (*partial gastrectomy* or *total gastrectomy*) and chemotherapy. Complete removal of the stomach is generally not performed unless the entire stomach is involved (American Cancer Society [ACS], 2016a). When a portion of the stomach or the whole stomach is removed, storage space for food is lost. If the whole stomach is removed, the esophagus and small intestine are often joined. Consequently, in either instance, individuals need small, frequent meals. They may also experience discomfort after eating called *dumping syndrome* due to rapid gastric emptying into the small intestine. In addition, if the portion of the stomach that is necessary for the absorption of vitamin B_{12} is removed (or when the whole stomach is removed), individuals will require lifelong vitamin B_{12} supplementation.

Cancer of the Small and Large Intestines

Cancer can occur in either the small intestine or the large intestine, including the rectum. At this time there is no known cause for cancer of the intestines, it is thought to have a genetic component, but this has not been proven and it continues under study (ACS, 2016b). Cancer of the small bowel is often managed surgically with chemotherapy. The extent of small bowel removed depends on the cancer's location and type (ACS, 2016b). Identification of cancers of the large intestine has been greatly improved with use of *colonoscopy* and *sigmoidoscopy*,

in which a tube is passed into the intestine, allowing visual examination and early identification of precancerous or cancerous tissue. Cancer of the large intestine or rectum is often curable when detected early (Maxwell & Isenberg, 2012). Management of colorectal cancer usually involves both surgical removal of the tumor and some resection of the colon itself, carried out through an incision in the abdomen. In many instances, the cancerous part of the bowel can be removed and the two remaining ends joined together (**anastomosis**), enabling the individual to retain regular bowel function. When this is not possible, a colostomy may be performed.

Cancer of the Liver

The liver is an accessory organ of the gastrointestinal tract. Major risk factors for developing cancer of the liver (hepatocellular carcinoma) are infections with hepatitis B or hepatitis C virus and alcoholic liver conditions (Doig & Huether, 2014).

Identification of liver cancer is usually based on noninvasive imaging tests such as computed tomography (CT) scan or magnetic resonance imaging (MRI), sometimes in conjunction with liver biopsy. The type of intervention undertaken for management depends on the stage of the cancer and individual factors. In early stages of the condition, surgical resection of the liver is usually the intervention of choice (Doig & Huether, 2014). Other individuals may be candidates for liver transplantation (Doig & Heuther, 2014; Kalia, Grewal, & Martin, 2012). In other instances, special chemotherapeutic agents may be used alone or with other interventions.

CANCER OF THE LARYNX

Although many structures in the head and neck can be a site of cancer, one of the most common cancers of these regions is cancer of the **larynx** (voice box). Smoking and alcohol are two leading risk factors for laryngeal cancer and are synergistic in their effects (Akst, 2012; Mayo Clinic, 2015a; NIH, 2015).

The larynx includes the vocal cords. The most common manifestation of cancer of the larynx is alteration in voice quality or hoarseness. Other manifestations may include **dysphagia** (difficulty in swallowing) and cough (NIH, 2015).

Procedures used to identify problems of the larynx include *laryngoscopy*, in which a hollow tube is inserted into the larynx so that structures of the larynx can be inspected visually and function of the vocal cords assessed.

Management of Cancer of the Larynx

Although management of cancer of the larynx depends on a number of factors, it usually involves irradiation, surgery, or a combination of the two. Although traditionally management of advanced cancer of the larynx involved total removal of the larynx, nonsurgical approaches comprising chemotherapy and radiation are now frequently used instead of surgery (NIH, 2015). When the cancer is in early stages (stage T1 or T2, N0, and M0), radiation alone—rather than surgery—may be used to eradicate the cancer and save the voice (NIH, 2016c). Laser interventions, which destroy the tumor by intense light beams, may also be used to manage early-stage cancer of the larynx, but they continue under study (ACS, 2016c). If the cancer is discovered before extensive involvement of the surrounding tissues has occurred, only partial removal of the larynx may be required. This procedure is called *subtotal (partial) laryngectomy*. Both subtotal laryngectomy and laser intervention can preserve the capacity for regular speech, although they may affect voice quality to some degree.

When cancer is more advanced, it may be necessary to remove the larynx completely (**laryngectomy**). Usually, individuals who have undergone this type of surgery are unable to breathe or speak by regular mechanisms. After the larynx has been removed, the trachea is no longer connected either to the nasopharynx or to the nasal passages. A permanent opening in the individual's neck and trachea, called a **tracheostomy**, is created surgically (**Figure 22-1**). It is through this opening (laryngeostoma) that the individual breathes rather than through the nose and mouth. Although individuals are able to eat and drink as usual, with a tracheostomy, they breathe, cough, and sneeze through the tracheostomy. The sense of smell, and consequently taste, is diminished because air

Figure 22-1   Tracheostomy

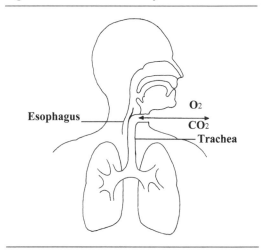

Esophagus — O_2 — CO_2 — Trachea

© Jane Tinkler Lamm.

flows through the opening in the neck instead of through the nose.

Functional Implications of Total Laryngectomy

Personal and Psychosocial Issues

Consequences of head and neck cancer, and cancer of the larynx in particular, can permanently alter individuals' quality of life, physical, psychological, social, emotional, nutritional, and communicative functioning (Eadie & Bowker, 2012). The psychosocial and vocational effects of laryngectomy can be profound. A healthy voice is important for effectiveness at work as well as personal and social interactions (Perry, Casey, & Cotton, 2015). Individuals immediately lose the ability to make vocal sounds for speech as well as the audible sounds of laughter or crying. Consequently, if management of the cancer of the larynx involves surgery, there is an attempt to maintain as much of the larynx as possible. When this is not possible, individuals must learn new techniques for speaking. There are new advances in equipment and speech therapy so these individuals can relearn to talk although their speech will sound different (ACS, 2016d).

Many techniques to improve the ability to speak after interventions for laryngeal cancer have been successful. Surgical techniques have evolved so that much of the larynx can be spared and does not have to be totally removed. Also, improved methods of voice rehabilitation after total laryngectomy have been developed. Three types of voice rehabilitation techniques after total laryngectomy are utilized:

- Tracheo-esophageal (shunt) speech
- Esophageal speech
- Electromechanical speech

In *tracheo-esophageal* techniques, a **fistula** (a passageway from one structure to another) is surgically constructed between the trachea and the esophagus, with a small prosthesis being placed in the fistula (ASA, 2016d; Perry et al., 2015). Closing the tracheostomy with the hand or fingers moves air from the trachea to the esophagus, thereby creating a *pseudovoice.* As a result, individuals are able to produce lung-powered speech of better quality than previously accomplished with other methods such as esophageal speech (discussed later in this section). The prosthesis in the fistula prevents food and liquid from entering the airway when the individual is eating. A limitation of the fistula is the need for periodic removal of the prosthesis for cleaning and replacement, and the need to use one hand to occlude the tracheostomy during speech. Special valves that fit into the opening are available so that the need for manual coverage of the opening is eliminated. During regular breathing, the valve remains open; however, when the individual begins to speak, because of increased expiratory pressure, the valve closes.

Esophageal speech is a technique of speaking that involves trapping air in the esophagus and gradually releasing it at the top of the esophagus to produce a pseudovoice. If the sounds produced by esophageal speech are too soft to be heard, a personal amplifier-speaker may be used to increase sound volume. Given that the air capacity of the upper esophagus is considerably less than that of the lungs, esophageal speech is typically limited in rate, volume, and duration (ASA, 2016d).

Electrolaryngeal (electromechanical) speech is another speech alternative that may be used by individuals with laryngectomy. It utilizes a battery-powered vibratory device called an artificial larynx. Several types are available; however, most are electronic, battery-operated devices that are held

against the throat to produce sound. Although the artificial larynx is relatively easy to use, the speech produced in this way has a mechanical, monotone sound that some individuals find objectionable (ASA, 2016d).

Regardless of the type of speech alternative that individuals use, *speech-language pathologists* are usually consulted for evaluation and possible interventions based on individuals' specific voice issues. Speech-language pathologists assess factors that affect voice production, identify any problem behaviors, and plan interventions to rectify the problem.

Activities and Participation

When individuals have a total laryngectomy, they must also adjust to the visible opening in the neck, the laryngeostoma. Any disfigurement, especially when related to a visible area, may damage individuals' self-concept and self-image (Perry et al., 2015). For cosmetic purposes, individuals may wear a scarf or other covering loosely around the neck. This covering also helps to keep dust and dirt out of the opening. Another type of covering available is a foam filter, which keeps moisture loss to a minimum, as well as prevents hair, shaving cream, or other particles from falling into the trachea during routine daily hygiene. Because the opening leads directly into the trachea and lungs, individuals must avoid activities such as swimming and water sports in which water could enter the opening. For showering, special laryngectomy shower collars that prevent water from running into the airway are available. With a laryngeostoma, individuals no longer have the benefit of having air humidified as it passes through the upper airway passages. Consequently, they may need to run a humidifier, especially at night, to keep the trachea moist.

Because the quality of speech is altered, individuals who have undergone laryngectomy may avoid social situations in which they have to speak, because they perceive their altered speech as distasteful and embarrassing. Although individuals can carry out most activities of daily living as usual, some may notice a decreased ability to lift heavy objects, because they cannot close the tracheostomy to build up internal pressure, as those persons without tracheostomy can do by compressing their lips and holding their breath. Individuals who have undergone a total laryngectomy should always carry an identification card or wear a medical identification bracelet to inform emergency personnel that they are a total neck breather.

Vocational Issues after Laryngectomy

Although most jobs can be resumed after laryngectomy, some individuals may not return to work because of fear of rejection by fellow workers or because of employers' misconceptions about their ability to perform. Those jobs performed in environments with extreme heat or cold, and those that expose individuals to extreme dust or fumes, should probably be avoided. Although the physical aspects of laryngectomy may not affect individuals' ability to work, the reliance on alternative modes of speech as part of employment can be of concern, especially if individuals' use of voice is a necessary component of work. Employers and coworkers may not be sure how to interact with individuals after laryngectomy, or may have difficulty finding them socially acceptable because of their speech and, therefore, avoid interactions with them. Educating employers and coworkers about laryngectomy as well as social support from friends, family, or participation in peer support groups such as the Lost Chord Club can help significantly in the adjustment process (Perry et al., 2015).

CANCER OF THE LUNG

An estimated 85% to 90% of all lung cancers are associated with cigarette smoking or passive smoke inhalation (Brashers & Huether, 2014); this incidence is related to the number of cigarettes smoked per day as well as the duration of smoking over the lifetime (Khuri, 2016). Other factors, such as exposure to environmental tobacco smoke and exposure to other carcinogens, such as asbestos fibers or beryllium, a metal used for alloys, can also contribute to the development of cancer. When these factors are combined with cigarette smoking, the risk of lung cancer almost doubles (Brashers & Huether, 2014; Khuri, 2016).

Lung cancers are divided into two major groups:

- Non-small-cell lung cancer (NSCLC), which is slower growing and accounts for most lung cancers
- Small-cell lung cancer (SCLC), which is noted for its aggressive growth and early metastasis

Manifestations of lung cancer are often not initially apparent, and consequently may be identified on a chest X-ray or exam that is conducted for other reasons (Doig & Huether, 2014). Lung cancer is usually identified through chest X-ray, CT scan, or *bronchoscopy*. A *needle biopsy* to obtain tissue is required to definitively identify type and stage of lung cancer so as to determine the appropriate intervention.

Management of lung cancer may consist of surgical resection, with removal of one lobe of the lung (**lobectomy**). Removal of an entire lung is called a **pneumonectomy**. The goal of surgery is to remove the tumor. This is usually the first approach to management to NSCLC, with possibility of the addition of chemotherapy and radiation, or a combination for persons with later-stage disease (ACS, 2016e). The extent of the surgery and other interventions chosen depends on the type of cancer, its location in the lung, and the presence (or not) of metastasis. Surgical management plays a major role in early NSCLC, however many individuals may not be candidates for surgery because of other comorbid conditions (Khuri, 2016). Chemotherapy and radiation therapy may also be used in NSCLC management, especially for those individuals in the later stages (Khuri, 2016). For individuals with SCLC, because of the propensity for rapid growth and metastasis, chemotherapy and radiation are more frequently used in management, with surgery occurring in only a small percentage of individuals (Khuri, 2016).

After having a portion of the lung removed, individuals may need to limit their physical activity to some degree, depending on the amount of lung removed and the functional capacity remaining. Given that cigarette smoking is frequently linked to lung cancer, emphysema may also coexist, further limiting respiratory capacity and, consequently, physical activity.

CANCER OF THE BONE

Primary bone cancers (**sarcomas**) are relatively uncommon, but metastic disease commonly affects the bone (Crowther-Radulwicz, 2014). When they do occur, however, they often result in amputation. For some types of bone cancers, it may be possible to remove only a section of bone and to avoid amputating the entire extremity. In some instances, bone cancers may be reduced by chemotherapy and then managed by radiation. More common is *metastatic cancer* to the bone, which contributes to fractures or pain.

CANCER OF THE URINARY SYSTEM

Cancer can develop in any organ of the urinary system, but the most frequent site of cancer in the urinary tract is the bladder. There is a high correlation between bladder cancer and cigarette smoking (Bajorin, 2016; Clark, 2012).

The most common manifestation of bladder cancer is **hematuria** (blood in the urine). When bladder cancer is suspected, the individual generally undergoes a procedure called *cystoscopy* in which a tube called a *cystoscope* is inserted into the bladder to visualize the inner surface of this organ and to take a biopsy for laboratory examination.

Bladder cancer is generally classified as either *superficial* (in which the cancer cells are confined to the lining of the bladder) or *invasive* (in which the cancer cells have penetrated other tissues). Cancer of the bladder may be managed in a variety of ways, depending on the stage and type of cancer involved.

Management of Superficial Bladder Cancer

Superficial bladder cancer may be managed with surgery as well as chemotherapy. A surgical procedure called *transurethral resection (TUR)* may be performed to identify bladder cancer as well as to remove cancerous tissue from the bladder. During this procedure, a *cystocope* is inserted into the bladder and cancerous tissue is removed. Individuals with superficial bladder cancer also receive *intravesical therapy,* in which chemotherapeutic agents are placed directly into the bladder through a catheter that has been inserted through the urethra into the bladder. Medications infused through the catheter work directly on the cells of the bladder. Although a number of agents can be used, after the bladder has had sufficient time to heal after the TUR, a substance called *bacillus Calmette–Guérin (BCG)* is commonly infused into the bladder through a catheter (Clark, 2012; Mayo Clinic, 2015b). Although BCG is related to tuberculosis (TB), when used therapeutically for bladder cancer, it does not cause TB but rather stimulates the immune system to fight cancer cells.

Management of Invasive Bladder Cancer

The most common surgical intervention for invasive cancer is **cystectomy**, a procedure in which the entire bladder is removed (Bajorin, 2016). When the bladder is completely removed, substitute methods for collecting and eliminating urine must be used. Surgical procedures for this purpose are called *urinary diversion.* Several different types of urinary diversion procedures can be used, depending on the individual situation. Some examples are described here:

- *Cutaneous uterostomy* is a procedure that brings the ureters to the surface of the abdomen through an opening called a **stoma**, where urine drains directly into an externally worn collection bag.
- *Ileal conduit* is a procedure in which a small reservoir is created from a segment of bowel that has been dissected and closed at one end, with the other end placed just under the abdominal wall. The other portion of the bowel is brought to the outside of the abdomen through an opening (stoma) (**Figure 22-2**) The ureters are connected to the internal pouch, where urine is collected and then eliminated through the stoma into a collection bag (*urostomy bag*), which is held in place either by adherent material placed on the skin or by a belt. The individual drains the bag as needed.
- A *continent urinary reservoir* is a pouch that has been surgically created from a portion of the intestine and has had the ureters connected to it so that urine drains directly into the internal pouch (see **Figure 22-3**). A portion of the intestine that forms the

Figure 22-2   Ileal Conduit

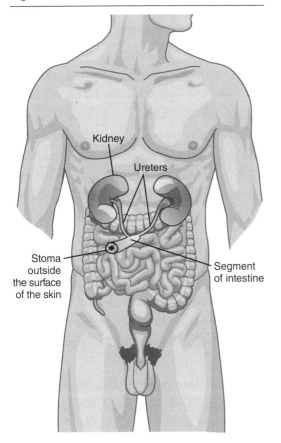

Figure 22-3   Continent Urinary Reservoir

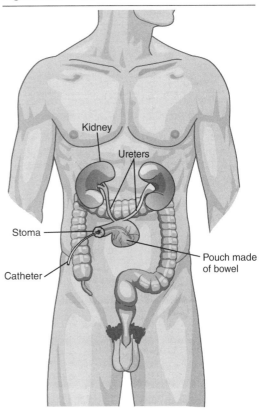

pouch is brought through an opening in the abdomen (stoma). Urine remains in the internal pouch until it is manually drained several times a day by placing a catheter into the opening. When it is not being drained, the opening is covered with a small bandage.

- *Ureterosigmoidostomy* is a less common form of urinary diversion in which the ureters are connected to the colon so that urine is excreted through the rectum. Because urine mixes with the contents of the colon, bowel movements are liquid, and frequent evacuation of stool is necessary.
- *Neobladder urinary diversion* is a procedure that is possible if the bladder alone has been removed and the urethra is still intact. In this instance, a reservoir may be constructed to replace the bladder and the individual will be able to excrete urine through the urethra almost as before.

Although surgery remains the intervention used most frequently for invasive bladder cancer, in some instances radiotherapy or a combination of chemotherapy and radiotherapy has been used as an alternative form of management (James et al., 2012).

Each type of urinary diversion procedure has its advantages and disadvantages. For individuals using internal urinary diversion procedures, risk of infection can be of concern. Individuals with urinary diversion methods that use an external pouch may be concerned about odor or leakage of the external bag, although proper techniques of bag use and cleansing can eliminate many of these concerns (Ali, Hayes, Birch, Dudderidge, & Somani, 2015).

Cancer of the kidney may be primary or metastatic in origin. Management of such cancer involves surgical removal of the tumor, partial removal of the kidney, or removal of the entirekidney (**nephrectomy**), often in combination with chemotherapy.

CANCER OF THE BRAIN OR SPINAL CORD

When malignant tumors of the brain are small and accessible, and if they have not invaded surrounding tissue, they may be surgically removed, followed by the administration of chemotherapy or radiation. If there are no complications from surgery, individuals may be able to return to active life, although some may experience neurological issues after surgery. If the tumor is embedded in the brain, or if it is located in a part of the brain that is inaccessible, however, surgery may not be possible without considerable risk. In these instances, chemotherapy or radiation alone may be instituted as a means of management or palliation. The degree or type of manifestations that result from a malignant brain tumor depends on the type of cancer, its size, and its location within the brain as well as any residual effects that might be experienced from surgery.

Cancers develop less often in the spinal cord than in the brain. Manifestations of a spinal cord tumor may be similar to those experienced with a spinal cord injury, including paralysis. Spinal cord tumors are usually managed surgically, with irradiation and chemotherapy playing roles as adjunct therapies.

LYMPHOMAS

Lymphoma is a term used to describe cancer of cells in the immune system. There are two general classifications of lymphomas:

- Hodgkin lymphoma (sometimes called Hodgkin's disease)
- Non-Hodgkin lymphoma

Hodgkin Lymphoma

Hodgkin lymphoma has the highest incidence in the United States, Canada, Switzerland, and Northern Europe (Connors, 2016). It is distinguished from other lymphomas by a characteristic neoplastic cell called the *Reed–Sternberg cell* (Connors, 2016; Schwartz & Rote, 2014). In this malignant, chronic, progressive condition, irregular cells gradually replace regular cells within the lymph nodes (Schwartz & Rote, 2014). The cause is unknown. Many individuals with Hodgkin's lymphoma have no manifestations until later stages of the condition, or they may have only peripheral **lymphadenopathy** (enlargement of lymph nodes). Hodgkin lymphoma is usually identified through an excisional biopsy of an affected lymph node.

Although many individuals' condition is advanced at the time it is identified, advances in interventions for management of Hodgkin lymphoma have made this disease mostly curable (Swartz & Rote, 2014). Management of Hodgkin lymphoma varies with the stage at which it is identified, but usually involves chemotherapy and radiation.

Non-Hodgkin Lymphoma

Non-Hodgkin lymphoma involves the proliferation of abnormal lymph cells, with the various types of this disease being classified according to their cell origin (e.g., *B-cell lymphoma, follicular lymphoma, peripheral T-cell lymphomas*). As is true for individuals with Hodgkin lymphoma, a common manifestation is lymphadenopathy (Swartz & Rote, 2014). Identification of non-Hodgkin lymphoma is made through examination of tissue that has been removed through excisional biopsy.

Non-Hodgkin lymphoma may progress slowly, or it may progress rapidly, depending on the classification of the cell and individual factors, such as age. Management of non-Hodgkin lymphoma is individual but generally includes chemotherapy, monoclonal antibodies, and radioimmunotherapy, depending on the subtype (Swartz & Rote, 2014).

MULTIPLE MYELOMA

Multiple myeloma is a slowly progressive cancer in which uncontrolled replication of irregular plasma cells leads to the destruction of the bone marrow and extends into the bone, resulting in anemia, bone pain, and **pathologic fractures** (fractures that occur because of conditions affecting the bone rather than from injury) (Rajkumar, 2016). Identification of multiple myeloma may be based on blood tests looking for anemia, radiologic examination of the skeletal system to identify bone destruction, or biopsy of the bone marrow itself. In some instances, individuals may also experience complications such as renal insufficiency and spinal cord compression (Swartz & Rote, 2014). Treatment for the individual with multiple myeloma will be a combination of chemotherapy, radiation therapy, and plasmapheresis (a removal of the plasma, cleaning it, and reinserting it).

Some individuals with multiple myeloma may be candidates for stem cell transplantation (Swartz & Rote, 2014). When stem cell transplantation is a management choice, it is usually performed in conjunction with chemotherapy. Not all individuals are considered good candidates for transplantation because of factors such as age, lack of an appropriate donor, or other chronic conditions that affect organ function (Rajkumar, 2016). Chemotherapy is a major intervention for multiple myeloma, especially for individuals who are not eligible for transplantation. Radiation therapy is often reserved for individuals who have not responded well to chemotherapy and those with severe bone pain. Since at present, multiple myeloma is considered incurable, the goal of management is to induce remission (Rajkumar, 2016).

Because inactivity results in additional breakdown of bone, it is recommended that individuals with multiple myeloma remain as active as possible, although they are cautioned to avoid activities that might result in trauma.

LEUKEMIAS

Cancers of tissues in which blood is formed are called *leukemias*. A number of types of leukemias exist. On a broad scale, leukemia can be classified as acute or chronic.

Acute Leukemia

In acute leukemia, there is an abnormal proliferation of cells that would normally become mature peripheral blood cells. Instead of differentiating and replicating at a regular rate, the malignant cells do not differentiate but proliferate in an uncontrolled manner, gradually replacing the bone marrow (Swartz & Rote, 2014). As a result, production of red blood cells, white blood cells, and platelets decreases. Consequently, individuals with acute leukemia may experience **anemia** because of the availability of fewer red blood cells, infection because of **neutropenia** (small number of mature white blood cells), and bleeding tendencies because of **thrombocytopenia** (small number of platelets). Irregular leukemic cells can also infiltrate other organs such as lymph nodes, liver, and spleen.

In most instances, there is no known cause of *acute leukemia*. Nevertheless, exposure to radiation, occupational exposure to certain chemicals, viruses, and genetic links have all been cited as possible contributing factors (Swartz & Rote, 2014). Subtypes of acute leukemia that are identified based on characteristics of cells include *acute myeloid leukemia*, *B lymphoblastic leukemia*, and *T lymphoblastic leukemia* (Appelbaum, 2016).

Acute leukemia is a rapidly progressing condition, so interventions are usually instituted immediately. The goal of intervention is to induce complete remission. Management usually consists of chemotherapy and, in some cases, bone marrow transplantation.

Chronic Leukemia

Chronic leukemia encompasses a broad spectrum of conditions, with two common types being *chronic myelogenous leukemia*, which occurs most frequently in midlife, and *chronic lymphocytic leukemia*, the most common leukemia, which occurs more frequently in older adults (Kantarjian & O'Brien, 2012). Chronic myelogenous leukemia involves unregulated growth of white blood cells in the bone marrow and accumulation of these cells in the blood. Chronic lymphocytic leukemia affects B cells and results in their unregulated growth and accumulation in the blood.

In both types of chronic leukemia, manifestations are often not present initially so that the condition is first discovered through blood tests during a routine health examination. Some individuals may experience enlarged lymph nodes (**adenopathy**) or **splenomegaly** (enlargement of the spleen). Identification of chronic leukemia is made through blood tests.

Advances in chemotherapy have greatly improved the degree to which chronic leukemia can be effectively managed (Jamieson, 2012). Some individuals may not require immediate intervention unless complications occur (Kantarjian & O'Brien, 2012).

CANCER OF THE BREAST

Breast cancer, like many other cancers, is not a single health condition but rather a large and complex family of health conditions (Lewis & Borgen, 2012). It is the second most common cause of death after lung cancer in women; it may also occur in men (Davidson, 2012; Phillippi, Latendresee, & McChance, 2014).

As with other types of cancer, early identification of breast cancer is most predictive of outcome and cure (Phillippi et al., 2014). Regular breast self-examination and screening mammography can lead to early detection, thereby permitting early intervention. Accurate and definitive identification of breast cancer, including the specific type, depends on laboratory examination of tissue obtained through needle biopsy.

The primary management options for breast cancer are selected based on the stage of the cancer at the time it is identified. Interventions may be local, regional, or systemic. Local/regional management usually involves surgery. Years ago either *mastectomy,* in which the total breast was removed, or *radical mastectomy,* in which the entire breast and its underlying tissue, including muscle and lymph nodes, were removed, was commonly performed to treat breast cancer. More recently, studies have shown that more conservative approaches *(breast conservation therapy [BCT])* are just as effective (Lewis & Borgen, 2012). Consequently, surgery for breast cancer now often consists of the following procedures:

- *Lumpectomy:* removal of the cancerous lesion itself and a small amount of surrounding breast tissue
- *Partial or segmental mastectomy:* removal of a quadrant of the breast
- *Mastectomy*: removal of all the breast tissue

The appropriateness of using more conservative surgical techniques that preserve as much of the breast tissue as possible depends on the size and location of the tumor. Lymph nodes in the axillary area may also be removed in some cases. In many instances, regardless of the type of surgery, radiation and chemotherapy are used as adjunct interventions (Mayo Clinic, 2015c). In addition, adjuvant *endocrine therapy,* such as *Tamoxifen,* which blocks estrogen, may be used as an intervention in *hormone-receptive* breast cancer.

Depending on the extent of surgery, individuals may experience some limitation in arm motion on the affected side. They may engage in physical therapy or other exercises to gain mobility and range of motion gradually. **Lymphedema** (swelling due to blockage of the lymph system) can occur, usually when the lymph nodes have been removed and the circulation of lymph fluid is slowed. If lymphedema is experienced, individuals may require use of a compression garment for their arm to reduce swelling.

Breast Reconstruction

Recent advances in cosmetic surgery have made breast reconstruction a viable option for some individuals, especially those who have experienced more radical surgical procedures. Breast reconstruction that transfers tissue from one part of the body to the other (such as a Transverse Rectus Abdominis Muscle [TRAM] flap, in which skin, fat, and muscle from the abdomen are used to create a reconstructed breast) has become more common in the last few years.

When much of the breast has been removed but breast reconstruction is not an option, or when the individual chooses not to have such a procedure, a permanent breast form called a *prosthesis* may be used. Breast forms vary in weight and are matched to the size and contour of the remaining breast. Breast prostheses are sold in surgical supply stores, or they may be available in the lingerie departments of large department stores.

Psychosocial Issues in Breast Cancer

Like other cancers, breast cancer frequently produces complex psychological changes that involve altered sense of self and changes in relationships (NIH, 2015). The psychological implications of breast cancer can be devastating for some women. The emotional impact of the loss of breast tissue varies from individual to individual. Not only are there concerns associated with the cancer itself but concerns also arise regarding changes in appearance. Breast cancer poses a dual threat, in the form of risk to life as well as threat to female self-image. The disfigurement that may be associated with loss of breast tissue is a constant reminder of a life-threatening condition. As a sexually associated structure and societally valued symbol of attractiveness, the breast is also closely linked to a woman's self-esteem.

The Reach to Recovery program of the American Cancer Society was established in 1969 as a means to help women adjust to breast cancer. In this program, volunteers who have fully recovered from breast cancer visit the individual and answer questions, provide tips, and offer encouragement. Breast cancer support groups have also been found helpful by some individuals.

GYNECOLOGIC CANCER

Types of Gynecologic Cancer

Gynecologic cancers include cancer of the ovary, uterus, or cervix, or the external genitalia. Regular screenings can be important in early recognition of gynecologic cancers and, consequently, early intervention and cure.

Ovarian cancer, used to be relatively rare, but the incidence has risen due to limited availability of early screening programs and no early detectable manifestations (Phillippi et al., 2014). Therefore, it may have metastasized by the time the cancer is identified. When ovarian cancer is identified, surgery is almost always required, with probable chemotherapy after surgery.

Endometrial cancer (cancer of lining of uterus) is the most common gynecologic cancer in the United States (Spriggs, 2016). Cancer of the endometrium is identified through biopsy. Early manifestations of endometrial cancer consist of abnormal uterine bleeding. Management usually consists of **hysterectomy** (removal of the uterus) with accompanying **oophorectomy** (removal of the ovaries).

Cancer of the cervix (the neck of the uterus, opening into the vagina) is detected through regular *Pap screening*—a type of test in which cancer cells can be identified microscopically. Although a variety of causes of cervical cancer have been suggested, recent findings have suggested that infection with the human papillomavirus (HPV) is a critical factor (Phillippi et al., 2014; Spriggs, 2016). In an attempt to reduce the risk of cervical cancer, an HPV vaccine has been developed to prevent cancer induced by this virus, although it appears to be most effective if received prior to first sexual contact (Spriggs, 2016).

Early-stage cervical cancer usually has no manifestations, so regular screening is important for early cancer detection. If cervical cancer is not managed, it can invade other organs and metastasize. In the case of early-stage cervical cancer, and especially if the woman wants to preserve fertility, the cancerous portion of the cervix may be excised, leaving the uterus. If the cancer is more advanced, both the cervix and the uterus are removed (*total hysterectomy*).

There are generally no physical limitations associated with gynecologic cancer and its management. However, individuals with advanced cancer, and those who undergo chemotherapy or radiation therapy in combination with surgery, may experience fatigue and other side effects directly related to the interventions.

Cancers of the *external genitalia* or *vagina* are rare, but are associated with HPV when they do occur (Phillippi et al., 2014). Management usually involves surgical resection and possibly chemotherapy or radiation.

Psychosocial Issues in Gynecologic Cancer

In addition to the stress caused by having cancer, the psychological issues associated with gynecologic surgery may cause some individuals significant distress. Gynecologic surgery because of cancer may produce changes in perception of body image, fertility, or sexuality. If the uterus or ovaries are removed and the woman is of reproductive age, issues regarding childbearing may be of concern. Removal of reproductive organs may have also emotional and psychological impact because of perceptions that sexual function will be diminished. These perceptions can, in turn, affect the woman's relationship with her partner.

Although surgery such as hysterectomy typically does not impair sexual function, considerable misinformation may surround gynecological surgery and can cause concern for the woman and her significant other. In instances where the cancer involves the external genitalia and necessitates its removal, the disfigurement and threat to body image may also produce significant emotional distress. Providing the individual and her partner with accurate information about the surgery and its implications can help to alleviate problems.

CANCER OF THE PROSTATE

The *prostate* is a gland that surrounds the urethra in males and secretes fluid that bathes and nourishes human semen. Prior to the late 1980s, the primary method of detecting prostate cancer was through digital rectal exam, which generally detected prostate cancer at later stages (Rodway & McChance, 2014). However, after a blood test that measured *prostate-specific antigen (PSA)* was developed, it was widely adopted for screening and detection of early-stage cancer (Rodway & McChance, 2014). More recently, studies have called into question the benefit and accuracy of PSA screening in terms of affecting overall outcome (NIH, 2012; Schröder et al., 2012). Consequently, the most effective way to identify prostate cancer remains controversial.

Manifestations of prostate cancer often consist of difficulties in urination owing to bladder outlet obstruction. Another condition, *benign prostatic hypertrophy (BPH)*, although not a malignancy, may cause similar problems. Biopsy of the prostate is generally needed to confirm the presence of cancer, although this procedure can be associated with bleeding, pain, and infection (NIH, 2016e; Rodway & McChance, 2014).

Interventions for prostate cancer, as with other types of cancer, are determined mainly by staging of the cancer. Some individuals may receive hormone therapy (*androgen deprivation*), surgery such as **prostatectomy** in which the prostate is removed, and postoperative radiation. Complications of surgery in some individuals with prostate cancer can include impotence and incontinence.

TESTICULAR CANCER

Testicular cancer is relatively rare (Rodway & McChance, 2014). Manifestations generally consist of testicular pain or a lump or growth in the testis. Testicular cancer is usually identified through examination and testicular ultrasound (Einhorn, 2016; Rodway & McChance, 2014). Depending on the stage of the cancer, management can consist of **orchiectomy** (removal of the testis) or chemotherapy.

In testicular cancer, if one testis is removed (*unilateral orchiectomy*), sexual function and ability to reproduce may be possible. If both testicles are removed (*bilateral orchiectomy*), sexual function as well as the ability to have children are affected. When both testes are removed, prosthetic implants may be inserted into the scrotum to provide a normal appearance of the genitals.

Personal and Psychosocial Issues in Testicular Cancer

Cancer of either the prostate or the testes can cause anxiety not only related to cancer but also related to body image and the potential effect on sexual performance, and in the case of testicular cancer, on reproduction. Nerve damage experienced during prostate cancer can contribute to impotence; if such nerve damage does not occur, however, sexual ability should remain intact. Nonetheless, many individuals may find concerns about sexuality to be a difficult topic to discuss. In some instances, the individual's emotional reaction may affect his sexuality more than the condition itself. Counseling and support to address specific questions and concerns may help to alleviate fears and anxiety.

Activities and Participation

In most instances, barring complications or advanced stages of the condition, individuals' functional capacity should not be affected by testicular cancer. However, myths about testicular cancer, negative attitudes, and stereotypes held by others may be a hurdle for individuals to return to full participation. Learning how to dispel myths and stereotypes as well as maintaining a sense of autonomy and control can bolster a sense of empowerment, which enables individuals to return to an active role of social participation.

SKIN CANCERS

Skin cancer is the uncontrolled growth and reproduction of irregular skin cells. Most skin cancers, if detected and treated early, can be cured. The number one risk factor associated with skin cancer is overexposure to the sun (McCann & Huether, 2014). Individuals with fair skin are at greater risk than individuals with darker skin. Prevention of skin cancer involves protection from ultraviolet exposure, using sunscreen, covering skin with clothing, and minimizing outdoor activities when the sun is the strongest.

Several types of skin cancer are distinguished. *Basal cell cancers* are the most common type of skin cancer and originate in the layer of cells that form the base between the **epidermis** (the top layer of skin cells) and the **dermis** (the lower level of skin cells). Less common are *squamous cell cancers*, which originate in the uppermost layers of skin. These types of skin cancers are called *nonmelanoma skin cancers*. Identification of basal cell and squamous cell cancers usually occurs through direct examination, but often biopsy and histological confirmation are undertaken.

Both types of nonmelanoma skin cancers usually do not spread and are easily cured if interventions— usually removal—are instituted promptly. Other types of interventions for nonmelanoma cancers may include *cryosurgery* (application of extreme cold—usually *liquid nitrogen*—to destroy abnormal tissue), radiation, or topical application of *antimetabolite medications* that disrupt cancer cell growth (McCann & Huether, 2014; Ortel & Bolotin, 2012).

The most serious type of skin cancer is *malignant melanoma*, a cancer that originates from the *melanocytes,* the cells that produce the skin's pigment or color. Early signs of melanoma usually consist of changes in shape, color, or surface of a pigmented area or mole (McCann & Huether, 2014). As with other cancers, the earlier malignant melanomas are identified and managed, the better the outcome. Identification usually consists of total excision of the mole and surrounding tissue,

which are then examined microscopically for cancer cells. Staging for melanoma is based on the TNM system as discussed in the "Introduction to Cancers: General Methods of Identification and Management" chapter. If lymph nodes are involved, **lymphadenectomy** (removal of lymph nodes) may be indicated. Some individuals may also receive chemotherapy (Petronic-Rosic, 2012).

GENERAL FUNCTIONAL IMPLICATIONS OF CANCER

Personal and Psychosocial Issues

Despite development of new interventions to effectively cure or manage cancer, individuals may find identification of cancer overwhelming, leading to feelings of anxiety, fear, and helplessness. Many persons with this diagnosis also feel vulnerable. Cancer may engender feelings of loss of control or helplessness, combined with initial reactions of depression, irritability, fear, withdrawal, anger and hostility, or denial (NIH, 2015b). Individuals, in an effort to assimilate the impact of identification of cancer, may attempt to minimalize or deny the fact as they attempt to marshal the emotional resources and coping skills needed to deal with the perceived threat. Clarifying ambiguity and uncertainty while permitting denial is at times a difficult balance for all concerned.

Reactions vary with the individual and are not always related to the type or extent of the cancer but rather to individuals' own preconceived perceptions, particular situation, and coping skills. For many in society, the word *cancer* continues to generate negative images; furthermore, for some individuals, having cancer is viewed as stigmatizing. As a result, individuals may fear rejection and isolation, or may perceive cancer as a threat to their mortality and to their future, regardless of their actual prognosis. Even when the prognosis is positive, concerns about outcome and fear of recurrence may linger, such that even routine follow-up with healthcare professionals becomes a source of anxiety.

Interventions for some types of cancers may be disfiguring and may affect body image. When disfigurement owing to surgical procedures accompanies the cancer, adjustment to the altered self-image tends to cause further stress and anxiety. Interventions that involve removal of a body part, such as mastectomy for breast cancer or removal of a limb as a result of sarcoma, may also require prosthesis use and subsequently serve as a source of self-consciousness for the individual, requiring a period of adjustment and adaptation. In some instances, there may be issues related to feelings of attractiveness or sexual issues.

Coping with cancer is not static, but rather a dynamic process, evolving over time (NIH, 2015a). Individuals may exhibit a wide spectrum of adaptive responses that may change over the course of the condition or over time. Through each phase of cancer, ranging from identification through intervention and remission, individuals face different stressors and utilize different coping skills in learning to live with their diagnosis. Their reactions can determine the level of functioning at each phase as well as the level of adherence to the management plan. Depression in individuals with cancer may not always be detected and may affect not only quality of life but also effective implementation of interventions (NIH, 2015b).

In addition to the initial distress experienced after identification of cancer, individuals may face a broad range of stressors related to interventions in terms of time demands, cost, or physical manifestations that can involve pain, fatigue, disfigurement, or other physical effects of cancer management. Even when individuals are in **remission** (free from cancer manifestations), they may still have feelings of uncertainty regarding the possibility of recurrence of the cancer or development of another cancer at a future date.

Some individuals cope by finding a general purpose or meaning to cancer so that a framework for events experienced can be established. Many individuals gain a sense of control by seeking as much information as possible about their cancer, being actively involved in management decisions, and assuming a leadership role, which in turn helps to generate positive feelings of empowerment. Although information can be an important tool in reducing anxiety, it must be acquired at a rate that is manageable for the individual (NIH, 2015a).

Coping with cancer is an ongoing effort in which the individual reacts to the condition and its implications. Issues for individuals vary across

a lifetime, as each life stage has its own opportunities and limitations. Individuals' reactions are influenced by outside forces as well as by their own intrinsic capabilities. Psychosocial support is important at all phases of cancer management. Openly talking about cancer and educating others about this condition can be anxiety relieving. Support groups can provide a nurturing atmosphere in which common experiences and feelings are shared.

Activities and Participation

Each type of cancer has its own unique impact on an individual's daily life. The extent to which cancer affects individuals' everyday activities depends on the type and location of the cancer and its management. Side effects of radiation therapy or chemotherapy, such as nausea, loss of appetite, or fatigue, may affect daily activities during interventions or for a short time after they are instituted. Certain surgical procedures for various types of cancer may also affect individuals' lifestyle to some degree. For example, amputation, colostomy, and laryngectomy all require some adaptation of certain daily tasks.

Sexuality

The effects of cancer on sexuality differ from person to person. Some individuals experience no difficulty with sexual functioning. Others experience a decrease in sexual desire because of fatigue, pain, depression, or anxiety. Some forms of cancer and its management may have direct impact on sexual activity; for example, surgery may directly affect the organs of sexual function. In addition, surgery may have indirect effects on sexual activity if it alters individuals' physical appearance, thereby influencing their body image and self-esteem. Regardless of whether cancer directly or indirectly affects individuals' ability to engage in sexual intercourse, the need for closeness and demonstration of affection, such as hugging, touching, or kissing, is usually unchanged.

Despite public education about the new healthcare advances that have rendered many cancers curable, the general public—and perhaps even family and friends of individuals with cancer—may still hold the unfounded belief that *cancer* is a synonym for *death*. Such misconceptions may lead to the emotional withdrawal of friends and acquaintances as they attempt to lessen the impact of loss before it occurs.

Some friends or family members may avoid individuals with a cancer diagnosis because of their own fears about cancer, or because they feel uncomfortable and do not know how to approach the individual. Others may have the mistaken notion that cancer is contagious and avoid close physical contact with affected individuals or shun them altogether.

In other instances, rather than being a source of alienation, cancer may engender a tendency in others to be overprotective of the individual or to enforce dependency, both of which can decrease individuals' sense of self-esteem and control. In other instances, denial on the part of family members or the inability to share feelings and concerns may create tension within the family group. Many challenges that confront family members of individuals with cancer are shaped by the quality of the family relationship prior to identification of cancer and the concurrent stressors those family members may be experiencing (NIH, 2015a). Because the course of cancer may change—being characterized by remissions, relapses, need for additional interventions, or just unpredictability—individuals' place and role in the family may also change and evolve, requiring different approaches over time (NIH, 2014).

The extent to which cancer affects social activities depends not only on the attitudes and acceptance of others but also on physical factors affecting the individual such as pain and fatigue. Myriad considerations, including time associated with various interventions, may at times supersede social and family activities. Special provisions that enable individuals with cancer to participate in social activities can decrease the disruption and the sense of conflict felt by these individuals and their families over time.

GENERAL VOCATIONAL ISSUES IN CANCER

A number of reports have described employment discrimination against, and lack of rehabilitation services for, persons with cancer (Cancer.net, 2015). One report cited a survey that found workers with cancer were fired or laid off five times as often as other workers (Arnold, 1999). Not only can the economic implications of cancer be great but work also takes on particular importance as a symbol of self-esteem, self-sufficiency, and an affirmation of life.

As with other conditions, the most significant barriers to employment following identification of cancer may be the attitudes of employers and fellow workers, who can have the same misperceptions about cancer that some other social groups hold. Attitudes of hopelessness related to cancer may be expressed in employers' reluctance to allow individuals with cancer to return to work, their unwillingness to make concessions for any associated limitations, or their rejection of special aspects of interventions for cancer management. In some instances, employers and coworkers may view cancer as a contagious condition. Employers may also express concern about the ability of these individuals to perform the same work-related tasks for which they had been previously responsible, and some may view individuals with cancer as a potential economic burden rather than as productive employees.

Although courts have argued about the status of individuals with cancer under the Americans with Disabilities Act (ADA), some have agreed that ADA provides important legal rights for individuals with this diagnosis (Cancer.net, 2015). As courts continue to discuss the definition of disability, educating and informing employers and individuals with cancer about the protections that ADA provides is an important step in advocacy and in helping individuals obtain or maintain employment for which they are qualified and that they desire (Cancer.net, 2015).

Vocational planning requires an awareness of the attitudes and prejudice that may exist in the work setting, as well as a specific knowledge about the condition and its management requirements, individuals' functional capacity, and demands of the work setting. Because of the variability of the functional capacity with the type and location of cancer, the importance of short-term versus long-term planning should be considered. It is also necessary to understand the multidimensional impact of cancer on individuals and their families. The degree to which individuals' former employment remains suitable takes many variables into account and must be examined realistically in the context of the demands and implications of returning to the former work setting, as well as the individual's own particular strengths and goals.

CASE STUDY

Mr. M. is a 56-year-old truck driver. He has been a heavy user of tobacco and alcohol for the last 40 years. After he had experienced consistent hoarseness for more than a year, he was been found to have cancer of the larynx. Subsequently, Mr. M. had a laryngectomy.

1. Which specific issues related to laryngectomy may be important to Mr. M.'s rehabilitation potential?
2. Which functional implications might Mr. M. experience after his laryngectomy?
3. Is it feasible for Mr. M. to continue in his current line of employment? If so, which specific factors might be important to consider?
4. Are there specific accommodations or assistive devices that may be helpful to Mr. M.?

REFERENCES

Akst, L. (2012). Hoarseness and laryngitis. In E. T. Bope & R. D. Kellerman (Eds.), *Conn's current therapy 2012,* (pp. 282–287). Philadelphia, PA: Elsevier Saunders.

Ali, A. S., Haves, M. C., Birch, B., Dudderidge, T., & Somani, B. K. (2015). Health related quality of life (HRQoL) after cystectomy: Comparison between orthotopic neobladder and ileal conduit diversion. *European Journal of Surgical Oncology, 41*(3), 295–299. doi:10.1016/j.ejso.2014.05.006

American Cancer Society. (2016a). *Stomach cancer.* Retrieved from http://www.cancer.org/cancer/stomachcancer/detailedguide/stomach-cancer-treating-types-of-surgery

American Cancer Society. (2016b). *Surgery for non-small cell lung cancer.* Retrieved from http://www.cancer.org/cancer/lungcancer-non-smallcell/detailedguide/non-small-cell-lung-cancer-treating-surgery

American Cancer Society. (2016c). *Laryneal and hypopharyngeal cancer.* Retrieved from http://www.cancer.gov/types/head-and-neck/hp/laryngeal-treatment-pdq

American Cancer Society. (2016d). *What happens after treatment for laryngeal or hypopharyngeal cancer.* Retrieved from http://www.cancer.org/cancer/laryngealandhypopharyngealcancer/detailedguide/laryngeal-and-hypopharyngeal-cancer-after-follow-up

Appelbaum, F. R. (2016). The acute leukemias. In L. Goldman & A. I. Schafer (Eds.), *Goldman-Cecil medicine* (25th ed., pp. 1239–1246). Philadelphia, PA: Elsevier Saunders.

Arnold, K. (1999). Americans with Disabilities Act: Do cancer patients qualify as disabled? *Journal of the National Cancer Institute, 91*(10), 822–825.

Bajorin, D. F. (2016). Tumors of the kidney, bladder, ureters, and renal pelvis. In L. Goldman & A. I. Schafer (Eds.), *Goldman-Cecil medicine,* (25th ed., pp. 1345–1351). Philadelphia, PA: Elsevier Saunders.

Brashers, V. L., & Heuthers, S. E. (2014). Alterations of pulmonary function. In K. L. McCance, S. E. Huether, V. L. Brashers, & N. S. Rote (Eds.), *Pathophysiology: The biologic basis for disease in adults and children,* (7th ed., pp. 1279–1286). St. Louis, MO: Elsevier-Mosby.

Cancer.Net. (2015). Cancer and workplace discrimination. *Journal of Clinical Oncology.* Retrieved from http://www.cancer.net/survivorship/life-after-cancer/cancer-and-workplace-discrimination

Clark, P. E. (2012). Malignant tumors of the urogenital tract. In E. T. Bope & R. D. Kellerman (Eds.), *Conn's current therapy 2012* (pp. 889–897). Philadelphia, PA: Elsevier Saunders.

Connors, J. M. (2016). Hodgkin lymphoma. In L. Goldman & A. I. Schafer (Eds.), *Goldman-Cecil medicine,* (25th ed., pp. 1268–1273). Philadelphia, PA: Elsevier Saunders.

Crowther-Radulewicz, C. L., (2014). Structure and function of muscular system. In K. L. McCance, S. E. Huether, V. L. Brashers, & N. S. Rote (Eds.), *Pathophysiology: The biologic basis for disease in adults and children,* (7th ed., pp. 1560–1565). St. Louis, MO: Elsevier-Mosby.

Davidson, N. (2012). Breast cancer and benign breast disorders. In E. T. Bope & R. D. Kellerman (Eds.), *Conn's current therapy 2012,* (pp. 1309–1317). Philadelphia, PA: Elsevier Saunders.

Doig, A. K., & Heuther, S. E. (2014). Structure and function of the digestive system. In K. L. McCance, S. E. Huether, V. L. Brashers, & N. S. Rote (Eds.), *Pathophysiology: The biologic basis for disease in adults and children,* (7th ed., pp. 1466–1427). St. Louis, MO: Elsevier-Mosby.

Eadie, T. L., & Bowker, M. S. (2012). Coping and quality of life after total laryngectomy. *Otolaryngologia Head Neck Surgery, 146*(6), 959–965.

Einhorn, L. H. (2016). Testicular cancer. In L. Goldman & A. I. Schafer (Eds.), *Goldman-Cecil medicine,* (25th ed., pp. 1365–1366). Philadelphia, PA: Elsevier Saunders.

James, N. D., Hussain, S. A., Hall, E., Jenkins, P., Tremlett, J., Rawlings, C., ... BC2001 Investigators. (2012). Radiotherapy with or without chemotherapy in muscle invasive bladder cancer. *New England Journal of Medicine, 366*(16), 1477–1488.

Jamieson, K. (2012). Chronic leukemias. In E. T. Bope & R. D. Kellerman (Eds.), *Conn's current therapy 2012,* (pp. 793–797). Philadelphia, PA: Elsevier Saunders.

Kalia, H., Grewal, P., & Martin, P. (2012). In E. T. Bope & R. D. Kellerman (Eds.), *Conn's current therapy 2012,* (pp. 493–501). Philadelphia, PA: Elsevier Saunders.

Kantarjian, H., & O'Brien, S. (2012). The chronic leukemias. In L. Goldman & A. I. Schafer (Eds.), *Goldman's Cecil medicine,* (24th ed., pp. 1209–1218). Philadelphia, PA: Elsevier Saunders.

Khuri, F. R. (2016). Lung cancer and other pulmonary neoplasms. In L. Goldman & A. I. Schafer (Eds.), *Goldman-Cecil medicine,* (25th ed., pp. 1303–1313). Philadelphia, PA: Elsevier Saunders.

Lewis, J., & Borgen, P. (2012). Breast disease. In E. T. Bope & R. D. Kellerman (Eds.), *Conn's current therapy 2012,* (pp. 1309–1317). Philadelphia, PA: Elsevier Saunders.

Maxwell, P. J., & Isenberg, G. A. (2012). Tumors of the colon and rectum. In E. T. Bope & R. D. Kellerman (Eds.), *Conn's current therapy 2012* (pp. 557–561). Philadelphia, PA: Elsevier Saunders.

Mayo Clinic Staff. (2015a). *Throat cancer.* Mayo Clinic. Retrieved from http://www.mayoclinic.org/search/search-results?q=cancer%20of%20throat or https://www.nlm.nih.gov/medlineplus/ency/article/001042.htm

Mayo Clinic Staff. (2015b). *Bladder cancer: Treatment and drugs.* Mayo Clinic. Retrieved from http://www.mayoclinic.org/diseases-conditions/bladder-cancer/basics/treatment/con-20027606

Mayo Clinic Staff. (2015c). *Breast cancer: Treatment and drugs.* Mayo Clinic. Retrieved from http://www.mayoclinic.org/diseases-conditions/breast-cancer/basics/treatment/con-20029275

Mayo Clinic Staff. (2016). *Liver cancer.* Mayo Clinic. Retrieved from http://www.mayoclinic.org/diseases-conditions/liver-cancer/home/ovc-20198165

McCann, S. A., & Huether, S. E. (2014). Structure, function, and disorders of the integument. In K. L. McCance, S. E. Huether, V. L. Brashers, & N. S. Rote (Eds.), *Pathophysiology: The biologic basis for disease in adults and children,* (7th ed., pp. 1641–1647). St. Louis, MO: Elsevier-Mosby.

National Institute of Health: National Cancer Institute. (2012). *Prostate-specific antigen (PSA test).* Retrieved from http://www.cancer.gov/types/prostate/psa-fact-sheet#q2

National Institute of Health: National Cancer Institute. (2014). *Coping with cancer.* Retrieved from http://www.cancer.gov/about-cancer/coping/survivorship

National Institute of Health: National Cancer Institute. (2015a). *Adjustment to cancer: Anxiety and distress—Health professional version.* Retrieved from http://www.cancer.gov/about-cancer/coping/feelings/anxiety-distress-hp-pdq

National Institute of Health: National Cancer Institute. (2015 b). *Feelings and cancer.* Retrieved from http://www.cancer.gov/about-cancer/coping/feelings

National Institute of Health: National Cancer Institute. (2016a). *Cancer.* MedlinePlus. Retrieved from https://www.nlm.nih.gov/medlineplus/cancer.html#summary

National Institute of Health: National Cancer Institute. (2016b). *Oral cancer.* MedlinePlus. Retrieved from https://www.nlm.nih.gov/medlineplus/oralcancer.html

National Institute of Health: National Cancer Institute. (2016c). *Laryngeal cancer treatment—Professional version.* Retrieved from http://www.cancer.gov/types/head-and-neck/hp/laryngeal-treatment-pdq

National Institute of Health: National Cancer Institute. (2016d). *Esophagus cancer.* MedlinePlus. Retrieved from http://www.cancer.org/cancer/esophaguscancer/detailedguide/esophagus-cancer-risk-factors

National Institute of Health: National Cancer Institute. (2016e). *Signs and symptoms of prostate cancer.* Retrieved from http://www.cancer.org/cancer/prostatecancer/detailedguide/prostate-cancer-diagnosis

Ortel, B., & Bolotin, D. (2012). Cancer of the skin. In E. T. Bope & R. D. Kellerman (Eds.), *Conn's current therapy 2012,* (pp. 201–205). Philadelphia, PA: Elsevier Saunders.

Perry, A., Casey, E., & Cotton, S. (2015). Quality of life after total laryngectomy: Functioning, psychological well-being and self-efficacy. *International Journal of Language and Communication Disorders, 50*(4), 467–475. Retrieved from http://eric.ed.gov/?q=laryngectomy&id=EJ1067604

Petronic-Rosic, V. (2012). Melanoma. In E. T. Bope & R. D. Kellerman (Eds.), *Conn's current therapy 2012,* (pp. 234–236). Philadelphia, PA: Elsevier Saunders.

Phillippi, J. C., Latendresse, G. A., & McChance, K. L. (2014). Alterations in the female reproductive system. In K. L. McCance, S. E. Huether, V. L. Brashers, & N. S. Rote (Eds.), *Pathophysiology: The biologic basis for disease in adults and children,* (7th ed., pp. 825–867). St. Louis, MO: Elsevier-Mosby.

Rajkumar, S. V. (2016). Plasma cell disorders. In L. Goldman & A. I. Schafer (Eds.), *Goldman-Cecil medicine,* (25th ed., pp. 1273–1284). Philadelphia, PA: Elsevier Saunders.

Rodway, G., & McCance, K. L. (2014). Alterations of the male reproductive system. In K. L. McCance, S. E. Huether, V. L. Brashers, & N. S. Rote (Eds.), *Pathophysiology: The biologic basis for disease in adults and children,* (7th ed., pp. 897–910). St. Louis, MO: Elsevier-Mosby.

Schröder, F. H., Hugosson, J., Roobol, M. J., Tammela, T. L. J., Ciatto, S., Nelen, V., ... Auvinen, A. for the ERSPC Investigators. (2012). Prostate-cancer mortality at 11 years of follow-up. *New England Journal of Medicine, 366*(11), 981–990.

Spriggs, D. (2016). Gynecologic cancers. In L. Goldman & A. I. Schafer (Eds.), *Goldman-Cecil medicine,* (25th ed., pp. 1360–1365). Philadelphia, PA: Elsevier Saunders.

Swartz, A., & Rote, N. S. (2014). Alteration of leukocyte, lymphoid, and hemostatic function . In K. L. McCance, S. E. Huether, V. L. Brashers, & N. S. Rote (Eds.), *Pathophysiology: The biologic basis for disease in adults and children,* (7th ed., pp. 1023–1030). St. Louis, MO: Elsevier-Mosby.

CHAPTER 23

Diabetes and Other Conditions of the Endocrine System

Revised by Kathy K. Hager, DNP, APRN, CDE

STRUCTURE AND FUNCTION OF THE ENDOCRINE SYSTEM

The *endocrine system,* as one of the body's two major communication systems, works together with the other communication system, the nervous system, to regulate or direct various body functions (Brashers, Jones, & Huether, 2014a). The endocrine system is composed of ductless glands *(endocrine glands)* distributed throughout the body. The endocrine glands produce chemical substances called *hormones* (see table 23-1), which are secreted directly into the bloodstream and act as messengers to target cells in other parts of the body. Endocrine glands include the following components of the body (see **Figure 23-1**):

- *Thyroid gland*—located in the neck, in front of and on either side of the **trachea** (windpipe).
- *Parathyroid glands*—small, bean-shaped glands buried under the thyroid gland.
- *Adrenal glands*—small glands lying on top of the kidneys. Each adrenal gland has two parts, the *medulla (middle of the gland)* and the *cortex (outer edge of gland).* Each part has a different function.
- *Pituitary gland*—located in the skull, just above the roof of the mouth, and connected to the brain by a slender stalk. It is divided into two parts, the *anterior lobe* and the *posterior lobe.*

- *Hypothalamus*—an area of the brain that coordinates the functions of the nervous-system and the endocrine system.
- *Islets of Langerhans*—special cells embedded in the pancreas that make insulin (lowers blood glucose) and glucagon (raises blood glucose).
- *Testes* in males and *ovaries* in females, responsible for sexual functioning.

The main function of the endocrine system is regulatory, with different hormones altering various body processes so that the body's internal balance (**homeostasis**) is maintained. The *kidney,* although not considered an organ within the endocrine system, plays an endocrine role, by secreting erythropoietin and renin, influencing the number of red blood cells produced and vasoactive properties of the blood vessels (constriction and dilation, respectively) responses (Sargis, 2016).

Although each gland has its own unique and independent function, the endocrine glands often work in concert. Hormones secreted by the endocrine system control and integrate a variety of body activities, establishing a delicate chain of communication between various body systems. Hormones influence and modify a number of physiologic processes throughout the body and regulate a number of body processes:

- Growth and development of the body and brain
- Reproductive maturity and function

Figure 23-1   The Endocrine System

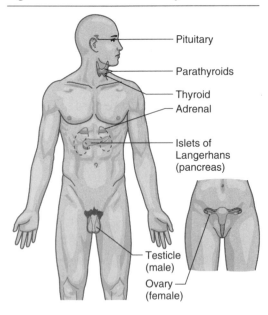

- Pituitary
- Parathyroids
- Thyroid
- Adrenal
- Islets of Langerhans (pancreas)
- Testicle (male)
- Ovary (female)

- Metabolism
- Adjustment to internal and external stress
- Water and electrolyte balance

Hormonal Feedback and the Neuroendocrine System

Overproduction or underproduction of one hormone can affect a number of other endocrine glands and a variety of body functions. Some hormones have the sole function of regulating the production and secretion of another hormone.

The *neuroendocrine system* refers to the interaction of the nervous system with the endocrine system to link activity of the nervous system with metabolic and hormonal activity. Key components of the neuroendocrine system are the hypothalamus and pituitary. The hypothalamus and pituitary function together to regulate a number of endocrine functions. For instance, *thyrotropin-releasing hormone (TRH)* produced by the hypothalamus stimulates the synthesis and release of *thyroid-stimulating hormone (TSH)* by the pituitary; TSH is then transported to the thyroid gland, which in turn produces and secretes *thyroid hormone.* The secretion of adequate amounts of thyroid hormone creates a feedback loop to the hypothalamus and pituitary gland inhibiting production of TRH and TSH, respectively.

Hormones of the Endocrine Glands

The hormone *thyroxine,* which is secreted by the thyroid gland, regulates the rate of metabolism, influences nervous system maturation, and has profound effects on the heart. When the level of the thyroxine in the blood is high, metabolism speeds up; when it is low, metabolism slows down.

The parathyroid glands (located in the neck, usually behind the thyroid gland), secrete parathyroid hormone, which regulates the concentrations of calcium and phosphate in the body. Excessive amounts of parathyroid hormone in the blood can result in the demineralization of bone, causing bones to become fragile so that they are easily broken. Insufficient amounts of parathyroid hormone in the blood can cause spasm and involuntary contraction of the muscles (**tetany**) from too little calcium.

The adrenal gland consists of two parts: the inner part, called the medulla, and the outer portion, called the cortex. The medulla secretes *epinephrine* and, to a lesser extent, *norepinephrine* at times of stress to prepare the body physiologically for emergencies. These hormones increase heart rate, increase muscle tone, and constrict blood vessels in times of stress. The cortex secretes hormones called *steroids,* which regulate many essential functions, such as electrolyte and water balance, metabolism, immune responses, and inflammatory reactions. The adrenal cortex is essential to life. If it is dysfunctional, death will occur within a few days unless the hormones that it usually secretes are replaced.

The pituitary gland, a component of the neuroendocrine system (as discussed previously), consists of two parts: the anterior lobe and the posterior lobe. The anterior lobe of the pituitary gland secretes thyroid-stimulating hormone, which is necessary for thyroid function. The anterior lobe also secretes growth hormone and hormones that control reproductive function. Finally, the anterior lobe secretes corticotropin, a hormone necessary for the function of the adrenal cortex. The posterior lobe of the pituitary gland stores hormones produced in the hypothalamus. *Antidiuretic hormone (ADH),* which increases water reabsorption by the kidneys, is produced by the hypothalamus but is stored in and secreted by the posterior lobe of the pituitary gland.

The function of the hypothalamus, which is also part of the neuroendocrine system, is complex and multidimensional. It regulates and controls a number of endocrine and, subsequently, body system functions.

The pancreas has both *exocrine* functions and *endocrine* functions. Endocrine functions of the pancreas are carried out by special cells *(beta cells)* located in an area of the pancreas called the islets of Langerhans. These cells produce the hormone *insulin,* which lowers blood glucose by promoting transport of glucose (sugar) into cells. Other special cells in the islets of Langerhans *(alpha cells)* produce the hormone *glucagon,* which raises blood glucose by stimulating the liver to convert *glycogen* to glucose. Insulin and glucagon are part of a regulatory system that keep blood glucose levels stable.

Hormones produced by the testes in the male and ovaries in the female are important for growth and development as well as for reproduction.

Table 23-1 summarizes the hormones secreted by various endocrine glands.

DIABETES MELLITUS

Defining Diabetes Mellitus

Diabetes mellitus—the most common of all endocrine conditions—is defined by the American Diabetes Association (ADA) (ADA, 2013d) as a *group* of metabolic conditions "characterized by hyperglycemia which results from defects in insulin secretion, insulin action, or both." Classification of diabetes is difficult. Although each condition classified as diabetes shares the common characteristic of **hyperglycemia** (high blood sugar), each type of diabetes has different mechanisms that cause blood sugar (glucose) to be elevated. Consequently, the type of interventions required for management of diabetes depend on both the type of diabetes and its underlying mechanism. (Different types of diabetes and specific interventions are discussed later in the chapter.)

Table 23-1   Hormones Produced by Endocrine Glands

Thyroid Gland
Thyroxine
Calcitonin
Parathyroid Glands
Parathyroid hormone
Adrenal Glands
Adrenal Cortex
Cortisol
Aldosterone
Adrenal Medulla
Epinephrine
Norepinephrine
Pituitary Gland
Anterior Pituitary
Luteinizing hormone (LH)
Follicle-stimulating hormone (FSH)
Adrenocorticotropic hormone (ACTH)
Growth hormone (GH)
Thyroid-stimulating hormone (TSH)
Prolactin
Posterior Pituitary
Oxytocin
Antidiuretic hormone (ADH)
Hypothalamus Gland
Corticotropin-releasing hormone (CRH)
Thyrotropin-releasing hormone (TRH)
Growth hormone–releasing hormone (GHRH)
Somatostatin
Gonadotropin-releasing hormone (GnRH)
Dopamine
Pancreas (Islets of Langerhans)
Insulin
Glucagon
Gonads
Testes—Male
Testosterone
Ovaries—Female
Estrogen
Progesterone

Significance of Diabetes Mellitus

The prevalence of diabetes has increased steadily throughout the last several decades (ADA, 2016a). The importance of this disease is highlighted by the fact that it affects every body system, and complications of diabetes can significantly affect functional capacity in a number of areas (Brashers et al., 2014b). Diabetes mellitus is a leading cause of *blindness, end-stage kidney disease,* and *nontraumatic amputation,* as well as a major risk factor for *hypertension* and *stroke, heart disease, peripheral neuropathy,* and *erectile dysfunction* in males (Brashers et al., 2014b; Crandall & Shamoon, 2016).

Mechanisms of Diabetes Mellitus

Depending on the type, diabetes mellitus results from either destruction *or* dysfunction of the cells in the pancreas that produce insulin, or the inability of cells in the body to use insulin *(insulin resistance)* (ADA, 2013a). Factors contributing to development of diabetes mellitus are varied and depend on the type of diabetes experienced.

Overall, diabetes mellitus involves an imbalance of the supply and demand of the hormone insulin (Brashers et al., 2014a), which is necessary for cells in the body to obtain and use glucose as an energy source for activities. Food ingested is eventually converted to glucose, which is then carried in the blood to be used by all cells in the body. Tissues such as muscle and fat require insulin so glucose can be used as a source of energy. When the supply of insulin is insufficient, or when cells are unable to incorporate glucose, large amounts of glucose accumulate in the blood (hyperglycemia).

As blood is filtered by the kidney, glucose is usually channeled back into the blood. Because individuals with diabetes mellitus have such a large amount of glucose in the blood, however, some glucose spills over into the urine (**glycosuria**). Owing to the large concentration of glucose in the urine, the kidney excretes large quantities of water, a manifestation called **polyuria**. As a result, individuals drink large quantities of water in an effort to replace the excess fluid lost (**polydipsia**).

The body's inability to use glucose means that food or energy available to body tissues is inadequate. To compensate for this condition, individuals with diabetes increase their food intake dramatically (**polyphagia**). Despite the increased food intake, lack of insulin prevents the body from using food as an energy source. Consequently, individuals begin to lose weight and become increasingly weak.

When the body's need for energy remains unmet, the body begins to metabolize its own stores of fat and proteins for energy. As a result, **ketones** (the by-products of fat metabolism) are formed. Usually, ketones are broken down and excreted. In individuals with diabetes mellitus, however, they accumulate more rapidly than they can be excreted. When ketone levels become toxic, a condition called **ketosis** or **ketoacidosis** (diabetic coma) occurs. Having too little or no insulin available for the amount of food ingested may also cause a diabetic coma (ADA, 2015a).

Types and Classifications of Diabetes Mellitus

The American Diabetes Association (2016a) recommends that diabetes mellitus be classified into four broad categories based on the cause of each type of diabetes:

- Type 1 diabetes
- Type 2 diabetes
- Gestational diabetes mellitus (GDM)
- Other specific forms of diabetes

Type 1 Diabetes

Type 1 diabetes accounts for approximately 5 to 10% of all cases of diabetes mellitus (ADA, 2016b). The cause of type 1 diabetes comprises a complex combination of genetic, environmental, and autoimmune factors (Brashers, 2014a; Crandall & Shamoon, 2016). It has been suggested that some individuals may inherit an immune system that is more responsive to environmental factors such as diet or exposure to a particular virus or toxin, such that it triggers an autoimmune response that destroys the insulin-producing cells in the pancreas (ADA, 2015a). A small percentage of those with type 1 diabetes do not have any markers for autoimmunity but do have a tendency to develop diabetic ketoacidosis (ADA, 2015a).

Individuals with type 1 diabetes produce little or no insulin, so that external sources of insulin are required for survival. Manifestations usually occur rapidly and include polyphagia, weight loss, polydipsia, polyuria, and fatigue. In some instances, the first manifestation is ketoacidosis.

Type 2 Diabetes

Type 2 diabetes is the most common type of diabetes mellitus, accounting for nearly 90% of all individuals with diabetes (Brashers, 2014a; ADA, 2013a). In type 2 diabetes, the body produces insulin, but either the amount is insufficient to meet the total body needs *or* the cells in the body are unable to use the existing insulin adequately *(insulin resistance)*. There may also be a component of abnormal glucagon production (Godoy-Matos, 2014). A major risk factor in development of type 2 diabetes is obesity (National Institute of Diabetes and Digestive and Kidney Diseases (NIDDK), 2014). Type 2 diabetes is often identified when elevated blood glucose is noted during a routine blood test.

Manifestations of type 2 diabetes may not be readily apparent because hyperglycemia develops gradually. Consequently, this disease may not be identified for years; even so, individuals are at risk for developing complications of diabetes (NIDDK, 2014), as discussed later in this chapter.

External sources of insulin may or may not be needed to manage the manifestations of type 2 diabetes, but survival does *not* depend on an external insulin source (ADA, 2013b; Crandall & Shamoon, 2016).

Gestational Diabetes Mellitus

Gestational diabetes is a condition in which high blood glucose levels are exhibited in pregnancy, despite no prior history of elevated blood glucose (NIDDK, 2014). After delivery, in most instances, the blood glucose level returns to normal. Women who develop gestational diabetes have a greater risk for developing diabetes mellitus in the future (Montella, 2016; CDC, 2015; NIDDK, 2014).

Other Specific Forms of Diabetes

Other classifications of diabetes are associated with other conditions or syndromes. For instance, diabetes can occur as a complication of other conditions, such as **pancreatitis** (inflammation of the pancreas), pancreatic damage, pancreatic tumors, or removal of the pancreas. It can also result from other endocrine conditions, such as Cushing's syndrome (discussed later in the chapter), or as a side effect of medications or other chemicals. In some instances, other severe conditions such as systemic infection or burns, can cause *stress hyperglycemia*. The correction of the underlying cause of other specific forms of diabetes may sometimes return blood glucose to normal levels, but in other instances, the manifestation of hyperglycemia will remain and necessitate permanent intervention for management (NIDDK, 2014).

Identification of Diabetes Mellitus

If individuals exhibit manifestations of diabetes, such as polydipsia, polyuria, polyphagia, and weight loss, a blood test that measures the levels of glucose in the plasma several hours after the person has eaten *(postprandial plasma glucose test [PPG])* will generally confirm that the individual has diabetes mellitus by demonstrating the glucose level is higher than would be expected in individuals without diabetes. Most diabetes, however, is identified through *fasting blood glucose (FBG)* (ADA, 2013a, 2013b), a test in which blood is drawn after the individual has not eaten for a number of hours or a Hemoglobin A1C (A1C). The FBG test compares the level of glucose in the individual's blood with the level expected in persons without diabetes mellitus under similar circumstances. The A1C test measures the amount of sugar stuck (adhering) to the hemoglobin in red blood cells. Because the red blood cells live about 120 days, the amount of sugar on the hemoglobin can be compared to the normal amount of glycosylation (sugar adhering to the red blood cell) in a person without diabetes. An estimated average daily blood sugar over a 3-month period can also be used to diagnose diabetes; the advantage is that no fasting is required (ADA, 2016a).

Presence of glucose in the urine (**glycosuria**), although an indication that further testing should be conducted, is not a definitive test in identifying diabetes mellitus. In some instances, individuals may also receive an *oral glucose tolerance test (OGTT)*, in which they are given concentrated glucose in liquid form to drink, and blood samples are drawn at 1-, 2-, and 3-hour intervals. The three tests make it possible to compare the individual's blood glucose level with the levels that would be expected in individuals without diabetes under the same conditions (ADA, 2016a).

Management of Diabetes Mellitus

There currently is no cure for diabetes mellitus, although landmark studies (Diabetes Control and Complications Trial Research Group, 1993, and the United Kingdom Prospective Diabetes Study), have demonstrated that strict control of blood glucose could significantly reduce or delay the microvascular complications of Type 1 and Type 2 diabetes (Nathan, 2014). Microvascular disease involves the very small blood vessels of the kidneys (nephropathy), eyes (retinopathy), and nerves (neuropathy). Medium and large vessel (macrovascular) disease, involving the heart and brain, are much more complex, with experts noting that tight blood sugar, in addition to other interventions are needed. Blood pressure control, ideal body weight, smoking abstinence or cessation, physical activity and normal levels of fats and cholesterol appear to also play a vital role in preventing or delaying heart attacks and strokes. Therefore, management of diabetes, regardless of type, is directed toward controlling levels of blood glucose as well as lifestyle interventions (Gugliucci, 2014; National Institute of Diabetes and Digestive and Kidney Diseases 2013).

Insulin

Insulin is a primary intervention for management of type 1 diabetes, although some individuals with type 2 diabetes may also use insulin as one of the interventions for management. Gastric juices inactivate insulin, so insulin cannot be taken orally but rather must be injected into a **subcutaneous** (fatty) layer of tissue in the body. Inhaled insulin is also available; its popularity is yet to be determined (Minz, 2014).

The goal of administering insulin as an intervention for management of diabetes is to maintain blood glucose levels as close to the recommended range as possible, thereby delaying or preventing complications of diabetes without causing low blood sugars. A number of commercial insulin preparations, which act in different ways, are available. The type, amount, and frequency of insulin injection are individually determined. Individuals have unique body-specific responses to insulin, absorption differences, and different levels of activity that affect insulin requirements. Individuals often require more than one insulin injection per day as well as a number of different types of insulin. Usually, the greater the number of injections taken per day, or the use of an insulin pump that delivers insulin hourly, and in bursts (based upon carbohydrate intake), the greater the person's flexibility is. The person is kept less to a tight schedule of eating and exercising, when the insulin lasts a short period of time, and can be given as needed (depending on exercise and food intake).

The various insulin preparations differ in the timing of their action. Classifications of insulin preparations are as follows:

- Rapid acting
- Short acting
- Intermediate acting
- Long acting

Each type of insulin preparation has a different onset of effect after administration, different peak effect, and different duration of action. For instance, rapid-acting insulin usually acts within 10 to 15 minutes after injection, with its effect peaking at 1 to 2 hours and lasting 1 to 4 hours, whereas long-acting insulin acts with 1 to 4 hours, has little or no peak, and produces an effect that lasts up to 24 hours (NIDDK, 2013) The amount and type of insulin are balanced with the number of calories consumed, the amount of physical activity performed daily, and the daily blood glucose measures (McCulloch, 2016).

Because insulin injected into the body must be balanced with the amount of glucose available, individuals cannot, after receiving insulin, decide to "skip a meal." Likewise, because physical exercise burns glucose for energy, a drastic increase in activity—even though adequate amounts of food were consumed—may mean that the rapid consumption of glucose for energy will leave too much insulin in the body for the amount of glucose left.

Conditions that increase the metabolism rate or cause the body to consume more of the available glucose—such as stress, fever, infection, and pregnancy—alter insulin requirements and, consequently, may necessitate a modification of an individual's insulin dosage. For this reason, individuals using insulin who have flu, fever, or other health conditions should consult their healthcare provider regarding adjustments to their usual insulin dosage.

Individuals must rotate the injection site to avoid a buildup of scar tissue, which can interfere with the absorption of insulin. An insulin syringe and needle may be used for insulin injections, or individuals may use a device called an *insulin injector,* which resembles a pen. The insulin injector consists of a cylinder into which a cartridge filled with a predetermined dose of insulin and disposable needles are placed. The advantage of this device is that it is relatively reliable and accurate in delivering the amount of insulin injected; it is also convenient. Such a device may be carried unobtrusively in a purse or pocket for use away from home. Individuals using the insulin injector do not need to carry extra syringes and insulin bottles. When at a social event, business meeting, or family outing, individuals can easily give themselves injections with minimal disruption.

For the most part, insulin no longer requires refrigeration for storage, but exposure to extremes in temperature and to intense light should be avoided. According to all three U.S. insulin manufacturers, it is recommended that insulin be stored in a refrigerator at approximately 36–46°F. Unopened and stored in this manner, these products maintain potency until the expiration date on the package (U.S. Food & Drug Administration, 2015).

Some individuals may choose an *insulin pump,* which provides a slow, continuous subcutaneous infusion of insulin throughout the day, thereby avoiding the need for numerous injections. Insulin pumps are also credited with improving glycemic control, decreasing episodes of low blood sugars and hospitalizations for diabetic ketoacidosis (Busko, 2013).

With this approach, insulin is delivered to subcutaneous (fatty) tissue in the abdominal wall through a needle and an open-loop delivery device consisting of a small insulin pump (about the size of a pager) that is worn 24 hours a day. Newer models of insulin pumps are now designed with glucose sensors and can suspend insulin when the blood sugars are low. This, in essence, prevents low blood sugars, and simultaneously allows tight blood sugar control (near normal), resulting in the prevention or delayed onset of the long-term complications of diabetic microangiopathy (McAdams & Rizvi, 2016). The advantage to insulin pumps also includes, as noted above, an improved flexibility in the schedule of the person with diabetes. When there are changes in the person's routine, the pump may simply be adjusted (less or more insulin delivered), depending on the activity, stress level, or food intake

Antidiabetic Agents

Although some individuals with type 2 diabetes may be able to control their blood glucose levels with exercise and weight loss or diet alone, in other instances *oral antidiabetic agents* (oral medications that are effective in lowering blood glucose or preventing the blood sugar from rising) may be needed. Several types of oral and injectable medications are available for this purpose. Individuals often use several oral medications in combination. Oral agents have different mechanisms of action. Some enhance insulin secretion, whereas others reduce glucose production by the liver (Skugor, 2014).

Some newer medications developed for use in type 2 diabetes have been called into question for various reasons including heart disease and fracture risks. The choice of whether to use these newer medications when older medications with less risk are available remains controversial (Nathan, 2014; Skugor, 2014). When oral medications do not adequately control blood glucose, individuals with type 2 diabetes may need to take supplemental insulin or a new class of injectable drugs called incretins or incretin-based therapies. Incretins are a group of metabolic hormones that decrease blood glucose levels by causing an increase in the amount of insulin released from the pancreatic beta cells of the islets of Langerhans after food intake (Skugor, 2014; Chon & Gautier, 2016).

Lifestyle Modification

Although different interventions are essential in management of different types of diabetes mellitus, lifestyle changes are significant aspects of the management of all types of diabetes. Specific lifestyle modifications related to management of diabetes include diet, physical activity, and self-management and monitoring of blood glucose and blood pressure levels.

Diet

A healthy diet is important to the well-being of all people, but to individuals with diabetes, dietary management is an integral part of the management of their condition (ADA, 2015c). The primary goal of diet as an intervention in diabetes is to optimize blood levels of glucose. Individuals with diabetes mellitus must consider, in addition to proper nutrition, the need to balance calories ingested with energy expenditure as well as the distribution of calories consumed throughout the day.

Individuals with type 1 diabetes use external sources of insulin. Consequently, they must match the number of calories consumed with the amount of energy expended, and the amount and type of insulin injected. Because a predetermined amount of insulin is injected, individuals need to match timing of meals with the action of the specific insulin. Although intensive individualized insulin protocols have greatly increased flexibility regarding timing and content of meals, calories need to be distributed appropriately throughout the day so that there is not a large concentration of calories at any one time. Individuals must learn how to compensate for any departures from the routine plan so that insulin doses or caloric intake can be adjusted appropriately. Because stress, infections, or other conditions can also affect glucose levels, persons with diabetes need to be aware of the necessity for careful monitoring and potential adjustment should these situations arise.

Individuals with type 2 diabetes may be able to manage blood glucose levels with diet alone or with a combination of diet and oral agents. Individuals who are overweight may be placed on a low-caloric reduction diet so that the body will need less insulin (McCulloch, 2016). In some instances,

external sources of insulin may also be needed if blood glucose levels cannot be maintained at an acceptable level. Individuals with type 2 diabetes may also have mobility issues associated with obesity, arthritis, or circulation problems (Pariser, Hager, Gillette, & Jackson, 2014). For individuals who are morbidly obese, bariatric surgery may be indicated (Harrar, 2015).

Diets for management of diabetes are individualized and based on many personal factors, such as weight, age, and type of daily activity (e.g., sedentary, moderately active, very active). For instance, due to growth needs, adolescents may be placed on a higher-caloric diet than an older individual of the same size. Individuals who remain mostly sedentary throughout the day may not require as many calories as individuals who are very physically active in their job or at home. Athletes who expend significantly more energy during a sports event than on a daily basis also need to adjust their caloric intake and insulin availability to meet these special needs. Given these concerns, counseling by a *dietitian* or *nutritionist* (an individual who studies and counsels individuals on the therapeutic use of food) is imperative in the diabetes management. Developing a diet based on individual needs and preferences can enhance the likelihood of dietary adherence. Lifestyle, family, religious, and cultural habits must all be considered as much as possible when dietary recommendations are made. The less flexible the dietary plan, the less likely the individual is to follow it. Consequently, emphasis is on maintaining an individualized healthy diet that the individual is more likely to follow (ADA, 2015c).

Physical Activity

Exercise is important for the general health and well-being of all individuals. For individuals with diabetes mellitus, however, calories must be balanced with the amount of activity performed as well as with the amount of insulin administered. Exercise, especially if it exceeds one hour, can rapidly reduce blood glucose levels; that effect is compounded if it coincides with peak action of insulin (the point at which the blood has the highest level of circulating insulin). Unplanned exercise that is not coordinated with caloric intake can also create an imbalance between the amount of insulin previously taken and the amount of glucose remaining available in the blood, resulting in **hypoglycemia** (insulin shock; discussed later in the chapter). Individuals using external sources of insulin must learn how exercise of a given intensity and duration affects their blood glucose levels and which adjustments must be made in eating patterns and insulin dosages to compensate for those variations (ADA, 2013c).

Self-Management and Monitoring

Effective management of diabetes often requires that certain changes be incorporated into the individual's daily routine and lifestyle and that the individual adhere to the management routine. Depending on the individual's lifestyle prior to identification of diabetes, adherence to the management routine may be more difficult for some persons than for others. Issues such as making healthy food choices, losing weight, increasing physical activity to enhance physical fitness, calibrating activity with food intake, eating regular meals, testing blood glucose levels, and general planning and problem solving require motivation and vigilance. Collectively, these considerations require that individuals be well informed and develop a certain degree of self-confidence in managing their condition, including being aware of changes or manifestations that warrant the attention of a healthcare professional.

Self-monitoring of blood glucose levels is important in the overall management of diabetes. Such monitoring helps to determine the efficiency of the current insulin dosage. Individuals who take insulin usually monitor their blood glucose levels at least several times each day.

It is important to vary the times of testing, even if done only once daily. If levels are drawn throughout the day the blood glucose levels can indicate how many hours of the day the blood is saturated with glucose (sugar). It is believed that sustained high blood glucose levels are toxic to the blood vessels and nerves, explaining the long-term complications of diabetes. Monitoring provides information about blood glucose levels and, consequently, suggests changes in management that may be appropriate. Medications can be adjusted to ensure that blood glucose levels return to normal as quickly after eating, as is possible. For instance, if the blood glucose level is too low, there may be the need for ingestion of a "quick-acting" sugar such as orange juice to prevent severe hypoglycemia. If the blood glucose level is consistently too high, the individual may need to inject additional insulin, decrease food intake (especially carbohydrates) or increase exercise. Sometimes, if the blood glucose is high the person must question what other factors could increase it. Stress of any kind can raise the blood sugar, as the body needs additional energy (glucose) to withstand the stress. The stress can be physical, like an infection, or emotional, like an argument, worry, or grieving.

Numerous techniques may be used to test blood glucose. Individuals may monitor their own blood glucose levels by lancing their finger and using a small portable machine called a *glucose meter* to assess the glucose content of the blood. Blood glucose monitoring is important because it helps individuals make decisions about food, exercise, amount of insulin needed, and if they are responding poorly or well to changes in their regimen.

Blood glucose may also be assessed through use of a *continuous glucose monitoring sensor.* This sensor is inserted just beneath the skin, usually on the abdomen. It is connected to a monitor, roughly the size of a cell phone, which is attached to a belt. The monitor provides information about trends in blood glucose fluctuation and alerts individuals when blood glucose levels are either too high or too low. Changes in insulin doses can then be based on the glucose readings (Crandall & Shamoon, 2016). During the period when the continuous monitoring device is in effect, the insulin pumps can self-adjust, and block insulin release when the blood glucose levels are below normal. Individuals may learn to alter their own insulin levels in accordance with their home blood glucose reading; however, such alterations should always be done with the advice and under the supervision of a healthcare professional (Vahist, 2013).

Transplantation and Artificial Pancreas

Pancreas transplantation continues to show promise as a treatment for diabetes mellitus, although currently it is an option only for people with diabetes who suffer kidney failure consequently, those receiving a kidney also receive the pancreas. These recipients are then given immunosuppressant medications to prevent their rejection of the organs (Kaufman, 2015). Transplantation of islet cells alone, the cells that produce insulin (and make up about 2% of the pancreas), shows promise and can result in insulin independence and good glucose control, although it is still considered to be experimental (going through clinical trials) and requires antirejection medications and a human donor (Norris, 2013).

Research is currently under way to develop an artificial pancreas, a device that links a glucose monitor embedded under the skin to an insulin pump so that the pump automatically infuses insulin based on the glucose monitor reading (Karoff, 2016). Two of the major goals and outcomes for any of these systems is to gain improved levels of blood glucose and to decrease or eliminate dangerously low blood glucose levels.

Hyperglycemia and Hypoglycemia

Careful management of blood glucose is important to prevent complications of diabetes (as discussed later in this chapter). Another important reason for careful management of glucose concentration is prevention of the potentially fatal, acute conditions characterized by either extremely high levels of blood glucose (hyperglycemia, diabetic coma, diabetic ketoacidosis) or extremely low levels of blood glucose (hypoglycemia, insulin shock),

Diabetic ketoacidosis (DKA) is a condition that occurs when the circulating glucose in the blood reaches a potentially lethally high level (usually occurs when the blood glucose levels are above 250mg/dL) and the body begins to break down fat as an energy source. This level can vary in the individual; usually people with type 1 are much more prone to DKA because they have an absolute insulin deficiency (people with type 2 usually do have some insulin). The muscle and fat cells of the body are insulin dependent (the cells need insulin to move the glucose out of the blood stream and into these cells); the sugar (glucose) cannot enter these cells without the presence of insulin. The insulin-dependent cells (muscle and fat which make

up most of the body) then experience a sense of starvation (none of the sugar is making it into these cells because of the insulin deficiency). This sense of starvation results in the body breaking down fat, which it can convert to sugar, is a final effort to provide these cells the sugar they need. The by-products of this fat breakdown are life threatening to the body. The body is perfectly capable of losing weight and handling the breakdown of fat. However, it cannot handle the rapid breakdown of fat, which can occur in people with type 1 diabetes (and occasionally in people with type 2) (ADA, 2015a).

Although DKA can be the first manifestation of diabetes, more frequently it occurs in individuals because of inadequate adjustment of insulin dosage, skipped insulin injection, or metabolic changes associated with infection or stress. The onset of DKA may be gradual, occurring over several days, or it may be more dramatic. Individuals may experience fatigue or lethargy with an increase in polydipsia and polyuria. The extreme thirst and large levels of urine output are related to the body's attempt to dilute and rid the body of toxically high levels of blood glucose. As blood glucose levels reach lethal levels, individuals may experience nausea and vomiting, difficulty breathing, flushed dry skin, confusion, and eventually unconsciousness. Many of these symptoms occur because of the dehydration that results when the body releases sugar (and water/urine to dilute the sugar) into the urine. Characteristically, the breath of individuals in diabetic coma has a fruity odor.

DKA can be a healthcare emergency that could result in death if appropriate management is not initiated quickly. Management is directed toward lowering the level of blood glucose through the injection of insulin and correcting dehydration and electrolyte imbalances through ingestion of fluids, or if treatment is too prolonged, the intravenous infusion of fluids (ADA, 2015a).

Hypoglycemia (Insulin Shock)

Hypoglycemia (low blood sugar level) is the most frequent complication of type 1 diabetes and is quite dangerous. It can occur any time, but is especially frightening at night when individuals are sleeping and thus unaware of severe lowering of their blood sugar. It can and does often occur in a person who has tight blood sugar control. Tight control means that the person's blood sugar (glucose) is near normal and that even the slightest factor may cause it to go low. For example, if a person got busy and skipped a meal, or if that person exercised more than usual the blood sugar may go too low, depriving the brain of its need for a constant continuous supply of sugar.

Hypoglycemia, or insulin shock, is a potentially life-threatening crisis if not immediately managed. Hypoglycemia is the opposite of diabetic coma, occurring when there is too little glucose in the blood relative to the amount of insulin present. It may result from injecting too much insulin, engaging in an unusual amount of exercise that burns up the glucose that is usually available, or failing to take in sufficient amounts of food for the amount of insulin injected.

Manifestations of hypoglycemia may consist of hunger, weakness, or feelings of anxiety. Individuals may perspire profusely, although their skin is cold to the touch. Confusion and personality changes may also occur during hypoglycemic episodes. If hypoglycemia is not identified so that appropriate interventions can be instituted, individuals may experience a seizure or lapse into unconsciousness, and brain damage and eventually death can occur (ADA, 2015b).

People with known diabetes and who take medicines that can lower the blood sugar should carry glucose monitors with them. When there is any reason to suspect hypoglycemia (feeling bad, confused, "different"), the blood sugar should be tested. If the blood glucose is below 70 mg/dL, the person may need to consume a small amount of carbohydrate.

Management of hypoglycemia is directed toward raising blood glucose levels. If individuals are conscious, simple sugars such as candy, orange juice, or honey may be ingested orally; tubes of gels or packaged tablets specifically designed for low blood sugar episodes are also available. The amount of these replacement foods should be about 15 grams. If the person's blood sugar remains below 70 mg/dL after 15 minutes, a second round of 15 grams may be given. If individuals are unconscious, glucagon injections should be available (providers order glucagon for all people with type 1 diabetes) and can be given in the buttocks, arms,

or legs. The person should be placed on his or her side if given glucagon, as it may cause nausea or vomiting. If any of these interventions are ineffective after 15 minutes, 911 should be called; glucose will be infused intravenously (ADA, 2015b).

Because hypoglycemia can occur at night during sleep, and because some people do not show or experience marked signs of low blood sugar, the use of service dogs that have been specially trained to recognize changes in scent that indicate hypoglycemia has been gaining in popularity. Service dogs recognizing the potential crisis, can wake the individual, alert family members, or trigger special emergency alarms that summon assistance (Nall, 2016).

Long-term Complications of Diabetes Mellitus

Long-term complications include those conditions that develop over a long period of time, usually at least 5 years. Because some people with type 2 diabetes can have very subtle symptoms (they usually do produce some insulin, so the body is not as acutely affected), for 5–6 years before diagnosis, people with type 2 diabetes should be evaluated for long-term complications at the time of diagnosis. Type 1 diabetes usually develops much more rapidly (because there is little or no insulin produced); for this reason, the person usually is evaluated for long-term complications, 5 years after diagnosis.

Individuals with diabetes mellitus, whether type 1 or type 2, are susceptible to these long-term complications. These complications can have a major impact on functional capacity (ADA, 2015b). These complications are typically divided into two types: microvascular (very small blood vessels perfusing the eyes, kidneys, and nerves) and macrovascular (medium-sized vessels perfusing the heart, brain, and gut). Exactly how diabetes causes complications in numerous body systems is a complex process that is not completely understood (Crandall & Shamoon, 2016). Research findings suggest that control of blood glucose levels can dramatically reduce or delay development of microvascular (those to the eye, kidney, and nerve) complications. Macrovascular complications can certainly be favorably affected by good blood glucose levels but are also influenced by blood pressure, high cholesterol levels, body weight, and smoking abstinence or cessation (Leontis & Hess-Fischl, 2016).

The degree to which individuals with diabetes mellitus will develop complications varies from person to person. Factors such as type of diabetes, age of onset, duration of the condition, and the extent to which individuals adhere to the management plan must be considered.

Complications Involving the Eye

Diabetic complications of the eye are many; all forms have the potential to cause vision loss and blindness. Retinopathy involves damage to the very small blood vessels of the retina, the nerve part of the eye that transmits pictures to the optic nerve and brain. When the blood glucose levels are too high for long periods of time (toxic), the blood vessels and nerves serving the retina are damaged. These blood vessels may hemorrhage or leak blood into the clear gel of the back of the eye, causing vision to be distorted. This condition is the leading cause of vision loss in the working-age population. There is a further complication of diabetic retinopathy that involves the central area of the retina and central vision called the *macula*; it is this part of the eye that is needed for straight-ahead vision, like reading and driving. Glaucoma, which can involve increased pressure in the eye and damage to the optic nerve, and cataracts, which involve a clouding the lens, occur in the general population, but often occur earlier and more frequently in the diabetes population (National Eye Institute [NEI], 2015).

Because so many eye conditions are seen in the diabetic population, it is vitally important that the person with diabetes have a dilated eye exam annually. The exams should begin at diagnosis for the person with type 2 diabetes (because it is believed that the person has probably had diabetes for 5–6 years prior to diagnosis), and 5 years after diagnosis for the person with type 1 diabetes.

According to the National Eye Institute (2015), early detection and treatment can reduce the risk of blindness by 95%. The importance of good blood glucose control, good blood pressure control, smoking abstinence/cessation, and low cholesterol levels cannot be understated; these lifestyle changes can be instrumental in preventing and delaying onset of eye disease. Once diagnosed, there are many treatment options and new medications/procedures that are proving very successful in delaying or preventing further damage to the eye, and often, improved vision. Treatments include laser surgery, where very small burns to the leaking blood vessels stop the leaking and hemorrhage. The blood leaking into the gel part of the eye and occluding vision, can also be removed, resulting in clearer vision. A novel approach to these abnormal vessels is an injection into the eye (called anti-vascular endothelia growth factor [anti-VEGF]) that slows down a growth factor responsible for these newly forming blood vessels. Annual dilated exams can result in early detection and best outcomes for people with diabetes (NEI, 2015).

Complications Involving the Kidney

Nephropathy refers to damage to the kidney. About 30% of people with type 1 diabetes and 10–40% of people with type 2 diabetes will experience kidney failure (National Kidney Foundation [NKF], 2015). The importance of annual monitoring is paramount to early detection and management of kidney failure. For people with type 2 diabetes, this annual monitoring should start at the time of diagnosis (their diabetes often started 5–6 years prior to diagnosis); for people with type 1 diabetes, the annual monitoring should begin 5 years after diagnosis. Kidney damage is greatly reduced or prevented when the diabetic person's blood glucose is tightly controlled. The closer the blood glucose is to normal, the less likely is the development of kidney disease. Lifestyle changes to normalize blood pressure, cholesterol, weight, and to stop or never smoke greatly decrease or delay chances of kidney failure (NKF, 2015).

The damage seen to the kidneys, very similar to the damage seen in the eyes, is related to blood vessels that supply the kidney; these vessels are damaged and do not filter the blood properly, allowing unneeded sodium (salt) and water to be retained, and sometimes allowing proteins that should stay in the blood, to escape into the urine. When this occurs, waste materials build up in the blood and needed protein is lost. Signs and symptoms include frequent urination (especially at night), swelling, weight gain, and high blood pressure;

as kidney failure advances, the person may feel ill with nausea, vomiting, appetite loss, weakness, fatigue, and anemia (NKF, 2015).

In addition to healthy lifestyles and maintaining near-normal blood glucose levels, there are specific medications that can slow down the progression of kidney disease. Special diets may also be necessary. If the disease progresses to late stages, exchange of fluids (dialysis) to rid the body of waste products normally accomplished by the kidneys, and kidney transplants may be performed. If the person has diabetes and complete kidney failure, he or she is much more likely to be offered both a kidney and pancreas transplant; any times organs are replaced, antirejection medication is needed (NKF, 2015).

Complications Involving the Nerves

Approximately 60–70% of people with diabetes have some form of nerve damage (neuropathy); the highest rate occurs in those people that have diabetes 25 years or longer. Nerves throughout the body can be damaged because of sustained high blood glucose levels; this high glucose level is toxic to the nerves. High blood pressure, high cholesterol, smoking, low insulin levels also contribute to the neuropathy. Damage to the peripheral nerves (**peripheral neuropathy**) may result in pain, tingling, or loss of sensation in the extremities (ADA, 2016b). With either pain or numbness in the lower extremities, mobility can be affected. In addition, if numbness occurs, the protective sensation of pain is absent, making extremities prone to injury and infection (NIDDK, 2013).

The *autonomic nerves* that control function of internal organs and sexual response may also be damaged by diabetes. As a result, damage to the nerves in the cardiovascular system can result in abnormal blood pressure and heart rate. Gastrointestinal manifestations such as nausea and vomiting, indigestion, constipation, or diarrhea may be experienced. There can also be difficulty with urination, such as the inability to empty the bladder fully, which in turn predisposes individuals to urinary infections. In some cases, individuals may be unable to retain bladder control, resulting in incontinence.

Sexual function can also be affected as a result of nerve damage causing erectile dysfunction in men and decreased genital sensation in women (NIDDK, 2013; ADA, 2014b).

Antidepressants, antiseizure medications, and regular pain medications are all used in the treatment and control of pain associated with neuropathies. In gastrointestinal disorders, diet adjustments, reflux medications, and antibiotics can be given to control indigestion, reflux, nausea, vomiting, constipation or diarrhea, dizziness and weakness. Physical therapy, diet changes, slow rising to a sitting or standing position, fluids and medications can be used to manage the problems. Erectile dysfunction can be treated with medication. Peripheral neuropathy requires frequent evaluation and protection of the feet. Protection includes keeping bath and shower temperatures regulated (as the person will not have the sensation of hot water), having toenails trimmed, wearing shoes whenever up (protects the feet if an object should fall or if the person stubs a toe), and inspecting the feet daily. Daily inspection is needed for early detection of injury; the person with neuropathy may not feel pain or pressure (NDDK, 2013).

Complications Related to the Cardiovascular System

According to the American Heart Association (AHA, 2016) at least 68% of people age 65 or older with diabetes will die from some form of heart disease and 16% will die of stroke. Individuals with diabetes are two to four times more likely to have heart disease or a stroke than adults with out diabetes (para. 1). Individuals who have risk factors in addition to diabetes, such as obesity, family history, or tobacco use, have an even greater chance of developing complications related to the cardiovascular system. Maintaining a heart-healthy diet, losing weight, increasing physical activity, and quitting smoking can help to diminish these risks (AHA, 2016).

Lower Extremity/Amputation

Diabetes is the leading cause of nontraumatic lower extremity amputations in the United States, and approximately 19% of patients with diabetes who develop a foot ulcer will require amputation (American Podiatric Medical Association [APMA], 2016). Approximately 60% of nontraumatic lower-limb amputations occur in individuals over 20 years of age and who have been diagnosed with diabetes. Individuals experiencing numbness in the foot due to peripheral neuropathy (in the lower extremities) have increased risk of injury and infection, which can in turn lead to amputation. Damage to the blood vessels, resulting in slowed or obstructed circulation, can occur from smoking, and from sustained high cholesterol, high blood pressure, and high blood glucose levels. Due to slow healing because of poor circulation, the injury, even though appearing minor, may become infected, leading to tissue **necrosis** (death) and subsequent amputation (APMA, 2016).

Inappropriate footwear is the most common source of trauma to the feet of individuals with diabetes, resulting in foot ulcers, which can lead to the need for amputation (APMA, 2016). Individuals with diabetes must be particularly vigilant about maintaining near-normal blood glucose levels, blood pressure levels, cholesterol levels, abstaining from smoking, performing meticulous foot care and providing foot protection (APMA, 2016).

Functional Implications of Diabetes Mellitus

Personal and Psychosocial Issues

Diabetes mellitus requires lifelong, multifaceted management, and the disease can have a significant impact on individuals' daily life and future, especially if complications develop. Motivation to follow the management recommendations is paramount in the management of diabetes mellitus (Song, Xu, & Sun, 2014).

Although some cases of diabetes are more difficult to manage than others because of physiological differences, both psychological and physiologic factors frequently determine the course of diabetes mellitus. Psychological factors, such as stress, may affect management of diabetes directly, by inducing metabolic changes that can alter blood glucose levels, or indirectly, by affecting individuals' motivation to consistently adhere to interventions related to medication, diet, and exercise (ADA, 2013d).

Diabetes mellitus is a hidden condition (Disabled World, 2015). Unless complications occur, manifestations are not generally visible. Others may see no indication of a chronic condition and may, therefore, have no understanding of alterations or changes that individuals need to incorporate into some aspects of their lifestyle or activity. If individuals with diabetes fear social nonacceptance or worry that because of adhering to their management plan they may not "fit in," they may attempt to hide their condition from others, ignoring dietary restrictions, or engaging in activities outside their management plan. For instance, some individuals may believe that following a diabetic diet draws attention to their condition and, therefore, may not closely adhere to the dietary plan. Others may feel self-conscious about checking blood glucose levels or self-administration of insulin so that self-monitoring is not performed consistently.

Studies suggest that depression is increased in people with diabetes, and that the chance of depression worsens with increased diabetic complications. Sadly, having depression with diabetes also increases the chances of complications; a vicious cycle evolves. It is vital that the person with diabetes realizes the importance of obtaining treatment for depression and in over 80% of the cases, symptoms can be alleviated (National Institute of Mental Health, 2015).

Activities and Participation

Lifestyle changes related to activity, especially for individuals using insulin, are part of the regular diabetes management. Diet and insulin dosage can be adjusted to accommodate different types of activities; however, advance planning and understanding of the relationship between exercise, food intake, and insulin requirements are needed (ADA, 2013c). For most individuals, activities, including exercise and meal times, should remain consistent from day to day; this is especially true if the person takes one or two injections per day. Eating on the run or skipping meals is not feasible unless appropriate alterations have also been made in calculating insulin dosage in relationship to caloric intake. If the schedule changes, food intake and insulin dosage must be changed accordingly. Traveling, especially across time zones, also requires alteration in management, as meal times and subsequent insulin administration times will differ. When traveling by plane, special meals need to be requested ahead of time, as well as making arrangements for them to be served at the time required for the dietary protocol. With multiple injections, or an insulin pump, much more flexibility is possible, as the person is able to dose the insulin, decreasing or increasing doses as food intake, exercise, or stress varies.

Activities such as eating in restaurants or in other people's homes need not be restricted. Individuals can learn to obtain appropriate meals in these situations by gaining an understanding of basic quantity and types of food, learning to judge calories and portions, and identifying which foods they should try to avoid or eat in smaller portions. Although intake of concentrated sweets and alcohol should usually be decreased, planning ahead can enable individuals to incorporate small quantities into the diet.

Family understanding and support are important in all chronic health conditions, and the same is true for diabetes mellitus. Because so much of the management in diabetes hinges on the degree to which the management plan is followed, social and family support can enhance the ability to adhere to the plan. Eating habits of family members, as well as their understanding of the importance of the dietary requirements of the individual with diabetes, can contribute to the individual's willingness to adapt to and follow the diet plan. Acceptance and understanding of diabetes and its requirements by friends and colleagues also contribute to individuals' self-concept and subsequent acceptance of their condition. Family acceptance and support of the individual's health condition depend to a great extent on the family composition, the family's usual coping mechanisms, the age of the individual at the onset of diabetes, the management plan itself, perceptions of future consequences, and functioning of the individual in the context of the family before the diabetes was identified (Miller & DiMatteo, 2013).

Although family support is important to the overall management plan, individuals with diabetes are ultimately responsible for becoming educated about and adept in carrying out the plan. In some instances, family members attempt to assume the responsibility for the plan so that the individual becomes excessively dependent. Family members who have assumed this responsibility may feel that they have new status and influence. If the individual attempts to become more independent and responsible for his or her own management plan, this shift in power can represent a source of conflict.

Effects of diabetes on other social relationships vary. In social situations where food and alcohol are the major focus of activity, individuals with diabetes mellitus may need to modify their participation, although they need not totally avoid such situations. Depending on the individual and others in the social setting, modifications may or may not affect the social relationship itself.

Sexuality

Results from worldwide epidemiological studies suggest that approximately 50% of men with diabetes experience erectile dysfunction. This dysfunction is usually associated with nerve dysfunction and inability of the penis to fill with blood. Women's sexuality is much more multifaceted, depending on nerve dysfunction (vaginal sensation), but also on other factors, including level of psychological wellness (absence of depression), lubrication, age, and menopause (Maiorino, Bellastella, Esposito, 2014).

At times, even though no complications associated with diabetes may have occurred, anxiety or stress brought about by having a chronic condition can affect sexual function and strain relationships. In either instance, open, clear communication between partners is important to avoid misunderstanding and build a basis for shared intimacy and closeness.

Neuropathy may be the cause of impotence in men and decreased genital sensation in women. Frequent vaginal infections in women with diabetes may also alter sexual activity because of the physical discomfort of the infectious condition. Discussion with a healthcare professional about potential interventions to counteract these problems may be helpful (ADA, 2014b).

In the absence of erectile dysfunction, reproductive function is not affected. Women with diabetes mellitus who become pregnant generally have more complicated pregnancies and need special healthcare attention to monitor progress of the pregnancy and to alter insulin and caloric requirements (CDC, 2014; CDC 2015b). The management of sexual dysfunction in men predominantly involves medications and devices that fill the penis with blood. The management of sexual dysfunction in women is focused on the cause, including antidepressants, lubricants, and counseling. The best treatment is prevention, including sustained normal blood glucose levels, blood pressure, cholesterol levels, smoking abstinence or cessation, and psychological well-being.

Vocational Issues in Diabetes Mellitus

Diabetes mellitus does not affect aptitude, motor, or cognitive abilities. In contrast, the type of diabetes, the demands of the job, the person's willingness and ability to carry out management recommendations, and the degree to which the management plan is effective in regulating glucose collectively determine any special needs of individuals with diabetes mellitus in the work environment. Certain modifications in employment may, in some instances, be necessary to accommodate needs associated with diabetes. In particular, the activity level should be consistent as much as possible, or activity should be planned so that it is balanced with food intake and insulin or dosage of oral diabetes medications. If at all possible, especially for individuals using insulin, rotating shifts or irregular schedules should be avoided because of the alterations in insulin and food schedules that would be required.

Work associated with a risk of even minor cuts and scratches, especially to the feet, should be avoided owing to the risk of infection. Comfortable, well-fitting shoes can help to eliminate the risk of foot injury that might otherwise lead to infection. If the individual experiences peripheral neuropathy so that sensation of the lower extremities is impaired, exposure to cold temperatures for long periods of time should be avoided to prevent possible complications such as frostbite.

Emotional stress has a direct impact on the blood glucose level. Consequently, individuals with diabetes mellitus should learn coping strategies that enable them to deal effectively with job stress or should avoid overly stressful job situations, if possible.

In most employment laws, diabetes is protected as a disability (ADA, 2015b); as such, it entitles people with diabetes to pursue their life goals, including the workplace, school and sports.

Despite the ability of many individuals to effectively manage their diabetes, discrimination in employment still occurs. Data is weak, but implies that discrimination suits for disability/illness comprise approximately 11% of the cases (ADA, 2014a, 2014b; Cann, 2015). Employers' perceptions of diabetic individuals as a safety risk because of fluctuations in blood glucose levels, which may cause unexpected incapacity, or concern about the potential of employees' developing complications because of their condition may create barriers to successful employment. Education of employers and assurance that individuals are able to handle situations that could occur with diabetes can help to counteract negative attitudes. Employers should generally be informed of the individual's diabetes so that misunderstandings about the need for regular meal schedules, glucose monitoring, routine activities, and avoidance of injury do not develop. In addition, employers should be alerted to the manifestations of diabetic coma or insulin shock so that appropriate action may be taken if either of these events should occur (ADA, 2014b).

Potential for complications should be considered in vocational planning. There is no guarantee that even strict adherence with the management plan will prevent all possible complications from occurring. Nevertheless, maintaining blood glucose levels can decrease the number of days lost from work because of minor complications and decrease the possibility of major complications. When complications do develop, alterations in employment are specific to the type of complication that the individual experiences. For example, individuals who develop diabetic retinopathy may require large screen computer monitors. Development of peripheral neuropathy of the upper extremities may interfere with sensation and manual dexterity. Amputation of a lower extremity may affect mobility (ADA, 2014b). Because of the possibility of diabetic coma or insulin shock, individuals with diabetes mellitus should not work in isolation.

OTHER CONDITIONS OF THE ENDOCRINE SYSTEM

Hyperthyroidism (Graves' Disease, Thyrotoxicosis)

Hyperthyroidism and thyrotoxicosis are terms used to describe excessive production of thyroid hormone by the thyroid gland. Depending on the author, both terms are considered the main grouping, with subtypes of excess thyroid hormone production, based on the cause, being the subgroups (Aleppo, 2015; Floyd, 2015). The terms *Graves' disease* and *thyrotoxicosis* describe forms of hyperthyroidism/thyrotoxicosis. Both are systemic conditions resulting from excessive thyroid hormone. Unmanaged hyperthyroidism can lead to cardiovascular complications including atrial fibrillation, cardiomyopathy, and congestive heart failure, as well as osteoporosis and fracture (Milas, 2014).

Graves' disease is the most common cause of hyperthyroidism/thyrotoxicosis, an autoimmune condition in which the individual's immune system attacks the thyroid gland, causing it to produce too much thyroid hormone. Other forms of hyperthyroidism/thyrotoxicosis could result from ingestion of excessive amounts of thyroid hormone, inflammation of the thyroid gland (thyroiditis) due to viral or bacterial infection, radiation-induced thyroiditis, thyroid and pituitary tumors, and tumors of the ovaries and testes (Lights, Solan, & Fantauzzo, 2015; Kim & Ladenson, 2016).

Manifestations of Hyperthyroidism

Hyperthyroidism results in *increased* metabolic rate, which in turn contributes to manifestations such as **palpitations** (sensation/awareness of heartbeat), **tachycardia** (fast heartbeat), restlessness, irritability, nervousness, difficulty concentrating, insomnia, and increased appetite with weight loss (Kim & Ladenson, 2016). The increased rate of metabolism causes intolerance to heat; thus environmental temperatures that seem comfortable to others may seem unbearably warm to individuals with hyperthyroidism.

Exophthalmos refers to a condition in which there is protrusion of the eyeball, causing changes in eye appearance, such as staring or wide-eyed gaze. The overactive thyroid gland may also be enlarged so that there is a visible swelling in the neck, called a *goiter* (Lights, Solan, & Fantauzzo, 2015).

Management of Hyperthyroidism

With early identification and appropriate management, hyperthyroidism usually causes no permanent consequences. Management is directed toward curtailing the secretion of the excess thyroid hormone. *Antithyroid medication* that blocks the production of the hormone may be used. Manifestations usually subside within weeks or months after management with medication. Medications do not alleviate exophthalmos, which can be a permanent manifestation of the condition; however, some surgical procedures have been used to reduce the effects (Mercandetti, 2016). Because Graves' disease is most likely an autoimmune disorder, lifelong follow-up is generally recommended (Yeun, 2015).

Iodine has an affinity for the thyroid gland; because of this affinity, radioactive iodine may also be used to destroy cells that produce the thyroid hormone. Manifestations usually subside within weeks or months. However, radioactive iodine causes some individuals to become **hypothyroid** (i.e., produce too little thyroid hormone); if so, they must take thyroid replacement medication for life.

Surgical intervention for managing hyperthyroidism is sometimes indicated. If surgery is indicated, usually a *subtotal thyroidectomy,* which involves removal of most, but not all, of the thyroid gland, is performed. Because some of the thyroid gland is left in place, replacement therapy with thyroid hormone may not be necessary (Milas, 2014; Kim & Ladenson, 2016.

Hypothyroidism (Myxedema)

Hypothyroidism can be classified as *primary hypothyroidism,* which is caused by dysfunction of the thyroid gland itself, (the most common cause) or *secondary hypothyroidism,* which results from deficient thyroid gland function due to inadequate stimulation of TSH. The inadequate stimulation of thyroid stimulating hormone can be due to insufficient or inactive TSH (which can be a congenital or acquired pituitary disorder). (Kim & Ladenson, 2016). Thyrotropin releasing hormone and thyroid stimulating hormone from the pituitary are necessary for adequate thyroid function, each responding to low levels of thyroid in the body by increasing its production. Likewise, if there is too much thyroid hormone, the hypothalamus and pituitary will respond by suppressing the release of thyroid hormone. In most cases of hypothyroidism, there is deficiency of thyroid hormone from lack of dietary intake of iodine needed to produce thyroid hormone (more common in children and in undeveloped countries), or from malfunction of the thyroid (primary), pituitary (secondary), or hypothalamus (tertiary) glands. A severe form of hypothyroidism is called *myxedema.*

The most common cause of hypothyroidism in developed countries is chronic autoimmune thyroiditis *(Hashimoto's thyroiditis),* in which an autoimmune response causes thyroid failure (Mathur, 2015).

Manifestations of Hypothyroidism

The manifestations of hypothyroidism are, in many ways, the opposite of those associated with hyperthyroidism. Individuals with hypothyroidism have a slowed metabolic rate and cold intolerance; they may feel tired, lack energy, and experience weight gain. Their hair becomes dry, brittle, and thin, and their voice may be slow, low-pitched, and coarse. Emotional responses are subdued and mental processes slowed.

Complications of hypothyroidism include the rapid development of atherosclerotic heart conditions including angina pectoris, myocardial infarction, and congestive heart failure from the slowed metabolism. Individuals with severe hypothyroidism can also develop psychosis, with associated paranoia and delusions, memory impairment, or dementia. Unless complications develop, however, appropriate management usually prevents any permanent consequences (Mathur, 2015).

Management of Hypothyroidism

The goal of management of hypothyroidism is to correct the thyroid hormone deficiency. Consequently, a primary way of managing hypothyroidism is with hormone replacement therapy. Individuals with hypothyroidism need to remain on this medication for life. In addition, their thyroid levels need to be checked

at least annually. Appearance and level of physical and mental activity usually improve gradually as the level of thyroid hormone rises (Mathur, 2015).

Cushing's Syndrome

Cushing's syndrome is the result of overexposure of tissues to the hormone *cortisol* over time. It can result from chronic use of *glucocorticoid hormones,* as *prednisone,* which has a similar effect on the body as the body's cortisol. It can also be caused by the body's overproduction of cortisol due to conditions such as tumors of the pituitary or adrenal gland (Mayo Clinic, 2016).

Manifestations of Cushing's Syndrome

Manifestations of Cushing's syndrome include puffiness and a rounded moon face, obesity of the trunk of the body, fat pads at the back of the neck (buffalo hump), and weakness. The skin becomes thin and fragile, bones become brittle, wound healing may be poor, and the person may experience frequent bruising. Cushing's syndrome is usually accompanied by **hypertension** (high blood pressure) and *insulin insensitivity (more than the normal amount of insulin is required for the body's work).* Women with Cushing's syndrome may demonstrate menstrual irregularities and facial hair growth. Men may experience decreased libido or impotence. Mood changes such as depression and anxiety may be experienced, and mental acuity may be altered. Diagnosis usually includes testing a battery of hormone levels (Mayo ClinicStaff, 2016).

Management of Cushing's Syndrome

Management of Cushing's syndrome depends on the cause. If Cushing's syndrome is due to use of steroids, management focuses on decreasing the amount of steroid taken or discontinuing steroids altogether if possible. If the cause is due to a tumor, management can involve surgical intervention to remove the tumor or pituitary irradiation. In most instances, intervention can cure the condition (Mayo Clinic, 2016).

Adrenal Insufficiency (Addison's Disease)

Adrenal insufficiency results when the adrenal cortex does not produce enough hormone *(cortisol* or *aldosterone).* Cortisol is crucial to life and regulates the body during periods of stress; aldosterone is responsible for fluid and electrolyte balance. Adrenal insufficiency can be primary, when there is damage to or disruption of the adrenal cortex itself *(Addison's disease),* or secondary, resulting from dysfunction of another endocrine gland that stimulates adrenal function (Macon and Yu, 2016).

Manifestations of Adrenal Insufficiency

Adrenal insufficiency can be acute or chronic. Individuals with *acute primary adrenal insufficiency,* which comes on rapidly, may have severe, potentially life-threatening reactions such as extremely low blood pressure (**hypotension, from low blood volume**) and circulatory collapse. In contrast, individuals who have *chronic adrenal insufficiency,* which develops more slowly over time, may have manifestations of weakness, fatigue, darker skin pigmentation, weight loss, loss of appetite, or development of unusual food preferences, such as craving salt (Macon and Yu, 2016).

Management of Adrenal Insufficiency

Intervention for acute adrenal insufficiency consists of immediate administration of steroids (Cortisol/prednisone and aldosterone). Intervention for chronic adrenal insufficiency consists of daily hormone replacement. Replacement therapy with synthetic corticosteroids now enables individuals with adrenal insufficiency to live full lives if replacement medication is taken daily. Careful monitoring for the development of the manifestations of excessive corticosteroid ingestion is also necessary (Macon and Yu, 2016).

Diabetes Insipidus

Diabetes insipidus is an uncommon condition in which either there is decreased production of the ADH, which helps in the body's water regulation, or the amount of ADH is sufficient but the kidneys do not respond to the hormone. Inadequate production of ADH, which is produced and stored in the brain, is called *central diabetes insipidus;* resistance of the kidneys to ADH is called *nephrogenic diabetes insipidus.*

Although diabetes insipidus has a number of causes, trauma (such as with head injury) is a common etiology for central diabetes insipidus. Other causes of central diabetes insipidus include brain infection and tumor.

Nephrogenic diabetes insipidus can be caused by mutations that affect the kidney's ability to respond to ADH. Alternatively, it can be acquired as a side effect of medications used as interventions in other conditions, such as lithium prescribed for bipolar disorder (Mayo Clinic Staff, 2016).

Manifestations of Diabetes Insipidus

Because ADH is not secreted or the kidneys are unable to respond to it in diabetes insipidus, excessive water is "lost" by the kidneys, leading to excretion of large volumes of dilute urine (polyuria). The normal person makes less than 3 liters of urine/day; the person with diabetes insipidus may make 15 liters. Excessive and constant thirst (polydipsia) is present, with individuals consuming as much as 30 quarts of water per day (Mayo Clinic Staff, 2016).

Management of Diabetes Insipidus

Depending on the cause, different hormonal preparations (including synthetic forms of ADH) may be used to correct central diabetes insipidus or to manage manifestations of this condition. In the kidney-related form, sodium restrictions and specific kidney-targeted medications are available, as well as adequate fluid intake to offset fluid loss is necessary (Mayo Clinic Staff, 2016).

THE ENDOCRINE SYSTEM AND BEHAVIOR

In 1936, the *British Journal of Psychiatry* noted that there was a relationship between psychoses and endocrine disturbances (Hutton & Steinburg, 1939). A number of health conditions result from endocrine dysfunction and constitute major health problems. Because manifestations of endocrine conditions are often similar to those associated with a number of psychiatric conditions, some endocrine conditions may go unrecognized or be incorrectly identified as psychiatric conditions. Likewise, administration of hormones in management of an endocrine deficiency may have side effects similar to the manifestations associated with some psychiatric conditions. Clearly, the endocrine system, in addition to regulating internal body functions and maintaining homeostasis, has a role in human behavior and emotions (Nelson, 2016).

GENERAL FUNCTIONAL IMPLICATIONS OF ENDOCRINE CONDITIONS

Personal and Psychosocial Issues

Changes in hormonal patterns associated with conditions of the endocrine system may cause behavioral changes that result in misinterpretation of manifestations, delay in initiating interventions, and unnecessary hardships for individuals. Manifestations of endocrine conditions may not be recognized as such, but instead may be labeled as resulting from a psychiatric condition. Consequently, individuals may receive interventions for management of a psychiatric condition rather than the interventions actually needed to manage their endocrine condition.

Endocrine conditions can cause a broad range of emotional and psychiatric manifestations (Nelson, 2016). For example, individuals with thyroid conditions may experience emotional outbursts, irritability, or manifestations of anxiety and depression that are not always recognized as manifestations of their condition. Older adults with a thyroid condition may demonstrate memory difficulties that are misidentified as Alzheimer's disease or other forms of dementia, such that interventions appropriate to the endocrine condition are not instituted. In most cases, changes in behavior are temporary and steadily improve as the endocrine condition is corrected (Nelson, 2016).

In children, unrecognized endocrine conditions can cause permanent consequences, such as lesser intellectual development. Recognition of the role of the endocrine system and various hormones in cognitive development of children has resulted in earlier recognition and management of endocrine conditions in childhood, in many cases preventing permanent consequences due to hormonal insufficiency from occurring (Bernal, 2015).

Changes in physical appearance, such as the exophthalmos associated with Graves' disease and the physical changes associated with Cushing's syndrome, can disturb individuals' body image, causing subsequent emotional reactions (Mercandetti, 2016). Management of many endocrine conditions involves long-term or lifelong ingestion of medications. For some individuals, taking medication daily creates frustration and resentment, leading to nonadherence with management interventions and the development of subsequent complications or a recurrence of the condition (Bask, McCaffrey, Bentley, Przybyla, 2014).

Activities and Participation

For most individuals, after the endocrine condition has been stabilized and barring complications, primary lifestyle changes involve remembering to take medications at the same time every day. The exception is, of course, diabetes mellitus, in which lifestyle changes are a significant part of the management of the condition and are often necessary for survival.

Many social issues associated with endocrine conditions depend on the specific condition involved. For example, individuals with hyperthyroidism may experience social isolation because of associated behavior changes that occur before appropriate interventions are instituted. Physical changes caused by endocrine conditions, such as those associated with Cushing's syndrome, may lead to self-consciousness and cause individuals to withdraw from social activities. The demands of diabetes mellitus can also cause stress in families, especially in siblings of children with Type 1 diabetes, causing isolation and resentment.

GENERAL VOCATIONAL ISSUES IN ENDOCRINE CONDITIONS

In most instances, individuals with conditions of the endocrine system, as long as they have been identified and are being appropriately managed, have no special vocational needs. When hormone replacement therapy is part of the management, however, the importance of adherence with the management plan cannot be overstated. This is especially true of individuals with diabetes mellitus, the vocational implications of which were discussed earlier in the chapter.

CASE STUDY

Mr. J. is a 52-year-old cabinetmaker. He is moderately overweight. Mr. J. has recently experienced blurring of vision and learned that he has type 2 diabetes. Mr. J. is concerned about how his health condition may affect his ability to continue in his current line of employment.

1. Are there issues resulting from Mr. J.'s health condition that may affect his rehabilitation potential? If so, which issues should be considered?
2. Which other factors might be important for Mr. J. to consider when developing a plan for the future?
3. Which issues in Mr. J.'s current line of employment may be important to consider?

REFERENCES

Aleppos, Grazia. (2015). Hyperthroidism overview. Retrieved from http://www.endocrineweb.com/conditions/hyperthyroidism/hyperthyroidism-overview-overactive-thyroid

American Diabetes Association (ADA). (2013a). Diagnosis and classification of diabetes mellitus. *Diabetes Care, 36*(1). Retrieved from http://www.diabetes.org/living-with-diabetes/know-your-rights/discrimination/employment-discrimination/S67-74. doi:10.2337/dc13-SO67

American Diabetes Association (ADA). (2013b). American Diabetes Association Releases New Guidelines – Retrieved from http://www.diabetes.org/newsroom/press-releases/2013/american-diabetes-association-releases-nutritional-guidelines.html

American Diabetes Association (ADA). (2013c). *Blood Glucose and Exercise*. Retrieved from http://www.diabetes.org/food-and-fitness/fitness/get-started-safely/blood-glucose-control-and-exercise.html

American Diabetes Association (ADA). (2013d). *Stress*. Retrieved from http://www.diabetes.org/living-with-diabetes/complications/mental-health/stress.html

American Diabetes Association (ADA). (2014a). *Common reasonable accommodations for individual with diabetes*. Retrieved from http://main.diabetes.org/dorg/PDFs/Advocacy/Discrimination/fact-sheet-reasonable-accommodations.pdf

American Diabetes Association (ADA). (2014b). *Sexual Implications of Emotional Health*. http://www.diabetes.org/living-with-diabetes/treatment-and-care/men/sexual-implications-emotions.html

American Diabetes Association (ADA). (2014c). *Your rights on the job*. Retrieved from http://www.diabetes.org/living-with-diabetes/know-your-rights/discrimination/employment-discrimination/your-rights-on-the-job.html

American Diabetes Association (ADA). (2015a). *DKA (Ketoacidosis) and ketones*. Retrieved from http://www.diabetes.org/living-with-diabetes/complications/ketoacidosis-dka.html

American Diabetes Association (ADA). (2015b). *Hypoglycemia (Low blood glucose)*. Retrieved from http://www.diabetes.org/living-with-diabetes/treatment-and-care/blood-glucose-control/hypoglytcemia-low-blood.html

American Diabetes Association (ADA). (2015c). Classification and diagnosis of diabetes. *Diabetes Care, 38*(1), S8–S16. doi:10.2334/dc15-S005. Retrieved from http://care.diabetesjournals.org/content/38/Supplement_1/S8.extract

American Diabetes Association (ADA). (2016a). *Statistics about diabetes*. http://www.diabetes.org/diabetes-basic/statistics

American Diabetes Association (ADA). (2016b). ADA standards of medical care in diabetes. *Journal of Clinical and Applied Research and Education, 39*(1).

American Heart Association (AHA) (2016). *Cardiovascular disease & diabetes*. Retrieved from http://www.heart.org/HEARTORG/Conditions/Diabetes/WhyDiabetesMatters/Cardiovascular-Disease-Diabetes_UCM_313865_Article.jsp#.WA-lXsldNP8

American Podiatric Medical Association (APMA). (2016). *Diabetic wound care*. Retrieved from http://www.apma.org/Learn/FootHealth.cfm?ItemNumber=981

Basak, R., Mccaffrey, D. J., Bentley, J. Pl, Przybyla, S. M., West-Strum, D., & Banahan, B. F. (2014). Adherence to multiple medications prescribed for a chronic disease: A methodological investigation. *Journal of Managed Care & Specialty Pharmacy, 20*(8), 815-825.

Bernal, J. (2015). *Thyroid hormones in brain development function*. Retrieved from http://www.thyroidmanager.org/chapter/thyroid-hormones-in-brain-development-and-function/

Brashers, V. L., Jones, R. E., & Huether, S. E. (2014a). Mechanisms of hormonal regulation. In K. L. McCance, S. E. Huether, V. L. Brashers, & N. S. Rote (Eds.), *Pathophysiology: The biologic basis for disease in adults and children* (7th ed., pp. 689–715). St. Louis MO: Elseiver-Mosby.

Brashers, V. L., Jones, R. E. & Huether, S. E. (2014b). Alterations of hormonal regulation. In K. L. McCance, S. E. Huether, V. L. Brashers, & N. S. Rote (Eds.), *Pathophysiology: The biologic basis for disease in adults and children* (7th ed., pp. 717–759). St. Louis, MO: Elseiver-Mosby.

Busko, M. (2013). *Insulin pump therapy bests injection therapy in large study*. Retrieved from http://www.medscape.com/viewarticle/809615

Cann, M. (2015). *Prevalence of discrimination in the workplace*. Retrieved from http://thebigidea.co.uk/prevalence-discrimination-workplace/

Centers for Disease Control and Prevention (CDC). (2014). Diabetes complications. http://www.cdc.gov/diabetes/statistic/complications_national.htm

Centers for Disease Control and Prevention (CDC). (2015a).*Crude and age-adjusted rates of diagnosed diabetes per 100 civilian, non-institutional population, United States 1980–2014.*

Retrieved from http://www.cdc.gov/diabetes/statistics/prev /national/figage.htm

Centers for Disease Control and Prevention (CDC). (2015b). *Diabetes and pregnancy.* Retrieved from http://www.cdc .gov/pregnancy/diabetes.html

Chon, S. & Gautier, J. F. (2016). An update on the effect of incretin-based therapies on β-cell function and mass. *Diabetes Metabolism Journal, 40*(2), 99–114.

Crandall, J. & Shamoon, H. (2016). Diabetes Mellitus. In L. Goldman & A. I. Schafer (Eds.), *Goldman-cecil medicine,* (25th ed., pp. 1527-1547). Philadelphia, PA: Elsevier Saunders.

Diabetes Control and Complications Trial Research Group. (1993). The effect of intensive treatment of diabetes on the development and progression of long-term complications in insulin-dependent diabetes mellitus. *New England Journal of Medicine, 329*(14), 977–986.

Disabled World. (2015). *Invisible disabilities: List & information.* Retrieved from http://www.disabled-world.com /disability/types/invisible/

Floyd, J. L. (2015). Thyrotoxicosis imaging. Retrieved from http://emedicine.medscape.com/article/383062-overview

Godoy-Matos, A. F. (2014). The role of glucagon on type 2 diabetes at a glance. *Journal of Negative Results in Biomedicine, 6.* doi:10.1152/phyrev.00045.2011

Gugliucci, A. (2014). *Diabetes and complications.* Warwick Medical School. Retrieved from http://www2.warwick .ac.uk/fac/med/research/tsm/mvhealth/proteindamage /physiology/diabetes

Harrar, S. (2015). Is weight loss surgery the answer for diabetes. *Endopcrineweb.* Retrieved from http;//www.endocrineweb .com/news/diabetes/15573-weight-los-surger-answer-diabetes

Hutton, J. H., & Steinburg, D. (1936). Endocrinopathies and psychoses. *British Journal of Psychiatry, 82*(341), 773–784. doi:10.1192/bjp.82.341.773

Inzucchi, S. E., & Sherwin, R. S. (2012a). Type 1 diabetes mellitus. In L. Goldman & A. I. Schafer (Eds.), *Goldman's Cecil medicine,* (24th ed., pp. 1475–1489). Philadelphia, PA: Elsevier Saunders.

Inzucchi, S. E., & Sherwin, R. S. (2012b). Type 2 diabetes mellitus. In L. Goldman & A. I. Schafer (Eds.), *Goldman's Cecil medicine,* (24th ed., pp. 1489–1499). Philadelphia, PA: Elsevier Saunders.

Kaufman, D. B. (2015). Pancreas Transplant. *Medscape.* Retrieved 4-30-16 from http://emedicine.medscape.com /article/429408-overview

Karoff, P. (2016, January). Artificial pancreas system aimed at type 1 diabetes mellitus. HARVARDgazette. Retrieved from http://news.harvard.edu/gazette/story/2016/01/artificial -pancreas-system-aimed-at-type-1-diabetes-mellitus

Kim, M., & Ladenson, P. (2016). Thyroid. In L. Goldman & A. I. Schafer (Eds.), *Goldman-Cecil Medicine,* (25th ed., pp. 1500–1514). Philadelphia, PA: Elsevier Saunders.

Leontis, L. M., & Hess-Fischl, A. (2016). Type 2 Diabetes complications. *Endocrineweb.* Retrieved from http://

www.endocrineweb.com/conditions/type-2-diabetes /type-2-diabetes-complications

Lights, V., Solan, M. & Fantauzzo, M. (2016). What is hyperthyroidism? *Healthline.* Retrieved from http://www.endocrineweb. com/conditions/type-2-diabetes/type-2-diabetes-complications

Macon, B., L. & Yu, W. (2016). Addison's Disease. *Healthline.* Retrieved from http://www.healthline.com/health /addisons-disease#Overview

Maiorino, M. I., Bellastella, G., & Esposito, K. (2014). Diabetes and sexual dysfunction: Current perspectives. *Diabetes Metabolic Syndrome Obesity, 7,* 95–105.

Mathur, R., (2015). Hypothyroidism. *MedicineNet.* Retrieved from http://www.medicinenet.com/hypothyroidism/article.htm

Mayo Clinic. (2016). *Cushing syndrome symptoms and causes.* Retrieved from http://www.mayoclinic.org/diseases-conditions /cushing-syndrome/symptoms-causes/dxc-20197177

Mayo Clinic Staff. (2016). Diabetes insipidus. Retrieved from http://www.mayoclinic.org/diseases-conditions /diabetes-insipidus/home/ovc-20182403

McAdams, B. H., & Rizvi, A. A. (2016). An overview of insulin pumps and glucose sensors for the generalist. *Journal of Clinical Medicine, 5*(5). doi:10.3390/jcm5010005

McCulloch, D. K. (2016). *Patient information: Diabetes mellitus type 1: Insulin treatment (Beyond the Basics).* Retrieved from http://www.uptodate.com/contents/diabetes-mellitus -type-1-insulin-treatment-beyond-the-basics

Mercandetti, M. (2016). Orbital Decompression for Graves. Disease *Medscape.* Retrieved from http://emedicine .medscape.com/article/878672-overview

Milas, K. (2014). Surgery of thyperthroidism. *EndocrineWeb.* Retrieved from http://www.endocrineweb.com/conditions /hyperthroidism/surgery-hyperthroidism

Miller, T. A., & DiMatteo, M. R. (2013). Importance of family /social support and impact on adherence to therapy. *Diabetic Metabolic Syndrome Obesity, 6,* 421–426.

Minz, M. (2014). Is inhaled insulin a "game changer"? *Medscape Diabetes & Endocrinology.* Retrieved from http:// www.medscape.com/viewarticle/828463

Montella, K. R. (2016). Common medical problems in pregnancy. In L. Goldman & A. I. Schafer (Eds.), *Goldman-Cecil medicine,* (25th ed., pp. 1610–1623). Philadelphia, PA: Elsevier Saunders.

Nall, R. (2016). Service dogs that can monitor their owners' diabetes. *Healthline.* http://www.healthline.com/health /type-2-diabetes/dogs#Overview1

Nathan, D. M. (2014). The diabetes control and complications trial/epidemiology of diabetes interventions and complications study at 30 years: Overview. *Diabetes Care, 37,* 9–16. doi:102337/dc13-2112

National Institute of Diabetes and Digestive and Kidney Diseases (NIDDK). (2014). *Causes of diabetes.* Retrieved from https://www.niddk.nih.gov/health-information/diabetes/causes

National Eye Institute (NEI). (2015). *National Institute of Health, National Eye Institute. Facts about diabetic eye disease.* Retrieved from https://www.nei.nih.gov/health /diabetic/retinopathy

National Institute of Diabetes and Digestive and Kidney Diseases (NIDDK). (2013). *Diabetic neuropathies: The nerve damage of diabetes.* Retrieved from https://www.niddk.nih.gov /health-information/diabetes/preventing-diabetes-problems /nerve-damage-diabetic-neuropathies

National Institute of Mental Health. (2015). Diabetes and depression. *PsychCentral.* Retrieved from http://psychcentral .com/lib/diabetes-and-depression/2/

National Kidney Foundation (NKF). (2015). *Diabetes—A major risk factor for kidney disease.* Retrieved from http://www .kidney.org/atoz/content/diabetes

Nelson, R. J. (2016). *Hormone & Behavior.* Retrieved from http://nobaproject.com/modules/hormones-behavior

Norris, J. (2013). For Type 1 Diabetes, Islet Transplantation gains momentum. *University of California.* Retrieved from https://www.ucsf.edu/news/2013/11/110271 /type-1-diabetes-islet-transplantation-gains-momentum

Pariser, G., Hager, K, Gillette, P., & Jackson, K (2014). Active steps for diabetes: A community-campus partnership addressing frailty and diabetes. *Diabetes Educator, 40*(1), 60–67. doi:10.1177/014572171314281

Sargis, R. M. (2016). About the endocrine system essentials. *EndocrineWe*b. Retrieved from http://www.endocrineweb .com/endocrinology/about-endocrine-system

Skugor, M. (2014). Diabetes mellitus treatment. *Cleveland Clinic-Disease Management.* Retrieved from http://www.clevelandclinicmeded.com/medicalpubs /diseasemanagement/endocrinology/diabetes-mellitus -treatment/Default.htm

Song, E., Xu, T-Z., Sun, Q-H. (2014). Effect of motivational interviewing on self-management in patients with type 2 diabetes mellitus: A meta-analysis. *International Journal of Nursing Sciences, 1*(3), 291–297.

U.S. Food & Drug Administration (2015). *Information regarding insulin storage and switching between products in an emergency.* Retrieved from http://www.fda.gov/Drugs /EmergencyPreparedness/ucm085213.htm

Vahist, S. K. (2013). Continuous glucose monitoring systems: A review. *Diagnostics (Basel). 3*(4), 385–412. doi: 10.3390 /diagnostics3040385 Retrieved from https://www.ncbi.nlm .nih.gov/pubmed/?term=diagnostics+(basal)++continuous +glucose+monitoring+systems%3A+A+review

World Health Organization (WHO). (2016). Diabetes programme: About diabetes. Retrieved from http://www.who .int/diabetes/action_online/basics/en/index4.html

Yeun, S-C. J., (2015). Graves disease treatment & management. *Emedicine Medscape.* Retrieved from http://emedicine .medscape.com/article/120619-treatment.

CHAPTER 24

Structure, Function, and Common Conditions of the Musculoskeletal System

THE SKELETAL SYSTEM

The skeletal system, which serves as the general framework of the body, consists of 206 bones. The largest bone in the body is the *femur* (leg bone), and the smallest are the *ossicles* in the ear. The skeletal system supports surrounding tissues and assists in movement by providing leverage and attachment for muscles (see **Figure 24-1**). It also protects vital organs, such as the heart and brain. The tough outer covering of bone is called the *periosteum*. Bones also have a network of sensory nerves and a network of tiny vessels to supply blood. Bones serve many functions other than support, movement, and protection.

Composition of Bone

Bone is a living, growing material that stores calcium and other mineral salts. New bone is constantly being produced and old bone replaced, a process called *remodeling*. The process of remodeling preserves bone mass and maintains bone strength. Remodeling takes place through the processes of *resorption* and *formation* (*ossification*). These two processes, in combination, maintain equilibrium within the body in terms of healthy bone and are important for bone restoration when a bone fracture occurs.

Resorption is a process of bone dissolution; it is counterbalanced by the process of formation, which results in new bone. The cells responsible for bone formation are stimulated by a variety of hormones—parathyroid hormone, thyroxine, and growth factors. If these processes become imbalanced so that resorption of bone exceeds formation, significant bone loss results.

In addition to providing structure to the body, bone has metabolic functions. Dietary intake and absorption of key minerals (e.g., calcium, magnesium, phosphate) are important in bone formation. The process of remodeling creates a dynamic relationship between calcium in the bone and calcium in the blood, thereby ensuring that calcium is available for a number of bodily functions, such as muscle contraction and nerve conduction.

Bone also plays an important part in formation of blood cells. Red blood cells, white blood cells, and platelets are manufactured in the red bone marrow in the bone by the process of *hematopoiesis*.

Types of Bone

Bones are classified according to their shape. Long bones are found in the arms and legs (e.g., the humerus and the femur). Short bones are found in the

Figure 24-1a   Anterior View of the Skeleton

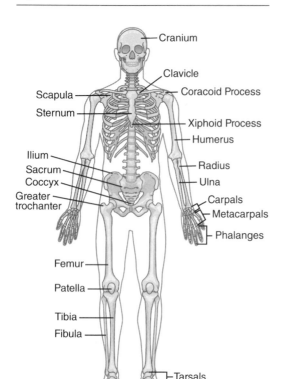

Figure 24-1b   Posterior View of the Skeleton

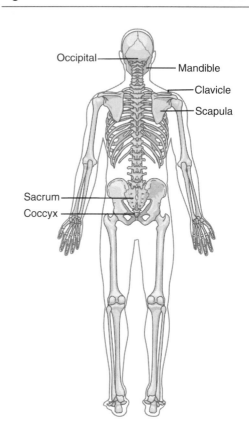

hands and feet (e.g., the carpals and the tarsal). Flat bones include those in the skull (*cranium*) and ribs, while irregular bones have differing shapes, such as those of the vertebrae and *mandible* (jaw bone).

The *vertebrae* (a series of irregular bones that surround the spinal cord) support the head and trunk of the body, protect the spinal cord, and enable bending and flexing. The 7 vertebrae at the neck and upper back are called *cervicalvertebrae*. The 12 vertebrae that extend from the upper to lower back are called *thoracic vertebrae*. In the lower back, there are 5 *lumbar vertebrae*; a bony prominence called the *sacrum*, which consists of fused bone; and the *coccyx,* or small residual "tail bone," which extends from the end of the sacrum.

Connective Tissue

Connective tissue supports and (as its name implies) connects other tissues and tissue parts. Ligaments, tendons, and cartilage are examples of connective

tissue. *Ligaments* are tough bands of fiber that connect bones at the joint site and provide stability during movement. *Tendons* are bands of tissue that connect muscle to bone, enabling muscle movement. *Cartilage* is a dense type of connective tissue that creates form, maintains structure, and can withstand considerable tension. Several different types of cartilage exist. Cartilage is found between the vertebral disks of the spine and in the joint of the knee to absorb shock and prevent friction. In addition, the cartilage in the external ear and nose provides form to these structures.

Another type of connective tissue is called a *bursa*. This small sac of tissue is lined with a *synovial membrane* that secretes *synovial fluid*. Bursae are commonly located between tendons and bones, tendons and tendons, or bones and skin; they help decrease friction and relieve pressure where two surfaces rub together.

Vertebrae are connected by ligaments. Between the vertebrae, which surround the spinal cord, are disks of cartilage (*intervertebral disks*) that cushion the spinal cord against shock. The tough, fibrous outer portion of the disk is called the *annulus,* and the spongy inner portion is called the *nucleus pulposus.*

Joints

A *joint* is a place where two or more bones are bound together. The coming together of two bones at a joint is called **articulation**. Some joints, such as those in the skull, *are fibrous* (fixed), meaning that they provide no movement. Other joints, such as the *pubis symphysis* (pubic bone) in the pelvis, are *cartilaginous* (contain cartilage) and provide slight movement.

Synovial joints, which account for most of the joints of the body, are freely movable, enabling both motion and change of position. These joints are surrounded by an *articular capsule,* which encloses two bone ends. The capsule is composed of connective tissue, reinforced by ligaments, and continuous with the periosteum. The inner layer of the articular capsule is lined with a synovial membrane that secretes synovial fluid. Synovial fluid acts like a lubricant to facilitate joint movement and helps cushion the joint against the shock produced by joint movement. *Articular cartilage,* which lines the end of each bone, absorbs shock, and receives its nourishment from the synovial fluid (see **Figure 24-2**).

Figure 24-2   A Synovial Joint

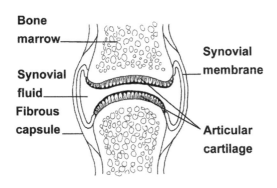

Bone marrow

Synovial fluid

Fibrous capsule

Synovial membrane

Articular cartilage

© Jane Tinkler Lamm.

Joint Movements

Synovial joints are capable of many types of movements (see **Figure 24-3**):

- **Circumduction**: circular movement
- **Eversion**: movement in which a body part is turned outward
- **Inversion**: movement in which a body part is turned inward
- **Flexion**: bending movement
- **Extension**: straightening movement
- **Abduction**: movement of a body part away from the midline of the body
- **Adduction**: movement of a body part toward the midline of the body
- **Ulnar deviation**: lateral movement of the hand away from the body
- **Radial deviation**: lateral movement of the hand inward, toward the body
- **Pronation**: turning movement of a body part downward
- **Supination**: turning movement of a body part upward
- **Dorsiflexion**: backward movement of a body part

The type of motion of a particular synovial joint depends on the type of joint:

- *Circular motion* is provided by ball-and-socket joints, such as those in the hip and shoulder.
- *Back-and-forth motion* is provided by hinge joints, such as those in the elbow and knee.
- *Gliding motion* is provided by joints of the vertebrae.
- *Pivotal motion* is provided by vertebrae that connect the head and the spine.

THE MUSCULAR SYSTEM

Several types of muscles are found in the body. *Involuntary muscles* work automatically, such as the cardiac muscle (**myocardium**) of the heart and the *smooth muscle* found in the digestive tract. In contrast, *striated* (skeletal muscle), which makes up 40% to 50% of an individual's body weight, is under *voluntary* control.

A *muscle sheath* (a hard band of connective tissue) contains blood vessels and nerve fibers and surrounds every muscle. Each of the two ends of

Figure 24-3   Movement of Synovial Joints

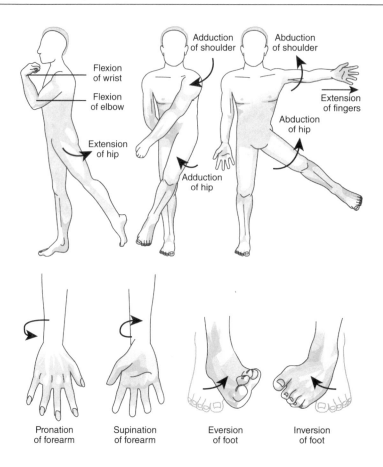

the muscle is attached to a different bone. The muscle attachment closer to the midline of the body is called the *origin* of the muscle, while the attachment of the end farther from the midline of the body is called the *insertion.*

Muscles produce movement through the contraction of opposite muscle groups. They are classified by their function:

- **Flexors**: muscles that bend a limb
- **Extensors**: muscles that straighten a limb
- **Abductors**: muscles that move a limb laterally, away from the body
- **Adductors**: muscles that move a limb closer to the body
- **Dorsiflexors**: muscles that bend a body part backward

Because of the continuous nerve stimulation of muscle, muscles maintain a partial state of contraction (tone) even at rest, when they are not being used.

CONDITIONS OF THE MUSCULOSKELETAL SYSTEM DUE TO INJURY

Fractures

Bone fractures result in pain and immobility. Depending on which bone is fractured and which type of fracture occurs, functional capacity may be altered either temporarily or, in some cases, permanently. Individuals with chronic conditions may be especially vulnerable to fractures if immobility associated with their condition increases demineralization of bone or because of physiological processes involved in the condition itself, such as in osteoporosis and certain types of cancer (Weber, 2016).

Types of Fractures

Any break or disruption in the continuity of bone is termed *a fracture*. Several types of fractures are distinguished, with varying levels of severity (see **Figure 24-4**):

- *Closed (simple) fracture* is an uncomplicated break in a bone with no breaking of skin.
- *Open (compound) fracture* is a break in a bone in which the skin is broken so that the bone protrudes through it.
- *Complete fracture* is a break in a bone that extends through the bone from one side to the other, including the periosteum (outer cover of the bone).
- *Incomplete (partial) fracture* is a break that does not extend all the way through the bone.

- *Transverse fracture* is a fracture that extends straight across the bone.
  - *Oblique fracture* is a fracture across the bone at a slant angle.
  - *Spiral fracture* occurs in a spiral around the bone and is usually caused by a twisting injury.
  - *Impacted fracture* is a break in which one portion of the bone is impacted, or forcibly driven, into another portion of the bone.
  - *Comminuted fracture* is a break in which the bone has been shattered, leaving fragments of bone at the site of the break.
  - *Displaced fracture* refers to a break in a bone in which the two ends of the bone are separated.

Figure 24-4   Types of Fractures

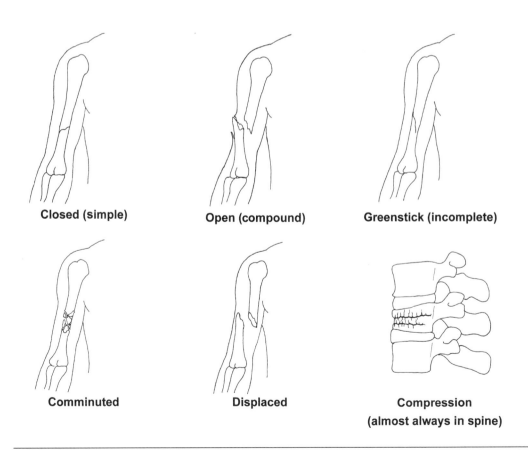

Closed (simple)   **Open (compound)**   **Greenstick (incomplete)**

Comminuted   **Displaced**   **Compression (almost always in spine)**

* *Complicated fracture* refers to a break in a bone in which the tissue surrounding the bone, such as blood vessels and nerves, is also injured.
* *Compression fracture* refers to a break in which the ends of the bones are pressed against each other. Compression fractures often occur in the vertebrae.
* *Pathologic fracture* refers to a break in a bone owing to changes in the bone that are associated with another condition.
* *Colles' fracture* refers to a break in a bone near the wrist.
* *Stress fracture* is a small break in a bone that occurs as the result of prolonged or unaccustomed activity.

Management of Fractures

Some fractures may be managed by *closed reduction,* a procedure in which bone fragments are realigned manually, without surgery, and immobilized with a plaster cast. Other fractures must be treated by *open reduction,* a procedure in which bone fragments are realigned and stabilized surgically. *Traction* may be used in combination with either closed or open reduction.

Many fractures heal well and result in no permanent functional incapacity. However, complications can occur, leading to significant impact on functional capacity. For example, bone edges or fragments of a compound, displaced, or comminuted fracture may injure tissue or nerves in the surrounding area, causing permanent damage. In fractures of large bones, such as the femur, blood loss can be significant. Open or compound fractures can become infected, leading to **osteomyelitis** (infection of the bone). When an individual with a chronic condition fractures a bone that affects mobility, there may be greater risk of complications related to immobility.

Dislocation

Displacement or separation of a bone from its regular joint position is called a **dislocation**. If the bone is not totally separated from the joint, the condition is called a **subluxation**. In addition to causing extreme pain, a dislocation causes a partial loss of movement at the joint and can impede blood supply to the surrounding tissue.

Dislocations can result either from trauma or from a congenital weakness or irregularity of the joint that predisposes it to dislocation. The shoulder and the hip are common sites of dislocation, although any joint can become dislocated.

Prompt intervention to correct joint dislocation is important to prevent complications, such as nerve damage or injury due to the decreased blood supply. The bones can usually be slipped back into place manually. If no damage has occurred to the nerves, blood vessels, or surrounding tissue, the injury does not usually have any permanent functional consequences. If dislocations recur in the same joint, however, individuals may need to avoid movements that precipitate the dislocation. When dislocation recurs frequently, surgical fixation of the joint may be necessary.

Contusions

Musculoskeletal injuries may not always involve bone; sometimes the injury involves underlying structures, such as the soft tissue under the skin. A **contusion** is a soft-tissue injury that results from a blunt, diffuse blow. Although the skin is not usually pierced and no bones are broken, local hemorrhage with associated bruising, swelling, and damage to the deep soft tissue under the skin occurs. Bleeding under the skin is responsible for the purplish discoloration at the site of injury—the bruise (**ecchymosis**). When a major vessel or a muscle is injured, a **hematoma** (a sac filled with accumulated blood) may develop under the skin.

Strains and Sprains

Although the terms *strain* and *sprain* are often used interchangeably by the general public, they actually refer to two different types of injuries. A **strain** is an overstretching or overuse of tendons and muscles, while a **sprain** is an injury or overstress of a ligament and its attachment site.

Strains may be acute, resulting from a sudden twisting or wrenching movement, or they may occur with unaccustomed vigorous exercise. Chronic strain may be the result of repetitive muscle overuse. Strains may be managed with analgesics, muscle relaxants, or anti-inflammatory drugs. One goal of intervention is to increase muscle strengthening. Consequently, immobilization is usually not recommended.

Sprains are categorized as mild, moderate, or severe (first-, second-, or third-degree sprains). First- and second-degree sprains are usually managed with analgesics, anti-inflammatory agents, or muscle relaxants. Management of second-degree sprains may also include immobilization of the injured joint and therapeutic exercises and physical therapy to promote an early return to motion. A severe sprain can tear a ligament completely from its attachment and may require surgical repair. Most sprains heal spontaneously with rest and support of the body part affected (Biundo, 2016).

Lacerations

Any injury that results in a tear or cut to the skin and underlying tissues is referred to as a **laceration**. *Puncture* and *penetration* injuries (such as a stabbing injury or gunshot wound) generally have a small entrance wound but cause extensive damage to tissues under the skin.

The degree of functional consequence experienced with lacerations, puncture wounds, or penetration wounds depends on the injury's location; the amount of damage to the underlying tissues, such as nerves, blood vessels, and internal organs; and any associated complications, such as infection. The risk of infection depends on the source and circumstances of the injury.

Bursitis, Tendonitis, and Tenosynovitis

Bursa can become inflamed with trauma or from overuse, or it can become infected, (**bursitis**), causing swelling and pain of the bursa (Biundo, 2016). Although any synovial joint may be affected, it commonly occurs in the shoulder, elbow, wrist or hand, hip, or knee. Acute episodes of bursitis may last for days to weeks and may recur. Management usually consists of splinting and rest of the joint, and/or nonsteroidal anti-inflammatory drugs (NSAIDS) (Biundo, 2016).

The term **tendinitis** describes a condition characterized by an inflammation of a *tendon*. The term **tenosynovitis** describes a condition in which the *sheath of tissue* that surrounds the tendon becomes inflamed. The two conditions usually occur simultaneously. Conditions involving the tendons frequently result from overuse, such as when a tendon repeatedly bears more of a load than it can withstand (Biundo, 2016). Although the exact cause is unknown, tendinitis may be associated with trauma, strain, or unaccustomed exercise. Its primary manifestation is pain on motion at the site of inflammation. Tendinitis usually subsides with appropriate management, although surgery may be indicated on rare occasions.

Carpal Tunnel Syndrome

Nerves (including the *median, ulnar,* and *radial* nerves) travel from the spinal cord to innervate the hands. These nerves are contained in small "tunnels" that may become narrowed, compressing the nerves. *Carpal tunnel syndrome* is a condition in which there is compression of the *median nerve* in the wrist, causing pain and **paresthesia** (a tingling, pricking sensation) in the hand. This condition is classified as a *compression* or *entrapment neuropathy* (Gillig, White, & Rachel, 2016).

Carpal tunnel syndrome can be associated with various autoimmune conditions, such as rheumatoid arthritis; metabolic conditions, such as diabetes; heredity conditions; or obesity. Activities involving rapid repetitive movement of the hands with few rest periods, or awkward or forceful movements, may contribute to the development of carpal tunnel syndrome or to a different condition called *repetitive-strain injury* (Gillig et al., 2016).

Confirmation of carpal tunnel syndrome is made through positive findings on physical examination and nerve conduction studies that indicate median nerve damage irregularities (Shy, 2016).

Manifestations of Carpal Tunnel Syndrome

With carpal tunnel syndrome, muscle strength in the hand may be weakened to such an extent that opening jars or twisting lids becomes difficult. Dull and aching pain may be present, or pain may radiate into the forearm. Individuals may complain of waking at night because the affected hand is numb.

They may also complain of numbness in the hands in the morning, feeling they have to shake their hands to get the circulation back. Manifestations may be mild and acute, or chronic.

Management of Carpal Tunnel Syndrome

In mild cases of carpal tunnel syndrome, wearing a wrist splint at night may be sufficient to relieve manifestations, along with medications such as NSAIDs (Shy, 2016). If the splint does not interfere with activity, individuals may also wear it or another type of wrist support during the day. Corticosteroids are sometimes injected into the area if the splint is unsuccessful at relieving manifestations; however, any improvement may be only temporary. If the hand becomes weakened or manifestations become intolerable, surgery to relieve pressure on the nerve may be indicated (Shy, 2016).

Vocational Issues in Carpal Tunnel Syndrome

Repetition, force, and posture are risk factors that can contribute to the development of carpal tunnel syndrome, although other factors, such as diabetes, arthritis, and obesity, may pose greater risk for its development (Shy, 2016).

Carpal tunnel syndrome can become severe enough to limit individuals' ability to work. It can be of particular concern to individuals who rely on sign language as a major form of communication. With continued exposure to risk factors without adequate care or rest, permanent damage to the soft tissue and nerves can result.

When carpal tunnel syndrome is related to activity, both the nature of the work and the amount of time spent on a task contribute to the potential for injury. For individuals with carpal tunnel syndrome aggravated by work-related activity, the factors in the work environment may need to be modified. For example, office workers using computer keyboards may need to take periodic rest breaks throughout the day. Ergonomic modifications such as forearm support, adjusting the height of the keyboard, or positioning the hands differently may be indicated. Assuming different body positions and using good posture may help reduce muscle fatigue and prevent exacerbation of manifestations of carpal tunnel syndrome.

CONDITIONS OF THE MUSCULOSKELETAL SYSTEM DUE TO BONE OR JOINT DEGENERATION

Osteoporosis

Osteoporosis is a metabolic condition in which the bone mass is reduced, causing bones to become weakened, fragile, and susceptible to fracture (Weber, 2016). In some instances, even in the absence of bone fracture, individuals may experience aching in various bones and often have chronic backache. Vertebral fractures—a serious consequence of osteoporosis—can lead to acute and chronic back pain as well as structural irregularity of the spine (Weber, 2016).

Individuals with osteoporosis commonly have no manifestations until a bone is broken as a result of minimal or no trauma. Frequent sites of bone fractures include the hips, especially in older or frail individuals, and the wrist (*Colles' fracture*). Crush or compression fractures may occur in the vertebrae (**Figure 24-4**).

Risks for Osteoporosis

Osteoporosis commonly occurs in individuals after middle age. Nevertheless, *secondary osteoporosis* may occur as a result of a number of other chronic conditions, including endocrine disorders, cancer, nutritional and gastrointestinal disorders, disorders of the blood, side effects of some medications, or overuse of alcohol (Weber, 2016). Individuals with chronic conditions in which they are nonambulatory or with conditions that require immobilization are also at higher risk of developing osteoporosis (Weber, 2016).

Management of Osteoporosis

Osteoporosis is a progressive condition, but appropriate interventions may slow the deterioration process. Prevention is a key component in management of osteoporosis. Prevention strategies include daily intake of adequate amounts of dietary calcium; weight-bearing exercise throughout life; avoidance of long-term use of steroid medications, which promote bone loss; and avoidance of falls (Weber, 2016).

When osteoporosis does occur, analgesics, heat, or rest can be used for relief of pain. In some instances, braces or splints may be used to provide support and stability. Individuals may find that exercise to strengthen muscles, which provides additional support, is beneficial. Although maintaining some level of physical activity is recommended, heavy lifting or any activity that increases the risk of falls should be avoided.

Pharmacologic interventions such as bisphosphonates and calcium supplements, supplemental vitamin D, or in some cases, for women, hormonal supplements may be used in management of osteoporosis (Weber, 2016).

Osteoarthritis

Osteoarthritis is a local joint condition characterized by joint pain and functional loss. Although some inflammation of the joint may be present, it is not associate with systemic inflammation such as is rheumatoid arthritis. Although repeated trauma or stress to a join can predispose individuals to developing osteoarthritis, the prevalence of osteoarthritis increases substantially with aging, and also obesity (Block & Scanzello, 2016). Although any joint may be involved, joints in the knees, hips, and hands, are most frequently affected (Block & Scanzello, 2016).

Because osteoarthritis is not a systemic condition, manifestations occur only around the affected joint. Bone spurs (**osteophytes**) may develop on the surface of the joints, eroding the cartilage so that it can no longer serve as a cushion or shock absorber. Consequently, ends of the bones at the joint rub against each other, causing pain and inflammation. Weight-bearing joints, such as the knees, hips, and spine, are frequently affected. In addition, finger joints are often involved. When osteoarthritis affects the knees or hips, it may interfere with mobility.

Osteoarthritis is generally unremitting. Overuse of the affected joints, exposure to cold and damp weather, and many other factors may intensify manifestations. Functional consequences of osteoarthritis depend on the type and magnitude of joint damage, the number of joints involved, the particular joints involved, and the daily activity of the individual.

Management of Osteoarthritis

Management of osteoarthritis is directed toward increasing function and preventing further immobility and discomfort. Specific exercises, including range-of-motion and strengthening exercises, are often part of the management plan to meet this goal. It may be necessary to balance resting of the joint with its use.

The use of assistive devices, such as canes or crutches, may prevent undue weight bearing on joints. If individuals with osteoarthritis are obese, weight reduction may help to remove undue pressure on the joints. Oral administration of aspirin or NSAIDs, as well as injection of steroids into the joint, may also be implemented. In cases of severe joint damage, total joint **arthroplasty** (joint replacement) can help to restore many individuals to pain-free functional independence (Mackenzie & Su, 2016).

Vocational Issues in Osteoarthritis

Osteoarthritis can have a long-term effect on function, although the degree to which it affects function depends on the specific joints affected. Individuals with osteoarthritis of the knees, for instance, may be unable to walk long distances or stand for long periods of time. They may also have difficulty with bending or stooping. Individuals with osteoarthritis of the upper extremities or vertebrae of the spine may have difficulty lifting, turning, and reaching. When fingers are affected, individuals may be unable to perform tasks that require significant motion of the hands.

BACK PAIN AND RELATED CONDITIONS

Back pain can be caused by a variety of conditions, most of which are mechanical, emanating from the spine's structural elements (Barbano, 2016) (see **Table 24-1**). It can produce a number of manifestations in addition to pain, depending on its location. Because of the subjective nature of pain and the different meaning of pain to different individuals, identification of the cause of back pain and the most appropriate form of management may be difficult. Although muscle strain is frequently identified as a cause of back

Table 24-1   Causes of Back Pain

Cause	Example
Degenerative conditions	**Osteoarthritis**
Congenital conditions	Spinal stenosis
Structural irregularity	Scoliosis
Muscle conditions	Spasm
Metabolic conditions	Osteoporosis
Injury	Compression fractures of vertebrae, muscle trauma
Cancer	Tumor, multiple myeloma, metastasis
Inflammatory conditions	Ankylosing spondylitis, rheumatoid arthritis
Infection	Meningitis
Referred pain (pain experienced in Aneurysm of the aorta, conditions involving the back but caused by another source)	Abdominal organs
Psychological causes	Anxiety, malingering

pain, underlying conditions of the spine may also be responsible for this manifestation (Barbano, 2016). It is important that the cause of back pain be established so that appropriate interventions can be implemented.

Back pain is classified as mild, moderate, or severe. Given that pain is a subjective measure, the extent of impaired function associated with back pain is often an indicator of the severity.

Types of Back Pain

Low Back Pain

Low back pain is one of the most common health-related conditions experienced. It is defined as pain in the lumbar or sacral region of the lower back. It may be experienced in the erect, non-moving spine (*static pain*) or during movement (*kinetic pain*). Low back pain may result from any of the following causes:

- Mechanical problems due to poor posture, such as **lordosis** (swayback posture)
- Poor body mechanics at work, causing sprain or strain
- Injury due to falls, motor vehicle accidents, or sports
- **Spondylolisthesis** (forward slippage of a vertebrae)

- **Spondylolysis** (breakdown or degeneration of a vertebrae)
- Arthritis or osteoporosis
- Infection of the bones of the spine or tissue between vertebrae
- Tumors in the spine, or metastasis of cancer originating outside the spine
- Herniation of an intervertebral disk
- *Referred pain* from other organs of the body, such as the kidneys or uterus

Back pain may be accompanied by sciatica, or it may occur alone. **Sciatica** is a syndrome of pain that radiates from the lower back into the hip and down the leg. It may be accompanied by numbness, tingling, and muscle weakness. Sciatica can accompany a number of conditions of the lower back, with herniated disk being the most common.

Chronic Back Pain

Low back pain persisting for 6 months or longer is considered *chronic back pain*. Chronic back pain may be an extension of manifestations due to injury or may result from osteoporosis, *degenerative spondylolisthesis* (discussed later in this section), or a narrowing (**stenosis**) of the spinal canal, which can be either congenital or acquired (Alleva, Hudgins, Belous, & Kristin Origenes, 2016).

Specific Conditions Contributing to Back Pain

Herniated or Ruptured Disk (Herniated Nucleus Pulposus)

Rupture of the soft, inner portion of the intervertebral disk (*nucleus pulposus*) through a tear in the tougher outer portion of the disk (annulus) is called a herniation (**Figure 24-5**). A sprain or strain of the back or any condition that weakens the annulus may cause herniation of a disk. This condition results in back pain, often accompanied by spasms of the back muscles. Protrusion of the herniated disk exerts pressure on the nerves that surround the area. Pressure on the nerves can cause a partial loss of sensation or weakness in lower extremities. In severe cases, pressure on the nerves can cause problems with bowel or bladder function.

Pain experienced with a herniated disk is frequently exacerbated by straining, coughing, or lifting. Manifestations may be intermittent at first but later progress to continuous pain or loss of sensation. Physical therapy and the use of anti-inflammatory medication may help to manage or eliminate pain. When surgical intervention for herniated disk is necessary, **diskectomy** (removal of the disk) and/or spinal fusion may be required (Deyo & Mirza, 2016).

Spondylolisthesis

Spondylolisthesis is characterized by slippage of a vertebral body into the one below it. This condition is associated with degeneration and narrowing of the involved disk. The major manifestation is back pain, especially with bending, lifting, or twisting. Individuals may also complain of leg pain or may have neurologic signs.

One intervention that may be part of the management plan is flexion exercises. Some individuals find corset support to be helpful. In addition,

Figure 24-5   Vertebral Herniation

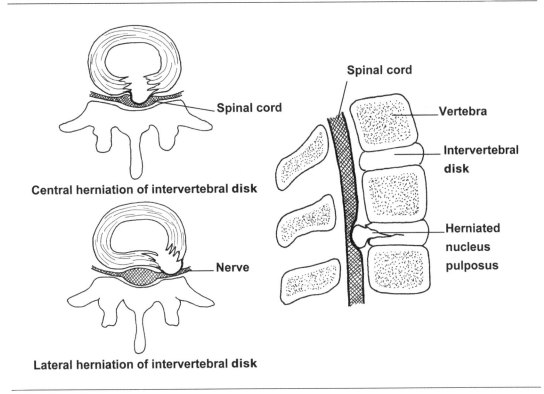

Central herniation of intervertebral disk

Lateral herniation of intervertebral disk

Spinal cord

Nerve

Spinal cord

Vertebra

Intervertebral disk

Herniated nucleus pulposus

NSAIDs may be utilized as part of the management plan. The most important measures are lifestyle changes such as avoidance of repetitive bending, heavy lifting, or twisting of the trunk of the body. *Spinal fusion surgery* (spinal **arthrodesis**), in which two disks are fused, may also be necessary for management of instability and structural irregularity of the disk.

Scoliosis

Scoliosis is a lateral, S-shaped curvature of the spine (see **Figure 24-6**), which can be either **congenital** (present at birth) or a complication of amputation or another condition that alters posture, such as poliomyelitis or cerebral palsy. Scoliosis can be corrected with early recognition and proper intervention. If the spinal irregularity becomes fixed, however, the condition is difficult to reverse. In severe cases, scoliosis can diminish respiratory capacity and can cause pressure on organs in the thoracic or abdominal cavity, thereby interfering with organ function.

Identification of Back Pain

The cause of back pain is identified through history of manifestations, observation of individuals in various body postures and activities, and physical examination. Although X-rays can be helpful in identifying bony irregularities of the spine, other conditions—such as ruptured disk, for example—may not be seen on a regular X-ray. Other tests may involve *electromyography (EMG),* which

Figure 24-6   Scoliosis

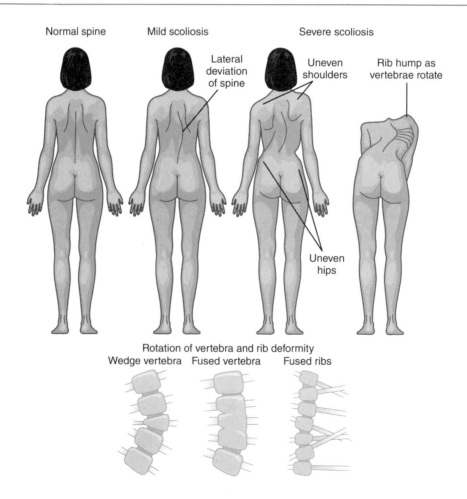

provides information about nerve function and nerve damage. *Computerized tomography (CT)* scan or *magnetic resonance imaging (MRI)* may also be used for identification of disk degeneration or ruptured disk.

Management of Back Pain

Exercise is an important part of both prevention and management of back pain. Interventions for back pain often involve controlled physical activity, medications such as NSAIDs, and muscle relaxants (Borenstein & Balagué, 2012). Maintaining activity is dependent on the demands of the individual's regular activities, such as the need for heavy lifting. Individuals are usually encouraged to maintain physical activities as tolerated.

Chronic back pain may be managed either nonsurgically or surgically. Management interventions for chronic back pain may include exercise, biofeedback, stress management, and medications such as muscle relaxants or steroids to reduce inflammation and nonnarcotic analgesics to reduce pain. The surgical intervention employed varies, depending on the cause of the pain.

Preventive measures, such as *conditioning of the muscles* of the back or use of *proper body mechanics*, are interventions that can help individuals avoid recurrences. Unfortunately, maintaining adherence to specific exercise routines after manifestations have subsided may be difficult. Although most back pain subsides spontaneously, overreaction to the condition can result in drug-seeking behavior, which can precipitate a more serious consequence of substance dependency.

Vocational Issues in Back Pain

Acute back pain caused by strain or sprain may significantly impair function for a period lasting from days to weeks. Pain is precipitated by repeated twisting or lifting, prolonged sitting, or operating vibrating equipment. Individuals may have difficulty standing erect and may need to change position frequently. Many individuals with acute back pain are able to return to work within 6 weeks (Deyo & Mirza, 2016).

Prevention is the best way to reduce back injury. Education about good body mechanics and conditioning can help to reduce the chance of further injury. Individuals who are the least physically active are more likely to have acute lower back injury; consequently, exercises that increase strength and muscle tone can help prevent injury. Modification of the workplace to reduce mechanical stresses may also be important to decrease both the frequency and the cost of lower back injuries.

Individuals whose jobs require lifting or heavy physical work may need mechanical assistance devices or tables to allow lifting from the waist. Regular rest breaks may be needed as well as instruction regarding good lifting techniques. Ergonomics review of the workstation and equipment can help assure that individuals are sitting and moving in ways that reduce the risk of strain. As much as possible, any equipment that causes whole-body vibration should be modified to reduce the amount of vibration. Individuals using equipment with significant vibration should schedule frequent rest periods or should rotate among workstations so that they also perform less strenuous tasks.

OTHER CONDITIONS OF THE MUSCULOSKELETAL SYSTEM

Osteomyelitis

Osteomyelitis is a bacterial infection of the bone that ultimately causes bone destruction, and is common in individuals with diabetes and peripheral neuropathy and those with vascular insufficiency (Matteson & Osmon, 2016). In these instances, bacteria from an ulceration, often on the foot, infect underlying bone. In other instances, bacteria from an infection in another part of the body enter the blood (**bacteremia**) and infect a bone at a different location. In still other instances, bacteria may enter the bone directly through an injury, such as an open or compound fracture in which the broken bone fragment has penetrated the skin, allowing pathologic organisms to enter and invade the bone.

Manifestations of Osteomyelitis

Osteomyelitis can be acute, but more often becomes chronic, requiring ongoing management. Manifestations usually involve localized pain over the affected bone and sometimes swelling (**edema**) and reddening (**erythema**).

Management of Osteomyelitis

Osteomyelitis is often difficult to cure. Interventions for its management may be either nonsurgical or surgical. Nonsurgical interventions consist of the administration of antibiotics and bed rest until the infection has been eradicated. Surgical interventions may be indicated to remove infected tissue, replace a portion of bone with a graft, or replace an infected prosthetic joint. In some instances, amputation may be indicated (Matteson & Osmon, 2016).

Fibromyalgia

Fibromyalgia is a condition in which individuals experience chronic, widespread pain, which is thought to be due from abnormal sensory processing with in the central nervous system, referred to as *central sensitization* (Bennett, 2016)

Manifestations of Fibromyalgia

Widespread pain and stiffness are the key manifestations of fibromyalgia. Discomfort associated with fibromyalgia is diffuse, involving the neck, shoulders, lower back, and hips, as well as other sites. Fibromyalgia is not a progressively degenerative condition and does not cause damage to bones or joints. Manifestations often also involve easy fatigability from activity as well as sleep disturbances, such that even with hours of sleep the individual remains tired. Due to chronic pain for which there seems to be no cure, many individuals with fibromyalgia also experience depression (Bennett, 2016).

Identification of Fibromyalgia

There are no definitive laboratory or radiographic tests available to definitively identify fibromyalgia. Thus identification is based on individuals' self-reports of history and types of manifestations, with the presence of pain being noted in at least 11 out of 18 specific points on the body when manually palpated (Bennett, 2016).

Management of Fibromyalgia

Management of fibromyalgia manifestations involves a comprehensive team approach, as well as helping the individual gain self-management skills. Medications such as antidepressants, anticonvulsants, and sedatives are sometimes used in management of manifestations. Psychosocial interventions, which assist individuals in improving internal locus of control and problem solving as well as cognitive-behavioral therapy and deconditioning, may also be useful (Bennett, 2016).

If individuals are experiencing stress or have other underlying psychological factors that exacerbate sleep disturbances or pain perception, then stress management, relaxation, or counseling may be needed to help them cope with the condition. Some individuals also find support groups useful. It is important that individuals remain physically and socially active, and efforts should be made to identify and eliminate stresses or environmental disturbances that may exacerbate manifestations.

Psychosocial Issues in Fibromyalgia

Psychological manifestations of anxiety and depression frequently accompany fibromyalgia. Adjustment to the manifestations of this chronic condition may be more difficult due to the uncertainty associated with it. Fibromyalgia can interfere with individuals' quality of life and may cause interpersonal difficulties when manifestations occur. Individuals often find it helpful to be reassured that the condition is "real." Legitimizing individuals' experience of manifestations can help reestablish self-control and self-esteem, enabling them to cope with their condition.

Vocational Issues in Fibromyalgia

Individuals with fibromyalgia may have repeated absenteeism at work because of pain, fatigue, or both. The direct effect on individuals' ability to work depends on a number of factors, including the nature of the job, the person's motivation to follow suggested lifestyle changes, and the presence of any underlying psychological factors.

Many individuals with fibromyalgia must learn how to pace themselves, as certain physical activities may take longer than before the condition arose. Very active individuals may have to cut back on activities. Individuals should be encouraged to remain active but not to push themselves beyond their limit.

Flexibility in scheduling may be beneficial as well. Some job modification and restructuring may be necessary to prevent overuse or overexertion of muscle groups. Any physical stressors identified should also be avoided. Because sleep disturbance is an accompanying manifestation, individuals may have difficulty concentrating while at work. Because of the vague nature of manifestations and the lack of a definitive test with which to identify fibromyalgia, individuals may be subject to the scrutiny of coworkers or employers, who may question the legitimacy of their condition and its manifestations. Individuals may be labeled as malingerers, and resentment from coworkers may result. Education of employers and coworkers can help to dispel myths and misinformation.

GENERAL MANAGEMENT OF CONDITIONS OF THE MUSCULOSKELETAL SYSTEM

Medications

Pain and inflammation are manifestations of many musculoskeletal and connective tissue conditions. *Salicylates* (e.g., aspirin) are commonly used to reduce pain and inflammation. *Nonsteroidal anti-inflammatory drugs* may also be used to reduce the pain and inflammation associated with musculoskeletal conditions. Both salicylates and NSAIDs can irritate the stomach lining, causing pain and, in some instances, bleeding if used in large amounts.

Corticosteroids can produce dramatic short-term anti-inflammatory effects, but they do not prevent progression of joint destruction and, because of their potency and subsequent side effects, can be used only on a short-term basis. Side effects of prolonged steroid use may include cataracts, demineralization of bone, delayed wound healing, poor resistance to infection, and manifestations similar to those observed with Cushing's syndrome (see the "Diabetes and Other Conditions of the Endocrine System" chapter). More serious systemic effects may involve severe adrenal insufficiency following withdrawal. Steroid use should always be carefully monitored, and these medications should never be discontinued suddenly. Although steroids for musculoskeletal conditions are generally taken

orally, they are sometimes injected directly into an inflamed joint for the temporary suppression of the inflammation.

Hyperbaric Oxygen Therapy

Hyperbaric oxygen therapy is an intervention in which 100% oxygen is given at two to three times the atmospheric pressure at sea level while the individual is in a special chamber called a pressure chamber. Hyperbaric oxygen therapy is used for a number of conditions, such as carbon monoxide poisoning and decompression sickness, but it has also been used in combination with other interventions for some conditions of the musculoskeletal system such as osteomyelitis (Yu et al., 2011) and foot and leg ulcers associated with diabetes (Goldman, 2009).

Hyperbaric oxygen therapy enhances the body's defenses against infection and promotes healing. Hyperbaric chambers are not available at all healthcare facilities, however.

Physical Therapy

Physical therapy is an intervention used in many types of musculoskeletal conditions to develop, restore, or preserve physical function. The type of physical therapy used depends on the particular musculoskeletal condition. Physical therapy may be directed toward increasing or maintaining a joint's range of motion, increasing muscle strength, preventing **atrophy** (shrinking of the muscles), relieving pain or muscle spasms, or teaching techniques for ambulation.

Some physical therapy interventions involve therapeutic exercise, which may be either passive or active. In **passive exercise**, the physical therapist or a mechanical device exercises the body part. In **active exercise**, the individual independently performs a specified exercise protocol under the direction or supervision of the physical therapist or physical therapy assistant.

Other physical therapy interventions may involve application of heat or cold or the massage of muscles for relaxation or relief of pain. Heat may be applied through hot packs, hot soaks, infrared radiation, or whirlpool baths. Another procedure for applying heat is *diathermy*, a process in which the temperature of the body part is raised through high-frequency ultrasonic waves. Because cold has a numbing effect, it may also be used to relieve pain; that is, cold packs or chemical packs may be applied to the painful area. *Massage*—the manipulation of muscles through rubbing or kneading—may be used to relax muscles, improve muscle tone, relieve muscle spasm, or increase blood flow to the area.

Casts

Another intervention used in the management of a variety of musculoskeletal conditions is casting. Although casts may be synthetic, they are more commonly made of plaster of Paris. Casts provide immobilization and support for a body part while it is healing. They may also be used to prevent or correct various musculoskeletal irregularities. The type and size of cast depend on the condition and the purpose of the casting. In addition to casts used on extremities, *spica casts*, which extend over the entire length of the lower extremity from the middle of the trunk of the body, may be used. In some instances, a full body cast is necessary.

Assistive Devices

Individuals with musculoskeletal conditions may use assistive devices to aid in ambulation, prevent undue strain on a body part, or restore or enhance functional capacity. Assistive devices may be used therapeutically in the healing period after musculoskeletal injury, or they may be used on a continuing basis. Examples of assistive devices that aid in ambulation or prevent excessive weight bearing on a lower extremity include canes, crutches, and walkers.

Orthosis

Devices used to straighten or correct an irregularity of a body part (**orthosis**) are applied to the body to control the motion of joints and the force or weight distribution to a body part. A brace, for example, is an orthotic device used to provide support or to prevent or correct an irregularity. The type of device used depends on the purpose of the bracing and the condition itself. An *orthotist* is an individual who constructs orthotic devices to meet individual needs.

Orthoses may be used for any musculoskeletal area, depending on the nature of the condition. For example, *lower limb orthoses* include orthopedic shoes and orthoses for the foot, ankle, knee, or hip. *Spinal orthoses* may be used to relieve compression forces on the spine, restrict movement of the spine, or modify the alignment of the spine.

At least 50 types of spinal orthoses are distinguished based on the level of application. Cervical orthoses may be used for a wide variety of problems, ranging from whiplash to fracture of the cervical spine. The *Taylor, Jewett Hyperextension TLSO,* and *C.A.S.H.* spinal orthoses restrict trunk flexion and rotation or provide hyperextension and reduce flexion in the thoracic–lumbar spine. *Lumbar–sacral spinal orthoses*, such as the *Knight Chairback* and *Williams,* are used primarily for low back pain and may consist of flexible or semi-rigid corsets that provide support and protection. The *Milwaukee brace* is an orthotic device used as an intervention for scoliosis (lateral S-shaped curvature of the spine).

Orthotic devices may also be used for the upper extremities. In these instances, they are most frequently used because of injury. Upper-extremity orthoses may be applied to the shoulder, elbow, or wrist/hand.

Newer orthotic devices, called *fracture orthoses*, are designed to allow early ambulation on fractures of the lower extremity. These devices permit functional use of the extremity much earlier than does conventional casting. Recently, fracture orthoses have also been used as interventions for some upper-extremity fractures.

Traction

Individuals with a variety of musculoskeletal conditions may benefit from *traction*, a therapeutic method in which a mechanical or manual pull is used to restore or maintain the alignment of bones or to relieve pain and muscle spasm. It may be applied in several ways. When traction exerts a constant pull, it is said to be *continuous*. If the pull is relieved periodically, the traction is said to be *intermittent*. Traction may be applied externally or internally.

Skin traction is applied by fastening straps, belts, or other external devices around the body and then to a source of countertraction (see **Figure 24-7**). In contrast, *skeletal traction* is applied internally; metal wires (*Kirschner wires*), pins (*Steinmann pins*), or

Figure 24-7   Skin Traction

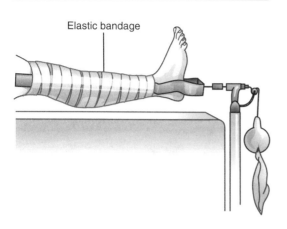

Elastic bandage

tongs (*Crutch-field tongs*) are inserted through the bone surgically and attached to a source of countertraction outside the body. Kirschner wires and Steinmann pins are typically used to reduce (align) fractures of the long bones of the extremities so as to promote bone healing or to stabilize the fracture until surgical intervention can be undertaken to correct

the fracture (**Figure 24-8**). Crutchfield tongs are inserted into the skull for injuries of the cervical spine.

The use of traction may reduce the need for surgical intervention in some cases, and it offers more freedom of movement than does a cast. However, there may be a risk of complications, such as osteomyelitis.

Surgical Management

Individuals with musculoskeletal conditions may require surgical interventions to correct, remove, or replace injured or damaged structures. Surgery may be performed on an emergency basis in the case of traumatic injury or on an elective basis in the case of damage attributable to a chronic condition or an old traumatic injury. Several types of surgical interventions are possible:

- *Open reduction:* Surgical alignment of the fractured bone.
- *Internal fixation:* Placement of screws, pins, wires, rods, or other devices through the bone to hold the bone fragments together.

Figure 24-8   Skeletal Traction

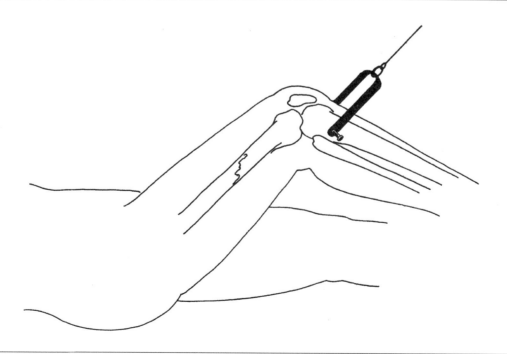

- *Arthroplasty:* Replacement of all or part of a joint with a prosthetic device to relieve pain or to restore function. Common sites of arthroplasty are the hip, shoulder, knee, and elbow. Reasons for arthroplasty include a broken hip (total hip replacement) and arthritis.
- *Arthrodesis:* Surgical fusing (joining) of two joint surfaces, making them permanently immobile. This procedure was once commonly performed to relieve joint pain. With the introduction of improved arthroplasty procedures, arthrodesis has become less common.
- *Synovectomy:* Surgical removal of the synovial membrane surrounding a joint. This procedure prevents recurrent inflammation, thereby reducing joint pain and further joint destruction.
- *Laminectomy:* Surgical removal of a portion of a vertebra, exposing the spinal cord. It is usually performed to facilitate the removal of any source of pressure on the spinal cord (e.g., to remove bone fragments from spinal cord injury; to remove tumor from the spinal cord).
- *Spinal fusion:* Grafting of bone from another area of the body into the disk interspace after a surgical procedure on the spine (e.g., laminectomy). After spinal fusion, mobility at the point of the fusion is lost.
- *Carpal tunnel repair:* A surgical procedure in which the median nerve is decompressed by the transection of surrounding ligaments. It is performed when the manifestations of carpal tunnel syndrome are severe, with progressive sensory loss in the fingers and hand.

GENERAL FUNCTIONAL IMPLICATIONS OF CONDITIONS OF THE MUSCULOSKELETAL SYSTEM

Personal and Psychosocial Implications

Most musculoskeletal conditions cause pain or discomfort to some degree. Pain, in turn, can cause anxiety or depression and alter individuals' responses to others in their family and social environment. Likewise, responses of others to the individual may be influenced by the individual's responses. Emotional factors and attitudes of others can affect the amount of discomfort that individuals perceive and how they respond to their condition.

Musculoskeletal conditions may also interfere with the physical movement and speed needed to accomplish a task, which can further contribute to anxiety and depression. If, for example, an individual used running as a way to reduce stress in the past, but now has to limit the activity due to an injury, increased stress may result. In other instances, individuals may be unable to continue activities related to work or daily activities at home. Depending on the circumstances and resulting hardship, additional emotional stress may be experienced as a result of these restrictions.

Discomfort and pain perception is related not only to various personality factors, but also to factors such as worker's compensation, litigation, or other benefits that may decrease individuals' motivation to reduce pain or restore function.

Activities and Participation

The degree to which activities are affected by a musculoskeletal condition depends on the nature of the condition, its associated manifestations, and the individual circumstances. Although many conditions of the musculoskeletal system require only short-term intervention and restrictions on activity are temporary, some conditions require greater adaptation. Sometimes, such as with osteoporosis, fear of fracture may lead to limitation of activity, which can in turn affect quality of life and contribute to depression. Restrictions on body movement resulting from pain, such as in osteoarthritis or back pain, may alter the individual's activities of daily living, social activities, and recreational activities. Individuals may need alternatives to activities that reduce the amount of stress placed on the joints.

Conditions affecting the ankles or the feet may require special shoes for joint protection and for comfort. Conditions such as carpal tunnel syndrome may require ergonomic devices to enable the individual to perform activities.

Lifestyle changes including dietary modifications may be necessary in some conditions of the musculoskeletal system. Obesity places extra strain on joints; consequently, a weight-reduction program may be needed. Many conditions of the musculoskeletal system require some form of exercise to restore strength or joint motion, or prevent structural irregularities. Such exercise programs must be incorporated into the daily routine.

Depending on the extent of discomfort and limitation of motion, individuals may be unable to perform all of their previous tasks, making it necessary for other family members to share household chores and duties. Their willingness or reluctance to accept necessary alterations in home life can affect how individuals adjust to their condition. When work or social activities are significantly altered by the individual's musculoskeletal condition, social identity may change as well. In some instances, if friendships initially developed around specific activities that now must be either abandoned or modified because of the condition, individuals may feel a sense of social isolation and "no longer fitting in."

Family and friends may have difficulty in coping with the feelings expressed by individuals because of pain or increased dependency, or in the case of fibromyalgia, the lack of definitive verification of the condition. Others may view individuals with musculoskeletal conditions as demanding, manipulative, and difficult. Depending on premorbid functioning of the family and the degree and quality of communication between family members, family dynamics can represent an increased source of tension.

Individuals with musculoskeletal conditions, especially those involving ongoing pain, are especially vulnerable to unorthodox, unproven "miracle cures." Although alternative and complementary practices have a place in management of musculoskeletal conditions, some unscrupulous individuals seek to take advantage of individuals' vulnerability by marketing and selling restorative methods that are of dubious value. In addition to the burden imposed by their expense, many of these fraudulent measures have dangerous side effects. Even in the absence of side effects, individuals may use these methods in place of recommended interventions, thereby losing the benefits of conventional interventions. When complementary and alternative methods are adopted by individuals for musculoskeletal conditions, the safety of the method and the legitimacy of the individual providing it should always be determined prior to use.

Sexuality

Most conditions of the musculoskeletal system do not hamper sexual activity. Nevertheless, pain, structural irregularities, decreased range of motion of joints, or alteration in body image may affect sexual function. Positioning may be difficult or painful, as in the case of low back pain. In some instances, medications used for management of musculoskeletal conditions can affect sexual function. Steroids used for a number of musculoskeletal conditions may decrease libido, and pain may inhibit sexual desire.

GENERAL VOCATIONAL ISSUES IN CONDITIONS OF THE MUSCULOSKELETAL SYSTEM

Musculoskeletal conditions represent one of the most common conditions affecting the workforce (Denis, St-Vincent, Imbeau, Jetté, & Nastasia, 2008). Although the restrictions associated with such conditions can interfere with work, the functional consequences of musculoskeletal conditions are a multifactorial, including factors in the workplace, the healthcare system, and the compensation system (Loisel et al., 2005).

Musculoskeletal conditions are not always associated with physically demanding jobs and are not always related to physical activity. They can also be related to emotional factors and psychological stress. Time pressure or stress at work can cause muscle tension, which can in turn contribute to discomfort or injury.

How a particular musculoskeletal condition impacts vocational function depends on the type of job previously held, individual factors related to job history and motivation, and the specific condition. Pain or limitation of range of motion or mobility may interfere with the individual's ability to work and can reduce productivity. The amount of sitting, bending, stooping, or lifting that the job requires must also be considered, and possibly modified. Generally, it is important that individuals return to work and daily activities as soon as possible to maintain good work habits.

Injured-worker programs and work-hardening programs have grown in popularity as means to help individuals return to work. These programs use a systemic approach of case management, evaluation, and other interventions that prepares workers for successful and safe reentry into the workforce after injury.

In injured-worker programs, individuals' physical capacity or level of function is evaluated as they progress through a graded series of job simulation tasks. Evaluation provides objective data regarding individuals' physical and functional capacity so that goals and a management plan can be established. Services are provided on an outpatient basis. Work-tolerance screening focuses on individuals' musculoskeletal strength, endurance, speed, and flexibility. Functional capacity evaluation documents individuals' ability to return to work from a physical, behavioral, and ergonomic perspective.

Work conditioning (work hardening) prepares individuals to return to competitive employment. Its goal is to increase work tolerance, increase work rate, help individuals learn to control manifestations of their condition, increase confidence and proficiency, and teach individuals to use work adaptations and assistive devices. Such a program is highly structured and, in addition to including simulated or real work tasks, instills expectations for the real-world environment, such as promptness, attendance, and appropriate dress.

Overuse of damaged joints owing to musculoskeletal conditions should be avoided. For example, individuals with osteoarthritis of the knees should avoid excessive walking; those with carpal tunnel syndrome should avoid repetitive activities with the hands. Occasionally, barriers such as financial disincentives, the status of legal claims, and other compensation protocols can interfere with effective rehabilitation.

Prevention through education and ergonomic strategies is a major way to diminish the occurrence of musculoskeletal conditions in the workplace. Likewise, emotional and psychological factors must be considered.

CASE STUDY

Ms. L. is a data entry specialist at a local industry. Her work requires her to use the computer most of the day. After experiencing pain in her left hand as well as numbness, she consulted with her healthcare provider and learned that she has carpal tunnel syndrome.

1. How might her health condition affect Ms. L.'s ability to continue her current line of employment?
2. Are there any workplace modifications, accommodations, or assistive devices that may be of use to Ms. L. in her work? If so, which types of modifications or devices may be useful?

REFERENCES

Alleva, J., Hudgins, T., Belous, J., & Kristin Origenes, A. (2016). Chronic low back pain. *Disease A Month, 62*(9), 330–333. pil:S0011-5029(16)30047.5 doi:10.1016/j.disamonth.2016.05.012

Barbano, R. L. (2016). Mechanical and other lesions of the spine, nerve roots, and spinal cord. In L. Goldman & A. I. Schaffer (Eds.), *Goldman-Cecil medicine,* (25th ed., pp. 2370–2382). Philadelphia, PA: Elsevier Saunders.

Bennett, R. M. (2016). Fibromyalgia, chronic fatigue syndrome, and myofascial pain. In L. Goldman & A. I. Schafer (Eds.), *Goldman-Cecil medicine,* (25th ed., pp. 1817–1823). Philadelphia, PA: Elsevier Saunders.

Biundo, J. J. (2016). Bursitis, tendinitis, and other periarticular disorders and sports medicine. In L. Goldman & A. I. Schafer (Eds.), *Goldman-Cecil medicine,* (25th ed., pp. 1749–1754). Philadelphia, PA: Elsevier Saunders.

Block, J. A., & Scanzello, C. (2016). Osteoarthritis. In L. Goldman & A. I. Schafer (Eds.), *Goldman-Cecil medicine,* (25th ed., pp. 1744–1749). Philadelphia, PA: Elsevier. Saunders.

Borenstein, D., & Balagué, F. (2012). Spine pain. In E. T. Bope & R. D. Kellerman (Eds.), *Conn's current therapy 2012* (pp. 39–43). Philadelphia, PA: Elsevier Saunders.

Denis, D., St-Vincent, M., Imbeau, D., Jetté, C., & Nastasia, I. (2008). Intervention practices in musculoskeletal disorder prevention: A critical literature review. *Applied Ergonomics, 39,* 1–14.

Deyo, R. A., & Mirza, S. K. (2016). Clinical practice: Herniated lumbar intervertebral disk. *The New England Journal of Medicine, 374*(18), 1783–1792.

Gillig, J. D., White, S. D., & Rachel, J. N. (2016). Acute carpal tunnel syndrome: A review of current literature. *Orthopedic Clinics of North American, 47*(3), 599–607.

Goldman R. (2009). Hyperbaric oxygen therapy for wound healing and limb salvage: A systematic review. *American Journal of Physical Medicine and Rehabilitation, 15,* 471–489.

Loisel, P., Falardeau, M., Baril, R., José-Durand, M., Langley, A., Sauvé, S., & Gervais, J. (2005). The values underlying team decision-making in work rehabilitation for musculoskeletal disorders. *Disability and Rehabilitation, 27*(10), 561–569.

Mackenzie, L. R., & Su, E. P. (2016). Surgical treatment of joint diseases. In L. Goldman & A. I. Schafer (Eds.), *Goldman-Cecil medicine,* (25th ed., pp. 1828–1833). Philadelphia, PA: Elsevier Saunders.

Matteson, E. L., & Osmon, D. R. (2016). Infections of bursae, joints, and bones. In L. Goldman & A. I. Schafer (Eds.), *Goldman-Cecil medicine,* (25th ed., pp. 1805–1810). Philadelphia, PA: Elsevier Saunders.

Shy, M. E. (2016). Peripheral neuropathies. In L. Goldman & A. I. Schafer (Eds.), *Goldman-Cecil medicine,* (25th ed., pp. 2527–2537). Philadelphia, PA: Elsevier Saunders.

Weber, T. J. (2016). Osteoporosis. In L. Goldman & A. I. Schafer (Eds.), *Goldman-Cecil medicine,* (25th ed., pp. 1637–1645). Philadelphia, PA: Elsevier Saunders.

Yu, W. K., Chen, Y. W., Shie, H. G., Lien, T. C., Kao, H. K., & Wang, J. H. (2011). Hyperbaric oxygen therapy as an adjunctive treatment for sternal infection and osteomyelitis after sternotomy and cardiothoracic surgery. *Journal of Cardiovascular Surgery, 17*(6), 141.

CHAPTER 25

Rheumatoid Arthritis, Lupus, and Other Rheumatic Conditions

Rheumatic conditions are disorders that produce manifestations that affect the joints, connective tissues, and muscle and are generally characterized by pain, inflammation, fatigue, and loss of motion. These disorders can be either noninflammatory or inflammatory. **Arthritis** is a general term used to describe an inflammation of the joints (Crowther-Radulewicz, 2014). **Myositis** refers to inflammation of muscle.

More than 116 conditions are classified as rheumatic conditions. Many are also considered to be *autoimmune conditions*, which are mediated by a physiological response in which the immune system attacks tissues as if they were considered foreign. The cause of most rheumatic conditions is unknown.

Rheumatic conditions may have manifestations that are acute or chronic, mild or severe, but most often involve pain and interference with daily activities. Manifestations are often unpredictable, so individuals with rheumatic conditions can never predict when pain, stiffness, or structural irregularity may strike.

RHEUMATOID ARTHRITIS

Rheumatoid arthritis (RA) is a progressive, chronic, systemic, inflammatory autoimmune disease distinguished by joint swelling and tenderness. It affects the synovial joints as well as other body system. The occurrence of RA has decreased over the past 5 decades due to earlier diagnosis and treatment, but the frequency increases with age (Crowther-Radulewicz, 2014; O'Dell, 2016). It has an unpredictable and fluctuating course characterized by

remissions, in which manifestations subside for a period of weeks to years, and *exacerbations*, in which manifestations become more severe. The exact cause of rheumatoid arthritis is unknown, but it appears to be triggered by a complex interaction of genetics and environmental factors that stimulate the immune system (Crowther-Radulewicz, 2014).

Although rheumatoid arthritis is a progressive condition, not all individuals are affected to the same degree. Some persons may experience rapid and severe exacerbations with progression of manifestations that affect functional capacity permanently, whereas others remain in a state of remission for years, continuing their regular employment and full activity.

Manifestations of Rheumatoid Arthritis

Rheumatoid arthritis is characterized by red and swollen joints with concurrent pain, and often accompanying stiffness and inability to move the joint in a normal manner. Synovial tissue is a thin vascular connective tissue that surround joints; the tissue secretes a thick liquid, which is a lubricant and nutrient for the joints. It is the primary focus of the autoimmune inflammatory response associated with rheumatoid arthritis. Because it is a systemic condition, individuals may also experience fatigue, weight loss, fever, or weakness combined with joint pain (Crowther-Radulewicz, 2014).

During an exacerbation of the condition, individuals develop **synovitis** at the joint in which synovial tissue becomes inflamed, with redness (**erythema**) and swelling (**edema**). In addition, synovial tissue produces excessive amounts of synovial fluid. As a result, individuals experience pain. A layer of inflammatory granulation tissue (*pannus*) that is derived from the synovial membrane interferes with the provision of nutrients to the cartilage of the joint, thereby leading to erosion and contributing to destruction of the cartilage. With each exacerbation, joints may sustain increased damage so that they never return to their regular state, even during remissions. Over time, with subsequent exacerbations, joint destruction and irregularity result. In some instances, scar tissue may become so tough and fibrous that **ankylosis** (stiffness and fixation of the joint) occurs, impeding movement of the joint.

Rheumatoid arthritis may not affect all joints, or it may affect different joints at different times. Occasionally, shoulders, hip, and cervical joints are involved. Most commonly, however, the joints involved include the following:

- Wrists
- Ankles
- Knees
- Elbows
- Fingers and toes

Joints are usually affected symmetrically. For example, both knees—rather than just one knee—will be affected. Joint pain and stiffness are generally worse in the morning, subside somewhat during the day, and again become painful at night.

Hands are frequently involved, with associated joint destruction and irregularity resulting in loss of function (**Figure 25-1**). Feet and large joints such as those in the knee and hip can also be affected, causing problems with mobility (Arthritis Foundation, n.d.a; Mayo Clinic, 2016a). Individuals with rheumatoid arthritis can develop carpal tunnel syndrome and peripheral neuropathy, which can further affect function.

Because rheumatoid arthritis is a systemic condition, other organ systems can also be affected. Although involvement of the cardiovascular system is rare, individuals with rheumatoid arthritis have a higher incidence of coronary artery conditions (Crowther-Radulewicz, 2014), although this incidence may often be attributed to the sedentary lifestyle due to joint pain and immobility. Individuals may also experience manifestations related to the respiratory system, including changes in the lungs, including nodules. Other systemic manifestations associated with rheumatoid arthritis include dry eyes and dry mouth.

Identification of Rheumatoid Arthritis

Early identification of rheumatoid arthritis is important to prevent or delay joint destruction as

Figure 25-1   Hand Affected by Rheumatoid Arthritis

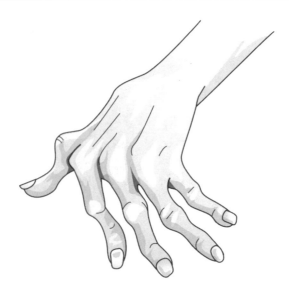

much as possible. Identification is usually based on a number of findings. Individual history of bilateral joint pain with redness and swelling are important first steps in identification. Laboratory tests that are positive for anemia as a result of chronic inflammation, rheumatoid factor (RF), and C-reactive protein (CRP) may, in association with the individual's history and manifestations, be used to help establish the presence of the condition. In some instances, aspiration of synovial fluid with microscopic examination may be used as well, although no one single test or factor can be used as the definitive confirmation of the presence of rheumatoid arthritis.

Management of Rheumatoid Arthritis

Nonsurgical Management

Rheumatoid arthritis is a lifelong condition with no known cure (O'Dell, 2016). Its management is directed toward suppressing the condition, alleviating pain, decreasing or preventing joint destruction, maintaining joint function, optimizing quality of life, and avoiding complications associated with management (Crowther-Radulewicz, 2014; Kavanaugh & Cherukumilli, 2012).

Medications

Medications are a mainstay of management in rheumatoid arthritis. They are used to reduce inflammation, thereby also reducing pain. Medications used for rheumatoid arthritis are often used in combination and are characterized into four main classes (Foltz-Gray, n.d. a; Mayo Clinic, 2016b):

- Nonsteroidal anti-inflammatory drugs (NSAIDs)
- Disease-modifying antirheumatic drugs (DMARDs)
- Glucocorticoids
- Biologic agents

NSAIDs (such as aspirin, ibuprofen, and naproxen) provide partial relief of pain and stiffness and help to reduce inflammation, but they do not slow joint destruction. Because they do not slow progression of rheumatoid arthritis, they are typically used in combination with DMARDs. Long-term administration of these medications can, however, result in stomach irritation or gastric bleeding.

DMARDs (such as methotrexate) are a mainstay in the management of rheumatoid arthritis (Crowther-Radulewicz, 2014; Kavanaugh & Cherukumilli, 2012). They are used to reduce manifestations and retard or halt progression of the condition by suppressing inflammation. DMARDs, however, are not without potentially serious side effects, such as bone marrow suppression and liver toxicity. Consequently, monitoring through laboratory tests to measure blood cell levels and liver function is needed regularly.

Glucocorticoids (such as prednisone) are added to the management plan because of the rapidity with which they suppress the inflammatory response while slower-acting drugs, such as DMARDs, are beginning to work. Not only do they help to reduce manifestations, such as pain and swelling, but they also decrease the rate of progression of rheumatoid arthritis. Because of potentially serious side effects, such as hyperglycemia (high blood sugar), cataracts, osteoporosis, and hypertension, glucocorticoids are rarely used on a long-term basis but rather are administered during acute exacerbations. After inflammation is controlled and slower-acting DMARDs begin to take effect, glucocorticoids are gradually withdrawn.

Over the past two decades, advances in the understanding of the pathophysiology of the condition lead to the development of biologic DMARDs, which have revolutionized the management of rheumatoid arthritis. These agents, especially when used in combination with methotrexate and other DMARDs have shown great efficacy in improving clinical and structural outcomes in this condition (Smolen, Aletaha, & McInnes, 2016).

Exercise

Exercise is an important component of management of rheumatoid arthritis. It is directed toward improving mobility and strength as well as improving psychological well-being. Generally, this intervention consists of specific range of-motion exercises for joints and exercises to promote muscle strength that are to be performed on a daily basis. In addition, dynamic and aerobic conditioning exercises may be recommended (Mayo Clinic, 2016c).

When individuals' joint destruction or ir-regularities compromise activities of daily living, physical therapy or occupational therapy may be recommended to educate individuals regarding use of assistive devices or alternative means of accomplishing various tasks so as to increase functional capacity.

Rest

In some instances, complete bed rest may be recommended for short periods during the acute phases of rheumatoid arthritis. In other instances, rest periods throughout the day may be recommended. Splinting of specific joints may be used to help reduce local inflammation. If used, splints are typically applied only at night and at rest to maintain the joints in extension. Splints are a temporary measure because their long-term use can promote structural irregularities due immobilization of affected joints.

Thermal Intervention

Thermal intervention (applications of either heat or cold) may be used to relieve pain. Interventions may include hydrotherapy, such as a whirlpool bath, or paraffin baths, in which the affected body part is placed in a bath of hot paraffin and then removed. As the paraffin cools externally, warmth to the body part is held in, reducing both pain and inflammation (Laufer & Dar, 2012).

Complementary and Alternative Therapies

Complementary and alternative medicine (CAM) is a term that describes a diverse range of products and practices for promoting health and preventing or managing conditions outside the mainstream of Western health care. Although some CAM practices have been researched and found to be beneficial, not all products or practices have been studied, and questions remain about these measures' safety and effectiveness (Offit, 2012). The effectiveness of CAM in management of rheumatoid arthritis has not been clearly established (National Center for Complementary and Integrative Health, 2016).

The types of alternative therapies used for rheumatoid arthritis range from topical ointments to dietary supplements to acupuncture (Mayo Clinic, 2016b). Alternative therapies such as massage, tai chi, yoga, and hypnosis are also used in the management of rheumatoid arthritis (Swann, 2007).

Surgical Management of Rheumatoid Arthritis

Most individuals with rheumatoid arthritis manage their condition with a combination of medication, exercise, and rest. At times, because of severe joint inflammation, severe damage, or structural irregularity of the joint, surgical procedures are necessary to relieve severe pain or improve function of a severely damaged joint, through either repair or replacement (Mayo Clinic, 2016b). The following surgical procedures may be performed in cases of severe rheumatoid arthritis:

- **Arthroscopy** is a procedure in which an endoscope is inserted into the joint space to inspect the joint or to repair damage.
- **Synovectomy** is the surgical removal of the synovial membrane surrounding a joint. It prevents recurrent inflammation, thereby reducing joint pain and further joint destruction.
- **Arthroplasty** (surgical replacement, formation, or reformation of a joint) may be necessary when the joint has become nonfunctional because of destruction, or when movement of the joint becomes so painful that activity is severely hampered.
- **Osteotomy** involves partial removal of a damaged bone.

Although joint replacement with prosthetic joints can improve quality of life, these replacements sometimes fail, necessitating additional surgery. Causes for failure include infection, dislocation, or fracture, either of the prosthesis itself or of the surrounding bone (Tande & Patel, 2014).

Functional Implications in Rheumatoid Arthritis

Personal and Psychosocial Issues

The consequences of rheumatoid arthritis and associated pain can affect individuals' ability to work or fulfill responsibilities at home as well as curtail their social life and ability to engage in recreational activities (Foltz-Gray, n.d.b; Silver, 2016). Living with pain is a factor to which individuals with rheumatoid arthritis must adjust.

Awareness of the lack of a cure and the progressive nature of the condition may lead to feelings of hopelessness. Individuals with rheumatoid arthritis may also experience sleep disturbances, which may increase fatigue and contribute to depression and irritability (Bosworth & Manning, 2014; Putre, n.d.).

In its early stages, before structural irregularities of joints occur, rheumatoid arthritis may be essentially an invisible condition. Its hidden nature may lead to misunderstandings on the part of family and friends, who may perceive individuals as merely seeking attention with their complaints of pain or attempting to avoid work or other activities rather than acknowledging the manifestations as real. The unpredictable nature of rheumatoid arthritis not only contributes to this misunderstanding but can also cause stress for individuals who are unsure on a day-to-day basis whether they will be able to participate in various activities.

Individuals may develop learned helplessness as a result of the unpredictable, chronic, and incurable nature of the condition (Camacho, Verstappen, Chipping, & Symmons, 2013). Helping individuals gain a feeling of control by increasing self-management of arthritic pain and the ability to cope with the vagueness of the condition can improve both social functioning and overall quality of life.

Activities and Participation

Independence is a critical issue for individuals with rheumatoid arthritis. Loss of the ability to perform certain tasks or associated role changes may require significant adjustment. For homemakers with rheumatoid arthritis whose partners must now assume some of the housekeeping duties, adjustment may be difficult for both parties. Conversely, individuals with rheumatoid arthritis who once prided themselves on being self-sufficient and strong may view having someone else perform what they consider simple tasks as a sign of weakness.

If individuals have to leave their jobs because of rheumatoid arthritis, their social identity may be threatened. Family roles may also be changed, with other family members taking over tasks once performed by the individual. As rheumatoid arthritis progresses and individuals become more dependent on others or on assistive devices, they may feel a loss of control, which can lead to poor self-esteem (Leach, 2015).

Also contributing to poor self-esteem is altered body image, resulting from structural irregularities of joints or the need for assistive devices that accompanies joint changes (Arthritis Foundation, n.d.c). Use of devices can, however, help individuals to gain independence and overcome feelings of helplessness. For grooming needs, individuals may use devices such as adaptive handles for combs and brushes or toothbrushes. They may use a long-handled sponge that has a compartment to hold a bar of soap. Devices such as a zipper pull or button aid may be of help with dressing.

Some individuals may be resistant to using an assistive device, viewing it as "giving up" or fearing that if they use the device rather than their joint, they will lose their ability to perform the task. Others may be concerned about appearances or fear that using the assistive device will call attention to their condition. Thus the use of assistive devices can be an emotionally charged issue. The degree of support from family and friends can make a difference in the individual's willingness to use such a device.

Vocational Issues in Rheumatoid Arthritis

Individuals with rheumatoid arthritis experience a number of work barriers, ranging from physical barriers (such as the need to handle items, writing, and energy-related barriers) to psychosocial barriers (such as lack of understanding by others in the workplace). Because not all individuals with rheumatoid arthritis are affected in the same way, vocational implications vary with the severity of the condition and its progression (Prior, Bodell, Amana, & Hammond, 2014). Not all individuals with rheumatoid arthritis will become totally incapacitated, but most individuals will experience reductions across a broad spectrum of activities (CDC, 2016).

A major limitation associated with rheumatoid arthritis is its unpredictability—that is, not knowing when the condition will change and whether additional functional loss will occur. Occupations characterized by significant physical demands may be more difficult for individuals to maintain than those that are sedentary or require light activity. Even when individuals are still able to perform moderate physical function in their work, the progressive nature of the condition and its potential for affecting mobility should be considered. Pain on motion, limited motion, and muscle weakness may all affect individuals' ability to perform tasks. Tasks requiring manual dexterity or pinch grip may also be difficult, if not impossible, if structural irregularity of the hands has occurred. Work that places stress or strain on joints may exacerbate the condition and should be avoided.

If joints in the lower extremities are involved, the ability to stand for long periods of time or walk for long distances may be affected (Arthritis Foundation, n.d.a). Individuals may have difficulty with climbing, stooping, bending, reaching, and kneeling. They may find it uncomfortable or difficult to remain in one position for long periods of time and may need to change position frequently. If they spend long periods of time traveling in a car, they should take frequent stops; if they travel on trains or planes, they should walk around frequently.

Individuals may need to organize and plan tasks as much as possible to conserve energy, protect joints, and minimize fatigue. They may attempt to do as much as they can while seated. If cervical joints are affected, individuals should avoid working with their neck bent over. They may use a slanted or elevated table or desk to avoid neck flexion.

Individuals should set priorities, giving up activities of least importance. They may consider alternating more difficult tasks with those requiring less energy. In all cases, they may need to learn to pace themselves, stopping to rest occasionally rather than persisting with the task until they are exhausted.

If individual manifestations are increased by temperature and humidity, an indoor, climate controlled environment may be preferable. In most instances, sudden, frequent changes in environmental conditions will prove more bothersome than the exact level of temperature or humidity itself. Consequently, going in and out of excessively cold or warm environments is generally to be avoided.

Effects of rheumatoid arthritis are more far-reaching than simply affecting one aspect of the person's life: all activities of daily living are affected. Consequently, individuals may require extra time to get ready for work or perform tasks at home, which can in turn affect their work schedule (CDC, 2016). The need for specific periods of rest and exercise must also be considered, both at home and in the work environment. A variety of environmental alterations may assist individuals with rheumatoid arthritis in maximizing their functional capacity, whether at work or at home. The need for reaching and bending can be reduced with modifications such as storage of heavy objects on lower shelves and use of pullout shelving or baskets to retrieve them. Pullout shelves can also be used to minimize bending and stretching for hard-to-reach items. Counters can be raised or lowered, either permanently or with adjustable components.

Assistive devices can help individuals manage their work environment as well as essential daily activities more easily and should be used as appropriate. Devices may enhance muscle strength, endurance, range of motion, manual dexterity, and mobility. Assistive devices such as long-handled reachers may be used to open cabinets. Knobs can be replaced by levers so that the whole hand can be used. This may be helpful if manual dexterity or hand strength is affected. Individuals with moderate to severe rheumatoid arthritis may use a motorized wheelchair to increase mobility and to conserve energy.

Although intellectual functioning or cognitive ability remains intact with rheumatoid arthritis, the effect of pain on individuals' ability to concentrate is a consideration. The combination of pain, functional incapacity, and changes in appearance associated with rheumatoid arthritis may result in depression, which in turn can affect work capacity. Management of depression, when identified, as well as interventions to enable individuals to decrease their pain and cope more effectively, may be beneficial in increasing their capacity for maintaining their vocational status.

SYSTEMIC LUPUS ERYTHEMATOSUS

Systemic lupus erythematosus is an autoimmune condition that produces inflammation and structural changes in multiple organs and organ systems in the body, including skin, musculoskeletal system, renal system, cardiovascular system, pulmonary system, gastrointestinal system, hematologic system (blood), and nervous system (Crowther-Radulewicz, 2014). It most commonly affects young women. Although the exact etiology is unknown, this disease is believed to be caused by a combination of genetic susceptibility; environmental triggers, such as microbial infection, sunlight, or drug interaction; and altered immune system function (Crow, 2016; Crowther-Radulewicz, 2014). It may progress rapidly or slowly, or it can become chronic with associated remissions and exacerbations.

Manifestations of Systemic Lupus Erythematosus

Manifestations vary from individual to individual, but most individuals experience *skin manifestations* such as a characteristic "butterfly rash" on the face and increased sensitivity to sunlight. Gastrointestinal manifestations may include loss of appetite with associated weight loss and, in some instances, abdominal pain or, in severe cases, **necrosis** (tissue death) of the intestine, which can cause perforation. Many individuals also experience *musculoskeletal manifestations* such as painful joints and irregularity of joints due to joint damage. Muscle inflammation may be present, resulting in *myositis*, or centralized changes may occur, resulting in *fibromyalgia*, which in turn contributes to fatigue and depression (Mayo Clinic, 2014a).

Other manifestations of systemic lupus erythematosus may involve vital organs and tissues such as the brain, heart, blood, or kidney and can be mild or severe (Mayo Clinic, 2014a). These conditions include *kidney disease*, which can be mild or severe (Hinshaw & Lawrence-Hylland, 2012); cardiac involvement, such as *pericarditis* and premature *atherosclerosis*; and pulmonary manifestations, such as *pleuritis* resulting in pain on respiration. Individuals also often experience *anemia* and *lymphadenopathy* (swollen lymph nodes). When the nervous system is involved, individuals may experience cognitive dysfunction, seizures, and stroke.

Although the extent to which pregnancy causes exacerbation of systemic lupus erythematosus is uncertain, women with lupus experience increased complications with pregnancy including gestational hypertension and increased chance of premature delivery and fetal loss (Crow, 2016).

Management of Systemic Lupus Erythematosus

Systemic lupus erythematosus requires individualized lifelong management. The goal is to improve or maintain organ function and to prevent permanent organ damage (Mayo Clinic, 2014a). When manifestations do not include organ systems, the condition may be managed with NSAIDs, low doses of corticosteroids, or antimalarial drugs (such as hydroxychloroquine) to limit progression of lupus (Crow, 2016).

When manifestations involve major organs or organ systems, the type and location of manifestations determine the intervention used. If major organs such as the heart or kidney are involved, management is directed toward preserving function and preventing organ failure.

Functional Implications of Systemic Lupus Erythematosus
Personal and Psychosocial Issues

The degree of psychosocial distress resulting from the condition depends, to some degree, on the severity of the manifestations. Although identification of systemic lupus erythematous alone may cause emotional reactions and psychological issues, some psychological manifestations may be manifestations of the condition itself. In either case, there is need for emotional support. Not only is systemic lupus erythematosus a potentially fatal condition, but most individuals affected are in young adulthood, when the psychosocial and vocational impact of the condition can have a profound effect. In addition, because of risks associated with pregnancy, the decision of whether to have children may be a difficult one for women with systemic lupus erythematosus.

Activities and Participation

Individuals with systemic lupus erythematosus may need additional rest, which may be difficult to obtain due to their other responsibilities. The ability to participate in activities is determined by the type of manifestations experienced. Individuals with joint involvement who have pain and joint damage may have their mobility affected, whereas individuals with cognitive dysfunction or seizures resulting from central nervous system involvement may have activities and participation affected in a different way. In all instances, the unpredictability of exacerbations and remissions may cause anxiety and depression, further affecting activities and relationships.

Vocational Issues in Systemic Lupus Erythematosus

Fatigue is a challenge for many individuals with systemic lupus erythematosus (Agarwal, 2015) so that more than the regular amount of rest is needed. Consequently, work schedules may need to be altered to accommodate the need for additional rest. Overexertion and stress can cause exacerbation of the condition, so they should be avoided.

Individuals with systemic lupus erythematosus are often sensitive to sunlight, which may trigger manifestations. Consequently, individuals should avoid excessive exposure to the sun, wear protective clothing, and use sunscreen routinely. If musculoskeletal system manifestations are present, environmental conditions that are cold and damp may make manifestations worse (Agarwal, 2015).

While this condition is in remission, if there is no associated permanent organ damage, individuals with systemic lupus erythematosus may have few restrictions with regard to work.

GOUT

Gout is a metabolic, inflammatory joint condition that results from *hyperuricemia*—that is, buildup of uric acid in the body (Crowther-Radulewicz, 2014; Edwards, 2016). Uric acid is a waste product of the metabolism of purines, which are found in a variety of foods. It is usually carried in the blood until it is excreted by the kidneys. In gout, uric acid levels in the blood increase, either because the kidneys are not excreting uric acid at a high enough rate or because the body is making too much uric acid. Excess uric acid is transformed into *urate crystals,* which then settle in the joints.

Manifestations of Gout

Manifestations of gout usually consist of rapid development of erythema (redness), edema (swelling), and excruciating pain in one or two joints, commonly in the lower extremities, especially the toe. Over the years, joints of the upper extremities, such as the wrists and elbows, can also become involved (Arthritis Foundation, n.d.b). Exacerbations of the condition can last for several days. Individuals with gout are more likely than are other persons to develop kidney stones (*urolithiasis*) (Mayo Clinic, 2015).

Management of Gout

The major goal of initial management of acute gout flare-ups is relief of pain and incapacitation caused by intense inflammation (Mayo Clinic, 2015). Over time, longer-term management is directed toward preventing urate crystal deposits in the joints and reducing acute flares of the condition (Edwards, 2016).

During acute attacks, the affected joint is placed at rest and NSAIDs are used along with the anti-gout drug, *colchicine.* Prevention of further attacks may require daily use of medications to lower the level of uric acid in the blood (such as *allopurinol*) or to increase its excretion by the kidneys (such as *probenecid*) (Edwards, 2016; Mayo Clinic, 2015).

Vocational Issues in Gout

Because gout can cause significant pain in affected joints, individuals may be unable to work during an exacerbation. When joints in the toes or other joints in the lower extremities are affected, mobility may be severely compromised. The extent of absences from work depends on the frequency and severity of the attacks. Not all joints are affected. Consequently, the degree of functional consequences that occur with any resulting joint damage or loss of motion depends on the joint involved and the degree to which that joint is crucial to job performance.

ANKYLOSING SPONDYLITIS AND OTHER SPONDYLOARTHROPATHIES

Ankylosing spondylitis is one of several inflammatory rheumatic conditions also referred to as *spondyloarthropathies* (SpA). Some other spondyloarthropathies include *Reiter's syndrome* and *psoriatic arthritis*. Although the cause of these conditions is unclear, a genetic predisposition, in conjunction with environmental factors, appears to affect their development. Spondyloarthropathies are more common in young men, although females can also be affected (Crowther-Radulewicz, 2014; Inman, 2016).

Manifestations of Ankylosing Spondylitis and Other Spondyloarthropathies

The spondyloarthropathies are characterized by joint involvement, particularly of the spine and lower extremities, and associated pain. Ankylosing spondylitis is a progressive condition that primarily affects the spinal and pelvic skeleton; it is characterized by persistent back pain, beginning in the lumbar area, often radiating to the buttocks. The inflammatory process around these joints, in addition to causing pain, can result in fusing of the joints (**ankylosis**), with subsequent loss and/ or restriction of motion and a permanent postural manifestation called **kyphosis** (humpback) (Crowther-Radulewicz, 2014). In addition, individuals with ankylosing spondylitis may experience *uveitis* (inflammation of the iris, ciliary body, and choroid layer of the eye) and inflammatory bowel disease (Crowther-Radulewicz, 2014).

The course of ankylosing spondylitis and its severity is highly variable (Inman, 2016). There may be occasional flare-ups when the manifestations become worse, but there may also be long periods with no manifestations (National Ankylosing Spondylitis Society, 2016).

Reiter's syndrome (also called *reactive arthritis*) occurs subsequent to an infection in another part of the body, often the gastrointestinal tract or genitourinary tract (Inman, 2016; Mayo Clinic, 2014b). In addition to arthritis (joint inflammation), it consists of a combination of **urethritis** (inflammation of the urethra) and **conjunctivitis** (inflammation of the conjunctiva).

Psoriatic arthritis is a condition that can occur in patients with *psoriasis*. Individuals may experience manifestations similar to those observed with ankylosing spondylitis or Reiter's syndrome (Mayo Clinic, 2014c).

Management of Ankylosing Spondylitis and Other Spondyloarthropathies

NSAIDs, including indomethacin, are commonly used in the management of the spondyloarthropathies, in addition to corticosteroids and DMARDs to help prevent joint destruction and fusion (Reveille, 2012). Management also focuses on maximizing function through physical therapy and exercise. Exercises are designed to strengthen supporting muscles and to maintain good posture and function. Good posture is essential to prevent spinal irregularity, thereby preserving the chest's ability to expand. Joint *arthroplasty* may be needed when individuals develop severe joint irregularity or fusion.

Vocational Issues in Ankylosing Spondylitis and Other Spondyloarthropathies

Individuals with spondyloarthropathies experience no limitation in cognitive skills or motor coordination. Nevertheless, because of the stiffness and potential fusing of joints, especially of the spine, twisting and turning motions as well as lifting may be limited. Walking is usually unaffected unless hips and knees are affected. Individuals who work in a sedentary setting may need periodic rest breaks to stretch. Joint irregularity or fusion, such as in kyphosis, can alter body image and may be accompanied by embarrassment and a reluctance to work in situations involving contact with the public.

GENERAL FUNCTIONAL IMPLICATIONS OF RHEUMATIC CONDITIONS

Personal and Psychosocial Issues

Pain and immobility are common characteristics of many rheumatic conditions. The quantity and quality of pain are experienced at different levels by different individuals and depend on the perception of pain as well as on the nature and degree of stresses that pain precipitates. Although pain can be a major stressor in and of itself, other stressors present as a result of rheumatic conditions can affect adjustment and adaptation as well.

Mobility issues can contribute to feelings of dependence, which in turn can be a source of emotional distress, especially in instances where individuals have taken pride in their self-sufficiency. Depending on the extent of immobility, there may be a sense of powerlessness, leading to anger, hostility, and later depression (Arthritis Foundation, n.d.a). Pain or joint irregularity may necessitate decreasing or in some instances giving up a valued activity. In some instances, other activities may be substituted, but in other instances, individuals may grieve for the inability to participate in activities once enjoyed.

Coping with the long-term nature of rheumatic conditions may also be a source of stress. The chronic nature of these conditions, combined with the periods of remissions and exacerbations associated with many rheumatic conditions, presents issues of unpredictability and uncertainty that many individuals find stressful (Davis, 2015). The inability to plan definitively and awareness of the possible need to change an activity if an exacerbation occurs can be stressful for many persons.

Physical changes in terms of joint irregularity, posture, or the need for assistive devices can alter individuals' body image and subsequently their self-esteem. The value and subjective meaning of appearance can influence individuals' reactions to any alteration of their appearance, such that concerns about acceptance of family, friends, and acquaintances can preoccupy their thoughts.

Interventions used in the management of many rheumatic conditions can also be a source of stress. Some medications, although necessary for management of the condition, have side effects that cause discomfort. Individuals undergoing surgery, such as joint replacement, may experience a mixture of fear and anticipation regarding the extent to which the surgery will restore function.

Education regarding the condition and interventions, assistive devices to enhance functional ability, and stress management are important aspects of total management of rheumatic conditions.

ACTIVITIES AND PARTICIPATION

Restrictions on body movement resulting from a loss of muscle strength, irregularity of joints, or pain may alter the individual's activities of daily living, social activities, and recreational activities (Mayo Clinic, 2016b & c). Using assistive devices or sitting while performing many tasks, such as meal preparation, may enable individuals to participate more fully in many tasks. Conditions affecting joints of the hands may require use of assistive devices such as hooks, zipper pulls, special openers, or other self-help aids so that individuals may perform activities of daily living independently. Adaptive handles for combs and brushes may be of help for grooming. Soft lead pencils and felt-tipped pens may be useful for decreasing pressure on finger joints when writing.

At home, work centers may be established where all items needed for a specific task are kept within easy reach. It may be necessary to lower tables and cabinets so individuals can be seated while they work or to raise beds, toilet seats, and chairs to facilitate sitting and arising. Organizing and planning daily activities can help to reduce strain and fatigue.

Many rheumatic conditions require some form of therapeutic exercise to maintain joint function, restore strength and joint motion, or prevent structural irregularities. Such exercise programs must be incorporated into individuals' daily routine (Arthritis Foundation, n.d.a). In addition, because fatigue is characteristic of many rheumatic conditions, a pattern of specified rest periods may need to be scheduled during the day.

Understanding and support of family and friends as well as reassurance that any associated physical changes are unimportant are important to affected individuals' self-esteem and confidence.

Depending on the extent of discomfort, limitation of motion, and structural irregularity, individuals may be unable to perform all of their previous tasks, making it necessary for other family members to share household chores and duties. Their willingness or reluctance to accept necessary alterations in home life can affect how individuals adjust. When work or social activities are significantly altered, social identity may be altered. Such role changes may be a source of stress.

Sexuality

Sexuality is an important but often neglected area in individuals with rheumatic conditions, and frequently is not addressed by healthcare providers. Manifestations of rheumatic conditions can impair sexual functioning because of physical issues including pain or structural difficulties, emotional issues, or condition-related stressors. Chronic pain, fatigue, or diminished self-esteem can further reduce sexual activity. Interventions to address specific issues and counseling can be important to improve sexual function and quality of life.

Vocational Implications of Rheumatic Conditions

The impact of rheumatic conditions on individuals' ability to continue work depends on the type of work, severity of the condition, and individual factors. The amount of sitting, bending, stooping, or lifting required as part of the job must be considered in many instances. Modifications of the work environment, such as raising or lowering of worktables or chairs, or establishment of specific rest periods may be needed. Because many rheumatic conditions may be affected by temperature, environments that are wet or cold may need to be avoided. In specific conditions, such as systemic lupus erythematosus, direct exposure to sunlight for extended periods of time may also need to be avoided.

The unpredictability of exacerbations and remissions in many rheumatic conditions may necessitate flexible work schedules. Although many individuals with rheumatic conditions are able to continue their current employment with no specific alterations, overuse of affected joints should be avoided, as should activities that produce overexertion, stress, and fatigue.

CASE STUDY

Ms. K., a 42-year-old cosmetologist, has been experiencing increasing discomfort in her hip joints and hands due to rheumatoid arthritis. Although she has been using a number of medications to manage inflammation, exacerbations of her condition appear to be occurring more frequently.

1. How might specific manifestations of rheumatoid arthritis affect Ms. K.'s functional capacity as a cosmetologist?

2. Are there specific workplace modifications that may be helpful to Ms. K.? If so, which modifications might be helpful?

3. Which other issues might be important for Ms. K. to consider?

REFERENCES

Agarwal, N. (2015). Lupus: Vocational aspects and the best rehabilitation practices. *Journal of Vocational Rehabilitation, 43*(1), 83–90. doi:10.3233/JVR-150757

Arthritis Foundation. (n.d.a). *About arthritis.* Retrieved from http://www.nras.org.uk/invisible-disease-rheumatoid-arthritis-and-chronic-fatigue-report

Arthritis Foundation. (n.d.b). *Gout.* Retrieved from http://www.arthritis.org/about-arthritis/types/gout/

Arthritis Foundation. (n.d.c). *Doctors should watch for depression in rheumatoid arthritis patients.* Retrieved from http://www.arthritis.org/living-with-arthritis/comorbidities/depression-and-arthritis/arthritis-and-depression.php

Bosworth, A., & Manning, J. (2014). Invisible disease: Rheumatoid and chronic fatigue. *National Rheumatoid Arthritis Society.* Retrieved from http://www.nras.org.uk/invisible-disease-rheumatoid-and-chronic-fatigue-report

Camacho, E. M., Verstappen, S. M. M., Chipping, J., & Symmons, D. P. M. (2013). Learned helplessness predicts functional disability, pain and fatigue in patients with recent-onset inflammatory polyarthritis. *Rheumatology.* doi:10.1093/rheumatology/des434

Centers for Disease Prevention and Control. (2016). Disability and limitations. Retrieved from http://www.cdc.gov/arthritis/data_statistics/disabilities-limitations.htm

Crow, M. K. (2016). Systemic lupus erythematosus. In L. Goldman & A. I. Schafer (Eds.), *Goldman-Cecil medicine,* (25th ed., pp. 1769–1777). Philadelphia, PA: Elsevier Saunders.

Crowther-Radulewicz, C. L. (2014). Structure and function of the Musculoskeletal System. In K. L. McCance, S. E. Huether, V. L. Brashers, & C. L. Rote (Eds.), *Pathophysiology: The biologic basis for disease in adults and children,* (7th ed., pp. 1568–1572). St. Louis, MO: Elsevier-Mosby.

Davis, J. (2015). *Stress and worry affect RA.* Arthritis Foundation. Retrieved from http://www.arthritis.org/living-with-arthritis/comorbidities/depression-and-arthritis/stress-rheumatoid-arthritis.php

Edwards, N. L. (2016). Crystal deposition diseases. In L. Goldman & A. I. Schafer (Eds.), *Goldman-Cecil medicine* (25th ed., pp. 1811–1816). Philadelphia, PA: Elsevier Saunders.

Foltz-Gray, D. (n.d.a). *Fight arthritis pain without pills.* Arthritis Foundation. Retrieved from http://www.arthritis.org/living-with-arthritis/pain-management/tips/arthritis-pain-relief-alternatives.php

Foltz-Gray, D. (n.d.b). *Relationships.* Arthritis Foundation. Retrieved from http://www.arthritis.org/living-with-arthritis/life-stages/relationships/keep-relationships-strong.php

Hinshaw, M., & Lawrence-Hylland, S. (2012). Autoimmune connective tissue disease. In E. T. Bope & R. D. Kellerman (Eds.), *Conn's current therapy 2012,* (pp. 567–570). Philadelphia, PA: Elsevier Saunders.

Inman, R. D. (2016). The spondyloarthropathies. In L. Goldman & A. I. Schafer (Eds.), *Goldman-Cecil medicine,* (25th ed., pp. 1762–1769). Philadelphia, PA: Elsevier Saunders.

Kavanaugh, A., & Cherukumilli, V. S. (2012). Rheumatoid arthritis. In E. T. Bope & R. D. Kellerman (Eds.), *Conn's current therapy 2012,* (pp. 591–595). Philadelphia, PA: Elsevier Saunders.

Laufer, Y., & Dar, G. (2012). Effectiveness of thermal and athermal short-wave diathermy for the management of knee osteoarthritis: A systematic review and meta-analysis. *Osteoarthritis and Cartilage, 20*(9), 957–966. doi:10.1016/j.joca.2012.05.005. Retrieved from http://www.sciencedirect.com/science/article/pii/S1063458412008199

Leach, M. Z. (2015). The impact of RA on self-esteem. *Rheumatoid Arthritis.net.* Retrieved from https://rheumatoidarthritis.net/living/the-impact-on-self-esteem/

Mayo Clinic Staff. (2014a). *Lupus.* Mayo Clinic. Retrieved from http://www.mayoclinic.org/diseases-conditions/lupus/basics/definition/CON-20019676

Mayo Clinic Staff. (2014b). *Ankylosing spondylitis.* Mayo Clinic. Retrieved from http://www.mayoclinic.org/diseases-conditions/ankylosing-spondylitis/basics/definition/CON-20019766?p=1

Mayo Clinic Staff. (2014c). *Psoriatric arthritis.* Mayo Clinic. Retrieved from http://www.mayoclinic.org/diseases-conditions/psoriatic-arthritis/basics/definition/con-20015006

Mayo Clinic Staff. (2015). *Gout: Complications.* Mayo Clinic. Retrieved from http://www.mayoclinic.org/diseases-conditions/gout/basics/complications/con-20019400

Mayo Clinic Staff. (2016a). *Rheumatoid arthritis.* Mayo Clinic. Retrieved from http://www.mayoclinic.org/diseases-conditions/rheumatoid-arthritis/home/ovc-20197388

Mayo Clinic Staff. (2016b). *Arthritis: Treatment.* Mayo Clinic. Retrieved from http://www.mayoclinic.org/diseases-conditions/arthritis/diagnosis-treatment/treatment/txc-20169117

Mayo Clinic Staff. (2016c). *Exercise helps ease arthritis pain and stiffness.* Mayo Clinic. Retrieved from http://www.mayoclinic.org/arthritis/art-20047971

National Ankylosing Spondylitis Society. (2016). *Flares and burn out.* Retrieved from http://nass.co.uk/about-as/just-diagnosed/flare-ups-and-burn-out/

National Center for Complementary and Integrative Health. (2016). *Rheumatoid arthritis in depth.* National Institutes of Health. Retrieved from https://nccih.nih.gov/health/RA/getthefacts.htm

O'Dell, J. R. (2016). Rheumatoid arthritis. In L. Goldman & A. I. Schafer (Eds.), *Goldman-Cecil medicine,* (25th ed., pp. 1754–1762). Philadelphia, PA: Elsevier Saunders.

Offit, P. A. (2012). Studying complementary and alternative therapies. *Journal of the American Medical Association, 307*(17), 1803–1804.

Prior, Y., Bodell, S., Amanna, A., & Hammond, A. (2014). Rheumatoid arthritis patients' views of a vocational rehabilitation intervention provided by rheumatology occupational therapists. *Rheumatology, 53*(1), 121–122. doi:10.1093/rheumatology/keu106.008. Retrieved from http://rheumatology.oxfordjournals.org/content/53/suppl_1/i121.3

Putre, L. (n.d.). *Rheumatoid arthritis and sleep.* Arthritis Foundation. Retrieved from http://www.arthritis.org/living-with-arthritis/comorbidities/sleep-insomnia/rheumatoid-arthritis-sleep.php

Reveille, J. D. (2012). Ankylosing spondylitis. In E. T. Bope & R. D. Kellerman (Eds.), *Conn's current therapy 2012,* (pp. 565–567). Philadelphia, PA: Elsevier Saunders.

Silver, J. M. (2016). Psychosocial factors and rheumatic disease (abstract). *UpToDate.* Retrieved from http://www.uptodate.com/contents/psychosocial-factors-and-rheumatic-disease

Smolen, J. S., Aletaha D., & McInnes, I. B. (2016). Rheumatoid arthritis. *The Lancet, 388*(10055), 2023–2038. pii:S0140-6736(16)30173-8 doi.10:1016/S0140-6736(16)30173-8

Swann, J. (2007). Rheumatoid arthritis: Coping strategies. *Nursing & Residential Care, 9*(6), 269–272.

Tande, A. J., & Patel, R. (2014). Prosthetic joint infection. *Clinical Microbiology Reviews, 27*(2), 302–345. doi:10.1128/CMR.00111-13. Retrieved from http://cmr.asm.org/content/27/2/302.full.pdf

CHAPTER 26

Amputation

DEFINING AMPUTATION

The general term used to describe loss of all or a portion of a body part is **amputation**. Amputation can occur for several reasons. The cause of the amputation can affect function, activity, and adjustment.

Although usually associated with the loss of an extremity, the term *amputation* is also used to describe loss of other body parts, such as loss of a breast through mastectomy for cancer or loss of an ear or the nose as a result of frostbite. Amputation can be performed surgically as an intervention to manage a condition, or it can result from trauma. Amputation may also refer the congenital absence of limbs at birth.

SPECIFIC CAUSES OF AMPUTATION

Traumatic Amputation

Traumatic amputation refers to the severance of a body part due to sudden severe trauma such as a motor vehicle accident, armed conflict in which a limb is severed in an explosion, mangling of an extremity in a machine, or severance of a body part by a sharp object. Traumatic amputation is most common in younger, predominately male adults (Tarim & Ezer, 2012). While amputation of any body part may result from trauma, causes of upper extremity amputations are often more often due to accidents, burns, explosions, or other types of traumatic injury.

Peripheral Vascular Disease

Peripheral vascular disease refers to condition in which there is poor circulation, usually affecting the lower extremities. It is the most common cause of lower extremity amputation, and is often associated with complications of diabetes in which tissue death has resulted from poor supply of oxygen to tissues in the lower extremities owing to poor circulation (Cox, Williams, & Weaver, 2011; Jindeel & Narahara, 2012).

Infections

Long-standing infections of the bone (such as in osteomyelitis) and other tissues (such as gangrene) may necessitate amputation if there is no chance of restoration of function or if there is danger of systemic infection (septicemia).

Malignant Tumors

Cancers of the bone such as sarcoma may require amputation to prevent metastasis. Depending on the location of the cancer, surgical intervention may involve major surgery and reconstruction.

Thermal Injuries

Thermal injuries can result from either heat or cold. In severe burns, amputation may be necessary because tissue damage is so severe that survival or restoration of the body part is not possible. Likewise, freezing injuries, such as frostbite, may result in tissue death that necessitates amputation of the body part affected.

Elective Amputation

In some instances, individuals who have a body part that has been previously injured so that it is no longer of use, or a limb that has such severe irregularities that is no longer functional, may find the extremity to be cumbersome or obstructive, hindering activity, or challenging well-being. In these instances, individuals may choose to have an elective amputation.

LEVELS OF EXTREMITY AMPUTATION

Amputation of an extremity may be performed at different levels. To provide for maximal length of the stump of the extremity and, therefore, maximal function with a prosthesis, surgeons usually perform an amputation as **distal** (farthest from the center of the body) as possible. Amputations are usually classified relative to the nearest joint (see **Figure 26-1**).

In the case of lower extremity amputation, it is especially important to retain the maximal length of the stump because the amount of energy required to use an artificial limb increases with the height of the amputation (Asano, Rushton, Miller, & Deathe, 2008; Brown, Crone, & Attinger, 2012). Newer prosthetic devices have been developed that

decrease the energy expenditure required to some degree (Kaufman et al., 2008).

Upper Extremity Amputation

Levels of upper extremity amputation are defined as follows:

- *Forequarter or interscapular–thoracic amputation:* the most severe upper extremity amputation, in which the entire arm, clavicle, and scapula are removed
- *Shoulder disarticulation (S/D):* removal of the arm at the shoulder joint
- *Above the elbow (A/E):* removal of the arm anywhere between the shoulder and the elbow joints
- *Elbow disarticulation (E/D):* removal of the arm at the elbow joint
- *Below elbow (B/E):* removal of the arm anywhere between the elbow and the wrist
- *Wrist disarticulation (W/D):* removal of the hand at the wrist
- *Partial hand:* amputation of one or more fingers or the loss of a portion of the hand

Figure 26-1   Levels of Upper and Lower Extremity Amputation

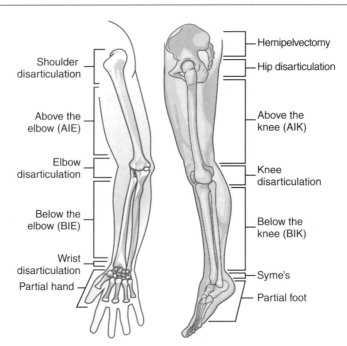

Lower Extremity Amputation

The following levels of lower extremity amputation are distinguished:

- *Transpelvic amputation or hemipelvectomy:* the most severe lower extremity amputation, in which the entire lower limb and half of the pelvis are removed
- *Hip disarticulation (H/D):* removal of the leg at the hip joint
- *Above the knee (A/K):* removal of the leg anywhere between the hip and the knee joints
- *Knee disarticulation (K/D):* the removal of the lower leg at the knee
- *Below the knee (B/K):* the removal of the lower leg anywhere between the knee and the ankle
- *Syme's amputation:* the removal of the foot at the ankle
- *Transmetatarsal* or *partial foot:* the removal of a portion of the foot

MANAGEMENT OF AMPUTATION

Surgery

When the viability of an extremity is in doubt, whether due to trauma, infection, or vascular insufficiency, the first priority is an attempt to save it. Use of antibiotics and control of other complications have allowed for more success in salvaging limbs than previously would have been possible.

When tissue damage, regardless of the cause, is too severe or when underlying conditions such as cancer or severe infection threaten well-being, amputation may be inevitable. The type of surgical amputation, the postoperative course, and type of rehabilitation depend to a great extent on the circumstances surrounding the amputation and the individual's general condition. Individuals who undergo amputation because of an underlying condition, such as diabetes, may be at risk for subsequent amputations due to complications from the condition. Individuals who undergo amputation due to injury may have other injuries that must be stabilized prior to surgery.

Replantation

Replantation (commonly known as *reimplantation* or *reattachment surgery*) refers to reattachment of an amputated body part, using neurovascular and musculoskeletal structures to salvage the limb and its function. With the evolution of surgical techniques and scientific technology, replantation procedures have resulted in better outcomes. Functional outcomes vary with the level of injury (Nanda et al., 2011). The degree of success depends on the general condition of the individual, the availability of rapid transportation to a replantation center, and appropriate care of the severed body part prior to replantation.

Prostheses

A **prosthesis** is a fabricated substitute for a missing body part, such as an artificial limb that replaces an amputated limb. Prosthetic devices may enable individuals to regain independent function, or they may be used only for cosmetic purposes. The type of prosthesis, its purpose, and its maximal use depend on the reason for the amputation, the type and level of the amputation, the presence of any underlying conditions, the development of any complications, and, most importantly, the needs of the individual and his or her motivation to use the prosthesis.

Needs of the individual are evaluated so that the prosthesis is constructed to meet the individual's daily activities, occupation, and cosmetic needs. The prosthesis is fabricated by a *certified prosthetist* (an individual who specializes in making prosthetic devices). Prosthetists design, construct, and fit prosthetic devices so that individuals are comfortable and obtain maximum function with the device.

Lower Extremity Prostheses

In some instances, an individual may receive a temporary prosthesis on the stump of a lower extremity immediately after surgery. In this case, a rigid total-contact dressing is applied to the stump in the operating room, and a *pylon* or adjustable rigid support structure is attached. An ankle–foot assembly is then attached to the lower end of the pylon. The immediate placement of a temporary prosthesis may have a psychological benefit for individuals, fostering a sense of independence and optimism as soon as they wake from surgery. It also promotes ambulation, reducing the risk of complications associated with immobility after surgery. Immediate placement of a temporary prosthesis is contraindicated when the individual has a severe underlying condition, such as diabetes or infection, or when the individual has experienced extensive damage as a result of injury. It is also contraindicated for individuals with limited mental capabilities, who may not be able to understand instructions or to regulate the weight placed on the stump in the early postoperative period.

When immediate prosthetic fitting is not advisable, individuals receive a temporary prosthesis 2 to 3 weeks after their surgery. Placement of a temporary prosthesis is necessary whether the fitting is immediate or delayed so that **edema** (swelling) can subside and the stump can shrink before the permanent prosthesis is fitted. A permanent prosthesis can usually be placed within 3 months.

As much as possible, lower extremity prostheses are designed to enable ambulation. The individual's walking ability after lower limb amputation is determined by many factors, including the presence of other conditions that may affect general health and the person's physical capacity (van Velzen, van Bennekom, van der Woude, & Houdijk, 2006). Generally, the lower the level of amputation, the easier the use of the lower extremity prosthesis. The ankle–foot attachment may be either immovable or movable. A commonly used ankle–foot mechanism is the *solid ankle–cushion heel foot (SACH)*. In above-the-knee amputations, the prosthesis must also replace knee function, providing a joint that is stable for both standing and walking. Good alignment and fit of the socket of the prosthetic device are crucial for optimal balance and support. Because proper alignment varies with the heel heights of shoes, individuals who wish to wear shoes with different heel heights on occasion may need several removable prosthetic feet designed to accommodate the varying heel heights.

Prosthetic devices for use after *hemipelvectomy* (transpelvic amputation) may be more difficult to use. The degree to which the prosthesis is useful for function as well as cosmetic effect is dependent to some extent on the individual's age and general health (Houdek, Dralovec, & Andrews, 2014). The increased energy needed for ambulation may make ambulation with a prosthetic device after hemi-pelvectomy more difficult for some. In some instances, individuals may use the prosthetic device after transpelvic amputation to maintain proper posture while sitting in a wheelchair. Although some individuals after hemi-pelvectomy may choose to use crutches or a wheelchair for their daily activities, with advances in prosthetic design, many individual wear the prosthesis most of the day (Kralovec et al., 2015)

Upper Extremity Prostheses

Upper extremity prostheses vary in type and purpose and are custom made according to individual need. Complex function of the hand cannot be replaced, but functions such as lifting, grasping, and pinching can often be restored with a prosthesis. A *terminal device* is a prosthesis that substitutes for a hand. The level of amputation and the individual's needs determine the type of terminal device used. In general, the better the cosmetic appearance of the device, the lesser its functional capacity.

The hook is the most simple type of terminal device, is lightweight, durable and cost effective, but because of its low cosmetic appeal, may have lower social acceptability (O'Keefe, 2011). Individuals who need grasping, holding, or lifting actions may, however, find a hook more beneficial as a prosthesis for work, opting for a more cosmetic device for other occasions.

Body-powered and cable-controlled devices use forces generated by joints near the amputation site to control movement of the terminal device. For instance, flexion or extension of an elbow may be used to open a prosthetic hand. Many devices have allowed the individual to either grasp or release, although both movements are helpful for certain tasks, most individuals would prefer to be able to use both actions. Consequently, devices in which individuals can choose to switch between the two modes of action, depending on the task appear to be more utilitarian than devices which provide one action or the other (Sensinger, Lipsey, Thomas, & Turner, 2015).

The electrically powered and controlled prosthesis use small light weight motors, which drive the required function of the prosthesis with power provided by small rechargable batteries imbedded in the prosthesis.

A frequently used electrical control device is the myoelectrical prostheses, the function of which is activated by electrical potentials produced by muscles. In this prosthetic device, electrodes are placed over the skin of the muscles to be used. The electrodes pick up electrical impulses from the muscles, transferring them to a motor in the prosthesis, which then stimulates the hand to open and close. Function of the electric prosthesis does not, however, approximate function of regular hand movement and dexterity. Myoelectrical prostheses are best suited for individuals with below-the-elbow prostheses. They are heavier because of the battery and motor that they contain, and they are more expensive than regular prosthetic devices.

The cosmetic appearance of the prosthetic hand may be more important to some individuals than the prosthetic hand's functional capacity in some instances. In these cases individuals may have one terminal device used for performing work-related tasks and a second cosmetic prosthesis for social occasions.

Because activation of function of a prosthesis is achieved by using the muscles in the remaining portion of the limb, prosthesis for a high upper extremity amputation may have more limited function. A prosthesis placed after a shoulder disarticulation or an interscapular–thoracic amputation, for example, may be mostly cosmetic with little, if any, functional capacity (O'Keefe, 2011).

Although the cosmetic appearance of terminal devices are important, functional capacity is also importance in order to assist individuals obtain a fuller degree of independence and self-sufficiency. Emerging biotechnologies are developing multijoint hands that include more coordinated and independent finger function in addition to having cosmetic appeal (O'Keefe, 2011).

COMPLICATIONS OF AMPUTATION

Complications may develop after either upper or lower extremity amputation. Coexisting conditions, such as peripheral vascular disease or diabetes, may increase the risk of developing complications (Robbins, Vreeman, Sothmann, Wilson, & Oldridge, 2009). It is essential that the prosthesis fit well and that there be no undue pressure or rubbing that could lead to ulceration. All individuals—but especially those whose amputation was made necessary by underlying peripheral vascular disease—must be careful to avoid skin ulceration, which could become infected and necessitate a higher level amputation.

Edema

Swelling (edema) of the stump after the permanent prosthesis has been placed can not only interfere with the proper fit of the prosthesis but also increase pressure and restrict the blood flow to the stump, contributing to the likelihood of ulceration. An improperly fitting prosthesis, rubbing, or swelling of the stump should be immediately brought to the attention of healthcare personnel and the prosthetist so that the prosthesis can be adjusted appropriately.

Ulceration

Ulceration of the stump may occur because of excessive pressure or rubbing from the prosthesis or because of edema. If the ulceration becomes contaminated, infection can occur. Keeping the stump clean and dry and avoiding ill-fitting prostheses are important to prevent ulceration and infection.

Individuals who have undergone amputation, especially loss of a lower extremity because of a chronic condition such as diabetes, must be especially careful to guard against injury and infection to the stump, which could result in the need for reamputation (Kono & Muder, 2012; Malhotra, Bello, & Kominsky, 2012). Consequently, skin care is a vital part of rehabilitation. Bathing in the evening, rather than in the morning, is advisable, as damp skin may swell and stick to a prosthesis, causing irritation and rubbing.

Contractures

Individuals undergoing amputation must also concentrate on preserving the range of motion in the remaining joints of the amputated limb. **Contractures**—deformities in which permanent contraction of a muscle makes a joint immobile—may occur because of improper positioning or limited activity of remaining joints. Contractures may impede or prevent effective use of the prosthetic device. These complications are easier to prevent through regular range-of-motion exercises of joints than they are to cure. When contractures develop, they may be corrected with extensive physical therapy and, occasionally, surgery.

Bone Spurs and Scoliosis

Other complications of amputation may include *bone spurs* and *scoliosis*. Bone spurs or bone overgrowth may develop at the end of the stump, changing its shape and causing pain. *Scoliosis* (an S-shaped lateral curvature of the spine) may occur after a lower extremity amputation because of the improper alignment of the body or because of improper use of the prosthesis. Whether or not scoliosis occurs, lower back pain may also be experienced with lower extremity prosthesis use (Devon, Carman, Hendrick, Ribeiro, & Hale, 2015; Yoder, Petrella, & Silverman, 2015). After a higher upper extremity amputation, scoliosis may develop if the prosthetic device creates an imbalance in the trunk. In both instances, scoliosis can be prevented by making sure that the prosthesis is in good alignment. Individuals who have had an upper extremity amputation may also perform exercises to strengthen the muscles that support the prosthesis.

Phantom Sensation and Phantom Pain

Although all individuals who have had an amputation experience some degree of **phantom sensation** (a sensation that the amputated extremity is still present), this sensation usually diminishes over time. Some individuals, however, experience chronic, severe pain sensation in the amputated extremity called **phantom limb pain** (Hsiao et al., 2012; Knotkova, Crucian, Tronnier, & Rasche, 2012). Phantom limb pain may gradually diminish over time, but it sometimes becomes incapacitating. In some instances, interventions to block the nerves that serve the amputated extremity may alleviate the pain. Individuals with chronic phantom pain may need chronic pain management.

Neuromas

At times, **neuromas** (bundles of nerve fibers) embedded in the scar tissue of the stump may cause pain and can be removed. This measure may not totally alleviate phantom limb pain, however.

FUNCTIONAL IMPLICATIONS OF AMPUTATION

Personal and Psychosocial Issues

Reaction to the loss of a limb is individual and based on a variety of factors, including age; educational, intellectual, and emotional status; economic status; and the individual meaning and circumstances of the loss. Individuals with amputation must make permanent behavioral, social, and emotional adjustments to cope with the multiple problems that can arise from this condition (Senra, Oliveira, Leal, & Vieira, 2012; Walsh et al., 2016). Amputation requires a major adjustment not only to a change in body image but also to a change in functional capacity (Akarsu, Tekin, Safaz, Göktepe, & Yazicioglu, 2012). When individuals are fitted with a prosthetic limb, they are immediately confronted with the irrevocable fact that they have lost a limb as well as the need to learn how to incorporate the prosthesis into daily function.

Traumatic amputation produces psychological and social effects that can be overwhelming if not addressed openly and candidly. The earlier that psychosocial intervention can be implemented, the more likely that psychological factors will not impede functional outcome. Individuals whose amputation was due to chronic condition may find it less difficult to adjust to the loss, especially if the body part amputated had been a source of pain or immobility prior to the amputation. Individuals who have who lost a body part suddenly—for example, because of traumatic injury—may have more difficulty with adjustment because they have had inadequate time to prepare for the loss (Kratz et al., 2010; Messinger, 2010).

Regardless of the reason for the amputation, it is important to understand individuals' interpretation of the loss (Cater, 2012). Individuals' ability to adapt to amputation depends on the circumstances surrounding the amputation, the usefulness of the prosthetic device, and individuals' perception of their condition. Some individuals who have lost a limb no longer consider themselves whole. They may fear that they will never again be able to function as they did prior to the amputation. For these individuals, a prosthesis is a reminder of perceived inadequacy rather than restoration of function. In some instances, loss of a limb is comparable to the loss of a loved one. Individuals may need sufficient time to grieve and adjust to their loss.

Activities and Participation

The extent of activity in which individuals can participate depends to some extent on the level of the amputation. Most individuals with lower extremity amputation can bicycle, swim, dance, and participate in many athletic activities with adaptive equipment. Driving a car is usually not a problem, although automatic transmissions may allow individuals to drive more easily. Activities such as climbing, squatting, and kneeling may be more difficult; however, even these tasks are mastered by some individuals. Individuals with upper extremity amputation may require other assistive devices in addition to the prosthesis to perform a number of activities of daily living.

While family can be of great assistance in helping individuals reintegrate their body image, family members may also have individual reactions to amputation. Reactions may also differ depending on the circumstances surrounding the amputation. Some family members may direct anger toward the individual if they believe amputation could have been avoided had the individual managed his or her underlying condition more carefully. In other instances, anger may be directed toward others if the amputation resulted from an accident in which it is perceived another person is at fault. Family members may be uncomfortable looking at the stump, which in turn influences individuals' self-esteem.

Sexuality

Although the amputation of an extremity has no direct effect on sexual activity, psychological factors or the reaction of sexual partners to the amputation may alter sexual function (Connell, Coates, & Wood, 2015). Reaction of individuals' partners to amputation may be either supportive or nonsupportive. The stability of the relationship prior to amputation as well as communication and understanding are important components to adjustment and, consequently, to the quality of the relationship.

VOCATIONAL ISSUES IN AMPUTATION

Individuals with amputation who wear a prosthesis may need to avoid hot, humid environments that can cause skin breakdown or contribute to the deterioration of the prosthesis. Dust or grit can be abrasive to the skin, exacerbating skin problems, and can interfere with the functioning of the movable parts of the prosthesis.

In the case of lower extremity amputation, physical demands of a job, such as the need for walking, climbing, or pushing, should be evaluated and altered, if necessary. The increased energy expenditure required for the use of a prosthesis should also be considered part of the physical demands of the job. Individuals in professional or managerial careers may have fewer functional consequences following the amputation of either an upper extremity or a lower extremity. Those with upper extremity amputation may have a greater need for a cosmetic-oriented prosthesis, however, than do those workers whose jobs require the prosthesis for tasks such as lifting.

CASE STUDY

Mr. R., a grain farmer, experienced an above-the-knee amputation of his left leg in a farming accident. He has been fitted with an above-the-knee prosthesis. He manages and works the farm on his own.

1. How might Mr. R.'s amputation affect his work?
2. Which types of modifications or assistive devices might be helpful to Mr. R.?
3. Are there any factors regarding prosthesis use that might be important to consider?

REFERENCES

Akarsu, S., Tekin, L., Safaz, I., Göktepe, A. S., & Yazicioglu, K. (2012). Quality of life and functionality after lower limb amputations: Comparison between uni- vs. bilateral amputee patients. *Prosthetics and Orthothotics International, 37*(1), 9–13.

Asano, M., Rushton, P., Miller, W. C., & Deathe, B. A. (2008). Predictors of quality of life among individuals who have a lower limb amputation. *Prosthetics and Orthotics International, 32,* 231–243.

Brown, B. J., Crone, C. G., & Attinger, C. E. (2012). Amputation in the diabetic to maximize function. *Seminars in Vascular Surgery, 25*(2), 115–121.

Cater, J. K. (2012). Traumatic amputation: Psychosocial adjustment of six army women to loss of one or more limbs. *Journal of Rehabilitation Research and Development, 49*(10), 1443–1456.

Connell, K. M., Coates, P., & Wood, F. M. (2015). Sexuality following traumatic injury: A literature review. *Burns and Trauma,* 2.20020061 doi:10.4103/2321-3868.130189

Cox, P. S., Williams, S. K., & Weaver, S. R. (2011). Life after lower extremity amputation in diabetics. *West Indian Medical Journal, 60*(5), 536–540.

Devon, H., Carman, A. B., Hendrick, P. A., Ribeiro, D. C. & Hale, L. A. (2015). Perceptions of low back pain in people with lower limb amputation: A focus group study. *Disability and Rehabilitation, 37*(10), 873–883.

Houdek, M. T., Kralovec, M. E., & Andrew, K. L. (2014). Hemi-pelvectomy: High level amputation surgery and prosthetic rehabilitation. *American Journal of Physical Medicine and Rehabilitation, 93*(7), 600–608.

Hsiao, A. F., York, R., Hsiao, I., Hansen, E., Hays, R. D., Ives, J., & Coulter, I. D. (2012). A randomized controlled study to evaluate the efficacy of noninvasive limb cover for chronic phantom limb pain among veteran amputees. *Archives of Physical Medicine and Rehabilitation, 93*(4), 617–622.

Jindeel, A., & Narahara, K. A. (2012). Nontraumatic amputation: Incidence and cost analysis. *International Journal of Lower Extremity Wounds, 11*(3), 177–179.

Kaufman, K. R., Levine, J. A., Brey, R. H., McCrady, S. K., Padgett, D. J., & Joyner, M. J. (2008). Energy expenditure and activity of transfemoral amputees using mechanical and microprocessor-controlled prosthetic knee. *Archives of Physical Medicine & Rehabilitation, 89*(7), 1380–1385.

Knotkova, H., Crucian, R. A., Tronnier, V. M., & Rasche, D. (2012). Current and future options for the management of phantom limb pain. *Journal of Pain Research, 5,* 39–49.

Kono, Y., & Muder, R. R. (2012). Identifying the incidence of and risk factors for reamputation among patients who underwent foot amputation. *Annals of Vascular Surgery, 26*(8), 1120–1126.

Kralovec, M. E., Houdek, M. T., Andrews, K. L., Shives, T. C., Rose, P. S., & Sim F. H. (2015). Prosthetic rehabilitation after hip disarticulation or hemipelvectomy. *American Journal of Physical Rehabilitation and Medicine, 94*(12), 1035–1040.

Kratz, A. L., Williams, R. M., Turner, A. P., Raichle, K. A., Smith, D. G., & Ehde, D. (2010). To lump or to split? Comparing individuals with traumatic and non-traumatic limb loss in the first year after amputation. *Rehabilitation Psychology, 55*(2), 126–138.

Malhotra, S., Bello, E., & Kominsky, S. (2012). Diabetic foot ulcerations: Biomechanics, Charcot foot, and total contact cast. *Seminars in Vascular Surgery, 25*(2), 66–69.

Messinger, S. D. (2010). Getting past the accident: Explosive devices, limb loss, and refashioning a life in a military medical center. *Medical Anthropology Quarterly, 24*(3), 281–303.

Nanda, V., Jacob, J., Alsafy, T., Punnoose, T., Sudhakar, V. R. & Iyasere, G. (2011). Replantation of an amputated hand: A rare case report: Acknowledgment of a multidisciplinary team input. *Oman Medical Journal, 26*(4), 278–282.

O'Keefe, B. (2011). Prosthetic rehabilitation of upper limb amputation. *Indian Journal of Plastic Surgery, 42*(2), 246–252.

Robbins, C. B., Vreeman, D. J., Sothmann, M. S., Wilson, S. L., & Oldridge, N. B. (2009). A review of the long term health outcomes associated with war related amputation. *Military Medicine, 174*(6), 588–592.

Senra, H., Oliveira, R. A., Leal, I. & Vieira, C (2012). Beyond body image: A qualitative study on how adults experience lower limb amputation. *Clinical Rehabilitation, 26*(2), 180–191.

Sensinger, J. W., Lipsey, J., Thomas, A. & Turner, K. (2015). Design and evaluation of voluntary opening and voluntary closing prosthetic terminal device. *Journal of Rehabilitation Research and Development, 52*(1), 63–76.

Tarim, A., & Ezer, A. (2012). Electrical burn is still a major risk factor for amputations. *Burns.* Retrieved from http://www.ncbi.nlm.nih.gov/pubmed/22853969

van Velzen, J. M., van Bennekom, C., van der Woude, L. H. V., & Houdijk, H. (2006). Physical capacity and walking ability after lower limb amputation: A systematic review. *Clinical Rehabilitation, 20,* 999–1016.

Walsh, M. V., Armstrong, T. W., Poritz, J., Elliott, T. R., Jackson, W. T., & Ryan, T. (2016). Resilience, pain interference, and upper limb loss: Testing the mediating effects of positive emotion and activity restriction on distress. *Archieves of Physical Medicine and Rehabilitation. 97*(5), 781–787.

Yoder, A. J., Petrella, A. J., & Silverman, A. K. (2015). Trunk-pelvis motion, joint loads, and muscle forces during walking with a transtibial amputation. *Gait and Posture. 41*(3), 752–762.

CHAPTER 27

Chronic Pain

In any given year, approximately 100 million people in the United States experience pain. While some pain is short term, resulting from injury or injury, approximately 9–12 million people experience chronic or persistent pain with debilitating consequences (Califf, Woodcock, & Ostroff, 2016).

Pain is a multidimensional, complex human experience with physical, psychological, spiritual, cultural, and social components that can have a dramatic effect on quality of life (Milks, 2012). Although the concept of pain is universally understood, because of its subjective nature, it is difficult to quantify

The purpose of pain is mainly protective: it can be a means of protecting against more serious injury, such as removing one's hand from a hot stove, or it can serve as a warning that an area of the body requires attention, such as pain associated with appendicitis. Pain can also be on going and chronic, when associated with chronic medical conditions.

THE EXPERIENCE OF PAIN

Although the concept of pain may be universal, the experience of pain is highly individual. The degree of incapacitation experienced with pain varies from individual to individual. The experience of pain is related to the nature of the pain, the individual's response to it, and the response of others in the individual's environment.

Individual response to pain is determined in part by each individual's *pain perception, pain threshold*, and *pain tolerance.*

Pain perception refers to recognition or awareness of the sensation of pain. Individuals' perception of pain and its severity can be influenced by a number of factors, including comorbid mood disorders, such as depression; personality traits, such as catastrophizing; environmental stressors; family relationships; social support; and cultural beliefs (McCarberg, Stanos, & Williams, 2012). Severity of pain is also influenced by the intensity, frequency, and duration of the pain stimulus, as well as by fear, anxiety, and expectations of the pain experience. For instance, although one needle prick may not be perceived as severely painful, continued or multiple needle pricks may be, especially if the individual is led to believe that successive needle pricks will be additionally painful. Anticipation of additional needle pricks usually results in increased fear and anxiety, heightening the perception of pain.

Pain threshold refers to the point at which pain is perceived. Not all individuals exposed to the same stimuli perceive the stimuli to be painful at the same point. For instance, some individuals may perceive a slight injury to be uncomfortable but not necessarily painful, whereas others with the same injury may perceive it to be painful, debilitating, and may require administration of analgesics.

Pain tolerance, refers to the point at which pain is perceived to be unbearable. Individuals have different levels of pain tolerance. Individuals with low pain tolerance may perceive the pain to be incapacitating and in need of treatment almost immediately, whereas individuals with heightened pain tolerance, although perceiving some discomfort, may continue with activities until the pain becomes more severe.

Pain intensity refers to the severity of the pain; however it is subjective. Observers often judge pain severity based on the individual's response to pain (*pain expression*) (i.e., grimacing, moaning, etc.). Pain intensity, as demonstrated by the reaction of the individual, is not however, always a reliable index of the seriousness of the condition.

Individual's response to pain is influenced by a number of factors, including the individual's physical and psychological state, cultural background and beliefs, and previous pain experience, as well as the location of the pain and the response of others. For instance, understanding and electively agreeing to a painful experience such as amputation of an extremity due to severe and prolonged infection may make the experience more tolerable, though still painful so that reactions may be more muted; by comparison, individuals experiencing amputation because of a sudden unexpected injury may have a more intense pain response. The same individual may endure pain less quietly if fatigued or in poor general health than when rested and well.

Distractions can also affect pain perception and response to pain (Carr, 2007). For example, individuals with rheumatoid arthritis may not perceive joint pain to be as severe when occupied with activities or when participating at a happy social event, as compared to at night when alone in the quiet of their home.

Individuals' cultural background also contributes to the way they experience and respond to pain. For instance, some cultural customs encourage a stoic response to pain, whereas other cultures permit free expression of feelings in response to pain. Upbringing, age, and circumstances all affect the response. Although the response to pain incorporates cultural components, individual responses within the same culture can also vary remarkably, so that stereotyping should be avoided. Even so, there should also be an awareness that nonresponse to pain does not necessarily mean that the individual is not experiencing discomfort.

CLASSIFICATION OF PAIN STATES

Pain states can be classified according to duration, location, and cause. Pain duration is classified as *acute* or *chronic*, and effective pain management is dependent on accurate differentiating between the two.

Pain classification based on origin is described as *somatic* or *visceral*. *Somatic pain* results from injury to or disease of the musculoskeletal system, joints, or skin, such as pain experienced in rheumatoid arthritis, or from a cut. *Visceral pain* results from injury, inflammation, or disease of the internal organs. Examples of conditions that cause visceral pain are kidney stones or bowel obstruction. Visceral pain is often more diffuse than somatic pain, which tends to be more localized.

Pain classification due to cause can be described as *neuropathic*, *nociceptive* or *mixed*. *Neuropathic pain* is the result of irritation or injury to tissue in the central or peripheral nervous system, such as pain associated with phantom limb pain or peripheral neuropathy associated with diabetes. *Nociceptive pain* refers to pain resulting from irritation of pain receptors due to in somatic structures such as skin, ligaments, joints, or bone. Pain experienced with bone fracture is an example of nociceptive pain. In some instances, pain is caused by a complex combination of nociceptive and neuropathic components. *Mixed pain states* refer to pain that is both neuropathic and nociceptive. Cancer pain, whether due to the cancer itself or pain associated with therapy, is an example of a mixed pain state.

ACUTE VERSUS CHRONIC PAIN

Acute pain usually is the result of injury or inflammation, is protective in that it promotes behaviors that minimize additional injury, and is often self-limiting and of short duration (Cohen & Raja, 2016). Examples of conditions causing acute pain include tooth ache, appendicitis, and muscle sprain. As healing occurs or the cause of the pain is corrected or removed, the pain usually decreases within an established course of time.

Acute pain management focuses on identifying and managing the underlying cause, alleviating the manifestations, and resolving the pain. If the underlying cause cannot be eradicated, or if interventions are not effective in relieving or managing the source of pain, acute pain can transition into chronic pain.

Chronic pain is considered as a pathological condition that serves no useful purpose and persists beyond the expected period of healing in most instances, longer than 3 to 6 months (Cohen & Raja, 2016). Chronic pain is one of the most debilitating medical conditions (Volkow & McLellan, 2016).

It has no biologic function of signaling injury, and it imposes psychological and physical stress on those who experience it. Individuals experiencing chronic pain may develop *chronic pain syndrome*, a condition characterized by physical, social, and behavioral consequences. Individuals with chronic pain syndrome often have marked alteration of behavior, as shown by depression or anxiety, restriction in daily activities, excessive use of medications, and frequent use of healthcare services. Pain becomes a central issue in their lives and interferes with both life activity and emotional functioning (Vellucci, 2012).

MANAGEMENT OF CHRONIC PAIN

Because pain is a complex multifaceted experience involving not only physiological components but subjective perceptions, emotions, and sociocultural influences, management of chronic pain involves a number of different modalities. The goal of chronic pain management is not only to reduce pain but also to improve functional status, mood, social interactions, and overall quality of life (Cohen & Raja, 2016). Total alleviation of pain may not be a realistic goal in many instances. Consequently, management of chronic pain incorporates multiple modalities, including pharmacologic, physical, and psychological interventions, often used in combination, to help individuals cope with the pain.

No one modality is effective for all individuals. Since the experience of pain is highly subjective, one of the most important components of pain management is determining which interventions are acceptable to and effective for the individual. Individuals' age, previous personal experiences, culture, and coexisting conditions (e.g., depression) are all variables that can influence the type and combination of interventions that may be the most beneficial.

Pharmacological Interventions

The type of medications used in pain management, depends on the cause and type of pain, as well as the individual's response the medication. No one medication has been found to be universally effective in managing chronic pain, and often medications are used in combination with or in addition to other interventions, as discussed later in this section.

Antipyretic medications, such as aspirin or acetaminophen, or nonsteroidal anti-inflammatory drugs (NSAIDs) are widely used as analgesics, although their effectiveness as stand-alone medications for severe pain is usually ineffective. In addition, side effects, such as bleeding or ulceration in the gastrointestinal tract make long-term use of these medications impractical.

Anticonvulsant and *antidepressant* medications, even when depression or seizures are not present, have been found to significantly reduce pain in some individuals and have less risk of serious side effects, such as tolerance or addiction (Moore, Wiffen, & Kalso, 2014). However, they appear to be more effective when the pain is neuropathic (Cohen & Raja, 2016).

Corticosteroids used for management of some chronic medical conditions, such as rheumatoid arthritis, may also relieve pain associated with the condition, however long-term use exclusively for pain management alone is generally contraindicated due to associated side effects such as gastrointestinal bleeding, elevated glucose levels, and development of osteoporosis.

Although *opioid analgesics* such as morphine and oxycodone are important tools for managing pain associated with cancer, or in short-term management of acute pain such as experienced in sickle cell crisis or pain experienced postsurgery, overall long-term use for management of chronic pain associated with other conditions is generally discouraged due to the risk of abuse, addiction, and other adverse effects (Requnath et al., 2016)

Long-term use of opioids have been found to be associated with *tolerance* in which there is decreased effectiveness of the opioid with repeated administrations so that higher or more frequent doses are needed to relieve pain. Long-term use of opioids has also been related to physical dependence in which individuals experience unpleasant physical manifestations such as insomnia, diarrhea, nausea, or muscle aches if the medication is continued. Over the last decade, overreliance on opioids to manage chronic pain has also resulted in increased individuals experiencing overdose as well as addiction (Volkow & McLellan, 2016).

Physical Interventions

Noninvasive Interventions

Physical Therapy

Physical therapy may be used to help alleviate or reduce pain as well as to enhance function. Interventions are directed toward evaluating and addressing specific factors that contribute to pain and providing education and procedural treatments to correct or reduce those factors. The goal is to help individuals with chronic pain gradually increase their exercise tolerance and activity level, as well as prevent additional injury. Interventions in this category may include exercises, correction of gait and postural irregularities, and application of hot or cold packs, infrared heat, or ultrasound.

Electrical Nerve Stimulation

There are several forms of electrical stimulation that can be used to manage pain. The most common form is *transcutaneous electrical nerve stimulation (TENS)*. In this technique, electrodes of a small, battery-operated device are placed over the painful area. When the unit is turned on, electrical current is used to stimulate nerve fibers at the site, providing a counter irritation that in turn blocks pain impulses. The intervention itself is painless.

The success of TENS depends to some extent on individuals' understanding of the technique and their motivation to use it. The degree and duration of pain relief with TENS units vary. For some individuals, the effects wear off after a few months. Other persons may use the TENS unit successfully for a longer period of time. Owing to the expense of using a TENS unit, long-term or permanent use of the unit is rarely feasible.

Biofeedback

Biofeedback is a technique in which individuals are able to gain awareness of physiological processes and consequently learn how to voluntarily modify or control those responses. Biofeedback has many uses and can be used to measure basic involuntary physiologic functions such as heart rate, blood pressure, skin temperature and muscle tension. One of its many uses is as a component in pain management.

Chronic pain creates complex biopsychosocial consequences including stress responses such as anxiety and muscle tension that can magnify or contribute to pain. Biofeedback helps individuals gain an awareness of stress responses so that they can learn to control them, therefore decreasing pain. The biofeedback device is a tool that is sensitive to very small changes in body functions. By measuring body changes and translating these changes into easily recognizable signals, individuals receive real time feedback that in turn enables them to voluntarily alter their response.

During a biofeedback session sensors are placed on the skin over localized muscles; wires from the sensors are then attached to an electromyogram machine, which measures electrical activity of the muscles. Individuals receive real-time feedback about the activity through signals in the form of sound or light. Through monitoring body responses through these cues, individuals become aware of body responses and can apply learned techniques, such as muscle relaxation, to alter them.

After learning techniques to reduce muscle tension, individuals are also able to monitor the effectiveness through the feedback system. With practice, they can learn to reduce the stress response at will without the benefit of physiologic monitoring.

Invasive Interventions

Acupuncture

Acupuncture is a key component of traditional Chinese medicine that has gained increased acceptance in Western Culture as a form of alternative medicine, especially in the management of chronic pain (Patil et al., 2016; Vickers & Linde, 2014). Acupuncture involves insertion of long, fine needles into selected points (trigger points) of an individual's body to eliminate the pain sensation.

There is no simple explanation for the mechanisms underlying the analgesic effects of acupuncture. Although considered an invasive technique, it is associated with few, if any, complications when performed under sterile conditions by individuals who have been appropriately trained and certified in acupuncture techniques.

Nerve Blocks

Nerve blocks eliminate pain locally. They are used during surgical procedures as well as in the intermediate-term management of chronic pain. This procedure involves injecting local anesthetics close to nerves, blocking their ability to conduct the painful stimuli. In some instances, corticosteroids are added to the local anesthetics to reduce inflammation which further contributes to pain. Generally, nerve blocks are given for the temporary relief of pain; however intermediate pain relief may facilitate the individual's participation in rehabilitation. In cases of severe pain, such as in terminal cancer, nerve blocks may be performed so that the effects are irreversible.

Neurosurgical Procedures

Neurosurgical procedures in which surgeons sever sensory nerves supplying the painful area may be used when severe pain cannot be ameliorated or controlled by other means. Cutting the nerves removes not only the sensation of pain but also the sensations of pressure, heat, and cold. Consequently, individuals who have undergone these procedures must be aware of the necessity of protecting the area from injury.

The type of neurosurgical procedure used depends on the type and location of the pain. For example, *sympathectomy* involves the autonomic nervous system; *neurectomy*, either the cranial or the peripheral nerves; and *rhizotomy* and *chordotomy*, the nerves close to the spinal cord.

Psychological Interventions

Psychological interventions as part of the multidisciplinary approaches to management of chronic pain assists the individual to achieve reduction in stress, gain increased self-management skills, improve coping ability, and reduce emotional distress. Skills gained through psychological interventions can empower the individual to become a more active participant in management of their pain.

A number of psychological interventions, including counseling and psychotherapy are used in pain management (Roditi & Robinson, 2011).

Some of the common psychological interventions used in pain management are discussed below.

Stress Management

Stress management can be an especially beneficial tool in the management of chronic pain. Stress experienced with chronic pain causes tension and anxiety, which in turn causes physiological changes that can exacerbate pain. When individuals are tense, the heart beats faster, blood pressure rises, and muscles tighten, contributing to more intense pain and more pronounced perception of pain. Decreasing stress reduces tension and anxiety and can, consequently, reduce pain and perception of pain intensity.

Stress management includes teaching individuals specific procedures that are designed to reduce stress and promote relaxation.

Guided Imagery

Guided imagery can be used to promote relaxation, manage pain, promote healing, or help individuals reach goals specific goals. The technique uses instruction or descriptive narrative provided by a trained professional to help individuals direct their thoughts to a relaxed, focused state. This intervention uses the individual's imagination to help the body respond to what he or she is imagining.

In the case of pain management, the individual may, for instance, be helped to imagine their pain as something over which they have complete control, or they may be helped to create a mental image of pain and then transform it into something more manageable.

Relaxation Therapy

Relaxation therapy is a technique used for a number of medical conditions but also a cornerstone of pain management. It is aimed at assisting individuals to learn the relaxation response, which decreases blood pressure, heart rate, oxygen consumption, and alpha wave (a type of brain wave) activity on electroencephalography (EEG). This technique, which can be learned through practice, may include both breathing techniques and progressive relaxation, thus reducing tension and anxiety.

Individuals who undergo progressive relaxation training are taught to tighten and relax different muscle groups gradually. This procedure promotes relaxation, decreases anxiety, and lessens muscle tension. When such techniques are used on a daily basis, they can help the individual cope with stress, and consequently decrease pain.

Cognitive-Behavioral Therapy

Cognitive-behavioral therapy (CBT) is a broad term that incorporates a number of strategies—including education, cognitive restructuring, coping strategies training, problem solving, and goal setting—that influence the individual's cognition, affect, and behavior. CBT is an individualized and collaborative effort between the individual and health professional based on the individual's goals (Freeman & Morgillo Freeman, 2016). Although used in a number of medical and psychosocial conditions, CBT has become recognized as an important intervention in pain management through combining a biopsychosocial and holistic approach, which seeks to assist individuals change their pain-related behaviors (Volkow & McLellan, 2016).

Meditation

Meditation is an intervention that also has been found to be useful in the management of chronic pain (Salomons & Kucyl, 2011). It is a technique that helps individuals achieve a relaxed state by concentrating on a variety of other processes such as breathing, chanting a repetitive phrase, or forming a visual image. The goal, in addition to achieving a state of relaxation, is to direct the individuals focus away from the painful sensation.

Hypnosis

Hypnosis is a procedure by which individuals are induced into a trance-like state, during which suggestion is used to alter attitudes, perceptions, or behaviors. The hypnotic state is attained through focusing on a soothing image or situation, purposeful relaxation of voluntary muscles, and controlled breathing. For individuals with chronic pain, hypnosis may be used to alter the reaction to painful stimuli or the perception of pain (Artimon,

2015). Skilled hypnotherapists may help individuals distract their thinking about pain through posthypnotic suggestion. Hypnosis should be conducted only by trained, certified individuals.

Operant Conditioning

As a behavioral technique designed to decrease the functional consequences associated with chronic pain, *operant conditioning* does not seek to cure or reduce the pain itself but rather alters the individual's behavioral response to the pain (Viaeyen, 2015). This technique is based on theories of *learning* and *conditioning*. The pain experience often results in a series of behaviors that communicate discomfort (e.g., grimacing, guarding, limping) and usually elicit responses from others in the form of sympathy, decreased expectations for performance or success, or even monetary compensation. Behavioral responses to pain may also be reinforced by the fact that they may help individuals avoid activities that they find unpleasant. Such reinforcement of pain behaviors may condition individuals to display them and, as a result, may increase the functional consequences associated with the pain behaviors. Operant conditioning involves withdrawing reinforcement for "pain" behaviors and reinforcing "well" behaviors.

Pain Groups

Chronic Pain Anonymous (CPA) was founded in 2004. The CPA model borrows from Alcoholics Anonymous (AA) and is based on the concept that similar psychological and emotional experiences arise with alcoholism and intractable benign pain: both disrupt personal and work relationships, cause loss of control and isolation, involve obsession, and are chronic conditions. CPA uses the same 12 steps as AA, substituting the word *pain* for the word *alcohol*. CPA groups help individuals learn to live with their pain when no other technique or intervention has proved successful for managing pain.

Other chronic pain support groups consist of a community of individuals with chronic pain who provide a forum for support, validation, and education in basic pain management. Individuals in the group share experiences and information.

FUNCTIONAL IMPLICATIONS OF CHRONIC PAIN

Personal and Psychosocial Issues

Chronic pain is a complex and distressing experience that can be expected to have some effect on personality. Irritability, preoccupation with pain, resentment, and depression are commonly associated with many chronic medical conditions. Individuals with chronic pain may exhibit the same characteristics. It has been estimated that between 30 and 60% of individuals with chronic pain experience manifestations of depression (Cohen & Raja, 2012). For some people, pain is unrelenting and persists at intolerable levels despite analgesic medication and futile attempts to manage it, resulting in feelings of hopelessness. In such cases, some individuals seek interventions that have not been shown to be effective and, in some instances, may be harmful. In other instances, depression can lead to abandoning interventions that, over time, can reduce pain (Padua et al., 2012).

Long-standing pain and associated depression can place limitations on pleasure and capabilities, leading to feelings of anger, guilt, and loss of self-esteem. Strain and conflict may arise in relationships with family, friends, and employers. As a consequent of deterioration of relationships and isolation from social and work activities, individuals may become fixated on their pain, amplifying its manifestations. In some instances, chronic pain can predispose individuals to engage in self-destructive behaviors.

Activities and Participation

In general, returning to regular activity as early as possible is important to prevent depression and to help individuals achieve pain reduction. Multidisciplinary pain clinics and multidisciplinary pain centers employ a wide variety of health professionals who can provide interventions that address many of the components of chronic pain and assist individuals to cope and live with the pain they are experiencing. For many individuals, a major impediment to effective management is access to healthcare professionals who are specifically trained in pain management; the cost of services may also present an obstacle to pain management (Pizzo & Clark, 2012). In multidisciplinary pain centers, the interventions and intensity of interventions are calibrated to each individual. When such centers or specialists in pain management are not available, pain management may be less effective due to health professionals' lack of knowledge or training in pain management as well as their concern about the possibility of addiction

VOCATIONAL IMPLICATIONS OF CHRONIC PAIN

The vocational impact of chronic pain, like chronic pain itself, is highly individualized and dependent on many factors. Comprehensive evaluation of the individual's abilities and needs and the type of assistive devices or accommodations needed can improve employment outcomes. Usually, early return to work helps individuals gain confidence, improves self-esteem, and increases motivation of the individual to remain employed. If constraints on physical activity are necessary, work limits should be defined and appropriate work modification instituted. At times insurance issues, worker's compensation, or other legal concerns may be a deterrent to successful return to work. An involved employer may reinforce individuals' motivation and enhance employment opportunities.

CASE STUDY

Case I

Ms. M., a 60-year-old relator recently was treated for malignant melanoma on her shoulder. The procedure involved removal of lymph nodes from under her right arm. Although the surgeon believes the surgery was successful, and there is no evidence the cancer has spread, Ms. M. continues to experience debilitating pain. Her general physician has prescribed OxyContin for her, which she states is the only thing that enables her to return to work. The physician has expressed concern about continuing to prescribe the medication. Ms. M. states she will be unable to continue employment without it.

1. What factors may be contributing to Ms. M.'s perception of pain?
2. What other modalities may be useful in helping Ms. M. to cope with her perceived pain?

Case II

Mr. H., a 38-year-old electrical engineer, received a back injury playing touch football with his colleagues while attending a company picnic. Despite physical therapy and a period of bed rest, his pain has persisted. MRI of the spine shows no fracture or herniation. The pain becomes more intense while sitting. Mr. H. states that he has increasing difficulty with concentrating during work and has become irritable and withdrawn.

1. Which specific issues regarding Mr. H.'s pain might be addressed?
2. Which issues might either help or hinder Mr. H.'s ability to continue working?
3. What specific interventions or services might Mr. H. find helpful?

REFERENCES

Artimon, H. M. (2015). Hynotherapy of a pain disorder: A clinical case study. *International Journal of Clinical and Experimental Hypnosis, 63*(2), 236–246.

Califf, R. M., Woodcock, J. & Ostroff, S. (April 14, 2016). A proactive response to prescription opioid abuse. *The New England Journal of Medicine, 374*, 1480–1485. doi: 10:1056/NEJMsr160137

Carr, E. (2007). Barriers to effective pain management. *Journal of Perioperative Practice, 17*(5), 200–208.

Cohen, S. P., & Raja, S. N. (2016). Pain. In L. Goldman & A. I. Schafer (Eds.), *Goldman-Cecil Medicine* (25th ed., pp. 133–143). Philadelphia, PA: Elsevier Saunders.

Freeman, A. & Morgillo Freeman, S. E. (2016). Basics of cognitive behavior therapy. In I. Marini and M. A. Stebnicki (Eds.), (pp 191–196). New York, NY: Springer Publishing Company.

McCarberg, B. H., Stanos, S., & Williams, D. A. (2012). Comprehensive chronic pain management: Improving physical and psychological function (CME multimedia activity). *American Journal of Medicine, 125*(6), S1.

Milks, J. W. (2012). Pain. In E. T. Bope & R. D. Kellerman (Eds.), *Conn's current therapy 2012* (pp. 24–31). Philadelphia, PA: Elsevier Saunders.

Moore, A., Wiffen, P., & Kalso, E. (2014). Antiepileptic drugs for neuropathic pain and fibromyalgia. *JAMA, 312*, 182–183.

Padua, L., Aprile, I., Cecchi, F., Molino, L. R., Arezzo, M. F., & Pazzaglia, C. (2012). Pain in postsurgical orthopedic rehabilitation: A multicenter study. *Pain Medicine, 13*(6), 769–776.

Patil, S., Sen, S., Bral, M., Reddy, S., Bradley, K. K., Cornett, E. M., Fox, C. J., & Kaye, A. D. (2016). The role of acupuncture in pain management. *Current Pain and Headache Reports, 20*(4), 22. doi:10. 1007/s11916-0552-1

Pizzo, A. A., & Clark, N. M. (2012). Alleviating suffering 101: Pain relief in the United States. *New England Journal of Medicine, 366*(3), 197–199.

Requnath, H., Cochran, K., Cornell, K., Shortridge, J., Kim, D., Akbar, S. . . . Koller, J. P. (2016). Is it painful to manage chronic pain? A cross-sectional study of physicians in-training in a university program. *Missouri Medicine, 112*(1), 72–78.

Roditi, D., & Robinson, M. E. (2011). The role of psychological interventions in the management of patients with chronic pain. *Psychology Research and Behavior Management, 4*, 41–49.

Salomons, T. V. & Kucyl, A. (2011). Does meditation reduce pain through a unique neural mechanism? *The Journal of Neuroscience, 31*(36), 12705–12707.

Vellucci, R. (2012). Heterogeneity of chronic pain. *Clinical Drug Investigation, 32*(Suppl. 1), 3–10.

Viaeyen, J. W. (2015). Learning to predict and control harmful events: Chronic pain and conditioning. *Pain,* (Suppl 1), S86–93.

Vickers, A. J. & Linde, K. (2014). Acupuncture for chronic pain. *JAMA, 311*, 955–956.

Volkow, N. D. & McLellan, A. T. (March 31, 2016). Opiod abuse in chronic pain: Misconcept6ions and mitigation strategies. *The New England Journal of Medicine, 374*:1253–1263. doi:10.2056/NEJMra1507771

CHAPTER 28

Cardiovascular Conditions

STRUCTURE AND FUNCTION OF THE CARDIOVASCULAR SYSTEM

The cardiovascular system consists of the following components:

- The *heart,* which pumps blood throughout the body
- The *coronary circulation,* which supplies the heart muscle with blood
- The *pulmonary circulatory system,* which carries blood to and from the lungs
- The *systemic circulatory system,* which carries blood throughout the body

Each system consists of networks of blood vessels through which oxygen and nutrients are distributed to tissues, wastes are removed, and deoxygenated blood is returned to the lungs to be oxygenated. The blood vessels in the circulatory system are classified as follows:

- *Arteries:* vessels that carry *oxygenated* blood *away* from the heart
- *Veins:* vessels that carry *unoxygenated* blood *to* the heart
- *Arterioles:* small branches of the artery, which carry oxygenated blood and transport it to a capillary
- *Venules:* small veins that carry unoxygenated blood from the capillary, transporting it to a larger vein
- *Capillaries:* minute blood vessels that connect arterioles and venules

The Heart

The heart—the principal part of the circulatory system—is a robust, strong, and powerful muscle located to the left of the center of the chest. It consumes more energy than any other organ in the body, beating approximately 100,000 times per day and pumping approximately 5,500 gallons of blood through the blood vessels of the body.

The heart muscle is called the **myocardium**; it is a unique type of muscle that has the ability to work continuously with only brief periods of rest between contractions. This *resting phase*, when the heart is relaxed and the chambers are filling, is called **diastole**. The *contraction phase*, when the heart muscle pumps blood out of the chambers, is called **systole**.

Diastole and systole produce different pressure gradients. The ratio of these two gradients is called *blood pressure*. The amount of pressure produced depends on the force with which the heart pumps and the degree to which the blood vessels resist blood flow. Blood pressure is expressed numerically as a fraction in which the systolic reading is the numerator and the diastolic reading is the denominator. For instance, in a blood pressure reading of 120/80 (measured in units of millimeters of mercury, or mm Hg), the systolic pressure is 120 mm Hg and the diastolic pressure is 80 mm Hg.

The heart contains four chambers. The two upper chambers are the right and left **atria**, and the two lower chambers are the right and left **ventricles**. Four valves help blood move from chamber to chamber in one direction without backflow. The right atrium receives deoxygenated blood from the systemic circulation through a large vein called the *vena cava.* The right atrium pumps blood through the *tricuspid valve* into the right ventricle. From the right ventricle, deoxygenated blood is pumped through the *pulmonary semilunar valve* into the *pulmonary artery*, where it is carried to the lungs for exchange of oxygen and waste (*pulmonary circulation*) (**Figure 28-1**). Oxygenated blood from the lungs is then pumped through the *pulmonary vein* into the left atrium, which then pumps through the *mitral (biscuspid)* valve into the left ventricle. From the left ventricle, blood is pumped through the *aortic semilunar valve* into the *aorta* to be carried to the general circulation.

The heart is enclosed in an outer covering (the **pericardium**) consisting of two layers. The space between the two layers of the pericardium contains a small amount of fluid to lessen friction between the two surfaces as the heart beats. The inner surface of the heart is called the **endocardium**.

Coronary Circulation

Like all muscles, the myocardium requires oxygen and nutrients to survive. A separate circulatory system, *coronary circulation,* consists of a network of blood vessels called the *coronary vessels*, which supply the myocardium with blood.

The coronary circulation consists of the *coronary arteries*, which carry oxygen and nutrients *to* the heart muscle, and *coronary veins*, which carry blood used by the heart muscle and containing wastes *away from* the heart muscle. This coronary circulation is essential to the heart's ability to pump blood to the entire body.

Pulmonary Circulation

Deoxygenated blood from the general body circulation is pumped by the *right ventricle* through the

Figure 28-1   The Heart

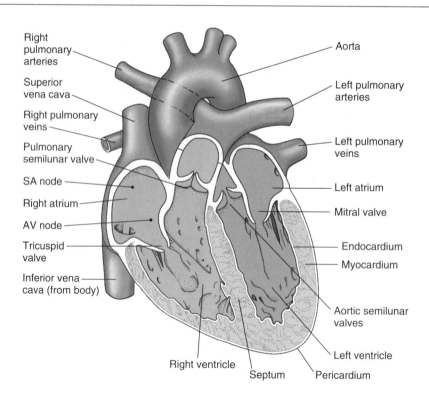

pulmonary artery into the lungs. The pulmonary artery is the only artery in the body that carries deoxygenated blood.

In the lungs, wastes, in the form of carbon dioxide, diffuse from the blood and are excreted from the lungs. Atmospheric oxygen diffuses into the blood from the lungs, and the newly oxygenated blood is pumped back to the left ventricle of the heart through the *pulmonary vein* (the only vein in the body that carries primarily oxygenated blood). (See **Figure 28-2**.)

Systemic Circulation

The heart pumps oxygenated blood into the *aorta*, through which blood moves to arteries in the systemic circulation. The network of arteries diminishes in size to arterioles, which then branch into capillaries. The capillary walls are very thin, allowing oxygen and nutrients from the blood to diffuse through the capillary membrane into body tissues. Waste products from body tissues in turn diffuse through the capillary membrane into the blood. Blood containing waste products is carried back to the heart through small venules, which then branch into veins that increase in size until they reach the larger *vena cava*, which returns deoxygenated blood to the heart. Within the heart, blood is pumped into the pulmonary circulation for reoxygenation.

Electrical System of the Heart

A special nerve network in the heart generates electrical activity and maintains the regular, rhythmic beating of the heart. Special cells, located within the right atrium, compose the *sino-atrial (SA) node* (also called the "pacemaker" of the heart), which initiates heart contractions. Impulses from the SA node spread over both atria, causing them to contract simultaneously.

The impulse then reaches special cells, the *atrioventricular (AV) node,* in the lower right

Figure 28-2   Pulmonary Circulation

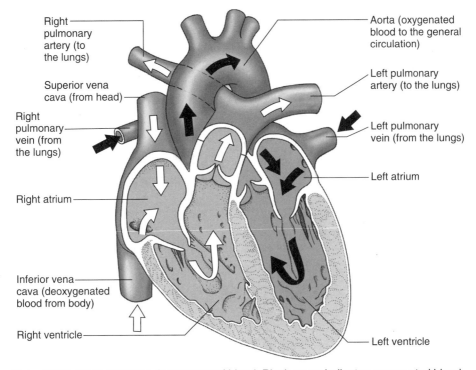

Right pulmonary artery (to the lungs)

Superior vena cava (from head)

Right pulmonary vein (from the lungs)

Right atrium

Inferior vena cava (deoxygenated blood from body)

Right ventricle

Aorta (oxygenated blood to the general circulation)

Left pulmonary artery (to the lungs)

Left pulmonary vein (from the lungs)

Left atrium

Left ventricle

Note: White arrow indicates deoxygenated blood. Black arrow indicates oxygenated blood.

atrium, From the AV node, impulses are transferred to special muscle fibers (*bundle of His*) located on the right (*right bundle*) and left (*left bundle*) sides of the septum separating the two ventricles. The bundles branch out to *Purkinje fibers*, which spread over both ventricles, causing them to contract. At this point, the cycle starts over.

Coordinated contraction and relaxation of the heart at a normal rate is called a *normal sinus rhythm*. Conduction of nerve impulses throughout the heart occurs involuntarily, When the system is working well, communication from the autonomic nervous system adjusts the heart rate automatically according to the body's changing need for oxygen, increasing the rate when more oxygen is needed, such as with exercise, and decreasing the rate when less oxygen is needed.

OVERVIEW OF CONDITIONS OF THE CARDIOVASCULAR SYSTEM

Cardiovascular conditions are those conditions that affect the heart or vascular system; they encompass a variety of health conditions with a wide range of manifestations. Such conditions are the third leading cause of incapacitation and can affect physical, psychological, and vocational function (Lloyd-Jones, 2016). Cardiovascular conditions may be either acquired or congenital, and include conditions such as stroke, hypertension, coronary artery disease, peripheral vascular disease, and congenital heart conditions. A number of risk factors have been shown to contribute to the development of acquired cardiovascular conditions (O'Donnell & Nabel, 2011). The greater the number of risk factors, the greater the likelihood of developing a cardiovascular condition. Although many of these risk factors can be modified to prevent development of cardiovascular conditions, some risk factors cannot (**Table 28-1**). Even when individuals have nonmodifiable risks for development of cardiovascular conditions, however, mitigating those risk factors that can be modified can significantly lower overall probability of an incapacitating or fatal cardiovascular event.

Table 28-1   Factors for Cardiovascular Disease

Modifiable	Nonmodifiable
Smoking	Age
Obesity	Gender
Physical inactivity	Ethnicity
	Family history

ATHEROSCLEROSIS

Overview of Atherosclerosis

Atherosclerosis is a chronic inflammatory response to accumulation of *lipids* (a type of fat) in the arterial walls and is the most common cause of coronary heart conditions and stroke (Lloyd-Jones, 2016). It develops over decades in response to a number of risk factors (Borissoff, Spronk, & Ten Cate, 2011; Hansson & Hamsten, 2016; Nabel & Braunwald, 2012). The buildup of plaques, which consist of fat and infiltrate from the inflammatory process, causes **stenosis** (narrowing) of the vessel, thereby impeding blood flow.

Atherosclerosis is generally associated with elevated cholesterol levels (**hyperlipidemia**). Cholesterol is a substance that is manufactured naturally in the body; in addition, the body receives cholesterol through dietary intake of food high in lipids. Although a strong link exists between cholesterol and heart disease, not all people with high cholesterol level develop conditions of the cardiovascular system; likewise, some people develop cardiovascular conditions even though they do not have elevated cholesterol levels.

Buildup of plaque inside an artery wall can contribute to physical manifestations resulting from lessened blood flow to tissues. Plaque accumulation can also provoke formation of a **thrombus** (blood clot) within the narrowed vessel, interrupting blood flow. This flow may be interrupted on a temporary basis so that manifestations are intermittent (such as angina pectoris, discussed later in the chapter); alternatively, the impediment may be permanent, so that **necrosis** (tissue death) occurs, as in myocardial infarction.

In some instances, the thrombus does not obstruct blood flow but rather is dislodged from the vessel wall, becoming an **embolus** and traveling in the bloodstream to another part of the body. (The term *embolus* can also refer to other substances traveling in the blood, such as an air bubble, fat globule, or other foreign matter.) The embolus can lodge in a blood vessel too small to allow its passage, occluding blood flow there. The effects of an *embolism* depend on the body part affected. For example, an embolism of the brain results in *stroke*, whereas an embolus lodging in the lungs would be called a *pulmonary embolus*. In all instances, embolism can result in severe tissue damage and can be fatal.

Manifestations of Atherosclerosis

Manifestations of atherosclerosis develop slowly and may be nonexistent unless blood flow becomes diminished to the extent of **ischemia** (inadequate oxygen supply to tissue), resulting in pain, fatigue, or altered function in the area affected. If blood flow and consequently oxygen supply are severely diminished necrosis can occur, as discussed earlier.

Specific manifestations vary depending on the extent of stenosis of the vessels and the location of the impeded blood flow. For example, stenosis of the *carotid arteries* (vessels carrying blood to the brain) can result in diminished cognitive function due to the decreased oxygen supply to the brain. Stenosis of vessels providing blood flow to the kidneys may contribute to kidney damage and chronic renal failure. Diminished blood flow to the heart may cause **angina pectoris** (chest pain) or, if blood flow is severely restricted, myocardial infarction. Stenosis of the aorta is associated with high mortality (Kodali et al., 2012; Makkar et al., 2012).

Management of Atherosclerosis

Management of atherosclerosis is directed toward preventing complications associated with the condition—namely, myocardial infarction, stroke, and kidney failure. A variety of medications, including *statins*, are in widespread use to lower blood cholesterol levels. Although it is generally recognized that response to lipid-lowering medications varies among individuals, there appears to be growing controversy regarding the extent to which statins, in particular, eliminate cardiovascular risk (Goldfine, 2012; Nabel & Braunwald, 2012).

When narrowing of the carotid arteries due to atherosclerosis occurs, either *carotid endarterectomy* or *carotid artery stenting* may be performed to remove the obstruction or widen the passage of vessels leading to the brain, thereby increasing blood flow and oxygen supply to the brain (Furlan, 2006). When narrowing of coronary arteries that supply blood and oxygen to the heart is identified prior to myocardial infarction, surgical procedures to widen these vessels may also be used—specifically, *coronary artery bypass graft (CABG)* or *percutaneous coronary intervention (PCI)*, both of which are discussed later in this chapter. Because nicotine further constricts already-narrowed vessels, tobacco use is contraindicated in individuals with atherosclerosis.

HYPERTENSION

Defining Hypertension

Individuals with **hypertension** (elevated blood pressure) have a sustained elevation of pressure in the arteries. Both systolic and diastolic pressures may be elevated. Hypertension in and of itself is not incapacitating, but prolonged elevated blood pressure is a major risk factor for myocardial infarction, heart failure, stroke, peripheral vascular disease, and renal failure—all of which can cause significant incapacitation (Victor, 2016).

Blood pressure normally fluctuates with physical activity, becoming lower at rest and higher with changes in posture, exercise, or emotion. When blood pressure remains high even at rest, it puts increased strain on body organs and increases the risk for development of other complications as mentioned earlier.

The most common type of hypertension is *primary (essential) hypertension*, in which a single reversible cause cannot be identified; factors such as obesity, excessive alcohol consumption, smoking, and excessive intake of sodium have been found to contribute to elevated blood pressure, however (Adrogué, 2012). A small percentage of

452 Chapter 28 • Cardiovascular Conditions

individuals have *secondary hypertension*, which results from other conditions, such as hyperthyroidism or kidney disease (e.g., *renal artery stenosis*). A less common, but more severe type of hypertension is *malignant hypertension*, which has an abrupt onset and is characterized by extreme blood pressure elevation. Malignant hypertension is a healthcare emergency and requires immediate attention (Victor, 2016).

Identification of Hypertension

Accurate measurement of blood pressure and verification of elevated blood pressure on several occasions are the accepted procedures for identifying hypertension. Hypertension is most accurately identified when blood pressure is measured under similar conditions over a period of time. Because blood pressure fluctuates throughout the day, and because it may be higher when measured in a healthcare setting than at home, 24-hour blood pressure monitoring is gaining recognition as a more accurate appraisal of blood pressure throughout the day (Victor, 2016).

Often, primary hypertension is initially identified during a routine physical examination. Manifestations of hypertension are often nonexistent, so this condition may go undetected until complications such as myocardial infarction, stroke, or visual changes such as retinal bleeding arise (Adrogué, 2012).

Management of Hypertension

The primary goal of management of hypertension is to lower blood pressure and reduce the risk of complications. In mild cases, lifestyle modifications, such as maintaining a proper body weight, exercising, reducing alcohol intake, ending tobacco use, limiting dietary intake of fats and sodium, and reducing calories consumed, may be sufficient to lower blood pressure (Victor, 2016). While stress alone may not directly cause primary hypertension, it may induce physiologic changes that may lead to elevated blood pressure. Learning to reduce stress or avoid chronically stressful situations may also be important in the overall management of hypertension.

When lifestyle modifications are insufficient to lower blood pressure or when blood pressure is too high to manage with lifestyle modification alone, medication may be required. A variety of classes of medications, called *antihypertensives*, may be used in the management of hypertension (Victor, 2016). Antihypertensives can also cause numerous side effects, such as dry cough with angiotensin-converting enzyme (ACE) inhibitors or erectile dysfunction with diuretics. Side effects can sometimes interfere with individuals' willingness to take their medications in accordance with the healthcare plan.

Psychosocial Issues in Hypertension

Individuals with hypertension frequently experience few manifestations, so they may not recognize the seriousness of their condition or the potential for the development of complications that can be severely incapacitating. Consequently, they may be less motivated to adhere to interventions to manage their condition. Management also often involves lifestyle changes—such as weight loss, smoking cessation, or exercise—that individuals may find difficult accomplish. Identifying potential problems that may contribute to nonadherence, and working toward solutions to overcome them, can be beneficial in managing hypertension and preventing complications.

Vocational Issues in Hypertension

There are usually no specific limitations associated with hypertension per se; however, isometric activities such as pushing, lifting, or carrying heavy objects can increase blood pressure during the activity and may need to be avoided. Although some degree of emotional stress is inherent in many jobs, individuals need to recognize that chronic, sustained stress may have a detrimental effect on blood pressure. Individuals may need to learn to manage stress experienced at work or seek ways of modifying the work environment to make it less stressful. The major impact that hypertension has on employment results from complications, such as stroke, myocardial infarction, or other complications that cause incapacitation. Consequently, reinforcement of adherence to the management plan is of major importance to ongoing employment.

ANEURYSM

Overview of Aneurysm

An **aneurysm** is the dilation or ballooning out of a weakened arterial wall. The weakened wall of the artery, if under increased pressure (e.g., due to hypertension), may burst and lead to hemorrhage. Common sites of aneurysms are in the brain and the aorta (the major trunk of the arterial system of the body). A *dissecting aneurysm* is a tear in the inner wall of the vessel that allows blood to leak between the layers of the wall of the vessel, moving longitudinally to separate the layers along the length of the vessel rather than rupturing into an open body space. Although atherosclerosis is a major contributor to aortic aneurysm, smoking is the strongest risk factor associated with development of this condition (Lederle, 2016).

Manifestations of Aneurysm

Manifestations experienced as a result of an aneurysm vary according to its location. In some instances, no manifestations become apparent until the aneurysm becomes large enough to create pressure, causing pain at the site. In other instances, there are no manifestations until the aneurysm ruptures, which could result in sudden death.

Identification of Aneurysm

Because there are often no manifestations to suggest the presence of an aneurysm, it is generally recommended that individuals who have smoked or have a family history of aneurysm be screened for this condition (Lederle, 2016). Aneurysms are usually identified through *abdominal ultra-sonography* or *computed tomography (CT) scan* (Neschis, 2012).

Management of Aneurysm

Aneurysms may be managed surgically if they are identified early or if surgery is not contraindicated because of associated health conditions. Surgical procedures to correct aneurysms involve removal of the weakened area of the artery, followed by connection of the two remaining ends (**anastomosis**). A *graft* to join the two remaining ends is used if a large portion of the vessel has

been removed. Controlling hypertension, if present, is an important aspect of continuing management after surgery.

CORONARY ARTERY DISEASE

Coronary artery disease is a condition in which the coronary arteries that supply blood and oxygen directly to the myocardium become narrowed. It is usually caused by atherosclerosis, in which plaque builds up on the inner walls of the coronary vessels. As a result, the myocardium receives an inadequate supply of blood (ischemia) and, consequently, a diminished supply of oxygen to meet its needs. Depending on the extent of blockage of blood supply to the heart muscle, individuals may experience either unstable angina pectoris or myocardial infarction (*acute coronary syndrome*) (Stone et al., 2011).

Angina Pectoris

Overview of Angina Pectoris

When there is a mismatch between the amount of oxygen a muscle needs and the amount of oxygen available, pain results. Insufficient supply of oxygen to the heart muscle results in chest pain, called **angina pectoris**. The most common cause of angina pectoris is coronary atherosclerosis (Tobin & Eagle, 2012).

The heart muscle's need for oxygen is greatest when demands are placed on the heart. Consequently, angina is often triggered by physical activity. Decreasing activity, and therefore decreasing the workload of the heart, often causes chest pain to subside. This type of angina is predictable and called *stable angina*. When chest pain occurs at rest, with no precipitating activity, or when pain is more severe, more frequent, or more prolonged, individuals are said to have *unstable angina*.

Manifestations of Angina Pectoris

The most common manifestation of stable angina is heaviness or pain in the middle of the chest that is associated with physical exertion or activity, emotional stress, or exposure to the cold. The duration of pain or discomfort with stable angina is usually brief and usually subsides with rest or medication, such as *nitroglycerin* (Boden, 2016). Individuals with unstable angina experience chest pain or discomfort even in the absence of exercise.

Identification of Angina Pectoris

Identification of angina is based on history of manifestations, laboratory evaluations, and non-invasive tests such as electrocardiogram, ambulatory monitoring, stress electrocardiogram, or stress echocardiogram, and in some instances a more invasive test, cardiac catheterization.

The *electrocardiogram (ECG)* is a graphic representation of electrical activity in the heart. It is useful in suspected angina pectoris to determine whether the cardiac muscle is receiving an adequate oxygen supply. *Ambulatory monitoring* may be used to provide a continuous graphic reading of the heart's function and alteration of function as individuals go about their daily activities. In ambulatory monitoring, a small portable device, such as a *Holter monitor*, is worn by the individual to check the heart's function with levels of activity. The *stress electrocardiogram* is a noninvasive exercise test in a laboratory setting in which an ECG reading is taken while an individual walks on a treadmill. A stress ECG provides a graphic record of the heart's activity during forced exertion and determines the extent of cardiac disease. A *stress echocardiogram*, performed in much the same way as the stress electrocardiogram, uses ultrasound to record the size, motion, and composition of the heart and large vessels, thereby determining the extent of vessel occlusion.

In some instances, *cardiac catheterization* may be used to define the location and severity of narrowing of the coronary vessels. Cardiac catheterization is an invasive procedure in which a catheter is inserted into a vessel, often in the groin area, and then threaded into the arteries of the heart to obtain X-ray images of the coronary arteries and cardiac chambers (*angiography*).

Management of Angina Pectoris

Management of angina pectoris is directed toward reducing manifestations, increasing functional capacity, preventing myocardial infarction, and, in some instances, taking steps to correct the cause. Management includes modification of ongoing risk factors, medication, and evaluation regarding the need for surgical intervention to alleviate coronary artery stenosis. Cessation of tobacco use, management of hypertension, and weight loss, if obesity exists, are important ways to modify risk (Tobin & Eagle, 2012). Angina pectoris may also be helped by administration of nitroglycerin, a medication that dilates the coronary arteries, enabling the heart muscle to receive more oxygen, thereby relieving pain.

When pain associated with angina occurs so frequently that limitation of activity becomes severely incapacitating or when occlusion of the coronary arteries becomes so pronounced that myocardial infarction is imminent, surgery such as percutaneous coronary intervention or coronary artery bypass graft, both of which are discussed later in the chapter, may be indicated.

Myocardial Infarction

Whereas angina pectoris describes a condition in which there is *diminished* blood supply and consequently diminished oxygen to the heart muscle, **myocardial infarction** (heart attack) describes a condition in which there is *total occlusion* of an a coronary artery so that part of the myocardium receives *no* oxygen (**anoxia**), and necrosis (tissue death) occurs. Not all individuals with angina go on to develop myocardial infarction, and not all people with myocardial infarction have first experienced angina.

Total occlusion of a coronary vessel can occur for the following reasons:

- Atherosclerosis, in which the coronary arteries become totally occluded
- Formation of a thrombus (blood clot) in a coronary artery, occluding blood flow
- Lodging of an *embolus* (a blood clot, a particle of bacterial growth from an affected valve, or other foreign material that has traveled through the bloodstream) in a coronary artery, occluding blood flow

Once a portion of the heart muscle has been destroyed, it cannot regenerate. The ability of the heart to continue functioning effectively as a pump is directly related to the amount of heart muscle damage that has occurred, and the location of the damage.

Manifestations of Myocardial Infarction

Most individuals with acute myocardial infarction experience prolonged chest pain and pressure that may radiate to the arms, neck, or back and may be accompanied by nausea, **dyspnea** (difficulty breathing), and **diaphoresis** (sweating). Some individuals, however, may not experience typical manifestations but rather experience manifestations that may be interpreted as caused by another condition, such as indigestion. Acute myocardial infarction is an emergency that requires immediate healthcare attention.

Identification of Myocardial Infarction

Myocardial infarction is identified through assessment of manifestations, ECG, resting echocardiogram, and, in some instances, cardiac catheterization as described earlier. Laboratory tests may also be used to determine whether tissue damage has occurred (Reeder & Prasad, 2012).

Management of Myocardial Infarction

The focus of emergency healthcare management for myocardial infarction is on assessment, stabilizing the condition, relieving pain, and preventing sudden death (Anderson, 2016). After emergency management, individuals are usually admitted to the *coronary care unit* (CCU), where the goal is to limit heart damage, initiate electrical stability of the heart, and promote comfort.

After experiencing myocardial infarction, individuals usually undergo cardiovascular risk factor assessment. Fundamental steps to reduce risk include lowering blood pressure, increasing exercise, dietary modifications, and smoking cessation. In addition, medications are often used to reduce blood coagulation. Individuals may also undergo surgical intervention, such as percutaneous coronary intervention or coronary artery bypass graft, as well as *cardiac rehabilitation*, all of which are discussed in the next section.

Management of Coronary Artery Disease

Surgical Interventions for Coronary Artery Disease

When the coronary arteries are partially or totally occluded, *surgical revascularization procedures* may be required to relieve obstruction and restore blood flow (Weintraub et al., 2012). One of two *revascularization* procedures may be used: percutaneous coronary intervention (PCI) or coronary artery bypass graft (CABG) (Cohen et al., 2011). The procedure used is individually determined, and each surgical option has relative advantages and disadvantages (Teirstein & Lytle, 2016).

Percutaneous Coronary Intervention

PCI or *angioplasty* is a minimally invasive procedure used to widen narrowed coronary vessels (Aversano, Lemmon, & Liu, 2012; Park et al., 2011). The procedure consists of inserting a hollow needle into an artery in the groin area (usually the femoral artery) and, under radio-graphic guidance, advancing a guidewire over which a special catheter can be threaded into the occluded artery. Angioplasty can involve several methods. In *balloon angioplasty*, a thin catheter (tube) with a balloon at its tip is threaded through the blood vessel to the affected artery. The balloon is then inflated, flattening the plaque against the artery wall. Another method involves placement of a *stent* (a small metal or mesh tube) in the vessel (Shahian, Meyer, Yeh, Fifer, & Torchiana, 2012). The stent is left in place to widen the artery and to maintain blood flow. Some stents contain medication to decrease the risk of blood clot formation (Curfman, Morrissey, Jarcho, & Drazen, 2007), although the use of medicated stents versus nonmedicated stents remains controversial (Teirstein & Lytle, 2016). A procedure now rarely used, *atherectomy*, which is similar to angioplasty, involves insertion of a catheter with a device on the end that removes plaque at the site.

PCI can reduce manifestations of angina and increase functional ability. In some individuals, restenosis occurs, requiring repeated revascularization procedures at a later time (Teirstein & Lytle, 2016). In addition, some individuals may be at higher risk for myocardial infarction due to PCI, although the extent of this risk is currently controversial (Prasad & Herrmann, 2011).

Coronary Artery Bypass Graft

CABG is a surgical procedure used to restore blood flow to the myocardium due to narrowing or occlusion of the coronary arteries (Grover, 2012). The procedure involves using a graft—usually a vein taken from the individual's leg—to bypass the obstructed artery. When several coronary arteries are constricted, additional grafts are needed.

The CABG procedure, although not a cure, is intended to alleviate manifestations of atherosclerotic heart disease, prevent myocardial infarction from occurring, or, if myocardial infarction has occurred, prevent additional damage (Lamy et al., 2012). Potentially serious complications after CABG include stroke (Selnes et al., 2012; Teirstein & Lytle, 2016) and renal failure (Grover, 2012).

Medication Management in Coronary Artery Disease

Management of coronary artery disease often involves medication. Medications such as nitroglycerin, which dilates blood vessels, thereby increasing the supply of blood to the myocardium, may be used by individuals with angina pectoris to relieve chest pain. Individuals with either angina or myocardial infarction may take *antiplatelet medications* such as *aspirin* to reduce the possibility of thrombus formation (Roe & Ohman, 2012). *Anticoagulants,* such as *heparin,* which also prevent clot formation, may be used as well. Because anticoagulants can cause bleeding, individuals' blood levels of these agents are carefully monitored. In addition, because of the possibility of bleeding while taking anticoagulants, activities that could result in injury should be avoided.

Cardiac Rehabilitation in Coronary Artery Disease

Functional capacity in angina and myocardial infarction is determined not only by physical aspects of the condition, but also based on psychological, social, and vocational factors. Although an important part of management for both angina and myocardial infarction involves medication, lifestyle modification, and possibly surgical intervention, an important intervention in helping individuals achieve optimal functional capacity is cardiac rehabilitation, which considers all of these factors. Cardiac rehabilitation is discussed in more detail later in the chapter.

Functional Implications of Coronary Artery Disease

Personal and Psychosocial Issues

Conditions that involve the heart, and especially manifestations in angina pectoris, are indicative of the potential of a more serious consequence—namely, myocardial infarction and sudden death. Pain associated with angina pectoris, as well as fear and anxiety regarding the potential for myocardial infarction, can be incapacitating, limiting participation in activities at home, at work, and for recreation. Limitation of activities can contribute to lowered self-esteem and depression. In some instances, reactions may involve denial of manifestations or limitations, so that individuals jeopardize their well-being by engaging in activities beyond their functional capacity.

Depression and depressive manifestations are common after major cardiac events, such as myocardial infarction (Milani & Lavie, 2007). The degree of stress experienced after myocardial infarction ranges from mild to devastating. The possibility of sudden death as a result of myocardial infarction as well as the unpredictability of this condition can be a continuing source of fear and anxiety, which can be incapacitating and sometimes lead to denial of the seriousness of the condition so that lifestyle modifications for the management of the condition are largely ignored.

Early interventions to provide education, to offer emotional support, and to reduce stress can be helpful in enabling individuals to cope with their feelings and plan for the future in a realistic and positive manner.

Activities and Participation

The life-threatening nature of myocardial infarction may cause a variety of reactions in family members, which in turn affect individuals' adjustment to their condition. Overwhelming anxiety about the possibility of another myocardial infarction occurring can result in family members' overprotection of individuals, inhibiting their return to their full functional capacity. The extent to which family members believe individuals contributed to the development of their condition by engaging in activities viewed as precursors of heart disease, such as smoking, improper diet, or obesity, may further influence relationships. Family members may express anger, resentment, or frustration, placing blame on the individuals for their behavior. In turn, individuals who have had a myocardial infarction may experience guilt, low self-esteem, and self-blame.

Sexuality

Depression and lowered self-esteem may both contribute to sexual dysfunction. In addition, some medications may impair sexual function. Individuals or their partners may be especially anxious about engaging in sexual activity after a heart attack, fearing the stress of sexual activity may precipitate another heart attack and possibly sudden death. Education and appropriate counseling, as well as reassurance, may be necessary to help the individuals and their partners alleviate these fears.

Vocational Issues in Coronary Artery Disease

Both physical and emotional factors should be considered prior to return to the work environment. After appropriate cardiac rehabilitation, most individuals are able to return to moderate levels of activity. Activity level is determined through appropriate evaluation of the energy cost of activities. Work activity should not exceed individuals' limits; thus, in some instances, some modifications may need to be made in the work environment. For the most part, isometric activities should be avoided because of the additional stress they place on the heart. Likewise, because of the stress that extreme temperatures place on the heart, work environments with controlled temperature may be preferable. Both the amount of stress experienced on the job and the individual's response to it should be considered as well.

The emotional stress associated with employment should also be considered, and steps taken either to reduce the stress associated with work or to help the individual develop strategies to cope with it. In some instances, stress involves misconceptions of the employer about return to work after a cardiac event. Exploration of attitudes and alleviation of misperceptions by providing information

about the individual's condition can help to create a positive, productive atmosphere.

HEART FAILURE

Heart failure describes a condition in which the myocardium is weakened or damaged to the extent that it cannot pump an adequate amount of blood to meet the demands of the body. Any condition that causes heart damage or produces chronic pressure or volume overload can cause heart failure. Coronary heart disease is the major cause of heart failure in developing countries (O'Connor & Rogers, 2016). Heart failure can also result from damage from cardiotoxic drugs, excessive alcohol intake, or hypertension. Although valvular dysfunction (discussed later in the chapter) can contribute to heart failure, interventions to correct valve-related irregularities have decreased the incidence of this condition significantly.

Heart failure is classified according to its severity. The various classes include individuals who are at risk for developing heart failure (i.e., those who have structural changes indicating heart failure but experience no manifestations), those individuals who experience manifestations, and those persons whose manifestations are severe (McMurray & Pfeffer, 2016).

Left-Sided Versus Right-Sided Heart Failure

Most individuals with heart failure have left-sided heart failure, resulting from dysfunction of the left ventricle. Although left-sided heart failure can be caused by irregularities of the left ventricle, most often it is due to atherosclerotic changes in the peripheral vessels that have become narrowed, leading to increased resistance as the left ventricle pumps blood into the aorta and the general circulation. When the left ventricle consistently must work harder to pump, over time it becomes enlarged (**hypertrophies**) and ineffective in its pumping action. As a result, blood backs up into the left atria and pulmonary veins so that the lungs become congested (*pulmonary edema*).

Right-sided heart failure (*cor pulmonale*) results in dysfunction of the right ventricle due to sustained increased work of the right ventricle to pump blood. This type of heart failure can result from right ventricular damage, lung conditions such as emphysema, or valvular dysfunction. The most common cause of right-sided heart failure, however, is *pulmonary hypertension* that results from left-sided heart failure (O'Connor & Rogers, 2016).

Manifestations of Heart Failure

Due to congestion of the lungs, individuals with left ventricular dysfunction (heart failure) may experience dyspnea (difficulty breathing) with activity, **orthopnea** (difficulty breathing associated with lying down), or **paroxysmal nocturnal dyspnea** (short periods of severe shortness of breath, waking individuals after several hours of sleep). As the right ventricle is unable to pump blood effectively into the lungs, fluid backs up into the peripheral circulation causing *peripheral edema*, **ascites** (fluid in the abdomen), and gastrointestinal manifestations such as **anorexia** (loss of appetite) and nausea.

Decreased pumping action of the heart and congestion in the lungs results in inadequate supply of oxygen to the rest of the body, causing individuals to experience fatigue and physical weakness. If oxygen supply to the brain is inadequate, cognitive deficits may occur.

Management of Heart Failure

Management of heart failure depends on the type, cause, and severity. Management in the early stages is directed toward prevention for those individuals at risk and prevention of progression or correction of the causes of heart failure in those individuals demonstrating structural changes in the heart but who are experiencing no manifestations. Management in later stages of heart failure is directed toward controlling or alleviating manifestations.

Medications play a major role in management of heart failure. A wide variety of medications designed to lower blood pressure (antihypertensives) are used to decrease vascular resistance, thereby decreasing the amount of work that the heart must perform to circulate blood. Medications to help the heart muscle work more efficiently by increasing

its pumping action (e.g., *digitalis preparations*) may also be used. The management plan may also include use of *diuretics* (medications that help rid the body of excess fluid) (Fonarow, 2011).

Nonpharmacologic interventions in management of heart failure are also important to reduce manifestations and increase functional capacity. Salt restriction, weight loss, smoking cessation, stress reduction, exercise to prevent deconditioning, and learning strategies of energy conservation can all help to decrease manifestations associated with heart failure (Winkel & Kao, 2012).

More advanced stages of heart failure may necessitate use of cardiac resynchronization therapy (CRT) or a device such as an implantable cardioverter–defibrillator. Severe heart failure may precipitate the need for a heart transplant. When a donor heart is not immediately available, a surgically implanted ventricular assistive device (VAD) can be used to take over the function of the failing heart. This pump is used to sustain the individual until a donor for transplant can be found (Baughman & Jarcho, 2007; Chapman, Parameshwar, Jenkins, Large, & Tsui, 2007). CRT, implantable cardioverter–defibrillators, and heart transplant are all discussed later in the chapter.

Functional Implications of Heart Failure

Personal and Psychosocial Issues

Although many manifestations of heart failure may be managed and progression of the condition slowed, severe heart failure signifies the end stage of cardiovascular disease. Individuals with heart failure may experience depression and anxiety about their present and future situations. Manifestations such as shortness of breath, fatigue, and edema of the extremities can cause discomfort, provoke anxiety, and limit individuals' ability or willingness to participate in daily activities. The ensuing increased dependency on others may lower self-esteem.

Because heart failure is often the result of gradually deteriorating function of the heart, individuals also live with the knowledge that their condition can result in increasing incapacitation. If they are candidates for cardiac transplant, uncertainty about whether a donor heart will be found before the condition deteriorates even more may be another source of continuing stress for individuals and their families.

If a ventricular assistive device is used, body image disruption may occur due to the incision and scarring from implantation of the device. In other instances, individuals may feel as if the device is an intrusion because of the noise and vibrations emitted from the device. Fear of potential device failure may be balanced with the hope that the device brings for bridging the time to transplant (Miller et al., 2007).

Activities and Participation

In the early stages of heart failure, individuals may have little restriction on their activity. Much is determined by the degree of distress individuals experience with exertion. A structured exercise program can improve functional ability as well as emotional well-being. Lifestyle modification such as weight loss, intake of small frequent meals, smoking cessation, and avoidance of excessive alcohol intake are important aspects of management that can improve functional status. Many individuals may find adherence to such lifestyle changes difficult, however.

Education regarding the condition and interventions that can improve function and quality of life are important not only for the individual, but also for the family, who may influence the individual's adherence. Family members may feel overwhelmed with the lifestyle changes or, in later stages of heart failure, with the interventions necessary for management of heart failure. Family members may also experience stress if a device such as an implantable cardioverter–defibrillator, CRT, or cardiac transplant is considered, or if heart transplant is imminent. Supporting the family can enable them to provide the support needed by the individual with heart failure.

Sexuality

Although sexual activity need not be restricted in heart failure, especially if manifestations are effectively managed, dyspnea as well as fear of a sudden cardiac event may cause anxiety, causing individuals to be reluctant to engage in sexual behavior. In some instances, medications, or anxiety

itself, can contribute to erectile dysfunction in men. Open discussion of strategies for energy conservation during sexual activity as well as discussion with health professionals regarding potential side effects of medications are important steps to maintaining sexual function.

Vocational Issues in Heart Failure

The extent to which individuals are able to continue to function in the work environment depends on the severity of manifestations experienced and the nature of the work. Individuals in sedentary occupations requiring limited activity will be able to function longer than individuals in occupations in which strenuous activity is required.

In general, emotional stress and physical demands on the job should be minimized as much as possible. Extremes in temperatures can put additional strain on the heart, so temperature-controlled environments are better tolerated.

CARDIAC ARRHYTHMIAS

Types of Arrhythmias

To function effectively, the human heart contracts with a regular rhythm and rate, both of which are coordinated by an intricate electrical network within the heart (Fishman, 2016). The term **arrhythmia** is used to describe an irregularity of the heart's rate or rhythm due to dysfunction of the heart's electrical system. Dysfunction in the system may cause irregularities, causing the heart to beat too fast (**tachycardia**), too slow (**bradycardia**), or irregularly (**dysrhythmia**). Irregularities may consist of premature beats (*extra systole*) from either the atrium (*premature atrial contraction [PAC]*) or the ventricle (*premature ventricular contraction [PVC]*).

There are many different types of arrhythmias and many different causes. Individuals with myocardial infarction or heart failure may develop an arrhythmia as a consequence of their condition (Moss, 2010); in other instances, no specific underlying health condition can be identified as the cause of the arrhythmia. Some arrhythmias may be relatively minor, requiring little or no intervention; some may require more sustained intervention; and others, such as *ventricular fibrillation*, may be life threatening (Bardy, 2011).

Arrhythmias are usually named for the type of electrical irregularity or the part of the electrical impulse system that is affected. For example, *sinus bradycardia* indicates that there is an abnormally slow rhythm arising in the *SA node* in the atrium (Zimetbaum, 2016), whereas *ventricular arrhythmias* describe arrhythmias that originate below the atrioventricular node or the His-Purkinje system (Garan, 2016).

A common arrhythmia, *atrial fibrillation*, was once thought to be benign, but is now believed to increase the individual's risk of stroke (ACTIVE I Investigators, 2011; Connolly et al., 2011; Healey et al., 2012; Saffitz, 2006). Consequently, interventions such as anticoagulants to prevent clots from forming in the atria and traveling to the brain are now often instituted to prevent complications such as stroke (Fye, 2006).

Manifestations of Arrhythmias

The manifestations experienced depend on the type and extent of the arrhythmia. Some individuals may experience no or only vague manifestations, whereas others may experience **palpitations** (awareness of heartbeat), **exertional dyspnea** (shortness of breath with activity), fatigue, **vertigo** (dizziness), or **syncope** (sudden loss of consciousness) (Olgin, 2016; Rho & Page, 2012). Severe or prolonged arrhythmia can result in sudden *cardiac arrest*, in which there is sudden loss of consciousness due to the absence of blood flow as a result of diminished cardiac pumping action. Without immediate intervention, central nervous system damage or death can occur (Myerburg, 2016).

Management of Arrhythmia

Management depends on the underlying condition and focuses on identifying and managing any precipitating underlying condition, managing any manifestations of the arrhythmia, if present, and preventing complications such as stroke, heart failure, or cardiac arrest.

Medications

Medications called *antiarrhythmics* regulate the heartbeat and are often a central part of management,

as well as other medications used in the management of any contributing conditions, such as antihypertensive medications. Because certain types of arrhythmia (e.g., atrial fibrillation) can contribute to thrombus formation and possibly embolus, some individuals may also need to be on anticoagulant medications (Fye, 2006).

Pacemakers, Cardiac Resynchronization Therapy, and Implantable Defibrillators

When the heart's ability to maintain an effective rate or rhythm is altered, an artificial cardiac pacemaker may be used to stimulate the electrical activity of the heart and maintain its function (Lamas, 2012). The pacemaker consists of a battery-operated pulse generator and a lead wire with an electrode tip. One end of the lead wire is inserted into a vessel and advanced into the individual's heart; the other end is connected to the generator. The generator sends out an electrical stimulus to the heart muscle. The generator may be external if the need for pacing is only temporary. If the pacemaker is to be permanent, a small battery-operated generator is placed under the skin and fatty tissue of the upper chest or lower thoracic area.

A variety of pacemakers are available. These devices are usually classified according to the chamber of the heart that is being stimulated, the chamber of the heart that is being monitored, and the response that the pacemaker is expected to deliver.

When the individual's own conduction system in the heart falls below a specific rate, the artificial pacemaker initiates its activity accordingly. The mode of pacing is determined on an individual basis according to the individual's specific arrhythmia. For most individuals, even permanent pacemakers may be inserted under local anesthesia with mild sedation.

In more severe arrhythmia, a procedure called *electrical cardioversion* may be indicated to return the heart to a normal rhythm. The procedure is performed under anesthesia and consists of delivering an electric shock through electrodes that have been placed on the chest. In individuals with a severe, recurrent arrhythmia that could result in a life-threatening arrhythmia (e.g., ventricular tachycardia, which can become ventricular fibrillation), a device called an *implantable cardioverter–defibrillator*

(ICD) may be surgically implanted. ICD placement involves creating a 3- to 4-inch incision into the left chest wall. The ICD produces visible scarring as well as a bulge around the implant site, which some people find objectionable because it shows under clothing (Sowell, Kuhl, Sears, Klodell, & Conti, 2006). The implanted defibrillator delivers an electric shock automatically to the heart when an arrhythmia occurs.

Cardiac resynchronization therapy (CRT) is a procedure in which a small device that sends out electrical impulses to both ventricles to help them beat in synchrony is implanted. CRT appears to be of most benefit to individuals with heart failure or specific types of ventricular arrhythmias (Tang et al., 2010). It may be used alone or in conjunction with an ICD.

Functional Implications of Arrhythmias

Personal and Psychosocial Issues

The psychosocial impact of arrhythmia can be significant, especially if manifestations are experienced. Fearful of triggering a potentially fatal arrhythmia, individuals may curtail many activities related to both work and leisure in an effort to prevent such an occurrence. In many instances, the fear and anxiety experienced by individuals with arrhythmia may be more incapacitating than the arrhythmia itself.

Activities and Participation

Not all arrhythmias necessitate modification of activities. However, if syncope is a manifestation, it could pose a danger to other individuals during activities such as driving, which would be contraindicated.

Individuals who have devices such as a pacemaker or an implantable defibrillator should at all times wear identification, such as a MedicAlert bracelet, or carry a card providing information about the device in case of health emergency. Electromagnetic interference with permanent pacemakers and implantable defibrillators may have deleterious effects (Santucci, Haw, Trohman, & Pinski, 1998). Although the shielding around devices has been improved significantly, individuals should be aware of possible interference from external electrical signals in the environment such as microwave, radar, and airport metal detectors.

Vocational Issues in Arrhythmias

Any activity that has been identified by the individual as triggering arrhythmia should be avoided. Avoiding excessive emotional stress as well as learning to manage stress may be an important component of the individual's ability to continue to perform adequately at work without danger of precipitating an arrhythmia. Individuals using anticoagulants as part of the management plan may need to be aware of the potential for excessive bleeding should injury occur. Excessive anxiety about precipitating an arrhythmia can become incapacitating, immobilizing individuals and preventing them from carrying out normal tasks and activities. Individuals may develop chronic depression, which can further interfere with their ability to work.

Individuals with pacemakers or implantable defibrillator devices may need to avoid activities that could potentially cause the device to become dislodged or malfunction. Referral to a counselor may be indicated to help individuals deal with their fears and enhance their ability to perform work activities.

VALVULAR CONDITIONS OF THE HEART

The valves of the heart, as discussed earlier in the chapter, permit blood to flow from one chamber of the heart to the other when open, and prevent backward flow of blood between chambers when they are closed. Impairment of the valves can lead to inefficient heart function and contribute to ventricular dysfunction, heart failure, and in some instances sudden death (Carabello, 2016).

Valvular conditions may consist of stenosis (narrowing) of a valve, which obstructs blood flow from one chamber to another, or weakening of a valve, which allows blood to be regurgitated from one chamber into another. In both instances, the heart must pump harder either to overcome the obstruction or to compensate for volume overload of the blood being regurgitated. Valvular irregularities may be congenital, may result from inflammation of the inner membrane of the heart (**endocarditis**), or may be caused by an immune response that occurs in conditions such as *rheumatic fever* (discussed later in the chapter). Valvular conditions are classified according to the nature of the irregularity of the affected valve.

Types of Valvular Conditions

Aortic Stenosis

Aortic stenosis refers to the narrowing of the aortic valve between the left ventricle and the aorta. When the aortic valve becomes narrowed, increased pressure arises in the left ventricle as it attempts to pump blood through the smaller-diameter valve. Initially there may be no manifestations; however, over time as pressure builds, fluid can back up into the lungs, resulting in *dyspnea*, and the left ventricle may become thicker and less efficient, which can result in *chest pain*.

If individuals are not experiencing manifestations, usually no interventions are instituted (Carabello, 2016). When manifestations, such as dyspnea or chest pain are present, surgical aortic-valve replacement with a prosthetic valve is usually performed (Gilard et al., 2012; Lazaar, 2010).

Mitral Stenosis

The most common cause of mitral stenosis is *rheumatic fever* (discussed later in the chapter) (Carabello, 2016). *Mitral stenosis* refers to narrowing of the mitral valve, which obstructs the blood flow from the left atrium to the left ventricle. There may be no manifestations until the valve restriction is reduced to approximately one-third of its regular size (Carabello, 2016). When restriction of flow is severely impeded through the valve, manifestations may consist of *dyspnea with exertion*, *orthopnea*, and *paroxysmal nocturnal dyspnea*. When no manifestations are present, no interventions are usually instituted. If dyspnea is mild, medications such as diuretics may be used.

When manifestations become more severe, surgical intervention in the form of either *balloon valvotomy* to dilate the valve area, *open commissurotomy* in which the valve is surgically opened, or *valve replacement* may be performed.

Mitral Regurgitation

Approximately 80% of individuals have some valve leakage, but mild regurgitation rarely leads to incapacitation or the need for intervention (Otto & Verrier, 2011). Severe mitral regurgitation, however, is associated with progressive left ventricular dysfunction and subsequent heart failure (Feldman et al., 2011). When manifestations of left-sided heart failure are mild, medications such as vasodilators may be used. Although medications may alleviate manifestations, they do not alter progression; thus surgical intervention is often indicated (Carabello, 2008).

Mitral Prolapse

In another valvular condition, *mitral prolapse*, floppy valve leaflets of the mitral valve lead to inadequate closure of the mitral valve during ventricular contraction so that blood to flows backward into the atria (Foster, 2010; Jacobson & Rahko, 2012). Most individuals with mitral prolapse experience no manifestations, and no interventions are needed. When manifestations such as palpitations are present, medications may be indicated to relieve them. If the condition progresses to severe mitral regurgitation, surgery may be necessary.

Other Valvular Irregularities

Tricuspid regurgitation and *tricuspid stenosis* are conditions similar to the regurgitation and stenosis conditions described earlier, but occur on the right side instead of the left side of the heart. The same process may affect the pulmonary or aortic valves.

Management of Valvular Conditions

Specific interventions for valvular irregularities depend on the nature and severity of the condition. Manifestations of some conditions may necessitate avoidance of strenuous activity. Others require no intervention or limitations. Damaged or prosthetic valves are more susceptible to infection. Consequently, prophylactic antibiotics may be given to prevent endocarditis (discussed later in the chapter) when there is a risk of a generalized bacterial infection, such as after a dental extraction.

Severe damage to or irregularity of a valve may require surgery to widen the opening, correct the damage, or replace the valve. When valves are replaced, either artificial (mechanical) valves or valves made of tissue may be used. Mechanical valves are made entirely from synthetic materials, while tissue valves may be made from a combination of synthetic and biological tissues. Mechanical valves require long-term anticoagulant therapy to prevent thrombus formation (Carabello, 2016). Although tissue valves decrease the risk of clot development, they may not have the long-term durability of mechanical valves. Because prosthetic valves are more vulnerable to infection, individuals may need to take antibiotics before procedures in which infection is a risk (e.g., dental work) are performed.

CONGENITAL HEART CONDITIONS

Congenital heart conditions include anatomic or physiologic irregularities of the heart present at birth. Many congenital heart conditions are identified in infancy or childhood; some, however, are not identified until adulthood.

In the past, many individuals with congenital heart conditions did not survive to adulthood. More recently, greater understanding of the conditions as well as the development of a number of surgical interventions to correct irregularities have enabled many more individuals to survive into adulthood (Marelli, 2016).

Septal Defects

Two types of *septal defects* are distinguished. An *atrial septal defect* is an opening (hole) located in the *septum* (wall) that separates the two atria; it is commonly known as *patent foramen ovale*. A *ventricular septal defect* is an opening in the septum that separates the two ventricles. Normally the septum provides a barrier to prevent mixing of deoxygenated blood from the right side of the heart with oxygenated blood from the left side of the heart. When there is an opening in the septum, the blood on the two sides of the heart becomes mixed.

The degree of manifestations depends on the size of the defect. Adults with a small defect may have no significant manifestations aside from a sound indicating a *heart murmur*. Larger defects may result in **cyanosis** (bluish appearance of the skin due to lack of adequate oxygen supply). Larger defects are usually corrected surgically.

Coarctation of the Aorta

Coarctation of the aorta (narrowing of the aorta) may not be identified until adolescence or young adulthood, with the first manifestation being hypertension. Although management consists of surgical repair, residual hypertension and long-term effects of surgical intervention require lifelong follow-up and periodic magnetic resonance imaging.

Tetralogy of Fallot

Tetralogy of Fallot and another congenital heart condition, transposition of the great arteries (discussed next), are classified as *cyanotic defects*, because cyanosis is one of the primary manifestations of both conditions. Tetralogy of Fallot consists of four irregularities of the heart, including *ventricular septal defect*, *narrowing of the pulmonary artery*, *right ventricular* hypertrophy (enlargement), and *overriding aorta* that has shifted to the right ventricle (Lange & Hillis, 2012). Adults with surgically corrected tetralogy of Fallot may have no significant manifestations.

Transposition of the Great Arteries

In *transposition of the great arteries*, the aorta comes from the right ventricle rather than the left, and the pulmonary artery comes from the left ventricle rather than the right. This condition is usually identified shortly after birth and surgically corrected, but individuals also require lifelong follow-up and monitoring. Depending on the intervention to correct complete transposition of the great arteries, adults may experience exercise intolerance, palpations, and possibly right ventricular failure (Marelli, 2016).

INFLAMMATORY CONDITIONS OF THE HEART

Endocarditis

Endocarditis is inflammation of the membrane that covers the inner layer of the heart (*endocardial surface*). Bacterial infection is the most common cause of this inflammation. Endocarditis is characterized by deposits of "vegetation" on the inner lining of the endocardium and, most frequently, on the valves, resulting in valve damage.

Rheumatic fever (discussed later in the chapter) was historically the major risk factor for endocarditis. However, with the advent of early recognition and management of rheumatic fever, other risk factors, such as mitral valve prolapse and prosthetic cardiac valves, have become more prevalent. Other significant risk factors include contamination through injection of illicit drugs and infection that results from healthcare procedures and devices, such as dialysis, intravenous catheters, or pacemakers (Fowler, Bayer, & Baddour, 2016).

Manifestations may be insidious at first, mimicking the flu. As the disease progresses, manifestations become more pronounced, and may include muscle pain and chest pain. Identification of the condition is based on history and manifestations, blood culture, and echocardiogram. Management consists of the administration of appropriate antibiotics to eradicate the infection before serious complications develop (Wang, 2012).

Complications of endocarditis may include embolism, damage to heart valves, or damage to distant organs in the body. Any organ or part of the body can be affected. Depending on the part of the body affected and the extent of damage, embolism can sometimes result in death.

Pericarditis

Inflammation of the outer layer of the heart (pericardium) is known as *pericarditis*. Most commonly, it is caused by a virus from a secondary condition. Viruses can also be introduced during healthcare procedures such as coronary angiography or placement of a pacemaker or defibrillator (Leal, 2012).

When inflamed, the pericardial layers can adhere to each other, creating friction as their surfaces rub together during cardiac contraction. The most common manifestation of pericarditis is chest pain, which is aggravated by position change and breathing because of the rubbing together of the two inflamed surfaces. A low-grade fever may also be present.

Identification of pericarditis is often based on manifestations, physical examination, and, at times, electrocardiogram. Management of pericarditis is directed toward alleviating pain caused by the inflammation. Medications such as nonsteroidal anti-inflammatory drugs (NSAIDs) are commonly used for this purpose.

Severe inflammation of the pericardium can result in accumulation of excessive fluid within the pericardial sac, a condition known as *pericardial effusion*. Excess fluid in the sac surrounding the heart may constrict the myocardium, causing cardiac dysfunction. If constriction of the heart is severe because of increasing amounts of fluid, *cardiac tamponade* (severe constriction of the heart that prevents it from filling and emptying properly) may occur. A procedure called **pericardiocentesis**, in which a needle is inserted into the pericardial sac and the fluid drained, may be performed to relieve the constriction (Little & Oh, 2012).

Rheumatic Heart Disease

Rheumatic heart disease is a heart condition caused by *rheumatic fever*, an inflammatory complication of group A *Streptococcus* infection, such as strep throat (Hahn, Knox, & Forman, 2005). Although recovery from rheumatic fever may be complete with no residual effects, some individuals experience permanent damage to the heart valves. Rheumatic fever is the most common cause of *mitral stenosis* (Carabello, 2016). The risk of rheumatic fever is decreased when there is adequate management of strep throat with early antibiotic intervention.

VASCULAR CONDITIONS

Lower-Extremity Peripheral Arterial Disease

Description, Manifestations, and Management

Lower-extremity peripheral arterial disease is a common manifestation of atherosclerosis and is associated with an increased risk of incapacitation in combination with cigarette smoking (White, 2007). When atherosclerotic changes have narrowed or occluded the larger peripheral vessels, an adequate blood supply cannot reach tissues in the extremities.

Manifestations experienced depend on the extent of the obstruction, the vessels involved, and the formation of any alternative blood supply routes, called *collateral circulation*. Exercise requires increased demand for oxygen by muscles. Therefore, individuals who have deficient blood supply to the muscles because of peripheral arterial disease may, with activity such as walking, experience aching, cramping, or fatigue of the muscles in the legs—a condition known as *intermittent claudication*. Stopping to rest decreases the muscles' demand for oxygen and consequently relieves the pain. If the condition progresses, however, pain in the extremities may occur even at rest. In severe cases, the feet may become numb and cold, and ulcerations of the foot may appear.

Management is directed toward reducing risk factors, with recommendations including regular exercise and smoking cessation. Individuals who are severely incapacitated due to lower limb *ischemia* may be candidates for *revascularization* surgery to relieve manifestations, or surgery such as *percutaneous transluminal angioplasty (PTA)*, in which the vessel is widened.

Owing to the diminished blood supply in peripheral atherosclerotic disease, even tiny injuries in the extremities may become infected and not heal properly. If circulation becomes so severely impaired that necrosis (tissue death) results, amputation of the extremity may be necessary to prevent complications, such as the spread of infection throughout the body.

Vocational Issues in Lower-Extremity Peripheral Vascular Disease

Peripheral arterial disease in the lower extremities can be significantly incapacitating, affecting work, depending on the activities required. Individuals with peripheral arterial disease may be unable to stand for long periods of time or may be unable to walk without pain or muscle fatigue. Stamina in relation to these activities should be evaluated. Environmental conditions, such as cold temperatures, or other factors that reduce blood supply to the extremities should be avoided. The potential for infection in the lower extremities because of inadequate blood supply necessitates avoidance of work environments containing hazards that could cause trauma to the feet or legs.

Thromboangiitis Obliterans (Buerger's Disease)

Thromboangiitis obliterans is a rare condition of the small- and medium-sized arteries and superficial veins of the extremities that causes diminished blood flow to the affected area. In contrast to *peripheral atherosclerotic disease,* thromboangiitis obliterans occurs predominantly in individuals between the ages of 20 and 40 who do not have significant atherosclerosis. Manifestations include numbness, tingling, and pain in the upper or lower extremities. Although its exact cause is unknown, thromboangiitis obliterans occurs almost exclusively in individuals who smoke. Consequently, the major intervention in management of the condition is smoking cessation. If individuals continue to smoke, the condition continues to progress and can ultimately require the amputation of affected extremities.

Raynaud's Phenomenon

Raynaud's phenomenon is a condition in which spasms of the vessels in the fingers or toes impair the blood flow to those areas, resulting in blanching of the skin from severe vasoconstriction, followed by cyanosis (bluish appearance). The digits may become numb and painful. As vasoconstriction abates, there is marked vasodilation increasing blood flow to the area, resulting in red color of the skin in the digit that may be accompanied by throbbing.

Primary Raynaud's phenomenon describes vasospasm that is precipitated by exposure to cold or emotional stress, but there is no additional underlying cause. *Secondary Raynaud's phenomenon* is associated with other condition.

In primary Raynaud's phenomenon, management is directed toward prevention, such as limiting exposure to cold and smoking cessation. Biofeedback or the use of relaxation techniques may also be helpful in reducing exacerbations of the condition. If Raynaud's phenomenon is secondary to another condition, management is directed accordingly (Olgin, 2016).

Phlebitis and Thrombophlebitis

Phlebitis is the inflammation of a vein. **Thrombophlebitis** is the inflammation of a vein with associated clot formation. Although phlebitis and thrombophlebitis can occur in any vein, they frequently occur in the lower extremities.

In health conditions in which activity is limited, thrombophlebitis can be a serious complication causing additional incapacitation or potentially death. Individuals with thrombophlebitis may experience pain and tenderness, especially in the calf area of the leg. Individuals with loss of sensation as a result of spinal cord injury may be unaware of the condition, and consequently they may not receive prompt intervention to manage the condition. Other manifestations may include swelling and redness of the affected part. If thrombophlebitis is unrecognized or inadequately managed, clots can break off and travel to the heart, lungs, or to other parts of the body, where they can lodge in a vessel, occluding blood supply to the body part. Depending on the location of the occlusion, individuals can experience stroke, myocardial infarction, or massive damage to whichever body part is affected.

Management of phlebitis and thrombophlebitis is directed toward decreasing inflammation and preventing or dissolving clots through use of anticoagulants, antithrombotic agents, or anti-inflammatory agents. Bed rest is usually prescribed during the acute period, along with medications that decrease clotting.

Varicose Veins

When blood cannot be returned efficiently to the heart, backup of blood may cause distention and congestion of the veins, called *varicose veins.* Anything causing stricture or pressure on the veins—such as prolonged standing, obesity, or constriction of the leg by circular garters—can aggravate this condition. Manifestations may include a sensation of heaviness in the legs, fatigue, and pain, as well as cosmetic manifestations.

In mild cases, management may consist of application of compression stockings that lend support and facilitate blood return. Other procedures that may be used include *sclerotherapy,* in which injections of a solution into the veins help

to close them so that they gradually fade; *laser surgery,* which closes the veins; and *vein stripping,* in which the vein is removed.

CARDIAC REHABILITATION

Cardiac rehabilitation is a comprehensive and individualized program for individuals with a variety of cardiac conditions. The goals of cardiac rehabilitation are to assist individuals to safely return to and maintain regular daily activities and work; to promote prevention measures, including healthy lifestyle; and to make psychological and social adjustments (Bybee & Kopecky, 2007).

Cardiac rehabilitation has been described by the U.S. Department of Health and Human Services (1995) as a program consisting of the following components:

- Health evaluation
- Prescribed exercise
- Education
- Counseling

Programs in cardiac rehabilitation use a multidisciplinary approach, incorporating exercise training, dietary consultation, smoking cessation, patient education, and counseling. Programs are designed to optimize individuals' physical and psychosocial functioning. Education and increasing awareness of the underlying condition and aspects of the prevention of future cardiac events serve as a cornerstone of cardiac rehabilitation programs. Because some individuals with cardiac conditions become incapacitated because of excessive fear, anxiety, or depression, interventions directed toward helping individuals and their families deal with these feelings are integral to the total rehabilitation program.

Psychological and vocational counseling are important components of cardiac rehabilitation programs as well.

CARDIAC TRANSPLANTATION

When heart damage is so severe or the heart condition so advanced (*end-stage heart disease*) that standard management interventions are no longer effective, quality of life has diminished, or survival is severely threatened, cardiac transplantation is considered. Individuals who undergo successful transplantation not only increase their chance for survival, but also increase their chance to return to a normal, productive life.

Pretransplant Considerations

Prior to cardiac transplant, individuals undergo a complete physical, immunologic, and psychosocial evaluation to identify any contraindications to transplantation. The individual and family undergo extensive assessment of their coping skills, family support, and motivation to follow the rigorous management plan that is required following this procedure. The evaluation period can be extremely stressful, with individuals becoming fearful they may be found unsuitable for transplant.

Not all individuals with heart disease are candidates for cardiac transplantation. Selection is based on factors such as general physical condition, absence of other systemic conditions that would in themselves limit survival, the ability to return to normal function after surgery, and the ability to adhere to the complex management plan that follows transplantation. Usually conditions such as active or recent cancer, HIV infection, and severe psychiatric conditions are contraindications to transplant (Mancini & Naka, 2016).

To be eligible for transplant, an individual's physical condition must be strong enough to survive the transplant procedure, and he or she must be able to adhere to the complex management plan required after surgery. Individuals accepted for transplant are placed on a waiting list. A 24-hour national computer network links all organ procurement centers in the United States. When a donor organ is identified, a computer search identifies potential recipients for the best match. The donor–recipient match is based not only on blood type but also on body and heart size.

When a donor heart has been identified and the matching of donor–recipient blood types has been confirmed, the transplant can be performed. The heart of the recipient is removed and the donor heart transplanted. Immunosuppressant therapy to block the body's natural response to foreign tissue begins immediately.

Posttransplant Considerations

Recovery from cardiac transplant requires a hospital stay for approximately 5 to 10 days, during which immunosuppression therapy continues. After discharge from the hospital, individuals are required to have frequent checkups, including biopsy of the transplanted heart, and monitoring of blood to assess immune status. If signs of rejection are observed, additional medications that augment immunosuppression are indicated.

Individuals undergoing cardiac transplantation must follow a complex management plan to prevent rejection of the donor organ and other complications. Because the body never really ceases its efforts to reject the donor heart, immunosuppressants must be taken indefinitely. These medications are a necessary part of management, but they have serious side effects, including increased risk of malignancy and increased susceptibility to infection (Mancini & Naka, 2016).

With advances in immunosuppression, overall survival after one year is 87.7%. Of those individuals, 90% report no functional limitations (Mancini & Naka, 2016).

The costs associated with heart transplantation can be staggering. There are significant charges for the transplant surgery and hospitalization and the continuing immunosuppressant medication, as well as costs associated with travel to and from the transplant center for checkups, food and lodging for family while the individual is hospitalized, and other support services that may be needed when the individual returns home.

Functional Implications of Cardiac Transplantation

Personal and Psychosocial Issues

The pretransplant period may be extremely stressful for individuals and their families as they wait for a donor to be identified. Many individuals will put their lives on hold while waiting for a transplant. In addition, the pressure of uncertainty as to whether or when a heart will become available can create severe stress in family relationships. Individuals and families have no control over when surgery will occur and, in the interim, the individual's condition may continue to deteriorate. Feelings of anxiety and depression are common.

Organ preservation time is limited from the time of procurement to the time of implant (approximately 4 hours), so individuals awaiting a transplant must be readily available for surgery at short notice. Thus, if individuals do not live near a transplant center, they may need to relocate to be closer to the facility. This relocation can be an additional source of stress not only for the individual but also for the family

Depression and anxiety are also issues in individuals after transplant. Individuals must learn to live with the possibility of rejection and infection. Some evidence suggests that individuals may experience grieving due to the loss of their own heart and take time to accept the donor heart on an emotional level (Kaba, Thompson, Burnard, Edwards, & Theodosopoulou, 2005). In addition, they may experience guilt because receiving a heart is dependent on the death of another person or they may have feelings of indebtedness to the donor.

Activities and Participation

Cardiac transplantation involves life-altering changes both for the individual and for the family. Individuals who had been in the terminal phase of heart failure and severely incapacitated may, after heart transplant, progress to an active lifestyle. This process may cause the individual and family members to experience a number of emotional issues.

After cardiac transplantation, many individuals are able to resume many of the same activities they engaged in prior to transplant. Driving is usually resumed in approximately 12 weeks. Because individuals no longer experience the manifestations they had with heart disease, such as chest pain and dyspnea, they may be more willing to participate in activities and events that they had previously avoided.

Sexuality

When individuals resume sexual activity depends on the individual and his or her unique circumstances. In some instances, medications may affect sexual desire and function. In other instances, anxiety about exertion and its effect on the newly transplanted heart may inhibit sexual activity. Frank and open discussion between partners as well as reassurance and information from healthcare professionals can help to alleviate any concerns.

Vocational Issues in Heart Transplant

When individuals return to work after transplant depends on the individual as well as the type of employment. Although many individuals are able to be physically active and return to work after transplant, they may require assistance in making the transition from their pretransplant state to one in which they return to employment. One barrier to employment is prejudicial attitudes of employers, who may have concerns about insurability and individuals' needs for continuing health care and follow-up after transplant. Although any functional limitations experienced by persons after transplant are individually determined, some restrictions on heavy lifting or aggressive exercise are likely.

After transplant, individuals' immune status is compromised due to the continuing use of immunosuppressant therapy to prevent rejection of the transplanted heart. As a result, they may be more prone to infection. Consequently, situations in which there is exposure to contagious infections should be avoided.

Psychological factors may also be a barrier to individuals' successful return to work. Prior to receiving the transplant, individuals may have been out of work for some time because of their condition. The adjustment to returning to employment after an extended absence may be a difficult psychological transition. Individuals may also have difficulty with body image, or they may fear that work-related activity could interfere with their new heart's effective functioning. Fear of contracting an infection or anxiety about potential rejection of the transplant may also be psychologically incapacitating, interfering with individuals' ability to work.

GENERAL FUNCTIONAL IMPLICATIONS OF CARDIOVASCULAR CONDITIONS

Personal and Psychosocial Issues

The heart has been given symbolic significance for centuries. Consequently, individuals' reactions to conditions involving the heart can have far-reaching implications. Given the association between sudden death and cardiac malfunction, fear and anxiety are common reactions to most cardiac conditions. Although many chronic conditions trigger these reactions, the heart is considered by many people as the most vital organ, and by some as the "seat of the soul." Thus any condition involving the heart can have significant emotional ramifications.

Most individuals come to accept their condition and its management as well as any associated restrictions. In other instances, however, individuals' responses may adversely affect their condition and its management. Reactions of anger, anxiety, and depression can be the most incapacitating factors in cardiovascular conditions, and can contribute to inactivity, social isolation, or self-destructive behaviors.

Individuals may be immobilized by fear, subsequently restricting their activities more than necessary. Excessive concern that additional stress or exertion may lead to a cardiac event may cause individuals to alter job, recreational, and family activities. If significant modifications in lifestyle or employment are necessary, some individuals may experience a sense of loss and bereavement.

Denial is part of the normal psychological defense that can be used to cope with a severe threat. Although denial can be an effective mechanism for reducing anxiety, it can be detrimental if it interferes with management of the condition. If the individual is in denial, manifestations may be ignored or trivialized, physical incapacity denied, or management plans and recommended lifestyle changes ignored. As a result, complications or progression of the condition may occur. The magnitude and type of the response may reflect the individual's unique personality, past experience, and personal situation at the time.

Activities and Participation

Not all cardiovascular conditions require significant lifestyle changes, but modifications in diet, decrease in alcohol intake, elimination of tobacco use, and establishment of a regular exercise program are often required. Even when recommended changes are minimal, individuals may perceive changes as having a negative effect on their quality of life. Depending on their relationships with family and friends, individuals may feel pressure to continue to engage in activities even though they are considered detrimental to their condition. In other instances, individuals may fear losing friends or social standing if behaviors are altered.

The various degrees to which stress contributes to development of cardiovascular conditions are unknown. Stress is not always associated with overcommitment and activity. For some individuals, reducing activity or involvement may be more stressful than continuing as before. Learning ways to cope with the stress that may result from activities and involvement may be more beneficial than abandoning those activities altogether.

To some degree, reactions of others influence how well individuals cope with any chronic condition. The quality of individuals' interpersonal relationships at the time of the cardiac event and the presence or absence of social supports can be major determinants of individuals' reaction to their condition.

Cardiovascular conditions can produce profound effects on family dynamics. Depending on the condition and extent of incapacitation, there may be a shifting of family roles and role reversal. Owing to the invisible nature of many cardiac conditions, some family members may not understand that individuals cannot sustain the activity level they engaged in prior to the condition. Lack of understanding may breed resentment or anger.

Family members may be a source of support and consolation; however, they may also contribute to individuals' fear and anxiety by being overly protective or showing anxiety out of proportion to the condition. Qualified professionals should discuss reactions and their potential impact on individuals' return to function with family members.

Although individuals with cardiovascular conditions may continue most forms of recreation, extremely rigorous activities or contact sports may need to be curtailed. When restrictions are placed on recreational activities that had previously been a social outlet, social isolation and depression may result unless another recreational activity can be substituted.

Sexuality

After a cardiac condition has been identified, sexual activity may be a special source of anxiety both for individuals and for their partners. In most instances, sexual activity can be maintained or resumed; however, associated fear and anxiety can hamper both enjoyment and performance, altering self-esteem and contributing to depression. Often, lack of information contributes to fear and misperceptions. Specific information regarding continuing or resuming sexual activity can relieve anxiety and enhance quality of life.

GENERAL VOCATIONAL ISSUES IN CARDIOVASCULAR CONDITIONS

For most individuals, work is both a source of pride and a financial necessity. The degree to which a cardiovascular condition inhibits the return to regular employment can influence individuals' reactions to the condition. In some instances, attitudes of employers represent formidable barriers to the successful return to work. Employers may be reluctant to employ or reemploy individuals with a cardiovascular condition because of fear of liability or responsibility for healthcare costs if the condition should worsen.

Each job must be viewed in relation to the individual's physical and emotional abilities and the effect that the job has on the individual's health status. In some instances, a job change may be necessary, which can be an additional source of stress. In other instances, individuals can return to their former jobs with little or no modification.

After healthcare evaluation, generally the degree and type of activity in which individuals with a cardiovascular condition may safely engage is specified. Most individuals with heart conditions are able to engage in light to moderate activity.

Because of their effects on the cardiovascular system, environmental conditions such as excessive heat or cold should be avoided. Isometric exercise elevates blood pressure and places an extra burden on the heart; consequently, any exertion that involves muscular activity against a fixed, unmoving resistance should usually be avoided. If individuals have a specific cardiac device, such as a

pacemaker, they should be aware that certain types of equipment may interfere with device function.

In most instances, once cardiovascular conditions are stabilized and an appropriate management plan is instituted, functional decline is slow or minimal. The greatest barrier to productive vocational activity may be the individual's unwillingness or inability to make the recommended lifestyle changes or nonadherence with the management plan.

CASE STUDY

Mr. C. is 50 years old and has his own landscaping business, which he started after graduating from community college 30 years ago. He experienced a myocardial infarction at the age of 40; however, he went through intensive cardiac rehabilitation and has returned to most of his former functional capacity. Over the past year, however, he has had increasing fatigue and shortness of breath. After a health evaluation, Mr. C. was found to be in the beginning stage of heart failure. Although his manifestations are currently managed with medication, if his cardiac condition continues to deteriorate, he may need a heart transplant within the next 5 years.

1. How would you approach Mr. C. about his rehabilitation potential?
2. Is there additional health information that would be helpful in establishing Mr. C.'s rehabilitation potential?
3. Is it feasible for Mr. C. to continue in his current line of work? If so, which modifications might be considered?
4. What would Mr. C.'s potential for maintaining his current line of work be if he has a cardiac transplant?

REFERENCES

ACTIVE I Investigators. (2011). Irbesartan in patients with atrial fibrillation. *New England Journal of Medicine, 364*(10), 928–938.

Adrogué, H. E. (2012). Hypertension. In E. T. Bope & R. D. Kellerman (Eds.), *Conn's current therapy 2012* (pp. 436–445). Philadelphia, PA: Elsevier Saunders.

Anderson, J. L. (2016). ST segment elevation acute myocardial infarction and complications of myocardial infarction.

In L. & A. I. Schafer (Eds.), *Goldman-Cecil Medicine* (25th ed., pp. 441–456). Philadelphia, PA: Elsevier Saunders.

Aversano, T., Lemmon, C., & Liu, L. (2012). Outcomes of PCI at hospitals with or without on-site cardiac surgery. *New England Journal of Medicine, 366*(19), 1792–1802.

Bardy, G. H. (2011). A critic's assessment of our approach to cardiac arrest. *New England Journal of Medicine, 364*, 374–375.

Baughman, K. L., & Jarcho, J. A. (2007). Bridge to life: Cardiac mechanical support. *New England Journal of Medicine, 357*(9), 846–849.

Boden, W. E. (2016). Angina pectoris and stable ischemic heart disease. In L. Goldman & A. I. Schafer (Eds.), *Goldman-Cecil Medicine* (25th ed., pp. 420–432). Philadelphia, PA: Elsevier Saunders.

Borissoff, J. I., Spronk, H. M. H., & Ten Cate, H. (2011). The hemostatic system as a modulator of atherosclerosis. *New England Journal of Medicine, 364*(18), 1746–1760.

Bybee, K. A., & Kopecky, S. L. (2007). In R. E. Rakel & E. T. Bope (Eds.), *Conn's current therapy* (pp. 417–426). Philadelphia, PA: W. B. Saunders.

Carabello, A. A. (2008). The current therapy for mitral regurgitation. *Journal of the American College of Cardiology, 52,* 319–326.

Carabello, B. A. (2016). Valvular heart disease. In L. Goldman & A. I. Schafer (Eds.), *Goldman-Cecil Medicine* (25th ed., pp. 461-473). Philadelphia, PA: Elsevier Saunders.

Chapman, E., Parameshwar, J., Jenkins, D., Large, S., & Tsui, S. (2007). Psychosocial issues for patients with ventricular assist devices: A qualitative pilot study. *American Journal of Critical Care, 16*(1), 72–81.

Cohen, D. J., Van Hout, B., Serruys, P. W., Mohr, F. W., Macaya, C., den Heijer, P., . . . Synergy between PCI with Taxus and Cardiac Surgery Investigators. (2011). Quality of life after PCI with drug-eluting stents or coronary artery bypass surgery. *New England Journal of Medicine, 364*(11), 1016–1026.

Connolly, S. J., Eikelboom, J., Joyner, C., Diener, H. C., Hart, R., Golitsyn, S., . . . AVERROES Steering Committee and Investigators. (2011). Apixaban in patients with atrial fibrillation. *New England Journal of Medicine, 364*(9), 806–817.

Curfman, G. D., Morrissey, S. A., Jarcho, J. A., & Drazen, J. M. (2007). Drug-eluting coronary stents: Promise and uncertainty. *New England Journal of Medicine, 356*(10), 1059–1060.

Feldman, T., Foster, E., Glower, D. G., Kar, S., Rinaldi, M. J., Fail, P. S., . . . EVEREST II Investigators. (2011). Percutaneous repair or surgery for mitral regurgitation. *New England Journal of Medicine, 364*(15), 1395–1406.

Fishman, G. I. (2016). Principles of electrophysiology. In L. Goldman & A. I. Schafer (Eds.), *Goldman-Cecil Medicine* (25th ed., pp. 339–344). Philadelphia, PA: Elsevier Saunders.

Fonarow, G. C. (2011). Comparative effectiveness of diuretic regimens. *New England Journal of Medicine, 364*(9), 877–878.

Foster, E. (2010). Mitral regurgitation due to degenerative mitral-valve disease. *New England Journal of Medicine, 363*(2), 156–165.

Fowler, V. G., Bayer, A. S., & Baddour, L.M. (2016). Infective endocarditis. In L. Goldman & A. I. Schafer (Eds.), *Goldman-Cecil Medicine* (25th ed., pp. 474–483). Philadelphia, PA: Elsevier Saunders.

Furlan, A. J. (2006). Carotid-artery stenting: Case open or closed? *New England Journal of Medicine, 355*(16), 1726–1729.

Fye, W. B. (2006). Tracing atrial fibrillation: 100 years. *New England Journal of Medicine, 355*(14), 1412–1414.

Garan, H., (2016). Ventricular arrhythmias. In L. Goldman & A. I. Schafer (Eds.), *Goldman-Cecil Medicine* (25th ed., pp. 367-374). Philadelphia, PA: Elsevier Saunders.

Gilard, M., Eltchaninoff, H., Iung, B., Donzeau-Gouge, P., Chevreul, K., Fajadet, J., . . . & Laskar, M. for the FRANCE 2 Investigators. (2012). Registry of transcatheter aortic-valve implantation in high-risk patients. *New England Journal of Medicine, 366*(18), 1705–1715.

Goldfine, A. B. (2012). Statins: Is it really time to reassess benefits and risks? *New England Journal of Medicine, 366*(19), 1752–1754.

Grover, F. L. (2012). Current status of off-pump coronary artery bypass. *New England Journal of Medicine, 366*(16), 1541–1543.

Hahn, R. G., Knox, L. M., & Forman, T. A. (2005). Evaluation of poststreptococcal illness. *American Family Physician, 71*(10), 1949–1954.

Hansson, G. K., & Hamsten, A. (2016). Atherosclerosis, thrombosis, and vascular biology. In L. Goldman & A. I. Schafer (Eds.), *Goldman-Cecil Medicine* (25th ed., pp. 417–419). Philadelphia, PA: Elsevier Saunders.

Healey, J. S., Connolly, S. J., Gold, M. R., Israel, C. W., Van Gelder, I. C., Capucci, A., . . . ASSERT Investigators. (2012). Subclinical atrial fibrillation and the risk of stroke. *New England Journal of Medicine, 366*(2), 120–129.

Jacobson, K. M., & Rahko, P. S. (2012). Mitral valve prolapse. In E. T. Bope & R. D. Kellerman (Eds.), *Conn's current therapy 2012* (pp. 454–457). Philadelphia, PA: Elsevier Saunders.

Jaff, M. R., & Bartholomew J.R. (2016). Other peripheral arterial diseases. In L. Goldman & A. I. Schafer (Eds.), *Goldman-Cecil Medicine* (25th ed., pp. 504-511). Philadelphia, PA: Elsevier Saunders.

Kaba, E., Thompson, D. R., Burnard, P., Edwards, D., & Theodosopoulou, E. (2005). Somebody else's heart inside me: A descriptive study of psychological problems after a heart transplantation. *Issues in Mental Health Nursing, 26,* 611–625.

Kodali, S. K., Williams, M. R., Smith, C. R., Svensson, L. G., Webb, J. G., Makkar, R. R., . . . PARTNER Trial Investigators. (2012). Two-year outcomes after transcatheter or surgical aortic-valve replacement. *New England Journal of Medicine, 366*(18), 1686–1695.

Lamas, G. (2012). How much atrial fibrillation is too much atrial fibrillation. *New England Journal of Medicine, 366*(2), 178–180.

Lamy, A., Deveraux, P. J., Prabhakaran, D., Taggart, D. P., Hu, S., Paolasso, E., . . . CORONARY Investigators. (2012).

Off-pump or on-pump coronary-artery bypass grafting at 30 days. *New England Journal of Medicine, 366*(16), 1489–1497.

Lange, R. S., & Hillis, L. D. (2012). Congenital heart disease. In E. T. Bope & R. D. Kellerman (Eds.), *Conn's current therapy 2012* (pp. 422–427). Philadelphia, PA: Elsevier Saunders.

Lazaar, H. L. (2010). Transcatheter aortic valves: Where do we go from here? *New England Journal of Medicine, 363*(17), 1667–1668.

Leal, M. A. (2012). Pericarditis and pericardial effusions. In E. T. Bope & R. D. Kellerman (Eds.), *Conn's current therapy 2012* (pp. 457–461). Philadelphia, PA: Elsevier Saunders.

Lederle, F. A. (2016). Diseases of the aorta. In L. Goldman & A. I. Schafer (Eds.), *Goldman-Cecil Medicine* (25th ed., pp. 492–497). Philadelphia, PA: Elsevier Saunders.

Little, W. C., & Oh, J. K. (2012). Pericardial diseases. In E. T. Bope & R. D. Kellerman (Eds.), *Conn's current therapy 2012* (pp. 473–481). Philadelphia, PA: Elsevier Saunders.

Lloyd-Jones. (2016). Epidemiology of cardiovascular disease. In L. Goldman & A. I. Schafer (Eds.), *Goldman-Cecil Medicine* (25th ed., pp. 257–262). Philadelphia, PA: Elsevier Saunders.

Makkar, R. R., Fontana, G. P., Jilaihawi, H., Kapadia, S., Pichard, A. D., Douglas, P. S., . . . PARTNER Trial Investigators. (2012). Transcatheter aortic-valve replacement for inoperable severe aortic stenosis. *New England Journal of Medicine, 366*(18), 1696–1704.

Mancini, D., & Naka, Y. (2016). Cardiac transplantation. In L. Goldman & A. I. Schafer (Eds.), *Goldman-Cecil Medicine* (25th ed., pp. 519–523). Philadelphia, PA: Elsevier Saunders.

Marelli, A. J. (2016). Congenital heart disease in adults. In L. Goldman & A. I. Schafer (Eds.), *Goldman-Cecil Medicine* (25th ed., pp. 405–417). Philadelphia, PA: Elsevier Saunders.

McMurray, J. J. V., & Pfeffer, M. A. (2016). Heart failure: Management and prognosis. In L. Goldman & A. I. Schafer (Eds.), *Goldman-Cecil Medicine* (25th ed., pp. 305–320). Philadelphia, PA: Elsevier Saunders.

Milani, R. V., & Lavie, C. J. (2007). Impact of cardiac rehabilitation on depression and its associated mortality. *American Journal of Medicine, 120*(9), 799–806.

Miller, L. W., Pagani, F. D., Russell, S. D., John, R., Boyle, A. J., Aaronson, K. D., . . . & Frazier, O. H. for the HeartMate II Clinical Investigators. (2007). Use of a continuous-flow device in patients awaiting heart transplantation. *New England Journal of Medicine, 357*(9), 885–896.

Moss, A. J. (2010). Preventing heart failure and improving survival. *New England Journal of Medicine, 363*(25), 2456–2457.

Myerburg, R. J. (2016). Approach to cardiac arrest and life-threatening arrhythmias. In L. Goldman & A. I. Schafer (Eds.), *Goldman-Cecil Medicine* (25th ed., pp. 352–356). Philadelphia, PA: Elsevier Saunders.

Nabel, E. G., & Braunwald, E. (2012). A tale of coronary artery disease and myocardial infarction. *New England Journal of Medicine, 366*(1), 54–63.

Neschis, D. G. (2012). Acquired diseases of the aorta. In E. T. Bope & R. D. Kellerman (Eds.), *Conn's current therapy 2012* (pp. 395–399). Philadelphia, PA: Elsevier Saunders.

O'Connor, C. M., & Rogers. J. G. (2016). Heart failure: Pathophysiology and diagnosis. In L. Goldman & A. I. Schafer (Eds.), *Goldman-Cecil Medicine* (25th ed., pp. 298–305). Philadelphia, PA: Elsevier Saunders.

O'Donnell, C. J., & Nabel, E. G. (2011). Genomics of cardiovascular disease. *New England Journal of Medicine, 365*(22), 2098–2108.

Olgin, J. E. (2016). Approach to the patient with suspected arrhythmia. In L. Goldman & A. I. Schafer (Eds.), *Goldman-Cecil Medicine* (25th ed., pp. 344–352). Philadelphia, PA: Elsevier Saunders.

Otto, C. M., & Verrier, E. D. (2011). Mitral regurgitation: What is best for my patient. *New England Journal of Medicine, 364*(15), 1462–1463.

Park, S. J., Kim, Y. H., Park, D. W., Yun, S. C., Ahn, J. M., Song, H. G., . . . Seung, K. B. (2011). Randomized trial of stents versus bypass surgery for left main coronary artery disease. *New England Journal of Medicine, 364*(18), 1718–1726.

Prasad, A., & Herrmann, J. (2011). Myocardial infarction due to percutaneous coronary intervention. *New England Journal of Medicine, 364*(5), 453–464.

Reeder, G. S., & Prasad, A. (2012). Acute myocardial infarction. In E. T. Bope & R. D. Kellerman (Eds.), *Conn's current therapy 2012* (pp. 399–406). Philadelphia, PA: Elsevier Saunders.

Rho, R. W., & Page, R. L. (2012). Atrial fibrillation. In E. T. Bope & R. D. Kellerman (Eds.), *Conn's current therapy 2012* (pp. 411–418) Philadelphia, PA: Elsevier Saunders.

Roe, M. T., & Ohman, E. M. (2012). A new era in secondary prevention after acute coronary syndrome. *New England Journal of Medicine, 366*(1), 85–87.

Saffitz, J. E. (2006). Connexins, conduction, and atrial fibrillation. *New England Journal of Medicine, 354*(26), 2712–2714.

Santucci, P. A., Haw, J., Trohman, R. G., & Pinski, S. L. (1998). Interference with an implantable defibrillator by an electronic antitheft–surveillance device. *New England Journal of Medicine, 339*(19), 1371–1374.

Selnes, O. A., Gottesman, R. F., Grega, M. A., Baumgartner, W. A., Zeger, S. L., & McKhann, G. M. (2012). Cognitive and neurologic outcomes after coronary-artery bypass surgery. *New England Journal of Medicine, 366*(3), 250–257.

Shahian, D. M., Meyer, G. S., Yeh, R. W., Fifer, M. A., & Torchiana, D. F. (2012). Percutaneous coronary interventions without on-site cardiac surgical backup. *New England Journal of Medicine, 366*(19), 1814–1823.

Sowell, L. V., Kuhl, E. A., Sears, S. F., Klodell, C. T., & Conti, J. B. (2006). Device implant techniques and consideration of body image: Specific procedures for implantable cardioverter defibrillators in female patients. *Journal of Women's Health, 15*(7), 830–835.

Stone, G. W., Maehara, A., Lansky, A., de Bruyne, B., Cristea, E., Mintz, G. S., . . . PROSPECT Investigators. (2011). A prospective natural-history study of coronary atherosclerosis. *New England Journal of Medicine, 364*(3), 226–235.

Tang, A. S. L., Wells, G. A., Talajic, M., Arnold, M. O., Sheldon, R., Connolly, S., . . . Resynchronization-Defibrillation for

Ambulatory Heart Failure Trial Investigators. (2010). Cardiac-resynchronization therapy for mild-to-moderate heart failure. *New England Journal of Medicine, 363*(325), 2385–2395.

Teirstein, P. S., & Lytle, B. W. (2016). Interventional and surgical treatment of coronary artery disease. In L. Goldman & A. I. Schafer (Eds.), *Goldman-Cecil Medicine* (25th ed., pp. 456–461). Philadelphia, PA: Elsevier Saunders.

Tobin, K., & Eagle, K. (2012). Angina pectoris. In E. T. Bope & R. D. Kellerman (Eds.), *Conn's current therapy 2012* (pp. 406–411). Philadelphia, PA: Elsevier Saunders.

U.S. Department of Health and Human Services. (1995). *Public Health Services AHCPR: Cardiac rehabilitation clinical practice guideline*. Rockville, MD: Author.

Victor, R. G. (2016). Arterial hypertension. In L. Goldman & A. I. Schafer (Eds.), *Goldman-Cecil Medicine* (25th ed., pp. 381–397). Philadelphia, PA: Elsevier Saunders.

Wang, A. (2012). Infective endocarditis. In E. T. Bope & R. D. Kellerman (Eds.), *Conn's current therapy 2012* (pp. 448–454). Philadelphia, PA: Elsevier Saunders.

Weintraub, W. S., Grau-Sepulveda, M. V., Weiss, J. M., O'Brien, S., Peterson, E. D., Kolm, P., . . . Edwards, F. H. (2012). Comparative effectiveness of revascularization strategies. *New England Journal of Medicine, 366*(16), 1467–1476.

White, C. (2007). Intermittent claudication. *New England Journal of Medicine, 356*(b12), 1241–1250.

Winkel, E., & Kao, W. (2012). Heart failure. In E. T. Bope & R. D. Kellerman (Eds.), *Conn's current therapy 2012* (pp. 432–436). Philadelphia, PA: Elsevier Saunders.

Zimetbaum, P. (2016). Cardiac arrhythmias with supraventricular origin. In L. Goldman & A. I. Schafer (Eds.), *Goldman-Cecil-Medicine* (25th ed., pp. 356–367). Philadelphia, PA: Elsevier Saunders.

CHAPTER 29

Chronic Obstructive Pulmonary Disease, Asthma, and Other Conditions of the Pulmonary System

STRUCTURE AND FUNCTION OF THE PULMONARY SYSTEM

The pulmonary system draws *oxygen* from the atmosphere, which is then incorporated into the blood and subsequently distributed to body tissues. The pulmonary system also removes *carbon dioxide*, a waste product of tissue metabolism, from the blood and tissues and returns it to the atmosphere. This process is accomplished by moving air into and out of the lungs through *breathing*. Dysfunction of the pulmonary system affects every system of the body. Diminished supply of oxygen *or* an excess of carbon dioxide not only affects body function but can also result in loss of consciousness and death.

The pulmonary system consists of the *nasooropharynx*, *trachea*, *bronchi*, and *lungs* (**Figure 29-1**). The *diaphragm* and *intercostal muscles* of the chest cavity (**thorax**) also contribute to movement of air into and out of the lungs.

Breathing is an involuntary activity under the control of the *breathing center* in the brain. Changes in levels of carbon dioxide and oxygen in the blood bring about automatic changes in rate and depth of breathing. As the concentration of carbon dioxide in the blood increases, breathing rate increases to hasten elimination of the waste product. When oxygen levels in the blood are sufficient, the breathing rate slows.

Ventilation refers to breathing air into and out of the lungs. **Inspiration** is the act of breathing in, whereas **expiration** is the act of breathing out. **Respiration** is a physiologic process that refers to the actual diffusion of gases (*oxygen* and *carbon dioxide*) within the lungs, and eventually within all tissues of the body.

Air first enters the pulmonary system through the nose during inspiration. Air entering the nostrils comes in contact with the mucous membranes, which warm and moisten it. Tiny hairs within the nostrils trap dust particles and organisms before they reach the **pharynx** (throat), which serves as a passageway for both air and food. At the bottom of the pharynx are two openings: one into the *esophagus* for the passage of food, and the other into the *larynx* (voice box) for the passage of air. The larynx contains the vocal cords, which are necessary for speech. A flap called the *epiglottis*, located on top of the larynx, closes over the larynx

Figure 29-1   The Pulmonary System

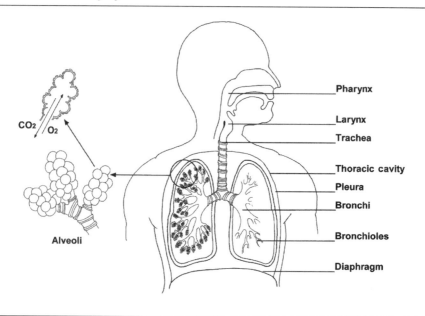

Pharynx
Larynx
Trachea
Thoracic cavity
Pleura
Bronchi
Bronchioles
Diaphragm
CO_2 O_2
Alveoli

© Jane Tinkler Lamm.

when food is ingested to prevent food from entering the pulmonary system.

Following inspiration, air passes through the larynx into the main airway to the lungs, the *trachea* (windpipe). The trachea is a cartilaginous tube lined with special hair-like projections called *cilia*. The cilia are part of the body's defense against foreign objects, such as bacteria or other particles that have not been filtered out by the upper part of the pulmonary system. With a rhythmic motion, cilia project mucus or other particles up toward the pharynx, where they can be expectorated.

After entering the chest cavity, the trachea divides into two branches, called the right and left *bronchi*. Each bronchus, which also contains cilia, enters a lung and continues to branch into smaller segments called *bronchioles*. The bronchioles terminate in tiny sacs called *alveolar sacs*. Within the alveolar sacs are small balloon-like structures called *alveoli*, which make up most of the lung's mass. It is within the alveoli that the exchange of oxygen and carbon dioxide takes place through tiny blood vessels called *capillaries*.

External respiration is the process of exchanging oxygen and carbon dioxide in the *lungs* and the atmosphere. The exchange of oxygen and carbon dioxide at the tissue level is called *internal respiration*. Oxygen diffuses through the alveolar walls into capillaries, through which it is distributed to the general circulation and delivered to tissue throughout the body. Body cells release carbon dioxide into the blood, which then carries it to capillaries in the alveoli. Here carbon dioxide diffuses across the alveolar wall and is expelled from the lungs through expiration.

The lungs are two sponge-like structures contained within the thoracic cavity. The left lung contains two lobes: the upper and lower lobes. The right lung contains three lobes: the upper, middle, and lower lobes. The heart is located between the two lungs. Pulmonary vessels carry blood to and from the lungs from the heart. The *pulmonary artery* carries *deoxygenated blood from* the heart *to* the lungs, whereas the *pulmonary vein* carries *oxygenated blood to* the heart *from* the lungs.

After delivering oxygen to the body tissues, deoxygenated blood containing carbon dioxide returns to the heart from the general circulation; it is then pumped from the right ventricle of the heart into the lungs, from which the carbon dioxide can be expelled through expiration. In the lungs, oxygen that has been taken in through inspiration diffuses into blood. The oxygenated blood then returns through the pulmonary vein to the heart, which in turn pumps the oxygenated blood into the general circulation to be distributed to the body tissues.

The thoracic cavity is lined with a thin membrane called the *pleura*, which secretes a thin layer of fluid to help minimize the friction created when the lungs expand and contract against the chest wall during ventilation. The thoracic cavity is surrounded by ribs. Muscles around the ribs (*intercostal muscles*) expand when air is inhaled and contract when air is exhaled. The thoracic cavity is separated from the abdominal cavity by the main pulmonary muscle, called the diaphragm.

Air is able to move into and out of the lungs because of pressure changes, which occur because of the contraction and relaxation of the *diaphragm* and intercostal muscles. The pressure within the lungs and the thorax must be less than the pressure in the atmosphere for inspiration to occur. As air is taken into the lungs, the diaphragm contracts, moving downward, increasing the size of the thoracic cavity, and lowering the pressure within the thoracic cavity. The lungs expand. Atmospheric air, which is at higher pressure, then flows into the lungs, bringing in oxygen as inhalation occurs. Next the diaphragm moves in the opposite direction, relaxing and moving upward, causing the thoracic cavity to become smaller, and thereby increasing intrathoracic pressure. As the lungs are compressed, air is forced out and carbon dioxide is exhaled.

OBSTRUCTIVE PULMONARY DISEASE
Overview of COPD

The term *chronic obstructive pulmonary disease (COPD)* describes a group of conditions characterized by obstructed airflow, including *chronic bronchitis* and *emphysema*. The principal cause of COPD is

smoking (Hanania & Sharafkhaneh, 2012; King, 2011; Niewoehner, 2016), although not everyone who develops COPD has a history of smoking. Other environmental exposures such as dust in certain work environments or air pollution can also contribute to the development of COPD (Hanania & Sharafkhaneh, 2012; Rabe, 2007).

COPD involves chronic inflammation of the airways, which subsequently results in destruction of functional lung tissue, hyperinflation, and increased mucus production (Washko et al., 2011). As inflammation continues, airways become narrowed, resulting in obstruction of airflow. The structure of alveolar walls is destroyed, causing permanent enlargement of the airspaces. Eventually, alveolar units become less functional, and the amount of lung area available for gas exchange is reduced.

COPD is generally progressive, although its course varies. In some cases, the condition develops slowly, with pulmonary function remaining relatively stable for years. In other cases, pulmonary function deteriorates rapidly. Ongoing exposure to cigarette smoke or other pollutants can facilitate the progression and severity of COPD.

Manifestations of COPD

Although chronic bronchitis and emphysema can be two distinct conditions, they frequently coexist. Both share similar pulmonary manifestations, including **dyspnea** (shortness of breath), especially on exertion; intermittent cough; sputum production; limitation of airflow; chronic inflammation of the lungs; and fatigue (Rabe, 2007). This combination of manifestations is a major contributor to incapacitation, with dyspnea in particular significantly altering quality of life. Fatigue is a common manifestation in most individuals with COPD. Dyspnea of COPD can affect individuals' ability to exercise or perform tasks of daily living. Individuals with early COPD may experience dyspnea after walking for short distances, while those in later stages of the condition may experience significant dyspnea with even minimal activity, such as brushing their teeth. COPD is marked by **exacerbations** (acute worsening of manifestations), which become more frequent and more severe as COPD progresses, and which appear to accelerate decline in lung function (Albert et al., 2011; Hurst et al., 2010; Tashkin, 2010).

Chronic Bronchitis

Acute bronchitis should be distinguished from chronic bronchitis. *Acute bronchitis* is a self-limited inflammation of the airways of the lung, usually of less than 3 weeks' duration, with a primary manifestation of cough (Wenzel, 2016; Davids & Schapira, 2012). *Chronic bronchitis* is clinically defined as a chronic cough with sputum, with abnormal enlargement of the mucous glands within the airways and a manifestation of COPD (Niewoehner, 2016).

Manifestations of chronic bronchitis consist of a persistent cough, especially in the early morning, accompanied by an excessive volume of mucus and expectoration. The lining of the air passages becomes irritated, swollen, and clogged with mucus. This mucus, in turn, obstructs airflow into and out of the alveoli. Sometimes the small muscles around the air passages tighten—a phenomenon called *bronchospasm*—which makes breathing even more difficult. Chronic bronchitis often leads to emphysema. Although bronchitis may predispose individuals to develop emphysema, it can also result from other conditions of the lung, such as *occupational lung diseases* and *cystic fibrosis*.

Emphysema

Emphysema is defined as a permanent enlargement of the alveoli caused by the overinflation of and destructive changes in the alveolar walls (Niewoehner, 2016). As a result, the alveoli have less surface area available for the exchange of oxygen and carbon dioxide, and the bronchioles close before exhalation is complete. As more and more alveoli are affected, the lungs lose some of their natural ability to stretch and relax, which diminishes the efficiency of expiration, as all of the air present in the lungs cannot be expelled. Airways become obstructed; stale air, which is high in carbon dioxide and low in oxygen, becomes trapped in the alveoli; and the lungs become hyperinflated (Washko et al., 2011).

Advanced COPD

Because of the airway obstruction that accompanies COPD, **hypoxemia** (decreased levels of oxygen in the blood) may occur. As COPD becomes more advanced and hypoxemia increases, oxygen supply to the brain may become inadequate, resulting in impaired judgment, confusion, or motor incoordination. A buildup of carbon dioxide (**hypercapnia**) may also occur because of inadequate gas exchange in the lungs, resulting in drowsiness or apathy. To counteract the low concentration of oxygen, the body's production of red blood cells increases, resulting in a condition called **polycythemia**. The increased number of red cells in the blood increases blood viscosity, which in turn can impede blood flow. When polycythemia is severe, periodic **phlebotomy** (removal of blood) may be performed to reduce the number of red blood cells, thereby decreasing the viscosity of the blood. As COPD advances, individuals may experience increased difficulty expectorating secretions; increased shortness of breath, especially upon exertion; and increased vulnerability to pulmonary infections. For individuals with this condition, pulmonary infections can be life threatening because they may further compromise an already-diminished gas exchange.

As a result of the obstruction of airflow in the lungs and the subsequent breakdown of the alveolar walls, many capillaries in the lungs are destroyed. The surrounding capillaries become constricted, as a compensatory mechanism for the lower concentrations of oxygen. Constriction of the capillaries channels additional blood flow to areas of the lungs that are better oxygenated; however, constriction of capillaries also creates a resistance to the blood being pumped into the lungs by the right ventricle of the heart. As a consequence, the right ventricle must pump against resistance and becomes hypertrophied (enlarged), losing its ability to pump effectively, a condition called *cor pulmonale*. Because of the inefficient pumping action of the enlarged right ventricle, blood returning to the right side of the heart from the general circulation begins to back up, causing **edema** (swelling) in other parts of the body. Organs of the digestive system may become engorged with fluid, causing nausea and vomiting. Edema may also develop in the lower extremities, predisposing individuals to skin ulcerations.

Identifying COPD

Most often, COPD goes unrecognized for years. Individuals usually seek health advice when they note shortness of breath with exercise or at rest. At this point, more than 50% of their lung function may already have been lost (Hanania & Sharafkhaneh, 2012).

Although history of smoking, cough, and excess mucus secretion may be indicative of COPD, *pulmonary function tests* are required to identify COPD and document the degree of loss of lung function. Rate and volume below the standard established for normal individuals indicate dysfunction of the lung (Scanlon, 2016).

Pulmonary function tests are used to detect irregularities in pulmonary function and to determine the degree of impairment. These tests involve breathing into a machine called a *spirometer*, which measures several types of pulmonary function. *Spirometry* assesses various aspects of airflow (e.g., air volume and flow rate of air). Pulmonary function tests are used to assess the volume of air that an individual can take in and expel from the lungs, as well as the ability to move air into and out of the lungs. They may be used to determine the cause of dyspnea, the extent to which the lung is affected, or the effectiveness of management of lung conditions. The results are then printed out in a graphic representation called a *spirogram*. Types of pulmonary function that are measured in terms of lung capacity are listed here and illustrated in **Figure 29-2**:

- *Vital capacity*: The maximum volume of air that can be inspired and expired.
- *Forced expiratory volume (FEV):* The volume of air that the individual can forcibly exhale at 1-, 2-, and 3-second intervals. Readings of the FEV are reported as FEV_1, FEV_2, and FEV_3, respectively.
- *Residual lung volume:* The amount of air left in the lungs after maximum expiration.
- *Maximum voluntary ventilation (MVV):* The maximum volume that an individual can breathe in 12 seconds, breathing in and out as rapidly and forcefully as possible.

Figure 29-2   Pulmonary Volumes

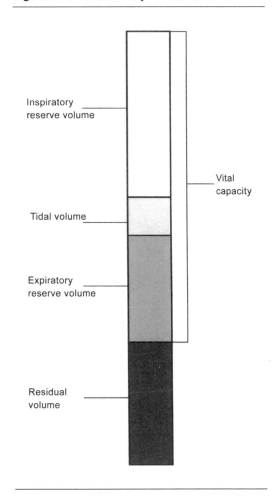

© Jane Tinkler Lamm.

- *Tidal volume:* The amount of air breathed in and out at rest.
- *Inspiratory capacity:* The volume of air taken in by maximal inspiration after normal expiration.
- *Functional residual capacity:* The volume of air remaining in the lungs after normal expiration.

The Global Initiative for Chronic Obstructive Lung Disease (GOLD, 2013) developed a –four stage classification for identification of the severity of COPD ranging from Mild (Stage I) to Very Severe (Stage IV). Stages are based on FEV reading as measured by spirometry, and on the type of of manifestations the individual is experiencing. (Garcia & Jenkinson, 2007).

Limitation of airflow is usually progressive in COPD, although the degree of progression and associated limitation of function varies from person to person. The degree to which COPD impedes the individual's function is determined by the severity of manifestations (such as breathlessness and exercise capacity) in addition to any other co-existing medical conditions, rather than the degree of airflow limitation (FEV reading on spirometry) alone.

Management of COPD

The major goals of management of COPD are relieving manifestations, improving health status, improving functional capacity, and reducing chance of complications (Niewoehner, 2016).

Smoking Cessation and Lifestyle Modification

An important aspect of management is smoking cessation. Unfortunately, many individuals with COPD fail to refrain from smoking (Hanania & Sharafkhaneh, 2012). A number of behavioral techniques, support groups, nicotine supplements, and other medications have been introduced as interventions directed toward assisting smoking cessation.

Exercise such as daily walking or other structured exercise program can help individuals build strength and endurance, maintain their physical condition, and improve work capacity (Spruit et al., 2012). Consuming a series of small meals throughout the day, rather than a few large meals, may facilitate breathing, as a distended stomach or abdomen can push against the lungs, interfering with breathing.

Medications

A variety of medications may be used in the management of COPD. *Bronchodilators,* which help to relax the airways, thereby increasing airflow, can help to relieve dyspnea. Bronchodilators are usually delivered through an inhaler such as a metered-dose inhaler or a nebulizer. To receive maximum benefit from the inhaler, individuals must use the correct technique, which some individuals may find difficult to coordinate. Inhaled steroids may be used, especially during exacerbations.

Vaccinations

Individuals with COPD are susceptible to pulmonary infections and pneumonia. Because these individuals already have reduced lung function, pulmonary infection that further compromises lung capacity may have serious consequences. Given this risk, vaccinations for influenza and pneumonia are usually recommended.

Breathing Techniques

Many individuals with COPD benefit from learning new breathing techniques that stress *abdominal, diaphragmatic breathing* (to reduce use of accessory muscles for breathing and to conserve energy) or *pursed-lip breathing* (to slow breathing rate and help remove trapped air from the lungs). A *resistive breathing device* may also be used in the home daily to "exercise" muscles of respiration.

Other interventions may include *postural drainage* or *chest physiotherapy* (to remove secretions from the lungs) or *resistive breathing devices* (to increase breathing capacity). Avoidance of pulmonary irritants, especially those produced by smoking, is of primary importance.

Oxygen

Supplemental home *oxygen therapy* may be required, depending on the amount of lung damage and the oxygen level in the blood. Often individuals with COPD have right ventricular failure, polycythemia, severe dyspnea, and sleep-associated hypoxemia. Oxygen administration during ambulation can reduce the effects of dyspnea and increase endurance and the ability to carry out daily activities. The use of oxygen therapy is highly individual and depends on the degree of hypoxemia experienced at rest or during exercise. Some individuals require oxygen only at night and during exercise, whereas others will require supplemental oxygen 24 hours a day.

Oxygen may be supplied through several different systems. When choosing a system, attributes such as weight, portability, ease of refilling, availability, and cost are taken into account. Stationary systems contain large amounts of oxygen and usually require an electrical source; the oxygen comes in large cylinders, which can weigh as much as 100 pounds. Stationary systems may be mounted near the bed to be used at night during sleep, or used as oxygen storage devices for filling smaller systems. Small portable devices contain a limited amount of oxygen and can be carried or wheeled on a cart or stroller to be used throughout the day. Many individuals use both stationary and portable systems.

Due to danger of combustion, individuals using oxygen should avoid close contact with individuals who are smoking and stay away from open flames. Combustible materials such as aerosol sprays, paint thinners, or petroleum-based products should also be removed from the area.

Surgical Intervention

The surgical intervention known as *lung-volume reduction surgery*, in which selected areas of hyperinflated lungs are resected, improves pulmonary muscle function and consequently exercise tolerance (Anzueto, 2010; Sciurba et al., 2010).

Lung transplantation in COPD is usually reserved for individuals who experience severe incapacitation as a result of COPD, and who have no other major chronic conditions (Cypel et al., 2011; Niewoehner, 2016). Lung transplantation may involve one or both lungs. As with other types of transplants, individuals who undergo this surgery must have ongoing immunosuppression after transplant, must be closely monitored for signs of rejection, and are at high risk for malignancy and serious infections that can be life threatening (Feller-Kopman & Decamp, 2016)

Pulmonary Rehabilitation

Pulmonary rehabilitation is an important aspect of COPD management and is directed toward optimizing functional capacity and enhancing quality of life. It consists of an individualized multidisciplinary program composed of breathing exercises, physical conditioning, energy conservation, physiotherapy, education, and nutritional, psychological, behavioral, and vocational interventions.

Individuals with COPD frequently become more sedentary as their condition progresses. This lack of activity contributes to muscular and cardiovascular deconditioning, which decreases endurance and further hampers activity. Pulmonary

rehabilitation helps individuals build endurance as well as learn skills to cope psychologically and physically.

Functional Implications of COPD

Personal and Psychosocial Issues

Shortness of breath can lead to anxiety and panic, whether or not it is associated with a health condition. Dyspnea associated with COPD may produce severe anxiety and contribute to avoidance of all activities that cause dyspnea as well as preoccupation with bodily complaints. Individuals may adopt an abnormally and potentially unnecessarily restricted lifestyle, even though they are physically capable of being more active. Because strong emotions naturally raise the breathing rate, fear of becoming short of breath may in itself increase dyspnea, creating a vicious cycle that can prove totally incapacitating.

Although oxygen use can increase functional capacity for some individuals, in others it can contribute to social isolation. Some individuals may be reluctant to use portable oxygen in public because they feel it is stigmatizing and calls attention to their condition. Others may become psychologically dependent on oxygen and be reluctant to venture out without the oxygen source, even when it is not required. In other instances, individuals may have concern that the portable oxygen source will become depleted and consequently be reluctant to leave their home. Psychological dependency on the oxygen may be more debilitating than the pulmonary condition itself.

Activities and Participation

Individuals with COPD may find themselves excluded from activities of their families and friends because of limited understanding of the condition and the amount of activity that can be achieved safely. In some instances, social activity and interaction may be made more difficult because of the individual's bouts of coughing and expectoration.

Although exertion can cause difficulty breathing, individuals with COPD are generally able to maintain some level of activity unless they have associated cardiac complications. Exercise programs can both improve self-esteem and reduce manifestations to some extent. If individuals experience dyspnea partly due to ineffective breathing patterns and partly from lack of conditioning, it is crucial that they work to increase exercise tolerance through daily breathing or conditioning exercises, in addition to participating in other exercise routines.

Individuals with COPD can learn to become accustomed to some dyspnea and to adapt to the sensation so that they can maintain an optimal level of activity without undue fear or anxiety. Finally, they may need extra time to accomplish tasks so that they can take rest periods. They may need to divide some activities into smaller tasks rather than trying to accomplish the entire task at one time.

Although an environment near sea level with a mild climate and minimal air pollution is ideal for individuals with COPD, it is not always possible to live in this type of setting. Individuals living in less moderate climates should avoid extremes in temperatures. Home and work temperatures should be kept cool. Radiant or baseboard heaters may be better than forced-air heating systems, as the latter have filters that need to be cleaned or changed regularly. If a humidifier is used, it should be cleaned regularly to inhibit mold growth. Fireplaces and wood-burning or coal-burning stoves should be avoided, as they are potential sources of air pollution.

Maintaining adequate hydration is important in COPD due to the overproduction of mucus. The environment should be well humidified, and a nebulizer or aerosol may be used periodically throughout the day to deliver humidity directly to the lungs. High levels of humidity may make breathing more difficult, however. For this reason, individuals living in hot, humid environments should have air conditioning to maintain the temperature and the humidity at acceptable levels. Filters on air conditioners should be changed on a regular basis.

Responses of family and friends to COPD may affect an individual's ability to cope with his or her condition. Family members may unintentionally place individuals in an "invalid" role, reducing expectations of them in the family structure or removing responsibility from them, even though individuals may be capable of engaging in a number of activities. Individuals with COPD may respond by using breathing difficulty to escape from life's demands, to receive emotional rewards, or to manipulate or control the behavior of others. In other instances, family members may overestimate individuals' abilities, not fully understanding the seriousness of the condition and its implications for function. Such reactions may push individuals to go beyond their functional capacity or to ignore management interventions for managing COPD.

As is true with other chronic conditions, the lifestyle changes required by COPD depend on the amount of lung damage and any additional complicating health conditions. In general, it is important for individuals to maintain good nutritional status and normal weight. Because of the increased burden that obesity or overeating can place on breathing capacity, individuals with COPD should be urged to avoid both of these practices.

Cessation of smoking is a necessary component of management. Many individuals consider this requirement to be the most difficult part of management. Even when they are aware that smoking exacerbates COPD, they may find it difficult to alter their behavior. Enrollment in specially designed smoking cessation programs may be necessary to help individuals stop smoking, although some individuals may continue to resist participation.

Counseling and support groups can help to increase self-esteem and help family members cope with the individual's condition. Education of both individuals with COPD and their family members is important. In addition, both the individual with COPD and family members should develop reasonable expectations of what can be accomplished with adequate management and be helped to understand the importance of adhering to the management plan.

Sexuality

Sexual difficulties may be a particular problem for individuals with COPD. These problems may stem from a fear of becoming short of breath rather than from any physical limitation attributable to the condition. Because both the rate and the depth of respiration are increased during sexual excitement, the fear of suffocation may cause some individuals to be reluctant or restrained when engaging in sexual activity. Although dyspnea may be uncomfortable, individuals with COPD with no complications can generally maintain sexual activity. They can often increase their tolerance for sexual activity through conditioning, or their partners may assume a more active role.

Concerns about dyspnea can inhibit sexual activity and affect intimate relationships. In some instances, sexual function may be negatively affected by depression. Discussion and education about sexual issues can provide reassurance and confidence, which in turn can enhance individuals' sexual function.

VOCATIONAL ISSUES IN COPD

The most limiting factor related to COPD is dyspnea. Chronic hypoxemia may cause neuropsychological deficits that diminish individuals' ability to perform a number of mental functions, which can further contribute to difficulties in the work setting.

In later stages of COPD, dyspnea may become so severe that walking and communicating become difficult. Individuals may need to learn energy conservation techniques and ensure that activities are planned and paced to improve performance within the limitations of their condition. They may need to change their methods of performing more energy-consuming activities so as to improve their energy efficiency. Proper attitude, breathing techniques, body mechanics, pacing, and relaxation can all increase work tolerance.

Although stress is a part of every job, when demands are too challenging, the muscles become tense, heartbeat increases, and breathing becomes more difficult; as a consequence, more oxygen is required. Learning to manage stress as well as reducing stress-provoking situations in the workplace as much as possible can help to reduce emotional strain that may contribute to dyspnea.

Sitting to do work (rather than standing) as much as possible requires less energy. Proper height of stools or chairs in relation to tables or desks and arrangement of equipment, tools, or supplies so that they are placed within easy reach can

minimize strain on breathing. Unnecessary motion or movements should be eliminated. Arranging work to make tasks simpler can increase functional ability. For example, pushing or sliding objects is easier than lifting them. Placing casters on items can facilitate movement. Pushing a wheelbarrow or cart with a light load of items is less strenuous than carrying items.

Individuals may also need to prioritize tasks. Distributing more difficult tasks throughout the day and breaking up activities into constituent parts, with periods of rest between the subcomponents, can enable individuals to accomplish tasks more easily. Individuals with COPD may be limited in how much they can use their arms and upper body because of the additional stress placed on accessory muscles of respiration. For this reason, they may need to avoid activities that involve lifting or reaching. Using special long-handled tools to access materials can also help individuals avoid stooping, bending, and reaching. With such accommodations, individuals may be able to continue in sedentary lines of work even in the later stages of the condition.

Transportation to and from work is another issue that should be considered. Although many people with COPD continue to drive, driving in crowded traffic conditions in which fumes and pollutants are present may be a detriment to their health. Planning to drive via alternative routes that are less congested, or driving earlier or later in the day, can help to conserve energy and decrease exposure to pollutants.

The work environment should also be relatively free of allergens as well as dust, fumes, or chemicals that are irritating to the airways. Generally, extremes such as heat, cold, wind, distance, and duration should be avoided. The work environment should be well ventilated and climate controlled so that the temperature is neither too hot nor too cold. If any type of breathing device or aid is used, the extent to which the device will be a hazard in the work environment must be considered. The tubing in some portable devices may become caught in machinery, for example, or cause falls. Oxygen, because of the danger of fire or explosion, should not be used in close proximity to an open flame.

ASTHMA

Overview of Asthma

Asthma is a condition characterized by reversible airflow obstruction, hyperresponsiveness of the bronchi, and airway inflammation (Tschumperlin, 2011). The prevalence of this condition has increased more than 45% since the late 1970s, with the greatest increase occurring in industrialized countries (Drazen, 2016). In addition to the discomfort experienced with the disease, asthma accounts for significant loss of school and work days, limitations in activities, and sleep disruption (Schatz, 2012), and can have life-threatening exacerbations (Smith, 2010).

Although the exact cause of asthma is unknown, it appears to have a genetic component and some association with environmental pollutants, including workplace exposure to dusts or chemicals (Moffatt et al., 2010). Asthma is worsened both by infection and, in sensitized persons, by allergen exposure (Grainge et al., 2011). The current theory regarding the cause of airway inflammation in asthma revolves around inflammation, which is due to an immune responses (von Mutius & Drazen, 2012).

Asthma can range from a mild condition with infrequent exacerbations to a severe condition in which exacerbations occur almost daily. Terms used to describe asthma often reflect situations that appear to trigger an exacerbation. When exacerbations occur spontaneously with no specific factor identified as a trigger, individuals are said to have *intrinsic asthma*. If a specific allergen has been identified as triggering exacerbations, the individual is said to have *extrinsic asthma*. When manifestations occur only with exercise, the individual is said to have *exercise-induced asthma*. Asthma brought on by occupational exposure to irritants is termed *occupational asthma*, whereas preexisting asthma that is exacerbated by workplace exposure is termed *workplace-exacerbated asthma*.

Manifestations of Asthma

During an acute exacerbation of asthma, individuals experience dyspnea, often accompanied by cough, wheezing, and anxiety (Drazen, 2016). Triggers of asthma exacerbations involve complex interactions with factors within the environment as well as individual factors. Factors such as exercise, emotional stress, inhalation of cold air, and exposure to pulmonary irritants such as fumes from paint or gasoline, cigarette smoke, or perfumes may precipitate an exacerbation. For some people, exacerbations are triggered by food preservatives or substances found in some medications, such as aspirin (*aspirin-exacerbated pulmonary disease*). Most triggers set off an allergic response, which causes the immune system to initiate an inflammatory response in which the airway swells and secretes excess mucus that clogs the passages. At the same time, the muscles that control air passages constrict and go into spasm, causing the airways to narrow. As a result, individuals have difficulty breathing and the lungs work less efficiently.

The severity of manifestations and the frequency of asthma exacerbations vary with the individual. Some individuals may experience only a slight cough and shortness of breath during an exacerbation, whereas others may be so restricted by cough and shortness of breath that they are unable to speak more than a few words at a time.

The severe, prolonged exacerbation known as **status asthmaticus** comprises a severe exacerbation of asthma that is unresponsive to management interventions and can be fatal. Status asthmaticus requires emergency healthcare intervention.

Management of Asthma

Management of asthma is directed toward the identification and avoidance of precipitating or aggravating factors; the relief of manifestations experienced in exacerbations; maintenance of activity, including work, school, and leisure; and the prevention of future exacerbations (Schatz, 2012). Interventions can involve short-term management for relief of manifestations during an acute exacerbation, or long-term management to modify the airway environment so that exacerbations occur less frequently.

Education

One of the most important aspects of management of asthma is education and monitoring. Individuals should be aware of how to recognize and manage exacerbations of the condition; they should also be able to identify and, if possible, avoid environmental triggers. Individuals should learn how to effectively use special devices (as described later in this section) for management or monitoring. Asthma self-management education is tailored to the need of the individual, taking into account cultural beliefs and practices.

Environmental Modifications

When *allergens* are responsible for precipitating exacerbations, attempts should be made to rid the environment of them. Home modifications may be necessary to reduce or eliminate exposure to common allergens such as animal dander, dust mites, mold, or pollen. In addition, individuals should seek to avoid or reduce exposures to other pollutants in the public and work environment.

Immunizations

Pulmonary infection in individuals with asthma can be more serious. Because of the high risk for developing complications after contracting influenza or pneumonia, individuals with asthma are encouraged to receive vaccinations for seasonal influenza and pneumonia (Drazen, 2016).

Medications

Several medications are commonly used to manage asthma. They can be used to reduce manifestations during an acute exacerbation, or for long-term management to decrease the frequency of exacerbations in individuals with severe asthma. Individuals with mild asthma who experience no manifestations between exacerbations may require medication only during an exacerbation, whereas individuals with more severe asthma may require medication on a daily basis.

Corticosteroids are one of the mainstays of management of asthma (von Mutius & Drazen, 2012). Individuals with mild persistent asthma may only use *inhaled corticosteroids* during exacerbations (Drazen, 2016). *Systemic corticosteroids* may be indicated for moderate or severe asthma, or for individuals with mild asthma if the exacerbation is severe. Ongoing long-term use of corticosteroids is contraindicated due to the potential side effects, such as cataract formation or bone loss (Drazen, 2016).

Medications called *bronchodilators* dilate the bronchioles by relaxing the muscles of their walls, thereby creating a larger opening for the passage of air. These agents may be inhaled, used in tablet or liquid form, or injected. Short-acting bronchodilators may be used for relief of manifestations during an acute exacerbation. Long-acting bronchodilators may be used on a regular basis for prolonged management and to decrease the frequency of exacerbations.

Special Devices

Some medications may be taken orally, but many medications used in the management of asthma are administered through special devices that deliver medication directly to the lungs. A *nebulizer* is one of several types of devices that convert liquid medication into tiny droplets that individuals then inhale into the lungs so that the medication acts immediately. Nebulizers do not require the same degree of precision and coordination as some of the other devices, so they are less difficult to use.

A *metered-dose inhaler* is a small handheld device that delivers a specific amount of medication in aerosol form directly into the lung. To receive the full benefit of the metered-dose inhaler, individuals must learn and use the proper technique when using it. *Spacer devices* may also be used with the metered-dose inhaler. This tube or bag is attached to the metered-dose inhaler at one end, with a mouthpiece for the individual to inhale through the other end. The spacer acts as a holding chamber, slowing down the delivery of the medication and allowing more efficient delivery.

A *dry-powder inhaler* is an alternative to aerosol-based devices such as the metered-dose inhaler. This handheld device delivers medication in a powdered form directly into the lungs as the individual inhales. To receive the maximum benefit from the device, individuals must be able to inhale with a certain force to extract the powder from the inhaler.

A *peak flow meter* is another handheld device that is used regularly by individuals to determine the severity of their asthma and to identify how well they are responding to management interventions. It can also be used during an exacerbation to determine how well short-acting medications are working. The individual blows forcefully into the device. The peak flow meter then measures the rate of airflow out of the lungs, providing an indication of the degree of narrowing of airways. The peak flow meter can indicate narrowing of airways well in advance of an exacerbation.

Monitoring and Assessment

Self-management is important in a variety of chronic health conditions; however, in asthma, regular self-monitoring, adherence to the medication schedule, an action plan for increased manifestations and exacerbations, and understanding when to seek urgent health care are crucial (Schatz, 2012). The severity of the condition and the appropriate management vary widely among individuals. Because an individual's condition can change over time, with new allergies developing or the severity of the asthma increasing or decreasing, periodic healthcare assessment is usually recommended.

Functional Implications of Asthma

Personal and Psychosocial Issues

Effective management of asthma requires adherence to the management plan to control exacerbations, but a variety of obstacles may impede individuals' ability to follow this plan. Asthma, unlike many other chronic conditions, has manifestations that, with appropriate intervention, are usually reversible and should only minimally affect daily living. As a result, when individuals are exacerbation free, they may become lax in following the management plan or monitoring their condition.

Individuals may also believe that monitoring and interventions necessary to reduce exacerbations draw attention to their condition or are stigmatizing. Consequently, they may not monitor as carefully as needed, or may not avoid situations, environments, or activities that could potentially trigger an exacerbation.

Emotional factors can compound the effects of physical manifestations of asthma. Anxiety or emotional upset may increase difficulty in breathing, causing more anxiety and leading to yet more difficulty in breathing. When it is possible to

identify situations that increase anxiety or stress, it is important to institute interventions to decrease anxiety so that the difficulty in breathing does not escalate.

Depending on the severity of asthma, a number of hospitalizations may be required. Hospitalization can contribute to feelings of dependency and can contribute to anxiety, which then becomes self-limiting. Fearful of experiencing additional exacerbations that could lead to future hospitalizations, individuals may withdraw from activities or social interactions, thereby becoming more socially isolated; this pattern can in turn lead to emotional reactions, such as depression or anger, which can trigger exacerbations.

Counseling and education regarding asthma, and support and guidance in self-management, can contribute to individuals' acceptance and adaptation to their condition as well as build confidence in their ability to effectively manage their condition.

Activities and Participation

Individuals who have had asthma since childhood may be especially vulnerable to social adjustment problems because of stressors experienced due to hospitalizations and restrictions, which may have impeded their social development. The degree of family support and the degree to which participation in social activities was encouraged may have a major impact on individuals' continued adaptation to their condition and social interactions in adulthood.

Unless individuals are actually experiencing an exacerbation, asthma is not usually recognized as easily as are conditions associated with visual cues, such as crutches or a wheelchair. Consequently, the expectations of others regarding individuals' ability to perform various activities may not be consistent with their functional capacity or their need to avoid certain activities or certain environments. Similarly, the lack of visual cues may enable individuals to deny their condition and avoid management interventions that are necessary to prevent exacerbations from occurring.

Individuals with asthma, as well as those around them, may become very anxious about participation in any type of physical activity that could potentially bring on an exacerbation. As a consequence, limitation of activity out of fear, rather than out of necessity, may prove incapacitating. Education regarding asthma and activity as well as understanding of specific factors that are more likely to precipitate an exacerbation can enhance individuals' ability to continue pursuing their optimal level of activity.

If factors in the home contribute to asthma, environmental modifications, such as removing any substances that precipitate an exacerbation, may be required. This change may be especially distressing if the trigger of exacerbation is animal dander from a pet. The environment should also be kept dust free. It may be necessary to install special filters to cut down on molds and household dust.

Financial constraints can be a source of anxiety for individuals with asthma. Obstacles such as lack of healthcare insurance coverage may result in episodic care and inadequate follow-up and monitoring. Out-of-pocket expenditures for health care and medication costs may impose an undue hardship on affected individuals and their families, making it difficult to obtain necessary medication and health care.

Access to necessary medications and health care are crucial to management of asthma and, in turn, to individuals' ability to fully participate in activities. When an effective management plan is in place, individuals are also able to learn how to make appropriate modifications that enable them to participate more fully in social and recreational activities.

Vocational Issues in Asthma

The degree to which individuals' work is affected by asthma can vary depending on the severity of the condition and the extent to which it is successfully managed. Because exposure to irritants and allergens can increase asthma exacerbations, substances that act as triggers for exacerbation should be avoided. Likewise, if exertion or exposure to extremes in temperature triggers exacerbations, then workplace modification may be needed so that precipitating factors can be decreased or avoided.

TUBERCULOSIS

Overview of Tuberculosis

Tuberculosis (TB) is an infectious condition caused by the organism *Mycobacterium tuberculosis* (the TB bacillus). It is transmitted from person to person in tiny microscopic droplets that are propelled through the air from a sneeze or cough from a person infected with the organism. Tuberculosis most frequently affects the lungs (*pulmonary tuberculosis*) but can also involve sites outside the lungs (*extrapulmonary tuberculosis*) including bones, joints, or any organ in the body (Ellner, 2016).

Infection occurs when the organism is propelled through the air from the cough or sneeze of an individual with active tuberculosis. Others who inhale the organism can then also become infected. Exposure to the TB bacillus may or may not lead to infection or to an active form of TB. Only 20 to 30% of individuals exposed to the TB bacillus become infected (Pasipanodya, Hall, & Gumbo, 2012). Whether infection or manifestations of TB develop depends on the individual's general physical condition and the intensity of the exposure. Ordinarily, tuberculosis is not contracted from brief exposure to a person with TB.

Many factors predispose individuals to develop TB. Lowered body resistance owing to inadequate rest and poor nutrition may be one predisposing factor. Persons with other chronic conditions—for example, diabetes, alcoholism, HIV infection, and conditions that affect the lungs (e.g., silicosis)—are also more likely to develop tuberculosis if they should come in contact with the TB bacillus (Ellner, 2016).

Tuberculosis can be *latent* or *active*. Usually the immune system in healthy individuals is able to contain the TB bacillus, and sometimes eradicate it completely. In some individuals, however, the bacillus becomes dormant in the body but causes no manifestations; this form of tuberculosis is called *latent tuberculosis*. Individuals with latent tuberculosis are not contagious and the immune system continues to hold the bacillus dormant. Should the immune system become compromised or less efficient, however, the tubercle bacillus can become active. Most cases of tuberculosis in the

United States involve reactivated latent tuberculosis (Horsburgh & Rubin, 2011).

Active tuberculosis denotes a condition in which the individual develops manifestations and can transmit the tubercle bacillus to others. Active TB damages infected organs and, if not adequately managed, can be fatal.

Individuals infected with TB for the first time are said to have a *primary infection*. Primary infections may remain dormant for years until the person's physical resistance is lowered. When the immune system is no longer able to contain the TB bacillus, it begins to multiply, damage organs, and cause manifestations. This form of tuberculosis is called *reactivation* or *secondary tuberculosis*.

Manifestations of Active Tuberculosis

Individuals with active TB or reactivated or secondary TB may experience initial manifestations of weight loss, **anorexia** (loss of appetite), and a slight elevation of temperature. Manifestations may then progress to cough, night sweats, and **hemoptysis** (blood-streaked sputum), and possibly chest pain.

Identification of Tuberculosis

Infection with the TB bacillus is identified through cultures of sputum, chest X-rays, and tuberculin skin tests. Skin tests can be a valuable screening tool to determine whether the individual has been infected with the TB bacillus. After being infected by the TB bacilli, the body develops an allergic response over time, resulting in tissue sensitivity. This sensitivity can be identified through the tuberculin skin test, which involves injection of a small amount of filtrate (*purified protein derivative [PPD]*) of the TB bacillus under the skin. If an individual has been exposed to and infected by the TB bacillus, a local skin reaction will occur at the injection site. Skin tests are interpreted for reaction at 24 hours and again at 48 to 72 hours after injection.

A positive reaction to a tuberculosis skin test (TST) indicates that the individual has been exposed to and infected with the TB bacillus, but it does not indicate whether the condition is active.

Individuals who have a positive skin test, but do not have any manifestations or other evidence of the active form of the condition on X-ray or sputum specimens, do not have the active form of tuberculosis and are not contagious to others. It is usually recommended that they receive interventions to eradicate the TB bacillus so as to prevent the possibility of tuberculosis becoming active at a later date (Horsburgh, 2004).

Definitive identification of TB is based on culture of sputum and chest X-ray (for pulmonary TB) or culture or biopsy of other body tissue if other organs are involved.

Management of Tuberculosis

The goals of management of TB are to cure the infection and to minimize transmission to others (Pasipanodya et al., 2012). Management of TB consists an intensive phase of medication intervention for several months, followed by 4 to 6 months of continued medication, after which another sputum or tissue culture is obtained and examined (Ellner, 2016).

It is essential that individuals being treated for TB take the medication accurately and consistently. Nonadherence with the medication plan has contributed to the development of TB bacilli that are resistant to once-effective medications. *Multidrug-resistant (MDR) tuberculosis* and *extensively drug-resistant (XDR) tuberculosis* have become global health problems (Nathanson et al., 2010; Small & Pai, 2010).

Functional Implications of Tuberculosis
Personal and Psychosocial Issues

Although anyone of any social class or educational level can be infected by the tubercle bacillus, development of TB is often associated with crowded conditions, poverty, alcoholism, substance abuse, and homelessness (Ellner, 2016). In many cultures, the social stigma attached to tuberculosis may contribute to individuals' denial that they have the condition and poor adherence to the management plan. Individuals with tuberculosis who remember the social stigma once associated with the condition may feel ashamed and embarrassed, try to hide their condition from others, or ignore or discontinue management interventions. Such reactions have serious consequences for both individuals with tuberculosis and those who may contract TB from them.

Close supervision of adherence to the management plan has been recommended. In addition, education, counseling, and support can be of benefit to individuals with regard to adaptation to their condition and its management.

Activities and Participation

The degree to which TB affects individuals' ability to participate in activities depends on whether the condition is active or latent and how severe the manifestations are. Individuals with latent TB often are unaware of their condition, experience no manifestations, and consequently continue their regular activities. In active TB, fatigue, cough, and fear of contagion may cause individuals to limit both activities and social contacts.

Due to the social stigma and misperceptions that are sometimes still associated with TB, individuals may find themselves isolated from others even after they are no longer contagious. Much of the stigma associated with this disease results from others' unfounded beliefs about transmission of the infection, fear of contracting TB, and general lack of knowledge about the condition. In addition to general public education about the condition, the most useful intervention to overcome stigma may be to empower the individual to resist the judgment of others while working to educate family and friends about the condition.

Vocational Issues in Tuberculosis

When TB bacilli are no longer present in the sputum, individuals are no longer considered infectious to others and are able to return to work (usually within 2 to 4 weeks). With effective management of TB, providing there have been no associated complications, the ability to return to work or to complete tasks performed previously should not be affected. Due to misinformation and stigma attached to tuberculosis, one of the major barriers to employment for persons with TB may be the attitudes of employers and fellow employees.

Providing employers and workers with accurate information about the condition can help to alleviate these concerns.

CYSTIC FIBROSIS

Overview of Cystic Fibrosis

Cystic fibrosis is a genetic, progressive, multisystem condition that affects the lungs, pancreas, liver, intestines, sweat glands, and reproductive system (Accurso, 2016). It is caused by genetic mutations that affect the mechanisms involving electrolyte (i.e., *sodium* and *chloride*) movement across cell membranes. Alterations cause the lining or passageways in many organs to retain increased amounts of sodium and chloride, which in turn draws water from the passageways. This results in thick, viscous mucus that obstructs the passageways and contributes to infection and eventual destruction of tissue (Accurso et al., 2010).

In the past, individuals with cystic fibrosis rarely lived beyond childhood; now, however, due to improvements in management, many individuals survive well into adulthood (Giusti, 2012). Although many organs are affected in cystic fibrosis, lung involvement is one of the most frequent causes of functional incapacitation and, if complications occur, can result in death (Accurso, 2016).

Manifestations of Cystic Fibrosis

Lung

Individuals with cystic fibrosis often experience a chronic cough, with thick purulent sputum, frequent pulmonary infections, and sinusitis. Pulmonary involvement occurs because of formation of thick mucus in the small bronchi, which can lead to severe *bronchitis* and *emphysema*. **Atelectasis** (collapse of the lung) is not uncommon. As the condition progresses, there is usually a gradual decline in pulmonary function.

Pancreas

The pancreas may become inflamed so that individuals develop *pancreatitis*. Because ducts of the pancreas are plugged by the thick mucus, enzymes produced by the pancreas that aid in digestion are unable to function in this capacity, leading to poor digestion of protein and fat. As a result, individuals experience chronic malnutrition and delayed growth.

Intestines and Liver

Intestines may become obstructed, resulting in abdominal pain and constipation. Although intestinal obstruction may be present in infancy, older adults with cystic fibrosis may also develop an intestinal obstruction—distal intestinal obstruction syndrome (DIOS)—that results in abdominal pain.

Ducts in the liver may also become plugged, resulting in **jaundice** (yellow discoloration of skin) and damage to the liver.

Sweat Glands

Individuals with cystic fibrosis have poorly functioning sweat glands, so that excessive loss of salt occurs. This phenomenon may result in **hyponatremia** (decreased concentration of salt in the blood).

Reproductive System

Cystic fibrosis affects the reproductive system, especially in males. Males with cystic fibrosis have an infertility rate of approximately 97% (Chotirmall et al., 2009). Although fertility for women is not as severely affected, pregnancy can require extra healthcare monitoring due to potentially poor nutrition and progressive decline of lung function as a result of cystic fibrosis (McArdle, 2011).

Identifying Cystic Fibrosis

Biochemical screening of newborns for cystic fibrosis occurs in all 50 states so that if the condition is present, early management interventions can be instituted (Accurso, 2016). In adults or children who did not undergo newborn screening, as well as in many newborn screening programs, *sweat testing* is used to confirm presence of cystic fibrosis. Because there is an increased concentration of sodium and chloride in the sweat of individuals with cystic fibrosis, the sweat test measures concentrations of chloride. The noninvasive procedure involves collecting and analyzing sweat from a small area of the individual's arm.

Management of Cystic Fibrosis

A major intervention in the management of cystic fibrosis is maintaining open airways and preventing lung infection (Welsh, 2010). Because mucus production is increased in individuals with cystic fibrosis, clearance of secretions is important so that organisms do not have an environment in which they can grow and thrive. Several interventions are available. *Chest physiotherapy* (*percussion therapy*) is used to clear lung secretions and prevent complications related to accumulation of mucus in the lungs. The procedure can involve either manual chest percussion or use of special devices that percuss the chest to mobilize secretions. Percussion is a form of massage in which the chest is repeatedly tapped or vibrated to loosen mucus and allow it to drain. Individuals may also use *daily inhalation therapy*, which includes *nebulized mucolytic agents* to reduce sputum viscosity. Another intervention involves hydration of airway surface fluid with hypertonic saline to facilitate clearance of airway mucus. Prophylactic inhaled antibiotics, inhaled corticosteroids, and oral anti-inflammatory medications are also often used (Giusti, 2012).

Dietary Management

If pancreatic ducts become blocked, supplemental enzymes may be taken at mealtimes to aid in digestion and prevent malnutrition. Despite use of supplemental enzymes, individuals with cystic fibrosis often experience delayed growth and malnutrition, and they are typically underweight. Owing to the increased salt loss characteristic of cystic fibrosis, dietary intervention may be necessary to ensure adequate salt intake. Adequate oral hydration also helps to liquefy secretions, and other dietary interventions may be needed to prevent nutritional deficiencies.

Lung Transplantation

If lung changes associated with cystic fibrosis progress to severe functional incapacitation, double-lung transplantation may be performed to halt progression of the condition and restore function. The lack of availability of suitable donor organs continues to be a limiting factor for this intervention (Giusti, 2012).

Functional Implications of Cystic Fibrosis

Personal and Psychosocial Issues

Because cystic fibrosis is a genetic condition, with manifestations usually present in childhood, issues of growing up with a chronic and potentially fatal condition can affect individuals' successful passage through normal growth and development. Attitudes of family, teachers, and peers are instrumental in helping children develop their self-concept, their view of their condition, and its impact on future function.

The psychological impact of cystic fibrosis in adulthood varies. Management of this condition requires time, energy, and resources to perform many of the home interventions such as chest physical therapy, dietary adjustment, monitoring for pulmonary infection, enzyme administration, and routine use of other medications such as bronchodilators and antibiotics. Special skills are required for monitoring manifestations, interpreting changes, and making decisions about the need to alter the management plan. Children who have been encouraged to assume more responsibility for their self-care will be more likely to grow into gradual independence.

During adolescence, behavioral responses to a chronic condition may be made more difficult by the need to "fit in" or by the attitudes of rebellion and defiance characteristic of that age. These factors may potentially result in health-compromising behaviors. Without appropriate support, individuals may be less able to adapt and cope with their chronic condition, resulting in isolation and altered relationships.

Individuals with any chronic condition may find adherence to the management plan difficult because of its long-term and complex nature. Adhering to the management plan is a daily reminder of the condition. Some individuals may feel that, given the likelihood of increasing deterioration and potential mortality, adherence is not worthwhile.

Activities and Participation

Exercise training programs for many chronic pulmonary conditions have been found to enhance functional exercise capacity and health status. The same has been demonstrated for cystic fibrosis (Decramer & Gossellink, 2006). Exercise rehabilitation programs can help individuals with cystic fibrosis become more able and confident in performing activities of daily living and enhance their activity levels as a whole.

Fertility problems in individuals with cystic fibrosis may bring an emotional toll. In addition to coping with the challenges of daily management of the condition, issues of infertility may be incorporated into their relationships with significant others.

Vocational Issues in Cystic Fibrosis

Cystic fibrosis is an incurable chronic condition. Nevertheless, depending on the type of work and work environment, individuals with cystic fibrosis can have productive careers, with minimal accommodations. In some instances, decrease in lung function can affect energy and exercise capacity (Williams, Burker, & Kazukauskas, 2011). For some individuals, even though they are healthy enough to work, fear of losing disability benefits may be a barrier to return to work (Williams, Burker, Kazukauskas, & Neuringer, 2012).

Because individuals with cystic fibrosis have heightened susceptibility to pulmonary infections, environments in which there is high potential for exposure to such infections should be avoided, and flu and pneumonia vaccinations obtained. Individuals should also avoid exposure to dust, toxic fumes, and other air pollutants.

Due to excessive loss of salt through sweat, hot, humid environmental conditions should be avoided and hydration maintained. In some instances, individuals may need time for airway clearance techniques during the workday, and may need brief times away from work when this therapy can be accomplished.

OCCUPATIONAL LUNG CONDITIONS

Occupational lung conditions include a wide variety of pulmonary conditions, many with manifestations similar to nonoccupational lung conditions, but which are associated with inhalation of particles, dust, or fumes in the occupational environment (deShazo & Weissman, 2012). Occupational lung conditions are classified based on the type of particles inhaled.

Pneumoconiosis

The term *pneumoconiosis* refers to a group of lung conditions in which there has been inhalation of particulate matter. Types of pneumoconiosis include *silicosis* and *asbestosis*.

Silicosis

Silicosis is an occupational lung condition caused by exposure to silica dust, the most common form being quartz, which is found in sand and most rocks. This condition may develop in people who work in quarries, metal mining, foundries, pottery making, sandblasting, or other occupations involving exposure to silica. Development of chronic silicosis generally takes 10 to 30 years of exposure, whereas acute silicosis can occur within weeks to a few years after intense exposure (deShazo & Weissman, 2012). When particles of silica enter the alveoli, special cells within the lungs engulf the foreign material and then die. In response, a special substance is released in the lung, resulting in **fibrosis** (fibrous tissue) within the lung. No pulmonary consequences may be apparent at this point, although initial damage in the form of nodules may be identified by X-ray.

In the early stages of the condition, individuals may show no manifestations. As damage continues, however, they may experience dyspnea accompanied by cough. Tobacco use worsens manifestations. Individuals with silicosis are at increased risk for developing pulmonary tuberculosis and consequently should receive tuberculosis testing (deShazo & Weissman, 2012).

Management of silicosis is based on manifestations, and is similar to management of other chronic lung conditions. Some individuals' lung condition may progress to COPD; in some instances, the condition may progress even further to end-stage lung disease, necessitating lung transplantation.

Asbestosis

Asbestosis is an occupational lung condition resulting from long-term inhalation of asbestos fibers.

Although the use of asbestos has declined, asbestosis remains a health problem due to the length of time between exposure to the material and development of manifestations (Tarlo, 2016). The inhalation of asbestos fibers can cause fibrinous changes within the lung. Manifestations usually consist of cough and dyspnea on exertion. Management involves interventions to relieve manifestations.

A complication of asbestosis is *mesothelioma*, a malignant tumor of the **pleura** (chest lining) or the **peritoneum** (lining of the abdominal cavity), which can occur several decades after exposure to asbestos. Individuals with asbestos exposure also have a risk of developing lung cancer. Cigarette smoking increases this risk sixfold (deShazo & Weissman, 2012).

Other Occupational Lung Conditions

Occupational asthma is a condition characterized by airway restriction and hyperresponsiveness of airways caused by an immune response to a sensitizing agent in the workplace. Work-exacerbated asthma is asthma that has not been caused by sensitizing agents in the work environment but rather is exacerbated by exposure to sensitizing agents in the workplace. If it is proven to be occupational in origin, this exposure must be reduced or avoided completely, depending on the severity of the condition. Manifestations and management of occupational asthma or work-exacerbated asthma are similar to those of nonoccupational-related asthma, as discussed earlier in the chapter.

Occupational COPD has the same manifestations as COPD that is not work related, but the condition is caused by exposure to dust, fumes, or other inhaled substances in the work environment. Management is the same as for individuals with nonoccupational COPD, as discussed earlier. Exposure to environmental pollutants should be minimized.

Functional Implications of Occupational Lung Conditions

The circumstances that surround the development of an occupational lung condition may elicit guilt on the part of the individual with the condition or anger on the part of family members. Because smoking increases the lung destruction associated with occupational lung conditions, individuals who have smoked heavily may feel guilty for having contributed to their condition. Family members may express anger, blaming the individual for smoking, or may be angry because of the individual's exposure to unrecognized hazards or, if hazards were identified, because of the employer's failure to take proper precautions to protect employees from them.

The legal implications of lung conditions that appear to be occupationally related may be barriers to continued employment. For individuals who are eligible for worker's compensation or other benefits, financial considerations may influence their motivation and cooperation with the management plan. In other instances, the employer's fear of liability may limit job opportunities for individuals with pulmonary conditions.

UPPER AIRWAY INFECTIONS: PHARYNGITIS AND LARYNGITIS

The upper pulmonary tract consists of the nose, the pharynx, and the larynx. **Pharyngitis** (sore throat) is a condition of the upper airway that may be caused by viral or bacterial infection. In this condition, the mucous membrane lining the throat becomes inflamed, which may cause manifestations such as sore throat, fever, or difficulty in swallowing. **Laryngitis** (inflammation of the larynx) is usually caused by a virus and can produce hoarseness, loss of voice, cough, and sore throat. Both pharyngitis and laryngitis are relatively minor and tend to be self-limiting.

PNEUMONIA

Overview of Pneumonia

Pneumonia is an acute condition caused by inflammation and infection, which affect the bronchioles and alveolar tissue in the lung. It is characterized by cough, chest pain, fever, and breathlessness. Pneumonia can be a life-threatening condition when it is superimposed on other chronic conditions, such as heart conditions, alcoholism, neuromuscular conditions (such as multiple sclerosis), chronic obstructive lung disease, spinal cord injury (especially quadriplegia), dementia, altered immune status, or swallowing abnormalities—all of which place individuals at high risk for developing pneumonia. Individuals with limited mobility or who are subject to prolonged inactivity owing to bed rest also have a particularly high susceptibility to this infection. Individuals who have difficulty swallowing, often due to a neuromuscular condition, or who have altered consciousness due to drugs, alcohol, or a neurological condition, may aspirate food, liquid, or other substances into the lungs, causing development of *aspiration pneumonia.* Aspiration of toxic materials such as oils, bile, gastric acid, or alcohol causes additional complications because of direct damage to the alveolar membrane, leading to *chemical pneumonitis.*

Generally pneumonia can be classified into: *community-acquired pneumonia, healthcare-associated pneumonia,* and *health care acquired* (Musher, 2016). Community-acquired pneumonia describes infectious pneumonia in which individuals have been exposed to bacteria (*bacterial pneumonia*) or a virus (*viral pneumonia*) in the community setting. Healthcare-associated pneumonia occurs when individuals who live in a skilled nursing facility, are hospitalized, have repeated contact with a medical facility, or are immunosuppressed and become infected with an organism. Healthcare-acquired pneumonia describes pneumonia that develops after the individual is hospitalized, when they had no evidence of pneumonia at time they were admitted to the hospital (Musher, 2016)

Usually the defenses of the pulmonary system are sufficient to ward off infection. However, when the body defenses are weakened due to another health condition, or when the causative agent is overwhelming, defenses in the pulmonary system fail and pneumonia develops. When pneumonia is caused by inactivity or immobility such that the lungs do not expand sufficiently, the condition is known as *hypostatic pneumonia.*

Manifestations of Pneumonia

Individuals with pneumonia experience cough, dyspnea, sputum production, and often chest pain. Inflammation and infection of the alveoli in pneumonia interfere with oxygen and carbon dioxide exchange in the lungs. The greater the extent of inflammation and infection, the greater the interference with respiration. Infection triggers changes in the capillary walls in the alveoli, causing fluid to flow into the alveoli, where it accumulates. The accumulation of fluid provides an excellent growth medium for additional organisms, exacerbating the infection. Accumulation of fluid in the lungs further interferes with the exchange of carbon dioxide and oxygen. When the infection becomes widespread, systemic infection becomes a risk; it is potentially life threatening.

Identification of Pneumonia

Pneumonia is usually identified through assessment of manifestations as well as via chest X-ray, which helps to detect the location and degree of lung involvement. Culture of sputum specimens may be conducted to identify the precise organism responsible for the infection so that management with the appropriate medication can be instituted.

Management and Prevention of Pneumonia

Once the cause of pneumonia is determined, management with medication is directed toward eradicating the specific organism causing the infection. Medications that facilitate removal of secretions from the lungs (expectorants) may also be administered. Because individuals with pneumonia may have lowered oxygen content in the blood (**hypoxia**) owing to poor gas exchange, oxygen may be administered. Manual chest physiotherapy may also be performed to facilitate drainage from the lungs.

Individuals at high risk for developing pneumonia must be especially vigilant to prevent infection that can precipitate pneumonia. Good nutrition, adequate hydration, and adequate sleep are all measures that help bolster immunity. Minimizing situations in which individuals are exposed to infection, especially during cold and flu season, and obtaining flu and pneumonia vaccines are especially important preventive measures. Individuals with limited mobility should have their position changed frequently to facilitate lung expansion and drainage. It is also important to avoid pulmonary irritants such as secondhand cigarette smoke or other pollutants that can make individuals more susceptible to infection.

Vocational Issues in Pneumonia

Pneumonia can cause significant morbidity and consequent loss of workdays, and be potentially life threatening. Because individuals with chronic conditions often have increased susceptibility to pneumonia, the steps mentioned previously to minimize development of pulmonary complications are especially important. Conditions in the workplace that can induce or aggravate lung conditions may require job modification or complete avoidance. Although risk of exposure may be present in a number of work situations, specific exposure to pulmonary irritants or to large numbers of people who may have pulmonary infections should be avoided as much as possible.

BRONCHIECTASIS

Bronchiectasis is a chronic condition characterized by chronic inflammation and dilation of the bronchi and bronchioles, leaving them permanently vulnerable to recurrent infection, and subsequent progressive lung destruction. In many cases, the cause of bronchiectasis cannot be identified, however some causes are pulmonary infection, anatomic abnormalities, immune and autoimmune disease, or genetics. (O'Donnell, 2016). Individuals with bronchiectasis experience cough and chronic sputum production, with **purulent** (pus-containing) material collecting in the dilated airways. Individuals may also experience fatigue, weight loss, loss of appetite, or hemoptysis (coughing up blood).

Identification of bronchiectasis is usually based on manifestations, chest X-ray, and, in some instances, a computed tomography (CT) scan to pinpoint the location and extent of damage. Pulmonary function tests may also be performed to determine the severity of airflow obstruction. *Bronchoscopy*, in which a hollow tube is inserted via the mouth into the bronchus, allows for visualization of the walls of the bronchus and identification of any irregularities.

Management includes administration of *antibiotics* for infection, *bronchodilators* to clear the airways, maintenance of general health through rest and nutrition, and avoidance of further infections. Individuals may also learn special techniques (*bronchopulmonary hygiene*) or receive other interventions (*chest physiotherapy*) to remove pulmonary secretions.

Damaged bronchi do not return to their pre-inflammatory state. If the inflammatory and destructive process continues, surgical removal of the affected part of the lung may be necessary.

OBSTRUCTIVE SLEEP APNEA

Overview of Obstructive Sleep Apnea

The term **apnea** refers to cessation of breathing. Apnea is associated with a variety of conditions. One of the more common conditions associated with apnea is *obstructive sleep apnea (OSA)*, in which repeated episodes of the cessation of breathing occur during sleep. This condition is more common in individuals who are overweight, although other anatomic irregularities may also predispose individuals to OSA (Basner, 2016).

Individuals with obstructive sleep apnea may be unaware that they stop breathing during sleep, but may experience excessive daytime drowsiness, difficulty with attention or concentration, and irritability because of the disruption of their sleep. Although individuals with sleep apnea may be unaware of their condition, sleep partners may complain of being awakened by the individual's loud snoring or sudden body movements during periods of apnea.

The consequences of OSA go beyond sleep disruption and daytime drowsiness. Individuals with sleep apnea have an increased risk of hypertension, heart failure, myocardial infarction, and stroke (Basner, 2016). Because of sleep deprivation, people with sleep apnea are also at increased risk of accidents.

Identification of Obstructive Sleep Apnea

The evaluation of sleep apnea (*polysomnography*) takes place in a sleep laboratory, where breathing during sleep over the course of an entire night is monitored and recorded. Portable monitoring systems can also be used outside the sleep laboratory, but the resulting data may not be as accurate.

Management of Obstructive Sleep Apnea

Obstructive sleep apnea may be treated behaviorally, with medication, or surgically. The type of intervention chosen depends on the individual's manifestations and the function of his or her cardiopulmonary system. Management goals are directed toward establishing normal breathing and oxygenation of the blood and toward eliminating disruption of sleep. Because alcohol consumption reduces muscle tone of the upper airway and increases the frequency of irregular breathing during sleep, limiting alcohol use is advised. Individuals who are obese are encouraged to lose weight to reduce obstruction. Exercise is not only helpful in weight reduction, but also has been associated with decreasing sleep apnea (Awad, Malhorta, Barnet, Quan, & Peppard, 2012). Some individuals have more difficulty with sleep apnea when lying on their back and may need to focus on sleeping on their side.

Some individuals with sleep apnea use a form of mechanical intervention called *positive airway pressure (PAP)* or *continuous positive airway pressure (C-PAP)* delivered through a mask. The machines used for this purpose weigh only about 5 pounds. These devices are used at night and fit on a bedside table. Individuals may use a mask that covers only the nose, nasal prongs, or a mask that covers both the nose and the mouth. The amount of positive pressure applied is determined through evaluation in a sleep laboratory. Some individuals choose oral appliances that are worn during sleep to help keep the airway open rather than using positive-pressure machines.

Surgical interventions can range from **tracheostomy** (in which a surgical opening is made through the neck into the trachea to enable the individual to breathe) to surgical correction of structural irregularities of the palate or the facial structure that contribute to obstruction.

Vocational Issues in Obstructive Sleep Apnea

Obstructive sleep apnea can cause significant vocational impairment. In addition to daytime sleepiness, individuals may experience irritability, impatience, or even depressive manifestations, which can affect their relationships with others at work. Individuals with obstructive sleep apnea may also experience cognitive consequences including difficulty with attention and concentration, visual/motor abilities, and difficulties with memory. Tasks involving planning, verbal fluency, or general intellectual performance may be impaired. As mentioned earlier, because of sleep deprivation, individuals with obstructive sleep apnea may be more accident prone.

If obstructive sleep apnea is identified and managed, its manifestations can be reversed. Unfortunately, in many cases the condition is not identified and a decrease in job performance is attributed to other causes.

CHEST INJURIES

Fractured ribs are a common chest injury. Although painful, they are usually managed relatively easily by wrapping a strap or binder around the chest for support. In some instances, however, a fractured rib punctures other organs, such as the lungs or heart, and the consequences are more serious.

An open wound to the chest, such as a puncture wound, may allow air to enter the thoracic cavity. This condition, called **pneumothorax**, may cause the lung on the affected side to collapse. Pneumothorax unrelated to trauma can occur secondary to a number of pulmonary conditions (*spontaneous pneumothorax*), such as COPD, asthma, or cystic fibrosis. Spontaneous pneumothorax is caused by a tear or rupture of air sacs in the lung, causing air to escape into the thoracic cavity. Pneumothorax is generally managed by insertion of a tube through the chest wall to facilitate expansion of the lung. Individuals who have experienced pneumothorax should avoid smoking, high diving, or flying in unpressurized aircraft, all of which can cause recurrence of the condition.

Escape of blood into the thoracic cavity because of an injury to the chest that damages vessels in the thoracic cavity is called **hemothorax**. It may also cause collapse of a lung. In the case of pneumothorax or hemothorax, the lung is compressed, hampering breathing. A large pneumothorax or hemothorax requires emergency intervention to remove air or blood in the chest and repair the injury.

The removal of fluid from the thoracic cavity is called **thoracentesis**. In this procedure, a needle is inserted into the thoracic cavity and fluid is then aspirated through the needle.

RESTRICTIVE PULMONARY CONDITIONS

Restrictive pulmonary conditions prevent affected individuals from receiving an adequate supply of air so that the volume of air taken into the lungs is diminished during inspiration. Conditions that cause restrictive pulmonary conditions may include skeletal problems such as **scoliosis** (lateral curvature of the spine) and **kyphosis** (forward curvature of the spine), both of which decrease chest expansion. Other conditions that may cause pulmonary restriction include nervous system conditions such as polio, spinal cord injury, and Parkinson's disease, in which the muscles that assist in respiration are hindered. Obesity also restricts lung expansion.

GENERAL FUNCTIONAL IMPLICATIONS OF PULMONARY CONDITIONS
Personal and Psychosocial Issues

Difficulty breathing can be a frightening and distressing experience. Associated fear and anxiety may lead to inactivity, which in turn may result in additional physical problems. For individuals who have been active and self-sufficient, the inability to engage in activities without breathing difficulty can lead to feelings of helplessness and depression. Individuals may begin to focus on activities in which they can no longer participate, at least not as vigorously, rather than attempting to attain the optimal activity level.

Emotional factors can compound the effects of physical manifestations of pulmonary conditions and contribute to breathing difficulties. When situations that increase anxiety or stress are identified, it is important to institute interventions to decrease responses to the situation so that breathing difficulty does not escalate.

Some individuals may use their breathing difficulty as a way to escape from life's demands, to receive emotional rewards, or to manipulate or control others. Awareness of how these reactions can hamper full inclusion and participation and learning alternative ways of coping can enhance relationships and participation.

Activities and Participation

Expectations of others regarding individuals' ability to participate in activities may not be consistent with a particular individual's functional capacity. In some instances, family members or others may overestimate individuals' abilities, not fully understanding the restrictions associated with the condition. As a result, individuals may be pushed beyond their functional capacity. Education of others regarding the condition, restrictions, and specific aspects of management can enhance understanding and positive interactions.

GENERAL VOCATIONAL IMPLICATIONS OF PULMONARY CONDITIONS

The extent to which individuals with pulmonary conditions continue regular employment depends on the type of work, the work environment, and the severity of the pulmonary condition. When individuals' work requires little physical exertion, they may be better able to continue work than individuals whose work is physically demanding. In other instances, modifications of tasks or the work environment can enhance the ability to maintain employment.

Environmental irritants and pollutants aggravate most pulmonary conditions. Consequently, steps to reduce exposure to these factors may enhance individuals' ability to continue work.

In some instances, legal and compensation implications of lung conditions—if they are occupationally related—may be barriers to continued employment.

CASE STUDY

Mr. L., a 55-year-old bartender in a large metropolitan area, has been a heavy smoker for 40 years. He discovered he had COPD 7 years ago. Mr. L. lives in the city and takes the city bus to work, although he still has to walk about 3 blocks to the bar where he works. He has found it increasingly difficult to walk the 3 blocks without stopping to rest at frequent intervals. At work, his manager has also expressed concern about the effect Mr. L.'s continuous coughing has on customers.

1. Is it feasible for Mr. L. to continue working as a bartender? Why or why not?
2. Which issues should Mr. L. consider regarding a rehabilitation plan?
3. Are there specific modifications regarding Mr. L.'s work that may be useful? If so, which modifications should be considered?

REFERENCES

Accurso, F. J. (2016). Cystic fibrosis. In L. Goldman & A. I. Schafer (Eds.), *Goldman-Cecil Medicine,* (25th ed., pp. 562–566). Philadelphia, PA: Elsevier Saunders.

Accurso, F. J., Rowe, S. M., Clancy, J. P., Boyle, M. P., Dunitz, J. M., Durie, P. R., . . . Ramsey, C. W. (2010). Effect of VX-770 in persons with cystic fibrosis and the G551D-CFTR mutation. *New England Journal of Medicine, 363*(21), 1991–2033.

Albert, R. K., Connett, J., Bailey, W. C., Casaburi, R., Cooper, J. A., Criner, G. J., . . . ClOPD Clinical Research Network. (2011). Azithromycin for prevention of exacerbations of COPD. *New England Journal of Medicine, 365*(8), 689–698.

Anzueto, A. (2010). Endobronchial valves to reduce lung hyperinflation. *New England Journal of Medicine, 363*(13), 1280–1281.

Awad, K. M., Malhorta, A., Barnet, J. H., Quan, S. F., & Peppard, P. E. (2012). Exercise is associated with reduced incidence of sleep disordered breathing. *American Journal of Medicine, 125*(5), 485–490.

Basner, R. C. (2016). Obstructive Sleep Apnea. In L. Goldman & A. I. Schafer (Eds.), *Goldman-Cecil Medicine,* (25th ed., pp. 638–642). Philadelphia, PA: Elsevier Saunders.

Chotirmall, S. H., Mann, A. K., Branagan, P., O'Donohoe, C., Lyons, A. M., Flynn, M. G., . . . McElvaney, N. G. (2009). Male fertility in cystic fibrosis. *Irish Medical Journal, 102*(7), 204–206.

Cypel, M., Yeug, J. C., Liu, M., Anraku, M., Chen, F., Karolak, W., . . . Keshaviee, S. (2011). Normothermic ex vivo lung perfusion in clinical lung transplantation. *New England Journal of Medicine, 364*(15), 1431–1440.

Davids, S., & Schapira, R. M. (2012). Acute bronchitis. In E. T. Bope & R. D. Kellerman (Eds.), *Conn's current therapy 2012,* (pp. 321–322). Philadelphia, PA: Elsevier Saunders.

Decramer, M., & Gosselink, R. (2006). Physical activity in patients with cystic fibrosis: A new variable in the health status equation. *European Respiratory Journal, 28,* 676–679.

deShazo, R. D., & Weissman, D. N. (2012). Pneumoconiosis. In E. T. Bope & R. D. Kellerman (Eds.), *Conn's current therapy 2012,* (pp. 363–365). Philadelphia, PA: Elsevier Saunders.

Drazen, J. M. (2016). Asthma. In L. Goldman & A. I. Schafer (Eds.), *Goldman-Cecil Medicine,* (25th ed., pp. 548–555). Philadelphia, PA: Elsevier Saunders.

Ellner, J. J. (2016). Tuberculosis. In L. & A. I. Schafer (Eds.), *Goldman-Cecil Medicine,* (25th ed., pp. 2030–2039). Philadelphia, PA: Elsevier Saunders.

Feller-Kopman, D. J. & Decamp, M. M. (2016). Interventional and surgical approaches to lung disease. In L. Goldman & A. I. Schafer (Eds.), *Goldman-Cecil Medicine,* (25th ed., pp. 642–647). Philadelphia, PA: Elsevier Saunders.

Garcia, J. A., & Jenkinson, S. G. (2007). Management of chronic obstructive pulmonary disease. In R. E. Rakel & E. T. Bope (Eds.), *Conn's current therapy,* (pp. 264–274). Philadelphia, PA: W. B. Saunders.

Giusti, R. (2012). Cystic fibrosis. In E. T. Bope & R. D. Kellerman (Eds.), *Conn's current therapy 2012,* (pp. 350–353). Philadelphia, PA: Elsevier Saunders.

Global Initiative for Chronic Obstructive Lung Disease (GOLD). (2013). Global strategy for the diagnosis, management, and prevention of COPD. Retrieved from http://www.goldcopd.org/guidelines-global-strategy-for-diagnosis-management.html

Grainge, C. L., Lau, L. C. K., Ward, J. A., Dulay, V., Lahiff, G., Wilson, S., . . . Howarth, P. H. (2011). Effect of bronchoconstriction on airway remodeling in asthma. *New England Journal of Medicine, 364*(21), 2006–2015.

Hanania, N. A., & Sharafkhaneh, A. (2012). Chronic obstructive pulmonary disease. In E. T. Bope & R. D. Kellerman (Eds.), *Conn's current therapy 2012* (pp. 343–348). Philadelphia, PA: Elsevier Saunders.

Horsburgh, C. R. (2004). Priorities for the treatment of latent tuberculosis infection in the United States. *New England Journal of Medicine, 350*(20), 2060–2067.

Horsburgh, C. R., & Rubin, E. J. (2011). Latent tuberculosis infection in the United States. *New England Journal of Medicine, 364*(15), 1441–1448.

Hurst, J. R., Vestbo, J., Anzueto, A., Locantore, N., Müllerova, H., Tal-Singer, R., . . . Evaluation of COPD Longitudinally to Identify Predictive Surrogate Endpoints (ECLIPSE) Investigators. (2010). Susceptibility to exacerbation in chronic obstructive pulmonary disease. *New England Journal of Medicine, 363*(12), 1128–1138.

King, T. E. (2011). Smoking and subclinical interstitial lung disease. *New England Journal of Medicine, 364*(10), 968–971.

McArdle, J. R. (2011). Pregnancy in cystic fibrosis. *Clinical Chest Medicine, 32*(1), 111–120.

Moffatt, M. F., Gut, I. G., Demenais, F., Strachan, D. P., Bouzigon, E., Heath, S., . . . GABRIEL Consortium. (2010). A large-scale, consortium-based genomewide association study of asthma. *New England Journal of Medicine, 363*(13), 1211–1221.

Musher, D. M. (2016). Overview of pneumonia. In L. Goldman & A. I. Schafer (Eds.), *Goldman-Cecil Medicine,* (25th ed., pp. 610–620.). Philadelphia, PA: Elsevier Saunders.

Nathanson, E., Nunn, P., Upleker, M., Floyd, K., Jaramillo, E., Lönnroth, K., . . . Raviglione, M. (2010). MDR tuberculosis: Critical steps for prevention and control. *New England Journal of Medicine, 363*(11), 1050–1058.

Niewoehner, D. E. (2016). Chronic obstructive pulmonary disease. In L. Goldman & A. I. Schafer (Eds.), *Goldman-Cecil Medicine,* (25th ed., pp. 555–562). Philadelphia, PA: Elsevier Saunders.

O'Donnell, A. E. (2016). Bronchiectasis, atelectasis, cysts, and localized lung disorders. In L. Goldman & A. I. Schafer (Eds.), *Goldman-Cecil Medicine* (25th ed., pp. 566–571). Philadelphia, PA: Elsevier Saunders.

Pasipanodya, J., Hall, R., & Gumbo, T. (2012). Tuberculosis and other mycobacterial diseases. In E. T. Bope & R. D. Kellerman (Eds.), *Conn's current therapy 2012* (pp. 375–381). Philadelphia, PA: Elsevier Saunders.

Rabe, K. F. (2007). Treating COPD: The TORCH Trial, *p* values, and the dodo. *New England Journal of Medicine, 356*(8), 851–854.

Scanlon, P.D. (2016). Respiratory function: Mechanisms and testing. In L. Goldman & A. I. Schafer (Eds.), *Goldman-Cecil Medicine,* (25h ed., pp. 539–545). Philadelphia, PA: Elsevier Saunders.

Schatz, M. (2012). Asthma in adolescents and adults. In E. T. Bope & R. D. Kellerman (Eds.), *Conn's current therapy 2012* (pp. 327–335). Philadelphia, PA: Elsevier Saunders.

Sciurba, F. C., Ernst, A., Herth, F. J. F., Strange, C., Criner, G. J., Marquette, C. H., . . . VENT Study Research Group. (2010). A randomized study of endobronchial valves for advanced emphysema. *New England Journal of Medicine, 363*(13), 1233–1244.

Small, P. M., & Pai, M. (2010). Tuberculosis diagnosis: Time for a game change. *New England Journal of Medicine, 363*(11), 1070–1071.

Smith, L. J. (2010). Anticholinergics for patients with asthma? *New England Journal of Medicine, 363*(18), 1764–1765.

Spruit, M. A., Pokey, M. I., Celli, B., Edwards, L. D., Watkins, M. L., Pinto-Plata, V., . . . Evaluation of COPD Longitudinally to Identify Predictive Surrogate Endpoints (ECLIPSE) Investigators. (2012). Predicting outcomes from 6-minute walking distance in chronic obstructive pulmonary disease. *Journal of the American Medical Directors Association, 13*(3), 291–297.

Tarlo, S. M. (2016). Occupational lung disease. In L. Goldman & A. I. Schafer (Eds.), *Goldman-Cecil Medicine,* (25th ed., pp. 588-595). Philadelphia, PA: Elsevier Saunders.

Tashkin, D. P. (2010). Frequent exacerbations of chronic obstructive pulmonary disease: A distinct phenotype? *New England Journal of Medicine, 363*(12), 1183–1184.

Tschumperlin, D. J. (2011). Physical forces and airway remodeling in asthma. *New England Journal of Medicine, 364*(21), 2058–2059.

von Mutius, E., & Drazen, J. M. (2012). A patient with asthma seeks medical advice in 1828, 1928, and 2012. *New England Journal of Medicine, 366*(9), 827–834.

Washko, G. R., Hunninghake, G. M., Fernandez, I. E., Nishino, M., Okajima, Y., Yamashiro, T., . . . COPD Gene Investigators.

(2011). Lung volumes and emphysema in smokers with interstitial lung abnormalities. *New England Journal of Medicine, 364*(10), 897–906.

Welsh, M. J. (2010). Targeting the basic defect in cystic fibrosis. *New England Journal of Medicine, 363*(21), 2056–2057.

Wenzel, R. P. (2016). Acute bronchitis and tracheitis. In L. Goldman & A. I. Schafer (Eds.), *Goldman-Cecil Medicine,* (25th ed., pp. 608–609). Philadelphia, PA: Elsevier Saunders.

Williams, L. W., Burker, E. J., & Kazukauskas, K. (2011). Cystic fibrosis and achieving vocational success: The key role of the rehabilitation counselor. *Journal of Applied Rehabilitation Counseling, 42*(4), 12–18.

Williams, L. W., Burker, E. J., Kazukauskas, K., & Neuringer, I. (2012). Lung transplant: Information and recommendations for rehabilitation counselors. *Journal of Applied Rehabilitation Counseling, 43*(2), 9–16.

CHAPTER 30

Chronic Kidney Disease and Other Conditions of the Urinary System

STRUCTURE AND FUNCTION OF THE KIDNEY AND URINARY TRACT

The kidney and urinary tract enable the body to eliminate by-products of metabolism, regulate body fluids and electrolyte content, and recover or reabsorb essential substances to prevent their elimination in the urine (Al-Awqati & Barasch, 2016).

The Urinary Tract

The term *urinary tract* refers to the collecting system for urine. The urinary tract consists of two ureters, the bladder, and the urethra. The *ureters* are tubes (one tube from each kidney) leading from the kidney to the bladder. The *bladder* is an expandable storage area that holds urine until it is eliminated. The *urethra* is a single tube leading from the bladder to an exterior opening called the *urinary meatus,* through which urine is eliminated (see **Figure 30-1**).

The Kidney

The two kidneys, each of which is about the size of a fist, lie behind the abdominal cavity (*retroperitoneal*) on either side of the vertebral column. They have multiple functions:

- Homeostasis: maintenance of the body's internal chemical balance
- Regulation of water content in the body
- Electrolyte balance (Electrolytes are charged particles, such as sodium and potassium, that

are important to many of the body's internal functions.)
- Excretion of metabolic waste products such as *urea, uric acid,* and *creatinine*
- Removal of foreign chemicals from the body (such as drugs and pesticides)
- Hormone secretion:
  - Renin stimulates production of a hormone called angiotensin, which in turn stimulates an endocrine gland, the adrenal cortex, to secrete a hormone called aldosterone, which influences how the kidney regulates potassium and sodium levels in the body, and consequently affects blood pressure.
  - Erythropoietin controls production of red blood cells.
  - Vitamin D regulates calcium absorption from the intestine and influences the calcium balance in the body.

Kidney Structure

A thin layer of white fibrous tissue called the *renal capsule* surrounds the kidney. The outer layer of the kidney is called the *cortex;* the inner portion is called the *medulla.* The *renal pelvis* is a funnel-shaped structure through which urine passes into the ureters. The *medulla* contains 10 to 15 triangular structures called *renal pyramids,* which serve as a portion of the renal drainage system.

The cortex and medulla contain units called *nephrons,* which are the functional units of the

Figure 30-1   The Urinary Tract

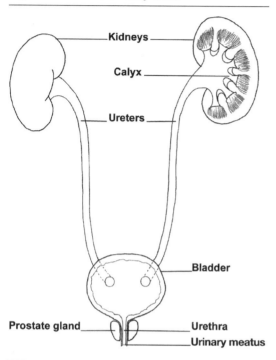

© Jane Tinkler Lamm.

kidney. There are approximately 1 million nephrons in each kidney. Each nephron contains an initial filtering system (*glomerulus*), which is itself surrounded by a *Bowman's capsule*. Glomeruli are loops of capillaries (*glomerular capillaries*). Extending from the glomerulus are the *renal tubules*, which end in a *collecting duct*. The collecting ducts from each nephron merge to empty into the renal pelvis. (See **Figure 30-2**.)

Kidney Function

The kidney filters a large volume of blood each day. Approximately 20% of the body's blood flows into the kidney through the renal arteries, at a rate averaging approximately 1 liter of arterial blood per minute. The remaining 80% of blood remains in the general body circulation and does not enter the renal circulation. Blood enters the kidney through the *renal arteries* and leaves from the kidney to enter the general body circulation through the *renal veins*.

Blood entering the kidney flows first to the glomerular capillaries, where it is filtered, and then to a second capillary bed surrounding the

Figure 30-2   Kidney and Nephron

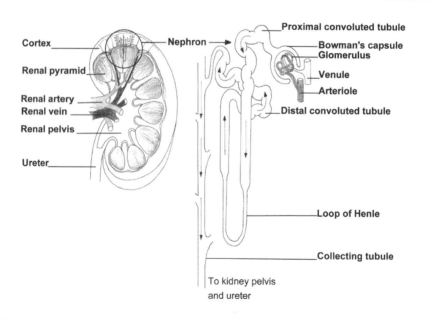

© Jane Tinkler Lamm.

tubules (*peritubular capillaries*), which form the veins through which blood leaves the kidney. The process by which the kidney removes waste products from the blood is called *glomerular filtration*. The level of kidney function is measured by the *glomerular filtration rate (GFR)*, the rate at which a given compound passes through the glomerulus in a given time (usually measured in milliliters per minute), or the filtration rate of blood through the renal glomerular capillaries into Bowman's capsule per unit of time.

Initial filtration occurs as the blood enters the glomerulus and some waste products are removed. As the glomerular filtrate continues to move through the tubules of the nephrons, substances are either reabsorbed into the bloodstream, continue through the tubules, or are added back to the *filtrate*. As the filtrate moves into the collecting system, it eventually drains into the *calyx* at the mouth of each pyramid and empties into the renal pelvis as urine. From the renal pelvis, urine drains into the ureters to the bladder, where it is stored until it is ready to be excreted through the urethra and urinary meatus.

Metabolic end products and toxic substances are removed from the blood through the filtration process, and are then subsequently eliminated from the body as urine. Conversely, other substances such as *sugar* and *amino acids* (the building blocks of protein) are reabsorbed into the bloodstream. Consequently, in healthy individuals, sugar and protein should not be found in the urine. *Electrolytes* (e.g., sodium and potassium) are also returned to the bloodstream along with 99% of the water in the filtrate.

Potassium is important to muscle contraction, nerve function, and heart function, whereas *sodium* is important to heart and nerve function as well as water balance. *Phosphorus* is important for regulating calcium in the body and for building strong bones. The amounts of water and electrolytes reabsorbed are variable, being regulated according to the body's specific needs; however, this internal chemical balance is crucial for the general function of most other organs. Consequently, adequate kidney function is crucial to the function of many organs and many body systems.

CONDITIONS OF THE URINARY TRACT AND KIDNEY

Urinary Tract Infections

The urinary tract and urine are typically sterile. If bacteria enter the urinary tract through the urinary meatus, however, infection and inflammation of the urinary tract can occur. The most common cause of urinary tract infection (UTI) is fecal contamination (Nicolle & Norrby, 2016)

Cystitis is a condition in which bacteria enter the bladder, causing it to become infected and inflamed. Although cystitis itself is generally not an incapacitating condition, it can be a serious problem for individuals with a chronic health condition and, if not adequately managed, could lead to worrisome complications.

Manifestations of cystitis usually develop rapidly and may include *frequency* (frequent urination), even though the bladder may not be full; **dysuria** (painful urination); *urgency* (a need to urinate immediately); pain in the lower abdomen or lower back; or **pyuria** (pus in the urine) or **hematuria** (blood in the urine). Cystitis is identified through reports of these manifestations and by examination of the urine for evidence of bacteria (**bacteriuria**), white blood cells, or other indications of infection or inflammation.

Early management of cystitis is important to reduce the risk of infection of the kidney (**pyelonephritis**) or infection that moves into the bloodstream (**urosepsis**) and can be life threatening. Management of uncomplicated cystitis includes the administration of medications, such as antibiotics (Nicolle & Norrby, 2016). If cystitis is recurrent, management may include identifying, removing, or correcting factors that contribute to the development of UTIs, such as structural irregularities or poor hygienic practices. Immobility or use of an external catheter can predispose individuals to develop cystitis.

If the bacteria move from the bladder to the kidney, pyelonephritis can occur. Pyelonephritis may be acute or chronic. Although individuals with *acute pyelonephritis* may be acutely ill with fever and chills, flank or abdominal pain, nausea, and vomiting, no long-term incapacitation usually occurs if this condition is adequately managed with antibiotics. A goal of management in acute pyelonephritis is to prevent chronic pyelonephritis from occurring (Nicolle & Norry, 2016). *Chronic pyelonephritis* can cause irreversible degenerative changes in kidney structure and function, leading to kidney failure (described later in the chapter). Identification of pyelonephritis is based on manifestations and laboratory examination of urine (Nicolle & Norrby, 2016).

Kidney Stones

Ranging in size from a stone as tiny as a grain of sand to a stone large enough to fill the inner portion of the kidney, kidney stones (also known as *nephrolithiasis* or *renal calculi*) can cause excruciating pain (*renal colic*) and obstruct urine flow. Some individuals appear to be more prone to developing kidney stones than others. In addition to structural or metabolic irregularities, prolonged immobility or bed rest, inadequate fluid intake, and a variety of chronic health conditions can predispose individuals to develop kidney stones.

As kidney stones form and grow, no manifestations may initially be present. When the stone moves from the renal pelvis into the ureter, however, individuals often experience severe pain in the flank or kidney area, and possibly hematuria (blood in the urine). Identification of a kidney stone is based on the manifestations, examination of the urine, and ultrasound and is confirmed with computerized tomography (CT) scan.

If a stone severely obstructs its flow, urine may back up to the kidney (**hydronephrosis**; discussed later), causing kidney damage. Most kidney stones pass through the urinary meatus spontaneously. If a stone does not pass spontaneously, it may have to be removed surgically. The type of surgery depends on the size and location of the stone. The least invasive approach is *extracorporeal shock-wave lithotripsy (ESWL),* in which high-frequency sound waves from an external source are used to fragment the kidney stone, and the fragments are then passed in the urine (Vartanian & Park, 2012). ESWL is usually performed in an acute care setting.

If the stone becomes lodged in the ureter, its removal can be attempted by using a *cystoscope,* an instrument that is inserted into the bladder through the urinary meatus, so that the stone can be broken apart or removed. Two other more invasive procedures—*percutaneous nephrolithotomy* and *nephrolithotripsy*—may be performed to remove the stone if other methods are not successful or if the stone is irregularly shaped (Bushinsky, 2016). In both procedures, the kidney is entered through a small incision in the back. An instrument called a *nephroscope* is used to visualize the stone. If the stone is removed through this instrument, the procedure is called *nephrolithotomy*. If the stone is broken into fragments and removed, the procedure is called *nephrolithotripsy*.

Hydronephrosis

An obstruction can occur anywhere in the urinary tract for a variety of reasons: a stone; a narrowing caused by an infection; an injury; a congenital abnormality; a tumor; or enlargement of the prostate gland (known as *benign prostatic hypertrophy [BPH]),* a condition seen in older men. Obstructions prevent urine from flowing through the urinary tract so that backflow of urine into the kidneys occurs. Because the kidneys continue to produce urine even though there is backup of urine from the urinary tract, the renal pelvis eventually becomes swollen and distended—a condition called hydronephrosis. Obstruction of the urinary tract and backflow of urine also predispose individuals to infection of the kidney (pyelonephritis).

The manifestations experienced by individuals with hydronephrosis depend on the location of the obstruction, the degree of blockage, and the duration of the blockage (Zeidel, 2016). Individuals with hydronephrosis may experience pain, or they may feel little discomfort. Identification of hydronephrosis is usually made through laboratory evaluation and CT scan.

To prevent permanent damage to the kidney, whatever is causing the obstruction must be removed. The degree of incapacitation experienced because of hydronephrosis depends on the degree of permanent damage to the kidney. In severe cases, this condition can result in kidney failure.

Nephritis, Glomerular Conditions, and Nephrotic Syndrome

Nephritis

Nephritis is a general term that refers to an inflammation of the kidney. It may involve the glomeruli, the tubules, or the kidney tissue surrounding the tubules or glomeruli. It can be caused by infection, by agents which are toxic to the kidney (nephrotoxins), hypersensitivity to drugs (which can include prescription drugs), or from an autoimmune disease (Neilson, 2016). Nephritis can be acute or chronic.

Glomerular Conditions

Glomerular conditions refer to a type of nephritis that results from inflammation or damage to the glomeruli (**glomerulonephritis**). Because glomeruli remove excess fluids, electrolytes, and wastes from the blood so they are secreted in the urine, when they are inflamed or injured and unable to perform this function adequately, fluid and wastes accumulate in the blood and individuals may experience manifestations such as swelling (edema) or high blood pressure (hypertension) because of water retention and electrolyte imbalance, as well as fatigue (Appel & Radhakrishnan, 2016).

Glomerulonephritis can result from structural and biochemical changes that occur in the glomeruli secondary to a condition such as diabetes (Harris, 2016), or it can result from an immunologic response to bacteria or viruses present elsewhere in the body (Appel & Radhakrishnan, 2016). Manifestations are variable, but often also include **hematuria** (blood in the urine) and **proteinuria** (protein in the urine). When the glomeruli are inflamed or damaged, excessive amounts of protein are eliminated in the urine, rather than being reabsorbed into the bloodstream during the filtering process. Glomerulonephritis can result in irreversible, permanent structural changes in the kidney leading to *chronic kidney disease* (*CKD*) (discussed later in the chapter). The extent of kidney damage depends on the cause of the glomerulonephritis and the speed and the effectiveness with which the process can be stopped through appropriate management. Management of glomerulonephritis focuses on relieving the manifestations and eliminating the underlying cause.

Nephrotic Syndrome

When individuals have *albuminuria* (large amounts of albumin in the urine), *edema,* and *hyperlipidemia* (high lipid or fat level in the blood), they are said to have *nephrotic syndrome.* Weight gain and *periorbital edema* (swelling around the eyes) often accompany nephrotic syndrome. Nephrotic syndrome may be primary or it may be secondary to a number of other chronic conditions, including diabetes mellitus (chapter 23), systemic lupus erythematosus (chapter 25), Hodgkin lymphoma (chapter 22), or sickle cell disease (chapter 18). It may also be secondary to infection, medication-related effects, or allergens (Appel & Radhakrishnan, 2016).

Polycystic Kidney Disease

Polycystic kidney disease (PKD) comprises a group a hereditary conditions characterized by the presence of many cysts in the kidneys. The most common form of PKD, *autosomal dominant polycystic kidney disease (ADPKD)*, accounts for approximately 10% of all cases of *end-stage renal disease (ESRD)* in the United States (Arnaout, 2016).

ADPKD progresses slowly over many years, often with few, if any, manifestations. This condition may be discovered by accident during a routine examination, or as cysts enlarge, manifestations such as **nocturia** (excessive urination at night), low back pain, hematuria, or hypertension may become evident. As the cysts become enlarged, renal tissue becomes compressed, placing functional kidney tissue under pressure, and the kidney becomes enlarged.

ADPKD is identified through family history, ultrasound screening, CT scan, or *magnetic resonance imaging (MRI)*. Management of early stage disease involves interventions for manifestations such as hypertension or recurrent UTI. If the condition progresses to ESRD, individuals may undergo dialysis or kidney transplantation (both of which are discussed later in this chapter).

Severe Kidney Damage

If the kidney has been severely injured from trauma, if renal calculi have caused severe damage or are too large to remove, or if the kidney is chronically infected or nonfunctional, the entire kidney may need to be removed (**nephrectomy**). Individuals can usually continue their regular activities with one functioning kidney, but they must guard against infection or injury that could compromise the function of the remaining kidney.

Acute Renal Failure

Acute renal failure (ARF; also called acute kidney injury [AKI]) has a sudden onset and can occur within hours or days as a complication of other health conditions, surgery, or trauma (Molitoris, 2016). Diminished blood volume (**hypovolemia**) due to hemorrhage or severe dehydration, extremely low blood pressure (*hypotension*), **septicemia** (bacteria in the blood), urinary tract obstruction, and **nephrotoxins** (substances harmful to the kidneys such as certain drugs, solvents, or metals) are all potential causes of acute renal failure.

Immediate management of ARF is necessary to prevent permanent kidney damage. Such management is directed toward correcting reversible causes, and restoring the body chemistry to its normal state. Depending on the cause, with immediate intervention, ARF can often be reversed with no permanent damage to the kidney. Dialysis may be instituted temporarily to take over kidney function until the cause of the kidney failure can be corrected, or to remove nephrotoxins (Schroeder, 2012)

CHRONIC KIDNEY DISEASE

Chronic kidney disease (CKD), also called *chronic renal failure (CRF)*, refers to conditions in which kidney function has declined due to a systemic health condition that damages the kidney (e.g., diabetes) or from conditions intrinsic to the kidney itself (e.g., polycystic kidney). There are many causes of CKD and ESRD, although diabetes mellitus (Harris, 2016) and hypertension account for the majority of cases (Crandall & Shamoon, 2016).

The course of CKD may span many years, over which time individuals have partially compromised

kidney function. When the kidney becomes so severely compromised that it fails to perform most functions, the condition is said to have progressed to *ESRD,* sometimes called *end-stage kidney disease (ESKD)*. The number of individuals with ESRD has grown steadily and will continue to grow in tandem with the prevalence of diabetes and as the general population ages (Harris, 2016).

Stages of Chronic Kidney Disease

Whereas acute renal failure occurs rapidly, CKD may progress gradually over time. Its severity can be classified based on the glomerular filtration rate (Landry & Bazari, 2016). (See the discussion of GFR earlier in this chapter under *Kidney Structure*.) Staging assists in evaluation, monitoring, and management of CKD; the stage of the CKD is based on the level of kidney function measured in terms of the GFR. Individuals are considered to have CKD when kidney function has diminished to the point that GFR falls below a specified standard.

Manifestations of Chronic Kidney Disease

Manifestations experienced with CKD depend on the stage of the condition. Because the kidneys have many functions important to the body, their dysfunction affects all organ systems.

Fatigue

In the early stages of CKD, manifestations may be barely perceptible. One of the first noticeable manifestations may be fatigue resulting from anemia or the buildup of toxic wastes (both of which are discussed later in this section) that accompanies kidney failure.

Proteinuria

An early sign of kidney damage, albeit one with no physical manifestations, may be proteinuria. Because protein is usually reabsorbed into the regular body circulation after being filtered through the kidney, the presence of protein in the urine is an indication of failure of this mechanism, and consequently a sign of kidney damage.

Red Blood Cell Production

The kidneys normally produce the hormone *erythropoietin (EPO),* which regulates red blood cell production in the bone marrow. As kidney function declines, less erythropoietin is produced and the production of red blood cells declines, causing anemia. With fewer red blood cells available to transport oxygen, the heart may work harder to compensate for decreased oxygen supply to the tissues. As a result, anemia in CKD can contribute to **cardiomyopathy** (disease of the heart), in which the heart becomes enlarged (Mitch, 2016). In addition to fatigue and potential heart involvement, anemia can be associated with changes in mentation and decreased physical stamina.

Elimination of Waste

CKD diminishes the kidneys' ability to adequately filter blood and remove wastes such as urea and creatinine, which are by-products of protein metabolism that are normally excreted in the urine. When these wastes cannot be filtered by the kidney, they accumulate in the blood, a toxic condition called **uremia**. The buildup affects the body's delicate internal chemical balance, in turn altering the function of numerous other body systems.

In later stages of CKD, uremia may cause manifestations such as loss of appetite, nausea and vomiting, and consequent weight loss. Changes in mental function, such as difficulty with concentration, development of shortened attention span, or change in sleep patterns, may be present as well. Waste accumulation in the blood also contributes to **pruritus** (overall itching).

Water Regulation

The kidney plays an essential role in water regulation through its ability to both excrete water by producing dilute urine and retain water by concentrating urine. When the kidney loses the ability to appropriately regulate urine concentrations, individuals may experience **polyuria** (overproduction of urine). In later stages of CKD, urine production may become severely diminished (**oliguria**) or nonexistent (**anuria**).

Electrolyte Imbalance

Internal body chemistry, including fluid content of body tissue, is regulated by electrolytes, such as sodium and potassium. In CKD, the kidneys are unable to excrete sodium. Elevated blood levels of sodium result in retention of fluid, with resulting **edema** and hypertension. Excessive fluid in the body also puts stress on the circulatory system, and especially the heart, potentially causing cardiac dysfunction and subsequent heart failure. Outward manifestations of fluid overload consist of weight gain, edema, and difficulty breathing (**dyspnea**).

Potassium regulates contraction and relaxation of muscles, including the heart and the muscles used for respiration. Normally most potassium taken in through the diet is excreted by the kidney; however, in CKD the kidney is unable to excrete potassium, so this electrolyte is retained, leading to subsequent high blood levels of potassium (**hyperkalemia**). Excessive amounts of potassium in the blood can adversely affect the heart, potentially causing cardiac arrest and death.

Bone Structure

Calcium in the blood is decreased below normal levels in CKD, partly because the kidney is unable to produce sufficient amounts of the active form of vitamin D, which is necessary for calcium absorption, and partly because calcium absorption in the intestine is decreased. Low calcium in the blood causes overactivity of the parathyroid glands, leading to calcium loss from the bone (**osteoporosis**), and contributing to bone pain and fractures.

Iron Deficiency

Iron deficiency results not only from the kidneys' inability to produce erythropoietin so that production of red blood cells is diminished, resulting in anemia, but also from a decline in the ability to absorb iron from the intestine. Iron deficiency in CKD contributes to manifestations of weakness and low exercise tolerance.

Peripheral Neuropathy

Uremia has toxic effects on nerves, especially the *peripheral nerves* of the hands and feet. It may, therefore, result in **peripheral neuropathy**, an incapacitating manifestation leading to weakness and loss of sensation in the upper or lower extremities. As a result of peripheral neuropathy, individuals may have both difficulty manipulating objects with their hands and difficulty walking.

Sexual Function

Due to both physical and emotional changes present in CKD, individuals may experience impaired sexual function. Hormonal changes, circulatory problems, changes in the nervous system, lack of energy, and side effects of medications may all contribute to diminished sexual desire or performance. Likewise, changes in self-concept and body image may hamper sexual interest and activity.

Identification of Chronic Kidney Disease

In the absence of a family history of conditions such as polycystic kidney disease, early CKD may not be identified until manifestations of fatigue or hypertension become apparent. When CKD is suspected, a variety of laboratory tests to measure GFR as well as to identify substances such as protein in the urine and blood chemistries may be indicated. Ultrasound examination of the kidneys and bladder may also be used to identify potential obstruction or enlargement of the kidney.

Management of Chronic Kidney Disease

Management of CKD is directed toward improving outcomes by controlling and delaying progression of kidney deterioration through management of high blood pressure, diabetes, and other primary processes involved in CKD (Harris, 2016). In very early stages, management may include restricting water to an amount equal to urine output, carefully monitoring body weight, and managing the diet to provide adequate nutrition without overtaxing the kidney with metabolic waste products. This effort may require a low-sodium diet, with restrictions on consumption of excessive amounts of protein, potassium, or phosphorus.

Medications may also be used to slow the progression of kidney disease. The kidneys can usually continue to function with as little as 10% of normal kidney function. Loss of function beyond this point requires *renal replacement therapy (RRT)* to survive. RRT consists of *hemodialysis, peritoneal dialysis,* or *kidney transplant* (all of which are discussed later in this chapter). Each type of renal replacement therapy has risks as well as benefits (Cohen & Valeri, 2016).

Diet

When kidney function is significantly reduced, individuals' diet and fluid intake must be regulated. Intake of protein, sodium, potassium, fluid, and calories must be carefully regulated and monitored to achieve the following goals:

- Minimize waste products in the body
- Maintain electrolyte levels in the body within normal limits
- Avoid too much or too little fluid in the body
- Maintain weight and adequate nutrition

Diets are tailored to the individual. Individuals with chronic kidney failure work closely with dietitians to develop a diet plan right for them. The type of diet is based on individual needs and the stage of kidney disease. When CKD is the result of another chronic health condition, such as diabetes, specific dietary needs for management of that condition must also be considered.

In CKD, the kidney is no longer able to filter out waste products of protein metabolism (urea), so dietary intake of protein must be controlled. Consequently, dietary intake of foods that are especially high in protein, such as meat, fish, eggs, poultry, and dairy products, is restricted.

Sodium is important in the regulation of fluid in the body as well as to maintain the body's internal chemical balance. Due to the kidneys' inability to excrete sodium effectively in CKD, dietary intake of sodium must be regulated. Sodium restrictions affect not only intake of salt

Table 30-1   Restricted Foods in CKD: Foods High in Sodium

Corned and chipped beef
Bacon
Ham
Cold cuts such as bologna
Pork sausage
Canned tuna, salmon, sardines
Pork sausage
Hot dogs
Cheddar and Swiss cheese
Snack foods such as pretzels, popcorn, potato chips
Some crackers
Most canned vegetables
Olives
Soft drinks

Table 30-2   Restricted Foods in CKD: Foods High in Potassium

Oranges and orange juice
Grapefruit, grapefruit juice
Bananas
Apricots
Cantaloupe
Kidney beans
Pears
Potatoes
Spinach
Tomatoes
Peaches
Strawberries
Raisins
Beets
Cabbage
Carrots
Celery
Many breakfast cereals
Many breads
Many nuts
Salt substitutes

Table 30-3   Restricted Foods in CKD: Foods High in Phosphorus

Beer
Ice cream
Pudding
Yogurt
Chocolate
Coffee
Fish and seafood
Ricotta cheese
Milk
Dried beans and peas

but also intake of a number of other foods high in sodium. Consumption of foods containing high levels of sodium must, therefore, be restricted (see **Table 30-1**).

Because of the kidneys' inability to excrete potassium, and the adverse and potentially fatal effects of elevated potassium level on heart and other muscles, hyperkalemia (elevated potassium levels) must be avoided. Dietary intake of foods rich in potassium (**Table 30-2**) must, therefore, be restricted. The more severe the loss of kidney function, the more carefully potassium levels must be regulated.

Phosphorus is necessary for regulating calcium and building strong bones and is present in many foods (Yu, 2016). The kidney excretes excess phosphorus which helps the body regulate a phosphate balance. In CKD, the kidney is unable to excrete excess phosphorus from the blood. High levels of phosphorus in the blood can cause loss of calcium from the bones, making them weaker and prone to fracture. In addition, high levels of phosphorus in the blood can lead to calcification in soft tissues, causing organ damage (Yu, 2016). Because phosphorus is contained in many foods, and the kidney, in CKD, looses the ability to excrete excess. intake of foods high in phosphorus may need to be reduced. Examples of foods high in phosphorus are listed in **Table 30-3**.

Calorie intake must also be monitored, as must weight gain. Due to food restrictions, individuals may have difficulty maintaining sufficient caloric intake and adequate nutrition. Foods low in sodium, potassium, and protein may be needed throughout the day as supplements to provide additional calories. For snacks between meals, specialized products with high calorie content but only small amounts of protein and electrolytes may be used.

Frequent monitoring of weight also serves as an indicator of fluid buildup and edema. Especially in later stages of CKD, the kidneys are unable to maintain fluid balance, so fluid intake may need to be restricted. Excessive weight gain may also be an indication of fluid retention due to excess sodium, which means that sodium intake may need to be reduced even further.

Medications

Use of antihypertensive medications to reduce blood pressure may prevent further damage to the kidney as well as prevent other complications related to hypertension. Medications such as vasodilators or diuretics may also be used in early stages of CKD to maintain renal blood flow and reduce fluid retention and edema.

Injections of *iron supplements* may be given to combat the anemia that is common in advanced CKD. In later stages of kidney disease, *erythropoietin* or *erthropoietic-stimulating agents* may be given to stimulate production of red blood cells (Bahrainwala & Berns, 2016).

Management of End-Stage Renal Disease

ESRD describes a condition in which CKD has progressed to the extent that the kidney is irreversibly damaged and unable to function such that the condition is life threatening. At this stage of the disease, RRT is instituted. RRT helps individuals compensate for absent kidney function and can consist of the following measures:

- Hemodialysis
- Peritoneal dialysis
- Renal transplantation

Hemodialysis

The primary goal of hemodialysis is to reproduce the fluid environment that is characteristic of kidney function. Hemodialysis is generally provided at an outpatient dialysis unit 3 times per week for 3–4 hours at each session, using a machine called a *dialyzer* (Cohen & Valeri, 2016). The dialyzer filters the blood that has been circulated outside the body to meet the following goals:

- Remove metabolic waste from the blood
- Maintain appropriate balance of body chemistry
- Remove excess fluid from the blood

In acute renal failure (discussed earlier in the chapter), hemodialysis may be a temporary measure until kidney function is restored. In ESRD, however, kidney damage is irreversible and permanent, so hemodialysis is needed on an ongoing basis for survival. If individuals with ESRD are suitable candidates for kidney transplantation, hemodialysis may be used until an appropriate donor kidney becomes available; however, not all individuals with chronic kidney failure are suitable candidates for kidney transplantation. If a transplant is not feasible, individuals with CKD must remain on dialysis for the rest of their lives.

Hemodialysis requires access routes through which blood is removed from the individual; this blood is then circulated through the dialyzer and ultimately returned to the individual's circulation. Access may be surgically created through a *synthetic arteriovenous graft,* an *arteriovenous fistula,* or an *internal jugular cannula* (Shakarchi et al., 2015). Access routes are created surgically, most often in the forearm. Another procedure, the *external arteriovenous shunt,* may be used if immediate and temporary access is needed, as in the case of acute renal failure. This procedure consists of surgical placement of a tube (*cannula*) under the skin to connect an artery to a vein.

Synthetic arteriovenous grafts involve surgical placement of synthetic material to connect an artery and a vein. Due to the higher rates of **thrombosis** (blood clot formation) and infection associated with such grafts, they are typically used for dialysis only if a fistula is not feasible, such as in peripheral vascular disease (Cohen & Valeri, 2016).

Figure 30-3   Access for Hemodialysis through a Fistula

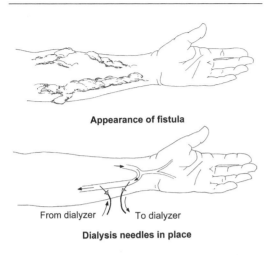

Appearance of fistula

From dialyzer   To dialyzer

Dialysis needles in place

© Jane Tinkler Lamm.

Figure 30-4   Access for Hemodialysis through a Subclavian Cannula

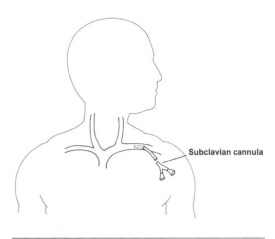

Subclavian cannula

© Jane Tinkler Lamm.

The arteriovenous fistula (**Figure 30-3**) is the most widely used venous access because it is more durable and associated with fewer complications. In this procedure, an artery is surgically joined to a vein (**anastomosis**) underneath the skin, establishing an opening called a **fistula** between the two. Shunting arterial blood into the vein causes the vein to become thickened and enlarged, allowing it to be used repeatedly as a point of access to the circulation for dialysis. It may take from two to six weeks for the fistula to become thickened and enlarged enough that it can be used for dialysis. In the meantime, temporary access may be maintained through the internal jugular vein (see **Figure 30-4**).

During dialysis, a large needle is placed into the artery side of the individual's access site and another large needle is placed in the vein side of the access. Tubes are then attached to the needles and connected to the dialysis machine. Blood moves from the first tube to the dialysis machine, which is composed of small artificial capillary tubes lined with a *semipermeable membrane*, a porous material that allows some substances to pass through the membrane while keeping other substances in the blood. The blood of individuals undergoing hemodialysis is on one side of the membrane, and a specially prepared solution called a *dialysate* is

on the other side of the membrane. Differences in concentrations of the blood and dialysate allow certain particles—but not others—to pass from the blood through the membrane and into the dialysate, where they can then be removed through dialysis. The cleansed and filtered blood is subsequently returned to the individual through the second needle in the vein (**Figure 30-5**).

Hemodialysis is usually performed from 3–4 hours per day, 3 times per week (Cohen & Valeri, 2016). It can take place at a kidney dialysis center or, in some instances, at home (Rydell, Clyne, & Segelmark, 2016). Because home hemodialysis requires a high degree of individual control, self-destructive tendencies in individuals, and unwillingness of family members or caregivers to participate in the procedure are contraindications for this procedure. Home dialysis requires someone (a family member, or someone who has been hired) who has been trained to assist with the procedure. The level of responsibility as well as the need to be always present at specified times of dialysis can cause stress for the helper, especially if he or she is a family member. Stress levels associated with home hemodialysis are usually evaluated and monitored before the implementation of such a program.

Figure 30-5   Hemodialysis Machine

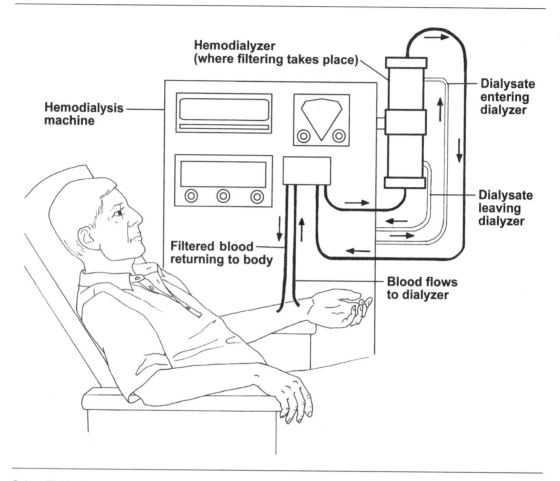

© Jane Tinkler Lamm.

The success of hemodialysis depends on individuals' level of motivation, the presence of other health conditions that may cause complications, and development of complications from the hemodialysis itself. Rapid changes that occur in fluid and chemical balances in the body during dialysis may cause some individuals to experience nausea, vomiting, headaches, or muscle cramps in association with hemodialysis. Potential complications *during* hemodialysis range from **hypotension** (low blood pressure) to the technical complication of air embolus, in which air enters the tubing, causing dyspnea, cough, or chest pain. Other complications may involve infection of the access route, which can develop into bacteremia (bacteria in the blood), a potentially life-threatening complication;

cardiac-related complications; and stroke or some other thrombolytic event. Because of the risk of clot formation in the access route, individuals on hemodialysis may receive *anticoagulant medication* during the procedure. Administration of this medication, however, may also increase the risk of bleeding. Some individuals may become anemic, and some experience sleep disturbances or mental cloudiness. Individuals on prolonged hemodialysis may develop changes in nerves of the extremities resulting in peripheral neuropathy (loss of sensation and weakness in the arms and legs).

Hemodialysis itself is painless, although some minor discomfort may occur when needles are inserted for dialysis. During this procedure, individuals remain stationary in the dialysis unit, but they can still read, use a computer, watch television, or sleep. Individuals with ESRD, especially after beginning dialysis, are unable to regulate fluid balance, so the amount of fluid taken orally may need to be restricted. Included in this measure of fluid intake are ice cubes, gelatin desserts, sherbet, or any other food that liquefies at room temperature. When individuals are on dialysis, the amount of fluid intake permitted is based on the individual's weight gain between dialysis interventions and may be severely restricted.

Hemodialysis can relieve many of the manifestations of kidney disease, but not all of them. Individuals receiving such therapy may develop secondary conditions that increase the risk of bone fractures, or the procedure may not adequately clear all wastes, leading to a feeling of weakness.

The degree of functional capacity varies from individual to individual. Many are able to continue regular activities, except for the interruptions required for dialysis.

Peritoneal Dialysis

Peritoneal dialysis also uses a semipermeable membrane, but in this case the **peritoneum** (the thin membrane that lines the abdominal cavity) in the individual's body acts as the semipermeable membrane through which wastes and fluid are removed. In peritoneal dialysis, a tube or catheter is surgically placed within the abdominal cavity. During peritoneal dialysis, dialysate from a bag is drained through the catheter into the abdominal cavity (**Figure 30-6**). The catheter **H** is clamped, and the dialysate is left in the abdominal cavity

Figure 30-6   Peritoneal Dialysis

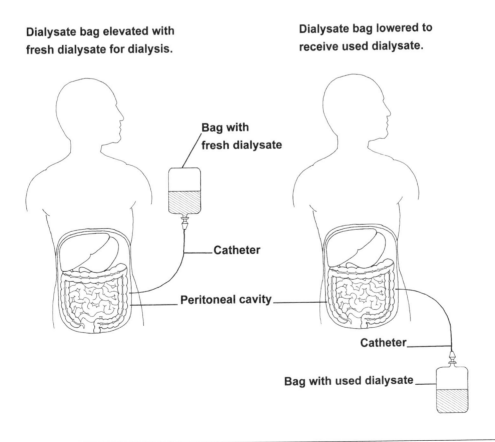

Dialysate bag elevated with fresh dialysate for dialysis.

Dialysate bag lowered to receive used dialysate.

Bag with fresh dialysate

Catheter

Peritoneal cavity

Catheter

Bag with used dialysate

for a specified amount of time. During this time, waste products and excess fluid pass from the blood through the peritoneal membrane and into the dialysate. At the end of the specified period, the catheter is unclamped and the dialysate, which now contains the waste products and excess fluid, is drained from the body through the catheter. The tube is again clamped and remains in place for the next dialysis session.

Peritoneal dialysis is performed at home, either manually or with a machine. Several methods of peritoneal dialysis are possible:

- Continuous ambulatory peritoneal dialysis
- Intermittent peritoneal dialysis
- Continuous cycling peritoneal dialysis

Regardless of the method used for peritoneal dialysis, the underlying principles remain the same. With *continuous ambulatory peritoneal dialysis (CAPD),* dialysate is instilled into the abdominal cavity manually, using gravity. A bag of dialysate solution is connected to the catheter. The individual then elevates the bag, causing the dialysate to flow into the abdominal cavity. The catheter is clamped, and the dialysate is left in place for 4 to 8 hours. The catheter is then unclamped and the bag lowered so that the dialysate drains from the abdominal cavity by gravity. When the bag is full, the individual detaches it from the catheter, attaches a new bag of dialysate, and begins the process again. Individuals change the dialysate manually four to five times per day. Each exchange takes approximately 30 to 40 minutes. Individuals using this type of peritoneal dialysis are able to continue their regular daily activities, stopping only for periodic intervals to drain the dialysate and attach a fresh bag.

Intermittent peritoneal dialysis (IPD) and *continuous cycling peritoneal dialysis (CCPD)* both use a machine. IPD is now infrequently used as a form of peritoneal dialysis, but when it is used it is performed 3 or more times a week, with each exchange lasting for 10 or more hours. With this approach, the catheter is connected to the cycling machine at night. The exchange takes place while the person sleeps; consequently, individuals are free to engage in their regular activities during the day.

CCPD also uses a cycling machine but is performed daily. With this approach, the catheter is connected to the cycling machine, which performs multiple solution exchanges while the individual sleeps. In the morning, the individual disconnects the catheter from the machine, sometimes leaving the last solution in the abdomen all day, while engaging in his or her regular activities.

Peritoneal dialysis may be chosen as the dialysis method for individuals who have, in addition to kidney disease, other health conditions that increase the risk of complications associated with hemodialysis. In other instances, it may be chosen because of its relative ease and the limited use of sophisticated equipment—both factors that enable individuals to use peritoneal dialysis in the home. Depending on the type of procedure used, individuals may have more mobility with peritoneal dialysis than with hemodialysis. If severe vascular disease interferes with the blood supply to the peritoneum or if there is an increased vulnerability to infection, however, peritoneal dialysis may be contraindicated.

Although generally a safe procedure, peritoneal dialysis can have a number of associated complications. The most common is **peritonitis** (inflammation of the peritoneum), which occurs when the peritoneum is contaminated with bacteria. If peritonitis develops, antibiotics may be used for the infection, or peritoneal dialysis may be discontinued and hemodialysis begun. Other potential complications include plugging or displacement of the catheter, development of hernias, and pain during dialysis. Over time, infection or the dialysate concentration itself may damage the peritoneum. Peritoneal dialysis is usually a limited procedure because of the loss of membrane function.

Kidney Transplantation

Kidney transplantation involves surgically placing a kidney from a *donor* into the body of an individual with kidney disease (the *recipient*). The nonfunctioning kidney is usually not removed from the individual receiving the kidney transplant, unless there is uncontrolled infection, uncontrolled hypertension, or a limitation of space. Transplants may be received from a family member (*living-related donor*), an individual who is not related to the individual (*living-unrelated donor*), or an individual who has recently died (*deceased donor*). Regardless of the status of the donor, the donor's blood must be the same type as that of the recipient and his or her tissues must closely match those of the recipient to decrease the chances of the recipient's body rejecting the transplant. In addition, donors must undergo in-depth psychological evaluation and verification that they have not been coerced into donation. Donation must be altruistic and totally voluntary.

Kidney transplant frees individuals from restrictions associated with dialysis, diminishes many manifestations of ESRD, and improves overall quality of life (Cohen & Valeri, 2016). Before being considered for kidney transplant, recipients undergo careful and thorough evaluation to see if they are suitable candidates. It is essential prior to transplant that the individual knows that transplantation is an intervention, not a cure. Individuals having the transplant may still have the chronic health condition, such as diabetes or hypertension, that caused the initial kidney damage, and consequently they must continue to effectively manage that condition to prevent damage to the new kidney.

When being considered for transplant, the recipient's general health—including the presence of other health conditions that may potentially affect the success of the transplant or make it impossible—is evaluated. Pretransplant evaluation also includes a thorough psychological evaluation. Discussion of the risk of rejection and infection and the lifelong need to use immunosuppressants with their corresponding risk is a part of the pretransplant protocol. In some instances, the ability to finance the procedure and the cost of medications needed after transplant may be assessed before someone is evaluated for eligibility for transplantation.

Expectations for the transplant are discussed with both the recipient and the living donor. Also evaluated is the recipient's ability to adjust to the transplant as well as his or her ability to adjust should the transplant fail. The degree of family and social support is assessed as well. Besides the cost of the kidney transplant itself, the costs associated with travel to the transplant center, lodging for family members, and lifelong medication needed after the transplant can be staggering. Consequently,

the social service evaluation includes the financial status of the candidate for transplant and identification of resources that can help to cover costs.

Scarcity of donors is the major factor that limits kidney transplantation (Cohen & Valeri, 2016). Whether the donor is living or deceased, compatibility of tissue type and blood type and a variety of other factors determine the success of the transplantation. Tissue typing is most important in decreasing the possibility of rejection. While the most desirable sources of kidneys for transplantation are closely related living donors, unrelated donors are now acceptable, and new protocols are being developed so that blood type–incompatible donors may be used as sources of organs.

At the time of transplant, both the donor and the recipient are hospitalized. The individual with ESRD has dialysis the day before the transplant. The donor has renal angiography to determine which kidney will be used for the transplant. The surgical procedure for the kidney transplant consists of removing the kidney from the donor and placing it in a surgically constructed pocket in the lower abdomen of the recipient. Once the donor kidney has been transplanted, it may begin to function immediately. Early functioning of the transplanted kidney is a good prognostic sign for success of the procedure.

The major complication of kidney transplantation is rejection, which can destroy the transplanted kidney. Rejection most commonly occurs within the first 3 months to 6 months after transplantation (Cohen & Valeri, 2016). The body's defense system—that is, the immune system—naturally attacks foreign substances in the body. Consequently, individuals must take immunosuppressant medications after transplant to block the body's immune response (Bamgbola, 2016). Immunosuppressants can cause a number of complications—namely, increased susceptibility to infection, formation of cataracts, degeneration of bone (**avascular necrosis**), and an increased rate of **malignancy** (cancer), especially skin cancer (Cohen & Valeri, 2016). Individuals need to be particularly careful to avoid contact with persons with communicable (infectious) conditions. After transplant, prophylactic antibiotics are usually taken prior to any dental work.

After transplant, the individual receiving the kidney may return to work within 6 to 8 weeks. Because of the extensive surgical procedure necessary for removing the kidney from the donor, the recovery time for the donor was considerably longer in the past. Today, however, the donor surgical procedure is frequently done with a laparoscopic approach, which has greatly decreased recovery time; even so, the donor should expect to be away from work for at least 4 to 6 weeks. Donors who undergo traditional flank incisions will have a longer recovery time than the recipient and should expect to be absent from work for 8 to 12 weeks.

Functional Implications of CKD/ESRD

Personal and Psychosocial Issues

CKD can profoundly affect all areas of an individual's life, causing psychological stress and altering quality of life. Psychological changes accompanying CKD vary and can be associated with both the emotional reactions to a potentially life-threatening condition and the physiological changes that occur with CKD. Elevated levels of toxic waste in the blood can produce cognitive changes, such as impaired judgment, drowsiness, and difficulty with concentration. Other possible cognitive changes include memory loss, speech impairment, and irritability.

In later stages of CKD, shock and realization of kidney failure and its ramifications may be immobilizing. Reactions vary in degree from severe depression to total denial. Mourning loss of part of body function, loss of control, feelings of disconnectedness, and anger are all emotional reactions commonly reported by individuals with kidney failure.

Additional stress may be experienced when kidney function has deteriorated to the extent that dialysis is necessary. The physical discomfort associated with dialysis—such as interrupted sleep patterns, nausea, lethargy, and shortness of breath—may increase the individual's psychological distress. Individuals who begin dialysis may have a period of adjustment. Although many individuals reach a stage of acceptance in which restrictions and complications of dialysis are incorporated into their daily lives, some persons experience significant emotional stress.

In the early sessions of dialysis, individuals may initially experience apprehension or uneasiness about the possibility that the machine may malfunction, although as they become more comfortable with dialysis, these fears generally subside. As they become aware of the immediate physical improvements they experience following dialysis, they may be hopeful, confident, and optimistic.

As the individuals continue with dialysis, they may become discouraged and disenchanted as they realize that kidney damage is irreversible, and that they are permanently dependent on dialysis for survival. Dependence on the dialysis may cause loss of self-esteem, feelings of helplessness or inadequacy, and fear of death. Individuals may also experience apprehension about continuing to live a life sustained by dialysis with its subsequent restrictions.

Individuals may have conflicting feelings of dependency and independence—even conflicting feelings about living and dying. Feelings may be expressed openly, but they may also be internalized as individuals on dialysis realize the degree of their dependence not only on a machine but also on family members and others who are involved in support.

Uncertainty can also be an issue in CKD. Management choices are not always final. In early stages of CKD, management may consist of dietary restrictions and medication. As kidney function deteriorates, however, other management interventions, such as dialysis, will be needed. Individuals who initially choose peritoneal dialysis rather than hemodialysis may need to switch procedures if complications from peritoneal dialysis occur. Individuals using hemodialysis may later consider a kidney transplant should an organ become available. Individuals eligible for kidney transplant may also experience stress while waiting for a transplant. Even after individuals receive a kidney transplant, uncertainty remains because there is always the chance that rejection of the transplant may occur.

Although some individuals with CKD take needed lifestyle modifications in stride, others may see these modifications as profound. Dietary restrictions may be viewed as stringent, and dialysis, even though lifesaving, may be viewed as a restriction on both time and freedom. Even if an individual receives a transplant that succeeds, the management plan both before and after the transplant may seem overwhelming.

The stress of dealing with such uncertainty, the demands of the management plan, and overall fear can lead to a variety of psychological reactions, including denial. Although denial can be a helpful mechanism to reduce stress levels, it can be life threatening if it leads to nonadherence with the management plan. Internalized feelings can be self-destructive if individuals rebel against the restrictions and protocol of the management plan and become nonadherent with the recommended diet, taking in too much fluid, skipping dialysis, or in other ways failing to cooperate with the management plan.

When transplantation is a management choice, individuals who are found to be eligible recipients of a transplanted kidney are often initially elated about the anticipated improvement in their quality of life after the transplantation. Despite anticipation and psychological preparation prior to transplantation, however, they may still experience postsurgical psychological responses for which they feel unprepared. If the donor is a family member or friend of the recipient, the relationship may be altered. At times the relationship is strengthened, but it may also become weakened. Recipients may experience guilt, anxiety, or depression because of the donation of the kidney they received. If potential donors felt pressure, either real or imagined, to donate a kidney, they may experience stress, conflict, or guilt, especially if they decided to decline, or resentment if they donated their kidney under duress. If the kidney was received from a deceased donor, recipients may have fantasies about embodying the spirit of someone who is dead. Whether the transplant was from a living or deceased donor, recipients may still feel that the kidney is foreign.

The chance of later rejection or the risk that infection will damage the transplanted kidney may be a source of anxiety. If the transplanted kidney is rejected, individuals can be devastated by the knowledge that dialysis will once again be required. Even if rejection does not occur and quality of life improves significantly, individuals with a transplanted kidney may express disappointment that long-term monitoring and evaluation are still necessary. In addition, they may be disappointed if transplantation does not restore them to the state of health that was theirs prior to the onset of CKD.

Activities and Participation

Early stages of CKD may not affect individuals' social or other regular activities. As CKD progresses, exercise can increase strength and endurance and reduce stress. Although individuals with CKD may be unable to tolerate as much physical activity as before they developed the condition, exercise programs individually tailored to individuals' specific needs and abilities are beneficial. Although many daily activities can be continued, flexibility is important given that physical tolerance for various activities may be unpredictable from day to day.

Physiologic changes, the demands of the management plan, and the chronic nature of CKD or ESRD affect not just individuals with the condition, but the entire family unit. Individuals with CKD/ESRD may withdraw from family and friends owing to feelings of inadequacy. They may struggle to resolve qualms about their dependence on dialysis and on others for assistance. Individuals with unresolved dependency conflicts may become uncooperative and ill tempered. Rather than confronting the individual, family and friends may excuse his or her behavior, reinforcing the sick role.

Family members' reactions and stability can either help or hinder individuals' acceptance of their condition. Some family members may be either over-solicitous or rejecting, making it more difficult for individuals to reestablish their own emotional balance and their role within the family. Although family, friends, and associates play an important supportive role in individuals' adjustment to kidney failure, an overindulgent attitude can impede individuals' return to the earlier level of independence. If there were previous problems in relationships, these may be amplified when individuals learn that they have CKD. The additional stress brought on by dialysis or the wait for transplantation may intensify discord if it exists.

If dialysis is conducted at home, the family member assisting with dialysis may feel burdened and strained by the added responsibility and protocol of the dialysis program, given that activities must be programmed around the schedule. Individuals' physical complaints, fatigue, and loss of interest in sexual activities may compound the problem. Although financial assistance for dialysis is usually available through government or private agencies, the overall financial burden imposed by healthcare bills, dialysis, and lost income if the individual with kidney disease is not able to continue working may put additional stress on relationships.

Kidney disease may become the focus of activities to the exclusion of family interactions. Individuals and families can work to develop a life that incorporates the condition into family structure rather than overwhelming it.

Food and drink are important parts of the modern social fabric. The food and fluid restrictions imposed by CKD/ESRD, however, may require adjustment in social activities that center on food and fluid intake. While many individuals with CKD/ESRD adapt to these changes and continue to participate in the social milieu, others may find the restrictions embarrassing or laborious and may avoid social events where food is a highlighted activity. Individuals may be reluctant to accept the dinner invitations of friends because of dietary restrictions, for example, or they may themselves give up entertaining because of limitations associated with their condition.

Individuals on dialysis may need to alter some activities because of the dialysis schedule. Whether peritoneal dialysis or hemodialysis is selected, traveling and vacations are still possible, but require careful planning and arrangements to be made in advance. For individuals on hemodialysis, dialysis units must be located near the vacation spot or travel destination, and arrangements must be made for dialysis at the center prior to departure. Peritoneal dialysis, although offering more flexibility, also requires planning for travel. Depending on the amount of time away and the method of travel, there may need to be prearranged shipment of dialysate or a cycling machine to the destination. Individuals with shunts should avoid any activity that could expose the shunt area to potential injury. Because heat intolerance is often associated with CKD, activities requiring long exposure to hot environments should be avoided.

Sexual Activity

Although there are no limitations or restrictions regarding sexual activity, desire for sexual activity may change in individuals with CKD/ESRD because of side effects of medications, because of physical manifestations of the condition, or because of emotional reasons, such as depression or anxiety. Some men with CKD experience impotence; women with CKD may experience decreased response to sexual stimulation. Reproductive capacity of both men and women on dialysis is severely diminished. Sexual function may improve after kidney transplant, however, and conception is possible. If the transplant is rejected or the individual is heavily medicated, sexual function may be impaired.

Vocational Issues in CKD/ESRD

As CKD progresses and manifestations become more pronounced, the impact on vocational function increases. Fatigue may necessitate a shortened workday or rest periods during the day. In addition, problems of impaired judgment, difficulty with memory, or irritability may interfere with adequate job performance. Peripheral neuropathy may make it difficult or impossible to perform tasks such as lifting or to complete tasks that require manual dexterity. Fatigue or the decreased ability to walk caused by peripheral neuropathy may necessitate a change to a more sedentary line of work.

Individuals on dialysis may need a flexible work schedule to accommodate the dialysis schedule. Many dialysis centers operate 24 hours each day, enabling individuals to arrange dialysis in their off-hours. Blood access routes, such as fistulas, require protection, so occupations that pose a potential threat of damage to the fistula should be avoided. Environmental issues should also be considered. Specifically, work that requires exposure to high temperatures should be avoided because of the heat intolerance associated with kidney diseases. Excess heat in the work environment should be avoided as well.

After transplant, many individuals are able to return to work. In other instances, complications related to immunosuppressant medications, such as infection or fatigue, may make returning to work more difficult. At times, financial disincentives or employer concerns about lost work time may also be barriers to employment.

The degree to which kidney disease affects employment depends on individuals' occupation, previous work history, management plan, and status of any secondary health conditions. Individuals with early stage kidney disease can generally continue their previous jobs, especially if the job is sedentary and does not require strenuous activity.Individuals with CKD may experience reduced work tolerance owing to impaired concentration and fatigue. If they are no longer capable of performing the physical activity that the work requires, a job modification or change may be necessary. Individuals with CKD who experience a decreased attention span or an inability to concentrate may require jobs that accommodate these limitations.

CASE STUDY

Ms. M. is a 29-year-old female who has worked as a grocery store manager for the last 9 years. She has had type 1 diabetes since she was 10 years old and also has hypertension. Her kidney function has continued to decline over the last few years, and recently Ms. M. has learned that she is in stage 3 renal failure. It is recommended that she begin hemodialysis.

1. Given Ms. M.'s type of work, which specific factors related to her health condition should she consider?
2. How might hemodialysis affect Ms. M.'s work or work schedule?
3. Are there special accommodations Ms. M. may need to continue in her current line of employment while still on dialysis?

REFERENCES

Al-Awqati, Q., & Barasch, J. (2016). Structure and function of the kidneys. In L. Goldman & A. I. Schafer (Eds) *Goldman-Cecil medicine* (25th ed., pp. 737–740). Philadelphia, PA: Elsevier Saunders.

Appel, G. B., & Radhakrishnan, J. (2016). Glomerular disorders and nephrotic syndromes. In L. Goldman & A. I. Schafer (Eds.), *Goldman-Cecil medicine* (25th ed., pp. 783–793). Philadelphia, PA: Elsevier Saunders.

Arnaout M. A. (2016). Cystic kidney diseases. In L. Goldman & A. I. Schafer (Eds.), *Goldman-Cecil medicine* (25th ed., pp. 816–822). Philadelphia, PA: Elsevier Saunders.

Bahrainwala, J., & Berns, J. S. (2016). Diagnosis of iron deficiency anemia in chronic kidney disease. *Seminars in Nephrology*, *36*(2), 94–98.

Bamgbola, O. (2016). Metabolic consequences of modern immunosuppressive agents in solid organ transplantation. *Therapeutic Advances in Endocrinology and Metabolism*, *7*(3), 110–127.

Bushinsky, D. A. (2016). Nephrolithiasis. In L. Goldman & A. I. Schafer (Eds.), *Goldman-Cecil medicine* (25th ed., pp. 811–816). Philadelphia, PA: Elsevier Saunders.

Cohen, D., & Valeri, A.M. (2016). Treatment of irreversible renal failure. In L. Goldman & A. I. Schafer (Eds.), *Goldman-Cecil medicine* (25th ed., pp. 841–847). Philadelphia, PA: Elsevier Saunders

Crandall, J., & Shamoon, H. (2016). Diabetes mellitus. In L. Goldman & A. I. Schafer (Eds.), *Goldman-Cecil medicine* (25th ed., pp. 1527–1548). Philadelphia, PA: Elsevier Saunders

Harris, R. C. (2016). Diabetes and the kidney. In L. Goldman & A. I. Schafer (Eds.), *Goldman-Cecil medicine* (25th ed., pp. 804–806). Philadelphia, PA: Elsevier Saunders

Landry, D. W., & Bazari, H. (2016). Approach to the patient with renal disease. In L. Goldman & A. I. Schafer (Eds.), *Goldman-Cecil Medicine* (25th ed., pp. 728–736). Philadelphia, PA: Elsevier Saunders

Mitch, W. E. (2016). Chronic kidney disease. In L. Goldman & A. I. Schafer (Eds.), *Goldman-Cecil medicine* (25th ed., pp. 833-840). Philadelphia, PA: Elsevier Saunders

Molitoris, B. A. (2016). Acute kidney injury. In L. Goldman & A. I. Schafer (Eds.), *Goldman-Cecil medicine* (25th ed., pp. 778-783). Philadelphia, PA: Elsevier Saunders.

Neilson, E. G. (2016). Tubulointerstitial nephritis. In L. Goldman & A. I. Schafer (Eds.), *Goldman-Cecil medicine* (25th ed., pp. 793–799). Philadelphia, PA: Elsevier Saunders.

Nicolle, L. E., & Norrby, S. R. (2016). Approach to the patient with urinary tract infection. In L. Goldman & A. I. Schafer (Eds.), *Goldman-Cecil medicine* (25th ed., pp. 1872–1876). Philadelphia, PA: Elsevier Saunders.

Rydell, H., Clyne, N., & Segelmark, M. (2016). Home- or institutional hemodialysis?—A matched pair-cohort study comparing survival and some modifiable factors related to survival. *Kidney and Blood Pressure Research*, *41*(4), 392–401.

Schroeder, K. (2012). Acute renal failure. In E. T. Bope & R. D. Kellerman (Eds.), *Conn's current therapy 2012* (pp. 873–877). Philadelphia, PA: Elsevier Saunders.

Shakarchi, J. A., Nath, J., McGrogan, D., Khawaja, A., Field, M., Jones, R. G., & Inston, N. (2015). End-stage vascular access failure: Can we define and can we classify? *Clinical Kidney Journal*, *8*(5), 590–593.

Vartanian, V., & Park, S. (2012). Renal calculi. In E. T. Bope & R. D. Kellerman (Eds.), *Conn's current therapy 2012* (pp. 904–906). Philadelphia, PA: Elsevier Saunders.

Yu, A. S. L. (2016). Disorders of magnesium and phosphorus. In L. Goldman & A. I. Schafer (Eds.), *Goldman-Cecil medicine* (25th ed., pp. 774–778). Philadelphia, PA: Elsevier Saunders

Zeidel, M. L. (2016). Obstructive uropathy. In L. Goldman & A. I. Schafer (Eds.), Goldman-*Cecil medicine* (25th ed., pp. 799–803). Philadelphia, PA: Elsevier Saunders.

CHAPTER 31

Conditions of the Gastrointestinal System

STRUCTURE AND FUNCTION OF THE GASTROINTESTINAL SYSTEM

The primary function of the *gastrointestinal system* is the conversion of nutrients, water, and electrolytes from food into energy that helps the body function, as well as temporary storage and excretion of undigested waste (Doig & Huether, 2014). The *gastrointestinal tract* (*alimentary canal*) consists of the mouth, esophagus, stomach, small and large intestines, rectum, and anus (**Figure 31-1**).

The Digestive Process

The digestive process begins in the mouth (*oral* or *buccal cavity*), where teeth break food into smaller particles. The teeth at the front of the mouth (*incisors*) provide a cutting action, while the teeth at the back of the mouth (*molars*) provide a grinding action. Breaking food into smaller particles not only facilitates passage of food into the stomach but also enlarges the surface area available for gastric juices to begin the digestive process when food reaches the stomach.

While still in the mouth, smaller particles of food are mixed with *saliva*, which lubricates and softens food, and facilitates its passage down the throat. Saliva, which is produced by the *parotid glands, submaxillary glands*, and *sublingual glands*, contains an enzyme that begins the breakdown of sugars.

Food passes from the *pharynx* (throat) into a muscular tube called the *esophagus*, which leads from the mouth to the stomach. The esophagus and *trachea* (windpipe) have a common opening at the pharynx. A flap called the *epiglottis* closes over the opening to the trachea when food is swallowed, ensuring that food will pass into the esophagus rather than the trachea. The esophagus moves food along via rhythmic, muscular movements called *peristalsis*.

The esophagus passes through a muscular wall called the *diaphragm*, which separates the *thoracic cavity* (chest cavity) from the *abdominal cavity*. The abdominal cavity contains the stomach, intestines, and other abdominal organs and is lined with a thin membrane called the *peritoneum*. The esophagus passes through the diaphragm to reach the stomach. Food enters the stomach from the esophagus through an opening called the lower esophageal sphincter, also known as the *cardiac sphincter*. Pressure gradients around this opening prevent the backflow of food and gastric juices into the esophagus from the stomach.

The stomach is a muscular organ that stores, mixes, and liquefies food. It contains gastric juices, which continue the digestive process. One component of gastric juice, *hydrochloric acid*, kills most organisms that enter the stomach. *Pepsin*, the primary enzyme of gastric juice, digests protein in the presence of hydrochloric acid. Also produced in the stomach is *intrinsic factor*, a substance that is necessary for the absorption of vitamin B_{12}. Gastric secretion is stimulated by the *vagus nerve* as well as by the presence of food in the stomach. The stomach lining is protected from irritation and action of the gastric enzymes by a thin layer of mucus, which is secreted by tiny glands within the

Figure 31-1 The Gastrointestinal System

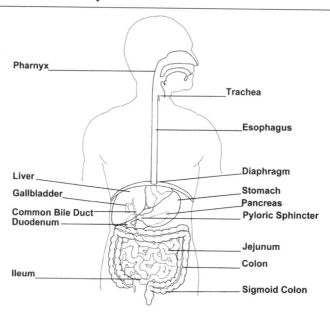

Pharnyx

Trachea

Esophagus

Diaphragm

Liver

Gallbladder

Common Bile Duct

Duodenum

Stomach

Pancreas

Pyloric Sphincter

Jejunum

Colon

Ileum

Sigmoid Colon

© Jane Tinkler Lamm.

stomach's lining. Although some alcohol, water, sugars, and drugs are absorbed in the stomach, most digestion and absorption take place in the small intestine.

From the stomach, food passes through an opening called the *pyloric sphincter* into the small intestine. The small intestine is approximately divided into three parts. The first part of the small intestine, the *duodenum*, is approximately 10 inches long and is connected to the stomach at the pyloric sphincter. The middle section, the *jejunum*, is approximately 8 feet long. The last part of the small intestine, the *ileum*, connects to the large intestine and is approximately 12 feet long. Digested food continues to move through these sections of the gastrointestinal tract by peristaltic movements. Most nutrients are absorbed in the small intestine. Although some fluid is also absorbed in the small intestine, most fluid is absorbed in the large intestine. Thus the contents of the small intestine tend to be liquid in nature.

The small and large intestines are connected by the *ileocecal valve,* which allows the contents of

the small intestine to flow into the large intestine but prevents their backflow. The large intestine (*colon*) is only approximately 5 feet long, but, like the small intestine, it is divided into parts. The part attached to the small intestine at the ileocecal valve is the *cecum*, to which the *appendix* is attached. The major portion of the large intestine is divided into the *ascending colon, transverse colon, descending colon*, and *sigmoid colon*. The sigmoid colon leads to the *rectum,* which leads to the *anus*, the opening through which solid waste is excreted from the body. The large intestine collects food residue and is the site of most water absorption from intestinal contents. Consequently, the waste products (*feces*) found in the large intestine are more solid. The brown color of feces is due primarily to *bile pigments* from the liver.

Accessory Organs of Digestion

The liver, gallbladder, and pancreas—sometimes called accessory organs of digestion—are located together in the upper abdominal cavity.

The Liver

The *liver* is the largest single organ in the body and is necessary for survival. In addition to aiding in digestion, the liver is important to *carbohydrate, protein*, and *fat* metabolism. This organ performs the following functions:

- Converts *glucose*, a product of carbohydrate metabolism, into an energy source, *glycogen*
- Stores glycogen until the body needs it
- Converts the end products of protein metabolism into *urea*, which is later excreted by the kidneys
- Manufactures and secretes *bile* for the digestion and absorption of fat
- Breaks down red blood cells
- Produces substances important in coagulation
- Acts as a detoxification center of the body, neutralizing poisonous chemicals and drugs

Two major blood vessels supply the liver with blood: the hepatic artery and the portal vein. The *hepatic artery* carries oxygenated blood to the liver. The *portal vein* carries blood containing nutrients and toxins from the pancreas, spleen, stomach, and intestine for processing, metabolism, or detoxification by the liver. Once blood has been filtered and processed, it returns to the systemic circulation through the *hepatic vein*, which joins the vena cava where it returns to the heart.

The Gallbladder

The *gallbladder*, a small sac that stores *bile*, is located on the underside of the liver. Bile leaves the liver via the *hepatic ducts* and enters the gallbladder through the cystic duct. When the gallbladder contracts, bile flows through the common bile duct into the small intestine. Bile, along with bile salts, contains *bilirubin*, an orange pigment formed from the breakdown of red blood cells. *Bile salts are important to fat digestion and absorption.*

The Pancreas

The *pancreas*, in addition to its *endocrine function* of producing the hormones *insulin* and *glucagon*, also plays an important *exocrine function* in digestion. The pancreas lies behind the stomach and produces *pancreatic juice*, which contains enzymes to digest *fats, carbohydrates*, and *proteins*. Pancreatic juices enter the *common bile duct* through the *pancreatic duct* and then continue to the small intestine.

CONDITIONS OF THE MOUTH

Although usually not a major cause of incapacitation, conditions of the mouth can contribute to the development of other more serious conditions, interfere with nutrition, and affect social functioning.

Dental caries (tooth decay) and **periodontal disease** (inflammation of the tissues that surround and support the teeth) can lead to the loss of the teeth, allow for the development of infection, and affect self-esteem and social participation. The early form of the periodontal disease **gingivitis** (inflammation of the gums), if not managed properly, can develop into the more severe gum condition known as **periodontitis**; this condition can, in turn, lead to the destruction of underlying tissues and subsequent tooth loss.

Loss of teeth has implications not only for cosmetic appearance but also for nutrition and general health. Moreover, periodontal disease has been implicated as contributing to a number of other systemic conditions, such as cardiovascular disease.

Inability to chew food adequately due to tooth loss may limit food intake and interfere with the initial digestive process. Dentures may enhance the ability to chew food and be important cosmetically, but they cannot match the effectiveness of natural teeth for chewing. Dental caries and periodontal disease are best managed through prevention, early detection, and early management.

Other conditions of the mouth that may interfere with proper nutrition include **stomatitis** (inflammation of the mouth) and **parotitis** (inflammation of the parotid glands). Stomatitis can be the result of infection, injury, toxic agents, or systemic health condition (Daniels,

2012). Parotitis can result from inactivity of the glands due to lack of oral intake; can be caused by infection, such as mumps; can arise as a side effect of medications; or may be related to another health condition such as HIV infection. Management of both stomatitis and parotitis is directed toward correcting or alleviating the underlying cause.

CONDITIONS OF THE ESOPHAGUS

General Conditions of the Esophagus

Dysphagia (difficulty in swallowing) is a major manifestation of a variety of conditions. One cause of dysphagia is **stricture** (narrowing) of portions of the esophagus because of injury or obstruction. When dysphagia is caused by narrowing or constriction of the esophagus, the goal of management is to widen the opening of the passageway. To do so, the opening may be dilated repeatedly with a dilating instrument, or surgical repair may be necessary. When narrowing is caused by a tumor, surgical removal of the tumor or part of the esophagus may be indicated. Dysphagia may also be caused by neurologic conditions, such as *stroke* or *multiple sclerosis.*

Achalasia (cardiospasm) is a type of dysphagia believed to be caused by degeneration of the nerves that innervate muscles of the esophagus. As a result, motility of the lower portion of the esophagus is decreased, and food is unable to pass into the stomach efficiently. Food accumulates in the lower esophagus, causing esophageal irritation (**esophagitis**) and regurgitation. Emotional upsets can aggravate the problem. In addition to the discomforts of esophagitis and the embarrassment of regurgitation, aspiration of undigested food particles into the lungs may occur, resulting in **atelectasis**.

Management of achalasia aims to reduce the amount of pressure at the lower end of the esophagus, thereby reducing the extent of the obstruction. The opening between the stomach and the esophagus may be dilated mechanically with a dilating instrument or, in more severe cases, by surgery, which involves cutting the muscle fibers of the sphincter of the lower esophagus.

Dyspepsia (indigestion or discomfort in the upper part of the abdomen) is a common manifestation of conditions of the esophagus. It may be experienced either alone or in combination with dysphagia. Among the causes of dyspepsia is **esophageal reflux**, in which stomach contents flow back into the esophagus, irritating the esophageal lining. Esophageal reflux may be managed with medications (e.g., antacids) that decrease acidity, avoidance of smoking, and avoidance of foods or beverages that seem to increase gastric acidity and discomfort. Interventions may include mechanical measures such as sleeping with the head of the bed raised to minimize the amount of reflux by gravity.

Hiatal Hernia (Esophageal Hernia, Diaphragmatic Hernia)

The esophagus passes through an opening in the diaphragm to the stomach. When that opening becomes stretched or weakened, the stomach may protrude through the opening in the diaphragm into the thoracic cavity. This condition, which is called **hiatal hernia**, allows gastric juices to come into contact with the esophageal wall, causing esophagitis (inflammation of the esophagus), dyspepsia (indigestion), and possibly ulceration of the esophagus. Individuals with a hiatal hernia may experience mild to severe pain and discomfort with the development of esophagitis.

A hiatal hernia may not cause extensive functional consequences, but the resulting discomfort and potential complications may nevertheless interfere with individuals' sense of well-being and subsequent productivity. If manifestations are mild, management of hiatal hernia may be similar to the management of esophageal reflux, as described earlier. To decrease the frequency of manifestations, individuals with a hiatal hernia may need to refrain from any activity that increases intra-abdominal pressure, such as strenuous exercise and bending. In addition, they may need to modify the timing and size of meals (such as having four to six small meals per day) to decrease the amount of gastric acid the stomach produces. Raising the head of the bed by approximately 6 inches while sleeping may also decrease gastric discomfort.

In other instances, hiatal hernia may have to be repaired surgically. Surgery returns the stomach to its regular position and makes the opening in the diaphragm smaller so that the stomach cannot again move above the diaphragm.

Gastroesophageal Reflux Disease (Reflux Disease)

Gastroesophageal reflux is a condition in which gastric contents move from the stomach to the esophagus, causing irritation and discomfort. Although reflux occurs in everyone, most individuals have no discomfort or associated damage from this phenomenon. When reflux causes damage or complications, such as erosion or ulceration of the esophagus, the condition is called *gastroesophageal reflux disease* (GERD) (Falk & Katzka, 2016). In most instances, GERD involves the *lower esophageal sphincter* (LES), which connects the esophagus and the stomach. During normal digestion, when food is swallowed, the LES opens to allow food into the stomach. After the food passes the sphincter, the LES usually closes to prevent food and stomach acids from coming in contact with the esophagus. If the sphincter becomes weakened, however, it may not close adequately, allowing stomach contents to flow backward (*reflux*) into the esophagus (*acid regurgitation*), which in turn causes inflammation of the esophagus (esophagitis). When this happens, individuals experience manifestations commonly known as heartburn or acid indigestion. These manifestations cause pressure and burning chest pain, often moving upward to the neck and the throat. Complications of GERD can include ulceration, fibrosis with stricture formation, and Barrett's esophagus (Roberts & Castell, 2012).

Numerous lifestyle and dietary factors have been implicated as playing roles in the development of GERD, although conflicting data have been gathered on the impact of most of these factors, including the role of alcohol and tobacco. Obesity can increase intragastric pressure, which then contributes to LES relaxation and predisposes individuals to GERD (Falk & Katzka, 2016), as may hiatal hernia.

Identification of GERD is based on manifestations and in some instances *endoscopy* (examination of the esophagus through a hollow tube). Short-term management of GERD usually consists of medications to inhibit gastric acid secretion, avoidance of foods that seem to aggravate the condition, consumption of smaller meals, avoidance of large meals later in the day, and weight loss if obesity is an issue.

Barrett's Esophagus

Barrett's esophagus is an acquired condition resulting from tissue changes in the lining of the esophagus due to injury to the mucosal lining, often from GERD. Smoking also contributes to Barrett's esophagus. Manifestations include, in addition to general discomfort, increased duration and severity of reflux manifestations, especially at night, and complications such as esophagitis or bleeding. Management generally consists of medications to relieve manifestations and promote healing; regular endoscopic monitoring; and, in some cases, surgical resection. Although the incidence of esophageal cancer in individuals with Barrett's esophagus is slightly higher than in persons without this condition, the overall cancer risk remains relatively low (Falk & Katzka, 2016).

CONDITIONS OF THE STOMACH
Gastritis

Gastritis is an inflammation of the lining of the stomach that can be caused by a variety of irritants or infectious organisms. *Acute gastritis* is of short duration, with manifestations of nausea, vomiting, and pain; it is generally self-limiting, requiring little intervention except for managing manifestations. *Chronic gastritis*, which is of longer duration, may consist of nondescript upper abdominal distress with vague manifestations. Extensive evaluation may be necessary to identify its causative factors. Chronic gastritis may be caused by irritation of the stomach from medications used to manage another condition (such as aspirin used in the management of rheumatoid arthritis), or it may be a complication of another condition, such as HIV infection. The most common cause of chronic gastritis is infection with the organism *Helicobacter pylori* (Lowe & Wolfe, 2012). If left unmanaged, chronic gastritis can progress to scarring of the stomach lining, ulceration, or hemorrhage.

Peptic Ulcer

Types of Peptic Ulcers

Peptic ulcer disease is a chronic, inflammatory gastrointestinal condition characterized by ulcer formation in the esophagus, stomach, or duodenum. Peptic ulcers in the upper portion of the small intestine are called *duodenal ulcers*; those in the stomach are called *gastric ulcers*. Duodenal ulcers occur more frequently than do gastric ulcers.

Ingestion of spicy food, stress, and lifestyle were once considered to be major causes of peptic ulcers. In the 1980s, the discovery of the bacterium *Helicobacter pylori* and its association with peptic ulcer disease significantly changed the approach to peptic ulcer disease (Lowe & Wolfe, 2012).

H. pylori breaks down the mucosal barrier of the gastric lining and seems to increase gastric acid secretions (Doig & Huether, 2014). Although not everyone who is colonized with *H. pylori* develops peptic ulcers, infection with this organism is a risk factor for individuals with other precipitating factors such as immune response, smoking, and stress (Kuipers & Blaser, 2012).

After infection with *H. pylori*, the second most common risk factor for developing a peptic ulcer is use of aspirin or nonsteroidal anti-inflammatory drugs (NSAIDs) (Kuipers & Blaser, 2012). Although some foods and beverages (e.g., alcohol and caffeine-containing beverages) increase gastric secretion and can irritate the lining of the gastrointestinal tract, there is no evidence to suggest that the intake of these substances alone causes ulcers (Kuipers & Blaser, 2012).

Another type of peptic ulcer, a **stress ulcer**, may develop after an acute physical crisis, such as a severe injury or a serious health condition. Major risk factors for stress ulcers include mechanical ventilation, **hypotension** (low blood pressure), and conditions such as liver or renal failure (Kuipers & Blaser, 2012). Special names are given to stress ulcers that develop with some conditions. For example, stress ulcers associated with burns are called

Curling's ulcers; those associated with head injury are called *Cushing's ulcers*. The reason that these ulcers develop is unknown; however, they develop rapidly, sometimes within 72 hours of the injury or serious health condition. Manifestations may not appear until the ulcer perforates and massive gastric hemorrhage occurs.

Manifestations and Complications of Peptic Ulcer

The most common manifestations of peptic ulcer are epigastric pain, a gnawing or burning pain located in the lower chest above the heart, and dyspepsia (disturbance in digestion), which may include nausea, bloating, or reflux.

Pain or discomfort usually occurs several hours after eating, when the stomach is empty, and is relieved by the ingestion of food, especially in the case of a duodenal ulcer. Bleeding of the ulcer may also occur, causing manifestations of **hematemesis** (vomiting of blood) or **melena** (black, tarry bowel movements). In some instances, blood loss may be enough to cause individuals to become anemic.

Peptic ulcers can be life threatening if complications develop. Two serious complications of peptic ulcer are *hemorrhage* and *perforation*, both of which are emergencies. In perforation, erosion of the ulcer through the gastric lining allows the contents of the gastrointestinal tract to escape into the *peritoneal cavity*, causing irritation of the peritoneal lining. The resulting inflammation of the peritoneum (Prather, 2012) can be fatal.

Identification of Peptic Ulcer

Identification of peptic ulcer disease is based on both manifestations and usually endoscopic examination to detect ulceration or erosion of the gastric wall. *H. pylori* infection can be determined by *biopsy, stool antigen test*, or *urea breath test*. With biopsy, a small tissue sample of the gastric lining is removed during endoscopy and then examined for the presence of *H. pylori*. The stool antigen test involves immunoassay of a fecal sample to detect the presence of this pathogen. For the urea breath test, the individual ingests urea that contains a small amount of radioactive material, which can be traced a short time later when the individual's breath is analyzed. This test is used both to identify the presence of *H. pylori* infection and, after intervention, to confirm eradication of the organism.

Management of Peptic Ulcer

The overall goals in the management of peptic ulcer are to identify and irradiate the cause, relieve discomfort, and heal the ulcer itself. *Antacids* can help to relieve discomfort, and medications to suppress stomach acid secretion such as *H_2 blockers* and *proton pump inhibitors (PPIs)* are major focuses of peptic ulcer management. Although decreasing gastric acid secretion with these medications helps the ulcer to heal, if *H. pylori* infection is present, unless the organism is eradicated ulcers will recur in 50 to 90% of cases (Kuipers & Blaser, 2012). Consequently antibiotic intervention to eradicate *H. pylori* is necessary.

Little evidence suggests that dietary intake causes peptic ulcer or that dietary control is useful in its management. Even so, individuals are generally encouraged to avoid foods that produce discomfort and to use alcohol and coffee only in moderation. Other substances that irritate the stomach lining, such as tobacco, aspirin, and NSAIDs, are generally discontinued as well. Individuals who must continue using aspirin—for example, in the management of arthritis—may be encouraged to use buffered aspirin or enteric-coated aspirin.

Although surgical management of peptic ulcer is rare today, if the ulcer does not respond to therapy or if complications such as uncontrollable bleeding or perforation occur, surgery is indicated.

Functional Implications of Peptic Ulcer

Personal and Psychosocial Issues

Stress had been viewed as a major contributor to development of peptic ulcer prior to the discovery of the organism *H. pylori* as a contributing factor in ulcer formation. Although treatment now focuses on management of the condition rather than lifestyle modification, the role of stress as a factor contributing to development of the peptic ulcers is frequently ignored, but cannot be dismissed. The effects of *H. pylori* and stress may be additive, promoting increased acid secretion (Lowe & Wolfe, 2012). Even though stress alone may not be a causative factor in development of

peptic ulcers, it can certainly worsen manifestations. Consequently, minimizing stress in general and learning stress-reduction techniques may be important parts of the overall management plan for many individuals with peptic ulcers.

Vocational Issues in Peptic Ulcer

In most instances, there are no long-term vocational consequences related solely to peptic ulcers. Because medications are now used predominantly in the management of peptic ulcers (rather than surgery), the incidence of major functional consequences has decreased significantly in recent years. Most individuals, with appropriate and timely management, will be able to continue in their employment. Individuals with additional chronic conditions, individuals who do not have access to appropriate health care, and individuals who are nonadherent to the management plan have a greater chance of experiencing reoccurrence and subsequent complications as a result of their condition.

CONDITIONS OF THE INTESTINE

Hernia

Protrusion of an organ through the tissues that usually hold it in place is called **hernia**. In addition to hiatal hernia (discussed earlier in this chapter), common types of abdominal hernias include *inguinal* and *femoral hernias*, in which the intestine protrudes through a weakened part of the lower abdominal wall. Men are more likely to develop inguinal hernias, whereas women are more likely to develop femoral hernias (Prather, 2012).

Manifestations of hernia are often mild, consisting of little more than a lump or swelling on the lower abdomen underneath the skin. The protrusion may appear when intra-abdominal pressure is increased, such as through coughing or lifting. Application of manual pressure over the hernia often pushes it back into place (reduces the hernia). If the hernia is not reducible, it is said to be *incarcerated,* and can be a discomfort. If the incarcerated hernia become swollen and constricted by the opening, it may become ischemic (lacking blood supply); this condition, called *strangulation*, leads to tissue death and is a surgical emergency.

Uncomplicated hernias have few long-term consequences, although it may be necessary to avoid activities such as lifting or pushing heavy objects. Even though there may be few significant activity-related consequences of hernia, because of the danger of hernia strangulation it is important for individuals to have the hernia evaluated, even though they have no pain. This is especially true if they engage in strenuous work.

The surgical procedure used to repair hernias is called **herniorrhaphy**. In this surgery, the intestine is pushed into place and the weakened abdominal wall repaired.

Inflammatory Bowel Disease

Inflammatory bowel disease (IBD) refers to two chronic lifelong conditions that cause inflammation of the bowel: *Crohn's disease* and *ulcerative colitis*. These conditions can occur at any age and are marked by *remissions* and *exacerbations*. The cause of inflammatory bowel disease is unknown, but three interacting factors—genetic predisposition, immune responses, and environmental antigens—are thought to contribute to its development (Lichtenstein, 2012).

Crohn's Disease

Crohn's disease primarily affects segments of the **ileum** (small intestine), although any part of the gastrointestinal tract may be affected (Swaroop & Podolsky, 2012). It is marked by remissions and exacerbations, and is characterized by abdominal pain, typically in the lower right quadrant; chronic diarrhea; weight loss; and fatigue. The condition's manifestations and unpredictable recurrence cause restrictions on lifestyle and can interfere with work attendance.

Crohn's disease may be complicated by obstruction of the intestine because of **stenosis** (narrowing) of the intestine or by the formation of *abscesses*. Bowel obstruction in Crohn's disease is an emergency. Other complications may include formation of an irregular, tube-like passage (**fistula**) between the small intestine and other parts of the abdominal cavity. In both of these instances, surgical intervention may be necessary.

Ulcerative Colitis

In contrast to Crohn's disease, which mainly affects segments of the small intestine, ulcerative colitis is an inflammatory condition of the **colon** (large intestine), beginning at the rectum or lower end of the colon and spreading upward, and at times involving the entire colon. The colon lining becomes **edematous** (swollen), thickened, and congested with small ulcers that ooze blood. Ulcerative colitis is also marked by remissions and exacerbations, with manifestations usually including cramping abdominal pain and bloody diarrhea.

Ulcerative colitis can include systemic manifestations that range from malnutrition to **arthritis** and **ankylosing spondylitis**. Because individuals with ulcerative colitis have an increased risk of developing cancer of the colon, regular cancer screening is essential (Lichtenstein, 2012).

Nonsurgical Management of Inflammatory Bowel Disease

Management of inflammatory bowel disease is directed toward reducing inflammation, promoting and maintaining remissions, preventing complications, and improving quality of life (Swaroop & Podolsky, 2012). The type of intervention used in management depends on the location and severity of the condition. During exacerbations, physical activity may be kept to a minimum. Individuals may continue working, but may need frequent rest periods. Individuals whose manifestations are severe may require extended bed rest.

Nonsurgical management of Crohn's disease is aimed at reducing manifestations, improving quality of life, and minimizing complications. In mild Crohn's disease, medications such as *sulfasalazine* may be used to prevent or control infection and reduce inflammation. During more intense exacerbations, medications such as *steroids* may be used on a short-term basis. When exacerbations are severe, hospitalization may be necessary, during which time individuals' oral intake is restricted and nutritional support is provided through *total parenteral nutrition (TPN)* (Lichtenstein, 2012).

Nonsurgical management of ulcerative colitis is dependent on the amount of colon affected and the location of ulceration. When only the rectum or the lower portion of the colon is affected, medication may be administered to the local area through suppository or enema. For more severe exacerbations, systemic therapies—steroids, anti-inflammatory medications, or medications that suppress the immune system—may be used (Swaroop & Podolsky, 2012). If individuals experience intractable diarrhea or severe blood loss, hospitalization may be necessary, along with provision of total parenteral nutrition.

Surgical Management of Inflammatory Bowel Disease

When nonsurgical management fails to resolve inflammatory bowel disease or if complications occur, surgery may be indicated.

In Crohn's disease, surgery is not curative but rather is indicated for complications such as obstruction or abscess formation (Lichtenstein, 2012). Surgical management of Crohn's disease may involve removing or resecting the affected portion of the intestine *(segmental resection)* and surgically connecting the two ends of the intestine. This surgical connection is called an **anastomosis**.

In ulcerative colitis, when exacerbations are recurrent and severe so that quality of life is affected, surgical intervention in the form of **colectomy** (removal of the colon) may be needed. For ulcerative colitis, colectomy is curative. Removal of the entire colon does, however, require a permanent **ileostomy** (see **Figure 31-2**) so that all fecal waste is eliminated through this opening rather than through the rectum.

Several different procedures and types of ileostomy may be performed after colectomy. The type of procedure is individually determined based on the individual's age, social circumstances, and general health factors.

In a regular ileostomy, a portion of the small intestine (ileum) is extended through a surgically created opening to the outside of the abdomen, creating a **stoma**, which is exposed to the outer surface of the abdomen. All fecal waste is then excreted through the stoma rather than the rectum. A small plastic bag (an *ostomy bag)* is placed over the stoma to collect fecal waste. A variety of products are also available that may be placed in the

Figure 31-2   Ileostomy

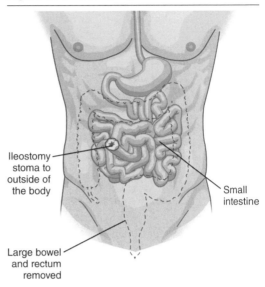

Ileostomy stoma to outside of the body

Small intestine

Large bowel and rectum removed

bag to neutralize odor. The bag is attached by a separate base plate that adheres to the individual's skin and fits snugly around the stoma. A skin barrier paste is typically applied to ensure a tight seal, thereby preventing leakage. Because the stoma of an ileostomy has no sphincter, individuals have no control over the elimination of wastes through it. Individuals with an ileostomy have more liquid and more frequent bowel movements because most liquid is normally removed from fecal matter in the colon. Consequently, they may have more difficulty regulating elimination.

Two other types of ileostomy are the continent ileostomy and ileoanal pouch (**Figures 31-3a & b**). With *continent ileostomy,* an intra-abdominal pouch *(Kock pouch)* is surgically constructed from a portion of the small intestine. Fecal waste collects in the pouch until the individual drains the pouch through the stoma with a catheter. Those persons who have such a pouch need not wear an external appliance. Individuals insert a catheter three or four times each day, as needed, to remove the waste.

With an *ileoanal pouch,* after the colon is removed, the small intestine is sutured to the anal opening. An internal pouch for storing feces is created from the ileum so that individuals are able to have bowel movements through the anus. A temporary ileostomy may be necessary until the

Figure 31-3a   Kock Pouch

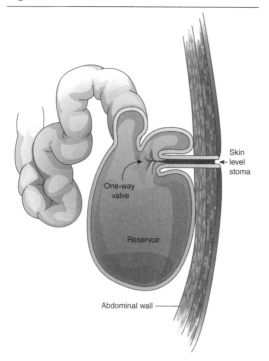

Figure 31-3b   Ileoanal Pouch

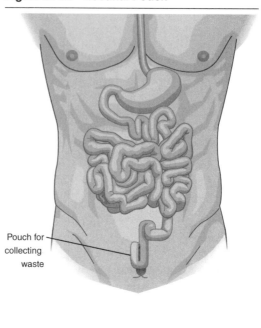

area around the ileoanal pouch heals, but after 2 to 3 months, the ileostomy may be closed and anal elimination resumed.

Functional Implications in Inflammatory Bowel Disease

Personal and Psychosocial Issues

The chronic nature of inflammatory bowel disease, along with its associated remissions and exacerbations, may cause stress due to the inability to predict flare-ups of the condition. Manifestations of the conditions can contribute to additional stress. Bouts of diarrhea and urgency to defecate, along with fear of fecal incontinence, may be stressful and make it difficult for individuals to function effectively in social or work settings.

If surgery is required, some individuals may feel newly liberated by no longer being encumbered with the manifestations and unpredictability of their condition. In other instances, altered body image may occur with the resulting ileostomy, due to the presence of an external stoma or because of the inability to control elimination. Individuals may fear the potential of odor or "embarrassing"

sounds during social interactions and thereby limit social interactions. Educational programs through which individuals receive support as well as practical interventions to alleviate these concerns are important interventions to enable individuals to overcome these fears.

Activities and Participation

For many individuals with inflammatory bowel disease, effective management of manifestations and decreasing remissions will enable them to continue a full and active life. When exacerbations are frequent and severe, however, activities and social interactions may become more limited. The reactions of significant others, family, and friends greatly influence individuals' adjustment to their condition. An atmosphere of acceptance and support is important to individuals' self-esteem and ability to adjust to their condition.

Vocational Issues in Inflammatory Bowel Disease

When in remission, inflammatory bowel disease should have few effects on function in the work setting. During an exacerbation, depending on the severity of manifestations, individuals may have repeated absences from work. In some instances, if the condition is severe, repeated hospitalizations may be needed.

Ileostomy should have no impact on the ability to work. Even so, individuals' own level of comfort (or discomfort) with ileostomy may be a major determinant of the extent to which they continue in their work.

Diverticulitis of the Colon

Diverticulosis of the colon refers to a condition in which small balloon-like sacs or pouches (**diverticula**) develop in the walls of the large intestine (**Figure 31-4**). The emergence of diverticulosis appears to be related to lack of intake of dietary fiber as well as obesity (Prather, 2012). Many individuals experience no manifestations from diverticula and are unaware they are present. Individuals with no manifestations usually experience few consequences and require no special interventions.

Individuals with diverticulosis can, however, develop a condition called **diverticulitis** in which the diverticula become infected and inflamed. In addition to causing manifestations of abdominal pain, **anorexia** (loss of appetite), and fever, diverticulitis can result in complications of abscess formation, intestinal obstruction, fistula formation, and, in some cases, intestinal perforation and hemorrhage (Prather, 2012). Intestinal perforation can result in inflammation of the peritoneum (**peritonitis**), which can be life threatening.

Uncomplicated diverticulitis may be managed with antibiotics. Surgery usually involves a *colon resection*, in which the portion of the bowel containing the inflamed diverticula is removed and the healthy portions of the bowel are rejoined (anastomosis). Individuals who undergo surgery for diverticulitis may be able to resume activities within 2 to 4 weeks after surgery.

Irritable Bowel Syndrome (Spastic Colon)

Irritable bowel syndrome (IBS) is a chronic, intermittent condition of the gastrointestinal tract in which individuals experience spasms of the large intestine; cramping abdominal pain; and

Figure 31-4   Diverticula

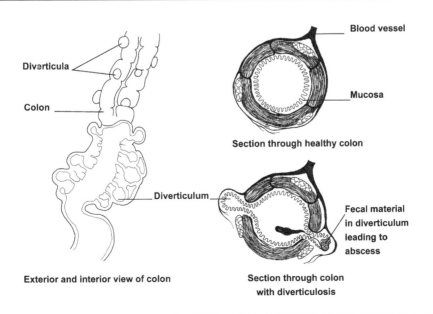

Exterior and interior view of colon

Section through colon with diverticulosis

diarrhea, constipation, or both (Pimentel et al., 2011). It is one of a number of gastrointestinal conditions categorized as *functional conditions*, meaning conditions for which there is no one identifiable organic cause (Mayer, 2012). Thus each functional condition is classified according to manifestations rather than cause. Although functional conditions have widespread differences in their manifestations, they share certain common features related to enhanced sensitivity to stress and heightened sensory perception of abdominal manifestations. Functional conditions also frequently coexist with a number of mental health conditions (Mayer, 2012).

Although there is no general agreement on how stress is related to manifestations of IBS, it has been suggested that in susceptible individuals, overactive autonomic nervous system responses to stimuli such as stress play a part (Mayer, 2012). In these individuals, exaggerated autonomic system response renders the intestine more sensitive to stimuli such as stress, causing heightened intestinal contraction and secretion responsible for manifestations. Although IBS does not cause significant functional consequences, it can affect quality of life and have a large economic impact on healthcare use and indirect costs as a result of absenteeism and decreased productivity in the workplace (Velasco & Fisher, 2012).

Manifestations of Irritable Bowel Syndrome

Although the manifestations and location of abdominal discomfort are highly variable, ranging from mild to very severe, many individuals experience cramping abdominal pain, typically in lower left quadrant of the abdomen, along with an urgent need to defecate, especially after meals. Abdominal manifestations are relieved by defecation, although relief may be temporary.

Identification of Irritable Bowel Syndrome

Minimal tests are advocated in the initial approach to identifying IBS. Identification of this condition is usually made through a detailed history of abdominal pain or discomfort associated with chronic altered bowel habits.

Management of Irritable Bowel Syndrome

Because no specific structural or biochemical-cause of IBS has been established, interventions to effectively manage IBS are limited and there is no cure (Doig & Heuther, 2014). Management is directed toward relieving manifestations and altering response to stress. Dietary modification may be indicated. Foods and beverages that appear to aggravate the manifestations should be avoided. Individuals who experience constipation may be helped by consumption of a high-fiber diet.

Medications such as laxatives for constipation or antidiarrheal medications for diarrhea may also be used, as may medications to reduce intestinal activity or to relieve tension and anxiety. Antispasmodics for pain and tricyclic antidepressants may be prescribed as well.

Educational programs directed toward increasing understanding of the condition and manifestations as well as cognitive-behavioral programs that focus on relaxation techniques and promotion of healthy behaviors may be used to give the individual a sense of control and help in adaptation to the condition.

Individuals with IBS always live with the potential for irregular function of the colon. If an individual is able to identify what triggers the manifestations—whether it is a certain food or a stressful situation—it may be helpful in controlling the occurrence of manifestations. Because the bowel responds to stress, individuals with this syndrome should maintain a healthy lifestyle that includes adequate nutrition, rest, exercise, and recreation.

Functional Implications of Irritable Bowel Syndrome

Personal and Psychosocial Issues

Irritable bowel syndrome can be incapacitating, significantly affecting individuals' quality of life. Individuals may, as a result of their condition, experience a number of concerns related to their social activities, home life, and work.

Manifestations may continue to be a focus of concern, causing individuals to limit their engagement in activities. Because of the frequent, intense need to use the restroom, individuals may be afraid to attend social events or to travel even short distances because of their special needs. There may be increased sensitivity to the physical discomfort they experience and preoccupation with restroom locations.

Learning to identify and avoid triggers of manifestations and to manage exacerbations and stress can increase confidence and support the ability to fully engage in activities of daily life.

Vocational Implications of Irritable Bowel Syndrome

Individuals with IBS have been reported to miss three times as many days from work as individuals without the syndrome (Velasco & Fisher, 2012). Although no specific workplace modifications are necessary, restroom accessibility in the workplace may help relieve anxiety. Learning how to manage stress is also important in overall management of the condition as well as in maintaining productivity in the workplace.

Colon Cancer

Colorectal cancer is the second most common cause of cancer death in the United States for men and women (Centers for Disease Control and Prevention, 2016). Individuals with Crohn's disease and ulcerative colitis (discussed earlier in this chapter)

are at increased risk for developing colorectal cancer (Blanke & Faigel, 2012). Manifestations of such malignancy include bleeding, change in bowel habits, and abdominal pain.

Although in advanced colorectal cancer, a *colectomy* with permanent ileostomy may be needed, more often only a portion of the colon is removed in surgery for this disease. In some instances, a segmental resection of the colon can be performed and the ends *anastomosed* (joined together) with no alteration of bowel function. In other instances, the lower portion of the colon and the rectum are removed and a colostomy created. In **colostomy**, an opening is made in the external surface of the abdomen, and the remaining portion of colon is extended through it to create a stoma through which solid wastes (**feces**) will be excreted. Colostomies may be either temporary or permanent. In some instances, if only a segment of the colon is removed, a temporary colostomy may be used to permit healing, after which the two remaining sections of the colon are again connected. If the lower section of the colon is removed, the colostomy is permanent (see **Figure 31-5a**).

Because the stoma of the colostomy has no sphincter, individuals have no control over elimination

Figure 31-5a   Colostomy

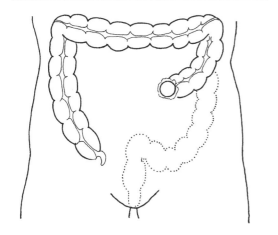

Figure 31-5b   Colostomy with Bag

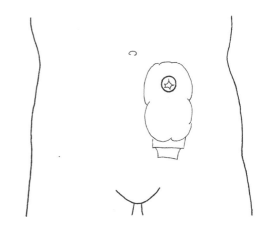

of waste through the stoma. As most liquid from digestion is removed from waste products in the colon, waste excreted through the colostomy is more solid; thus individuals with the colostomy may be able to control the timing of bowel movements through regular daily colostomy irrigation. Individuals with colostomy wear ostomy pouches, like those used with ileostomy. (See **Figure 31-5b**). Some of the same psychosocial issues experienced with ileostomy may be experienced by individuals with colostomy.

CONDITIONS OF THE ACCESSORY ORGANS OF THE GASTROINTESTINAL SYSTEM

Conditions of the Pancreas

Pancreatitis

Pancreatitis is an inflammatory condition of the pancreas that may be either acute or chronic. Pancreatitis begins with activation of digestive enzymes within the pancreas, which produce tissue injury and tissue **necrosis** (death). In addition to the localized damage to the pancreas and surrounding tissues, enzymes can be released into the systemic circulation, producing a systemic inflammatory response that results in multiple organ failure, including renal failure.

Acute Pancreatitis

The most common causes of *acute pancreatitis* in the United States are gallstones and alcohol abuse (Fisher, 2012). Acute pancreatitis may be mild or severe. Manifestations of acute pancreatitis include abdominal pain, nausea, and vomiting. Although most individuals with acute pancreatitis recover within several days without developing chronic pancreatitis, some individuals can develop complications such as pancreatic abscess, infection, or severe bleeding (Forsmark, 2016).

Acute pancreatitis is typically managed in the hospital with intravenous fluids and pain medications during the initial phase of the condition. If there are no complications and early interventions have been implemented, inflammation and manifestations usually subside with no long-term effects.

Chronic Pancreatitis

Chronic pancreatitis involves chronic inflammation of the pancreas with irreversible changes and destruction of tissue typically resulting in permanent loss of pancreatic function. Most cases are caused by alcohol abuse (Fisher, 2012). Manifestations of chronic pancreatitis may be similar to those of acute pancreatitis, including severe abdominal pain, often radiating to the back and frequently accompanied by nausea and vomiting. As the condition progresses and pancreatic function is lost, individuals may experience weight loss due to the pancreas's inability to produce enzymes needed in the digestive process. As pancreatic function continues to decline, *endocrine function* of the pancreas is affected, so secondary conditions such as *diabetes* occur.

Although damage to the pancreas will be permanent, interventions to manage chronic pancreatitis may involve hospitalization for control of pain. Abstinence from alcohol and tobacco is crucial, but does not reverse pancreatic damage. Because pancreatic enzyme production necessary for digestion is lost, individuals may require enzyme supplements as well as supplementation with vitamin D to prevent the development of *osteoporosis*. Individuals who develop diabetes as a result of chronic pancreatitis will also require interventions to manage that disease. Surgical interventions are usually reserved for only the most severe cases.

Pancreatic Cancer

Pancreatic cancer usually refers to ductal *adenocarcinoma*, the most common form of cancer of the pancreas (Tempero & Brand, 2012). Pancreatic neuroendocrine tumors (pNETs) are less common (Jensen, 2016). Risk factors for developing pancreatic cancer include cigarette smoking and genetic predisposition (Tempero & Brand, 2012).

Conditions of the Gallbladder: Cholelithiasis and Cholecystitis

One of the most common conditions of the gallbladder is the presence of gallstones, also called **cholelithiasis** (Caddy, 2012). Although most individuals with gallstones have no manifestations, in some instances gallstones may block the cystic duct, causing injury to the gallbladder and preventing the passage of bile that is stored there (Fogel & Sherman, 2016). As a result, the gallbladder becomes inflamed, a condition called **cholecystitis**. Although cholecystitis can occur in individuals with severe trauma or other critical health conditions even if they do not have gallstones, an obstruction of the cystic duct by a gallstone is the most common cause of this condition (Caddy, 2012).

Manifestations of cholecystitis include severe pain in the upper abdomen, often accompanied by nausea and vomiting. Initial management of this condition may begin with the elimination from the diet of fatty and highly seasoned foods that aggravate the condition. For uncomplicated cholecystitis, individuals may also receive intravenous fluids and antibiotics.

Possible complications of cholecystitis include infection and perforation of the gallbladder, damage to the liver, and pancreatitis. Obstruction of the bile duct with a gallstone can cause elevation of bilirubin in the plasma (**hyperbilirubinemia**), leading to **jaundice** (a yellowish appearance of the skin and the whites of the eyes) (Berk & Korenblat, 2012).

The curative intervention for cholelithiasis is surgical removal of the gallbladder, a procedure called **cholecystectomy**. Today cholecystectomy is often performed through a small incision and insertion of a tube called a *laparoscope*—a technique called *laparoscopic cholecystectomy*. This procedure eliminates the need for large incisions through the muscles of the abdominal wall. Consequently, cholecystectomy is often performed in an ambulatory surgical setting, with individuals going home 24 to 48 hours after surgery.

In instances in which only a single stone is present, extracorporeal shock wave lithotripsy may be performed to fragment the stone. However, only a small percentage of individuals meet this criteria (Fogel & Sherman, 2016).

CONDITIONS OF THE LIVER

Hepatitis

The term *hepatitis* refers to conditions characterized by inflammation of the liver, which can cause permanent liver damage. While *infectious* and *autoimmune hepatitis* are among the more frequent causes of liver damage, the liver may also be damaged by drugs, alcohol, or other toxic substances (**hepatotoxicity**). Although manifestations of liver inflammation and subsequent liver damage may be the same in hepatitis resulting from noninfectious causes and hepatitis resulting from infectious causes, noninfectious hepatitis does not require the same level of precaution to prevent its spread.

Acute Viral Hepatitis

Several viruses can cause *acute hepatitis*, including *hepatitis A virus (HAV)*, *hepatitis B virus (HBV)*, *hepatitis C virus (HCV)*, *hepatitis D virus (HDV)*, and *hepatitis E virus (HEV)*. These viruses are transmitted in different ways, but they all initiate an inflammatory process in the liver that interferes with its effective functioning. Hepatitis is categorized according to the cause.

Hepatitis A

Hepatitis A, caused by HAV, is a highly contagious type of infectious hepatitis and is usually transmitted by the oral–fecal route through ingestion of food or water contaminated with fecal material due to poor personal hygiene or poor sanitation. Affected individuals usually experience initial flu-like manifestations such as weakness, *malaise* (a feeling of general fatigue or discomfort), or body aches. Later, individuals may develop jaundice, along with **hepatomegaly** (enlargement of the liver) and **splenomegaly** (enlargement of the spleen).

Hepatitis A is identified through blood tests. There is no specific medication or intervention available that can eradicate the infection. Acute hepatitis A infection is usually self-limited (Wedemeyer & Pawlotsky, 2012). Usually, this disease resolves spontaneously after 1 to 2 months. During that interval, management is directed toward alleviating the manifestations and maintaining the individual's state of health. Rest and adequate nutrition as well as abstinence from alcohol during recovery are the cornerstones of management.

Individuals with hepatitis may generally return to work after their jaundice disappears and they feel sufficiently strong to resume their duties. Vaccination for hepatitis A is available for individuals at high risk for contracting this virus, such as travelers to areas where the rate of infection is high.

Hepatitis B

Hepatitis B, which is caused by HBV, is a major health problem. Initial manifestations may consist of flu-like manifestations, although sometimes individuals experience no manifestations with early-stage disease. Eventually, jaundice may appear because of an excess of bilirubin in the blood, with associated **pruritus** (itching of the skin).

The hepatitis B virus can live in all body fluids and is transmitted by contact with blood, semen, and vaginal fluids. This virus may be spread through injection with contaminated needles when injecting drugs and through tattooing, ear piercing, electrolysis, or acupuncture. It may also be transmitted through contact with contaminated body fluids during sexual intercourse and through sharing of personal care items such as razors or toothbrushes with someone with hepatitis B. Pregnant women who are positive for HBV may transmit the virus to their babies at birth. Hepatitis B is identified through a blood test. In some instances, interferon may be used in the management of this infection (Garber & Pratt, 2012).

There is no cure for hepatitis B. Once individuals are infected with HBV, they continue to be carriers of the virus. Consequently, individuals who are HBV positive should take steps to avoid transmission of the virus to others by using barrier protection during sexual intercourse, not sharing needles or other items, such as toothbrushes or razors, and not donating blood. Although there is no cure for HBV, it can be prevented. Prevention is based on vaccination. Many countries have established routine vaccination of infants and adolescents and vaccination of high-risk adults (Wedemeyer & Pawlotsky, 2012).

Hepatitis C

Hepatitis C, which is caused by HCV, is one of the leading indications for liver transplantation (Chung, 2012). This infection is contracted primarily through the transfusion of contaminated blood or blood products or from infected needles. Transmission through sexual contact and mother-to-fetus transmission can occur, but are not as common.

Individuals with hepatitis C may experience no manifestations, or they may develop flu-like manifestations, such as anorexia (lack of appetite), chills and fever, nausea and vomiting, or headache.

Management of hepatitis C may include a combination of medications such as *interferon* and *ribavirin* (Garber & Pratt, 2012). There is currently no immunization available to prevent hepatitis C infections. Consequently, the best prevention is avoidance of high-risk behaviors.

Hepatitis D

Hepatitis D, which is caused by HDV, is spread primarily through injection-drug use and sexual activity. Manifestations of the condition are similar to those seen with other forms of hepatitis. There is no specific intervention for the management of hepatitis D. Vaccination for HBV does, however, protect individuals from HDV infection (Wedemeyer & Pawlotsky, 2012).

Hepatitis E

Hepatitis E, which is caused by HEV, is acquired most frequently through exposure to food or drinking water contaminated with fecal material in countries in which hepatitis E is endemic. It is rarely transmitted from person to person. Manifestations of hepatitis E are similar to those for hepatitis A. There is no specific intervention or vaccine available for HEV.

Chronic Hepatitis

Chronic hepatitis describes a condition in which there is chronic inflammation of the liver. Although the major cause of chronic hepatitis is infection by HBV and HCV, chronic hepatitis may also be due to autoimmunity and chronic alcohol use (Pawlotsky & McHutchison, 2012). When liver inflammation persists for more than 3 to 6 months, individuals are said to have chronic hepatitis. This condition may lead to progressive fibrous changes in the liver or cirrhosis. The prognosis is variable, depending on the cause.

Toxic Hepatitis

Because the liver metabolizes and detoxifies many drugs as well as other toxic or poisonous substances, overexposure to or presence of **hepatotoxins** (substances that are harmful to the liver) can cause liver damage and chronic liver disease. Toxin-induced and drug-induced liver injury accounts for more than 50% of all cases of liver failure in the United States (Lee, 2012). The prognosis depends on the extent of the liver damage and the prevention of associated complications.

Fatty Liver Disease

Fatty liver disease refers to conditions in which lipid accumulation in the liver causes this organ to become enlarged. Two common types are *alcoholic fatty liver disease* and *nonalcoholic fatty liver disease*. Risk factors for alcoholic fatty liver disease include excessive alcohol consumption, whereas nonalcoholic fatty liver disease does not involve excessive alcohol intake but rather is related to obesity and diabetes. Alcoholic fatty liver is often reversible if there is total abstinence from alcohol, whereas development of *alcoholic hepatitis* carries a high mortality rate (Chalasani, 2012).

Nonalcoholic fatty liver disease is one of the most common causes of chronic liver disease in Western countries (Targher, Day, & Bonora, 2010). In nonalcoholic liver disease, lifestyle modification with dietary restriction of saturated fat, high sugar intake, and alcohol, along with weight loss and exercise, can reduce progression of the condition. Even so, nonalcoholic fatty liver disease can progress to cirrhosis and liver failure.

Cirrhosis

Cirrhosis is the final stage of liver disease from any cause. It is characterized by fibrosis of liver tissue and structural changes in which liver function becomes altered. Chronic viral hepatitis C and alcoholic liver disease (both discussed earlier in this chapter) are the most common causes of cirrhosis (Garcia-Tsao, 2016).

Many individuals with cirrhosis have no manifestations until the late stages of liver disease or until complications occur. Complications of cirrhosis include *portal hypertension* with accompanying development of varices and ascites. Blood flow to and from the liver depends on proper functioning of both the portal vein and the hepatic artery. When the liver is damaged, blood flow is altered so that the spleen and other organs that empty into the portal system become congested. The increased pressure causes veins in the abdominal wall to dilate and distend, a condition called **varices**. Varices can rupture, causing hemorrhage. **Ascites** refers to fluid accumulation in the abdomen. In cirrhosis, ascites results from portal hypertension due to changes in pressure that allows plasma to leak from the portal vein into the peritoneal cavity.

Management of varices includes medication to constrict blood vessels and, in some instances, if bleeding persists, surgical or radiologic placement of a shunt for decompression (Garcia-Tsao, 2016). Management of ascites consists of sodium and fluid restriction and diuretics. In severe instances, fluid may need to be drained from the abdomen, in a procedure called **paracentesis** (Kalia, Grewal, & Martin, 2012).

Liver transplantation is considered when end-stage liver disease has progressed to the point that the potential for survival without transplantation is low. The most common indications for liver transplantation in adults are chronic hepatitis C and alcoholic liver disease (Everson, 2016). Although much progress has been made in the field of liver transplantation, complications, including development of renal failure, remain a major risk (Weber, Ibrahim, & Lake, 2012). The outcome of cirrhosis depends on the stage of the condition and the development and severity of complications.

GENERAL MANAGEMENT OF CONDITIONS OF THE GASTROINTESTINAL SYSTEM

Medications

A variety of medications are used in management of conditions of the gastrointestinal system (Drugs. com, 2016). These agents may act on either muscular or glandular tissues. Medications frequently used in the management of gastrointestinal conditions are classified as follows:

- Antacids and acid inhibitors—to counteract excess acidity.
- Anticholinergics—to inhibit the action of the involuntary nervous system. In gastrointestinal

conditions, these medications may be given to reduce activity of the intestine or to decrease secretions.

- Antiemetics—to prevent nausea and vomiting. A side effect of these medications may be drowsiness.
- Antimicrobials (e.g., sulfonamides)—to inhibit the growth of microorganisms.
- Antidiarrheals—to prevent diarrhea.
- Digestive enzymes—to replace missing enzyme secretions when there is an enzyme deficiency in the gastrointestinal tract.
  - Laxatives and cathartics—to relieve constipation. Generally, laxatives have mild actions, whereas cathartics have stronger actions.
- Histamine H_2 receptor antagonists (e.g., cimetidine)—to inhibit cells in the stomach lining from producing acid.
- H. Pylori eradication agents—stomach acid inhibitor combined with antibacterial agent
- Proton pump inhibitors (PPIs)—inhibits gastric acid secretion; used for gastric and duodenal ulcers and gastroesophageal reflux disease.

Hyperalimentation (Total Parenteral Nutrition)

When individuals are unable to take nourishment by mouth, or when their nutritional status is compromised, it is possible to bypass the gastrointestinal tract to provide nourishment. Hyperalimentation entails the infusion of a special nutritional solution into a vein. Because of the nature of this solution, infusion usually involves a large vessel such as the *subclavian vein*, located in the upper body. Hyperalimentation may be used in the management of any condition that compromises the individual's nutritional status. It may also be used when there is a need to rest the gastrointestinal tract, as in inflammatory bowel disease, or when there is an obstruction or malabsorption problem in the bowel.

Stress Management

Although stress management may be helpful for a variety of conditions, it is often especially useful in the management of conditions affecting the gastrointestinal tract. Stress itself may not be a direct cause of many conditions of the gastrointestinal tract, but it may exacerbate or prolong an acute episode in some patients with an existing condition.

The body has a number of defensive mechanisms that take action in the face of threat or danger. When stress is encountered, a variety of physiologic reactions take place in the body, including in the gastrointestinal tract. The digestive system responds differently to different kinds of emotional stimuli. For example, it may become more or less active, and it may secrete more or less gastric juice. The intensity of the physiologic reaction depends on the individual and on the situation.

Stress management helps individuals to control their reactions to stress. Programs in stress management may vary from exercise to techniques that alter the body's response to stress, such as biofeedback.

GENERAL FUNCTIONAL IMPLICATIONS OF CONDITIONS OF THE GASTROINTESTINAL TRACT

Personal and Psychosocial Issues

Although they are not a causative factor in all instances, there appears to be at least some association between psychosocial factors and conditions affecting the gastrointestinal system. Factors that may significantly influence gastrointestinal conditions include nutritional and lifestyle behaviors, such as alcohol and tobacco ingestion. In some instances, gastrointestinal conditions may also be directly related to the management of another condition, such as intake of aspirin for management of rheumatoid arthritis, which in turn results in gastritis.

Conditions that affect the physical processes of eating and elimination have many psychological implications. Throughout life, eating is often associated with pleasure and social interaction. Management of gastrointestinal conditions frequently requires avoidance of substances that irritate the gastrointestinal tract or cause the excessive secretion of gastric juices. When certain types of food and beverages are restricted or when special diets are required, individuals may have difficulty giving up something that they enjoyed.

Elimination is associated with privacy and personal cleanliness. The modification of elimination habits is learned in childhood as part of the socialization process. Individuals with problems of elimination may fear embarrassment and social ridicule as a result of their condition. Those with an ileostomy or a colostomy may fear the loss of physical and sexual attractiveness because of odor or embarrassing sounds. Individuals who have inflammatory bowel disease accompanied by diarrhea may fear fecal incontinence and concomitant humiliation.

Other psychosocial responses to gastrointestinal system conditions are common as well. Individuals with hepatitis may fear transmitting the condition, whereas individuals with ulcerative colitis may be preoccupied with their increased risk of cancer. Depression is common in individuals with irritable bowel syndrome. The identification and resolution of these reactions may be crucial to rehabilitation.

Emotions affect the involuntary nervous system, which in turn affects the gastrointestinal tract. For example, anxiety may contribute to flare-ups of many conditions, such as inflammatory bowel disease. Although rest and relaxation are of prime importance in the management of many gastrointestinal conditions, individuals may find it difficult to modify their schedules, to adjust to new life patterns, or to alter stressful situations at home or work. Often, directions to "rest and relax" are useless, unless individuals are assisted with education on methods and techniques to do so.

Although many conditions of the gastrointestinal tract do not affect body image, individuals with an ileostomy or a colostomy may encounter problems with both body image and self-concept. Specifically, they may perceive themselves as being different from others. They may also visualize themselves as unattractive and believe that they must wear shapeless, dowdy clothes to hide the ileostomy or colostomy bag. It is often helpful if individuals are able to meet other persons who have a similar condition and are leading active lives.

Many conditions of the gastrointestinal tract require permanent alterations in lifestyle and constant control over emotional tension. At times, individuals with such conditions may exhibit manifestations of the condition that are out of proportion to the objective findings. Educational programs and support can help individuals make the recommended alterations and maintain as regular a lifestyle as possible.

Activities and Participation

Engagement in a healthy lifestyle, including adequate nutrition, rest, and exercise, in the face of any chronic condition contributes to individuals' ability to reach their optimal functional capacity. This is especially true of gastrointestinal conditions, because stress, fatigue, and emotions appear to have at least some direct effects on the digestive system. Individuals who are accustomed to performing in high-pressure, high-stress situations may need to learn ways to decrease the stressful aspects of their daily life or work and employ coping mechanisms that enable them to deal with stress.

Many gastrointestinal conditions carry notable nutritional implications; thus, in many situations, diet is the cornerstone of management. For individuals whose work or daily schedule is erratic, meeting these dietary demands may be difficult. Alterations and restrictions of diet are often based on avoiding foods that appear to cause distress. Food, however, is a part of celebration and socialization as well as a means of nourishment. When specific conditions of the gastrointestinal system prohibit individuals from eating or from having foods that have typically been part of their social milieu, their social interactions may be adversely affected. Depending on the meanings that these foods have for individuals, it may be difficult to abide by the restrictions. In most instances, eating well-balanced, regular meals is part of the management plan.

Alcohol intake is not necessarily always restricted in gastrointestinal conditions, but it may be limited. Tobacco use is restricted for many individuals with gastrointestinal conditions. Depending on individuals' former habits and the importance of alcohol and tobacco use to their social circle, both of these recommendations may be difficult to follow.

Social situations that are stressful for individuals with conditions affecting the gastrointestinal system may cause a flare-up of the disorder. To avoid such stress, some individuals with gastrointestinal manifestations may withdraw from many social activities. For individuals with an ileostomy or a colostomy, problems may arise if family members do not understand the need for a specific schedule or the care routines involved. The acceptance of the individual by family members and friends often determines to a great degree the acceptance of the condition by the individual.

Sexuality

In most instances, conditions of the gastrointestinal tract do not directly affect sexual function. Individuals may, however, be reluctant to engage in sexual activity if their gastrointestinal condition affects body image or if they fear fecal incontinence. Those with an ileostomy or a colostomy may have fears of defecation during sexual contact or may be self-conscious about the stoma itself. In some cases, men may become impotent as a result of nerve damage caused by the surgical procedure. Open discussion about such issues is important to uncover underlying fears and concerns, as well as to provide information that can help individuals and their partners deal with such issues.

GENERAL VOCATIONAL IMPLICATIONS OF CONDITIONS OF THE GASTROINTESTINAL TRACT

In most instances, special work restrictions are not necessary for individuals with gastrointestinal conditions. Those persons with a diverticular condition or hernia may need to avoid activities that increase intra-abdominal pressure, such as lifting or bending.

Modifications in the work environment or work schedule may occasionally be necessary for those individuals with other gastrointestinal conditions. For example, erratic or rotating schedules may make it difficult for individuals with peptic ulcer to eat regular, well-balanced meals, aggravating the condition. Work situations that cause undue stress may contribute to a flare-up of certain gastrointestinal conditions. If schedules or workload cannot be changed, individuals may need to learn different ways of expressing tension and coping with

stress. Special considerations, such as the ready availability of restrooms with adequate privacy in the workplace, may be necessary for individuals who experience diarrhea as a manifestation of a gastrointestinal condition or for those who have an ileostomy or a colostomy that may need attention during the day.

CASE STUDY

Mr. G. is a pharmacy technician who has experienced a number of remissions and exacerbations of ulcerative colitis. Over the past 6 months, exacerbations of the condition have interfered with his ability to maintain his regular work schedule. As a result of the worsening of his condition, Mr. G. has decided to have a colectomy.

1. Which specific issues may Mr. G. experience as a result of the surgery?
2. Are there specific factors that Mr. G. may need to consider when returning to employment as a pharmacy technician?

REFERENCES

Berk, P., & Korenblat, K. (2012). Approach to the patient with jaundice or abnormal liver tests. In L. Goldman & A. I. Schafer (Eds.), *Goldman's Cecil Medicine,* (24th ed., pp. 956–966). Philadelphia, PA: Elsevier Saunders.

Blanke, C. D., & Faigel, D. O. (2012). Neoplasms of the small and large intestine. In L. Goldman & A. I. Schafer (Eds.), *Goldman's Cecil Medicine,* (24th ed., pp. 1278–1289). Philadelphia, PA: Elsevier Saunders.

Caddy, G. R. (2012). Cholelithiasis and cholecystitis. In E. T. Bope & R. D. Kellerman (Eds.), *Conn's current therapy 2012,* (pp. 490–493). Philadelphia, PA: Elsevier Saunders.

Centers for Disease Control and Prevention (2016). Colorectal (Colon) Cancer. Division of Cancer Prevention and Control. Retrieved from http://www.cdc.gov/cancer/colorectal

Chalasani, N. P. (2012). Alcoholic and nonalcoholic steatohepatitis. In L. Goldman & A. I. Schafer (Eds.), *Goldman's Cecil Medicine,* (24th ed., pp. 996–999). Philadelphia, PA: Elsevier Saunders.

Chung, R. T. (2012). A watershed moment in the treatment of hepatitis C. *New England Journal of Medicine, 366*(3), 273–275.

Daniels, T. E. (2012). Diseases of the mouth and salivary glands. In L. Goldman & A. I. Schafer (Eds.), *Goldman's Cecil Medicine,* (24th ed., pp. 2449–2454). Philadelphia, PA: Elsevier Saunders.

Doig, A. K., & Huether, S. E. (2014). The digestive system: The structure and function of the digestive system. In

K. L. McCance, S.E. Huether, V. L. Brashers & N. S. Rote (Eds.). *Pathophysiology: The biologic basis for disease in adults or children,* (7th ed., pp. 1393–1413). St. Louis MO: Elsevier-Mosby.

Drugs.com. (2016). Gastrointestinal agents. Retrieved from http://www.drugs.com/drug-class/gastrointestinal-agents.html

Everson, G. T. (2016). Hepatic failure and liver transplantation. In L. Goldman & A. I. Schafer (Eds.), *Goldman-Cecil Medicine,* (25th ed., pp. 1031–1038). Philadelphia, PA: Elsevier Saunders.

Falk, G. W., & Katzka, D. A. (2016). Diseases of the esophagus. In L. Goldman & A. I. Schafer (Eds.), *Goldman-Cecil Medicine,* (25th ed., pp. 896–908). Philadelphia, PA: Elsevier Saunders.

Fisher, W. E. (2012). Acute and chronic pancreatitis. In E. T. Bope & R. D. Kellerman (Eds.), *Conn's current therapy 2012,* (pp. 479–486). Philadelphia, PA: Elsevier Saunders.

Fogel, E. L., & Sherman, S. (2016). Diseases of the gallbladder and bile ducts. In L. Goldman & A. I. Schafer (Eds.), *Goldman-Cecil Medicine,* (25th ed., pp. 1038–1048). Philadelphia, PA: Elsevier Saunders.

Forsmark, C. E. (2016). Pancreatitis. In L. Goldman & A. I. Schafer (Eds.), *Goldman-Cecil Medicine,* (25th ed., pp. 959–967). Philadelphia, PA: Elsevier Saunders.

Garber, J., & Pratt, D. (2012). Acute and chronic viral hepatitis. In E. T. Bope & R. D. Kellerman (Eds.), *Conn's current therapy 2012,* (pp. 486–490). Philadelphia, PA: Elsevier Saunders.

Garcia-Tsao, G. (2016). Cirrhosis and its sequelae. In L. Goldman & A. I. Schafer (Eds.), *Goldman-Cecil Medicine,* (25th ed., pp. 1023–1031). Philadelphia, PA: Elsevier Saunders.

Jensen, R. T. (2016). Pancreatic neuroendocrine tumors. In L. Goldman & A. I. Schafer (Eds.), *Goldman-Cecil Medicine,* (25th ed., pp. 1334–1339). Philadelphia, PA: Elsevier Saunders.

Kalia, H., Grewal, P., & Martin, P. (2012). Cirrhosis. In E. T. Bope & R. D. Kellerman (Eds.), *Conn's current therapy 2012,* (pp. 493–501). Philadelphia, PA: Elsevier Saunders.

Kuipers, E. J., & Blaser, M. J. (2012). Acid peptic disease. In L. Goldman & A. I. Schafer (Eds.), *Goldman's Cecil Medicine,* (24th ed., pp. 886–895). Philadelphia, PA: Elsevier Saunders.

Lee, W. M. (2012). Toxin- and drug-induced liver disease. In L. Goldman & A. I. Schafer (Eds.), *Goldman's Cecil Medicine,* (24th ed., pp. 979–984). Philadelphia, PA: Elsevier Saunders.

Lichtenstein, G. R. (2012). Inflammatory bowel disease. In L. Goldman & A. I. Schafer (Eds.), *Goldman's Cecil*

Medicine, (24th ed., pp. 913–921). Philadelphia, PA: Elsevier Saunders.

Lowe, R. C., & Wolfe, M. (2012). Gastritis and peptic ulcer disease. In E. T. Bope & R. D. Kellerman (Eds.), *Conn's current therapy 2012,* (pp. 513–522). Philadelphia, PA: Elsevier Saunders.

Mayer, E. A. (2012). Functional gastrointestinal disorders: Irritable bowel syndrome, dyspepsia, and functional chest pain of presumed esophageal origin. In L. Goldman & A. I. Schafer (Eds.), *Goldman's Cecil Medicine,* (24th ed., pp. 868–874). Philadelphia, PA: Elsevier Saunders.

Pawlotsky, J. M., & McHutchison, J. (2012). Chronic viral and autoimmune hepatitis. In L. Goldman & A. I. Schafer (Eds.), *Goldman's Cecil Medicine,* (24th ed., pp. 973–979). Philadelphia, PA: Elsevier Saunders.

Pimentel, M., Lembo, A., Chey, W. D., Zakko, S., Ringel, Y., Yu, J., . . . TARGET Study Group. (2011). Rifaximin therapy for patients with irritable bowel syndrome without constipation. *New England Journal of Medicine, 364*(1), 22–32.

Prather, C. (2012). Inflammatory and anatomic diseases of the intestine, peritoneum, mesentery, and omentum. In L. Goldman & A. I. Schafer (Eds.), *Goldman's Cecil medicine* (24th ed., pp. 921–928). Philadelphia, PA: Elsevier Saunders.

Roberts, J. R., & Castell, D. O. (2012). Gastroesophageal reflux disease. In E. T. Bope & R. D. Kellerman (Eds.), *Conn's current therapy 2012,* (pp. 520–522). Philadelphia, PA: Elsevier Saunders.

Swaroop, P. P., & Podolsky, D. K. (2012). Inflammatory bowel disease: Crohn's disease and ulcerative colitis. In E. T. Bope & R. D. Kellerman (Eds.), *Conn's current therapy 2012,* (pp. 533–538). Philadelphia, PA: Elsevier Saunders.

Targher, G., Day, C. P., & Bonora, E. (2010). Risk of cardiovascular disease in patients with nonalcoholic fatty liver disease. *New England Journal of Medicine, 363*(14), 1341–1350.

Tempero, M., & Brand, R. (2012). Pancreatic cancer. In L. Goldman & A. I. Schafer (Eds.), *Goldman's Cecil Medicine,* (24th ed., pp. 1289–1292). Philadelphia, PA: Elsevier Saunders.

Velasco, B. R., & Fisher, R. S. (2012). Irritable bowel syndrome. In E. T. Bope & R. D. Kellerman (Eds.), *Conn's current therapy 2012,* (pp. 548–551). Philadelphia, PA: Elsevier Saunders.

Weber, M. L., Ibrahim, H. N., & Lake, J. R. (2012). Renal dysfunction in liver transplant recipients: Evaluation of the critical issues. *Liver Transplantation, 18*(11), 1290–1301. doi:10.1002/lt.23522

Wedemeyer, H., & Pawlotsky, J. (2012). Acute viral hepatitis. In L. Goldman & A. I. Schafer (Eds.), *Goldman's Cecil Medicine,* (24th ed., pp. 966–973). Philadelphia, PA: Elsevier Saunders.

CHAPTER 32

Burn Injury and Other Conditions of the Skin

STRUCTURE AND FUNCTION OF THE SKIN

The skin is the largest organ of the body and has a number of functions:

- Protection of the body's inner structures from microorganisms, drying, and trauma
- Regulation of body temperature through evaporation of perspiration for cooling and constriction of superficial blood vessels to conserve heat
- Excretion of water and electrolytes through perspiration
- Sensory perception of touch, pressure, and pain

The skin consists of two layers: the outer layer, called the **epidermis**, and the inner layer, called the **dermis** (**Figure 32-1**). The epidermis protects the deeper tissues from drying, from invasion by organisms, and from trauma. The epidermis has several layers. Its deepest layer constantly produces new cells, which are pushed to the surface of the skin; there they die, are shed, and are replaced by new cells. Cells called *melanocytes,* located in the basal layer, contain the skin pigment melanin, which is responsible for skin color. Dark-skinned people have more melanin than light-skinned people.

The dermis lies beneath the epidermis. It contains blood vessels, nerves, lymphatics, hair follicles, and sebaceous and sweat glands, as well as various types of cells that promote wound healing. The dermis also contains major sensory fibers responsible for distinguishing pain, touch, heat, and cold.

With the exception of the palms of the hands and the soles of the feet, hair follicles are located in the dermis throughout the body, although they are more numerous in some areas, such as the scalp, axilla, and pubic area. Hairs are continually falling out and being replaced by new ones. When this process is excessive, thinning of hair or baldness results.

Sebaceous glands, contained within the dermis and surrounding hair follicles, produce an oily substance called *sebum* that protects the skin from excessive dryness. *Sweat glands*, also located in the dermis, are present all over the body, but are concentrated in the axilla, forehead, palms of the hands, and soles of the feet. They produce perspiration, which aids in regulation of the body temperature as well as excretion of water and electrolytes. When the environment is warm, evaporation of perspiration cools the body. When the environment is cool, constriction of superficial blood vessels conserves body warmth.

Interfacing with the dermis at its lower level is a **subcutaneous** (under the skin) layer of fat, called adipose tissue. This subcutaneous fat not only provides insulation for the body, but also gives shape and contour to the body over bone.

BURN INJURY

Any tissue injury resulting from direct heat contact, scalds, flame, chemicals, radiation, or electrical current is termed a *burn*. Management and outcomes of burn injuries depend on the cause or type of burn, the depth of burn, and the amount of

Figure 32-1   The Skin

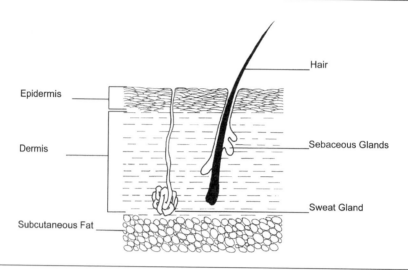

© Jane Tinkler Lamm.

body surface that has been burned, as well as the individual's age and general health condition. Individuals who are very young or very old are most vulnerable to the effects and complications of burns. Preexisting chronic health conditions, such as heart conditions, diabetes, lung conditions, or chronic abuse of drugs or alcohol, can further complicate recovery and severely affect recovery and outcome.

Individuals with burn injury undergo many dramatic physiologic and metabolic changes over the course of the injury, which is divided into four phases (Sheridan, 2016):

- Resuscitation phase (0–36 hours after the initial injury)
- Postresuscitation phase (2–6 days after injury)
- Inflammation and infection phase (7 days after injury until wound closure)
- Rehabilitation and wound-remodeling phase (up to 1 year after injury)

Types of Burn Injuries

Thermal Burns

The most common type of burns are *thermal burns,* which are caused by fire, hot liquids, or direct contact with a hot surface. In addition to causing direct injury to the skin, thermal burns can cause severe damage to underlying structures if the heat is intense or the exposure is prolonged.

Chemical Burns

Chemical burns result from direct contact with strong acids (e.g., sulfuric acid), alkaline agents (e.g., lye), gases (e.g., mustard gas), or other chemicals that cause tissue death. The extent of injury from chemical burns depends on the duration of the contact, the concentration or strength of the chemical, and the amount of tissue exposed to the chemical source. Some chemicals cause burns directly through the production of physiologic changes in the tissue with which they come into contact; other chemicals cause burns indirectly through the heat produced by their chemical reaction with the skin. In some instances, chemicals can cause freeze burns.

Freeze Injuries

Freeze injuries, such as frostbite to extremities, are also managed as if they were burns. Exposure to extremely cold temperatures may cause severe vasoconstriction (constriction of the blood vessels), with resulting **ischemia** (lack of blood supply) and potential subsequent **necrosis** (tissue death). Extremities, especially the toes and fingers, and appendages such as the nose and ears are especially susceptible to cold injury (Korley & Leikin, 2012). In addition to frostbite, chemicals such as propane and Freon can cause burn injuries.

Radiation Burns

The degree of damage caused by a *radiation burn* depends on the dose of radiation received. Sources of radiation burns may include ultraviolet radiation, such as that from the sun, and ionizing radiation, such as that from nuclear materials and X-rays. Localized skin reactions to low doses of radiation may cause discomfort, but usually heal spontaneously. Larger doses of local radiation may damage underlying tissues and organs, requiring more extensive management.

Electrical Burns

Electrical burns result from direct contact with electrical current or lightning. Injuries from these types of burns range from local tissue damage to sudden death because of cardiac arrest (Latenser, 2012). The effects of electricity on tissue depend on the current, the voltage, the type of current (e.g., direct or alternating), and the duration of contact (Sheridan, 2016). *Flash burns,* or low-voltage electrical injuries, often result in greater incapacitating effects that may include cognitive or behavioral changes as well as chronic pain. *High-tension injuries* (more than 1,000 volts) often result in amputation, larger areas of damage, or death.

Because the entry point of the electric current may be relatively small, electrical burns may appear to have caused little external damage. In fact, extensive internal damage may occur as the current travels through the body tissues, damaging nerves, blood vessels, and other major organs. The electrical current may also interfere with the electrical activity of the heart, causing it to stop *(cardiac arrest).* Electrical burns are generally full-thickness burns and, therefore, are associated with severe postburn conditions; these conditions may require multiple amputations owing to damage to blood vessels, nerves, bones, or muscle resulting from the injury (Tarim & Ezer, 2012). If clothing of the individual caught on fire as a result of exposure to the electricity source, thermal burns may be present as well. Individuals with electrical burns may also experience secondary injuries such as head injury, fractures, injury to other organs, or spinal cord injury because of falls associated with the injury.

Lightning injuries may be classified as mild, moderate, or severe. Being struck by lightning can, of course, be fatal; even so, a number of people survive such events. In mild cases, individuals may appear dazed and confused, having only mild physical injury. In more severe cases, individuals may experience sensory organ damage, such as rupture of the *tympanic membrane* in the ear or cataract formation in the eye; these types of injuries may not become evident for weeks, months, or years after the incident. If cardiac arrest occurred and the individual experienced **hypoxia** (decreased oxygen) before resuscitation could occur, the person could develop *brain damage* or a seizure condition.

Inhalation Injury

Inhalation injury to the respiratory tract is caused by inhalation of steam, toxic gases, or vapors. Smoke inhalation and carbon monoxide toxicity are the most common form of such injuries (Latenser, 2012). Individuals with inhalation injury experience cough, increasing hoarseness, shortness of breath, anxiety, wheezing, and potentially loss of consciousness. If cyanide is present in smoke, it is absorbed by the lungs, leading to systemic toxicity. Inhalation of noxious gases alone may lead to brain injury or death.

Upper or lower airways may be damaged from inhalation injuries that cause edema of the airways and compromise their patency. Management usually involves administrating 100% oxygen and maintaining an open airway (Sheridan, 2016). Inhalation injuries may sometimes necessitate **tracheostomy** (a procedure that creates a surgical opening into the trachea) to assist with breathing.

Burn Severity

The severity of a burn varies with the source of the burn as well as a number of other factors:

- Burn depth
- Percentage of body surface involved
- Location of burn

Burn Depth

Burn depth depends on the *temperature* of the burning agent and the *length of exposure.* Burn injuries may consist of only one burn depth, or a combination of different burn depths may be present. Based on their depth, burns are typically classified into one of four categories:

- *Superficial (first-degree) burn:* A burn that affects only the epidermis (outer layer of the skin). The skin becomes reddened and painful, but no underlying structures are damaged.
- *Partial-thickness (second-degree) burn:* A burn that affects both the epidermis and the dermis. The skin is reddened and blisters erupt, providing a portal of entry for organisms that can cause infection at the burn site.

Second-degree burns are very painful owing to the stimulation of sensitive nerve endings in this layer of the skin.

- *Full-thickness (third-degree) burn:* A burn that destroys the dermis and epidermis, as well as skin appendages, such as hair follicles, sebaceous glands, and sweat glands. There is little pain, because nerve endings have been destroyed. Full-thickness burns cannot heal spontaneously and are more susceptible to infection.
- *Fourth-degree burn:* A burn in which tissue damage extends to the underlying subcutaneous fat, muscle, or bone.

Percentage of Total Body Surface

Another factor determining burn severity, in addition to the source of the burn and the burn depth, is the *percentage of body surface* affected. A commonly used method of calculating the amount of body surface injured is the *Rule of Nines,* in which the body is graphically divided into areas that represent a different percentage of the total body surface (see **Figure 32-2**).

Figure 32-2   Rule of Nines

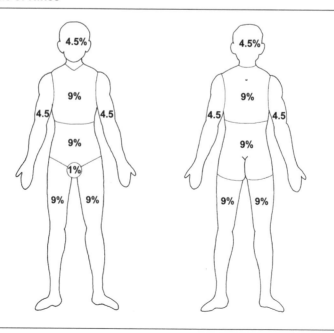

A more accurate method of estimating the total body surface burn is the *Lund and Browder method*. Recognizing that body proportions differ in children and adults, this method calculates the surface area of different body parts according to age. The chart used in the Lund and Browder model lists various body sections and the percentage of body surface each section represents for ages ranging from 1 year to adult. Each burned area is given percentage points based on the age of the individual; points are then added to estimate the total area of the body surface burned.

Burn Location

The *location* of the burn also affects burn severity. For example, persons with burns to the upper body, especially the head and neck, may be prone to respiratory complications because of possible smoke inhalation, heat damage to the respiratory structures, exposure to toxic by-products of the combustion of materials (e.g., from synthetic materials used in home furnishings), or restriction of air passages due to swelling caused by the injury.

For electrical burns, points of contact and the pathway that the current followed through the body are important considerations in determining the severity of tissue damage and the type of tissue and organs injured.

Manifestations after Burn Injury

Individuals experience a systemic response after major burns. Severe burns disrupt the body's internal balance. Because of tissue injury, plasma seeps from blood vessels into surrounding tissues, causing swelling and decreasing the amount of fluid in the general circulation. As a result, the body's general **homeostasis** (equilibrium) is lost, which can affect all body systems.

A second danger that negatively affects outcome for individuals with burns is *infection*, especially for those persons with partial-thickness or full-thickness burns. The degree of incapacitation experienced after burn depends on the extent and location of the burn. For example, burns involving the hand may result in loss or contracture of the fingers, limiting joint motion. Severe burns of a leg may impair ambulation or necessitate amputation. Burns around the head and face may involve loss of vision or loss of nose, ears, or hair. Scarring—especially *hypertrophic scars* (configurations of scar tissue that are out of proportion to the amount of scar tissue normally expected for wound healing)—may affect not only appearance but also function.

Phases of Burn Management

Individuals who have experienced burns undergo dramatic physiologic and metabolic changes over the course of the injury, which includes continuing changes as the process evolves. The type of burn management depends on the severity of the injury. Burn injury combined with other types of injuries, such as those associated with a vehicle accident, explosion, or fall, will necessitate a more complicated management plan as other injuries are also addressed.

Individuals with moderate or severe burn injury require hospitalization. Once at the hospital facility, most of these persons will be transferred to its *burn center*. Burn centers are specially equipped and have specially trained staff to provide both a multifaceted and multidisciplinary approach to management of moderate to severe burn injuries. Although the length of hospitalization varies with the extent, degree, and location of the burn, other factors that play a role in determining the duration of the inpatient stay include the presence of inhalation injury or other injuries, and the individual's age and general health prior to the burn injury.

Resuscitation Phase

In the resuscitation phase, the immediate concern of management is to alleviate any life-threatening breathing problems, stabilize the individual's general condition, restore fluid balance, and prevent complications. The major task for the individual during this phase is survival.

Postresuscitation Phase

In the postresuscitation phase, when the individual's condition has been stabilized, continued respiratory support and maintenance of fluid stability in the body are important aspects of management. During this phase, water loss through evaporation from the burn surface is a major concern.

Inflammation and Infection Phase

Because individuals who have been severely burned are vulnerable to infection, precautions must be taken to prevent exposure to harmful organisms. The greatest danger comes from organisms within the individual's own body. Nevertheless, some burn units may maintain a relatively sterile environment in which individuals with severe burns are placed in rooms equipped with special air filtration systems to screen out harmful organisms.

In some burn units, persons who provide care may wear caps, gowns, and masks to protect individuals with burns from infection. Visitors may be restricted or, when allowed to visit, may be asked to wear masks and gowns. As a result, individuals with burns may experience an increased sense of social isolation. Because of the stress imposed by these restrictions, and because of the growing evidence that risk of infection from outside sources is minimal, some burn units now restrict the environment much less—that is, caps and gowns are not worn by personnel or visitors, and the time frame for visiting is more liberal.

General Burn Management

Wound Management

Burn wounds are managed in different ways. Sometimes an exposure method is employed, in which no dressing or covering is applied to the wound. When this approach is used, more sterile conditions are essential to prevent infection. In other cases, the wound may not be covered, but topical medication, such as *silver sulfadiazine* to inhibit bacterial growth, may be applied. In some cases, burn wounds are covered with dressings that are changed daily. Methods of management depend on the type and extent of the burn wound, as well as on the general philosophy of the specific burn unit.

Daily hygiene is important to deter infection. Individuals may be asked to wash daily with antimicrobial soap as they would at home. **Eschar** (charred, dead tissue) may be **debrided** (removed) to prevent organisms from collecting and growing on the dead tissue, thereby reducing risk of infection and promoting wound healing. Debridement may be performed in the hospital room, or surgical debridement may be performed in the operating room if the area of tissue to be removed is more extensive.

Nutritional Support

The nutritional needs of individuals with severe burns are great. In the early postburn period, individuals may lose as much as 1 pound or more per day. A high caloric intake is, therefore, essential to meet the increased energy requirements during this period. In individuals with larger-surface-area burns, it is usually necessary to supply extra calories either via a tube in the esophagus or, rarely, intravenously. Tube feeding (known as *enteral feeding*) is often chosen as the means of nutritional support during this time to ensure appropriate caloric and nutritional intake.

Splinting

Certain parts of the body require special care when burned. When the hands, arms, legs, or neck have been burned, for example, special care is necessary to prevent the loss of function due to *scarring* or **contracture** (fixation of a joint in a position of nonfunction). Affected extremities and joints may be *splinted* in a position of function to prevent formation of contracture. Each type of splint is customized to the individual.

Pain Management

Pain resulting from burn injury is common and can be directly related to the burn wound or to interventions used in burn management. In the early stages of burn management, pain medications are administered with caution due to the physiologic changes and disruption of body equilibrium that ensues from the burn injury. In later stages, a number of medications can be used for pain, although alternative approaches to pain management may also be used. Many individuals with burns experience **pruritus** (a sense of itching), which can continue well after the healing period. Topical medications and laser therapy have been used with some success in management of pruritus associated with burns.

Rehabilitation and Wound Remodeling

Grafting

After the acute phase of burn management, *grafting procedures* usually begin. A *graft* is tissue that is transplanted to a part of the body to repair an injury or defect.

Biologic dressings may be used to cover a burn wound temporarily and prepare it for grafting. The types of biologic dressings include the following:

- *Xenograft* (heterograft): A graft taken from another species. Porcine (pig skin) grafts are often used for burn wounds.
- *Homograft* (allograft): A graft taken from the same species, but not the same person. Homografts may be taken from a living donor or from a cadaver skin bank. Another type of homograft is *amnion,* which consists of placental membrane.
- *Biosynthetic graft:* A graft that has been chemically manufactured. Synthetic skin substitutes are viable alternatives as temporary wound coverings. Such material is semitransparent and sterile. It adheres to the wound and prevents infection and can also help in debridement.

When the burn wound appears healthy, a skin graft is applied. An *autograft* is a section of the individual's own skin that has been removed from an uninvolved site. Depending on the size of the graft needed, the same donor site may be used repeatedly. A skin graft from another individual *(allograft)* may also be obtained from a skin bank.

Skin grafting may be performed in several ways. A *split-thickness graft* consists of the epidermis and part of the dermis and can be either a *sheet graft* or a *mesh graft.* A sheet graft consists of a single layer; a mesh graft contains many little slits that enable it to cover a larger area. A full-thickness graft, which includes both the epidermis and the dermis from the donor site, is thicker and is often used when the grafting is particularly important for cosmetic purposes.

When larger quantities of tissue are needed, a *flap* may be used. A flap is a tissue in which one area remains attached to the donor site and, consequently, has its own blood supply. The free end of the flap is then placed over the injury, sutured into place, and allowed to heal. Because flaps maintain their own blood supply, their use may offer better cosmetic results than grafts, which may not maintain natural skin color.

Scar Management

The healing burn area may be compressed with elastic dressings to prevent or decrease the formation of **hypertrophic** (overgrowth) scarring. Special elasticized garments, commonly called pressure garments, are available to be worn continually over the body part for a year or more to prevent this type of scar formation (**Figure 32-3**). The garments, such as gloves, vests, face masks, or neck garments, are customized to fit the specific body part involved. Individuals may need compression garments for 1 to 2 years after initial injury, and the garments must be worn 23 hours per day. Because they are unattractive and are hot and uncomfortable, individuals may have a difficult time adjusting emotionally to this phase of burn management.

If contractures have occurred as a result of the burn, physical therapy may be necessary to return mobility to a joint. When the measures are unsuccessful or if the contracture is severe, surgical intervention may be necessary.

Reconstructive Surgery and Cosmetic Interventions

Many individuals with severe burns require reconstructive or plastic surgery after the wound has healed, especially if there has been severe disfigurement or if contractures have formed so that movement of a joint is limited. Surgical interventions may also be performed to reconstruct a

Figure 32-3   Pressure Garments

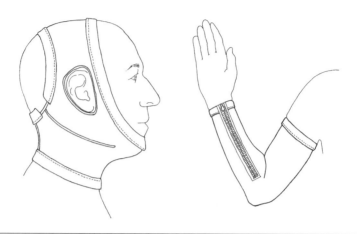

© Jane Tinkler Lamm.

body part, such as the nose or the ear, or to remove hypertrophic scar tissue. Many of these procedures take place over a number of years after the initial burn injury.

Corrective cosmetics (camouflage therapy) can also be used for skin discoloration or to minimize scars or suture lines. Corrective cosmetics differ from standard makeup in that they provide heavier coverage and adhere better to the skin. If individuals with severe burns experience major hair loss, wigs or toupees may be worn. In some instances, surgical placement of hair plugs may be used for scalp hair replacement, as well as surgical hair implants for eyebrows.

Most recently, a number of laser modalities, including fractionated carbon dioxide, pulse dye laser and intense pulsed light, have been developed to address various types of burn scars. Each of these treatment have shown enormous promise, but the protocols and guidelines for their use are still being developed (Hultman, Friedstat, Edkins, Cairns, & Meyer, 2014).

Functional Implications of Burn Injury

Personal and Psychosocial Issues

Experiencing a burn injury can have both physical and emotional effects that alter function. Responses to burn injury vary with the individual's premorbid personality traits, personal circumstances, type of burn injury, and psychological meaning of the injury to the individual. Some individuals with burn injury may experience posttraumatic stress syndrome, depression, or sleep disturbance, which can be incapacitating; others reach acceptance of the injury and focus on working toward returning to their regular activities. Any preexisting health condition that may have contributed to the burn injury, such as substance abuse or mental health condition, adds more complexity to the process of rehabilitation and adjustment.

Individuals who experience alterations in body appearance as a result of burn injury or scarring must make psychological adjustments not only to the change in appearance but also to the long-term course involved in reconstruction and plastic surgery. Although many individuals have realistic expectations regarding the degree to which reconstructive surgery can restore appearance, others may hold out false hopes and overly optimistic expectations, which if unfulfilled can result in disappointment and depression.

Changes in appearance or function associated with burn injury may require development of a new sense of self that differs from the self-concept held prior to injury. The extent to which this evolution is accomplished can be a determining factor in whether individuals reestablish themselves as functional members of the community or withdraw from social integration.

During the initial phases of burn injury, individuals often focus on survival and adaptation to the sudden changes invoked by the injury. In later phases, in addition to adjusting to the physical manifestations of the burn injury itself, individuals may experience stress related to interventions to burn management. Management of burn injury may involve isolation, pain, multiple operations, and procedures that take place over an extended period of time, leading to feelings of vulnerability and sorrow. Adjustment may be compounded by a variety of other situational factors, such as separation from family, friends, and other sources of gratification; the experience of pain; the disruption of future life plans; and concerns involving the impact the burn may have on established relationships.

As recovery progresses and individuals become more aware of their circumstances, they may regress, becoming overly dependent. Loss of independence, concern about appearance, and exposure to continuing interventions and procedures serve as a constant source of stress. Individuals may feel powerless over what is done to them and for them, leading to fear and frustration. Reactions may become generalized so that, even after the recovery period, individuals continue to experience anxiety about unknown or unrecognized dangers. Viewing the injury for the first time can also be stressful. Stress can be reduced through provision of reassurance and optimism as well as a realistic view of what can be accomplished with interventions during the rehabilitation process.

Because burn injuries are frequently associated with accidents, the circumstances surrounding the burn injury can contribute to individual reactions. If the injury resulted from negligence or actions of others, individuals may exhibit feelings of anger, guilt, regret, or resentment. If the injury was due to their own actions or inactions or if others were also injured in the incident, self-blame and guilt may intensify individuals' reaction to their injury.

Discharge from the burn unit does not mark the end of the stress. It is difficult psychologically for individuals who have experienced a change in appearance due to burn injury to reenter the community. Adjusting to the reactions of others, dealing with social stigma, and realistically accepting limitations are important psychological issues with which the individual with burns must deal. Support groups can help individuals learn strategies to discuss their injury with others and can promote confidence and self-esteem, thereby enhancing community reentry.

Activities and Participation

Most individuals with burn injuries are able to return to active and productive lives. Issues that arise in everyday activities in relation to burn injuries and the degree to which everyday activities may need modification depend on the extent, nature, and location of the burn itself. For example, severe burns of the hands can result in contracture of the hands and fingers, necessitating the use of assistive devices to carry out activities of daily living. Burns to the face that result in loss of vision may also make it necessary to use adaptive devices.

As noted earlier, individuals who have experienced severe burn injuries often must undergo a series of reconstructive operations over several years. Thus frequent hospitalizations may interrupt work and home activities. Relationships may be altered because of absences from the social environment necessitated by these repeated hospitalizations. Increased dependence and length of hospitalization due to burns can disrupt relationships within the family as well as other social relationships. Friends and family may be shocked at the sudden change in an individual's appearance after a burn injury. Reintegration into the community may require adjustment, especially if physical appearance or function has been affected as a result of the burn injury. Reactions of others may consist of pity and curiosity, stares, or insensitive remarks.

Depending on the circumstances of the accident, family members and friends may exhibit feelings of anger, guilt, or resentment, which can be manifested in a variety of ways. In an attempt to make sense of the injury and its aftermath, family members, friends, and coworkers may focus on the question of responsibility for the cause of the injury. Those who were present at the time of the injury may feel that they should have done more or that they were to blame. Others may wonder why they escaped the same type of injury. These feelings may affect reactions to the individual with burn injury as well as further social interactions. Family reactions can range from oversolicitude to emotional withdrawal. Concerns about financial considerations and altered social roles may cause additional family stress.

Support groups and burn camps that assist individuals in facing the challenges of their burn injury and management and allow individuals and their families to share common concerns may be helpful. Groups such as the National Phoenix Society, for example, can help individuals and their families cope with the ongoing difficulties of returning to society.

Sexuality

Issues related to sexuality are often a neglected part of management and rehabilitation for individuals with burn injury. Sexual concerns are important during acute phases of management in the burn unit as well as during discharge and ongoing rehabilitation. Sexuality encompasses much more than sexual activity or genital function: it encompasses the whole person and is an important part of identity, self-image, and self-concept. Changes of appearance associated with burn injury as well as reactions of others can challenge individuals' view of themselves as sexual beings, and can affect their adjustment and adaptation. Open discussion to address these concerns is an important aspect of rehabilitation and recovery.

Vocational Implications in Burn Injury

The ability of individuals experiencing burn injury to return to their former occupation depends not only on the occupation itself but also on the extent and location of the burn. At times, the main factor in determining how successful individuals can be in returning to their former position is the attitudes of others in the workplace. Acceptance of the individual in the workplace by fellow employees may be difficult for a variety of reasons. If the injury was work related, depending on the circumstances, coworkers may feel guilty, causing them to alter their approach to the individual. Others may feel uncomfortable because of the individual's appearance and avoid contact. In some instances, even though individuals who have experienced severe burn may not consider themselves incapacitated, others may attach labels to them that are unwarranted.

Emotional stress on the part of coworkers can preclude the individual's effective reentry at the workplace. Employers may not have confidence in individuals' ability to return to the former job or may be concerned about others' reaction to the altered appearance of the individual with burn injury. Discussion with coworkers and employers is sometimes necessary to provide a smoother transition for individuals returning to work after burn injury.

Individuals who require extensive reconstructive surgery may require intermittent hospitalizations over a 1- to 2-year period after the initial injury. Disruption to work activity associated with such hospitalizations should be considered before individuals return to regular employment. Those who have other conditions resulting from burns, such as contracture, loss of a limb, or loss of vision, have the vocational limitations noted for those persons with the same condition due to other causes (see the specific related chapters).

Individuals who wear compression garments may need to avoid extremely warm work environments because of the excessive warmth of the garment. Those who wear compression gloves also have decreased manual dexterity. A facial mask may be a cosmetic disadvantage if dealing with the public is a requirement of employment. The degree to which cosmetic appearance due to the burn itself is a factor in employment depends on the individual, the occupation, and the employer.

Skin that has been grafted may be more sensitive than normal skin. Consequently, grafts should not be exposed to extremes of temperature. If individuals are exposed to the sun, they should use sunscreen and wear sun-protective clothing. Because burns may have destroyed sweat glands, individuals' ability to regulate body temperature may be altered. In addition, less fat insulation may be present at burned areas than in healthy normal tissue, which affects the individual's ability to tolerate extremes of temperature. Extremely dry climates may exacerbate the itching that is often associated with the new skin growth of skin grafts. A more humid environment may be desirable in such cases.

Other residual issues related to burn injury may also affect the appropriateness of the work environment. For example, individuals who have experienced altered lung function as a result of inhalation injury should avoid work settings characterized by air pollution or exposure to smoke and dust. Individuals with burns to the lower extremities may have difficulty in standing for prolonged periods and may need more sedentary employment.

GENERAL SKIN CONDITIONS

Because the skin is in constant contact with the environment, it is vulnerable to injury and irritation. It is also vulnerable to changes in the internal body environment and may provide visible evidence of systemic conditions, such as *systemic lupus erythematosus*. Emotional factors can also precipitate or contribute to skin conditions. Skin conditions may be localized or may involve the entire body. They may cause mild discomfort or severe pain and disfigurement.

Dermatitis

The general term **dermatitis** describes a superficial inflammation of the skin. *Atopic dermatitis* is a chronic inflammatory skin condition involving a complex interrelationship of genetic, psychological, immunologic, and environmental factors (Ong, 2012). Although it is more common in childhood, it can be a lifelong condition. Depending on its location, atopic dermatitis can affect appearance, especially if on the face. Constant scratching of the skin can cause tenderness and bleeding. If the skin's protective outer layers crack, individuals are also at risk of infection. Management is directed toward correcting skin dryness, controlling the itch, and preventing infection.

Eczema is a type of dermatitis characterized by redness (**erythema**), swelling (**edema**), and itching (**pruritus**). In addition to managing the general dryness and controlling the itching, topical steroids are sometimes applied in cases of eczema.

Management of atopic dermatitis includes avoidance of prolonged contact with hot water (e.g., taking lukewarm showers rather than long, hot baths), avoidance of drying soaps, and use of moisturizers on the skin. Medications such as *antihistamines* or *steroid creams* and *ointments* may be used to control itching; however, prolonged use of steroid medications is contraindicated due to the potential for side effects. New medications called *topical immunomodulators* are also used. In severe cases, *phototherapy* (light therapy) or *photochemotherapy* (combination of ultraviolet light and special medication) may be used.

Contact dermatitis is a localized skin inflammation that results from contact with a specific substance. The manifestations occur at the site of contact. The substance may produce a localized allergic response (*allergic contact dermatitis*) as a result of a previous exposure, or the substance may be a primary irritant that causes a nonallergic skin reaction (*irritant contact dermatitis*) following exposure (Yiannias & Egnatios, 2012). Common causes of localized allergic contact dermatitis include chemicals, dyes, cosmetics, and industrial agents. Alkalis, acids, metals, salts, solvents, and various dusts may cause irritant dermatitis. Usually only skin that comes into contact with the substance is involved, so the area of skin affected is rather clearly demarcated. Manifestations generally disappear when contact with the substance is avoided. In addition to localized allergic reactions, individuals can experience generalized allergic reactions, as described next.

Allergic Reactions

An allergy is a hypersensitivity and overreaction of the immune system to harmless environmental allergens or to a specific substance or substance (Wasserman, 2016). Predisposed individuals may experience allergic reactions after exposure to innocuous substances (antigens) that stimulate an adaptive immune response. Sensitization to the substance may take days or weeks to occur. Once the response has been established, however, the next contact with the substance produces an allergic response.

Allergic responses may be external or systemic. External allergic reactions consist of manifestations such as hives (**urticaria**), redness, swelling, itching, or rash. Systemic allergic responses, usually caused by allergic reactions to medications or certain foods, may include skin manifestations in addition to generalized body manifestations, some of which can seriously compromise respiratory function. Management of allergy is usually directed toward avoiding contact with the substance, reducing sensitivity to the substance if contact cannot be avoided, or reducing or eliminating manifestations associated with the allergic response.

Psoriasis

Psoriasis is a chronic inflammatory autoimmune condition that affects the skin, scalp, and nails (Lim, 2016; Papp et al., 2012). As a result of the rapid formation of these cells, individuals develop noticeable skin lesions. Several variations of psoriasis exist, which are categorized as localized or generalized depending on the severity of the condition and its overall impact on the individual's quality of life and well-being. In addition, some studies have suggested that individuals with psoriasis may have an increased risk for cardiovascular disease (Armstrong, 2012).

Plaque psoriasis is characterized by plaques of *erythema* covered with silvery scales, which tend to shed. Patches or plaques may occur on localized areas, such as the elbows and knees, lower back, and the scalp, or they can cover the entire body. In some instances, individuals develop *pustular psoriasis,* in which small pustules are spread over the body and, in some instances, can lead to systemic infection. Some individuals with psoriasis develop *psoriatic arthritis,* which causes aching and deformity of joints.

Although the primary cause of psoriasis remains unknown, it is considered a genetically influenced, immune-mediated chronic condition (Lim, 2016). It is characterized by periods of **remission** (when manifestations become better) and periods of **exacerbation** (when manifestations become worse) of varying frequency and duration. Thus the course of the psoriasis is often unpredictable and can improve or worsen for no obvious reason. Emotional stress and anxiety may aggravate the condition. In some individuals, climate change or warm temperatures tend to make the condition worse.

Management of Psoriasis

Psoriasis is noncontagious and noncancerous. Although it is incurable, it is controllable (Puchalsky,

2012). The goal of management is to suppress the immune-mediated response, which causes manifestation (Waisman, 2012). Any aggravating factors should be identified and removed if possible. Given that injury to the skin can trigger flare-ups, trauma to the skin should be avoided as much as possible.

Management depends on the severity of the condition and the degree to which it affects the individual's quality of life (Puchalsky, 2012). Psoriasis can be managed with topical steroids as well as other topical medications.

If topical medications do not prove to be sufficiently effective, *phototherapy* may be used. Phototherapy consists of exposure to ultraviolet light in a light booth. It may be administered at a specific provider location, but home light units are also available. Phototherapy reduces activity of the immune system and promotes remission.

Some individuals do not respond to phototherapy or may be unable to receive it (e.g., because of the distance between the provider facility and the individual's home, or because of the individual's work schedule). In these instances, systemic medications may be used instead. Systemic medications such as *methotrexate, aceitretin,* and *cyclosporine* may be used for moderate to severe psoriasis. While all three of these medications are effective, they can also generate side effects such as liver damage, renal damage, increased blood lipids, and bone marrow suppression and, therefore, require frequent blood monitoring (Puchalsky, 2012).

Among the newer interventions for management of psoriasis are biological drugs—that is, proteins produced by recombinant DNA technology. Although they are effective, these agents cannot be used when individuals have an infection or malignancy, and their cost makes their use prohibitive for many individuals.

Psychosocial Impact of Psoriasis

Psoriasis ranges from a cosmetically annoying condition to a physically incapacitating condition (Leonardi et al., 2012). It does not affect the individual's general health, but the psychological and social stigma associated with an obvious unsightly skin condition may cause frustration and discouragement. Psoriasis can cause difficulty with work performance, problems with social rejection, sexual dysfunction, and depression. Itching may be mild or severe and can cause loss of sleep and general fatigue, which can contribute to irritability. The condition can be a burden in terms of the financial and time resources required to deal with it, can interfere with work, and can disrupt the individual's lifestyle. Although psoriasis is not infectious, it may be a source of stares, embarrassing questions or comments, or outright avoidance of the individual by others. The outcome depends on the extent and the severity of the condition. In general, the earlier the condition begins, the more severe its manifestations.

Infections

A number of organisms, including bacteria, fungi, parasites, and viruses, may infect the skin. Infection may be the primary cause of a skin condition, or it may be a secondary condition associated with another skin condition. The degree and length of incapacity associated with infections of the skin depend on the type and severity of the infection. Effective management requires the proper identification of the causative organisms and interventions appropriate to those particular organisms.

Acne

Acne is the most commonly encountered skin condition (Korman, 2016). It results from interaction between bacteria in the skin, excess oil production, and hormones. The face, neck, and trunk of the body are the body parts most frequently affected. Although acne is most common in adolescence, some individuals—especially women—have acne that continues into young adulthood. Acne in itself is not frequently thought of as an incapacitating condition, but it can have a devastating effect on the individual's self-image and self-esteem. The goal of management is to prevent the clogging of hair follicles, reduce inflammation, mitigate infection, and minimize scarring. Management usually consists of topical application of medication and, occasionally, systemic medication in severe or prolonged cases. In some instances, individuals with severe scarring from acne may choose to have cosmetic procedures such as *resurfacing* or

dermabrasion (a procedure in which scars, wrinkles, or other skin blemishes are worn away) to diminish the scarring once their acne is no longer active.

Varicella Zoster (Herpes Zoster; Shingles)

Varicella zoster (also called herpes zoster, or *shingles)* is a reactivation of the virus that caused chickenpox in individuals at a younger age (Korman, 2016). After the individual has had chicken pox, the virus remains dormant in the nervous system. When the individual's immune system becomes weakened because of aging, or because of health conditions such as organ transplantation, cancer, or HIV infections, the virus can become reactivated. **Vesicles** (fluid-filled blisters) erupt along a peripheral sensory nerve distribution. The blisters, which form a band along the nerve, are usually located on the trunk of the body, and cause pain, itching, burning, and tenderness along the nerve route. Although vesicles usually appear on the trunk of the body, they may also affect the face and eye. Pain in the affected area may be severe.

The goal of management for herpes zoster is to relieve pain, reduce potential complications, and shorten the duration of the manifestations. Antiviral medication, administered either orally or intravenously, is often required (Brice, 2012). Steroids or anti-inflammatory medications may also be used. Pain accompanying herpes zoster is often managed with analgesics.

Complications of herpes zoster can include prolonged pain at the site even after lesions have subsided. Other complications may include scarring, which may be quite disfiguring if it involves the facial area. If the eye is affected, another complication may consist of ulceration, which could result in blindness.

Skin Cancers

Cancer of the skin occurs more frequently than does cancer of any other organ. Because *basal cell carcinoma* is directly visible, it can be identified earlier and, therefore, has a high cure rate. *Malignant melanoma,* a cancer originating in the *melanocytes* (cells containing skin pigment), is far more dangerous and is potentially fatal because it may spread rapidly into deeper skin layers and metastasize to other body organs (Petronic-Rosic,

2012). Because of the seriousness of the condition, surgical removal of the melanoma itself, as well as portions of surrounding tissue, may be necessary to eradicate the cancer. This procedure may lead to significant deformity, depending on the location.

GENERAL MANAGEMENT OF CONDITIONS OF THE SKIN

Medications

Many skin conditions are managed with medications that are applied directly to the skin surface *(topical application)* in the form of lotions, creams, ointments, or powders. The type of medication chosen depends on the cause of the skin condition. For example, *antifungals* are used for fungal infections, *antibiotics* or *antibacterials* for bacterial infections, and *antivirals* for viral infections. Topical *antipruritics* may be applied to reduce the discomfort due to itching. Topical *corticosteroids* are often used to reduce local inflammatory responses.

Because topical medications can have side effects, prolonged use or overuse of medications such as corticosteroids should be avoided. Some skin conditions may be managed with systemic medications (i.e., medications that are injected or taken orally and, therefore, distributed throughout the body), such as antibiotics and corticosteroids. Although corticosteroids can produce dramatic improvements in skin conditions, they also have potentially serious side effects. Consequently, the use of corticosteroids requires careful monitoring.

Dressings and Therapeutic Baths or Soaks

Management of skin conditions in which there is excessive skin scaling or in which crusts have formed over lesions may include *wet soaks* or *therapeutic baths* to reduce the drying effects of air, relieve discomfort, or enhance the removal of scales and crusts so that healing may take place. In some instances, dressings are applied to skin lesions to protect the skin from injury and infection from the environment.

Phototherapy (Light Treatment)

Artificial light sources may be used for localized or generalized management of various skin conditions. Phototherapy is frequently accompanied by therapeutic baths or soaks, or it may be used in combination with topical medication to potentiate its effect.

Dermabrasion

Dermabrasion is a method of mechanically resurfacing skin so as to smooth out irregular contours caused by acne, tattoos, scars from trauma, burn injury, or other conditions. The procedure consists of buffing, or abrading, the top surface of the skin so as to reduce scarring.

Chemical Face Peeling

Chemical face peeling involves a controlled chemical burn that destroys the upper layer of the skin. It is generally performed for cosmetic purposes to remove fine lines or blemishes, but it can also be helpful in the management of acne and precancerous growths. Individuals with chemical face peeling need to avoid sun exposure and be aware that the skin will not tan evenly.

Plastic and Reconstructive Surgery

Plastic and reconstructive surgery involves correction of irregularities, restoration of function of parts of the body, or enhancement of physical appearance. It plays an important role in rehabilitation, not only to improve healing and establish or reestablish function but also to enhance individuals' self-image and minimize limitations.

Plastic surgery is, of course, important in cases involving conditions of the skin, but it can be performed on many parts of the body. For example, plastic surgery may be used to minimize or correct congenital anomalies such as *cleft lip* or *cleft palate.* It may be performed to restore function lost due to contractures (tightening of tissue around a joint, which then limits range of motion). Such surgery may also be undertaken to correct deformity and restore function after a hand injury or to promote healing and correct deformity resulting from complications such as

decubitus ulcers (pressure sores caused by immobility and lack of blood supply to tissue, such that tissue death occurs). In addition, plastic and reconstructive surgery may be performed to correct deformities that occur secondary to a variety of health conditions in which a large portion of tissue has been removed or deformity results, including cancer, and burns in which scarring, contractures, or loss of a body part due to the burn has been sustained.

Plastic and reconstructive surgery can help to restore function and minimize disfigurement, thereby assisting individuals' adjustment to their condition and reentry into the workplace and the community. The extent to which reentry is possible varies from individual to individual and depends on the part of the body affected, the extent of limitations that remain, and the person's own psychological characteristics.

GENERAL FUNCTIONAL IMPLICATIONS OF CONDITIONS OF THE SKIN

While not generally life threatening, skin conditions can have an adverse effect on quality of life, restricting work, social, family, leisure, and sexual activities (Bruckner-Tuderman, 2010). Healthy skin is correlated with higher self-esteem and better self-image. A skin condition that might seem trivial to others can have a major psychological impact on the individual who experiences it. Emotional responses to skin conditions can have a negative effect on individuals' self-image as well as adverse effects on interpersonal relationships.

Personal and Psychosocial Issues

The skin, which is exposed and, therefore, readily observable, determines to a great extent an individual's appearance to others, and it is through personal appearance that others build an image of the individual. Individuals, in turn, observe the reactions of others and incorporate them into their own self-image. Consequently, conditions affecting the skin can have considerable impact on self-esteem, perception and attitudes. Conditions or injury affecting the face may be particularly devastating. More than any other body part, the face is tied to personal identity. While clothing can cover other body parts, the face is left exposed so that disfigurement is readily observable. Our society places considerable emphasis on a clear, radiant appearance. When a health condition or injury alters this image, it is not surprising that the psychological impact on the affected individuals is considerable.

Acute skin conditions may be managed or prevented. Chronic skin conditions, in contrast, require ongoing intervention. Stress affects some skin conditions, and individuals with these conditions may need to learn ways to reduce the amount of stress in their environment or to alter their reaction to stress.

Activities and Participation

Necessary changes in lifestyle resulting from skin conditions depend on the severity of the condition and circumstances. Skin conditions resulting from exposure to or contact with certain substances within the environment make it necessary to avoid those substances. The discomfort associated with some skin conditions, such as itching, may affect daily activities to some degree. If special baths or dressings are required, these interventions must be incorporated into the individual's daily routine.

Disease or injury to the skin may isolate individuals perhaps more than any other condition. Some people, because they associate skin conditions with uncleanliness and contagiousness, may avoid individuals with skin conditions even though the associations are unfounded. Because of the reactions of others, individuals with skin conditions or injury may become very sensitive. Having experienced stares or other negative reactions, they may develop an accentuated state of awareness and assume that others are focusing totally on their appearance. They may become extremely self-conscious and withdraw from social contact.

Visible disabilities provoke greater discrimination and social stigma than do invisible disabilities. Physical attractiveness is highly valued in our society, where it is viewed as a salable commodity. Skin conditions, especially if they involve the face, may evoke even more profound responses from others. People may feel uneasy in the presence of individuals with disfigurement and uncertain about what to do or say. In social settings, individuals with disfigurement due to a skin condition or injury may encounter staring, feelings of pity, or repulsion. These reactions may cause individuals to limit or avoid social activities or to restrict their social interactions with others.

Enhanced self-esteem as well as techniques and coping skills for handling social situations can be fostered by support and educational programs in which these issues are discussed.

Sexuality

Although conditions of the skin may not affect sexual function directly, the emphasis frequently placed on physical attractiveness in society, especially when related to issues of sexual attractiveness, can affect individuals' self-confidence and self-esteem, thereby indirectly affecting sexual function. Skin conditions or disfigurement (particularly of the face), as well as the reactions of others, may alter individuals' feelings about their own desirability. The anxiety or depression that often accompanies skin conditions may further disrupt sexual function. Counseling and support, as well as encouragement of open discussion, can be beneficial in improving this aspect of sexuality.

GENERAL VOCATIONAL IMPLICATIONS IN SKIN CONDITIONS

Most individuals with skin conditions continue with employment with no special modifications. Those persons whose skin conditions are precipitated or exacerbated by exposure to substances in the work environment may require special considerations in choice of employment, or alteration of work tasks to minimize or alleviate exposure. If stress precipitates or exacerbates the skin condition, stress reduction techniques that improve the individual's reaction to stress may be helpful. In some instances, it may be necessary to alter the work site.

Because skin cancer appears to be related to exposure to the sun, those persons who work outside should take precautions to avoid excessive exposure to sunlight, such as wearing protective clothing or sun shields. Those who have had skin cancer or who have a propensity toward it should take additional precautions to avoid direct exposure to the sun as much as possible. Likewise, individuals who use medications that cause photosensitivity, and individuals who have new skin grafts, may need to avoid the sun.

Attitudes of employers and coworkers may create barriers to employment for individuals with skin conditions, especially when the condition alters their appearance. Coworkers may fear contagion or may be uncomfortable because of the individual's appearance. Consequently, education and strategies to alleviate misperceptions may be an important factor in facilitating the individual's successful reentry or continuation in the work setting.

CASE STUDY

Ms. H., a bank teller, experienced burn injuries when the small commuter plane in which she was a passenger crashed and caught fire. Although a bystander was able to pull her from the wreckage, Ms. H. experienced significant smoke inhalation and burns to her head, neck, and hands. As a result of the burns, she has significant facial scarring and amputation of the thumb and index finger of her right hand. She has undergone two reconstructive surgeries.

1. Which specific issues regarding Ms. H.'s injuries might have implications for her return to work at her job as a bank teller?
2. Which specific modifications or services might contribute to Ms. H.'s ability to return to work in her current line of employment?

REFERENCES

Armstrong, A. W. (2012). Coronary artery disease in patients with psoriasis referred for coronary angioplasty. *American Journal of Cardiology, 108*(7), 976–980.

Brice, S. L. (2012). Viral diseases of the skin. In E. T. Bope & R. D. Kellerman (Eds.), *Conn's current therapy 2012,* (pp. 269–277). Philadelphia, PA: Elsevier Saunders.

Bruckner-Tuderman, L. (2010). Systemic therapy for a genetic skin disease. *New England Journal of Medicine, 363*(7), 680–682.

Hultman, C. S., Friedstat, J. S., Edkins, R. E., Cairns, B. A., & Meyer, A. A. (2014). Laser resurfacing and remodeling of hypertrophic burn scars: The results of a large, prospective, before-after cohort study, with long-term follow-up. *Annals of Surgery, 260*(3), 519–532.

Korley, F. K., & Leikin, J. B. (2012). Disturbances caused by cold. In E. T. Bope & R. D. Kellerman (Eds.), *Conn's current therapy 2012,* (pp. 1120–1124). Philadelphia, PA: Elsevier Saunders.

Korman, N. J. (2016). Macular, popular, vesiculobullous, and pustular diseases. In L. Goldman & R. I. Schafer (Eds.), *Goldman-Cecil Medicine,* (25th ed., pp. 2671–2682). Philadelphia, PA: Elsevier Saunders.

Latenser, B. A. (2012). Burn treatment guidelines. In E. T. Bope & R. D. Kellerman (Eds.), *Conn's current therapy 2012,* (pp. 1115–1120). Philadelphia, PA: Elsevier Saunders.

Leonardi, C., Matheson, R., Zachariae, C., Cameron, G., Li, L., Edson-Heredia, E., . . . Banerjee, S. (2012). Anti-interleukin-17 monoclonal antibody ixekizumab in chronic plaque psoriasis. *New England Journal of Medicine, 366*(13), 1190–1199.

Lim, H. W. (2016). Eczemas, photodermatoses, papulosquamous (including fungal) diseases, and figurate erythemas. In L. Goldman & R. I. Schafer (Eds.), *Goldman-Cecil Medicine,* (25th ed., pp. 2662–2671). Philadelphia, PA: Elsevier Saunders.

Ong, P. Y. (2012). Atopic dermatitis. In E. T. Bope & R. D. Kellerman (Eds.), *Conn's current therapy 2012,* (pp. 190–193). Philadelphia, PA: Elsevier Saunders.

Papp, K. A., Leonardi, C., Menter, A., Ortonne, J. P., Krueger, J. G., Kricorian, G., . . . Baumgartner, S. (2012). Brodalumab, an anti-interleukin-17-receptor antibody for psoriasis. *New England Journal of Medicine, 366*(13), 1181–1189.

Petronic-Rosic, V. (2012). Melanoma. In E. T. Bope & R. D. Kellerman (Eds.), *Conn's current therapy 2012,* (pp. 234–236). Philadelphia, PA: Elsevier Saunders.

Puchalsky, D. (2012). Papulosquamous eruptions: Psoriasis. In E. T. Bope & R. D. Kellerman (Eds.), *Conn's current therapy 2012,* (pp. 239–243). Philadelphia, PA: Elsevier Saunders.

Wasserman, S. I. (2016). Approach to the patient with allergic or immunologic disease. In L. Goldman & R. I. Schafer (Eds.), *Goldman-Cecil Medicine,* (25th ed., pp. 1674–1677). Philadelphia, PA: Elsevier Saunders.

Sheridan, R. L. (2016.) Medical aspects of injuries and burns. In L. Goldman R. I. Schafer (Eds.), *Goldman-Cecil Medicine,* (25th ed., pp. 711–717). Philadelphia, PA: Elsevier Saunders.

Tarim, A., & Ezer, A. (2012). Electrical burn is still a major risk for amputations. *Burns.* Retrieved from http://www.ncbi.nim.nih.go/pubmed/22853969

Waisman, A. (2012). To be 17 again: Anti-interleukin-17 treatment for psoriasis. *New England Journal of Medicine, 366*(13), 1251–1252.

Yiannias, J. A., & Egnatios, G. L. (2012). Contact dermatitis. In E. T. Bope & R. D. Kellerman (Eds.), *Conn's current therapy 2012,* (pp. 205–208). Philadelphia, PA: Elsevier Saunders.

CHAPTER 33

Assistive Technology

INTRODUCTION

The International Classification of Functioning, Disability, and Health (ICF) presents a model for conceptualizing health conditions that deemphasizes limitations and emphasizes function in the context of what individuals actually do on a daily basis—rather than only what they have the ability to do (Scherer & Glueckauf, 2005). Changes in social philosophy as well as changes in policy and legislation have enhanced the ability of individuals with health conditions once considered "disabling" to live full and productive lives within the community (Peterson & Rosenthal, 2005). However, more active participation and independence have also been brought about through *assistive technology*, which facilitates independence and participation in activities related to home, social, recreational, and work environments (Berry & Ignash, 2003). Focus is on increasing individuals' function within the context of their own environment and personal goals, rather than simply increasing function per se (Blair, 2000; Kroll, Beatty, & Bingham, 2003; Scherer, Sax, & Glueckauf, 2005).

DEFINING ASSISTIVE TECHNOLOGY

Everyone uses assistive technology, whether or not a health condition is present. Informally, assistive technology can be thought off as any tool, apparatus, device, or machine used to accomplish some practical task or purpose in a home, work, or recreational setting (Blake & Bodine, 2002; King, 1999). Anyone who has used a calculator to balance a checkbook, a cell phone to link with friends, or a computer to play games has used assistive technology.

Assistive technology in some form—such as wheelchairs, Braille watches, and hearing aids—has been used by individuals with health conditions to meet their specific needs for many years. These devices were, however, often used in keeping with the *medical model*; that is, they were "prescribed" based on the standard presumed limitation associated with a health condition rather than resulting from individual goals and choice (Mendelsohn & Fox, 2002).

The importance of assistive technology being matched to the goals of the individual became more important as a result of legislation. The *Americans with Disabilities Act (ADA)*, enacted in 1990, established the right of individuals with disabilities to receive reasonable accommodations that would enable them to perform essential job functions. The role and importance of assistive technology for individuals with disability were affirmed with the *Assistive Technology Act of 1998,* which was reauthorized in 2004. The Assistive Technology Act of 2004 defines assistive technology as follows:

> Any item, piece of equipment, or product system, whether acquired commercially off the shelf, modified, or customized, that is used to increase, maintain, or improve functional capabilities of individuals with disabilities.

LEVELS OF ASSISTIVE TECHNOLOGY COMPLEXITY

Assistive technology enables people to achieve personal goals and to move toward future achievements in independent activities of daily living, education, employment, recreation, and full participation in society. The level of complexity and sophistication of the technology incorporated in assistive devices to meet individuals' needs in achieving their goals can vary greatly. Some devices are relatively easy to use, whereas others require training and practice before they can be used effectively. The most effective assistive device is one that the individual is comfortable using and that meets his or her own particular needs.

Assistive devices may be either "high tech" or "low tech." *High-tech* devices are technologically complex, require precise operations, and involve sophisticated materials, such as a *biomechanical prosthesis* for an upper extremity or *refreshable Braille displays* that provide tactile output of information on a computer screen for people with blindness or low vision. In general, the more sophisticated the device, the more complicated it may be to use. Although some individuals adapt to high-tech devices relatively easily, especially if they meet their individual needs, other persons may find such devices intimidating, leading to anxiety or hesitance about the device, and possibly resulting in abandonment of the device all together. In other instances, the cost of the high-tech device may make its use prohibitive.

Low-tech devices are constructed from readily available materials and are simple, inexpensive, and easy to use. They can include anything from simple do-it-yourself items such as a paint can opener when there is reduced hand strength, to a cane to assist in stability, to a rocker knife that enables individuals to cut food with one hand. Although they meet the needs and goals of some individuals and are less complex, inexpensive, and easier to use, low-tech devices may not be adequate to meet specific needs depending on the level and type of incapacitation.

Regardless of the sophistication of the assistive device, the most effective device is one that individuals are willing and able to use in their own environment to meet their own goals. Consequently, before any device is selected, it is important to consider individual goals and tasks within a given environment, psychosocial incentives and disincentives, personal characteristics, and abilities and preferences (Blair, 2000). Individuals should be actively involved in choosing their assistive devices and in assessing the devices' effectiveness. Having technology available does not necessarily mean that the resulting assistive device will be useful or that it will be used. Many factors aside from availability are relevant (Hasselbring & Glaser, 2000).

Individuals' use of assistive technology and the types of assistive devices used may change over time or as individuals age. If individuals have a condition marked by progressive levels of incapacitation, different assistive devices may be needed over the course of the condition to accommodate additional needs. In other instances, different devices may be required because an individual's lifestyle has changed. Human circumstances are not static. In turn, needs and goals change over time, and so may the type of assistive technology required by a particular individual.

USES OF ASSISTIVE TECHNOLOGY

Assistive devices are used to increase independence, save time and energy, and prevent injury. The type and use of assistive technology depend on the needs of the individual. Some common uses are listed here:

- Mobility, postural control, and transfers
- Transportation
- Self-help/personal care needs
- Home management/safety
- Communication/sensory needs
- Recreation
- Cognitive/memory/learning needs
- Workplace modification
- Accessibility

Mobility, Postural Control, and Transfers

Mobility refers to the ability to move within and around the immediate environment as well as the ability to travel outside the home. Mobility aids vary greatly in their type and use (Chen, Chen, Chen, & Lin, 2003). They can consist of low-tech aids such as a transfer board to help individuals get in or out of bed, bars to assist with getting on or off a toilet, and devices that maintain postural control while sitting or provide postural accommodation. They also encompass high-tech aids such as microcomputer-controlled powered wheelchairs and powered wheelchairs with puff and sip controls.

Different mobility devices may be needed for the same individual. Some individuals may require one type of wheelchair for indoor use and another type for sports or outdoor use. Lifts and stairway guides also increase individuals' mobility both in the home and away from home.

Transportation

Transportation is another important mobility need, both for getting to work and for achieving increased independence. Adapted personal vehicles, which include hand controls and steering devices for individuals with limited use of one or more extremities, may make it possible to drive standard motor vehicles. Van conversions and buses adapted to include wheelchair lifts enable individuals to carry wheelchairs or scooters, which can then be used at their point of destination.

Despite the availability of assistive devices for mobility, environmental constraints can remain a barrier. Wheeled mobility aids and transportation aids are maximally effective only when the environment accommodates their use. Both assistive devices and environmental modification are necessary for full mobility potential.

Self-Help/Personal Care Needs

Assistive technology for self-help or personal care needs facilitates completion of tasks of daily living such as eating, drinking, brushing hair, brushing teeth, putting on clothes, dressing, bathing, toileting, and tying shoes. These devices are generally low-tech aids. Although they are usually relatively inexpensive, they are nevertheless vital to independence and to reaching goals in other areas (Thyberg, Hass, Nordenskiod, & Skogh, 2004). Personal care devices may be as simple as an item purchased from a hardware store, or they can be specially manufactured to meet a specific need. Examples of devices that may be helpful for self-care include electric toothbrushes, button hooks, sock guides, and zipper aids.

The task to be performed and the environments in which the device is to be used determine the type of device needed for activities of daily living. Individuals' needs may change as they move to different environments. For example, devices used in the home for activities of daily living may not be appropriate on a business trip. The appropriateness of each device should be considered in the context of the setting in which it is to be used.

Home Management/Safety

A variety of devices used by individuals *without functional incapacitation* also increases the functional capacity of individuals *with functional incapacitation.* Devices such as microwave ovens, electric can openers, and other electronic devices may be convenience items for people *without* functional incapacity, yet can significantly increase the functionality and independence of people *with* functional incapacity. The increasing sophistication of computers, robotics, and other electronic devices may also offer more independence in activities of daily living for persons with functional incapacity in the future.

Assistive technology for home management or safety includes devices that assist with tasks such as cooking, cleaning, turning lamps on or off, locking/unlocking and opening doors, hearing the doorbell, writing checks, hearing a smoke alarm, and being aware of danger. Signaling and alerting devices, bottle and can openers, modified lighting, and automated closet adapters are examples of assistive devices that may increase individuals' ability to function more independently in the home (LoPresti, Brienza, Angelo, & Gilbertson, 2003).

Communication/Sensory Needs

Communication is a complex activity involving perception and integration of information. It includes speaking, writing, reading, hearing, signing, and nonverbal behaviors. Communication is vital to a number of tasks that many people take for granted, such as talking, hearing, speaking on the phone, making appointments, sending emails, and being able to explain a health problem to a healthcare provider. Assistive devices that enhance communication range from low-tech devices, such as books and pencils, to high-tech aids, such as augmentative and alternative communication (AAC) devices (Neumann et al., 2004). Whether individuals use low-tech or high-tech devices, a certain degree of cognitive and motor ability as well as training are required.

Communication devices can be manual or electronic. Examples of manual devices include communication boards, which contain line drawings, pictures, symbols, or other systems through which individuals spell out messages or indicate phrases to others. Electronic systems are often computer based and may filter or manipulate vocalizations or provide synthesized speech. For example, electronic voice-output communication aids (VOCAs) are computerized devices that produce synthetic or digitized speech output when activated. Individuals then point to visual-graphic symbols, which are used to represent messages. Because these devices provide speech output, they are more easily integrated into everyday environments with unfamiliar people (Miranda, 2001). Other types of devices that aid in communication include computer hardware and software applications that provide writing assistance, speech-generating devices, and the artificial larynx.

Because of the complexity of communication and the varying capabilities and needs of individuals in different situations, no one type of device is appropriate for everyone. The selection of the best assistive device to aid in communication is based on a systematic analysis of the individual's characteristics and environmental demands. In addition, a trial period of use is often necessary to determine whether the individual is able to use the device with ease and how well it meets the individual's needs (Sigafoos, O'Reilly, Ganz, Lancioni, & Schlosser, 2005). The device chosen to augment or enhance communication must be one that meets the unique specifications of the individual who will be using it. Because communication is such an individual and personal function, the individual using a device is best qualified to evaluate whether it improves communication outcomes.

Communication devices are also available for individuals who need to increase their functional capacity in sensory areas, including sight, hearing, touch, taste, and smell (Sokol-McKay, Buskirk, & Whittaker, 2003). Assistive devices to increase functional capacity in these areas may range from simple to complex. Examples of simple devices include eyeglasses, magnifiers, and a bath thermometer to prevent burns. Examples of more complex devices include voice recognition computers and optical-to-vibrotactile prostheses that make it possible for individuals who are blind to distinguish patterns of stimulation, enabling them to discriminate between certain properties of three-dimensional space. Assistive devices for individuals who are deaf or hard of hearing include amplification, vibrotactile prompts, hearing aids, and telecommunication display devices—all of which help individuals who are deaf or hard of hearing function more effectively in a hearing world.

Recreation

Recreational activities may range from gardening, playing cards, and reading to watching television, riding a bicycle, and climbing a mountain. Assistive devices needed for recreational activities vary with individual need, interest, and ability. Developers of assistive devices have already created sports equipment that enables athletes without functional incapacity to achieve far greater feats than previously had been expected. Some of the same types of technology have since been applied to recreational devices for individuals with functional incapacity, giving them new opportunities to engage in such activities that were not available to members of earlier generations.

The sophistication of the technology incorporated into recreational equipment varies with the activity. The technology required for assistance in card playing, for example, is much different from that required for assistance with downhill skiing. Individuals with functional incapacity have the same differing interests and skills related to recreational activities as persons without functional capacity. Unfortunately, one of the major barriers to participation in recreational activities of their choice for individuals with functional incapacity may be the bias of those around them, who may assume that their participation is inappropriate or impossible.

Cognitive/Memory/Learning Needs

Cognitive and learning disability may be either a primary or a secondary health condition. This type of disability can be acquired, such as with traumatic brain injury; the result of brain deterioration, such as in dementia; or congenital, such as intellectual disability. No matter what the cause, the individual's functional capacity is complex and unique and may change over time. Other areas of function, such as motor or behavioral function, memory, or learning, may also be affected. Assistive technology can aid individuals by enhancing performance of functional tasks as well as tasks related to cognitive function (Hammel, 2003; Scherer, 2005).

Memory function, regardless of the cause, can affect independent function. Although many techniques to increase memory performance have been developed, such improvements are often short-lived. Consequently, a number of assistive devices for memory enhancements have been developed, including record and playback devices, and voice-activated reminder calendars.

Functional ability in persons with cognitive disability is complex and multifactorial. In some individuals, the usefulness of an assistive device designed to address one area of function may be negated because of other areas of incapacity. For example, a small portable device designed to assist with memory may be helpful for that area of function, but is useless if the individual also has motor difficulty and cannot operate the device. In addition, sophisticated devices may be adequate for achieving greater functional capacity in some areas, but the individual may not have the cognitive capacity to learn to operate the device.

Workplace Modification

The American with Disabilities Act assured that reasonable accommodation would be afforded to individuals with disability so that qualified persons with disability could be employed. *Reasonable accommodation* was defined as a modification of a work site or job that did not impose financial hardship on the employer. The intent of job or workplace modification was to increase individuals' functional capacity, thereby enhancing their ability to perform the job.

Additional assistive devices may not be needed in the workplace if appropriate environmental accommodations can be made. For some individuals, modification of the environment through better lighting, air-temperature control, or removal of obstacles through architectural modifications or restructuring of the job may be all that is necessary to enable them to achieve functional capacity. In other instances, finding alternative ways to perform a job function or modifying existing devices may produce the same result. When assistive technology is needed, the necessary devices may be either low tech, such as reachers or extenders, or high tech, such as robotics (O'Day, Palsbo, Dhont, & Scheer, 2002).

Although computer technology can help individuals increase their functional capacity, some health conditions and associated limitations make computer use difficult, such that other assistive devices may be needed to enhance computer use. For instance, head controls and other adaptive computer aids can provide an alternative means to computer access (Fichten, Barile, Asuncion, & Fossey, 2000). Software has also been developed that automatically adjusts to the needs of the particular individual, especially if the health condition limits head or neck or movement of the upper extremities (LoPresti & Brienza, 2004). In addition, control mechanisms or switches may be used to operate computers or communication aids, thereby increasing functional capacity.

When assistive devices are needed in the workplace, as in other settings, the type of device is determined by the specific need and the individual's preference. As in other areas of the individual's life, high-tech devices are not always the most appropriate or effective way to meet an individual's need or to increase his or her ability to perform a specific function effectively. Focusing on individuals' ability (rather than their functional incapacity) and including them in the process of deciding what is needed are the most useful approaches to determining which, if any, assistive devices will be beneficial.

Accessibility

Accessibility can involve more than architectural structure. Assistive devices for use in the environment may also increase individuals' ability to function within their environment. Simple examples include a Braille labeler for assistance in identifying items, a talking location indicator, and verbal announcement of bus stops or elevator floors.

INDIVIDUAL ASSESSMENT

Both the physical and psychosocial environments affect the usefulness of any particular assistive device. Consequently, in addition to functional capacity and personal goals, the characteristics of the individual's unique environment must always be considered when determining the type and number of assistive devices needed (Blair, 2000; Hammel, 2003).

Few people function in only one setting. In turn, individuals with functional limitations may require certain types of devices for activities of daily living, different devices to be used at work, and still other devices to be used in social and recreational settings.

People with similar health conditions that result in functional limitation may not require the same type or the same number of assistive devices. The type of assistive device needed depends on the location where the equipment will be used, the tasks and activities in each environment, and the extent to which tasks would be enhanced by use of the device. Architectural accessibility and the amount of environmental support needed for the use of an assistive device are important considerations as well. The physical environment in which the assistive device is to be operated must be assessed, and obstacles that could interfere with the device's use must be identified. Sometimes environmental modification alone may increase the individual's ability to function. As society becomes increasingly aware of the need for universal design so that environments are more accessible for all individuals, design may change so that many of today's physical barriers no longer exist in the future.

The psychosocial environment also affects the usefulness of assistive devices. The amount of support and encouragement that individuals receive from others in their environment may be a major determinant of the degree to which an assistive device is used.

The cultural environment can also play a major role in the type of device obtained and the extent to which it is used. For example, not all individuals who are deaf or hard of hearing believe that they need to compensate for decreased auditory function. Individuals in the Deaf community have a strong cultural identity and may not be receptive to the technological advances currently available.

Before any assistive device is obtained, a thorough assessment of individual preferences and goals should be completed. If a certain type of device is inadequate to meet an individual's goals, it should not be assumed that no viable alternative exists. Likewise, it should not be assumed that individuals with the same health condition will always require the same type of device. Although high-tech devices may be useful for performing certain tasks, it should not be assumed that all individuals want to perform those tasks, or use a high-tech device to do so, or that other types of devices could not be equally useful.

Although access to consumer-responsive assistive devices and services is federally mandated, individuals differ in their goals, values, perspectives, motivations, and expectations—all of which can affect the use of assistive devices. All assistive devices should be matched to the individual's unique capabilities and temperament. The success of assistive devices is determined by the degree to which they match the goals and perspectives of the individual, rather than the devices' potential usefulness for any particular day-to-day activity.

SUPPORTS AND BARRIERS TO USING ASSISTIVE TECHNOLOGY

Assistive technology, whether high tech or low tech, is only as useful as the extent to which it meets the goals of the individual for whom it was designed. For some individuals, a barrier that prevents successful use of certain types of assistive technology is the amount of energy or work required to use it. In some instances, the problem may be remedied by a simple adjustment to the device, such as changing the location of a control. In other instances, because of the complexity of the device or the mechanics involved in its effective use, modifications cannot be made. When devices are too difficult to operate, user motivation and success rates decline (King, 1999).

Just as physical effort may reduce motivation and success in using assistive technology, so may the amount of cognitive effort required. Devices that require more complex thought processes or problem solving for effectiveness may be more difficult for some individuals to use.

The amount of time required to use an assistive device and the degree to which it meets the individual's goals also determine its effectiveness. Devices that require a number of steps, or that are slow to respond to commands, may be less acceptable to individuals than those devices that take relatively few steps to use and respond to commands immediately.

The cosmetic appearance of the device may also affect user motivation. Appearance is important to everyone. Devices that are more visually appealing are more likely to be utilized than devices perceived as creating a negative image (King, 1999). Individuals with functional incapacity may also be sensitive to the perception that the device makes them appear to others as being more incapacitated. For instance, an individual using a wheelchair who later also requires a hearing aid may fear that the latter device's use signals continued deterioration and incapacitation.

Cultural beliefs as well as the individual's personal philosophy regarding chronic health conditions or incapacitation and cultural expectations can also have an impact on the extent to which assistive devices are incorporated into the individual's daily life. Some individuals may have cultural objections to certain types of technology. Others may hold cultural beliefs or values regarding cultural roles and expectations that influence the degree to which assistive devices should be used.

Lastly, assistive devices must be durable and easily repaired. All mechanical or electrical devices can malfunction. The more complex the device, the more prone it may be to malfunction, and usually the more complicated and expensive it is to repair. Other maintenance-related issues regarding assistive device use may be whether the item must be shipped to the manufacturer for evaluation, how long the turnaround time for repair is, whether a loaner device will be available during the repair period, and what the repair will cost.

APPRAISAL OF ASSISTIVE DEVICES AND ALTERNATIVES

As new technologies become available, more choices of assistive devices will be offered to meet specific needs. Oddly enough, the large number of choices available may make it more difficult to choose the most appropriate device suited to the individual. Assistive devices must be assessed realistically. New devices on the market should have been appropriately evaluated, and performance results, safety data, and durability information for those items should be readily available.

The degree to which an assistive device can be upgraded or expanded as new technology becomes available should be assessed. In some instances, compatibility with other assistive devices may be important to determine. The initial cost of the assistive device, its maintenance costs, the availability of resources for repair and their associated costs, and the costs of replacement should all be assessed.

It is also important to consider the degree to which a device accurately reflects an individual's preferences, lifestyle, and values. The simplicity of less elaborate assistive devices should be weighed against the sometimes greater functionality of more elaborate devices in the context of the individual's specific needs. Whether a device is portable may determine whether an individual can use the device in more than one setting. The degree to which assistance is needed to learn to use a device and the extent to which the device can be used independently are other factors that affect use.

Although emphasis is placed on the degree to which a device increases functional capacity or quality of life, the aesthetics of the device cannot be ignored. The appearance of a device, its ease of use, and the disruption associated with its use in certain settings can determine individuals' willingness to use it. If individuals feel conspicuous using a device, believe it is stigmatizing, or feel that it interferes with social interaction, the device may be abandoned.

The physical and cognitive abilities needed to use an assistive device also are important considerations. Ergonomic aspects of the technology, as well as individuals' ability to learn to use a device and maintain it, should be explored. The best assistive device is not always the most expensive option. Locating the best assistive device requires closely examining the costs and benefits of the device (as opposed to just the available alternatives) and then matching the device to the individual's specific needs and resources.

To maximize the effectiveness of assistive devices, professionals working with individuals with functional incapacitation need to have comprehensive knowledge of the health condition and its associated limitations (Kroll & Neri, 2003; Wehman, Wilson, Parent, Sherron-Tagett, & McKinley, 2000), a good understanding of the multiple consequences of access barriers and barriers to service delivery (Bingham & Beatty, 2003; Neri & Kroll, 2003), and a knowledge of bureaucratic structure that could interfere with appropriate service delivery (Darrah, Magil-Evans, & Adkins, 2002; O'Day et al., 2002). Most of all, health professionals need to involve individuals in the decision-making process related to assistive devices and ask those individuals how they can best help them meet their goals and achieve optimal function and independence.

PSYCHOSOCIAL ISSUES

The usefulness of a device in helping individuals achieve their goals and functional capacity may be compromised if a number of psychosocial issues are not taken into consideration.

Stigma

Stigma—that is, the feeling of being devalued by others—is a common experience for many individuals with chronic health conditions (Parette & Scherer, 2004). Additional stigma may be experienced with assistive device usage (Zimmer & Chappell, 1999). An individual using an assistive device may feel that the device increases the visibility of the health condition, calling attention to it and emphasizing the individual's loss of functional capacity and increased vulnerability (Luborsky, 1993). Some individuals may believe that use of an assistive device brings about heightened evaluation and scrutiny of them in social settings, such that they feel an increased sense of alienation and isolation. As a result, use of these devices may affect self-image and result in lowered self-esteem if they perceive that others are treating them differently and that social interactions are negatively affected by the device. Rather than experience increased stigma, individuals may elect not to use the device at all, even though it could increase their functional capacity.

Aesthetics

An issue linked to self-image and self-esteem is the appearance of the assistive devices. In some cases, the aesthetic qualities of the device may determine the degree to which the device is used. Products that are designed to be more attractive and aesthetically pleasing may increase individuals' willingness to use them.

Cultural Factors

Varying cultural values, belief systems, and family structures can influence the extent to which assistive technology is incorporated into an individual's life. Chronic health conditions in general, and assistive technology in particular, may be viewed very differently by different cultures, and even in different subcultures embedded within the larger culture. Cultural philosophy regarding health and illness, their meaning, and the process of healing may have much to do with the success or failure of interventions to introduce assistive technology.

The culture of individuals may affect not only how they accept and adjust to their health condition but also their willingness to use assistive devices to increase functional capacity. Independence for an individual with functional incapacitation may not be viewed as important in some cultures in which it is expected that family and community will meet the needs of the individual. A high-tech device may be viewed as an extravagance and a luxury rather than as a useful tool needed to increase functional capacity. Use of an assistive device may have social consequences for individuals from different cultures. No matter how useful the device may appear to be in helping the individual increase function, unless cultural factors are considered, interest in and acceptance of assistive technology may not be sufficient to bring about positive outcomes regarding its use.

Age

Chronological age and developmental stage influence individuals' adaptation to chronic health conditions and functional incapacitation; likewise, they can affect receptivity to and acceptance of assistive devices designed to assist in achieving increased functional capacity. Although each individual is unique, age does, to some extent, define life tasks, expectations, and physical and mental preparedness of individuals in various stages of the life span. Just as the degree and types of chronic health conditions that individuals experience influence the rate of use of assistive technology, so the age of the individual and the tasks associated with his or her life stage may significantly affect the type of assistive device needed and the extent to which it is used. Older adults with the same chronic health condition and same limitations may have different assistive technology needs than do younger adults.

THE FUTURE OF ASSISTIVE TECHNOLOGY

The extent to which assistive technology is used to increase the function of individuals with functional incapacity is expanding rapidly. Further development of assistive technology and assistive devices will be affected by several factors:

- The shift from institutional care to community-based services
- Movement from the medical model to a social model
- Increased roles for individuals in selection and application of assistivetechnology (Cook, 2002)

The emphasis on helping individuals with functional incapacity function in their everyday life in the community in accordance with their goals will influence the type of assistive device utilized as well as the development of new technologies. Increased consideration is being given to the cultural and social effects of assistive technology. In addition, technology developers are investigating economic factors and means to increase accessibility. The concept of universal design emphasizes the creation of products and environments that are amenable to use by all people. It implies that environmental demands on all abilities should

be minimized. Seven basic principles underlie universal design:

1. Equitable use
2. Flexible use
3. Simple and intuitive use
4. Perceptible information
5. Tolerance for error
6. Low physical effort
7. Size and space for approach and use (Follette Story, 2011)

Equitable use refers to products that are useful and marketable to people with diverse abilities. Not only is the design appealing to all users but everyone can use the product in the same way so that individuals are not segregated or stigmatized by its use. Rather than requiring separate facilities for individuals with incapacity (such as toilet stalls), universal design provides ways of accommodating all people, regardless of their functional status. Curb cuts are an example of a design that is helpful to everyone crossing the street, from those with a stroller to those in a wheelchair.

Flexible use implies that the product accommodates a wide range of individual preferences and abilities. Individuals are provided with a choice in method of use. Elevators and automatic doors are examples of assistive technology that offer options and accommodate individual abilities. Sensor-activated faucets that have hands-free operation are another example of a design that provides flexibility in use.

Simple, intuitive design eliminates unnecessary complexity. Such a design is easy to understand regardless of the user's experience, knowledge, or language skills. Devices are able to accommodate a wide range of literacy and language skills and follow a predictable and intuitive mode of use. As an example, kitchen blenders with high-contrast on/off switches require no training and are relatively easy to use.

Perceptible information refers to effective communication of necessary information regardless of the individual's sensory abilities or the ambient conditions. Examples include use of different modes for presentation of essential information, such as using verbal or tactile modes, and providing compatibility with a variety of devices used by individuals who have sensory limitations.

Tolerance for error refers to designs that minimize hazards and the adverse consequences of accidents or unintended actions. For instance, arranging furniture to minimize hazards, providing warnings of potential hazards, and providing fail-safe features are all examples of this principle of universal design.

Low physical effort implies that the design can be used efficiently and comfortably with a minimum of sustained physical effort and with a minimum of fatigue. Lever door handles, as an example, do not require pinching, twisting, or grasping. Other examples include rocker light switches and sensor-activated doors that promote ease of performance, which can be beneficial to everyone.

The last principle—*size and space for approach and use*—refers to products that are designed so that approach, reach, manipulation, and use are appropriate regardless of body size. Examples include showers without thresholds, cabinets that may be used by seated or standing users, and accommodations in hand or grip size.

Making products and environments more usable by a wider range of individuals will reduce the currently higher cost of specialized products and the need for special environmental modifications. When individuals without functional incapacity and individuals with functional incapacity use the same products, the stigma once associated with use of special products is decreased. Products that are universally designed are also usually more aesthetically pleasing, which contributes to decreased stigma and enhanced motivation for use (Fozard, Rietsema, Bourna, & Graafmans, 2000).

REFERENCES

Americans with Disabilities Act of 1990. P.L. 101–336.

Assistive Technology Act of 1998. P.L. 105–394.

Assistive Technology Act of 2004. P.L. 108–364.

Berry, B. E., & Ignash, S. (2003). Assistive technology: Providing independence for individuals with disabilities. *Rehabilitation Nursing, 28*(1), 6–14.

Bingham, S. S., & Beatty, P. W. (2003). Rates of access to assistive equipment and medical rehabilitation services among people with disabilities. *Disability Rehabilitation, 25*(9), 487–490.

Blair, M. E. (2000). Assistive technology: What and how for persons with spinal cord injury. *SCI Nursing, 17*(3), 110–118.

Blake, D. J., & Bodine, C. (2002). An overview of assistive technology for persons with multiple sclerosis. *Journal of Rehabilitation Research and Development, 39*(2), 299–312.

Chen, Y. L., Chen, S. C., Chen, W. L., & Lin, J. F. (2003). A head oriented wheelchair for people with disabilities. *Disability Rehabilitation, 25*(6), 249–253.

Cook, A. M. (2002). Future directions in assistive technologies. In M. Scherer (Ed.), *Assistive technology: Matching device and consumer for successful rehabilitation* (pp. 269–280). Washington, DC: American Psychological Association.

Darrah, J., Magil-Evans, J., & Adkins, R. (2002). How well are we doing? Families of adolescents or young adults with cerebral palsy share their perceptions of service delivery. *Disability Rehabilitation, 24*(10), 542–549.

Fichten, C. S., Barile, M., Asuncion, J. V., & Fossey, M. E. (2000). What government, agencies, and organizations can do to improve access to computers for postsecondary students with disabilities: Recommendations based on Canadian empirical data. *International Journal of Rehabilitation Research, 23*(3), 191–199.

Follette Story, M. (2011). Principles of universal design. In W. F. E. Preiser & E. Ostroff (Eds.), *Universal design handbook* (pp. 152–168). New York, NY: McGraw-Hill.

Fozard, J. L., Rietsema, J., Bourna, H., & Graafmans, J. A. (2000). Gerontechnology: Creating enabling environments for the challenges and opportunities of aging. *Educational Gerontology, 26*, 331–345.

Hammel, J. (2003). Technology and the environment: Supportive resource or barrier for people with developmental disabilities? *Nursing Clinics of North America, 38*(2), 331–349.

Hasselbring, T. S., & Glaser, C. H. (2000). Use of computer technology to help students with special needs. *Future Child, 10*(2), 102–122.

King, T. W. (1999). *Assistive technology: Essential human factors.* Boston, MA: Allyn and Bacon.

Kroll, T., Beatty, P. W., & Bingham, S. (2003). Primary care satisfaction among adults with physical disabilities: The role of patient–provider communication. *Managed Care Quarterly, 11*(1), 11–19.

Kroll, T., & Neri, M. T. (2003). Experiences with care coordination among people with cerebral palsy, multiple sclerosis, or spinal cord injury. *Disability Rehabilitation, 25*(19), 1106–1114.

LoPresti, E. F., & Brienza, D. M. (2004). Adaptive software for head-operated computer controls. *IEEE Transactions on Neural System Rehabilitation Engineering, 12*(1), 102–111.

LoPresti, E. F., Brienza, D. M., Angelo, J., & Gilbertson, L. (2003). Neck range of motion and use of computer head controls. *Journal of Rehabilitation Research and Development, 40*(3), 199–211.

Luborsky, M. R. (1993). Sociocultural factors shaping technology usage: Fulfilling the promise. *Technology and Disability, 2*(1), 71–78.

Mendelsohn, S., & Fox, H. R. (2002). Evolving legislation and public policy related to disability and assistive technology. In M. J. Scherer (Ed.), *Assistive technology: Matching device and consumer for successful rehabilitation,* (pp. 17–28). Washington, DC: American Psychological Association.

Miranda, P. (2001). Autism, augmentative communication, and assistive technology: What do we really know? *Focus on Autism and Other Developmental Disabilities, 16*(3), 141–151.

Neri, J. T., & Kroll, T. (2003). Understanding the consequences of access barriers to health care: Experiences of adults with disabilities. *Disability Rehabilitation, 25*(2), 85–96.

Neumann, N., Hinterberger, T., Kaiser, J., Leins, U., Birbaumer, N., & Kubler, A. (2004). Automatic processing of self-regulation of slow cortical potentials: Evidence from brain-computer communication in paralyzed patients. *Clinical Neurophysiology, 115*(3), 628–635.

O'Day, B., Palsbo, S. E., Dhont, K. K., & Scheer, J. (2002). Health plan selection criteria by people with impaired mobility. *Medical Care, 40*(9), 725–728.

Parette, P., & Scherer, M. (2004). Assistive technology use and stigma. *Education and Training in Developmental Disabilities, 39*(3), 217–226.

Peterson, D. B., & Rosenthal, D. A. (2005). The International Classification of Functioning, Disability and Health (ICF) as an allegory for history and systems in rehabilitation education. *Rehabilitation Education, 19*(2 & 3), 95–104.

Scherer, M. J. (2005). Assessing the benefits of using assistive technologies and other supports for thinking, remembering, and learning. *Disability and Rehabilitation, 27*(13), 731–739.

Scherer, M. J., & Glueckauf, R. L. (2005). Assessing the benefits of assistive technologies for activities and participation. *Rehabilitation Psychology, 50*(2), 132–141.

Scherer, M. J., Sax, C. L., & Glueckauf, R. L. (2005). Activities and participation: The need to include assistive technology in rehabilitation counselor education. *Rehabilitation Education, 19*(2), 177–190.

Sigafoos, J., O'Reilly, M., Ganz, J. B., Lancioni, G. E., & Schlosser, R. W. (2005). Supporting self-determination in AAC interventions by assessing preference for communication devices. *Technology and Disability 17,* 143–153.

Sokol-McKay, D., Buskirk, K., & Whittaker, P. (2003). Adaptive low-vision and blindness techniques for blood glucose monitoring. *Diabetes Education, 29*(4), 614–618.

Thyberg, I., Hass, U. A., Nordenskiod, U., & Skogh, T. (2004). Survey of the use and effect of assistive devices in patients with early rheumatoid arthritis: A two-year follow-up of women and men. *Arthritis and Rheumatism, 51*(3), 413–421.

Wehman, P., Wilson, K., Parent, W., Sherron-Tagett, P., & McKinley, W. (2000). Employment satisfaction of individuals with spinal cord injury. *American Journal of Physical Medicine and Rehabilitation, 79*(2), 161–169.

Zimmer, Z., & Chappell, N. L. (1999). Receptivity to new technology among older adults. *Disability and Rehabilitation, 21,* 222–230.

CHAPTER 34

Aging with Disability

DEFINING AGING

Aging is a normal, lifelong process that begins at conception, evolves through the life cycle, and involves a constantly changing internal and external environment. Throughout the life cycle, each individual experiences physical, psychological, social, behavioral, and cognitive changes that are a normal part of growth, development, and aging. During the early portion of the life cycle, many changes are associated with growth and development. In contrast, in adulthood and later life, organs operate at reduced efficiency, and the capacity of the body to achieve physiological balance declines with age (Walston, 2016). Some changes associated with aging are readily observable, whereas other internal changes are less apparent. Not everyone undergoes changes at the same rate, nor do all body systems undergo change at the same rate. In general, changes that occur with age occur so gradually over time that they go unnoticed. The degree and level of age-related changes depend on a number of factors, including environmental, socioeconomic, lifestyle, cultural, and genetic influences.

Despite the natural changes associated with the aging process, many individuals remain active in older age with no major effect on daily function. Nevertheless, due to some of these changes, older adults become more vulnerable to chronic health conditions and manifestations that affect functional capacity.

The natural changes associated with aging and the implications of those changes occur not only in able-bodied individuals, but also in individual with chronic health conditions. As a result, the natural changes associated with aging may compound some of the manifestations that individuals with chronic health conditions already experience. In turn, as individuals with chronic health conditions age, certain body systems that have compensated for decreased function of other body systems in the past may experience increased potential for additional impact on functional capacity, or individuals may be at risk for developing new complications of their condition (Walston, 2016).

Although aging and associated changes are inevitable, some of these effects and associated manifestations can be slowed, enabling individuals to maintain optimal function and independence for a longer period of time (Newman & Cauley, 2016). Being aware of natural changes of aging and their effects on functional capacity, recognizing the manner in which natural changes combine with manifestations of chronic health conditions, and distinguishing between natural changes and those changes related to a new health condition are important steps to meet this goal.

AGING WITH A CHRONIC HEALTH CONDITION

Due to advances in health care and rehabilitation, many individuals with chronic health conditions who in the past might have succumbed to complications at a younger age are now living well into older adulthood. No matter during which period of the life cycle individuals experience a chronic health condition, the condition does not remain static over a lifetime. Age-related changes affect the manifestations of the chronic health condition and at times can contribute to individuals' increased susceptibility to complications (Rosso, Wisdom, Horner-Johnson, McGee, & Michael, 2011).

NATURAL CHANGES WITH AGING

The Cardiovascular System

The cardiovascular system includes the heart, blood, and blood vessels. Some individuals have a genetic predisposition toward development of chronic health conditions related to the cardiovascular system. The presence of risk factors such as elevated blood cholesterol, high blood pressure, obesity, tobacco use, and diabetes may also contribute to the development of cardiovascular-related health conditions.

Even when no risk factors appear to be present, a number of age-related changes in the cardiovascular system are likely to occur. Some heart muscle cells degenerate, some heart valves thicken and become less pliable, and the heart may pump less efficiently (Marks, 2016). The result may be a decreased ability to supply sufficient amounts of blood and oxygen to various parts of the body. The walls of the blood vessels also become thicker and less resilient over the course of a lifetime so that the heart works harder to force blood through vessels (Strait & Lakatta, 2012). In addition, areas around the heart's conduction system and changes in the natural pacemaker cells can affect the heart's rate and rhythm (Marks, 2016). In most cases, natural age-related changes alone have relatively little impact on individual's functional capacity. Because the heart becomes less efficient with aging, however, situations that place increased demands on the heart may make it difficult for this organ to respond effectively to the additional stress. A number of interventions—such as smoking cessation, management of high blood pressure, weight loss, and exercise—may help to maintain adequate cardiac function and reduce the risk of developing conditions such as stroke or myocardial infarction.

The Pulmonary System

The pulmonary system, which consists of the air passageways and lungs, declines in function to some degree with age (Ren, Li, Zhao, & Zhu, 2012). Ultimately, however, the extent to which it deteriorates depends on factors such as individual activity level, history of smoking, and exposure to environmental pollutants—all of which can in themselves contribute to functional changes in the lungs. In particular, these factors can cause the defense mechanisms usually present in the respiratory system to protect people from developing infections to be compromised.

For most older adults, the natural age-related changes in the respiratory system have little effect on functional capacity. Indeed, efficiency of the pulmonary system may be retained well into older age. Situations in which additional stress is placed on the lungs can, however, accentuate the lowered efficiency of the pulmonary system in older adults. As pulmonary function decreases, individuals may tire more easily. Moreover, in some instances, the oxygen supply to the brain may be reduced, resulting in manifestations of confusion.

The susceptibility of older adults to potentially serious pulmonary infections (Weinberger & Grubeck-Loebenstein, 2012) may be increased because of the decreased efficiency of defense mechanisms normally found in the pulmonary system. Consequently, annual influenza shots are an important protection against the development of severe pulmonary infections in older adults. Due to the decreased efficacy of the lungs with aging, prolonged bed rest can diminish pulmonary mechanics, further impeding lung function. In contrast, regular systematic exercise can increase or maintain pulmonary efficiency by promoting muscle tone and lung capacity. One of the most important interventions for maintaining pulmonary function is smoking cessation.

The Urinary System

The urinary system consists of the kidneys, ureters, bladder, and urethra. During the aging process, the kidneys shrink in size and become less efficient in excreting and reabsorbing substances from the blood. Consequently, decreased availability of substances important for red blood cell production and calcium absorption may make older individuals more prone to calcium deficiency and anemia. The kidneys also produce less of a substance that aids in intestinal absorption of calcium, a substance necessary for healthy bones. In addition, muscle tone in the urinary system diminishes and bladder capacity declines, both of which may contribute to urinary incontinence or urgency. If urinary incontinence has not been a problem in the past, frequency or incontinence due to age-related changes can be embarrassing and may contribute to social withdrawal.

The decreased adaptive ability of the kidney may increase individuals' risk of kidney failure should they develop a health condition or experience trauma. In addition, changes in the kidney due to natural aging make older individuals more susceptible to dehydration and urinary tract infections. The deceased efficiency of the kidneys may also delay excretion of medications, thereby contributing to the risk of medication overdose.

The Gastrointestinal System

The gastrointestinal system includes the mouth, esophagus, stomach, small and large intestines, rectum, and anus as well as the pancreas and liver, the accessory organs of digestion. As part of the natural aging process, both the number of taste buds and the production of saliva decline. Loss of muscle tone and slowing of movement of food through the intestinal tract may also occur (Grassi et al., 2011). Digestion and movement of digested food through the digestive system may take slightly longer. In addition, diminished blood flow to the intestines and liver may affect absorption of nutrients and the rate of metabolism for certain substances, such as medications and alcohol.

Usually age-related changes of the gastrointestinal system have little effect on overall functioning. However, these alterations in function may contribute to decreased absorption of nutrients, loss of appetite, consumption of smaller amounts of food, or skipping of meals—all of which can contribute to nutritional deficiencies (Moss, Dhillo, Frost, & Hickson, 2011).

Decreased muscle tone may also contribute to indigestion or constipation (Zuchelli & Myers, 2011), as both of these conditions may also be associated with poor eating habits.

Although diminished liver activity may not directly affect gastrointestinal function, it may contribute to serious side effects related to medication toxicity. Many medications are metabolized in the liver—and a less efficient liver may be unable to break down medications, allowing these pharmacologic agents to remain in the blood longer. If additional doses are taken, the potential

for medication buildup in the blood increases, as does the risk of medication overdose.

The Sensory System

The sensory system, in addition to encompassing organs related to smell, touch, and taste, includes the organs of sight and hearing. The most commonly experienced age-related changes involve vision and hearing. Specifically, natural changes resulting from aging cause diminished visual and hearing acuity. The degree to which there is loss of acuity of other senses is not well documented, although some decrease in the ability to taste and smell may occur.

Although a number of assistive devices, such as glasses and hearing aids, can be used to compensate for diminished visual and hearing function, age-related changes can also alter functional ability. Diminished visual acuity can affect night vision and the ability to see in dimly lit environments. In addition, diminished vision can contribute to falls that result in other types of injury.

Diminished hearing may lead to social isolation and have an impact on individuals' overall mental status. Individuals who experience difficulty in hearing may have problems in conversation and may become depressed and withdrawn. Inability to hear may also be misinterpreted by others as confusion, when in fact the individual simply cannot hear well.

The Skin

The skin consists of the epidermis and dermis, and contains sweat glands, sebaceous glands, and layers of fat. The largest body organ, it is the most exposed to the environment and, therefore, the most susceptible to environmental effects and factors. As part of the aging process, individuals experience a generalized thinning of the outer layer of skin, diminished function of oil production and sweat glands, and redistribution of fat (Levakov, Vuckovic, Dolai, Kacanski, & Bozanic, 2012). The skin and underlying structures become more fragile and less elastic. Fingernails and toenails become thickened and more brittle.

The skin of older adults becomes more prone to injury, yet healing of injuries is slower. Due to changes in sweat glands and redistribution of body fat, there is also diminished ability to maintain normal body temperature. Therefore, older adults are more sensitive to extremes of temperature. The most obvious age-related change in skin, of course, involves wrinkles.

The Immune System

The immune system protects individuals from invasion of foreign substances and, therefore, from infection. As part of the natural aging process, the effectiveness and efficiency of the immune system decline, rendering individuals more susceptible to infection (Dewan, Zheng, Xia, & Bill, 2012). In addition, decline in the efficiency of the immune system contributes to slower wound healing and a decreased ability to detect cell defects or foreign substances, which explains why the incidence of conditions such as cancer and autoimmune conditions increases with age.

The Musculoskeletal System

The musculoskeletal system consists of muscles, bones, and the structures connecting them. As aging occurs, individuals experience a loss of muscle mass and redistribution of body fat, with less lean muscle mass being available. Muscles become less elastic, and tendons and ligaments stiffen. Muscles regenerate less easily, and there is some reduction in bone mass. Changes in the musculoskeletal system alter body conformation and decrease stature. Bony landmarks become more pronounced. Although speed of movement is decreased, older adults maintain endurance. The rate of bone loss accelerates in older age, for both men and women; however, bone loss in postmenopausal women can be substantially higher, increasing the risk of fractures from falls (Weber, 2016).

The Nervous System

The nervous system consists of the brain, spinal cord, and nerves. With aging, sleep patterns change so that older adults sleep less and wake frequently throughout the night. There is a slowing of conduction of nerve impulses, and reflex action—although remaining constant with age—declines in terms of reaction time. In most instances,

natural changes in the nervous system associated with aging have minimal effect on function. Loss of cognitive function is not a direct result of the natural aging process, however, and is usually indicative of development of a health condition that needs attention.

POTENTIAL IMPLICATIONS OF NATURAL CHANGES OF AGING FOR INDIVIDUALS WITH CHRONIC HEALTH CONDITIONS

The Cardiovascular System

Depending on the nature of the health condition, maintaining a structured exercise program to increase the cardiovascular system's efficiency may be difficult for certain persons. Although not impossible, individuals with limited mobility, such as those with spinal cord injury or rheumatoid arthritis, may find maintaining an exercise program more difficult to achieve. In other instances when individuals already have a cardiovascular health condition, the increased demands placed on the heart with the natural changes of aging may increase their risk for developing cardiovascular complications. Thus reduction of risk factors, such as through smoking cessation, weight loss, and maintenance of a healthy lifestyle, may be even more important for individuals with health conditions as they age.

The Respiratory System

A number of health conditions, such as asthma and chronic obstructive pulmonary disease (COPD), may compromise pulmonary function on a long-term basis. When these deficiencies are combined with the additive effects of natural age-related changes, individuals with health conditions affecting the pulmonary system may be more vulnerable to complications such as pulmonary infections or compromised pulmonary function. Avoiding pollutants (including tobacco) and minimizing exposure to individuals with pulmonary infections are especially important steps to maintain health in such persons. Adequate sleep, good nutrition, and regular exercise are also important factors in preventing complications that could impair pulmonary function. CDC (2015) recommends influenza vaccine annually and pneumococcal vaccine at age 65 to reduce chance of getting influenza or pneumonia.

Individuals with decreased mobility, such as those with spinal cord injury, may also be more vulnerable to pulmonary conditions with aging. Because of decreased mobility, pulmonary function may be less efficient in such persons, increasing their risk of developing pulmonary infections.

The Urinary System

Some health conditions require various techniques of bladder management that can increase the risk of urinary tract complications. This risk is increased with natural changes of aging. For example, individuals with multiple sclerosis who use self-catheterization and individuals with health conditions in which bladder control has been lost so that a permanent catheter is in place may experience increased risk of such problems. If decreased mobility or motor incoordination makes regular toileting more difficult to accomplish, loss of muscle tone may perpetuate a tendency for incontinence unless appropriate interventions are implemented.

Many health conditions require multiple medications for management of the condition. With changes of natural aging in the kidney, individuals may be unable to tolerate the same dosage of medication as before, or complications related to medication dosage may not be noted. Awareness of the potential for different rates of medication excretion from the body owing to normal changes of aging and appropriate adjustment of medication dosage can help to prevent potential complications related to medication metabolism before they occur.

The Gastrointestinal System

Although maintenance of good nutrition is important for everyone, it is especially important for individuals with chronic health conditions, who may be especially prone to complications related to their health condition. Many older adults may need to alter their behavior or habits to adjust to changes in their oral and digestive systems as they age. Depending on the nature of their health condition, age-related changes may make it increasingly difficult to make the necessary changes. Moreover,

individuals with chronic health conditions may take multiple medications. Side effects of these therapies may sometimes contribute to appetite loss. In addition, because of altered liver function attributable to aging, dosages of medications may need to be adjusted to prevent overdose.

The Sensory System

Individuals with other health conditions may feel that diminished function in another area, such as sight or hearing, compromises or threatens the functional capacity that they have achieved with their original health condition. Individuals who experience blindness or health conditions that severely affect vision, for example, might feel that diminished hearing acuity creates additional challenges to function, as might individuals who are deaf and as a result of aging develop diminished visual acuity.

The Skin

Individuals who are immobile or tend to sit in one place all day are more prone to develop pressure sores, which may occur on the buttocks, heels, or elbows due to changes associated with aging of the skin and underlying structures. Pressure sores can become infected and, if not managed promptly and adequately, can lead to serious complications. Proper nutrition and hydration can help prevent skin complications.

In addition, due to hardened, brittle nails, older individuals may sustain injury when manicuring and pedicuring. If circulatory problems exist, such injury could result in serious infections that could necessitate amputation of an extremity.

The Immune System

Some individuals have conditions in which the immune system has become weakened as a result of interventions for management of the condition, such as therapies for some types of cancer, or have health conditions in which a weakened immune system is a manifestation of the condition, such as HIV infection. In these persons, the natural effects of aging on the immune system can accentuate declining immune function.

The Musculoskeletal System

Due to their relatively large number of bony landmarks, individuals with limited mobility may be more prone to experience pressure on bony prominences and, therefore, to develop pressure sores. Physiologic changes related to aging include decreased muscle strength, decreased range of motion of joints, decreased reaction time, and changes in the sensory system (Yang et al., 2012). When these changes are compounded by manifestations of a health condition that affects balance, such as Meniere's disease, individuals become more prone to falls, which can lead to fractures. In individuals with health conditions in which bones have become weakened, such as cancer and osteoporosis, this risk is increased even further.

The Nervous System

In individuals with a preexisting health condition that affects the nervous system, manifestations of cognitive dysfunction may sometimes be ignored because of prejudice and social misconceptions. In fact, changes in cognitive status should always be investigated. Cognitive status can be affected by many factors, some of which are reversible. Side effects or overuse of medications, alcohol abuse, malnutrition, vitamin or hormone deficiencies, dehydration, and poor physical health can all contribute to manifestations of confusion. Many of these causes can be reversed if they are properly identified and appropriate interventions instituted.

MEDICATIONS AND AGING

Individuals with health conditions frequently use a number of medications to manage their condition. Natural aging changes also alter the physiologic processes that affect absorption, distribution, metabolism, and excretion of medications. Age-related factors that contribute to changes in how the body handles medications include decline in kidney function, an increased proportion of fat cells in the body tissues, the effect of the chronic health condition itself, long-term use of medications, and general lifetime habits.

The simultaneous use of two or more medications is common in individuals with chronic health conditions. If an individual develops a secondary health condition in older age, additional medications may be needed to treat the new condition. Many types of medications can interact with one another and, in turn, increase, decrease, or change their intended actions. It is important that all medications used for all chronic health conditions be coordinated and monitored. Some medications may mask various manifestations that should receive attention but go unnoticed. In some instances, medications interactions and side effects may mimic manifestations of other conditions, leading to unnecessary intervention. Some medications can weaken body systems, leading to development of additional health conditions. Other medications may reduce adaptive functioning and increase dependence. Individuals should consider how medications might affect adaptive functioning, whether they will exacerbate a chronic health problem, whether they will interact with other medications, and how age-related changes will affect the medications' action.

PREVENTING AGE-RELATED COMPLICATIONS: SUMMARY

Although aging and disability are not synonymous, changes associated with aging can affect functional capacity. When a preexisting or coexisting health condition is present, the natural changes of aging can further compromise functional capacity as well as increase vulnerability to a number of potentially serious complications. Awareness of the natural aging process and its effects on various body systems can help individuals to implement measures to increase functional capacity and prevent development of complications that can seriously impede function and compromise general health.

Major barriers to the maintenance of function and independence in older adults frequently include the attitudes and myths endorsed by society, which attribute many potentially reversible manifestations to "old age." These stereotypes are often compounded when individuals have a preexisting health condition. Such misconceptions can interfere with appropriate evaluation and management of manifestations, resulting in potential deterioration.

REFERENCES

CDC, U.S. Department of Health and Human Services (2015). 2015 Recommended Immunizations for Adults: By Age. www.CDC.gov/vaccines

Dewan, S. K., Zheng, S. B., Xia, S. J., & Bill, K. (2012). Immunosenescence, aging, and systemic lupus erythematous. *Chinese Medical Journal, 125*(18), 3325–3331.

Grassi, M., Petraccia, L., Mennuni, G., Fontana, M., Scarno, A., Sabetta, S., & Fraioli, A. (2011). Changes, functional disorders, and diseases in the gastrointestinal tract of elderly. *Nutrition Hospitalaria, 26*(4), 659–668.

Lee, H. C., TI Huang, K., & Shen, W. K. (2011). Use of anti-arrhythmic drugs in elderly patients. *Journal of Geriatric Cardiology, 8*(3), 184–194.

Levakov, A., Vuckovic, N., Dolai, M., Kacanski, M. M., & Bozanic, S. (2012). Age-related skin changes. *Medicinski Pregled (Medical Review), 65*(5–6), 191–195.

Marks, A.R. (2016). Cardiac Function and Circulatory Control. In: L. Goldman & A. I. Schafer. (Eds.). *Goldman-Cecil Medicine*, (25th ed., pp 262-267). Philadelphia PA: Elsevier Saunders

Moss, C., Dhillo, W. S., Frost, G., & Hickson, M. (2011). Gastrointestinal hormones: The regulation of appetite and the anorexia of ageing. *Journal of Human Nutritional Dietetics, 25*(1), 3–15.

Newman, A. B. & Cauley, J. A. (2016). Epidemiology of aging: Implications of an aging society. In: L. Goldman & A. I. Schafer. (Eds.). *Goldman-Cecil Medicine*, (25th ed., pp 1637–1645). Philadelphia PA: Elsevier Saunders

Ren, W. Y., Li, L., Zhao, R. Y., & Zhu, L. (2012). Age-associated changes in pulmonary function: A comparison of pulmonary function parameters in healthy young adults and the elderly living in Shanghai. *Chinese Medical Journal, 125*(17), 3064–3068.

Rosso, A. L., Wisdom, J. P., Horner-Johnson, W., McGee, M. G., & Michael, Y. L. (2011). Aging with a disability: A systematic review of cardiovascular disease and osteoporosis among women aging with a physical disability. *Maturitas, 68*(1), 65–72.

Strait, J. B., & Lakatta, E. G. (2012). Aging-associated cardiovascular changes and their relationship to heart failure. *Heart Failure Clinics, 8*(1), 143–164.

Walston, J. D. (2016). Common clinical sequelae of aging. In: L. Goldman & A.I Schafer. (Eds.). *Goldman-Cecil Medicine*, (25th ed., pp 1637–1645). Philadelphia PA: Elsevier Saunders

Weber, T. L. (2016). Osteoporosis. In L. Goldman & A. I. Schafer. (Eds.). *Goldman-Cecil Medicine.* (25th ed., pp 1637–1645). Philadelphia PA: Elsevier Saunders

Weinberger, B., & Grubeck-Loebenstein, B. (2012). Vaccines for the elderly. *Clinical Microbiology and Infection, 18*(suppl. 5), 1–9.

Yang, X. J., Hill, K., Moore, K., Williams, S., Dawson, L., Borschmann, K., . . . Dharmage, S. C. (2012). Effectiveness of a targeted exercise intervention in reversing older people's mild balance dysfunction: A randomized controlled trial. *Physical Therapy, 92*(1), 24–37.

Zuchelli, T., & Myers, S. E. (2011). Gastrointestinal issues in the older female patient. *Gastroenterology Clinics of North America, 40*(2), 449–466.

Medical Terminology

All professions and sciences have their own terminology that provides for speed, precision, and economy of communication. The healthcare professions are no exception. The terminology used in health care can sometimes seem like a foreign language. Nevertheless, professionals working with individuals with chronic health conditions need to become familiar with commonly used terms so that they can communicate with other healthcare providers and have a better understanding of information contained in reports and records. Although each term could be looked up in a reference source,

that process would be time consuming. Memorizing some commonly used terms can certainly be helpful, but it is unrealistic to try to memorize all terms that you might encounter.

Becoming familiar with the prefixes and suffixes commonly found in healthcare terminology can help you translate unfamiliar terms and provides a framework from which you may be able to figure out a general meaning of a term. Following are commonly used prefixes and suffixes, along with some general terms that are frequently encountered.

PREFIXES

Prefix	Meaning	Prefix	Meaning
adeno	glandular	chondro	cartilage
angio	vessel	circum	around
ankyl	crooked, growing, together	craneo	skull
anti	against	cysto	bladder
arthro	joint	derma	skin
bi	double, twice	dis	negative
bili	bile	dors	back
brachy	short	duodeno	duodenum
brady	slow	dys	difficult, painful
broncho	bronchi	ect	outside
cardio	heart	endo	inside
cephalo	head	entero	intestine
cervico	neck	eryth	red
chole	gall, bile	ferro	iron
cholecyst	gallbladder	fibro	fibers

(continues)

PREFIXES (continued)

Prefix	Meaning	Prefix	Meaning
fore	before, in front of	ocul	eye
galacto	milk	odonto	tooth
gastro	stomach	oligo	few, little
gingive	gums	ophth, optic	eye
glyco	sugar	os	mouth
gyneco	female	oss, osteo	bone
hemato	blood	oto	ear
hemi	half	pan	all
hemo	blood	path	disease
hepato	liver	peri	around
histo	tissue	pharyng	pharynx
homo	same	phlebo	vein
hydro	water	photo	light
hyper	increased	pneumo	lung
hypo	decreased	pod	foot
hystero	uterus	post	after
iatr	physician	pre	before
idio	peculiar	procto	anus, rectum
inter	between	pseudo	false
intra	within	psych	the mind
jejuno	jejunum	pto	fall
laryngo	larynx	pyelo	kidney
latero	side	pyo	pus
leuko	white	pyro	fever
lipo	fat	quadri	four
lithio	stone	radio	radiation
macro	big, large	recto	rectum
mal	bad, poor, abnormal	retro	backward
masto, mammo	breast	rhino	nose
mega	great, large	sacro	sacrum
melan	black	salpingo	fallopian tube
meso	middle	sclero	hard or hardening
micro	small	skeleto	skeleton
mono	single	sten	narrow
muco	mucus	stomato	mouth
multi	many	sub	under, beneath
myelo	bone marrow, spinal cord	super, supra	above, extreme
myo	muscle	tachy	fast
narco	numbness	thermo	heat
neo	new, recent	thoraco	chest
nephro	kidney	thromb	clot
neuro	nerve	uretero	ureter
non	not	vaso	vessel
nos	disease		

SUFFIXES

Suffix	Meaning	Suffix	Meaning
algia	pain	ology	science or study of
ase	enzyme	oma	tumor
cele	tumor, swelling	osis	disease
centesis	to puncture	ostomy	new opening
cide	causing disease	otomy	incision, cutting
cyte	cell	pathy	sickness, disease
dynia	pain	penia	lack
ectasis	dilation	pepsia	digestion
ectomy	excision	pexy	fixation
emesis	vomiting	phage	ingesting
emia	blood	phylaxis	protection
esthesia	sensation	plasty	repair
gram	tracing, mark	plegia	paralysis
graphy	record, picture	ptosis	prolapse
iasis	condition, pathological state	rhagia	hemorrhage
itis	inflammation	rhea	flow, discharge
kinesis	motion	sclerosis	hardness
lithiasis	stones	scopy	visually examine
lysis	breakdown	sect	cut
mania	madness	statis	halt
megaly	enlargement	stenosis	narrowing
norexia	appetite	uria	urine
odynia	pain		

TERMINOLOGY RELATED TO POSITION AND DIRECTION

Term	Meaning	Term	Meaning
anterior	before or in front	plantar	pertaining to the sole of the foot
distal	far away from	posterior	behind or in back
dorsal	pertaining to the back	prone	lying face down
inferior	below	proximal	nearest to
lateral	to the side	superior	above
medial	to the center	supine	lying face upward
palmar	pertaining to the palm of the hand	volar	pertaining to the front or abdominal surface

TERMINOLOGY RELATING TO BODY AREAS

Term	Meaning	Term	Meaning
carpal	pertaining to the wrist	frontal	pertaining to the front
cervical	pertaining to the 7 vertebrae in the neck	pelvic	pertaining to the pelvis
costal	pertaining to the ribs	sternal	pertaining to the sternum or breastbone
cranial	pertaining to the skull	thoracic	pertaining to the 12 vertebrae in the upper portion of the back of the chest cavity
femoral	pertaining to the thigh		

PREFIXES OF QUANTITY

Prefix	Meaning	Prefix	Meaning
ambi	both	multi	many
bi	two	olig	few
di	two	poly	many
hemi	half	tri	three
mono	one	uni	one

GENERAL TERMS

chronic health condition: ongoing structural or functional change within the body judged to be atypical

complication: health condition concurrent with another health condition

diagnosis: determination of or naming of a health condition

etiology: study of the cause of health conditions; also, the cause of a specific health condition

history: written description of manifestations in a health record

idiopathic: cause unknown

incidence: measure of the number of individuals newly identified as having a specific health condition

manifestation: evidence of a health condition as perceived by the individual experiencing it; outward signs observed by others; laboratory irregularities

morbidity: rate of a particular health condition or proportion of individuals with a specific health condition living in a given locality; frequency of occurrence of a health condition within a population

mortality: proportion of deaths to the population of a region; the death rate from a particular health condition; measure of the number of people dying from a health condition in a given period of time

pathogenesis: development of a health condition; sequence of events that leads from the cause to structural irregularities and finally to manifestations of the health condition

pathology: study of health conditions

prevalence: number of people with a health condition at any given point in time

prognosis: probable outcome of a health condition

signs: physical observations made by the person examining an individual

syndrome: cluster of findings associated with a health condition

Glossary of Medical Terms

abduction movement of a body part away from the midline of the body

abductor muscle that moves a limb laterally, away from the body

abrasion scraping or rubbing off of the skin

accommodation change in the shape of the lens to help the eye focus for near or far vision

achalasia type of dysphagia in which motility of the lower portion of the esophagus is decreased and food is unable to pass into the stomach efficiently

acoustic nerve auditory nerve; eighth cranial nerve

acoustic reflex movement of the muscles attached to the malleus and stapes as a response to intense sound

acquired hearing loss hearing loss occurring after birth or later in life

active exercise individual independent performance of a specified exercise regimen under the direction or supervision of a physical therapist

adaptation chemical process in which the eye adjusts to see in the dark

Addison's disease condition involving underproduction of hormones by the adrenal cortex

adduction movement of a body part toward the midline of the body

adductor muscle that moves a limb closer to the body

adenopathy enlargement of lymph nodes

afferent nerves peripheral nerves that carry messages to the central nervous system

agnosia inability to interpret sounds or visual images or to distinguish objects by touch

agoraphobia fear of being in a situation or place from which it might be difficult or embarrassing to escape or in which no help may be available if a panic attack occurs

agranulocytosis marked reduction in the level of a specific type of leukocyte

agraphia loss of ability to write

akathisia extreme restlessness; inability to sit still for any length of time

akinesia complete or partial absence of movement

alexia loss of ability to read

allergen substance that causes an allergic response

allergy hypersensitivity to a specific substance or substances from previous exposure

allograft graft taken from the same species but not the same person; homograft

alopecia hair loss

alveoli air sacs in lungs in which exchange of oxygen and carbon dioxide takes place

Alzheimer's disease progressive, degenerative type of dementia

amblyopia loss of sight or dimness of vision

amino acids building blocks of protein

amnesia loss of memory

amputation removal of a body part

amyotrophic lateral sclerosis progressive condition in which degeneration of the nerve cells that convey impulses to initiate muscular contraction occurs

anaphylaxis severe systemic reaction resulting from sensitivity to a foreign protein

anaplastic term to describe cancer cells that take on abnormal characteristics and become less differentiated than the normal cells from which they are derived

anasarca generalized edema

anastomosis connection of two tubular structures, through surgery or through a pathological process

anemia condition in which a reduction in the amount of hemoglobin or the number of red blood cells occurs

aneurysm blood-filled sac formed by a dilation of the walls of an artery or vein

angina pectoris chest pain

anhedonia inability to experience pleasure

anhidrosis lack of sweating

ankylosing spondylitis systemic rheumatic disorder affecting the joints and ligaments of the spine

ankylosis immobility or fixation of a joint

anomia inability to name objects or remember names

anophthalmia congenital absence of the eye

anorexia appetite loss

anosmia loss of sense of smell

anosognosia one-sided neglect (e.g., condition in which individuals are unable to see objects on either the right or the left of the central field of vision)

anoxia no oxygen

antibody an immune substance produced within the body in response to a specific antigen

antigen a substance that causes the body to manufacture antibodies against a particular allergen

anuria condition in which the kidney is unable to excrete urine

aorta largest artery in the body

aortic semilunar valve valve through which blood is pumped from the heart into the general circulation

aphagia inability to swallow

aphasia inability to communicate through speech, writing, or signs due to brain dysfunction

apnea cessation of breathing

apraxia loss of ability to organize and sequence specific muscle movements to perform a task

apraxia of speech articulation disorder characterized by the inability to position and sequence the muscle movements involved in speech

arachnoid membrane middle, cobweb-appearing membrane that covers the brain and spinal cord

arrhythmia abnormality of the heart rhythm

arteriosclerosis thickening and loss of elasticity of arteries

arthritis joint inflammation

arthrocentesis aspiration of synovial fluid from a joint cavity

arthrodesis surgical fusing of two joint surfaces, making them permanently immobile

arthrogram radiographic study of a joint

arthroplasty surgical replacement, formation, or reformation of a joint

arthroscopy visualization of a joint through an arthroscope inserted into the joint

articulation coming together of two bones at a joint

ascites retention of fluid in the abdominal cavity

asphyxia suffocation due to decrease of oxygen and increase of carbon dioxide in the body

aspiration withdrawal of fluid or gas from a cavity by means of suction

aspiration pneumonia inflammation of the lung resulting from inhalation of foreign substances or chemical irritants

asthma chronic inflammatory disease of the airways

astigmatism distortion of the visual image resulting from an irregularity in the shape of the cornea or lens

asymptomatic without symptoms

ataxia impairment of muscle coordination

atelectasis collapse of the lung

atherosclerosis buildup of plaque on the inner walls of blood vessels

athetosis slow, writhing, purposeless movement

atonic lacking normal tone or strength

atresia narrowing or closing of a normal opening; often congenital

atria two upper chambers of the heart

atrophy shrinkage

attention deficit/hyperactivity disorder condition that appears before age 7 that is characterized by inattention, hyperactivity, and impulsivity

aura warning (flash of light or other unusual sensation) before a seizure

auricle visible portion of the outer ear

autistic disorder disorder of brain function with behavioral consequences, including impairment in reciprocal social interactions and impairment in verbal and nonverbal communication

autograft graft from the individual's own skin

autoimmune disease disease in which the immune system directs a response that attacks the body's own cells as if they were foreign substances

autonomic dysreflexia condition occurring in individuals with spinal cord injury, resulting from excessive neural discharge from the autonomic nervous system and characterized by sudden rise in blood pressure, profuse sweating, and headache

autonomic nervous system part of the peripheral nervous system that controls involuntary functions

avascular necrosis death of bone due to lack of blood supply

avolution inability to initiate or follow through with goal-directed activities

axon process emerging from the neuron that conducts electrical impulses away from the cell body

bacteremia presence of bacteria in the bloodstream

bacteriuria bacteria in the urine

basal ganglia gray matter embedded within the white matter of the brain

benign noncancerous

bicuspid valve mitral valve of the heart

biliary term applying to the gallbladder, liver, and their ducts

binocular vision coordinated use of both eyes to produce a single image

biopsy removal of a small portion of tissue from the body so that it may be examined microscopically (e.g., needle biopsy)

biosynthetic graft graft that has been chemically manufactured

blindness total loss of light perception

blood dyscrasias large group of disorders that affect the blood

body image individual's perception of his or her own physical appearance and physical function

bradycardia slow heartbeat

bradykinesia extreme slowness of movement

brain stem portion of the central nervous system located at the base of the brain between the cerebrum and the spinal cord

Broca's aphasia type of nonfluent aphasia characterized by misarticulation, laborious speech, hesitancy, and reduced vocabulary

Broca's area portion of the brain anterior to Wernicke's area and the major area of expressive function

bronchi branches leading from the trachea into the lungs

bronchiectasis dilation of the bronchi or bronchioles

bronchospasm tightening of small muscles around air passages

burr holes openings placed in the skull to relieve increased intracranial pressure

bursa sac that contains synovial fluid in the synovial joints

bursitis inflammation of the bursa

CABG coronary artery bypass graft

calculi stones

cancer cellular tumor; not one disease, but a broad term used to describe many diseases

candidiasis yeast infection

capillaries minute blood vessels connecting smallest arteries (arterioles) and veins (venules)

carbuncle a boil with infiltration into adjacent tissues

carcinogens chemicals or other substances that are thought to cause cancer

carcinoma cancer of the epithelial cells

cardiac tamponade severe constriction of the heart because of accumulation of fluid in the pericardial sac

cardiomegaly enlargement of the heart

cardiomyopathy disease of the heart

cardiospasm achalasia

carpal tunnel repair surgical procedure indicated for carpal tunnel syndrome

carpal tunnel syndrome painful condition involving compression of the median nerve in the wrist

carriers individuals who harbor organisms causing a disease and transmit the disease to others, while remaining well themselves

cataract clouding or opacity of the lens of the eye

cell body portion of the neuron

cellulitis inflammation of body tissue

central deafness hearing loss resulting from disorder of the auditory center of the brain

cerebellum portion of the brain located beneath the occipital lobe of the cerebrum

cerebral palsy developmental disability in which injury to the brain occurs during the fetal period, at birth, or in early childhood

cerebrospinal fluid fluid bathing the brain and spinal cord

cerebrovascular accident stroke

cerebrum largest portion of the brain

cerumen earwax

cervix neck of the uterus, opening into the vagina

cholecystectomy removal of the gallbladder

cholecystitis inflammation of the gallbladder

cholelithiasis gallstones

chorea jerky, involuntary movements

choreoathetosis abrupt, jerky movements

chronic manifestations of a condition that lasts indefinitely

chronic bronchitis defined clinically as a condition in which a chronic productive cough persists on most days for a minimum of 3 months in the year, for not less than 2 consecutive years

chronic obstructive pulmonary disease collection of diseases including emphysema, chronic bronchitis, and chronic asthma

cilia hairlike projections

circumduction circular movement

cirrhosis progressive disease of the liver in which liver function is altered because of fibrous changes in the structure of the liver

clonic pertaining to jerky movement of muscle

closed head injury injury in which the skull has not been fractured

coccyx tailbone

cochlea chamber of the inner ear

colectomy removal of all or part of the colon

collateral circulation alternative blood supply routes

colon large intestine

colostomy surgical opening in the outer wall of the abdomen through which a portion of the large intestine is brought to the external surface for elimination of fecal material

coma state of unconsciousness

compulsions persistent actions

concussion mild to moderate head injury in which a loss of consciousness occurs, with its timing varying from a few minutes to 24 hours after the injury

conductive hearing loss damage, obstruction, or malformation in the external or middle ear that prevents sound waves from reaching the inner ear

confabulation making up experiences to fill memory gaps

congenital present at birth

congenital hearing loss hearing loss present at birth

conjunctiva membrane that lines the inner eyelid and covers the front part of the eye

conjunctivitis inflammation of the conjunctiva

contracture deformity in which a permanent contraction of a muscle occurs, resulting in the immobility of a joint

contusion soft-tissue injury resulting from a blunt, diffuse blow in which the skin is not broken, nor are bones broken, but local hemorrhage occurs with associated bruising and damage to deep soft tissue under the skin

conversion disorder disorder in which physical function, often related to neurological function, is lost but no organic cause for the loss can be found

COPD chronic obstructive pulmonary disease

cor pulmonale right-sided heart failure

coronary angioplasty procedure to enlarge a narrowed coronary artery

coronary arteries vessels that carry blood directly to the myocardial muscle

coronary artery bypass graft procedure to relieve narrowing or constriction of coronary arteries

coronary artery disease condition in which arteries that supply blood directly to the myocardial muscle become narrowed or occluded

cortex gray matter that makes up the outer portion of the cerebrum

cranial nerves peripheral nerves that transmit messages directly to the brain

craniotomy surgical procedure in which the skull is opened to remove matter or to control bleeding

cranium skull; bony cover surrounding the brain

creatinine waste product eliminated by the kidney

Crohn's disease inflammation of segments of the small intestine

cross-tolerance demonstration of higher tolerances for related substances when tolerance for one substance has been developed

Curling's ulcer stress ulcer associated with burns

Cushing's disease condition involving overproduction of hormones by the adrenal cortex

Cushing's ulcer peptic ulcer associated with head injury

cyanosis bluish or gray appearance of skin resulting from lack of oxygen supply

cyclothymia mood disorder characterized by symptoms similar to those of bipolar disorder, including both hypomanic and depressive symptoms

cystectomy total removal of the urinary bladder

cystic fibrosis hereditary condition in which mucus-secreting organs in the body become obstructed by abnormal, thick mucus, resulting in degeneration and scarring of the organs involved

cystitis inflammation of the bladder

cytology study of cells

deafness inability to discriminate conversational speech through the ear

debride remove dead tissue

decibels (dB) sound intensity or loudness

decubitus ulcers pressure sores

delusions false beliefs

dementia deterioration of cognitive abilities

dendrite process emerging from the cell body of a neuron that is involved in transmission of electrical impulses to the cell body

dental caries cavities

dermabrasion procedure in which scars, wrinkles, or other skin blemishes are worn away to diminish scarring

dermatitis superficial inflammation of the skin

dermis inner layer of skin lying beneath the epidermis

diabetes insipidus condition involving inadequate secretion of antidiuretic hormone from the pituitary gland

diabetes mellitus chronic disorder of carbohydrate metabolism in which an imbalance of the supply of and demand for the hormone insulin occurs

dialysis artificial means to replace kidney function

diaphoresis excessive sweating

diaphragm muscular wall that separates the abdominal cavity from the thoracic cavity

diastole phase of heart activity when the heart is relaxed and the chambers are filling

diplegia paralysis affecting all limbs of the body

diplopia double vision

disability limitation or restriction of activity that results from an impairment

discography radiographic study of the cervical or lumbar disks

diskectomy removal of a portion of a disk

dislocation displacement or separation of a bone from its normal joint position

distal farthest from the center of the body

diuresis increased urinary output

diverticula small balloon-like pouches in walls of large intestine

diverticulitis infection or inflammation of diverticula

diverticulosis presence of numerous diverticula in the intestinal wall

DNA genetic material that is the blueprint for all the body's structures

dormant inactive

dorsiflexion backward movement

dorsiflexor muscle that bends a body part backward

duodenal ulcer peptic ulcer in the upper portion of the small intestine

duodenum first part of the small intestine

dura mater outer membrane of the brain and spinal cord

dysarthria impairment in the coordination and accuracy of the movement of the lips, tongue, or other parts of the speech mechanism

dyscalculia inability to perform mathematical calculations of functions

dysgraphia impaired writing ability

dyskinesia abnormal involuntary movements

dyslexia inability to understand written words

dysnomia inability to recall words correctly

dyspepsia indigestion

dysphagia difficulty in swallowing

dysphonia difficulty speaking

dyspnea difficulty in breathing

dysrhythmia irregularity of heartbeat

dysthymia chronic condition characterized by symptoms similar to those experienced in major depression but in a lesser degree

dystonia abnormal muscle tone

dystrophy progressive changes in tissue or organ due to faulty nutrition or metabolism

dysuria painful urination

ecchymosis purplish discoloration at the site of injury resulting from bleeding under the skin

eczema acute or chronic inflammatory condition of the skin with any of a combination of symptoms, including vesicles, scales, crusts, and redness

edema presence of abnormally large amounts of fluid in tissue spaces

edematous swollen

efferent nerves peripheral nerves that carry impulses away from the central nervous system

electrolytes electrically charged particles that are important to many of the body's internal functions (e.g., sodium and potassium)

embolus foreign particle or blood clot that travels in the bloodstream until it lodges in a blood vessel too small to allow its passage

emotional lability condition in which emotional reactions are inappropriate for the situation and usually unpredictable

emphysema permanent enlargement of the alveoli resulting from overinflation of and destructive change in the alveolar walls

encephalitis inflammation of the brain

end-stage renal disease disease or damage to the kidney to the point that it ceases to function

endarterectomy removal of plaque or clot in the carotid artery

endocarditis inflammation of the inner lining of the heart

endocardium lining of the inner surface of the heart

endometrium lining of the uterus

epidermis outer layer of skin

epidural pertaining to the space between the dura and the skull

epiglottis flap at the back of the throat that closes over the opening to the trachea when food is swallowed

epilepsy chronic neurological condition in which neurons in the brain create abnormal electrical discharges that cause temporary loss of control over certain body functions

epistaxis nosebleed

erythema redness

erythrocytes red blood cells

eschar dead tissue resulting from burns

esophageal reflux backflow of stomach contents into the esophagus

esophageal varices dilated tortuous veins of the esophagus

esophagectomy removal of the esophagus

esophagitis inflammation of the esophagus

eustachian tube tube connecting the throat and the tympanic cavity of the middle ear

eversion outward-turning movement

exacerbation time period when symptoms become worse

exertional dyspnea shortness of breath with activity

exophthalmos abnormal protrusion of the eyeball

expiration expulsion of air from the lungs

extension straightening movement

extensor muscle that straightens a limb

factitious disorder condition in which individuals voluntarily produce psychological or physical symptoms because of a compulsive need to assume the sick role

feces solid waste from the body

fetal alcohol syndrome toxic effects of alcohol on the developing fetus during pregnancy, resulting in deformity of the infant

fibromyalgia cluster of signs and symptoms in which individuals experience diffuse aching, pain, and stiffness in muscles or joints

fibrosis formation of fibrous tissue

fistula opening between two tubular structures

flaccid limp

flat affect showing little emotional responsiveness

flexion bending movement

flexor muscle that bends a limb

fluent aphasia receptive or sensory aphasia

frontal lobe portion of the brain located in the front part of each hemisphere

functional disorder disorder that has no readily identifiable organic cause

fused joined

gastric ulcer ulcer in the stomach

gastritis inflammation of the stomach

gastroenterostomy surgical procedure in which the bottom of the stomach and the small intestine are opened, and the two openings are connected to create a passage between the body of the stomach and the small intestine

gene unit of heredity that is composed of DNA and carries hereditary information about all characteristics of the organism

gingival hyperplasia gum overgrowth

gingivitis inflammation of the gums

glaucoma increase in intraocular pressure

global aphasia limited ability to communicate

glomerular filtration process by which the kidney removes waste products from the blood

glomerulonephritis inflammation of the glomeruli of the kidney

glomerulus small capillary located in the nephron of the kidney

glycosuria glucose in the urine

goiter swelling of the neck resulting from enlargement of the thyroid gland

grading system used to describe the structure of cancer cells

gray matter nonmyelinated nerve fibers in the central nervous system that receive, sort, and process nerve messages

Guillain–Barré syndrome acute and progressive condition characterized by muscular weakness usually beginning in the lower extremities and spreading upward

hallucinations sensory experiences without environmental stimuli

handicap disadvantage because of an impairment or disability that presents a barrier to fulfilling a role or reaching a goal

hearing impairment any degree and type of hearing disorder

hearing loss impairment in any part of the hearing system that interferes with hearing sound

hemarthrosis bleeding in the joint

hematemesis vomiting of blood

hematoma sac filled with accumulated blood

hematuria blood in the urine

hemianopsia loss of vision in half the visual field

hemiplegia paralysis on one side of the body

hemoglobin red pigmented protein that carries oxygen within the erythrocytes

hemolysis destruction of red blood cells

hemophilia chronic bleeding disorder characterized by a deficiency in or absence of one of the clotting factors

hemopoiesis process by which blood cells are formed

hemoptysis blood-streaked sputum

hemostasis cessation of bleeding from damaged vessels

hemothorax accumulation of blood in the pleural cavity

hepatitis inflammation of the liver

hepatomegaly enlargement of the liver

hepatotoxicity liver damage that has been chemically induced

hepatotoxin substance that is toxic to the liver

hernia (rupture) protrusion of an organ through the tissues in which it is normally contained

herniorrhaphy surgical procedure used to repair hernias

hertz (Hz) unit for measuring sound frequency or pitch

heterograft graft taken from another species; xenograft

hiatal hernia protrusion of the stomach through an opening of the diaphragm and into the thoracic cavity

histology study of the structure of tissue

Hodgkin's disease chronic, progressive disease in which abnormal cells replace normal elements within the lymph nodes

homeostasis maintenance of an internal chemical balance within the body

homograft graft taken from the same species but not the same person; allograft

Huntington's chorea slowly progressive, hereditary disease of the central nervous system characterized by jerky, involuntary movements and intellectual deterioration

hydrocephalus buildup of fluid in the brain

hydronephrosis buildup of urine in the kidney resulting from backup of urine and blocked outflow

hyperalimentation nourishment through infusion of a special nutritional solution into a large blood vessel

hyperbilirubinemia excess bilirubin in the blood

hypercapnia buildup of carbon dioxide

hyperglycemia accumulation of large amounts of glucose in the blood

hyperkalemia high levels of potassium in the blood

hyperlipidemia elevated cholesterol levels

hyperopia farsightedness

hyperproliferation overgrowth of cells resulting from a tumor

hyperreflexia increased reaction of reflexes

hypertension high blood pressure

hyperthermia increased body temperature

hyperthyroidism overproduction of thyroid hormone

hypertonic exaggerated muscle tone

hypertrophic scars ropelike configurations of scar tissue that form on the skin surface

hypertrophy enlargement

hyperuricemia buildup of uric acid in the body

hypochondriasis type of somatoform disorder characterized by preoccupation with physical illness

hypoglycemia decreased sugar in the blood

hyponatremia decreased concentration of salt in the blood

hypophonia weakened voice due to incoordination of muscles used in speech

hypotension low blood pressure

hypothyroidism insufficient production of thyroid hormone

hypotonic decreased muscle tone

hypovolemia diminished blood volume

hypoxemia decreased level of oxygen in the blood

hypoxia decreased oxygen supply

hysterectomy removal of the uterus

ileostomy portion of the small intestine brought through a surgical opening to the outside of the abdomen for drainage of fecal material

ileum last part of the small intestine

immune system complex organization of specialized cells and organs that distinguishes between self and nonself, defending the body against foreign materials

immunosuppression suppression of the immune system

impaction overloading; packed; as in feces in the bowels

impairment loss or abnormality of function at the body system or organ level

incisors teeth at the front of the mouth that provide a cutting action

incontinence loss of control of bladder or bowel

incus small bone in the middle ear

infarction death of tissue resulting from lack of blood supply

inflammatory bowel disease a group of disorders that cause inflammation or ulceration in the lining of the bowel

inspiration breathing air into the lungs

intermittent claudication aching, cramping, or fatigue of muscles in the legs when walking

internal fixation placement of screws, pins, wires, rods, or other devices through the bone to hold bone fragments together

intracranial hemorrhage bleeding within the cranium or skull

intracranial pressure pressure on the brain

intraocular pressure pressure within the eyeball

intravenous refers to an infusion directly into a vein

inversion inward-turning movement

iridotomy removal of a portion of the iris of the eye

irritable bowel syndrome chronic or intermittent condition of the gastrointestinal tract in which individuals experience spasms of the colon, diarrhea, constipation, cramping, and abdominal pain

ischemia inadequate blood supply

isotonic normal muscle tone

jaundice yellowish appearance of the skin and whites of the eyes resulting from an excess level of bilirubin in the blood

jejunum middle section of the small intestine

joint place where two or more bones are bound together

keratoplasty plastic surgery of the cornea

keratotomy incision in the cornea

ketoacidosis condition caused by an excessive level of ketones in the blood that increases the acidity of the blood to toxic levels

ketone metabolic product of fat metabolism

ketoacidosis acidosis accompanied by a buildup of ketone bodies in the blood (diabetic coma)

ketosis buildup of ketone bodies in the blood

kidney failure diminished functioning of the kidney

kyphosis (hump back) permanent postural deformity of the back

labyrinth inner ear

labyrinthitis inflammation of the labyrinth of the inner ear

laceration injury involving a tear or cut in the skin and underlying tissues

laminectomy surgical removal of the posterior arch of a vertebra

language set of symbols combined in a certain way to convey concepts, ideas, and emotions

laparotomy surgical incision into the abdomen

laryngectomy surgical removal of the whole or a part of the larynx

laryngitis inflammation of the larynx

laryngostoma surgical opening in the neck through which the individual breathes

larynx voice box

legal blindness central visual acuity not exceeding 20/200 in the better eye with correcting lenses or central field of vision limited to an angle of no greater than 20 degrees

lens small transparent disk enclosed in a transparent capsule and located directly behind the iris of the eye

lethargy listlessness

leukemia cancer of the tissues in which blood is formed

leukocyte white blood cell

leukocytosis white blood cell proliferation

leukopenia abnormal decrease in the number of white blood cells

ligaments tough bands of fiber that connect bones at the joint site

litholapaxy crushing of a kidney stone in the bladder

lithotomy surgical procedure to remove kidney stones

lobectomy removal of a lobe (e.g., of the brain; of the lung)

loosening of associations no logical progression of thought and rapid shifting from one unrelated idea to another

lordosis swayback

low back pain pain in the lumbar or sacral region of the lower back

lymph fluid clear fluid that bathes the body's tissue

lymph nodes small glands of the immune system that are located throughout the body and act as filters

lymphadenectomy removal of the lymph nodes

lymphadenopathy swollen lymph nodes

lymphatic system circulatory system separate from the general circulation and consisting of the lymph vessels, lymph fluid, and lymph nodes

lymphedema swelling resulting from blockage in the lymphatic system

lymphocyte white blood cell

lymphoma cancer of the lymphatic system

macrophage phagocyte that ingests dead tissue

macula spot on the retina that is the area of most acute vision

macular degeneration degeneration of the macula of the eye

melanin skin pigment that is responsible for skin color

melanocytes cells containing the skin pigment melanin

malignancy cancerous growth

malignant cancerous, harmful, virulent

malignant melanoma cancer that originates in the cells that contain skin pigment

malingering producing symptoms intentionally for secondary gain

malleus small bone in the middle ear

mandible jaw bone

mastectomy amputation of the breast

mastoid process bony prominence behind the outer ear

mastoidectomy surgical procedure for the removal of infected mastoid air cells located in the mastoid process

mastoiditis infection of the mastoid cells within the mastoid process located in the skull

megaloblastic anemia presence of large abnormal red blood cells

melanoma cancer of the pigment-producing cells

melena passage of dark, tarry bowel movement due to action of intestinal secretions of blood in the intestine

Meniere's disease disorder of the inner ear that includes symptoms of dizziness, hearing loss, and ringing in the ears

meninges membranes covering the brain and spinal cord

meningitis inflammation of the meninges

meningocele type of spina bifida in which membranes surrounding the spinal cord push out through an opening in the spinal column

metastasis movement of cancer cells from their original site to another part of the body

microcephaly abnormal smallness of the head

micrographia reduction in handwriting size

microphage a small phagocyte that ingests bacteria

micturition urination

mitral valve valve between the left atria and the left ventricle of the heart

mixed hearing loss hearing loss involving both conductive hearing loss and sensorineural hearing loss

molars teeth at the back of the mouth that provide a grinding action

monoplegia paralysis of one limb of the body

motor nerves peripheral nerves that carry impulses from the central nervous system to other parts of the body

multi-infarct dementia condition in which deficits in cognitive function result from small strokes in various locations of the brain

multiple myeloma cancer of plasma cells that is characterized by bone destruction

multiple sclerosis progressive disease of the central nervous system in which the myelin around message-carrying nerve fibers is destroyed in localized areas of the brain and spinal cord

mutation alteration or change of the DNA within the normal cell

myalgia muscle pain

myelin fatty sheath that surrounds the neuron

myelomeningocele most severe form of spina bifida

myocardial infarction death of a portion of the heart muscle

myocardium heart muscle

myopathy disease of the muscle

myopia nearsightedness

myositis inflammation of the muscle

myringoplasty type of tympanoplasty in which damaged eardrum is repaired

myringotomy incision into the eardrum to drain pus or fluid

necrosis tissue death

necrotic dead

neoplasm new and abnormal growth of cells that serve no useful function and may interfere with healthy tissue function

nephrectomy removal of the kidney

nephritis inflammation of the kidney

nephrolithotomy surgical entry into the renal calix

nephrosclerosis condition in which arteries of the kidney become thickened

nephrosis general term used to describe conditions, other than direct infection of the kidney itself, that damage the kidney

nephrotic syndrome collection of symptoms experienced in nephrosis

nephrotoxin substances that are harmful to the kidney

nerve bundle of fibers outside the central nervous system

neuroma bundle of nerve fibers

neuron functional unit of the nervous system

neuropathy general term to describe functional disturbances or changes in the nerves

neurotransmitter chemicals that help transmit nerve impulses between neurons

neutropenia small numbers of mature white blood cells

nocturia excessive urination at night

nocturnal dyspnea difficulty in breathing while lying down at night

nonfluent aphasia expressive or motor aphasia

non-Hodgkin's lymphoma proliferation of lymphoid cells that disseminate throughout the body

nystagmus involuntary eye movement

obsessions persistent thoughts

occipital lobe portion of the brain located in the posterior portion of each hemisphere

occult hidden

occupational lung disease group of lung disorders directly related to matter inhaled from the occupational environment

oliguria decreased production of urine

oophorectomy removal of the ovaries

open head injury injury in which the skull is fractured or penetrated

open reduction surgical alignment of fractured bone

ophthalmologist physician who specializes in conditions and treatment of the eye

opportunistic infection infection that would not occur in individuals with normal immune system function

orchiectomy surgical removal of a testicle

orthopnea difficulty breathing except in an erect position

orthosis any mechanical device applied to the body to control motion of the joints and to control force or weight distribution on a body part

orthostatic hypotension postural hypotension

orthotist individual who constructs an orthosis to meet individual needs

ossicles small movable bones in the middle ear

osteoarthritis local joint disease associated with degeneration of a joint

osteomyelitis infection of the bone

osteonecrosis bone death

osteopenia diminished bone tissue

osteophytes bone spurs

osteoporosis reduction in bone mass, causing bones to become weakened, fragile, and easily broken

osteotomy cutting into bone

otitis media infection of the middle ear

otoacoustic emissions measured reflections in the outer ear of mechanical activity in the cochlea

otolaryngologist physician who specializes in disorders of the ear and related structures

otosclerosis conductive hearing loss caused by fixing or hardening of the small bones in the middle ear that transmit sound impulses to the inner ear

ototoxic describes drugs or chemicals that destroy the hair cells of the inner ear or damage the eighth cranial nerve

oval window opening between the middle and inner ear

pain disorder preoccupation with pain that is severe enough to cause functional impairment in daily life

pain expression individual response to pain

pain threshold point at which sensation is perceived as pain

pain tolerance point at which an individual finds pain unbearable

palliative giving temporary relief of symptoms but no cure

pallor pale-appearing skin

palpitations awareness of beating of the heart

pancreatitis inflammation of the pancreas

panic attack episode in which the individual has feelings of intense anxiety or terror, accompanied by a sense of impending doom

paracentesis puncture of a body cavity with subsequent removal of fluid

paralytic ileus paralysis of the intestine

paraparesis partial paralysis of the lower extremities

paraphasia type of aphasia in which there is misuse of words

paraphrasia loss of ability to use words correctly and coherently

paraplegia paralysis of the lower extremities

parasympathetic nervous system part of the autonomic nervous system

paresthesia sensation of numbness or tingling in some part of the body

parietal lobe portion of the brain located in the middle of each hemisphere

Parkinson's disease slowly progressive disorder of the central nervous system involving extensive degenerative changes in the basal ganglia of the brain with associated loss of or decrease in levels of dopamine

parotitis inflammation of the parotid glands

paroxysmal nocturnal dyspnea short periods of severe shortness of breath, waking individuals from sleep

passive exercise exercise of a body part by a therapist or by a mechanical device

pathologic fractures fractures that occur because of disease of the bone rather than from injury

pathologist physician who specializes in the diagnosis of abnormal changes in tissues

peptic ulcer disease chronic inflammatory condition characterized by ulcer formation in the esophagus, stomach, or duodenum

percussion manual tapping or vibration of the chest or other body cavity

percutaneous transluminal coronary angioplasty (PTCA) procedure to enlarge a narrowed coronary artery

perfusion blood supply to an organ

pericardial effusion accumulation of excessive fluid within the pericardial sac surrounding the heart

pericardiocentesis puncturing of the pericardium to drain accumulated fluid

pericarditis inflammation of the pericardium of the heart

pericardium outer covering of the heart

periodontal disease disease of the tissues that surround and support the teeth

periodontitis severe form of gum disease

periosteum tough outer covering of bone

peripheral near the outside or surface of the body

peripheral nervous system all nerves extending from the brain and spinal cord

peripheral neuropathy disease of the peripheral nerves

peripheral vascular insufficiency inadequate blood flow to or from the lower extremities

peristalsis rhythmic, muscular movements that move food through the digestive tract

peritoneum lining of the abdominal cavity

peritonitis inflammation of the peritoneum

pernicious anemia complication of surgical resection of the stomach

personality disorder disorder characterized by inflexible or maladaptive behaviors that impair interpersonal or occupational functioning

pervasive developmental disorders conditions in which impairment occurs in several areas of development, including social interaction and verbal and nonverbal communication or stereotypical behavior

petechiae small purplish spots on the skin due to bleeding from small vessels

phagocyte cell that destroys and ingests foreign material

phagocytosis the process of cells ingesting other cells and foreign objects

phantom limb pain chronic, severe pain sensation in an amputated extremity

phantom sensation sensation that an amputated extremity is still present

pharyngitis sore throat

pharynx throat

phlebitis inflammation of a vein

phlebotomy removal of quantities of blood to reduce plasma volume

phobia fear and anxiety related to specific situations, persons, or objects

photophobia visual discomfort when exposed to bright light

photosensitive sensitive to the sun

pia mater inner membrane covering the brain and spinal cord

pinna visible portion of the outer ear

plasma watery, colorless fluid that makes up the liquid portion of the blood

pleura membrane lining the chest cavity

pneumonectomy removal of the lung

pneumothorax collapse of the lung resulting from air entering the thoracic cavity

poliomyelitis infectious disease that affects the nerve cells that control muscles

polycystic kidney disease hereditary disease characterized by the presence of many cysts in the kidneys

polycythemia increase in the number of red blood cells as well as in the concentration of hemoglobin within the blood

polycythemia vera form of polycythemia in which an overproduction of both red and white blood cells occurs

polydipsia excessive and constant thirst

polyphagia dramatic increase in food intake

polyuria excessive urination

postlingual hearing loss hearing loss that occurs after verbal language is obtained

posttraumatic stress disorder (PTSD) disorder that develops after experiencing or observing a traumatic or life-threatening event

postvocational hearing loss hearing loss that occurs after the individual has entered the workforce

poverty of speech diminished use of the spoken word

prelingual hearing loss hearing loss that occurs before the individual acquires language, usually before the age of 3 years

presbycusis hearing loss resulting from aging

presbyopia loss of the ability of the lens to accommodate to near and far images

pressure sores decubitus ulcers

prevocational hearing loss hearing loss that occurs after acquiring language but before entering the workforce

priapism sustained unwanted erection

prognosis prediction of the course and outcome of a disease process

pronation downward-turning movement

prostatectomy removal of the prostate gland

prosthesis fabricated substitute for a missing part for engaging in activities, occupation, and cosmetic needs

prosthetist individual who specializes in making prosthetic devices

proteinuria protein in the urine

pruritus itching of the skin

psoriasis chronic inflammatory disease of the skin in which epidermal cells in the basal layer of the skin are formed too quickly

psychogenic pain pain that persists for months or years but has no readily identifiable organic cause

psychosis loss of contact with reality

PTCA percutaneous transluminal coronary angioplasty

ptosis drooping

pulmonary artery vessel carrying blood from the heart to the lungs

pulmonary edema collection of fluid in the lungs

pulmonary embolus blood clot or other foreign substance that has traveled from another part of the body and become lodged in the lung

purpura condition in which hemorrhage into the skin or other tissue occurs

purulent pertaining to pus-containing material

pyelolithotomy surgical entry into the pelvis of the kidney

pyelonephritis infection of the kidney

pyloroplasty widening the opening between the stomach and the small intestine

pyuria pus in the urine

quadriplegia paralysis of all four extremities

radial deviation lateral movement of the hand inward toward the body

radiologist physician who specializes in radio-graphic procedures

radionuclide radioactive chemical

Raynaud's phenomenon spasms of the vessels in the fingers or toes that impair blood flow to those areas

recruitment hearing impairment characterized by an abnormal increase in the perception of loudness

reflex automatic response to stimuli

regurgitation backflow

remission period of weeks to years when symptoms subside

renal pertaining to the kidney

renal calculi kidney stone

respiration physiologic process that refers to diffusion of oxygen and carbon dioxide

reticular formation groups of cells within the brain stem

reticulocyte newly formed red blood cell

retina innermost coat of the eye that receives images formed by the lens

retinitis pigmentosa slow, progressive loss of peripheral vision

retinopathy disease or disorder of the retina

rheumatic disease condition that produces symptoms that affect joints, connective tissues, and muscle

rheumatic fever condition caused by the body's immune response against a specific organism

rheumatic heart disease condition in which the body undergoes a type of allergic response that can cause heart damage

rheumatoid arthritis chronic, progressive, and systemic disorder characterized by inflammation and swelling of the synovial joints, resulting in pain, stiffness, and deformity

sarcoma cancer of the bone, muscle, or other connective tissue

sciatica syndrome of pain that radiates from the lower back into the hip and down the leg

sclera white part of the eye

sclerosis hardening or scarring

scoliosis lateral S-shaped curvature of the spine

seizure temporary loss of control over certain body functions

self-concept an individual's perceptions and beliefs about his or her own strengths and weaknesses and beliefs about other people's perceptions of him or her

semicircular canals part of the vestibular system in the inner ear

sensorineural hearing loss hearing loss resulting from damage to the nerve pathways that transmit nerve impulses or damage to the areas of the brain in which sound is perceived

sensory nerves peripheral nerves that carry messages toward the central nervous system

sepsis widespread infection throughout the body

septicemia presence of toxins in the blood

sickle cell anemia severe anemia as a result of sickle cell disease; the most severe form of sickle cell disease

sickle cell crisis manifestation of sickle cell disease in which blood flow to a body part becomes obstructed by rigid, sickled red cells

sickle cell disease a chronic hereditary disorder characterized by abnormal hemoglobin

sickle cell trait abnormal gene causing the hemoglobin abnormality in sickle cell disease

social phobia phobic disorder in which the individual fears situations that may result in ridicule or humiliation

somatic nerves peripheral nerves that innervate body structures that are under voluntary control

somatoform disorder experience of physical symptoms for which no organic cause can be found

spasticity increased muscle tone, causing stiffness and awkward movements

speech verbal expression of language concepts

spina bifida congenital disorder of the spinal column in which one or more vertebrae are left open

spina bifida occulta the mildest form of spina bifida, which does not involve damage to the spinal cord

spinal fusion the grafting of bone from another area of the body into the disk interspace after laminectomy

spinal nerves peripheral nerves that connect and transmit messages directly to the spinal cord

spleen organ composed of tissue that disposes of worn-out blood cells

splenectomy removal of the spleen

splenomegaly enlargement of the spleen

spondylolisthesis forward slipping of a vertebra

spondylolysis breakdown of a vertebra

sprain injury to a ligament and its attachment site because of overstress

staging system to describe the extent to which cancer cells have spread

stapedectomy surgical procedure in which the stapes is removed and replaced with a prosthesis

stapes small bone in the middle ear

stasis stagnation

status asthmaticus severe, prolonged attack of asthma

status epilepticus continuous, uncontrolled seizures

stem cells cells that have the potential to become any type of cell in the body

stenosis narrowing of a duct or canal (e.g., a blood vessel)

stoma artificial opening

stomatitis inflammation of the mouth

strabismus disorder in which the eyes cannot be directed to the same object or one eye deviates from the central tract

strain injury to the tendons and muscles resulting from overstretching or overuse

stress ulcer peptic ulcer that develops after an acute medical crisis

stricture narrowing

subarachnoid space between the arachnoid membrane and the inner membrane covering the brain

subcutaneous beneath the skin; often refers to fatty tissue

subdural pertaining to the space beneath the dura

subluxation partial separation of a bone from a joint

supination upward-turning movement

sympathetic nervous system portion of the autonomic nervous system

synapse space between neurons where chemical transmission of electrical impulses takes place

syncope fainting

synovectomy surgical removal of the synovial membrane surrounding a joint

synovitis inflammation of the synovial tissue

systemic lupus erythematosus autoimmune disease of unknown cause

systole contraction phase of the heart's work

tachycardia fast heartbeat

tamponade pathological compression of a part

tardive dyskinesia abnormal muscle movements as a side effect of antipsychotic drugs

temporal lobe portion of the brain located under the frontal and parietal lobes

tendinitis inflammation of a tendon

tendon band of tissue that connects muscle to bone

tenosynovitis inflammation of the tendon sheath

tenotomy surgical division of a tendon

teratogenic development of abnormal structures in fetus

tetany involuntary contraction of the muscles

thalassemia group of inherited hemolytic anemias

thoracentesis removal of fluid from the thoracic cavity

thoracic refers to the chest area

thorax chest cavity

thromboangiitis obliterans rare condition of small and medium-sized arteries of the extremities in which blood flow is diminished to a body part

thrombocyte platelet

thrombocytopenia decrease in platelet number

thrombocytosis increase in platelet number

thrombophlebitis inflammation of a vein with clot formation

thrombosis formation of blood clot

thrombus blood clot

thymus lymphoid organ lying in the upper portion of the chest that produces a hormone important in controlling development of lymphocytes

TIA transient ischemic attack

tinnitus ringing in the ears

tolerance with regard to substance use, body adaptation to the substance such that larger amounts of the substance are needed to produce the same effects

tonic rigid

tonometry measurement of pressure in the eye

tophi deposits of crystals in the joints

trachea windpipe

tracheostomy surgical opening into the trachea

trachoma chronic infectious disease of the conjunctiva and cornea

traction therapeutic method in which a mechanical or manual pull is used to restore or maintain the alignment of bones or to relieve pain and muscle spasm

transient ischemic attack (TIA) temporary blocking of cerebral arteries, causing slight temporary neurological deficits

traumatic brain injury injury to the brain from an external physical force to the head

tricuspid valve valve between the right atrium and the right ventricle of the heart

triplegia paralysis of three limbs of the body

tuberculosis infectious disease caused by an organism called the tubercle bacillus

tumor new and abnormal growth of cells that serve no useful function and may interfere with healthy tissue function

tympanic cavity middle ear

tympanic membrane eardrum

tympanometry test of acoustic immittance in which the mobility or flexibility of the tympanic membrane is assessed by measuring how much sound energy is admitted into the ear as pressure is varied in the external auditory canal

tympanoplasty surgical procedure that involves the middle ear

ulcerative colitis inflammatory condition of the large intestine

ulnar deviation lateral movement of the hand away from the body

urea waste product eliminated by the kidney

uremia buildup of waste products (e.g., urea and creatinine) in the blood

ureterolithotomy surgical removal of stones from the ureter

ureterosigmoidostomy surgical procedure for urinary diversion in which the ureters are connected to the colon so that urine is excreted through the rectum

ureters tubes leading from the kidney draining into the bladder

urethra single tube leading from the bladder to the urinary meatus

urethritis inflammation of the urethra

urinary meatus outside opening through which urine is eliminated

urinary reflux backward flow of urine

urinary retention the inability to empty the bladder of urine

urinary tract collecting system for urine, including the ureters, bladder, and urethra

urosepsis septic poisoning due to retention and absorption of waste products in urine

urticaria hives

vagotomy cutting of the vagal nerve

valvuloplasty procedure to dilate a narrowed or stenosed valve of the heart

varices dilated and distended veins

varicose veins congestion of veins

vascular insufficiency inadequate blood and oxygen to a body part

vena cava large vessel carrying unoxygenated blood from the general circulation to the right atrium of the heart

venesection removal of quantities of blood to reduce plasma volume

ventilation process by which gases are transported between the atmosphere and the alveoli

ventricles small cavity, such as the cavity in each cerebral hemisphere of the brain or cavity that make up the lower two chambers of the heart

vertebrae bony covering of the spinal cord

vertigo illusion of spinning movement

vesicles fluid filled blister-like sac

vestibular system part of the inner ear that conducts impulses regarding body balance and movement

virus organism that cannot grow or reproduce outside of living cells

viscosity thickness

visual acuity ability to process visual detail; sharpness of vision

visual impairment any deviation of normal vision

visual–spatial deficit deficiency in depth perception, judgment of distance, size, position, rate of movement, form, and relation of parts to wholes

vitrectomy removal of the vitreous humor in the eye

Wernicke's aphasia type of fluent aphasia in which effortless speech, relatively normal grammatical structure, and increased verbal output occur, but with reduced information content

Wernicke's area portion of the brain located over the temporal and parietal lobes and the major area of receptive function

white matter myelinated fibers in the central nervous system that conduct electrical impulses

withdrawal experience of physical symptoms when the amount of a substance is decreased or absent

xenograft graft taken from another species; heterograft

Glossary of Medications

Medications are an important aspect of management of many health conditions. For this reason, it is important to be familiar with major types of medications used in management of health conditions and their biological and behavioral effects. At no time should a nonhealth professional advise an individual to stop taking a medication or to change the dosage of a medication. If questions or doubts arise regarding an individual's condition or an individual's reaction to a specific medication, a health professional should be consulted.

ROUTES OF ADMINISTRATION

Medications can be administered in a variety of ways. Knowing the different routes of administration can be helpful in planning effectively so that any special factors regarding medication that might affect an individual's rehabilitation plan can be considered. Routes by which medications can be administered are the following:

Oral

Ingested (swallowed)
Sublingual (under the tongue)
Buccal (on mucous membrane on the cheek or tongue)

Rectal

Suppository, inserted into the rectum
Liquid, given as a retention enema

Parenteral

Intravenous (into a vein)
Intradermal (into the skin)
Subcutaneous (into the fatty layer under the skin)
Intramuscular (into the muscle)

Other

Inhalation (breathing medication in)
Topical (on top of the skin)

FACTORS INFLUENCING MEDICATION DOSAGE

For a medication to be effective, it must be of sufficient concentration to produce the desired effect. The dosage is based on individual differences that influence how the medication is metabolized and, therefore, absorbed. Factors that influence dosage and metabolism include the following:

1. **Age.** Children are generally more sensitive to drugs than adults and, therefore, generally require smaller doses.
2. **Body weight.** The ratio of body weight to the amount of drug taken determines the concentration of the drug within the body and, therefore, affects its potency.
3. **Time of administration.** Oral medications are absorbed more rapidly if no food is present in the stomach and upper portion of the intestinal tract. However, drugs that irritate the stomach lining should be taken with food.

4. **Route of administration.** Medication injected directly into a vein has an immediate effect, whereas medication taken orally or injected into a muscle or subcutaneous tissue has a slower absorption rate, so it takes longer to reach a concentration in the body that will show an effect.

5. **Rate of excretion.** Some drugs build up in the body when they are not excreted or destroyed as fast as they are ingested. If a drug builds up in the body past a certain level of concentration, toxic symptoms can occur.

6. **Drug combinations.** Some drugs are taken in combination with other drugs to enhance their action. Not all drugs are compatible when taken together, however, and some can seriously affect the action of other drugs. Consequently, it is important that the healthcare provider is aware of all medications an individual is taking, even those prescribed by other healthcare providers.

7. **Pathology.** Certain conditions affect the absorption or excretion of different medications, rendering them ineffective or causing toxic manifestations.

8. **Allergies or other drug reactions.** Individuals are sometimes allergic to different medications or have an abnormal response to them. Once these medications are identified, individuals should be encouraged to inform their healthcare provider of the names of these drugs along with the reactions experienced.

9. **Adherence.** A medication for management of a specific health condition is only as effective as the individual's ability or willingness to take the medication according to the management plan.

METHODS OF CLASSIFYING MEDICATIONS

Medications may be referred to in three ways:

1. **Chemical name.** This is the precise description of chemical constituents of the medication. An example of a chemical name is N-methyl-4-carbethoxypiperidine hydrochloride.

2. **Generic name.** This reflects the chemical name for the medication, but is simpler. An example of a generic name is *meperidine*. Generic-name medications may be less expensive than the corresponding trade-name medications, but they may not always have all the components of the trade-name counterpart.

3. **Trade name.** This represents the brand name of the medication. The trade name is registered, meaning use of the name is restricted to the medication's manufacturer, which is the legal owner of the name. There may be many trade names for the same generic medication. An example of a trade name is *Demerol*.

THERAPEUTIC CLASSIFICATION OF MEDICATIONS

Medications can be placed into several categories based on the action or effect they are expected to produce. These categories are called *therapeutic classifications*.

EXAMPLES OF CATEGORIES OF THERAPEUTIC EFFECT

Ace Inhibitor	Dilates blood vessels to lowers blood pressure, reduce heart failure, and facilitate blood flow to kidneys
Analgesic	Reduces pain
Antacid	Neutralizes stomach acid
Antianxiety	Reduces symptoms of anxiety
Antiarrhythmic	Corrects abnormal rhythm of the heart
Antibiotic	Kills or inhibits growth of microorganisms
Anticoagulant	Lengthens the prothrombin time and helps to prevent clot formation
Anticholinergic	Inhibits action of the involuntary nervous system
Anticonvulsant	Prevents convulsions or muscle spasm
Antidepressant	Psychic energizers used to treat depression
Antidiarrhetic	Prevents diarrhea
Antiemetic	Prevents nausea or vomiting
Antifungal	Checks the growth of fungi
Antihypertensive	Lowers blood pressure
Antihistamine	Relieves symptoms of allergic reactions by preventing histamine action
Anti-inflammatory	Reduces inflammatory reactions such as redness and swelling
Antimicrobial (sulfonamide)	Inhibits growth of microorganisms
Antineoplastic	Prevents growth and spread of cancerous cells
Antipruritic	Relieves itching
Antipsychotic	Reduces psychotic symptoms and hallucinations
Antipyretics	Reduces fever
Antiseptic	Inhibits growth of microorganisms
Antispasmodic	Relieves muscle spasms
Antithyroid	Blocks thyroid hormone production
Antitussive	Sedative to prevent cough
Antiviral	Kills or inhibits growth of viruses
Astringent	Causes contraction of tissue and halts discharge
Beta Blocker	Reduces heart rate and increases blood flow to control high blood pressure and irregular heart rhythms
Bronchodilator	Opens airways to permit air to pass more freely in and out of the lungs
Calcium Channel Blockers	Relaxes and widens blood vessels, decreasing cardiac workload
Cardiotonic	Changes heart rhythm and rate and generally strengthens the heart
Cathartic	Relieves constipation

(continues)

EXAMPLES OF CATEGORIES OF THERAPEUTIC EFFECT *(continued)*

Cholinergic	Stimulates the effects of the parasympathetic nervous system
Corticosteroid	Produces dramatic short-term anti-inflammatory effects
Digestant	Supplements enzyme deficiency
Digitalis preparation	Increases pumping action of the heart muscle
Diuretic	Rids the body of excess fluid
Expectorant	Thins mucus to help expectoration
Histamine H_2 (receptor antagonist)	Blocks cells in the stomach lining from producing acid
Hypoglycemic agent	Oral medication that lowers blood sugar
Hypnotic	Induces sleep
Immunosuppressant	Blocks the body's natural response to foreign substances
Laxative	Relieves constipation
L-dopa	Decreases symptoms of Parkinson's disease
Nitrates	Dilates coronary arteries, enabling the heart muscle to receive more oxygen
Nonsteroidal Antiinflammatory (NSAID)	Reduces inflammation associated with bone and joint conditions
Proton Pump Inhibitor	Controls gastric reflux and gastric ulcer healing
Sedative	Produces calming, tranquilizing effect
Skeletal Muscle Relaxant	Reduces muscle tone, spasticity, and muscle pain
Statins	Lowers cholesterol
Thrombolytic Enzyme	Dissolves blood clots
Vasodilators	Dilates blood vessels and reduce blood pressure
Vasopressors	Contracts blood vessels and raise blood pressure

Glossary of Diagnostic Tests and Procedures

abdominal paracentesis procedure to remove fluid from the abdominal cavity through a hollow needle

abdominal sonography sonogram used to identify conditions of the pancreas, liver, gallbladder, or any other abdominal organ

acoustic immittance battery of tests to evaluate middle ear status

air conduction audiometry test of ability to hear sounds through the ear

alanine aminotransferase (ALT; formerly serum glutamic-pyruvic transaminase [SGPT]) blood test to identify liver disease

angiography (arteriography) injection of radiopaque contrast material into the arteries to visualize the vessels (see *arteriography*)

antinuclear antibodies (ANA) blood test that identifies the proteins or antibodies that are present with some autoimmune diseases

arteriogram (see *arteriography*)

arteriography (angiography) test performed to study the anatomy of vascular structures through injection of radiopaque material into the arteries; may be performed to evaluate the vasculature of vessels of the kidney, adrenal gland, brain, heart, or lower extremities

arthrocentesis insertion of a needle into a joint cavity for removal of synovial fluid for examination

arthrography X-ray study of a joint in which contrast material is injected into a joint, the joint is moved through its range of motion, and X-ray films are taken

arthroscopy direct visualization of a joint through insertion of a small instrument called an arthroscope into the joint

aspartate aminotransferase (AST; formerly serum glutamic-oxaloacetic transaminase [SGOT]) blood test to measure enzyme levels to identify possible coronary occlusive heart disease or liver disease

audiometric testing noninvasive procedure involving measurement of the degree of hearing loss through an electronic device called an audiometer

auditory brain stem response (ABR) record of electrical activity generated as sound travels from the auditory nerve through the auditory brain stem pathway to rule out auditory conditions

barium enema (lower GI series) X-ray examination of the lower gastrointestinal tract

barium swallow (upper GI series) X-ray study of the upper gastrointestinal tract

biopsy removal of a specimen of tissue from a specified site for examination

bleeding time blood test used to measure the length of time it takes for bleeding to stop after a puncture wound; determines how quickly a platelet clot forms

blood urea nitrogen (BUN) blood test that measures the level of a waste product of protein metabolism (urea) in the blood; used to evaluate kidney function

bone conduction audiometry test to determine whether hearing loss is sensorineural, conductive, or mixed; consists of placing a vibrator on the individual's mastoid process or the forehead through which calibrated tones are transmitted directly into the inner ear, bypassing the external and middle ear systems

bone marrow aspiration insertion of a needle into the marrow space of the bone and aspiration of a small sample so it may be examined microscopically for various abnormalities in the number, size, and shape of the precursors of blood cells

bone scan intravenous injection of radioisotopes that then concentrate in the bone, enabling the concentration to be measured by a special machine called a scanner, which produces a picture of the bone

brain scan infrequently used test that relies on radionuclides (radioisotopes) to identify changes in brain tissue, including tumors, infarction (death of tissue), or infection, or blockage of blood vessels in the brain

bronchoscopy visual examination of the bronchial tubes through a long hollow tube inserted through the mouth and into the bronchus

C-reactive protein test blood test used to identify inflammatory processes or tissue destruction

caloric test test to measure vestibular nerve function

cardiac angiogram (see *arteriography*)

cardiac catheterization invasive procedure in which a catheter is passed into the vessel of an arm or leg and then threaded into the heart; used to study the chambers, valves, and blood supply of the heart and to measure internal pressures

cardiac stress test noninvasive exercise test that provides a graphic record of the heart's activity during forced exertion

cerebral angiography invasive test in which a catheter is inserted into an artery and radiopaque dye injected, and a series of X-ray films is taken to visualize blood flow in the brain and identify blockage

chest roentgenography (X-ray) noninvasive radiographic procedure by which it is possible to visualize organs of the chest cavity on X-ray film

cholangiogram a study in which the bile ducts are visualized on X-ray film

cholecystography procedure in which the gallbladder is visualized on X-ray film to detect abnormalities, inflammation, or the presence of stones

colonoscopy procedure to examine the lining of the colon (large bowel) for irregularities by inserting a flexible tube into the anus and advancing it into the rectum and colon

complete blood count (CBC) blood test that evaluates a variety of components of the blood, including red and white blood cells (neutrophils, eosinophils, basophils, lymphocytes, monocytes), hemoglobin, and hematocrit

comprehensive eye exam examination of the external eye, including eye movements, size of pupils, and pupils' ability to react to light as well as visual acuity and visual field

computed tomography (CT scan; CAT scan) special X-ray procedure that produces three-dimensional pictures of a cross-section of a body part

creatinine clearance test test that compares the level of creatinine in the blood and the amount of creatinine excreted in the urine over a specified period of time

culture removal of a sample of exudate from body tissue, which is then implanted in a culture medium, where it is later examined for growth of organisms

cystoscopy insertion of a special tube called a cystoscope through the urethra and into the bladder to directly visualize the bladder wall

cytology study of cells that have been scraped from tissue surrounding an area (such as Papanicolaou [Pap] smear)

differential blood test to measure the proportion of each type of white blood cell

digital venous subtraction angiography invasive procedure in which a catheter is inserted into a vein, a contrast medium is injected, and a series of X-rays of the blood vessels in the head and neck are taken

discography X-ray study of the cervical or lumbar disks

echocardiography noninvasive ultrasound procedure in which the size, motion, and composition of the heart and large vessels are recorded

electrocardiography (ECG) graphic representation of electrical activity of the heart muscle

electrocochleography procedure in which stimulus-related electrical activity generated in the cochlea and auditory nerve is recorded to evaluate fluid in the inner ear

electroencephalography (EEG) noninvasive procedure producing a graphic representation of the electrical activity of the brain

electromyography (EMG) procedure in which electrical activity of certain muscles is evaluated to diagnose certain muscle diseases

electronystagmography procedure to monitor eye movement

ELISA enzyme-linked immunosorbent assay; initial blood test to screen for HIV antibodies

endoscopy (see *gastroscopy*)

enzyme immunoassay (see *ELISA*)

erythrocyte sedimentation rate (ESR; sed rate) blood test that measures the rate at which red blood cells settle in a special solution over a certain time period; detects tissue injury or inflammation

esophageal manoscopy (manometry) diagnostic procedure in which a catheter is placed through the individual's mouth into the esophagus to evaluate the function of the sphincter between the esophagus and the stomach

exploratory laparotomy surgical opening of the abdomen for the purpose of examination

fasting blood glucose (FBG) blood test to measure the glucose level in the blood when the individual has had nothing to eat

fluorescein angiography test used to detect changes in the blood vessels of the retina

free thyroxine test that estimates the amount of thyroxine circulating and unbound to protein in the blood to evaluate thyroid function

gastroscopy (endoscopy) diagnostic test in which a lighted, flexible tube called an endoscope or gastroscope is inserted through the mouth, into the esophagus, and into the stomach to enable the physician to visualize the walls of these organs

glucose tolerance test (GTT) blood test in which the individual, after fasting, is given concentrated glucose to drink and then blood samples are drawn at 1-, 2-, and 3-hour intervals

gonioscopy examination of the internal structures of the eye

Halstead–Reitan battery neuropsychological test battery

hematocrit blood test to measure the percentage or proportion of red blood cells in the plasma

hemoglobin blood test to evaluate the amount of hemoglobin content in erythrocytes

hemoglobin electrophoresis blood test used to make a definitive diagnosis of sickle cell disease or sickle cell trait

HIV viral load assay blood test that measures the amount of circulating human immunodeficiency virus (HIV) per unit of blood

Holter monitoring (ambulatory electrocardiography; event recorder) form of electrocardiography involving continuous recording of the heart's electrical activity; the individual wears the Holter monitor externally

incisional biopsy removal of tissue through an incision for examination

intravenous pyelogram (IVP) X-ray examination of the kidneys, ureters, and bladder in which a dye is injected into a vein in the arm and then X-rays are taken of the kidneys at intervals over approximately an hour to identify structural abnormalities as well as any problems with passage of the dye through the urinary system

KUB (kidney, ureters, and bladder roentgenography) X-ray of the kidney, ureters, and bladder to determine the size, shape, and location of these structures

laparoscopy procedure in which a hollow tube called a laparoscope is inserted into a body cavity through a small incision, and the contents of the body cavity are examined or surgical procedures are performed

laryngoscopy visual examination of the larynx through a tube called a laryngoscope that is inserted into the larynx; enables the physician to inspect the structure of the larynx as well as assess the function of the vocal cords

latex fixation (latex agglutination test) blood test to detect antibodies in response to certain health conditions such as rheumatoid arthritis

LE prep blood test that examines a specific cell in the blood; useful in the diagnosis of systemic lupus erythematosus

lumbar puncture (cerebrospinal fluid analysis; spinal tap) insertion of a needle into the subarachnoid space of the spinal column at the lumbar area so that cerebrospinal fluid may be aspirated and studied through laboratory analysis

Luria–Nebraska Neuropsychological Battery neuropsychological test battery

magnetic resonance imaging (MRI; nuclear magnetic resonance imaging [NMRI]) non-invasive procedure in which rapid detailed pictures of body tissue are produced; involves no ionizing radiation, but rather the pictures form when hydrogen atoms in a magnetic field are disturbed by radio-frequency signals

manometry diagnostic procedure to evaluate the function of the sphincter between the esophagus and the stomach

mean corpuscular hemoglobin concentration blood test that calculates the amount of hemoglobin in each red blood cell

mean corpuscular volume (MCV) blood test to calculate the volume of a single red blood cell

mental status examination structured interview used as a screening instrument in assessing cognitive impairment

Mini–Mental State Examination mental status test to evaluate orientation, memory, attention, and ability to write, name objects, copy a design, and follow verbal and written commands

Minnesota Multiphasic Personality Inventory (MMPI) objective personality test

myelography X-ray study of the spinal cord

needle biopsy test in which a needle is inserted into tissue and cells for examination are removed through the needle

nerve conduction velocity (electroneurography) procedure often performed in conjunction with electromyography; measures nerve activity at the nerve–muscle junction to assist in diagnosis of conditions that affect the peripheral nerves

neuropsychological tests procedures that are used to assess major functional areas of the brain

otoacoustic emissions measurement of reflections in the outer ear of mechanical activity in the cochlea; used for measurement of hearing in infants, individuals with dementia, and other persons who are difficult to test

paracentesis procedure in which a needle is inserted into a body cavity to remove fluid

partial thromboplastin time (PTT) blood test to evaluate the special part of the clotting mechanism not evaluated by prothrombin time

patch test application to the skin of small amounts of various substances to identify allergic responses

platelet count blood test to measure number of platelets in the blood

positron emission transaxial tomography (PET scan) radionuclear study in which biochemical

or metabolic activities of cells of body tissue are studied

postprandial plasma glucose (PPG) blood test in which the glucose level of the blood is measured several hours after eating

proctoscopy procedure involving direct visualization of the anus and rectum through a proctoscope inserted into the rectum

prothrombin time (PT; Pro Time) blood test to measure the length of time that a blood sample takes to clot when certain chemicals are added to it in the laboratory; tests for specific factors involved in clotting

pulmonary function tests procedures to assess the volume of air that can be taken in and expelled from the lungs as well as the ability to move air into and out of the lungs

pure-tone audiometry test of the ability to detect sound and pitch in each ear, whose results are then plotted on a graph called an audiogram

radionuclide imaging intravenous injection of a radioactive substance that localizes in a body tissue so that multiple views of the structure can be taken with a special camera and the images can be evaluated

red blood cell count (RBC) measurement of the total number of red blood cells

reticulocyte count blood test to assess bone marrow function by measuring production of immature red blood cells

retinal examination examination for retinal conditions through visualization of the retina

retrograde pyelogram procedure in which a small catheter is inserted through a tube that has been inserted into the bladder and then directed into the ureters to the pelvis of the kidney; dye is then injected through the catheter, and X-ray films are taken to visualize the structures and to detect any abnormalities

rheumatoid factor (latex fixation; agglutination test) blood test that determines whether an abnormal protein exists in the blood serum; assists in the diagnosis of rheumatoid arthritis or other rheumatic diseases

Rorschach inkblot test projective personality test

scrapings procedure in which scales of a skin lesion are scraped from the surface of the skin and examined under a microscope

serum creatinine measurement of the level of creatinine in the blood to evaluate kidney function

serum glutamic-oxaloacetic transaminase (SGOT) (see *aspartate aminotransferase*)

serum glutamic-pyruvic transaminase (SGPT) (see *alanine aminotransferase*)

serum thyroxine (T$_4$) blood test to measure level of thyroid hormone in the blood

Short Portable Mental Status Questionnaire (SPMSQ) mental status test to assess orientation, personal history, remote memory, and calculation

sickle cell prep blood test to detect the presence of irregular hemoglobin, but which cannot distinguish between sickle cell disease and sickle cell trait

sigmoidoscopy procedure in which there is direct visualization of the sigmoid colon through a sigmoidoscope inserted through the anus and rectum and into the colon

skull roentgenography X-ray of the skull to visualize bones of the skull and structures such as the sinuses to identify fractures or other abnormalities

slit-lamp exam evaluation of structures of the eye, including the cornea and iris, as well as screening for cataracts

smears tests in which exudate is obtained from body tissue, placed on a slide, and examined under the microscope

sonography (ultrasonography) test in which sound waves passed into the body are converted to a visual image or photograph of a body structure

SPECT single photon emission computed tomography; uses a computer and scanning camera rotating around the body to record images of the collection of radionuclides in areas of abnormality of the body

speech audiometry tests to measure the individual's ability to understand speech

speech discrimination threshold (word recognition test) test that measures the ability to understand words at a comfortable volume and distinguish between similar speech sounds

speech reception threshold test that identifies the lowest intensity or softest sound in decibels at which an individual first understands speech

Stanford–Binet intelligence test

Thematic Apperception Test projective personality test

thyroid-stimulating hormone (TSH) a blood test that measures the amount of thyroid-stimulating hormone in the blood and consequently serves as a measure of thyroid function

tonometry measurement of pressure of the eye

tympanometry technique used to measure the amount of sound energy admitted into the middle ear

ultrasonography (see *sonography*)

urinalysis examination of urine under a microscope or through other laboratory procedures to evaluate the concentration, acidity, and presence of components such as protein, sugar, blood, bacteria, or other types of cells in the urine

urine culture laboratory examination of sterile urine to determine whether infection is present, and if so, to identify the infectious organism

venogram X-ray study in which dye is injected into veins of a body part and X-ray films are obtained at timed intervals to visualize the structure of the venous system

ventilation/perfusion scan (lung scan) radio-graphic procedure that measures transport of gases between the atmosphere and alveoli of the lung or the degree to which blood is passed through the vessels into the lungs

Wechsler Adult Intelligence Scale-Revised (WAIS-R) intelligence test

Wechsler Intelligence Scale for Children-Revised (WISC-R) intelligence test

Wechsler Preschool and Primary Scale of Intelligence (WPPI) intelligence test

Western blot blood test that is performed as a confirmatory test for the HIV antibody

white blood cell count (WBC) measurement of the total number of white blood cells

Wood's light examination examination of the skin under an ultraviolet light to identify specific types of skin infections

Index

Italicized page numbers refer to figures, tables are noted with a *t*.

ITALY
Land of many dreams

Text by Rupert O. Matthews
CLB 1244
© 1986 Illustrations and text: Colour Library Books Ltd.,
   Guildford, Surrey, England.
Text filmsetting by Acesetters Ltd., Richmond, Surrey, England.
All rights reserved.
Published 1986 by Crescent Books, distributed by Crown Publishers, Inc.
Printed in Spain.
ISBN 0 517 46078 5
h g f e d c b a

Dep.Leg. B-2.259-86

ITALY
Land of many dreams

Text by
Rupert O. Matthews

CRESCENT BOOKS
NEW YORK

From the balcony of my hotel room, six or seven floors up, I had a bird's eye view of the seafront at Rimini, and of the wide promenade and the frenzy of activity there. A long row of large beach umbrellas, every one pristine white, had been set up and each was being worked on by an artist. Bright colours were slapped and sloshed onto the unusual 'canvases' and each artist was being cheered on by his or her enthusiastic supporters. My companion told me it was a lighthearted competition to select a design that would be used on beach unbrellas the following season. "It is not a serious competition, you understand," she said, "but just something for enjoyment. What you in England call 'a bit of fun', I think".

The memory of the Great Beach Umbrella Painting Competition has stayed with me for many years, and for all I know they still have their 'bit of fun' in Rimini each summer, turning a simple event into the expansive, explosive street theatre that is forever Italy.

I used to think that the entire country was a disorganised, anarchic mess, but that was long ago when I believed in the importance of newspaper articles. These articles worried about the latest economic or political crisis there, the most recent change of Government and the rumblings of unrest in Rome. Poor old Italy, I thought, having to bear the burden of such woes.

But then came more opportunities for visiting Italy. I managed to observe such events as the Rimini paint-sloshing grand prix; to become entangled in the choosing of a 'Miss Cinema' in Lido di Jesolo; to discover a spaghetti museum in a tiny town called Pontedassio; to explore the hill villages of Tuscany; to take the Highway of the Sun to the neglected south; to wallow in the emotional effect of Venice; to try to comprehend the artistic creations to be seen in such cities as Turin, Siena and Florence.

And I learned that Italians have, in reality, managed to get their priorities right. They leave the politicians to their posturings and get on with the important business of living each day to the full. "Choosing a good wine is much more important than choosing a good government," a Calabrian hotelier once assured me.

You may think such an attitude irresponsible, but on the whole I heartily approve of it. I like the fact that the Italians produce excellent food in their restaurants without making the song and dance about it that the French do. I like their dramatic *autostradas* – but shudder at the way they drive. I adore their old cities and their timeless countryside – but wish they'd take more care of them.

I don't expect I could live in such a style full time. But I look forward eagerly to every visit.

John Carter

The sun shines in Italy as it shines nowhere else on earth. The still heat is heavy with the scents of the flowers and shrubs which carpet the baked earth, and the deafening chirping of the crickets. By the dusty roadside, in the shade of some ancient arch, a group of locals sip wine. They wave their arms wildly, trying to emphasise an argument to which none of the others is really listening.

The Italians are amongst the most attractive, and infuriating, people in Europe. Cut off from the rest of Europe by the soaring Alps, the Italians have developed a culture and character unique to the peninsula which they inhabit. The national character of the Italian shines through the nation's history and present economic life.

No Italian responds well to discipline or to authority, and the resultant chaos has caused more than one headache for those unfortunate enough to try to govern them. It is thought, for example, that more than half of the Italians who should pay tax, don't. They manage this simply because they are not inclined to obey government edicts, and the local officials are not too concerned about the matter either. The whole national economy is in such a muddle, as far as officialdom is concerned, that while most people are kept busy and are doing rather well, the government figures paint a picture of unmitigated gloom.

Italians are also very taken with show, finery and style. The splendid uniforms and celebrated quick march of the crack riflemen are well known throughout Italy and excite the admiration of all. The *Carabinieri*, the elite police force, parade in splendid uniforms of another century, complete with epaulettes, lanyards, cocked hats and colourful plumes. Even when taking a fairly ordinary glass of wine on a street corner, an Italian may strike an elegant pose. Elegance has become synonymous with Italy, though it may sometimes be suspected that the average Italian puts too much emphasis on appearance and too little on substance.

At the same time, Italians are fiercely proud of their local communities. The expression *terra* may refer to any of a number of things, but is often taken to refer to the locality of an Italian. There are still very definitely Neapolitans, Sicilians and Milanese, among others, all of whom speak their own version of Italian and resent the fact that theirs was not chosen as the standard. Such regionality is hardly surprising, for little more than a century ago the Italian peninsula was divided into more than half a dozen independent countries, and sizeable areas were under the control of Austria. A few centuries earlier the situation was even more confused, with a proliferation of proudly independent city states. The heritage of these earlier Kingdoms, Duchies and Republics can still be felt powerfully throughout the country.

All these national characteristics came disastrously to the fore in 1848. In that year popular revolutions swept through Italy, throwing out despotic tyrants and Austrian domination in northeastern Italy. Troops from Naples, the Papal States and all the various small states joined the regular army of the Kingdom of Piedmont in a combined attack on the Austrians in the north. Before long, however, discipline began to break down and local jealousies to break out. Neapolitan troops refused to take orders from the Piedmontese generals, as did everyone else. Before long the alliance had collapsed and the Austrians easily defeated the Italians. It was largely left to the charismatic radical Garibaldi and his romantic force of a thousand 'Redshirts' to inspire the Italian spirit and bring about unification.

After the debacle of 1848 it may have seemed that Italy was destined to remain the mere 'geographical expression' that the Austrian Prince Metternich declared it to be in 1849. But greater things were afoot and the *Risorgimento* began to gain ground. Quite what this 'revival' was has been the subject of much debate. Some historians see it as an upper class movement of educated people, others as a mass movement of the population. Whatever may be argued, the *Risorgimento* had enormous effects upon Italian history and may be said to be the reason for the existence of the unified nation today.

The 'revival' can be traced back to the occupation of most of Italy by Napoleon in the early part of the century. The French brought many liberal ideas into the peninsula and their policy of unification spurred the ideas of nationalism amongst the educated Italians. The reactionary rule of the restored dukes and kings after the defeat of Napoleon in 1815 only intensified these ideas, and numerous secret societies sprang up. A series of liberal revolutions in 1831 were even less successful than the risings of 1848. By 1850 it was accepted that liberal revolts were useless and only the Kingdom of Piedmont held out any hope for the *Risorgimento*. In 1859 Piedmont manoeuvred Austria into the role of aggressor and, with French help, defeated her in a series of battles. The following peace brought much of northern Italy into the hands of Piedmont, and the moderate liberals would have been content with this success.

Garibaldi, however, was not content. He appealed to the romantic streak in the Italian nation and gathered together a thousand volunteers whom he dressed in striking red shirts. With this tiny force Garibaldi invaded Sicily, which he took in just three months with the aid of local rebels. To the consternation of the moderates he then invaded the mainland and forced the King of Naples to flee. Piedmont reacted by invading the Papal States and linked up with Garibaldi, who handed his conquests over to the King of Piedmont, who thereby became the King of Italy. Within ten years Venetia and Rome, with the exception of the Vatican, had been added to the new Kingdom and it only wanted the break up of the Austrian Empire, following the First World War, for Italy to reach, approximately, its present boundaries. The romantic movement of the *Risorgimento*, which had begun with such unworkable ideas, had finally succeeded in uniting a country once thought to be too disparate to work together.

If the Italians are not considered amongst the most organized nations in Europe, their leadership in the world of the arts has never been questioned. It is not just that they have produced some of the greatest painters and sculptors in history; the whole nation seems to have an innate sense of good taste. Nothing is too ordinary to warrant artistic attention, even the slabs of concrete which pave the footpaths are worked with elegant designs. The uniforms of the troops which failed to defeat the Austrians in 1848 were the most gorgeous and magnificent in the world. If the Austrians did not respect the Italians' organization, they must have envied those uniforms and their well-known ability to impress the *signorinas*.

Even a thousand years ago the talent of Italian craftsmen, particularly their armourers, was recognized throughout Europe and their work highly sought after. It was, however, with the Renaissance that the true Italian talent began to emerge in all its glory. Known to the Italians themselves as the *rinascimento*, or rebirth, the age was one of great excitement as the learning and culture of the ancients was rediscovered and adapted to the period. The Italians found themselves surrounded by the legacy of the Roman Empire. The numerous sculptures and bas reliefs, which were literally lying around, gave inspiration and precedents for artists eager to explore the new style. Those artists were fortunate to be living in Italy at that time. The whole country was split into innumerable city states, each jealous of its independence and proud of its heritage. The rich *signori* were keen to emphasise their power to their own people and to other *signori*. To do this they turned to art and spent lavishly on palaces and cathedrals which remain to this day as tributes to their wealth and taste.

The Renaissance was a comprehensive flowering of culture and thought. It was at this time that the Madrigal craze swept across Europe, having originated in Italy, and that Machiavelli first codified political thought. It is, however, the visual arts for which the Renaissance is best known and at which Italy shone. Throughout the country beautiful buildings adorned with magnificent sculptures and paintings were going up, to emphasise the glories of the rebirth of the grandeur that was once Rome. When Brunelleschi crowned the cathedral of Florence with a massive dome, the Renaissance really began. It was to produce such artists in Italy as Michelangelo, Donatello, Titian, Botticelli, Raphael and Leonardo da Vinci. The prominence which Italy gained during the Renaissance was not lost and the country stayed in the forefront of art and architecture for many years.

Today, however, the most popular aspect of Italian culture to spread across the modern world is that of the *dolce vita*. Italian cuisine has long been recognised as among the world's best. As far back as 1860 Mrs Beeton was extolling the values of pasta and declaring that the very best was that made in Naples and exported direct to Britain. The emigration of thousands of Italians to many parts of the globe has helped spread their cuisine and wines. The style of cooking typical of Italy dates right back to the Romans, and to the introduction of pasta from China. The Italians are probably the only nation to have mastered the use of cheese in cooking, and to have brought the use of garlic to fresh heights. Almost all Italian dishes, from spaghetti to pizza, should have these two vital ingredients, mixed in perfect proportion. In a country where there is little grazing land, the use of red meat has always taken second place to that of poultry, veal and fish. The Italians have devised far more light and appetising dishes from these basics than any other nation; dishes which seem particularly tasty beneath the warm, Mediterranean sun.

Italian wine can be very good and has a character all its own, which ideally suits the flavours of Italian cooking. It was not for nothing that the ancient Greeks named Italy *oenotria*, the land of wine; today she still produces more wine than any other country in the world, some 1,750 million gallons each year. The art of winemaking, like any art, is carried out to perfection in Italy; but in the most disorganized way. In France, wines are usually named after the region, or even vineyard, from which they come. Italy, however, has no such system and a bottle may carry the name of a district, grape type, local celebrity or even a purely mythical name of no relevance at all. The government is trying to introduce a more logical system which would increase sales abroad, but the confusion looks set to persist for many years.

Though modern archaeology may point to a much earlier date, the ancient Romans were adamant that their Eternal City was founded by Romulus in 753 BC. This first king led a highly adventurous life, which included killing his brother, Remus. After founding the city, Romulus is said to have had a successful military career before his death in 717 BC. He was followed by six legendary kings, the last of whom was such a tyrant that the Romans deposed him and founded the Republic. Under the Republic, Rome embarked upon an expansionist policy which, by 265 BC, gave her virtual control of the Italian peninsula.

At this time the growing territories of Rome ran into the well-established commercial empire of Carthage. The great North African city controlled huge areas of the Mediterranean and was seen as a threat by Rome, who decided to destroy it. In the first clash, which broke out in 264 BC, Rome had the upper hand and took sizeable territories from Carthage. During the second war of 218 to 201 BC the exploits of

Hannibal nearly brought Rome to its knees. In one battle, that of Cannae, Hannibal massacred 80,000 Roman troops and threw his enemy onto the defensive. In 211 BC, Hannibal advanced on Rome itself and, according to legend, hurled his spear at the gates. In truth the Carthaginians were already losing, and by 201 BC their power was broken. In 149 BC the Romans attacked again and, after a hard-fought, three-year siege, totally destroyed their rival. Of the population of a quarter of a million, only 50,000 Carthaginians remained alive to be sold into slavery.

With Carthage destroyed no other power could stand up to Rome and the way was open for her to build the largest Empire ever seen. At its furthest extent, in the second century AD, the Roman Empire stretched from Scotland to Egypt and from the Atlantic to the Caspian. As the capital for such an immense Empire, Rome grew in wealth, population and prestige. The mighty city became crowded with fine monuments as successive Emperors strove to outshine their predecessors and to impress the populace with their own invincibility. 'Bread and Circuses' were not in themselves sufficient to keep the people happy; they had to be continually reminded of the greatness of their city. It was for this purpose that the majestic buildings were erected, many of them surviving to the present day, despite the onslaughts of barbarians and time.

For the ancient Romans the most important part of their wonderful city was an area of land which, until the 6th century BC, had been a patch of marshy ground. The Forum, where markets, law courts and popular assemblies were held, was enlarged and embellished by Julius Caesar; a lead followed by Augustus and the emperors. Magnificent temples and triumphal arches were raised in fine marbles, making the Forum the epitome of Roman grandeur. After the collapse of the Empire the Forum fell into disuse and was actively destroyed as its buildings became a quarry for marble. By the year 1800 forty feet of rubble and refuse covered the Forum, but throughout the last century a series of projects has brought the finery of the area to light.

This small area of central Rome is resplendent with shattered pillars and partial entablatures. The great buildings of the emperors are marked out and their stones replaced as far as possible. But it is not just forlorn remnants which fill the Forum. The majestic Arch of Septimus Severus rises seventy feet into the air. The arch was built in AD 203 to celebrate that Emperor's victories over the Parthians. Nearby is another monument to military victory, Trajan's Column. Wound around the 125-foot-tall column is an 800-foot-long frieze of the Emperor's campaigns which is an important source of information on Roman military matters. The column was originally topped by a bronze statue of Trajan, whose tomb this was, but in 1588 a representation of Saint Peter replaced it. The best preserved arch in Rome is that of Constantine,

which stands to the east of the Forum. Built in AD 312 to commemorate yet another military victory, this arch incorporates much earlier sculpture and marble.

Of all the surviving monuments of Ancient Rome to be seen in the present city, the most famous and evocative is the Colosseum. Rising 150 feet, the four-storeyed arena is a stupendous sight with its monumental proportions and grand arcades. The 50,000 spectators which the Colosseum could hold entered by numbered arches and found their seats by climbing the appropriate staircase. The best seats, those nearest the arena, were reserved for the Emperor, senators and Vestal Virgins. The opening of the amphitheatre in AD 80 was celebrated by games which lasted for 100 days and involved 5,000 animals and 1,000 gladiators. The greatest games, however, called for the death of some 2,000 gladiators and condemned men were often thrown to wild animals in the arena. On other occasions the arena would be flooded and war galleys took part in mock naval engagements. The savage games were amongst the most popular pastimes with the pagan Romans. Although Constantine the Great banned gladiatorial fights in AD 325, they continued well into the fifth century. In the eighteenth century Pope Benedict XIV consecrated the building, dedicating it to the memory of the Christians who had been executed there, and erected a bronze cross.

The Colosseum and Forum are both ruined, as indeed are nearly all the relics of ancient Rome that can be seen today. But one of the finest buildings has managed to survive almost intact: the Pantheon. Built by Hadrian about AD 118 on the site of an earlier building, this remarkable structure is roofed by the largest dome built until modern times. Spanning 142 feet, the dome is open at the top to admit air and light. In 609 the pagan temple was converted into a Christian church and it is to this act that the structure probably owes its survival.

At the height of its prosperity, in the second century AD, ancient Rome had a population of over a million people. The Eternal City, however, had over-reached itself and soon began a slow decline. The centre of power for the Empire shifted from the city which had founded it to the provinces, which provided the majority of its wealth. In 330 the capital was moved to Constantinople and later the Empire was divided into East and West. In 410 the Western Emperor, Honorius, idled in Ravenna while Alaric and his barbaric Visigoths sacked Rome. The Vandals took Rome in 455 and the last Emperor was deposed in 476, by which time the city's population was down to a quarter of its highest level. A whole era had come to a violent end.

Misfortune followed misfortune in the succeeding centuries, and by 1360 the population of the city was down to just 20,000 souls. It was the residence of the Pope in Rome that saved the Eternal City from the fate of so many other important cities of antiquity which are now mere shattered ruins. With the cessation of the barbarian invasions and the return of relative stability to Europe, the popes played a dominant role in the conversion of the heathens. Rome still had a magic ring to its name for the kings of early medieval Europe, a fact which no doubt helped the Papacy to survive and expand.

A decline in prestige and the vicious rivalry of several Roman families drove Pope Clement V from Rome in 1309. After a stay in Avignon, France, and the traumatic Great Schism, the Papacy returned to Rome in 1420 in the shape of Martin V and embarked upon a course which gained momentum with the years and was to change the face of the Eternal City. The government of the city and the Papal States was reorganised along Renaissance lines and prosperity followed. The dirty, narrow streets of the medieval city were replaced by wide, impressive thoroughfares and the crumbling medieval structures replaced by magnificent Renaissance buildings. Even the ruthless sack of Rome in 1527 by the troops of the Holy Roman Emperor failed to check the artistic revival. By the mid-seventeenth century Rome was once again a prosperous and majestic city with a population of over 100,000. It is to this period, before the corruption and decline set in, that the truly great splendours of Rome belong.

St Peter's Basilica is possibly the most famous building in the tiny sovereign state of the Vatican. The first magnificently adorned basilica on the site of Saint Peter's tomb was begun around 330 by the Emperor Constantine the Great. A thousand years later, however, the building was in such a state of disrepair that in 1506 Julius II ordered a new church to be built. The project took more than a century to complete and the design was changed several times under a succession of architects. The popes were determined that the church should be the finest in the world and employed such men as Bramante, Raphael, Peruzzi, Michelangelo, Maderno and Bernini.

Today the basilica is approached across the thousand-foot-long Saint Peter's Square, built by Bernini after the church was completed. The 370 columns and pillars and the 140 statues of saints make this one of the most imposing approaches in Rome, set off magnificently by the Baroque facade of the basilica itself. The east front was added by Maderno and was one of the last parts of the church to be built. It was also Maderno who altered the ground plan of the basilica from Michelangelo's Greek cross to a Latin cross with one arm longer than the other three. Michelangelo's dome, to many the crowning architectural glory of the church, was also altered during construction and is now slightly taller than originally planned.

Quite apart from its architectural value, the church contains some of the finest works of art in the world. The sheer size of the interior is in itself staggering, but the excellence of the detail takes the breath away. Just within the door stands the Pietà created by Michelangelo in 1499, when he was just 25. Further into the cavernous interior is found the fine bronze statue of Saint Peter, which is dressed once a year in its bejewelled, regal finery. The statue came from the old basilica and probably dates back to the thirteenth century. Over the years pilgrims have continually rubbed and kissed the statue's right foot to such an extent that it has almost worn away. At the centre of the church stands the Papal Altar, which is covered by the magnificent bronze *baldacchino* with its gilded, spiral columns. Scattered throughout the basilica are the splendid tombs of several Renaissance and Baroque popes. Perhaps the finest of these monuments are those of Paul III, Urban VIII and Innocent VIII.

Beneath the floor of the present church is the *Sacre Grotte Vaticane* or crypt, on the level of the original basilica floor. In the the crypt are many papal tombs, including those of the most recent popes. Beneath this level are modern excavations of the *Necropoli Precostantiniana* which have culminated in the discovery of the tomb of Saint Peter.

Tucked away within the Vatican is the domestic chapel of the popes, the Sistine Chapel. Though far smaller than the basilica, the chapel, with its glorious frescoes, epitomises Renaissance art. Those along the side walls were begun as soon as the building was completed, in 1481, and were executed by the greatest artists of the day: Botticelli, Perugino and Ghirlandaio. It was almost thirty years before the ceiling was painted by Michelangelo. Depicting scenes from the Creation and Fall of Man, this is acknowledged as being amongst the master's greatest works. Twenty years later Michelangelo returned to the Sistine Chapel and painted the stupendous Last Judgement on the altar wall, a project which took nearly eight years to complete. The magnificent setting of the Sistine Chapel is still used for the election of a new pope by the cardinals.

Despite the glories of the Renaissance it took many years for Rome to climb back to its former size. As recently as 1870 Rome still had fewer inhabitants than when the last Emperor was deposed. In that year, however, troops of the King of Italy burst through the 1,600-year-old walls and turned the ancient city into the capital of Italy. The population grew rapidly and is now around three million, spreading the city out across 582 square miles. Vast, new building programmes and monuments have transformed Rome into a truly modern city. It is primarily an administrative and tourist city, where heavy industry or large-scale commerce finds little place. The beautiful city of churches, monuments and fountains depends for its livelihood upon its position as capital of Italy and inheritor of ancient splendour.

Spread across the face of Sardinia, the second largest island in the Mediterranean, are reminders of a unique culture older than Rome. Huge blocks of basalt stand in large truncated cones, known as *nuraghi*, which may have been fortresses, watchtowers or tombs. Thousands of them remain and they are almost always within sight of another. The Nuraghese were well known in the ancient world for attacking their enemies with stone balls. These builders of the *nuraghi* were a distinct people who may be represented by the features of the *vero Sardo*, sometimes seen amongst the people. With a language all their own, the Sards have been conquered throughout their history by Phoenicians, Carthaginians, Romans, Vandals, Byzantines, Saracens and Italians. Despite this, the island preserved its unique atmosphere and remains as culturally distinct from the mainland as it is politically united to it. The island has its own way of life, language and cuisine, including the famous pasta dish *malloreddus* and the baked *zuppa cuata*. It also has the vendetta.

Sardinia has always been poor, with meagre soil, few natural resources and rampant malaria. The peasant economy has kept going almost unaltered for centuries: cattle and goats are allowed to roam the hills freely, while sheep are herded to counter the foxes of the island, and along the coast a thriving fishing industry has long contributed to the economy. More recently the *Cassa per il Mezzogiorno*, a government fund for the development of the impoverished south, has helped Sardinia considerably. After the Second World War malaria was eradicated by exterminating the mosquito which spread the disease. Chemical works have been developed at Porto Torres and Sarroch and a coal mine at Carbonia. A business consortium headed by the Aga Khan, meanwhile, has taken advantage of the disappearance of malaria to develop a holiday resort at Arzachena, a lead followed by others.

Behind the beautiful beaches and their wonderful climate, the island has much to offer. Quite apart from the Nuraghic ruins there are many fine churches, some of the best of which were built by the Pisans when they were in control of the island. Saccargia di Santa Trinita, near Sassari, is typical of this type. The local people wear their colourful, traditional costumes in their everyday life about the towns of Oristano and Dorgali. It is the capital of the island, however, which best reflects the story of Sardinia. The site of Cagliari was inhabited in prehistoric times, but it was the Phoenicians who founded the city. During the Carthaginian occupation, before their defeat by Rome, Cagliari was their principal stronghold. After the collapse of the Roman Empire the city was independent for many years, until it came under the control of Pisa and subsequently Piedmont and Italy. The Pisans left three fine monuments of their overlordship: the Cathedral of Santa Cecilia and the two defensive towers of San Pancrazio and Elefante. The harbour of the town has been enlarged this century and now handles exports of lead, salt and zinc.

Sicily is in many ways similar to Sardinia, but in many other ways quite different. It is a land still dominated by an agriculture which is, unfortunately, inefficient. The coastal land is proverbially rich and modern methods of intensive vegetable and fruit growing are now developing its full potential. It is for wine, however, that the island is principally known. Though little of the output is good enough to warrant vintages, it is prolific in the extreme. The peculiar perfume of orange blossom which pervades the wine makes it indispensable for many dishes, especially the exquisite *vitello alla Marsala*. In addition to the evolving agriculture of the island the *Cassa per il Mezzogiorno* has helped to attract industry to the island, particularly petrochemicals around Gela and Syracuse.

Perhaps the most dramatic feature of the island is Mount Etna, the highest active volcano in Europe, which stands at the eastern end of the island. This violent mountain rises to over 10,000 feet and was known to the ancient Greeks as *Aitne*, 'I burn', from which the modern name derives. They believed that the mountain was the workshop of Hephaestus, the smith of the gods. The most violent eruption in historical times was in 1669, when nearly 100 million cubic yards of matter were ejected and a dozen villages destroyed. Eruptions have continued spasmodically, with twelve so far this century.

The Greeks did not just name Etna, they established important colonies upon the island. Some of the most important Greek remains are to be found on the island, particularly at Agrigento, near the south coast. Founded in the early 6th century BC, the city was ruled for a time by the tyrant Phalaris, who is best known for roasting men alive in a large brass bull. After being sacked, in turn, by the Romans and Carthaginians, the town became part of the Roman Empire in 210 BC. The site was deserted at the fall of the Roman Empire and many buildings have survived. There were originally seven temples on the site, all of which have survived in some form or anothr. The Temples of Hera and Concordia are the best preserved; the latter, lacking only the roof, is one of the most complete Doric temples in the world.

The capital of Sicily, Palermo, is at once Sicilian and cosmopolitan in character. The city was founded by the Phoenicians in the 8th century BC and flourished under later Carthaginian control. Under a succession of rulers – including Romans, Vandals, Byzantines and Arabs – the town languished until it reached its 'Golden Age' under the Normans in the 12th century. During this period the magnificent, domed cathedral was begun, together with the churches of San Giovanni degli Eremiti and Martorana and several splendid palaces. In the later Middle Ages Sicily slipped into decline once again and was always jealous of being controlled from Naples. The Sicilians eagerly supported Garibaldi when he arrived in 1860 and nearly a century later achieved autonomous government within the

Republic of Italy. Since 1950 the population of Palermo has leapt from 150,000 to 600,000 as new industry and port facilities have brought fresh prosperity to the region.

After the turn of the first millennium AD, Norman adventurers began arriving in southern Italy. They found that south of Rome the peninsula was divided up into numerous small, warring states. It was not long before the Normans found an outlet for their genius at war and began to seize lands. By 1130 the foot of Italy, south of Formia, and the island of Sicily had been welded into one solid, centrally organised state under Count Roger II. As King of Sicily, Count Roger formed his new domains into a powerful kingdom which would survive changes of dynasty, periods of misrule and foreign invasion for 720 years.

The 'toe' of Italy, which separates the Tyrrhenian and Ionian seas, is occupied by the region of Calabria. Despite help from the central government, Calabria continues to rely upon agriculture for its prosperity. The traditional produce – olives, cereals, sheep and goats – is now being replaced by cash crops such as citrus fruits, figs and chestnuts. The wine of the region, however, has continued unchanged; the exceptionally heady red Ciro and the dry white *Greco di Gerace* being among the most popular. It was in Calabria that Alaric, the chief of the Visigoths, died just a few months after sacking Rome in AD 410. His followers held him in such esteem that they buried him in the riverbed of the Busento, near Cosenza, so that his tomb could never be disturbed. It has never even been found.

The 'heel' of the nation, Puglia, is in many ways similar to the 'toe'. Indeed, the ancients called Puglia Calabria, the name later applied to the 'toe'. Both are rocky peninsulas which rely on agriculture for their income. In Puglia are produced the strongest wines in the country, which are generally used for blending purposes, together with those other crops which are common to Calabria and indeed the whole of the *Mezzogiorno*.

At the heart of the region of Campania stands the city which took over from Palermo as the capital of the southern Kingdom: Naples. This great city was founded around 600 BC by the Greeks and named by them *Neapolis*, the new town. Its Greek manners and way of life attracted the Romans in droves, and the city became a favourite of several emperors. Their palaces and homes adorned the area and it was here that Nero first performed on stage.

The Roman Naples has long since disappeared, but a glimpse of its splendour can be caught 12 miles to the southeast, at Pompeii. In AD 79 Pompeii was a prosperous provincial city with a population of some 20,000 people. Sixteen years earlier it had suffered a major earthquake and rebuilding work was still under way when nature again took a hand. In AD 79 a tremendous explosion shook Mount Vesuvius and Pompeii was buried beneath twenty feet of pumice and ash. The town remained buried until 1869, when excavations were begun which continue to this day. Some three quarters of the city are now laid bare, including some of the finest buildings. Fronting the Forum, or principal square, is the Temple of Apollo, complete with 48 Ionic columns, and the fine Basilica. Two theatres and an amphitheatre which could seat 20,000 spectators have also survived to the present day. Perhaps Pompeii's greatest attraction, however, is its preservation of the domestic and everyday. Dozens of houses, from mansions to hovels, are preserved and can be inspected. From this point of view the nearby town of Herculaneum is probably better preserved. The small town was engulfed by mud to a depth of nearly a hundred feet, a fact which ensured the survival of even wooden artifacts. The wealthier Herculaneum had finer houses than Pompeii, many with three storeys, and the furniture and statues are similarly more splendid.

The Bay of Naples, which stretches from the Isle of Ischia to the Isle of Capri, is one of the most beautiful in the world. Its sparkling blue waters are backed by the green hills and huddled towns, but dominating everything are the islands and Mount Vesuvius. To the north of the bay is the Isle of Ischia, which covers 18 square miles. Known principally for its wine, Epomeo, the island is rapidly becoming a holiday resort to rival its southern counterpart, Capri. Capri was inhabited by the Emperor Tiberius purely as a pleasure resort. He built a dozen villas here and refused to return to Rome even when he was dying. Today, even with the crowds of tourists, Capri keeps its magic. The famed Blue Grotto is a sea cave on the north shore of the island which, particularly in the morning, is suffused with an unearthly light. The strange light is caused by the bright sunlight diffusing into the cave through the water which covers the majority of its mouth.

Naples itself has long been recognised as a unique city. Its narrow, winding, steep streets are used almost as living-rooms by the thousands of citizens. After centuries of overcrowding, the Neapolitan way of life has adapted to make a blessing of what elsewhere would be a curse. Poverty has also been endured for centuries and the Neapolitans have learnt to cope with that, too.

Despite the poverty, Naples has long been a great cultural centre. Through the fourteenth to sixteenth centuries Naples was a centre for the artistic in Italy. This phase is reflected in the Capodimonte Gallery, which houses works by Botticelli, Titian, Bellini and Raphael, among others. The architecture of the city also reflects its past prosperity and grandeur. The Cathedral of San Gennarno at Olmo is a fine structure dating back to 1300, though the site is that of a temple to Caesar. The Castel Nuovo was first built in 1279, but was rebuilt in the 15th century when the magnificent marble arch was added. The castle grounds adjoin the Palazzo Reale, the 17th-century palace of the Kings of Naples which contains some government offices and magnificent State apartments. The palace fronts onto the Piazza del Plebiscito where a fine, semicircular colonnade was erected by Murat, one of Napoleon's generals who received the Kingdom of Naples in 1808. The colonnade is interrupted by the church of San Francesco di Paola, built by Ferdinand I when he regained his Kingdom after Murat was shot. All along the Via San Biagio dei Librai are run-down palaces with an air typical of Naples. The National Museum has many sculptures, bronzes and paintings from the Roman era, particularly examples from Pompeii and Herculaneum.

The long history of unity in southern Italy is not reflected in the more prosperous north. In the tenth century the Kingdom of Italy, which reached as far south as the Volturno, was ruled directly by the Holy Roman Emperor. As the years passed the Emperors' hold over northern Italy began to slip. The centre of Imperial power was in Germany and local nobles and cities in Italy gained increasing powers throughout the eleventh and twelth centuries. A long and bitter struggle was taking place between the popes and the emperors as they fought for dominance over each other. The rising families and communes in Italy were able to take advantage of the confusion to increase their own powers. By 1176 Milan was able to defeat an imperial army at Legnano and a hundred years later the Emperor's authority in northern Italy had virtually ceased.

The release from Imperial control came in fits and starts and each individual city or area achieved its own independence, which they proceeded to guard fiercely. The city states fought long and bitter wars over boundary disputes, commercial rivalry and long-standing dislike. Within the cities, powerful families struggled for control of government while the ordinary citizens, or *popolo*, tried to wrest power for themselves. All these struggles were made more murderous by the policy of the blood feud, or vendetta, which, together with intrigue, became a way of life. Despite this, the banking, commercial and trading interests of the states ensured their prosperity and survival. It was against such a background that the Renaissance arose. Each city and every faction turned to art to emphasise its prosperity and power. It is for this reason that the cities of northern Italy, many of which are tiny by modern standards, are so resplendent with architectural and artistic treasures.

Urbino is situated in the hills on the eastern slopes of the Apennines. Today it is a rather quiet university town but five hundred years ago it was a bustling centre of art and literature under its ruler Frederico da Montefeltro. The pride of Urbino is, undoubtedly, the Ducal Palace with its beautiful 15th-century architecture and fine artistic collection. In 1483

Raphael was born in Urbino, while soon afterwards the famous *Urbino maiolica* style of pottery began to be made. In 1626 the Duchy of which Urbino was the centre was taken over by the pope and the city's importance waned.

On the other side of the Apennines stands the town of Siena. Like Urbino, Siena lost its independence to a more powerful neighbour, but unlike the former it has retained its importance and is now a provincial capital. As the Roman town of Sena Julia, Siena was unimportant, but after freeing itself from Imperial control in 1115 the city gained in prosperity. The wealth was mainly based on merchants and bankers who did business as far afield as London and Champagne. In 1260 Siena reached the peak of success when its army smashed that of Florence at Montaperti. The Black Death struck the city in 1348, killing half of the 50,000 citizens, and thereafter the rising fortunes of Florence eclipsed those of Siena. In 1555 Siena fell to the Spanish after an heroic defence and the city was then given to Florence.

During its independent existence the city embellished itself with many beautiful buildings which remain to this day. The cathedral has a striking facade of red, black and white marble which dates from 1380. The cathedral itself was begun in 1229 but in 1339 a major rebuilding was decided upon to make it the largest in Italy. The Black Death ended such plans and the cathedral was never properly finished. The crenellated town hall, which fronts onto the Piazza del Campo, was completed in 1309, though the tower, which is its principal feature, was not finished until the year after the Black Death. It is in the Piazza del Campo that the annual *Palio* is held. Each year the seventeen districts of the old city join a parade in medieval costume and field a horse in a race around the piazza. The parade is awash with colour as bright uniforms and silk banners crowd the streets. Exhibiting all the grace and beauty of Italian design, the spectacular column winds through the streets accompanied by flag wavers who hurl streaming banners through the air. The district whose horse wins the race is awarded a *palio*, or banner, emblazoned with the Madonna.

The city state to which Siena lost its independence in the sixteenth century is one of the greatest of Italian cities. Attaining its freedom at the same time as Siena, Florence was soon ruled by its merchant families, the chief of which was the Medici. The Medici originated as peasants in the village of Cafaggiolo, north of Florence. In the twelfth century the family moved to Florence and by the end of the thirteenth they ranked amongst the most important in the city. By skilful banking and money changing the Medici increased their wealth to fantastic proportions. Then they turned to politics. After many years of manoeuvring, which resulted in execution, imprisonment and exile for various members of the family, Cosimo bribed and tricked his way into power. Using his money and influence Cosimo established undisputed power for himself without recourse to a title. The succession of power passed to his son Piero in 1464 and then to his grandson Lorenzo in 1469. Lorenzo, named the Magnificent, brought the Medici rule to the height of splendour. The Medicis had always associated themselves with the people and with the arts. He lavished unbelievable amounts of money upon architecture, painting and sculpture, making Florence into the finest city in Italy. The Medici family was firmly established in Florence, though political errors led to two brief exiles from power. In 1532 Alessandro Medici accepted a ducal crown, a move his ancestors had long avoided, and in 1569 a cadet branch of the family received the title of Grand Duke of Tuscany from the Pope. It was against this background of Florentine intrigue that Niccolò Machiavelli wrote his classic work *The Prince*.

As the centre of an expanding country, and with a ruling house intent upon displaying its wealth and power, Florence was bound to attract artists. Today the city has a collection of treasures which marks it out from any other city. Yet it is not a lifeless museum; there are prospering industrial areas and the city has a population of half a million. The indigenous population is swamped by the 1,700,000 visitors who come to the city each year. The attraction for the tourist is not the modern city, but the remains of the past.

The great museum of Florence is without doubt the Uffizi. Francesco Medici had the palace built in 1560-74 for the efficient band of civil servants through which he ruled Florence. He also began the collection of great paintings for which the palace is now famous. The Uffizi contains an almost complete record of Florentine painting, including some of the world's greatest masterpieces.

The Ponte Vecchio is, as its name suggests, the oldest bridge in the city and is lined with shops which jut precariously over the river. It dates back to 1345 and was the only bridge across the Arno to survive the Second World War. The nearby Cathedral is an amalgam of styles from 1296, when it was begun, down to the last century. The octagonal dome which dominates the city was built by Brunelleschi between 1420 and 1436 and is considered by many to be his masterpiece. The centre of the old city, however, is the Piazza della Signoria on which stands the Palazzo Vecchio, with its austere facade and fine sculptures. Florence was one of the most powerful city states and remains one of the greatest Italian cities.

The third of the famous trio of Tuscan cities is Pisa, now an elegant provincial city engaged in light industry. But in the 11th century Pisa was a bold and ruthless power. Her fleet was one of the most powerful in the Mediterranean and scored many victories over the Infidels and other rival powers. In 1284 the Pisan fleet suffered a decisive defeat at the hands of Genoa and two centuries of trading dominance were at an end. But the Pisans turned to industry, and an efficient wool trade tripled the population to 50,000 in just thirty years. The city then suffered a series of misfortunes: her harbour silted up, internal disputes became even more murderous and divisive than usual, and in 1348 the Black Death struck. By 1406 Pisa was so weak that she could not resist her larger neighbour and the city became subject to Florence. The town's prosperity recovered for a while under Florentine control but soon declined again, and by 1550 the population was down to just 9,000.

The great tourist draw of the city is its famous leaning tower, but this is just part of the Piazza del Duomo. Within the piazza are three beautiful, white marble buildings dating from Pisa's great days. The cathedral is the largest and was built after a spectacular naval victory over the Saracens in 1063. The circular baptistry was begun a century later and took 125 years to build. The Leaning Tower itself was the last of the trio to be built. A slight landslip during construction caused the famous lean, which is at present just over 5 degrees. It was from the leaning tower that Pisa's most famous son, Galileo, is said to have dropped weights to prove that they fell at the same speed.

Tuscany has not only cities to offer, the cuisine of the region is known throughout Italy. Minestrone originated here, as did *funghi alla Fiorentina* and the Florentines have a special way with steak. The countryside around the towns is particularly known for its Chianti wines, which may be either red or white and are amongst the best in the country.

Of all the city states that existed in Italy during the Renaissance only one has survived to the present day. The mountainous Republic of San Marino has its origins in AD 301, when Saint Marinus fled here to escape persecution. It gained its constitution in 1263 and is, therefore, the oldest as well as the smallest republic in the world. The country covers only 23 square miles and has a population of 19,000. It was probably because the country is so small and showed no inclination to expand that successive invaders, and the Italian Republic, have ignored it. The Republic has no natural resources and the economy rests on the citizens. Light industry, using imported materials, is the most important employer, followed by tourism, commerce and agriculture. The whole country is dominated by the bulk of Monte Titano with its three peaks. Each peak is topped by a medieval fortress which can be seen from many miles distant.

Of all the great Italian cities only Venice owes nothing to the Roman Empire. When Attila the Hun launched his great offensive into Italy in AD 452, having already devastated vast areas of Europe, one of the cities he destroyed was Aquileia. The citizens of this city, together with the coastal people of Venetia, sought safety on a group of islands in a lagoon. The town they founded became independent of Byzantium during the 8th century and found itself presented with fantastic prospects a century later. The whole situation in the Mediterranean had changed since the fall of Rome. The split between the Pope and the Eastern Church, the rise of the Arabs and the disruption of sea trade placed Venice in a unique position to exploit the riches of the Mediterranean. Galleys from Venice plied the sea, carrying the rich luxuries of the East to Europe and the grain and gold of Europe to the East. In 1380 the Venetian fleet smashed that of Genoa, which had earlier defeated Pisa, and established a trade monopoly over the area that was to last for centuries.

During those years Venice became the finest and most prosperous city in Italy, embellishing itself with many beautiful buildings. The city was ruled by the Doge, a kind of elected duke, who was advised by the city's nobles. Each year the Doge would row out into the lagoon in his fabulous state barge and symbolically marry the city to the sea by casting a gold ring into the waters. At the very height of her power, when the arts were flourishing as never before, two decisive blows were delivered to Venice. Vasco da Gama discovered a sea route to India and Christopher Columbus discovered America. Venice's position at the centre of world trade was lost, and by 1797 she had lost her independence and became a plaything of other powers.

The city, built on water, may be slowly sinking into the lagoon and the floodwaters may rise higher every year, but it still maintains its beauties and attractions in an atmosphere that is unique. Though the city has recently been linked to the mainland by both road and rail it is still essentially a canal city. Many of the canals, which follow the outlines of the original islands, are so narrow that even gondolas have difficulty in negotiating them. The Grand Canal, however, stands apart. It is never less than 120 feet wide and sweeps in broad curves through the city. It has always been important and is lined by 200 palaces and 10 churches.

The greatest palace and church, however, are beyond the end of the Grand Canal. Saint Mark's Basilica exemplifies the way in which Venice adapted the various styles to suit itself rather than merely adopting them. It was begun in 830, rebuilt in 976 and restyled along Byzantine lines two centuries later. Saint Mark became the city's patron saint in 829 when his body was brought from Alexandria under suspicious circumstances. The fine campanile was built in 1905 after the original collapsed. The Doge's Palace is said to have stood on the Piazza San Marco, beside the church, since 814, though the oldest remaining section dates only to 1309.

Venice is splendid with past glories and prosperity, but modern wealth is to be found in two cities to the west: Milan and Turin. The latter was the capital of the Kingdom of Piedmont and was therefore the centre for the *Risorgimento* after the defeats of 1848. After Italian unification the city served as the national capital from 1861 to 1865, but it has a much longer history than that. When Hannibal crossed the Alps he found a settlement of the Celtic Taurini tribe, which he destroyed. The site was later converted into a Roman military colony under the name of Augusta Taurinorum. After the fall of Rome Turin lagged behind the great cities of Italy, only coming to the fore after 1418. In that year the city passed into the main branch of the House of Savoy. Since the 15th, and more particularly the 17th century, Turin gained in importance as the star of the House of Savoy shone brighter.

The city is today one of the major industrial centres of the nation and has a population of well over a million. The economy of the thriving city rests on the great Fiat and Lancia works, aero-industries and ball-bearing production as well as a whole host of chemical, electrical and other light industries. Turin does, however, have its aesthetic attractions. The Palazzo Madama, the Royal Palace and the Church of San Lorenzo are fine examples of the peculiar and beautiful form the Baroque took in Piedmont. The church is topped by an unusual dome which dominates the skyline of the city. The Cathedral of the archbishop is faced with gleaming white marble which dates back five centuries. Behind the facade, black marble staircases lead to the Chapel of the Holy Shroud. The shroud is claimed to be that in which Jesus's body was wrapped after the Crucifixion.

Milan lies at the southern entrance to important trans-Alpine passes and, unlike Turin, has long been an important city. Around 600 BC the Gauls settled on the site and by the time the Romans took over in 222 BC Mediolanum, as it was called, was an important town. For a while the city became the administrative centre of the Western Empire, but in 452 Attila the Hun sacked the city and in 539 the Goths completed the work. During the early Middle Ages the city increased its prosperity and, after a bitter war, broke free of the Holy Roman Empire. The thirteenth century saw a struggle between rival factions within the growing city, which resulted in the dominance of the Visconti family.

It was in 1450, however, that the remarkable Sforza family came to the fore. Muzio Attendolo was the son of a farmer in the Romagna who decided that life held more than the annual round of sowing and reaping. He promptly left home and joined a band of mercenaries. By force of character and success on the battlefield Attendolo rose to the top of his profession and earned the nickname Sforza, which means 'force'. Muzio's equally remarkable son Francesco took over as *condottiere* of his father's mercenaries and married the daughter of the Duke of Milan. When the Duke died Francesco had to fight the forces of Venice, Naples, Savoy, Montferrat and Milanese Republicans to enforce his claim to the Ducal throne. Having enlisted the Medici, Sforza won recognition of his position and established a dynasty which would last until 1535, when Milan fell to the Hapsburgs. Even today the Sforzas are still in evidence, Carlo Sforza having been Italy's Foreign Minister earlier this century.

Milan stagnated during the Hapsburg rule, but in 1706 the city and its lands passed to Austria and the city began to grow larger, richer and more prosperous – a trend which has continued to the present day. There can be little doubt that Milan is the greatest industrial and commercial city in Italy today. Its population of nearly 2 million accounts for some 12 per cent of the nation's economic potential. Industries which predominate include cars, aeroplanes, electrical equipment, textiles, chemicals, publishing and banking. Of all the fine buildings in this prosperous city the two most magnificent are the cathedral and La Scala. The former was begun in 1386, but work proceeded slowly. The dome was completed around 1500 and the facade in 1809, while the massive bronze doors were not hung until late this century. The rich exterior is decorated with 135 pinnacles and well over 2,000 marble statues. Inside are 52 massive pillars topped not by capitals but by a ring of statues. La Scala did not take anywhere near as long to construct. It opened in 1776, having been built by the Empress of Austria, and is now one of the leading half dozen opera houses in the world. Unlike most of the others, La Scala specialises in lesser-known works, though popular works are also presented.

The great cities of northern Italy all lie on the broad lowlands centred around the River Po. Fertile land and easy communications have led to the concentration of population in this relatively small area of Italy. To the north, west and east of the lowlands rise the majestic Alps, whose snow-capped peaks form a boundary between Italy and the rest of Europe. The mountains have long held a fascination for those seeking quiet or adventure. The latter have often taken to climbing, and the Matterhorn is surely one of the finest peaks for such exercise. The 14,691-foot mountain straddles the border with Switzerland and remained unconquered until 1865. On July 14th of that year Edward Whymper climbed the peak from the Swiss side and three days later a party from Valtournanche scaled the more difficult Italian face.

The Alps, however, are not just an area of mountains; there are numerous lakes as well. Used by the Italians as health and holiday resorts, the lakes are remarkably free of tourism. The largest, and probably best known of the lakes, is Lake Garda, which has a surface area of 143 square miles. The narrow northern end of the lake belonged to Austria until 1919 when it was surrendered to Italy. The towering cliffs that line the northern shores give way as the lake widens to reveal richly vegetated lands where olives, vines and citrus fruits grow in abundance. A gentle steamer cruises the lake in summer, offering splendid views of the surroundings. The climate of the lake is warm and mild and is characterised by two winds: the *sover* from the north in the mornings and the *ora* from the south in the afternoons. Lake Como is similar in many ways,

being more mountainous in the north and having a similar daily shift in wind direction. Como has the added attraction of excellent fishing for trout and *agoni*, a type of herring.

As well as the scenic beauties of the crystal clear lakes and the romantic valleys, the Italian Alps have much to offer the visitor. In recent years various parts have been developed as sports areas. These are mainly based in Piedmont and Valle d'Aosta and cater for visitors from all over Europe. Sestriere has more than 70 ski runs available from November to May and many fine hotels. Not all the resorts in Piedmont centre on winter sports; Acqui and St Vincent are spa towns and the latter has a famous casino.

The lower foothills, away from the commercialised ski runs and the lakes, are as romantic as anybody could wish. The steep-sided valleys are flanked by precipitous hills on which are perched tiny towns. The narrow streets and sheer buildings seem to be left over from medieval days, when bands of mercenaries led by *condottieri* marched through the balmy valleys. Even today the people have not abandoned their mountain-top towns, though the prospect of climbing the slopes would daunt many. They carry on their lives as if little had changed in the world outside, for little has changed within the towns, except perhaps a new invention to help with the wine production. Towering above even the mountain towns are the really tall, scrub-covered peaks where the ruins of a neglected castle stand in mute testimony to more warlike days.

It is perhaps in the northwest of Italy that the excellent cuisine of the country reaches its most delicious. The cheeses of the area are famed throughout the world and include such names as Gorgonzola, Bel Paese, Stracchino and Crescenza. The long, crunchy breadsticks that are served in Italian restaurants around the world originated here, where they are known as *grissini*. Minestrone is made here with a special flair, while pasta is eaten in the shape of *agnolotti*, squares stuffed with spinach or cheese. The red wines of the region are probably the best in Italy. Barolo, Sasello and Barbaresco are full-bodied reds which complement the food perfectly. The white wine which is exported internationally is Asti Spumante, which has made a name for itself by undercutting the French Champagnes. It was also in this inventive region that, in 1786, a certain A.B. Carpano invented a process of blending wines, herbs and spices to produce vermouth.

Many people cross the border from France, discover the wonderful cuisine, wines and resorts of the northwest and go no further. The rest of Italy, however, has much to offer to both the visitor and resident alike. The magnificent treasures of the past that can be found throughout Italy blend with present vitality and charm to create a wonderful atmosphere which is unique.

The Matterhorn, or Monte Cervino, which straddles the border between Switzerland and Italy.

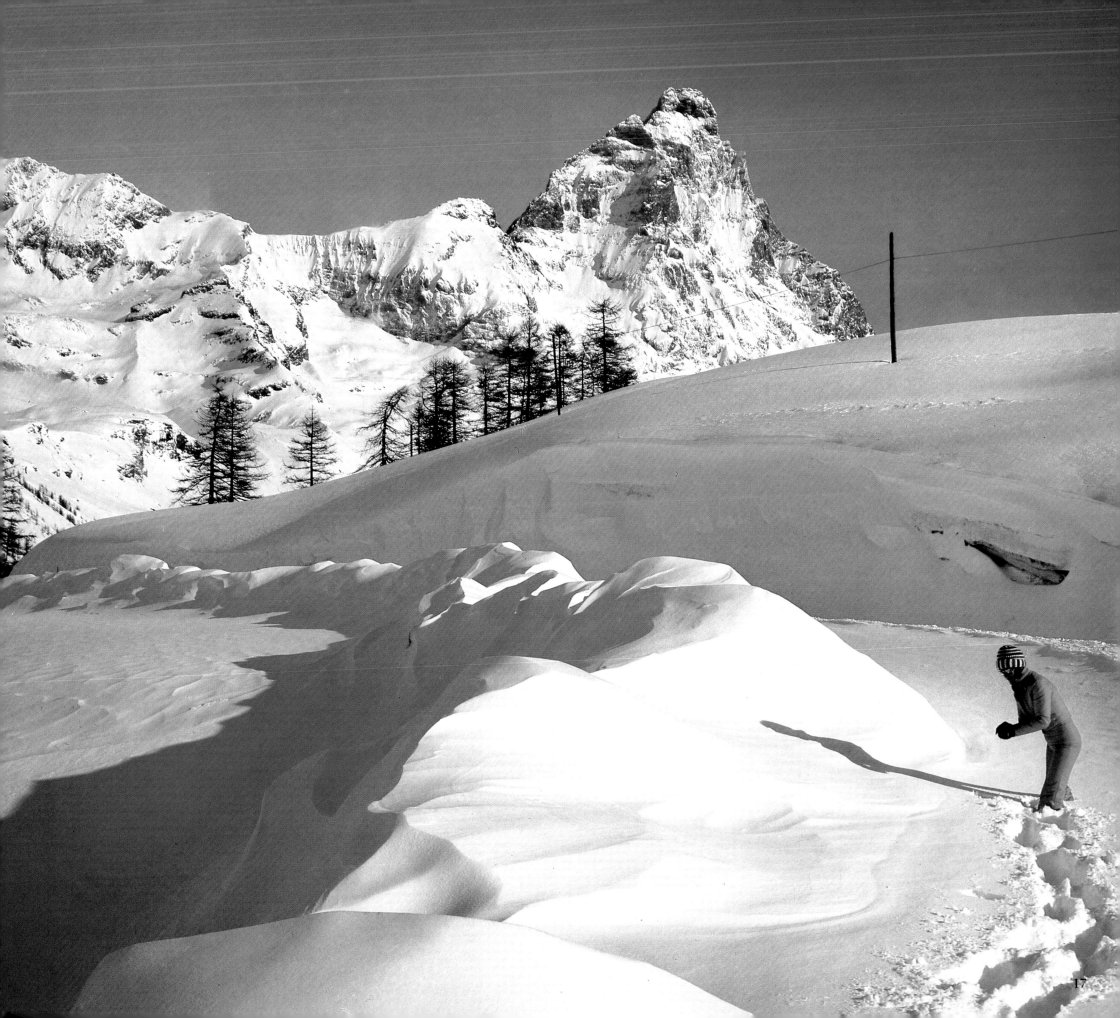

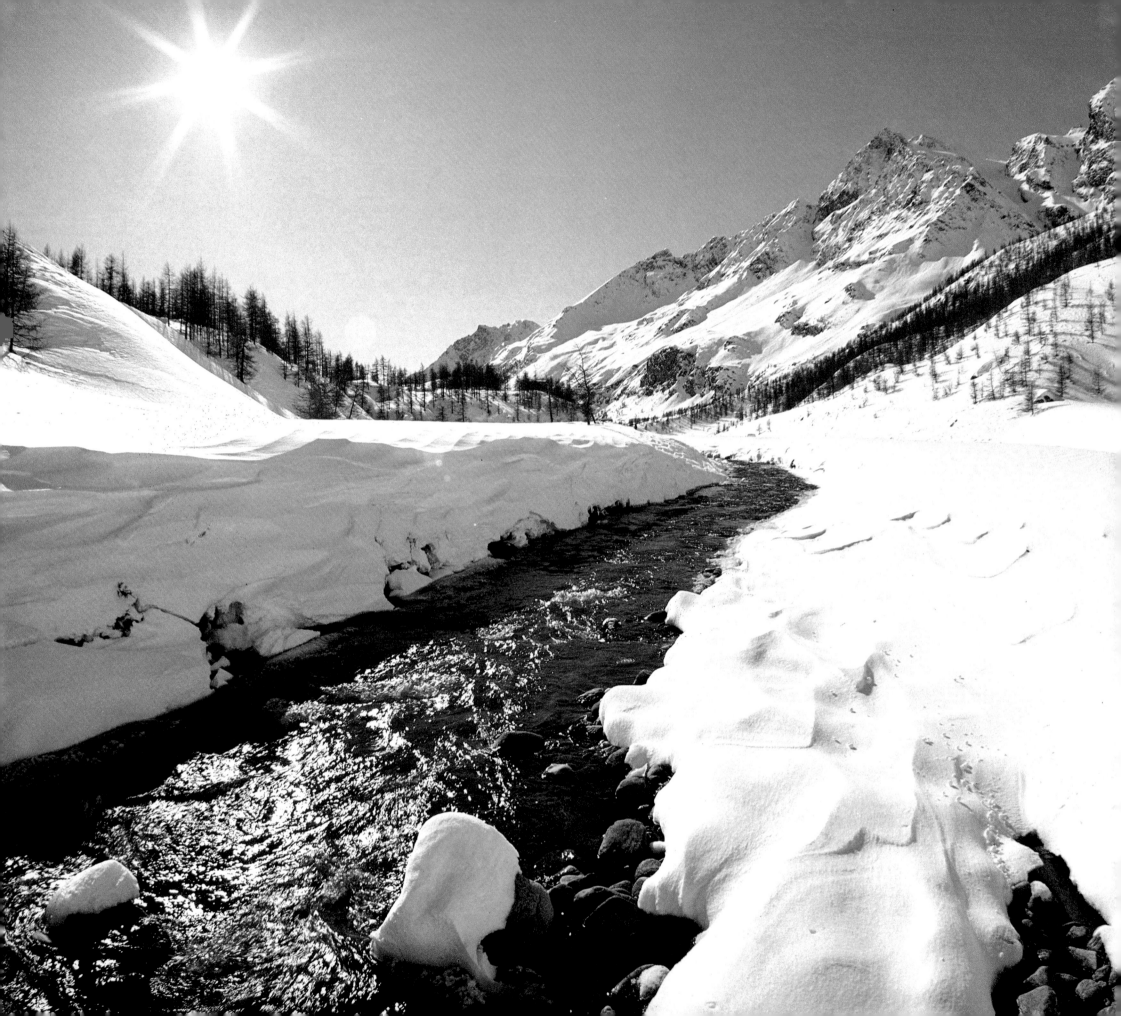

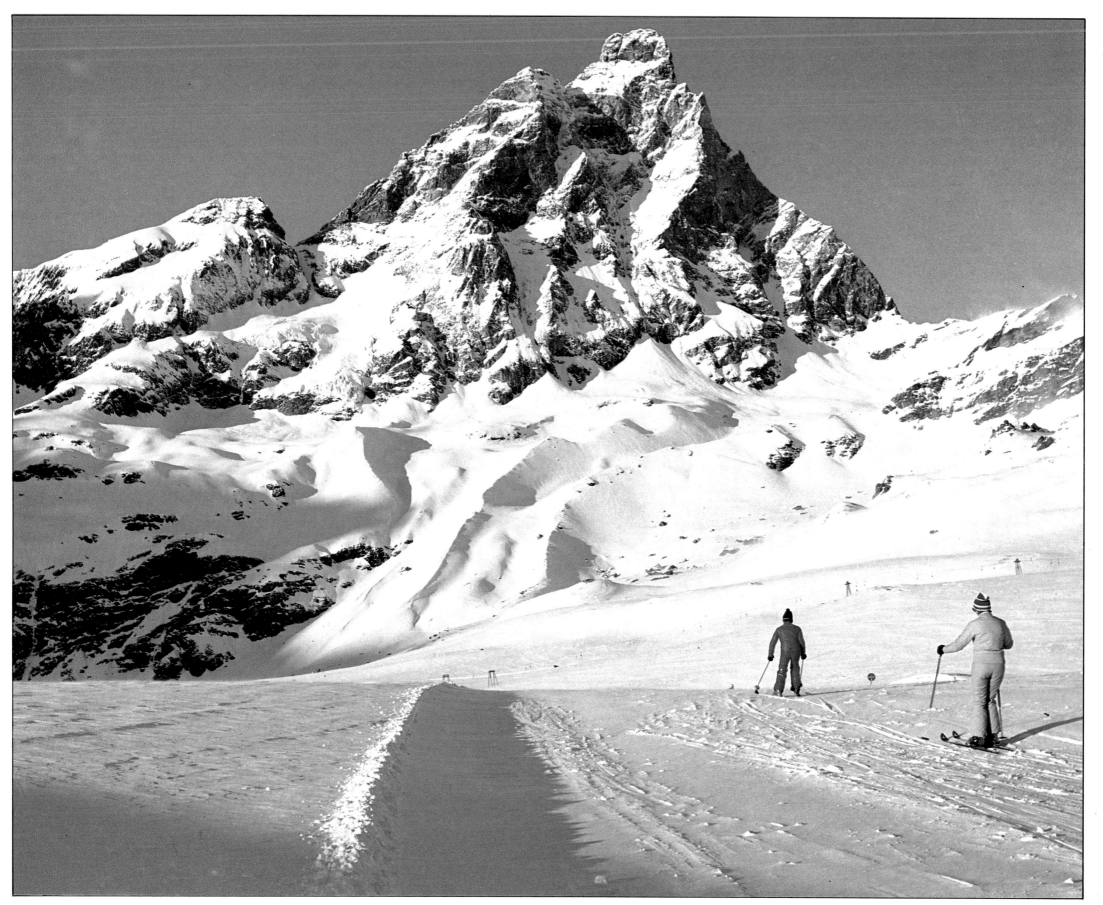

Facing page: a mountain river near Breuil Cervinia, in the Piedmont and (above) 14,691-foot-high
Monte Cervino, first scaled from the Italian side by a group of climbers from the village of
Valtournanche, led by the Italian guide Giovanni Antonio Carrel. Overleaf: (left) Alpine slopes near
Breuil Cervinia and (right) a narrow mountain road below the Passo di Pordoi in the Dolomites.

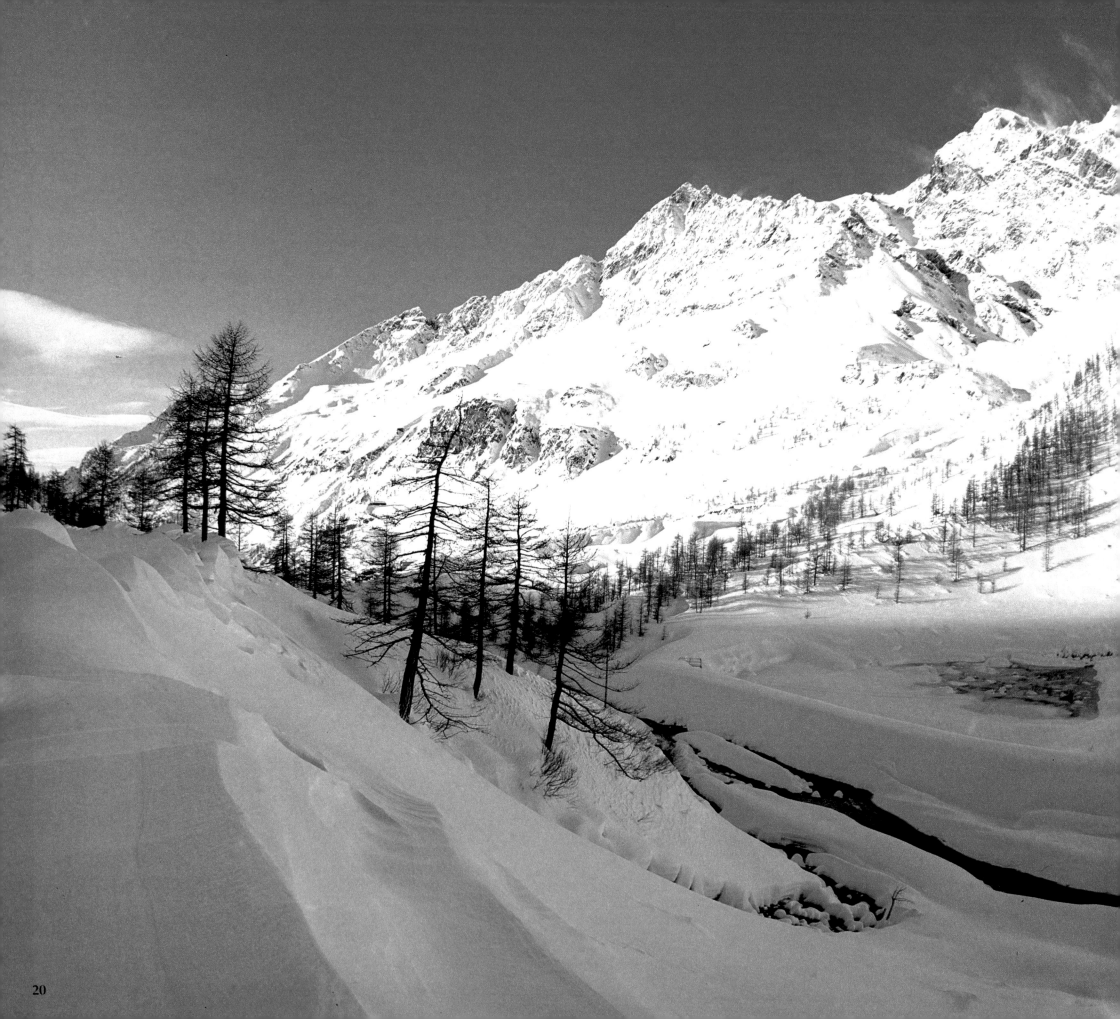

20

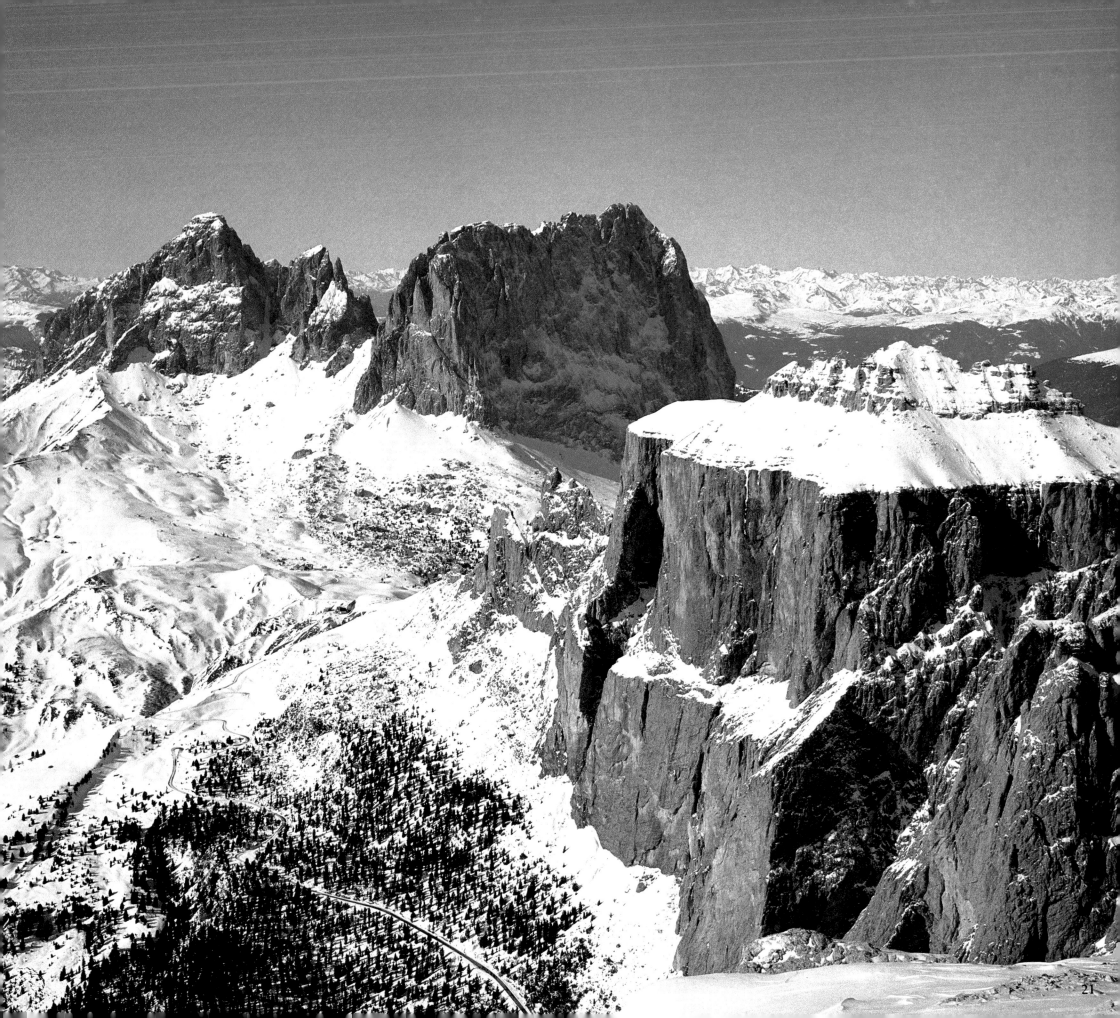

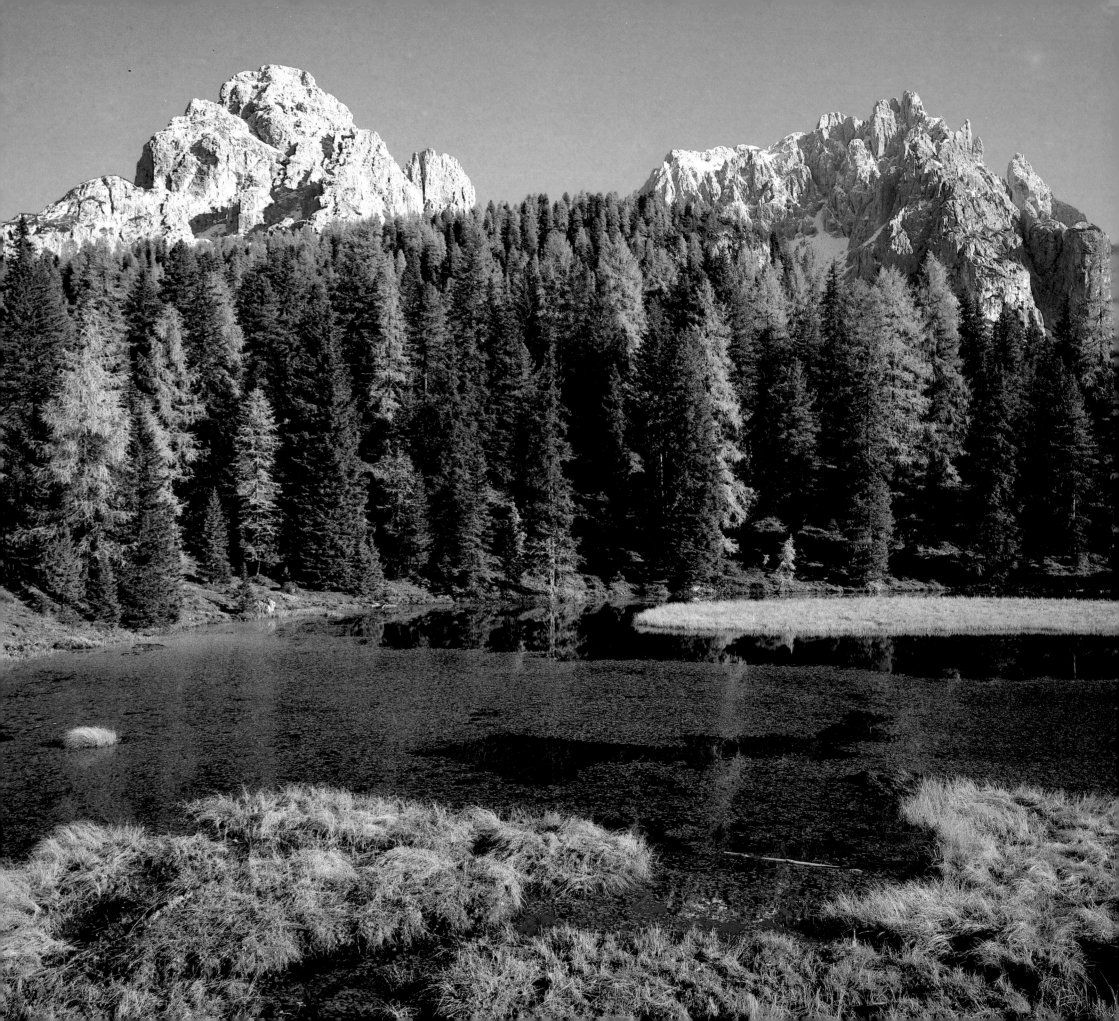

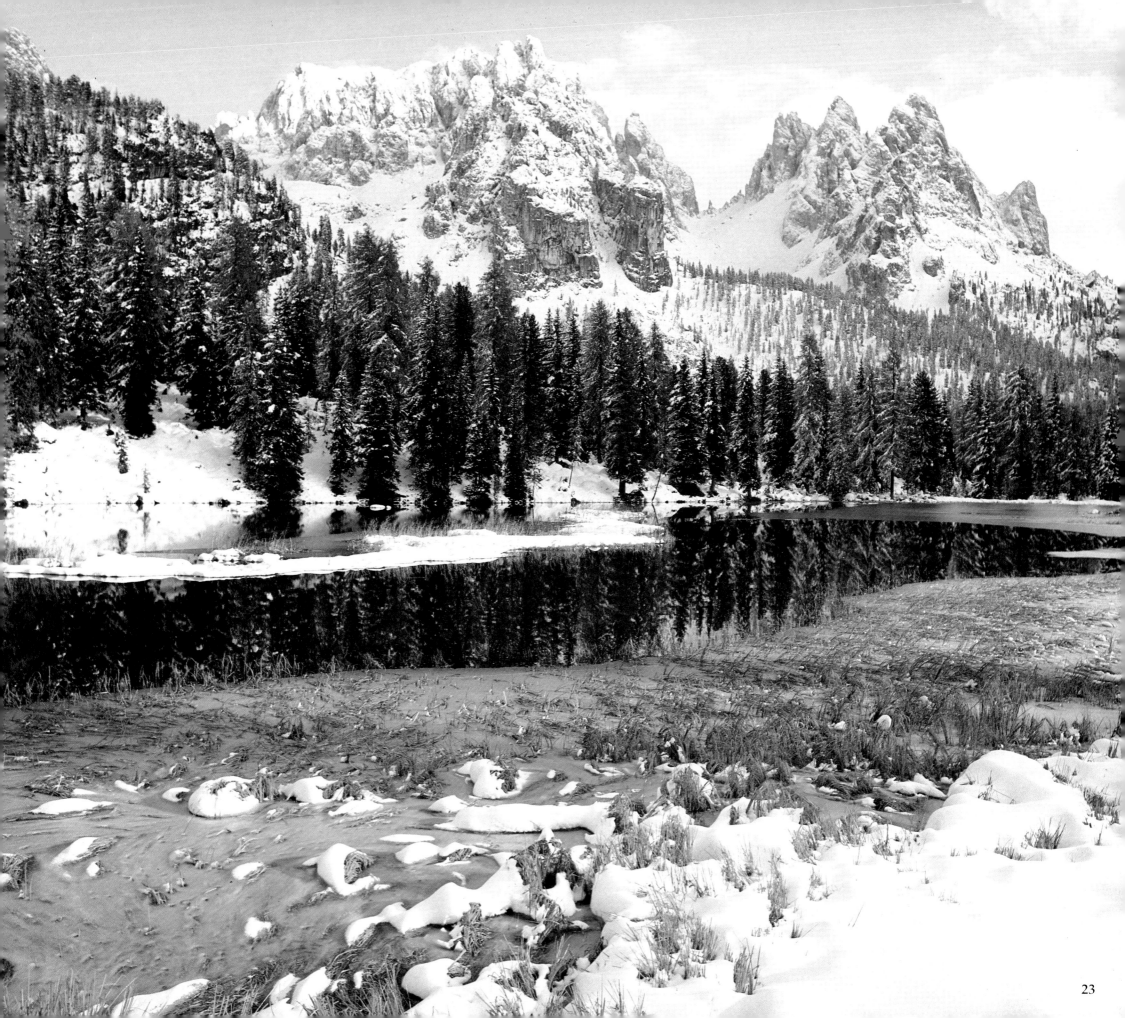

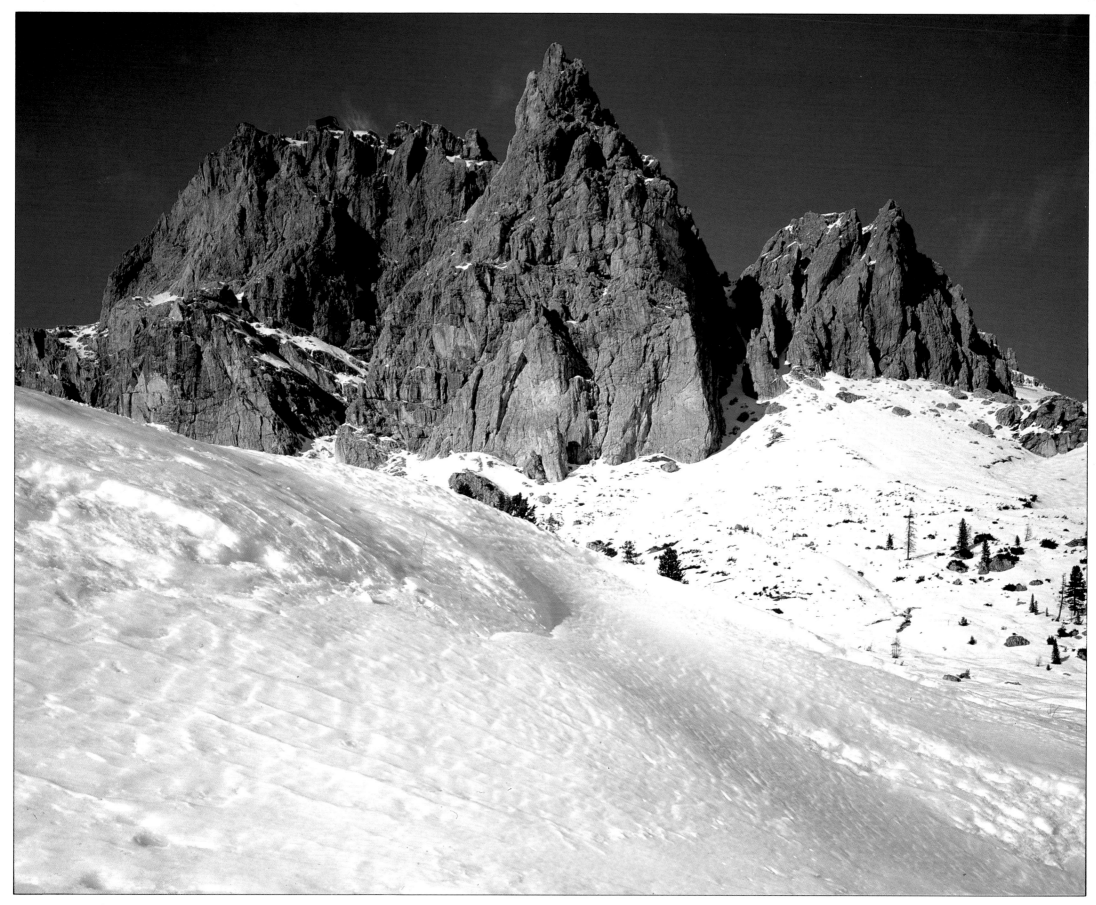

Previous pages: autumn (left) and winter (right) on a lake near Misurina in the Dolomite Mountains, and (above) the nearby peaks of the Tre Croci. Facing page: the town of Livigno, close to the border with Switzerland. Overleaf: (left) Cortina d'Ampezzo, in a gentle, green basin surrounded by Dolomite peaks and (right) the Sella Massif, formed of sharply-eroded limestone.

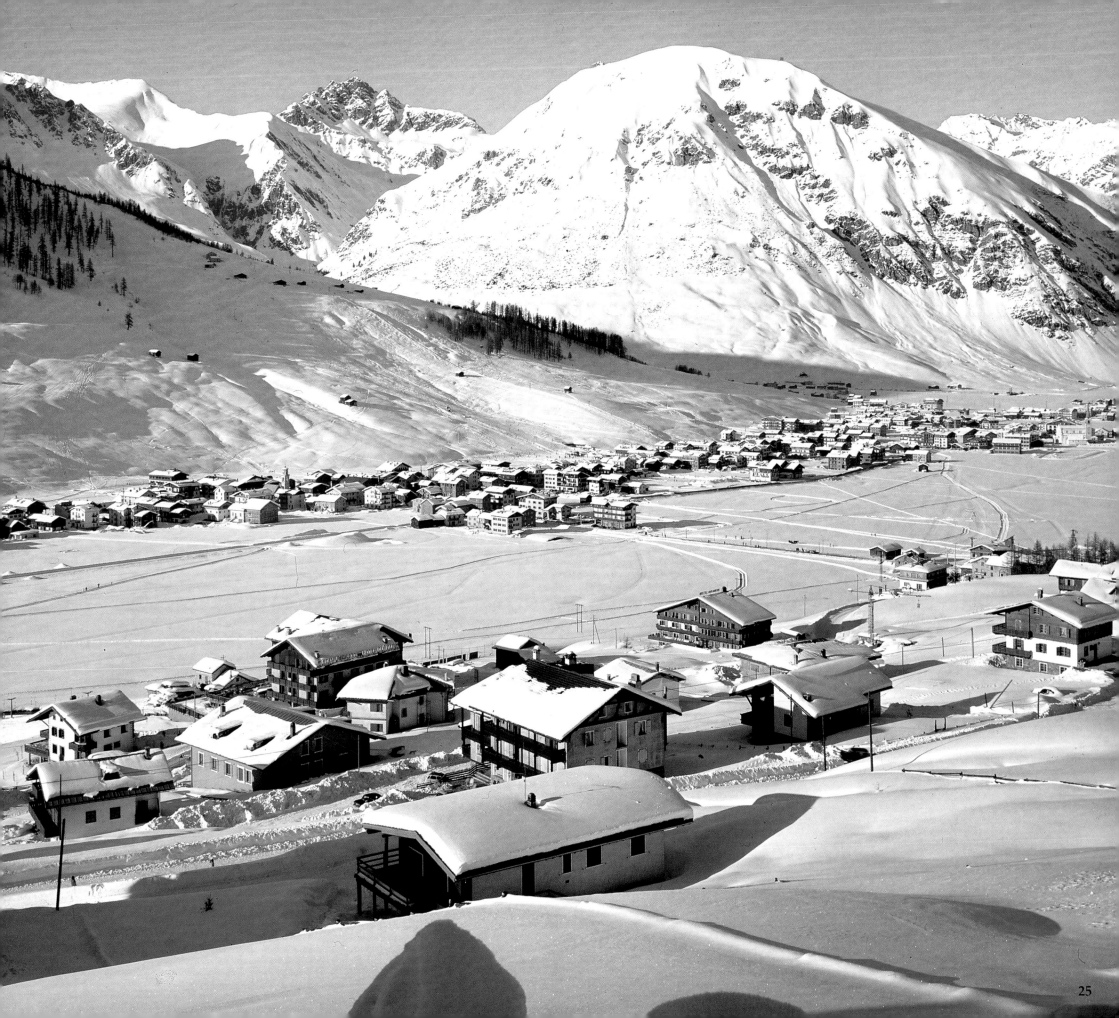

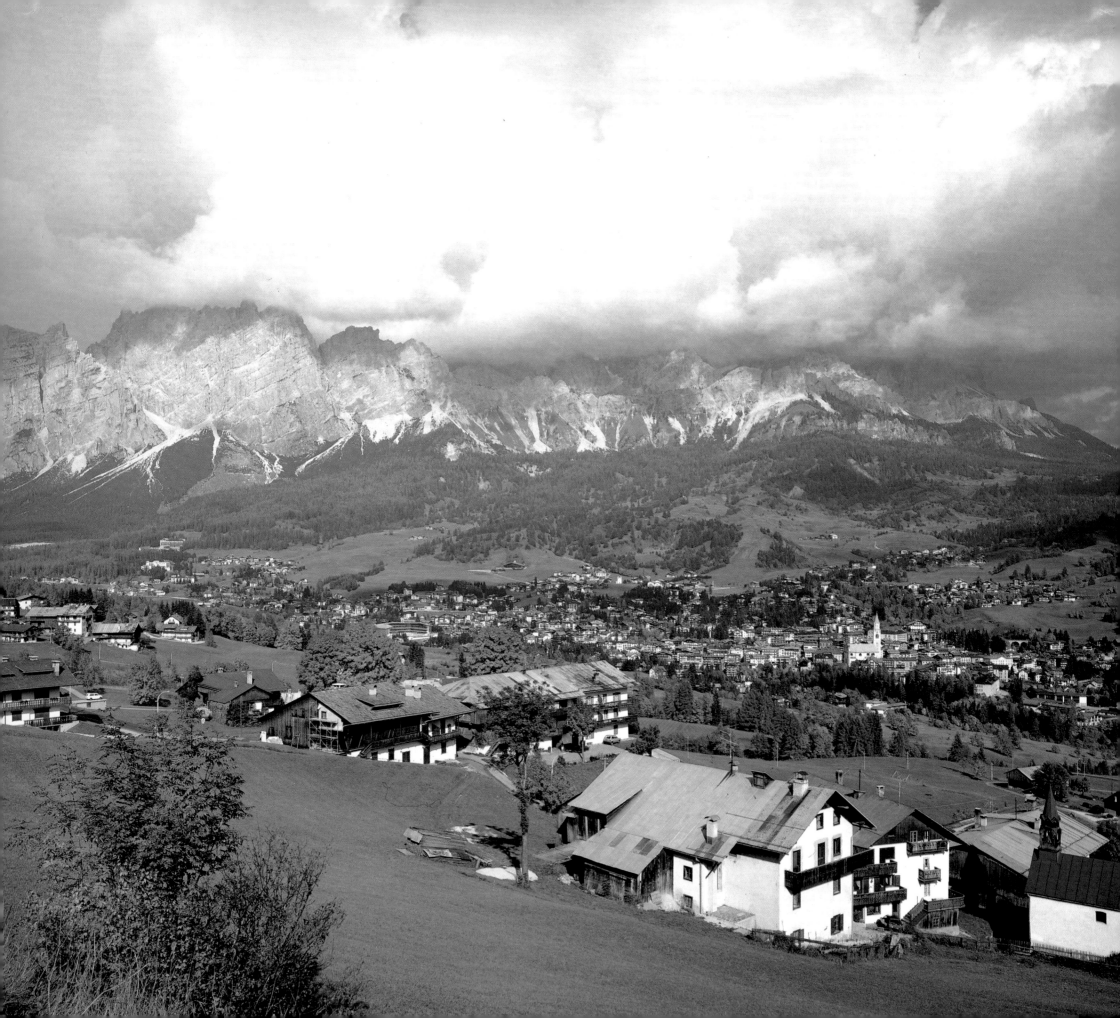

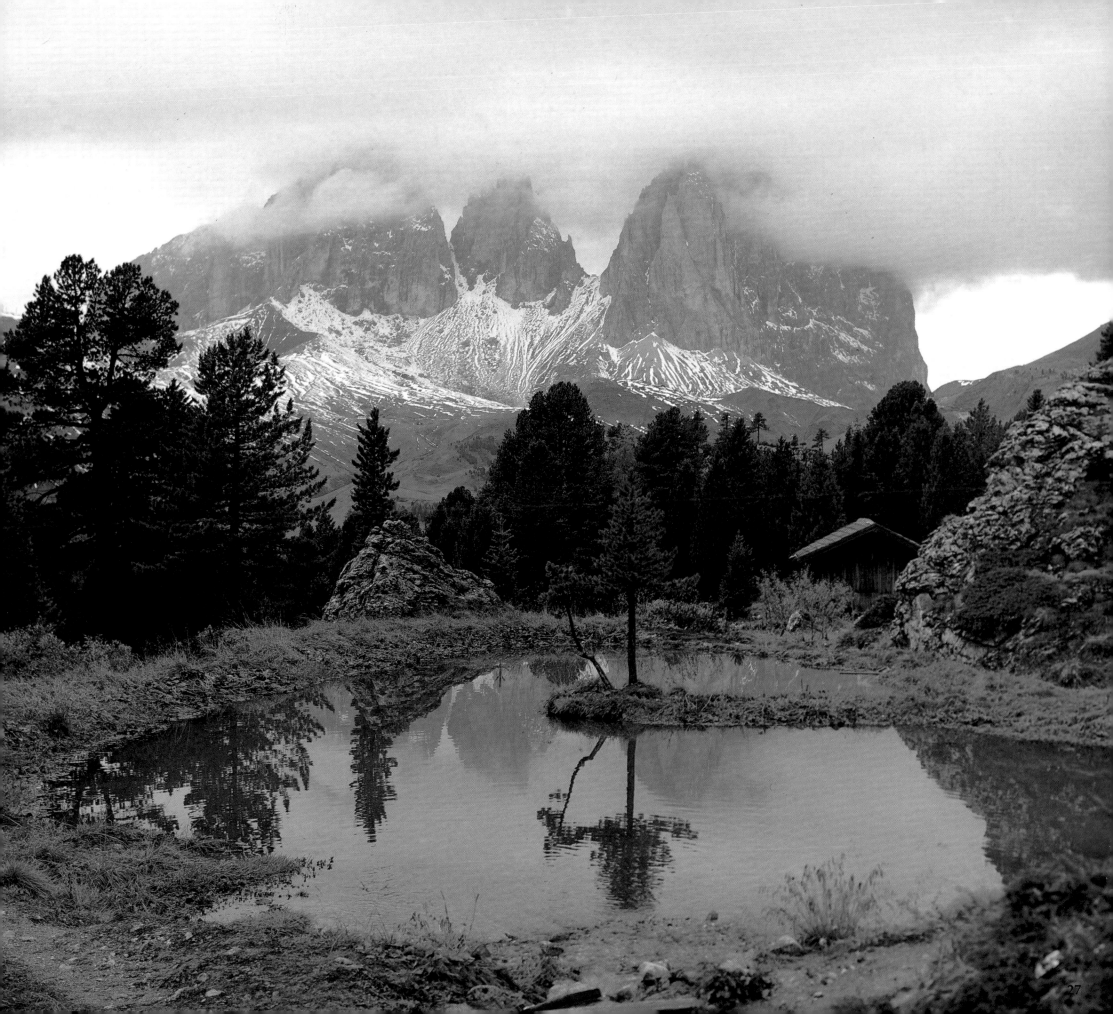

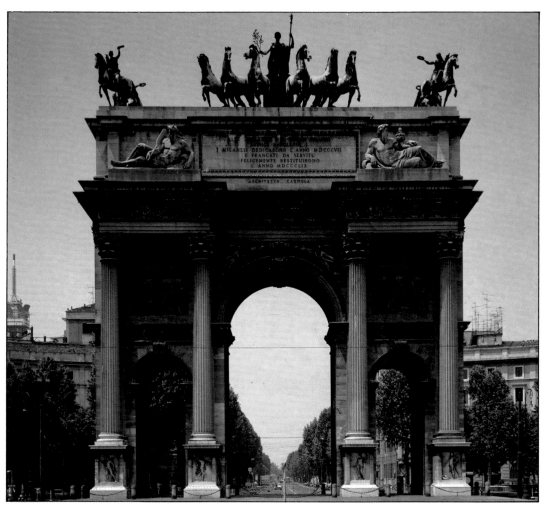

Left: the Arco di Pace in Milan, and (below) the 1st-century Roman amphitheatre in Verona. Bottom left: Lago d'Idro, and (bottom) Lago di Garda. Facing page: the restored, 13th century castle of the Scalingers in Sirmione, and (overleaf) Lazise harbour (right) on Lago di Garda (left).

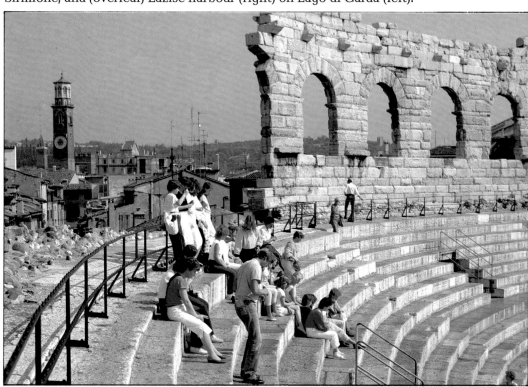

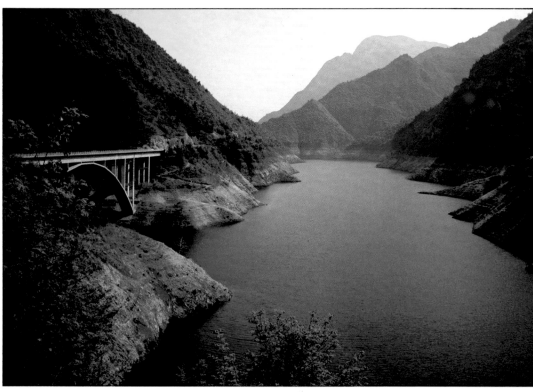

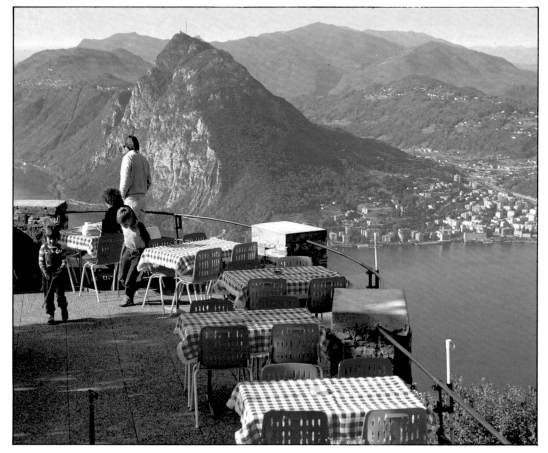

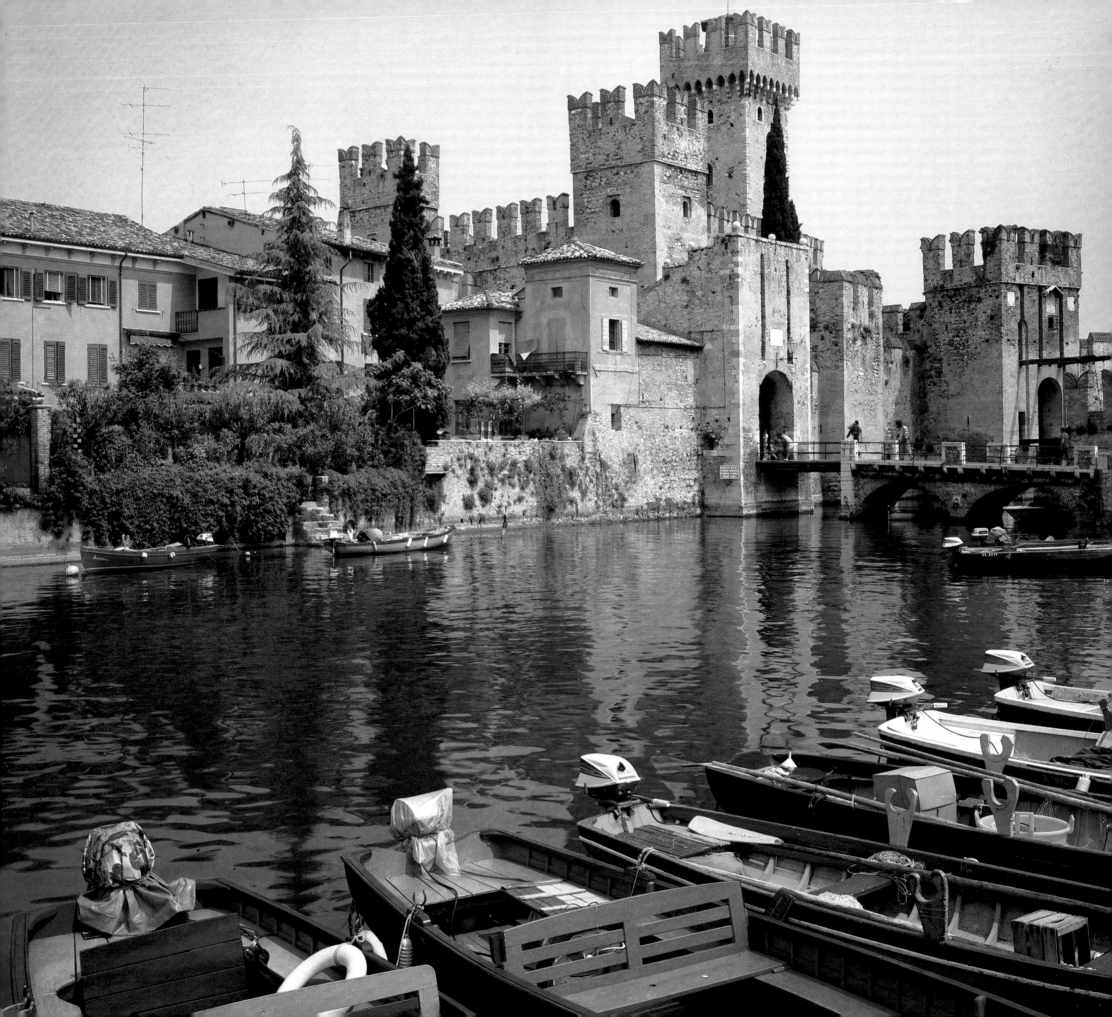

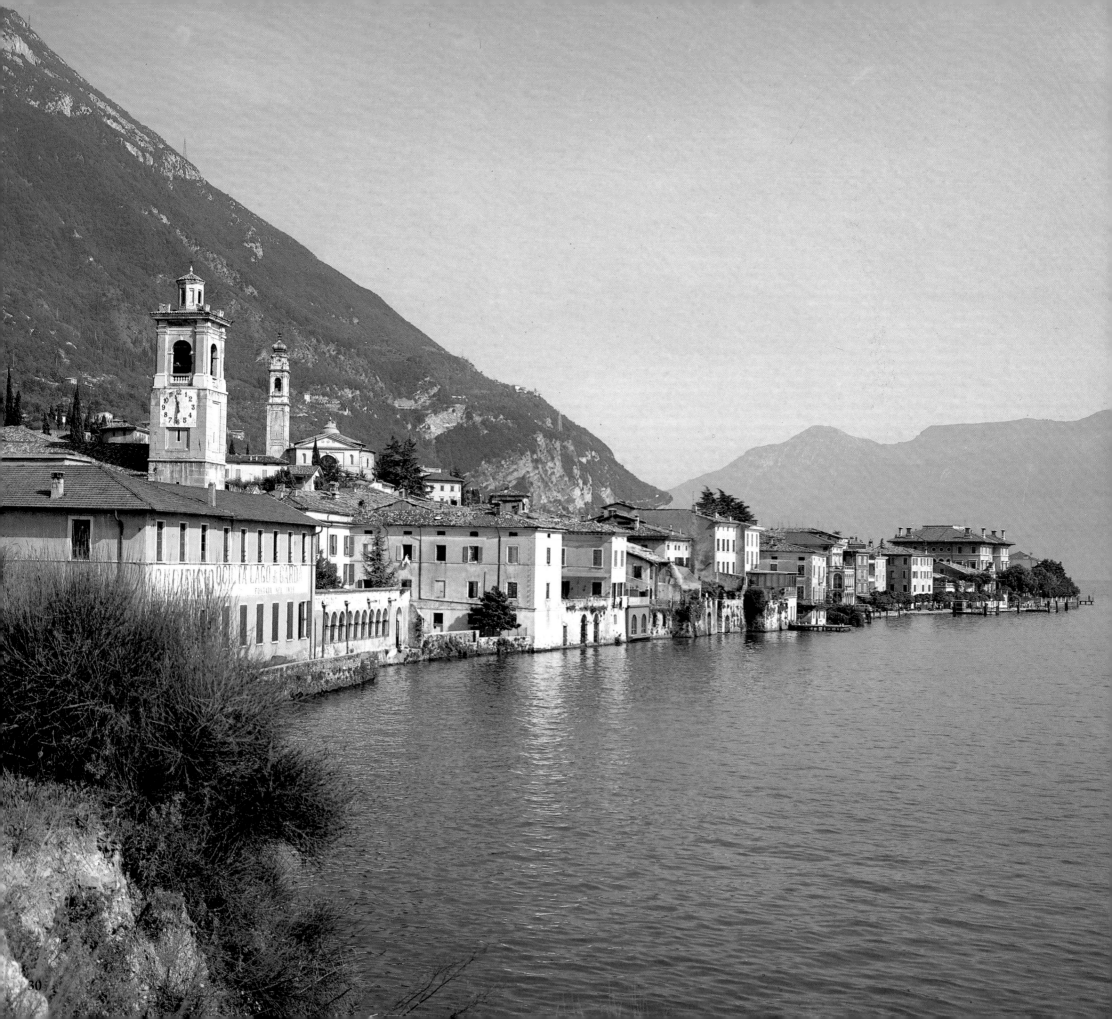

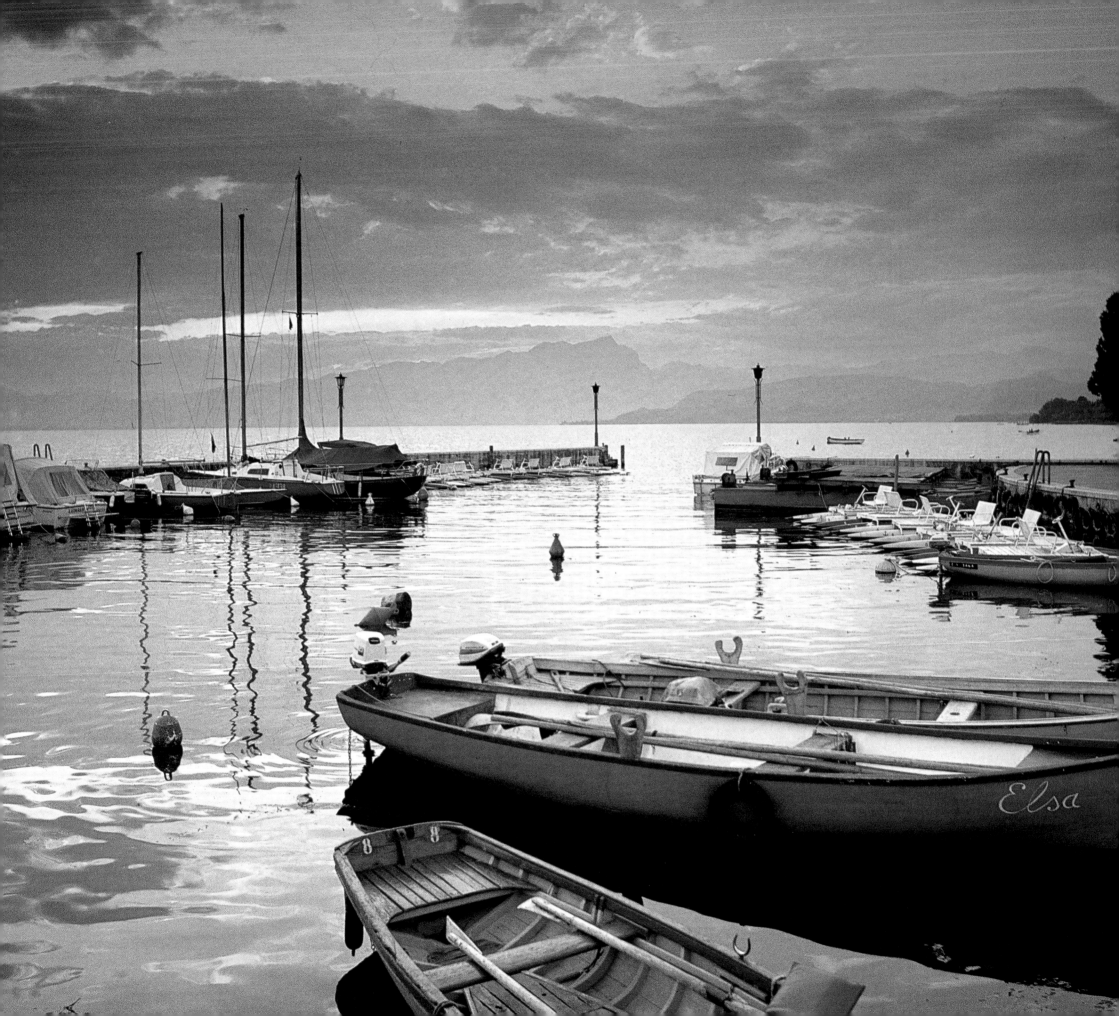

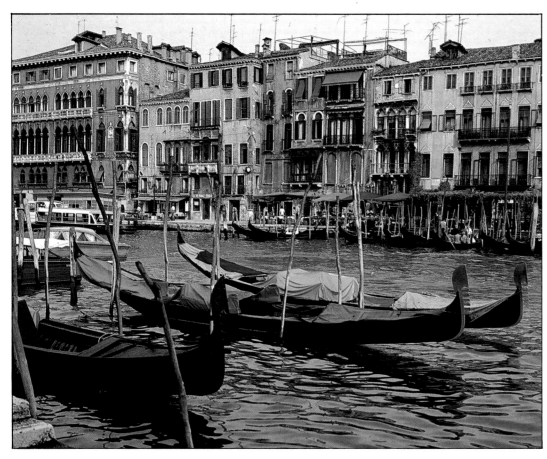

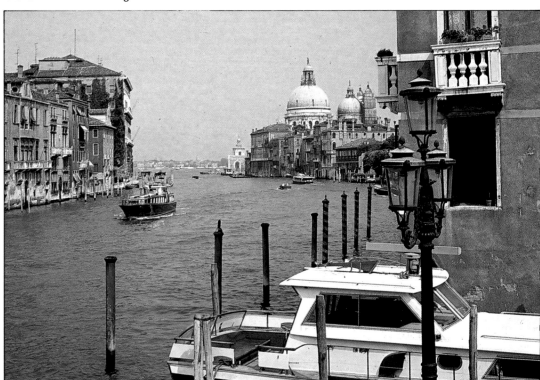

Left, bottom and facing page: Venetian gondolas, (bottom left) the Grand Canal, and, beyond, the white domes of Santa Maria della Salute (below). Overleaf: arched windows and wrought iron and marble balconies, seen (left) from the Rialto Bridge.

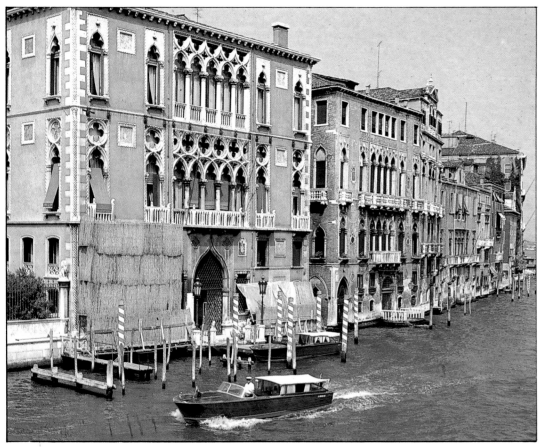

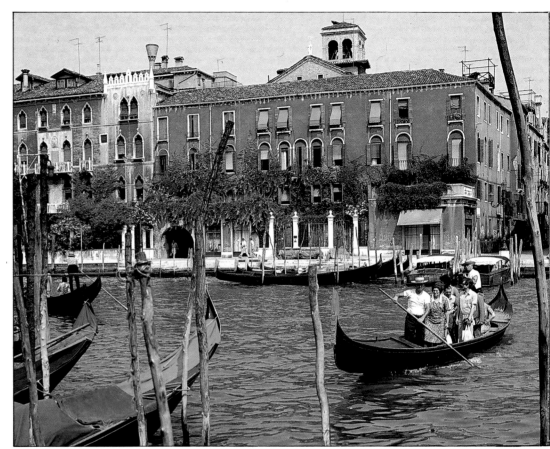

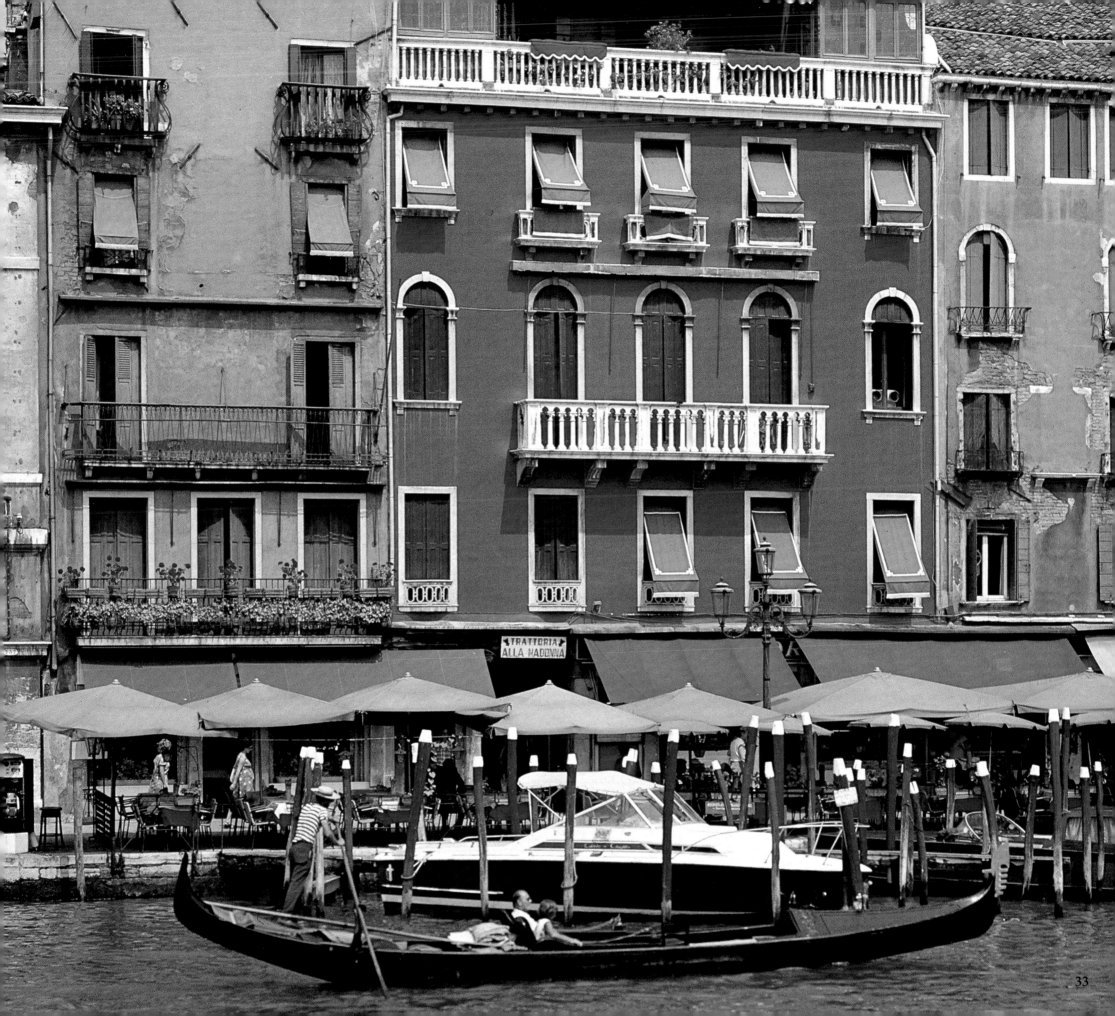

33

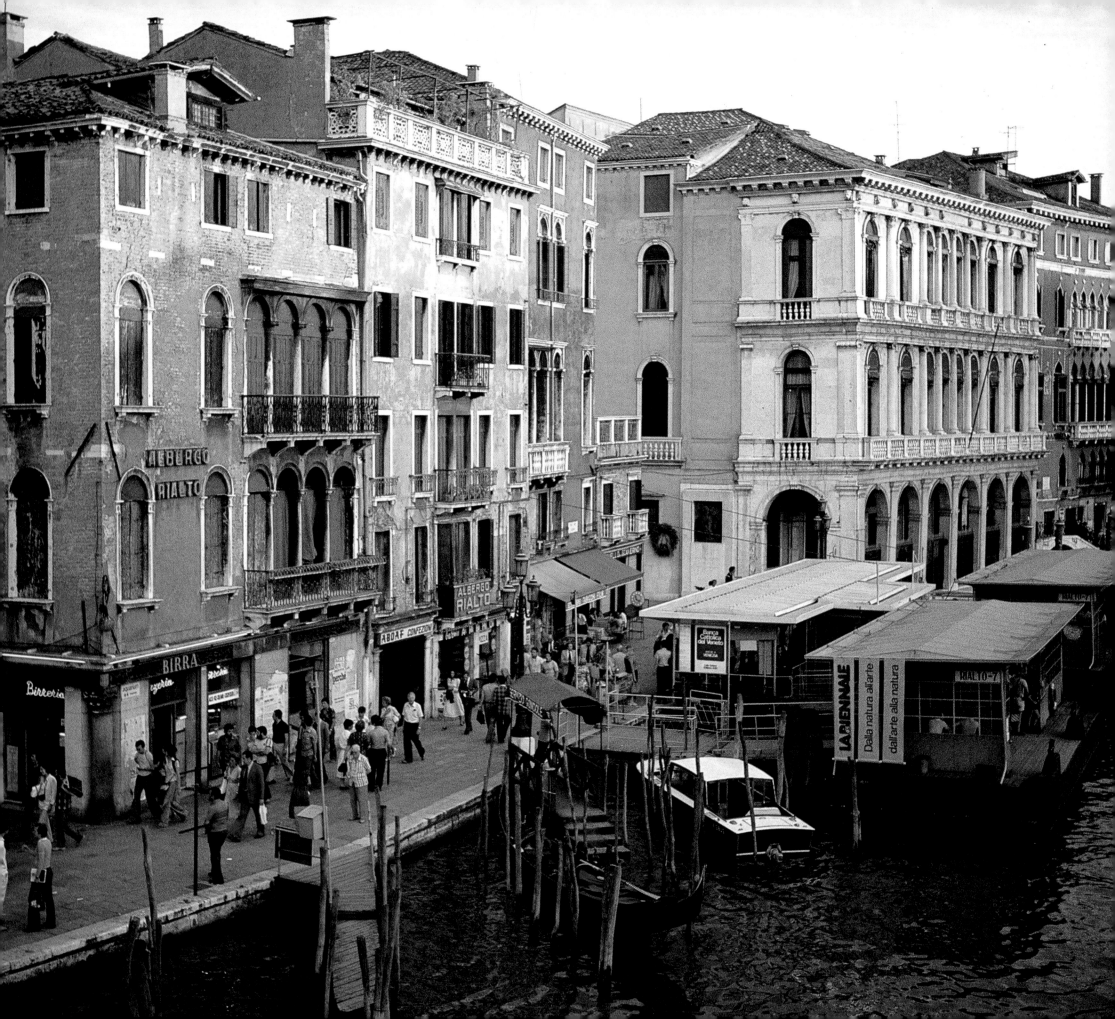

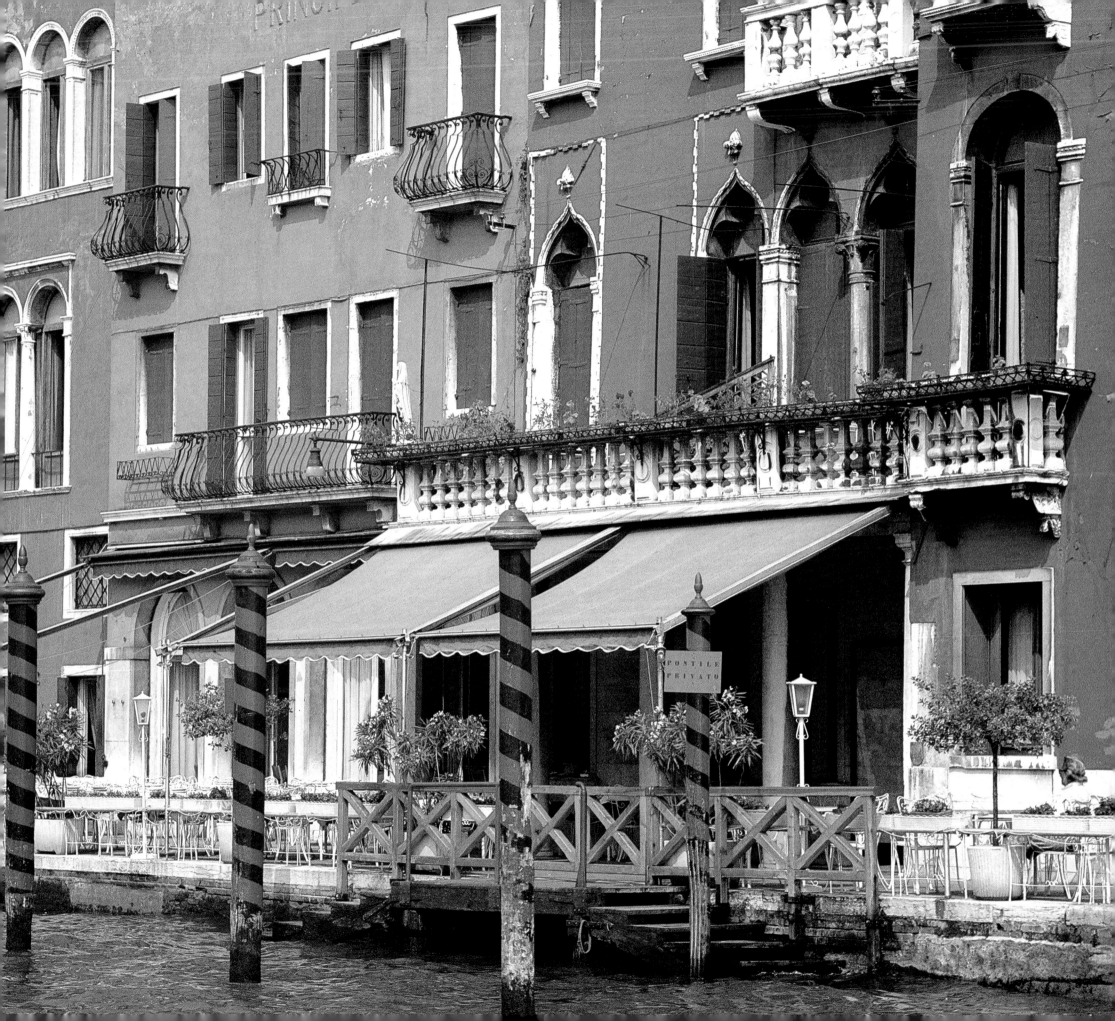

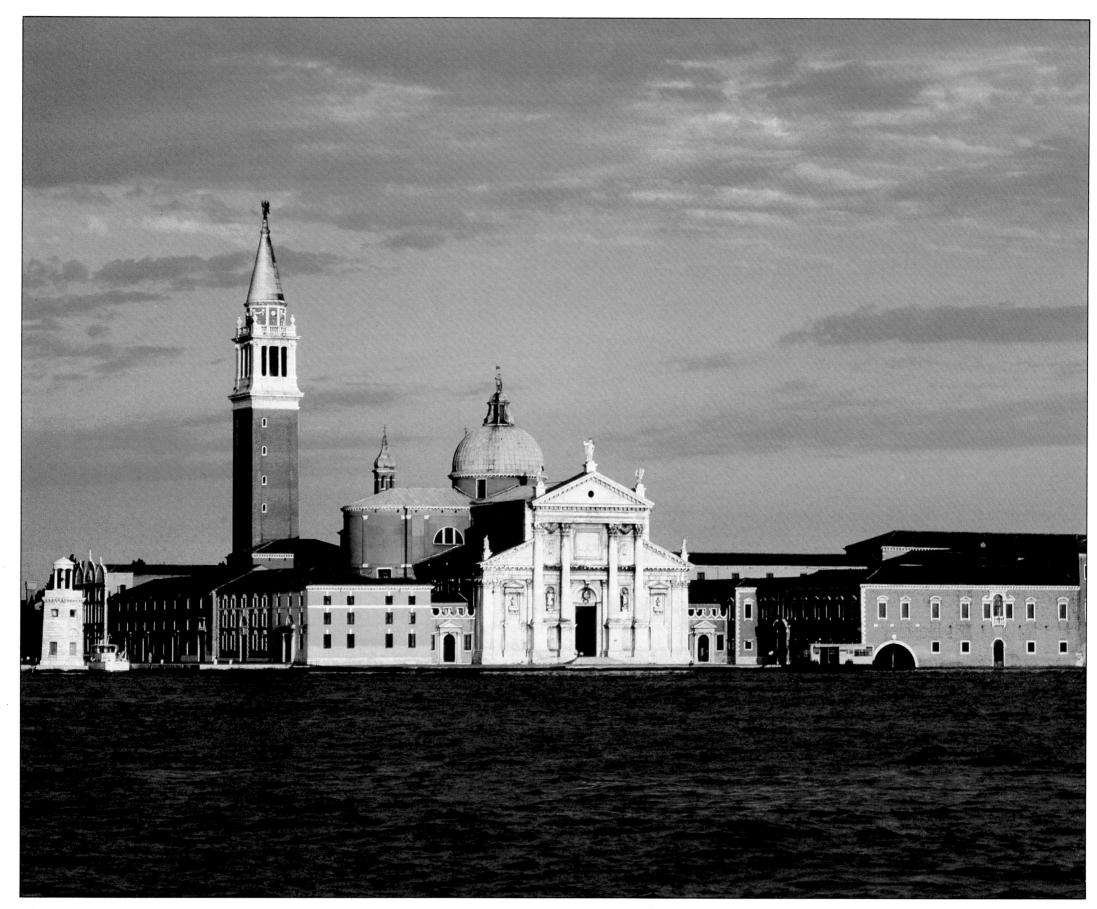

Above: the church and campanile, or bell tower, of San Giorgio Maggiore. Facing page: the green-roofed campanile and the pink and white marble tracery of the Palazzo Ducale, on the Piazza San Marco. Part of the Marciana Library, which fronts the Canale di San Marco, was built to be the Ducal Mint between 1537 and 1545. Overleaf: (left) regatta on the Grand Canal and (right) Santa Maria della Salute, built by Baldassare Longhena between 1631 and 1681 as a symbol of hope following the devastation of a year of plague.

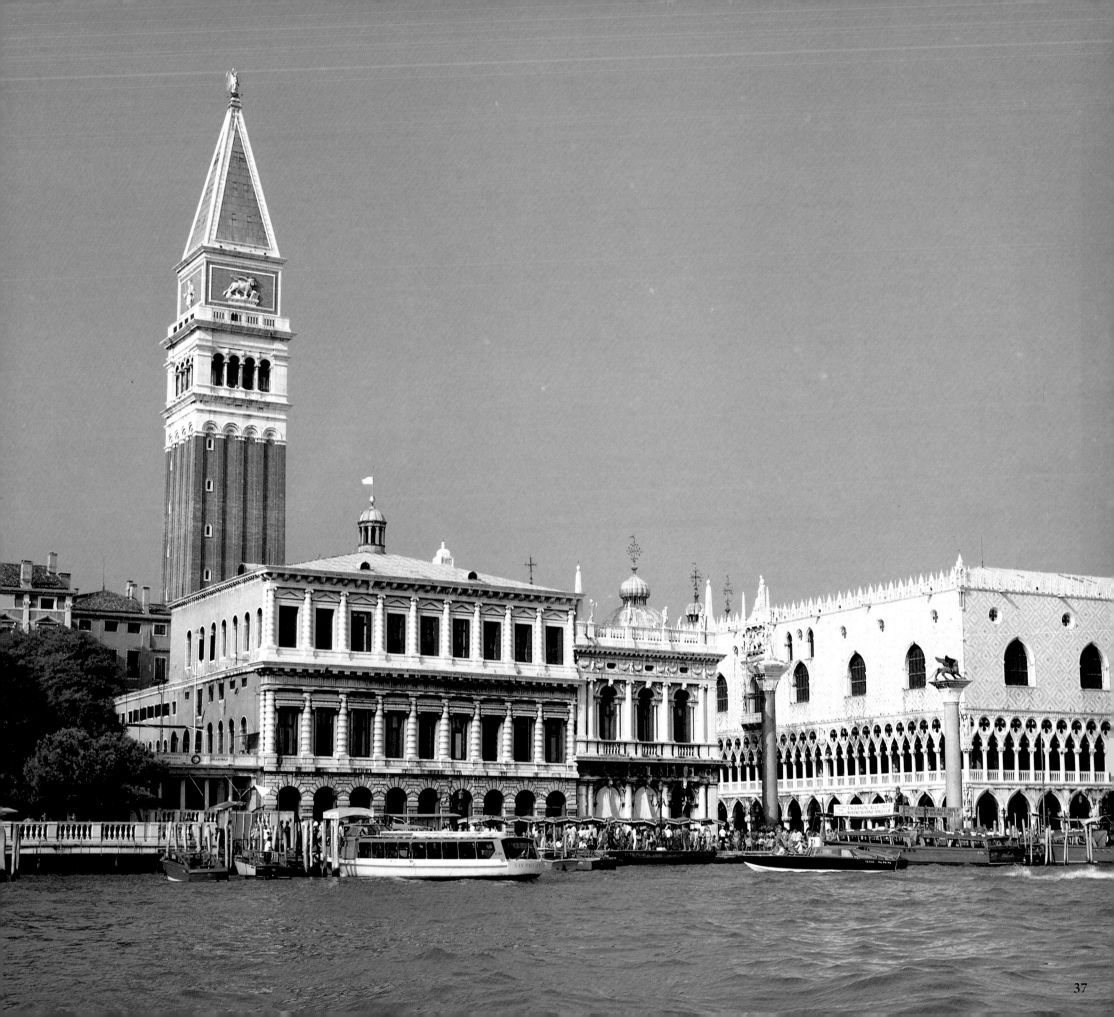

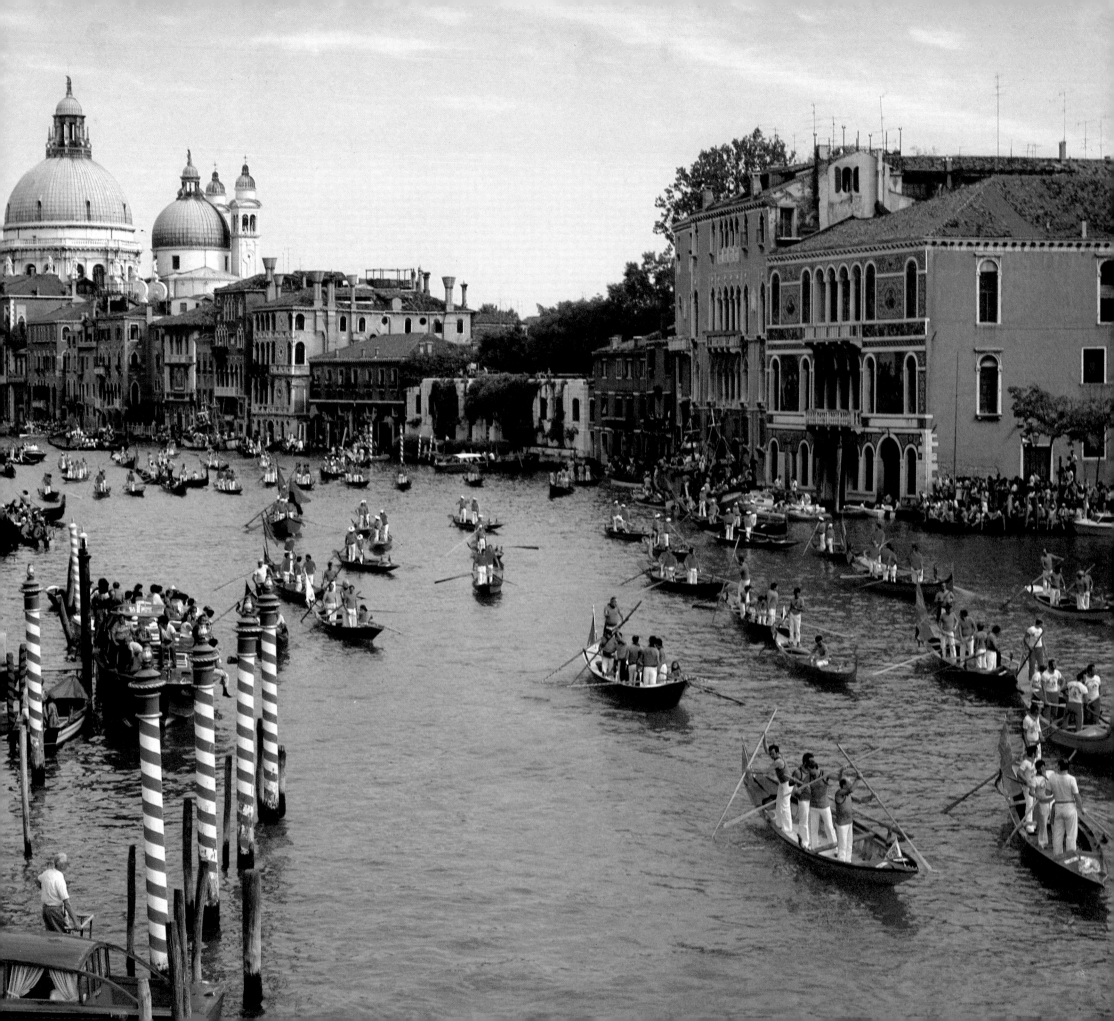

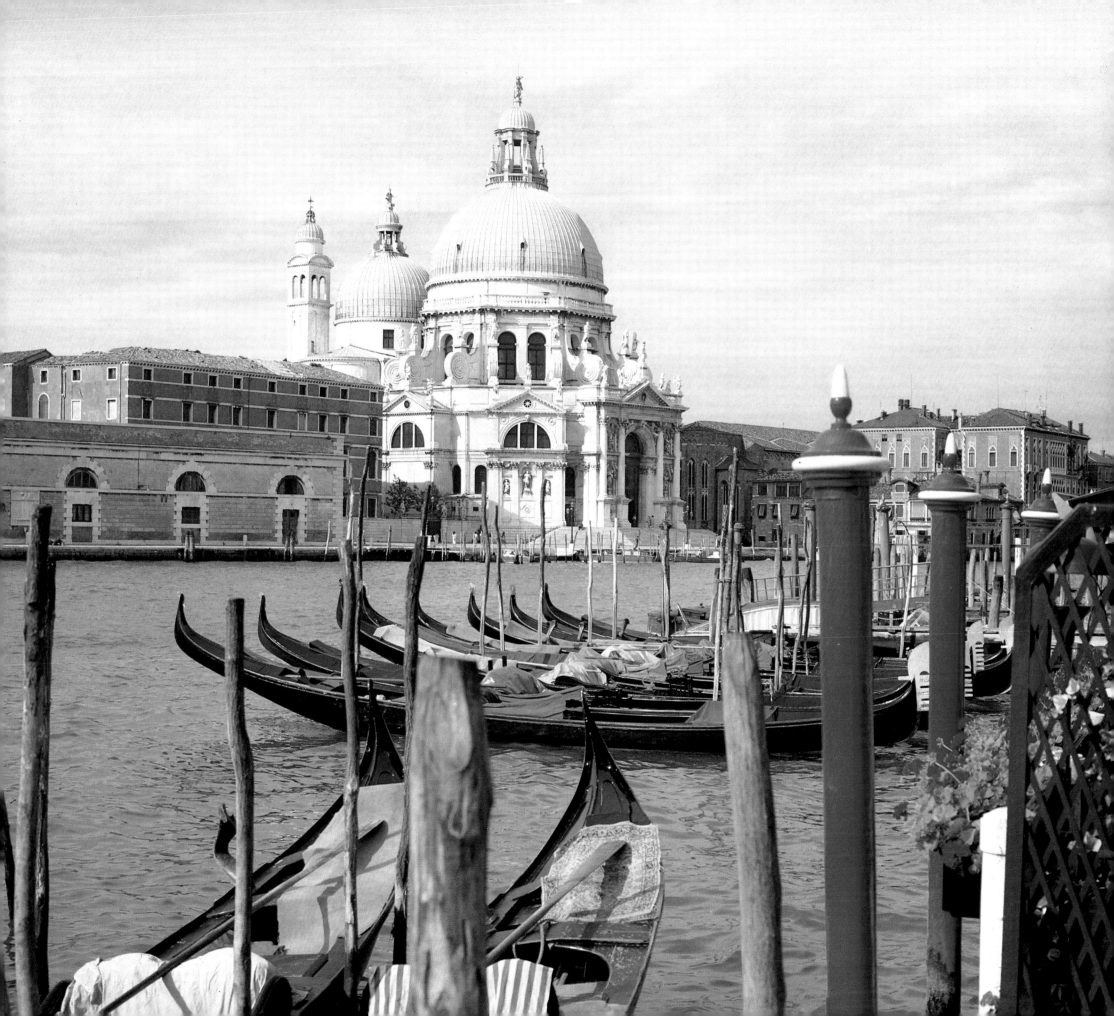

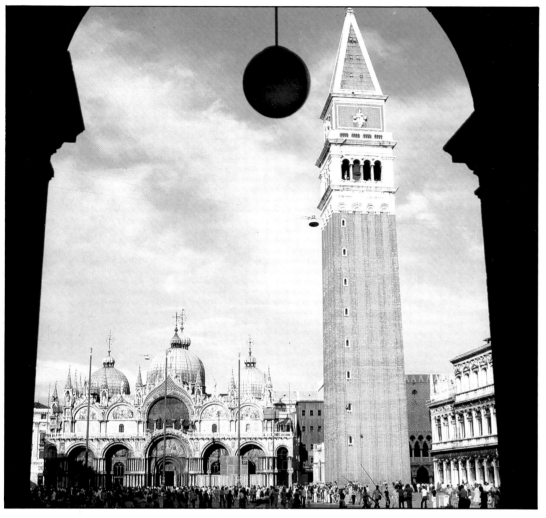

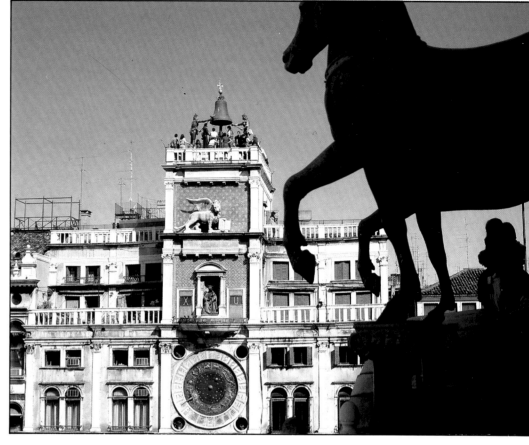

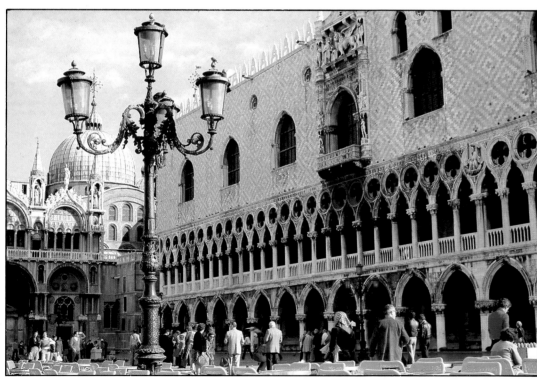

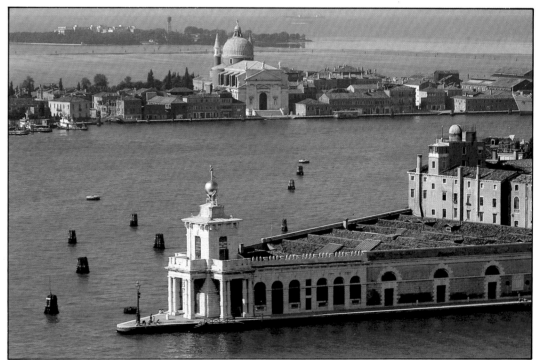

Top left: the campanile, rebuilt in 1912, and the Byzantine-influenced Basilica San Marco, consecrated in 1094. Top: the great gilded and enamelled clockface of the Torre dell'Orologio, built on the Piazza San Marco in 1496. Left: the Palazzo Ducale, and (above) the Punta della Dogana da Mar, where the tower of the Customs House supports a gilded sphere symbolising Fortune. Facing page: the Rialto Bridge.

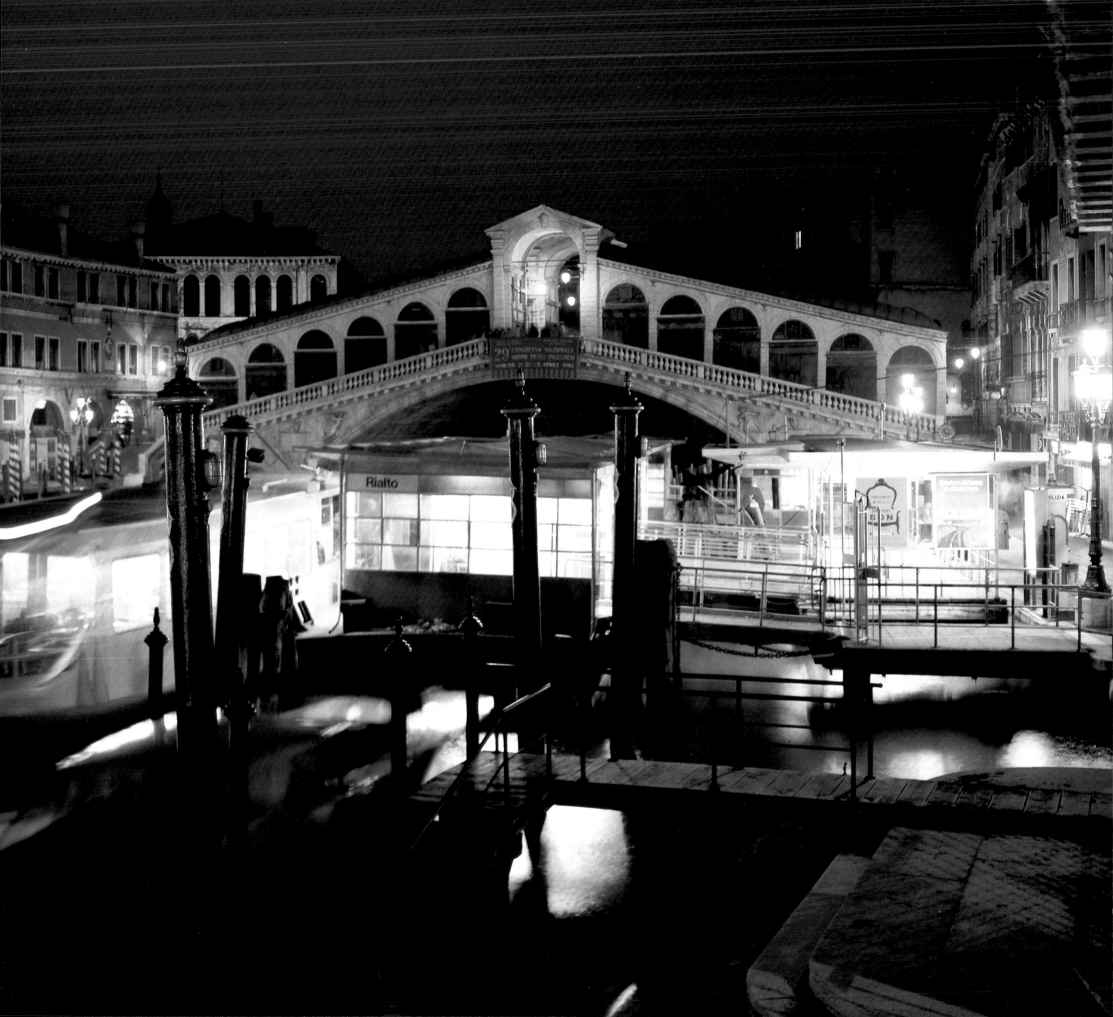

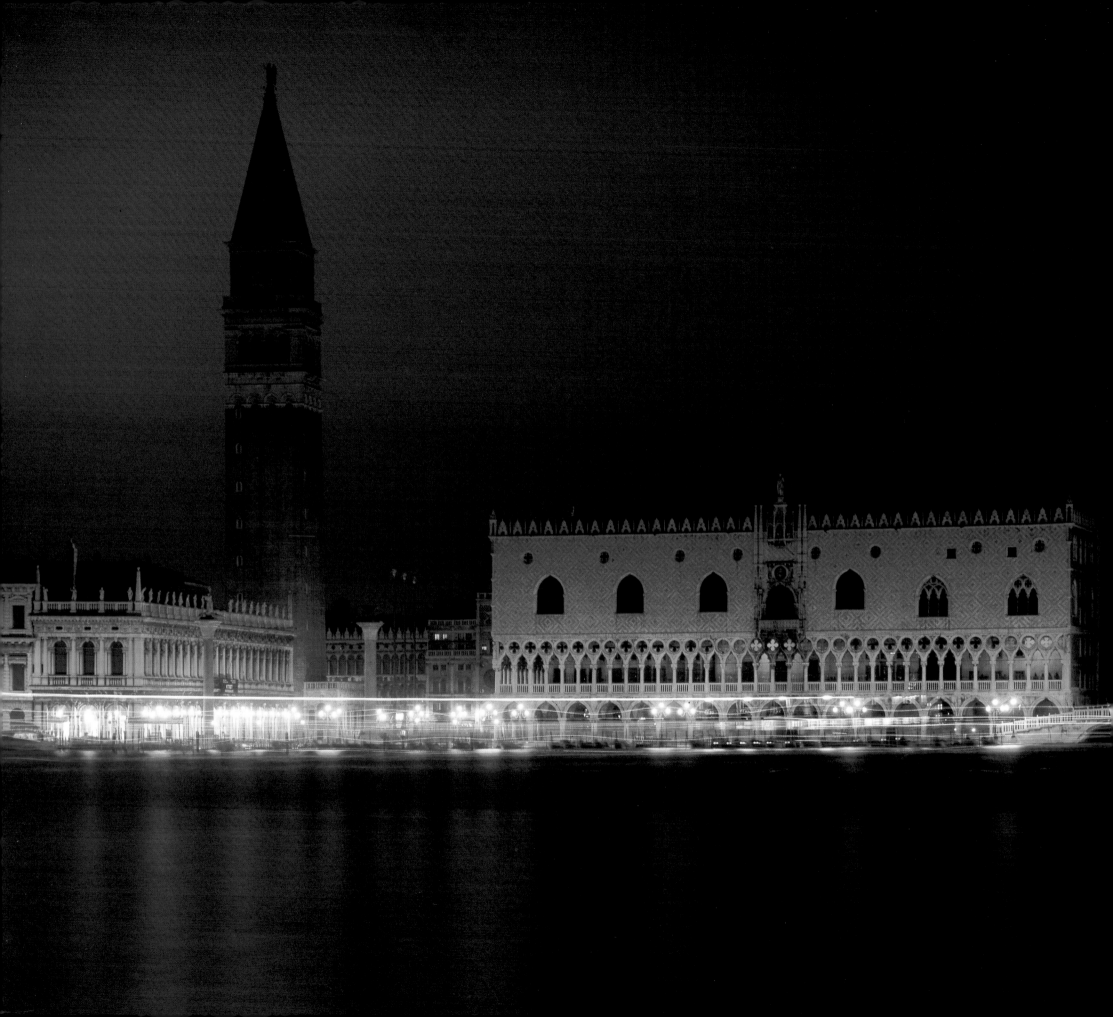

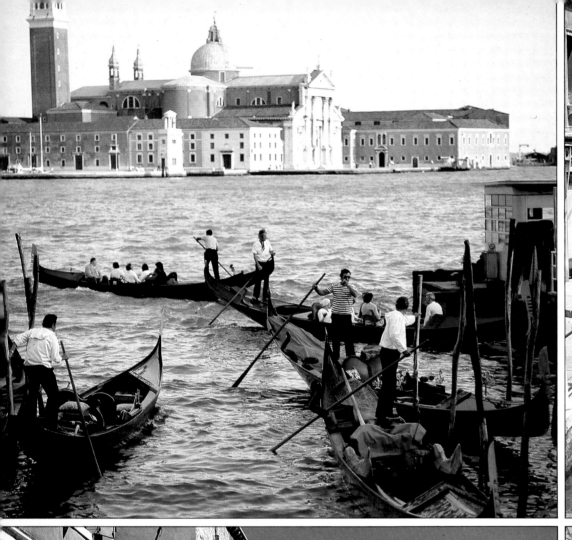
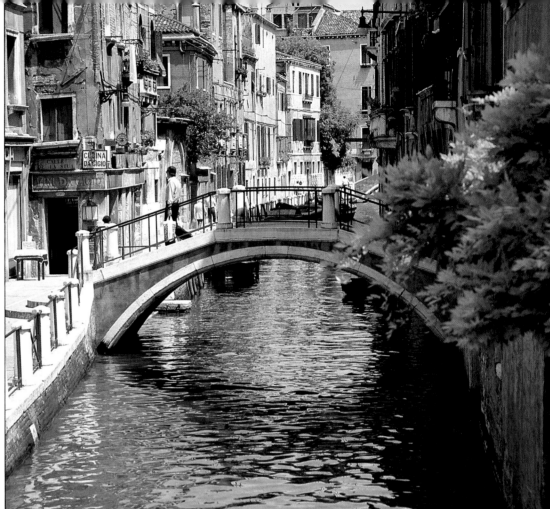
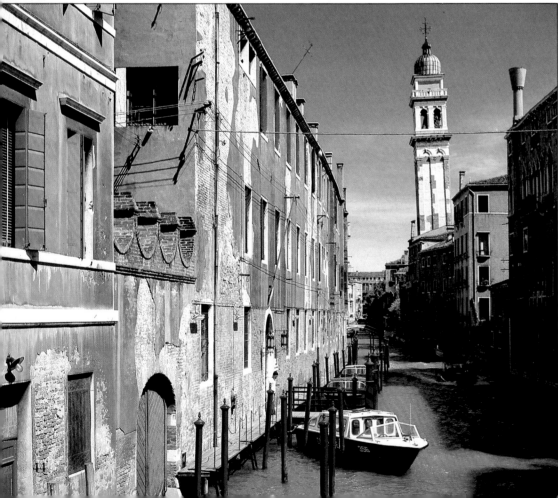
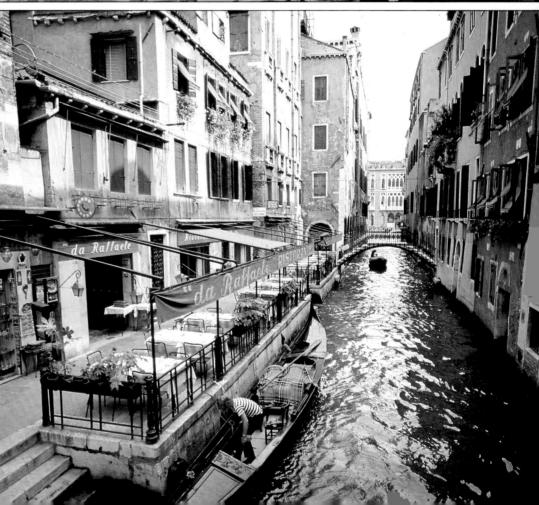

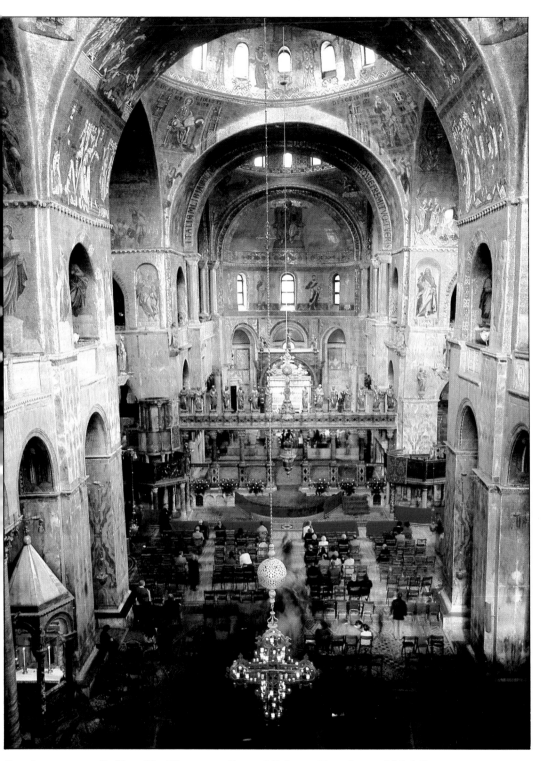

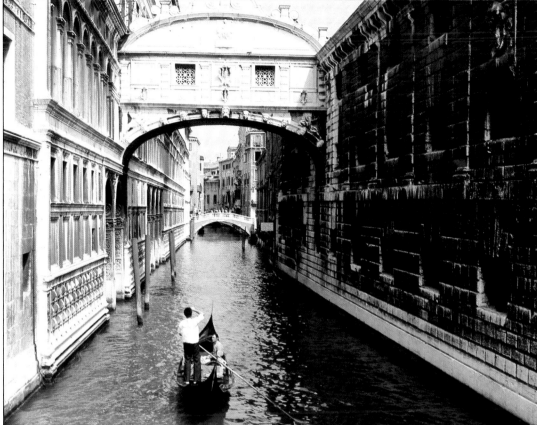

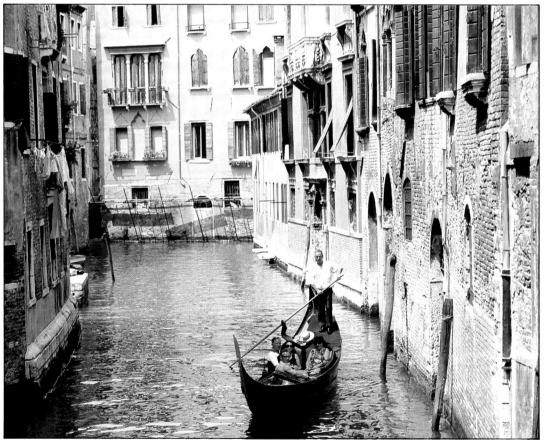

Previous pages: (left) softly-lit campanile and Palazzo Ducale, and (right) sunrise behind Santa Maria della Salute. Facing page: (top left) the church of San Giorgio Maggiore beyond the Canale di San Marco, and (bottom left) the tilted bell-tower of San Giorgio di Greci. Top right and bottom right: small bridges among the maze of narrow canals behind the Piazza San Marco. Above: rare marble and blue-based mosaics against gold face the entire interior of the Basilica San Marco. Right: individualised window-shapes. The covered Bridge of Sighs (top right), which links the east wing of the Palazzo Ducale to the Pozzi Prison, gave prisoners a last sight of the outside world through dense, stone latticework.

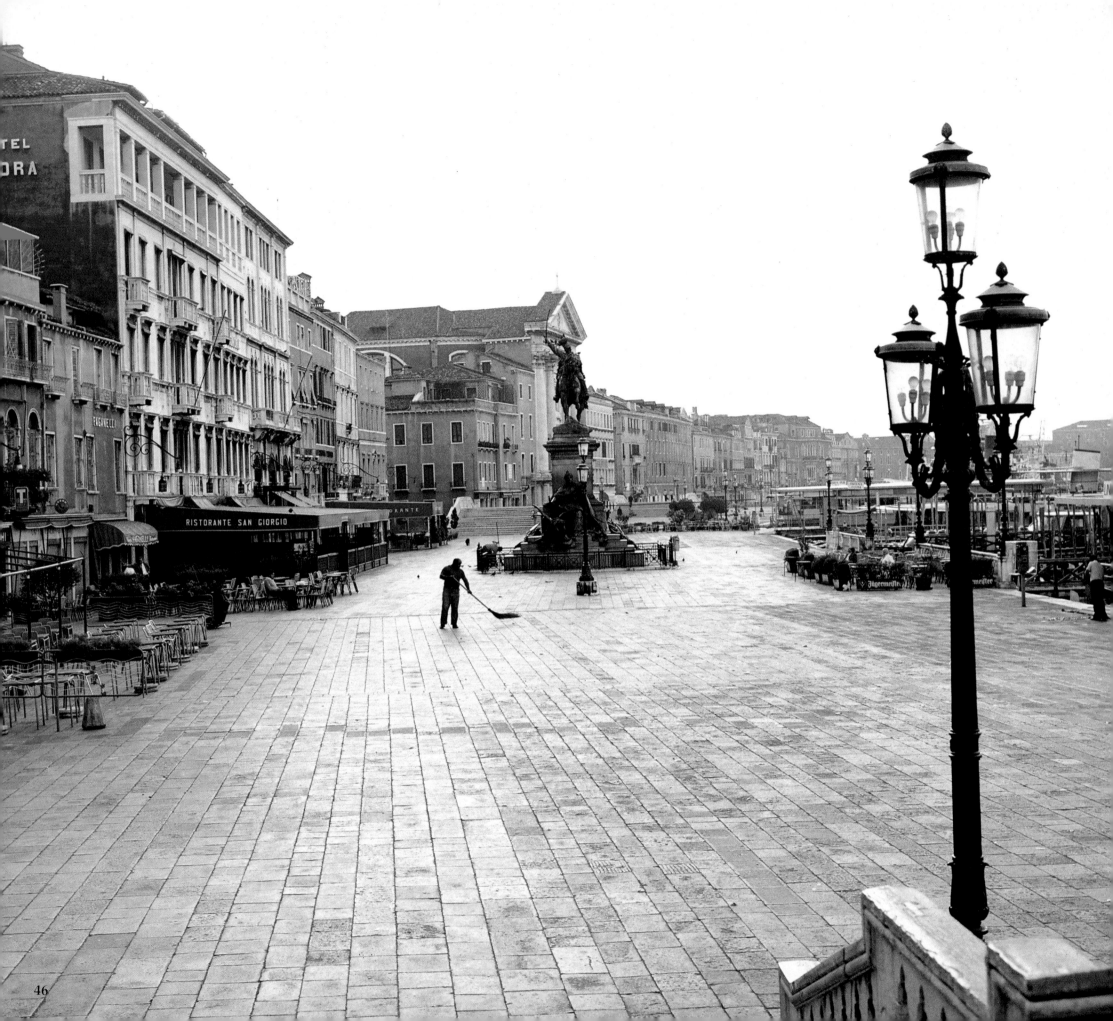

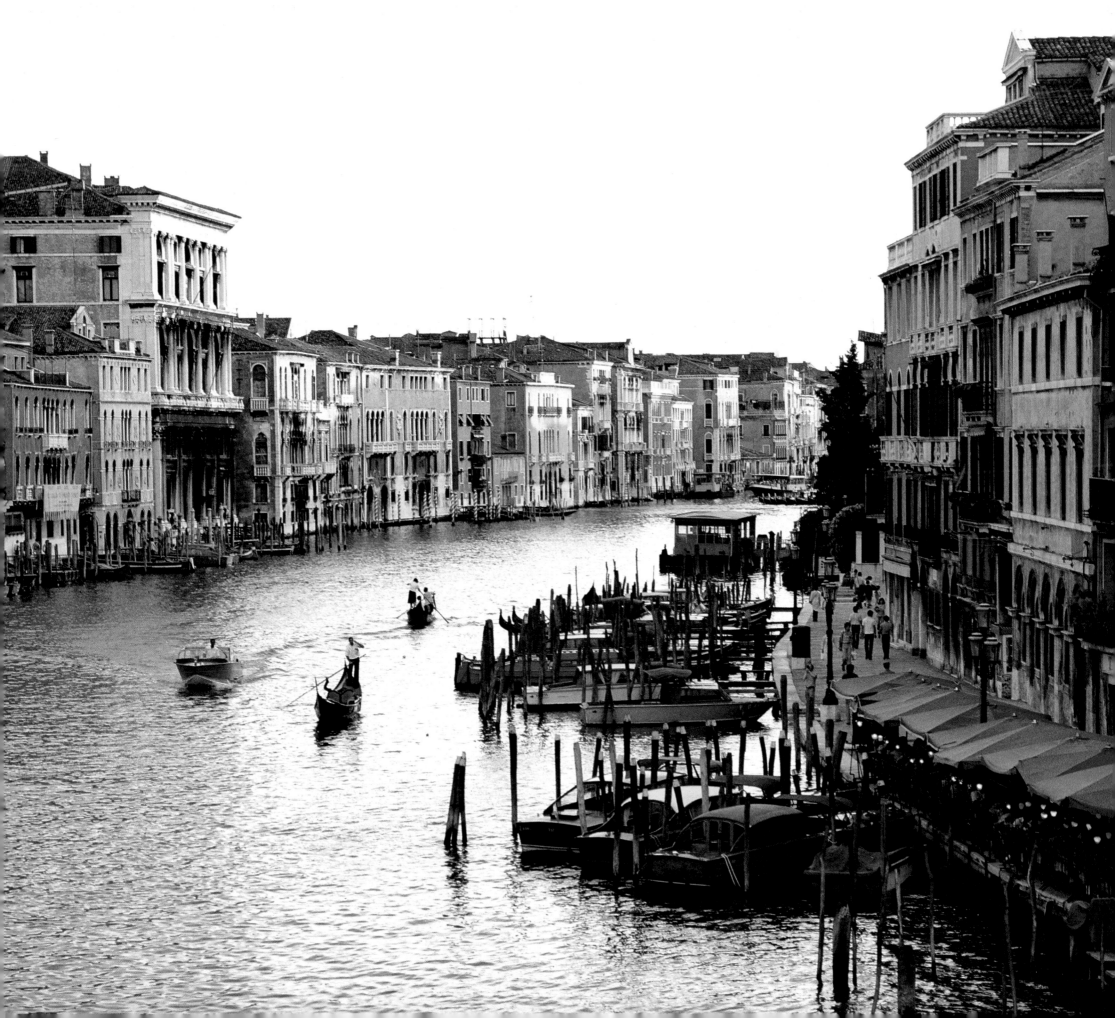

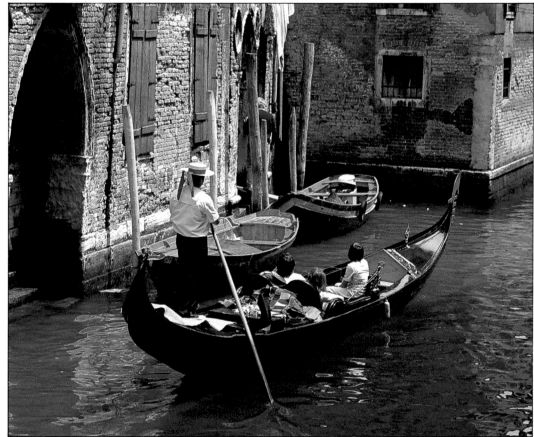

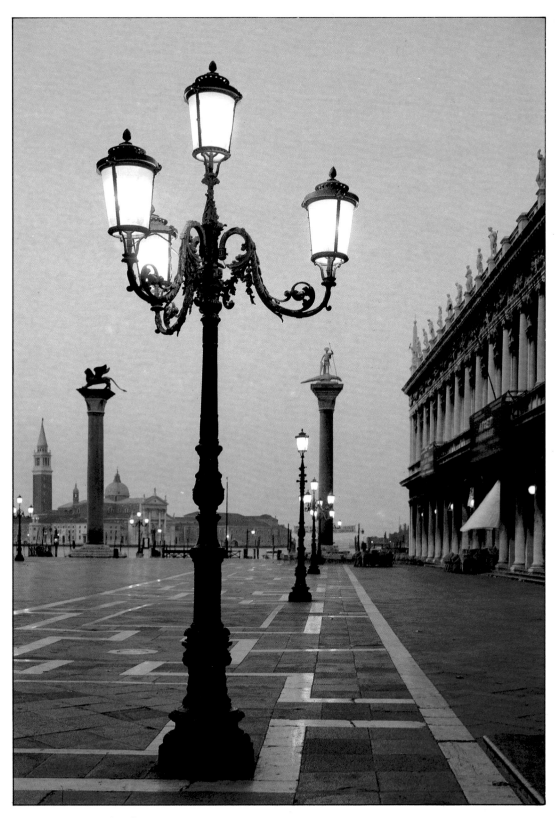

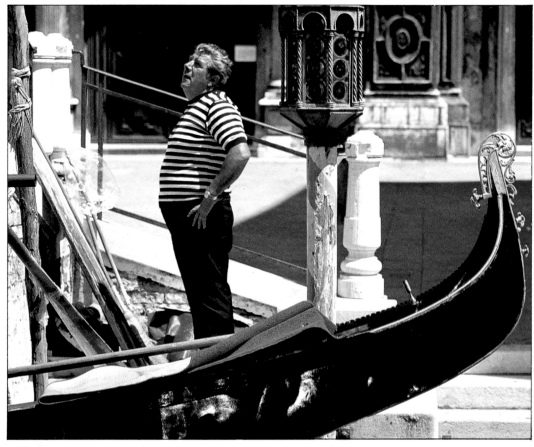

Previous pages: (left) early morning on the Riva Degli Schiavoni, and (right) the three white-pillared storeys of 16th-century Grimani Palace, facing onto the Grand Canal. Above: empty Piazzetta San Marco at morning, and (facing page) evening in the Piazza proper. Top right and right: gondoliers, and (overleaf left) gondolas moored along the mole. Overleaf: (right) guided tours of the Piazzetta San Marco.

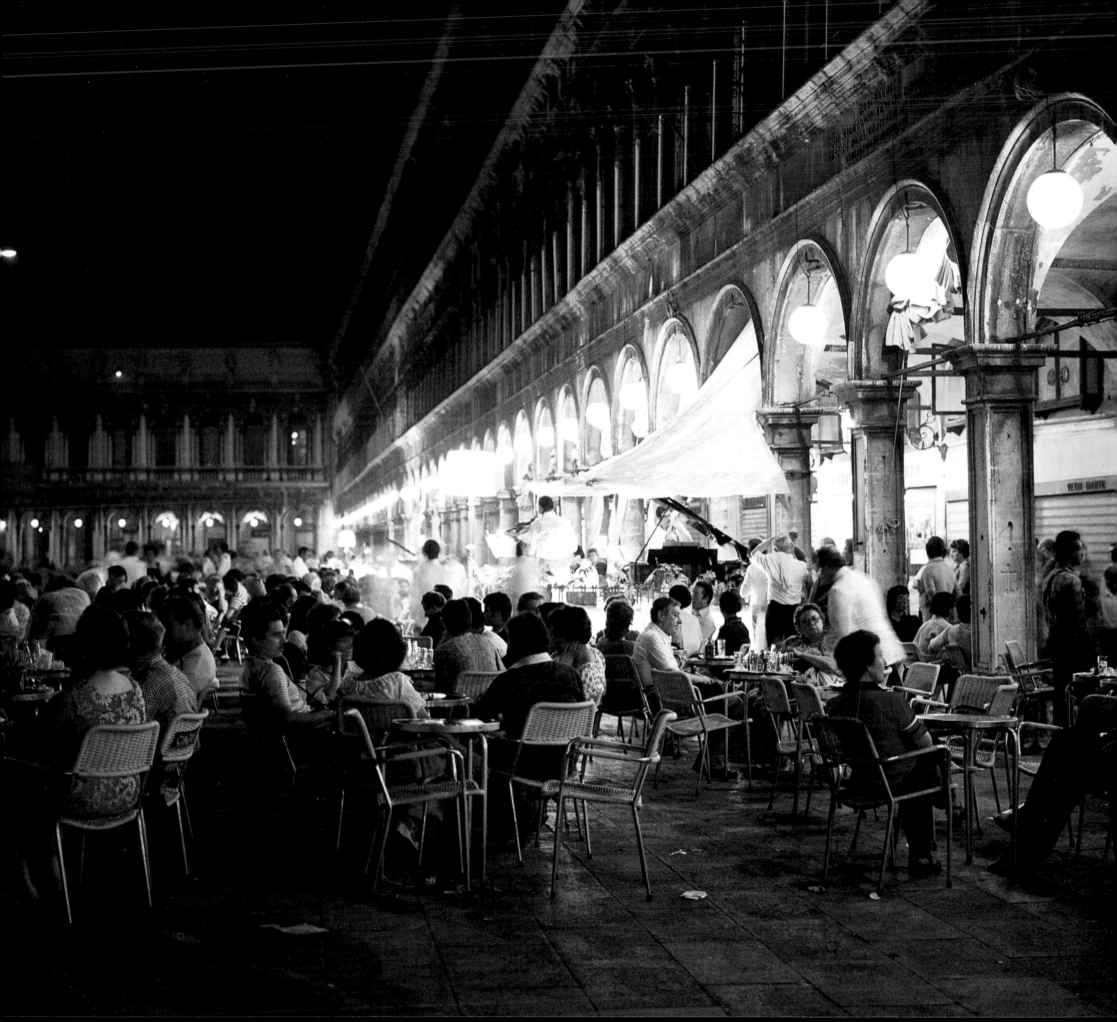

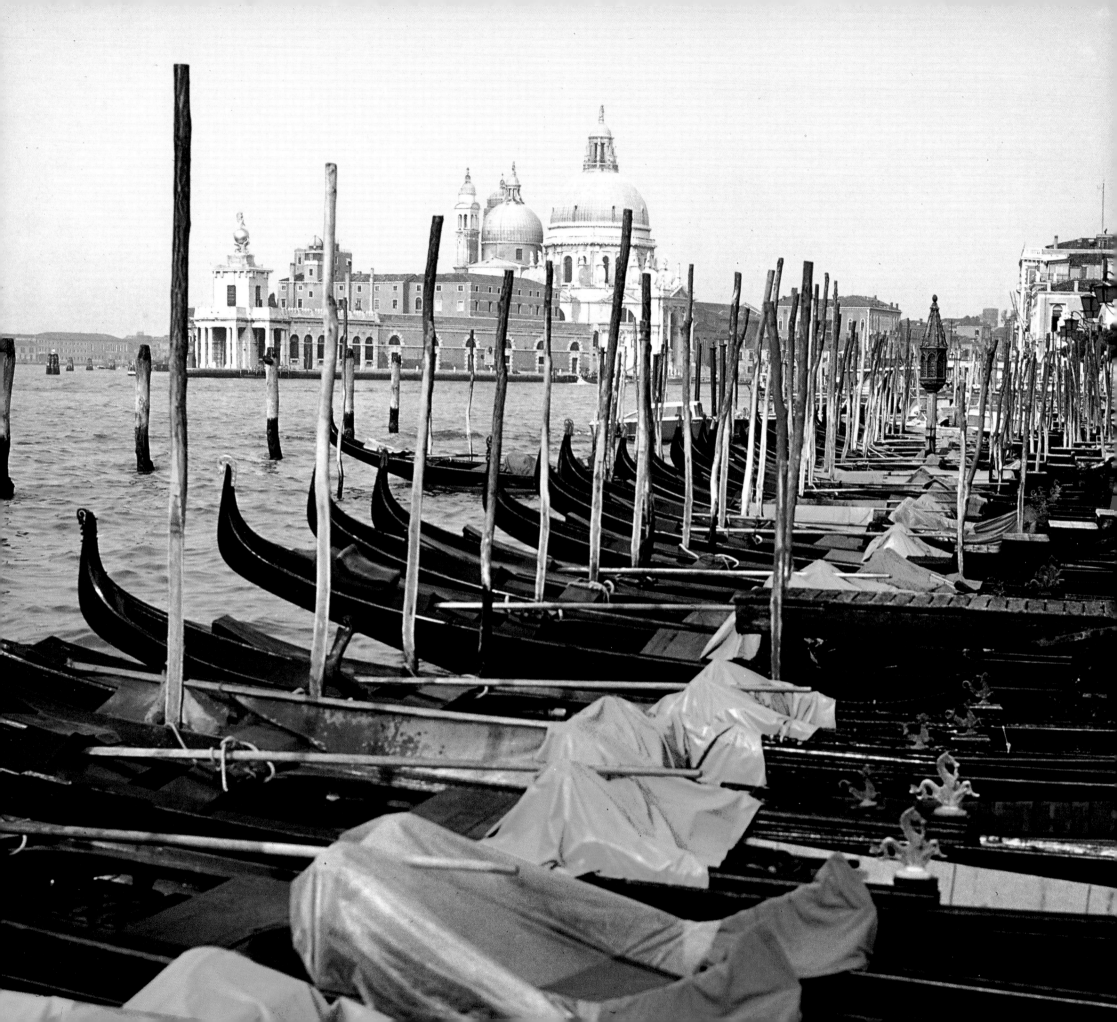

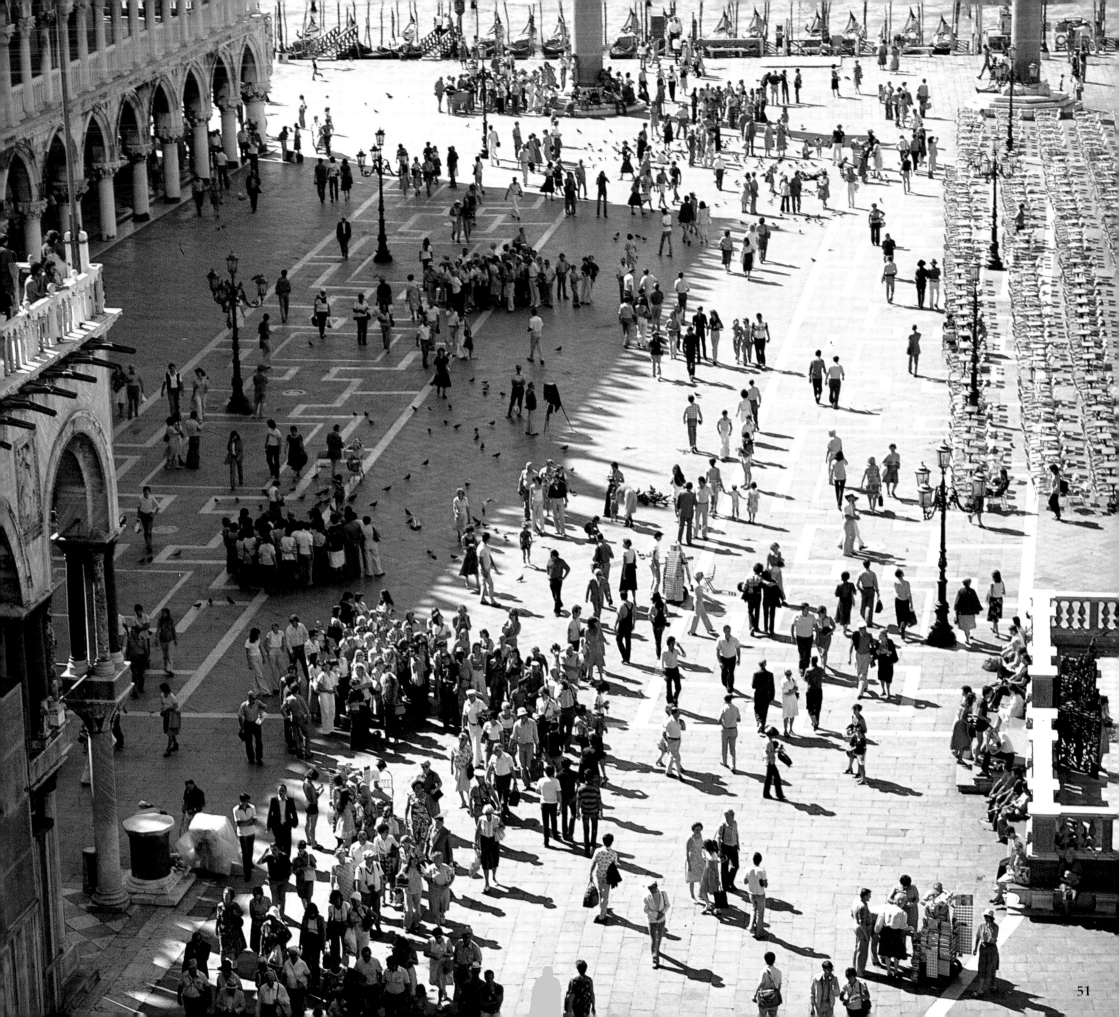

51

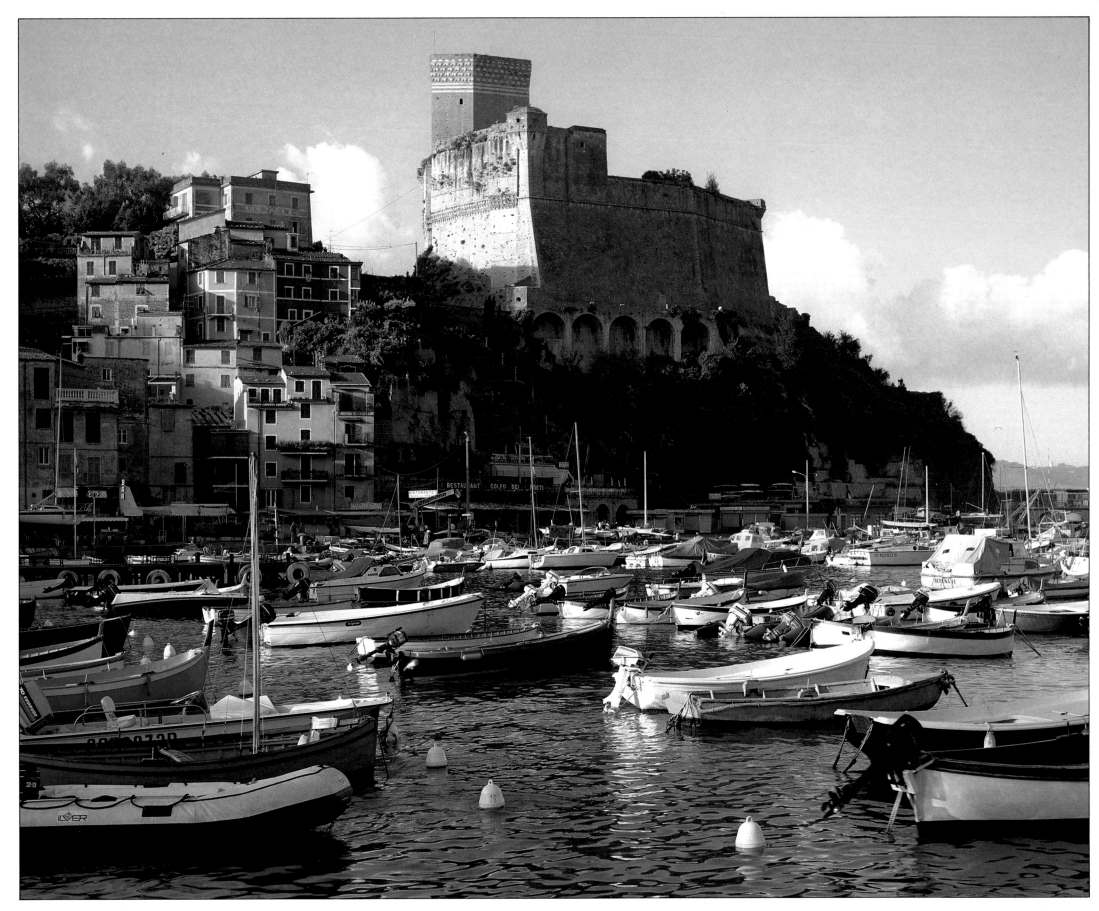

Above: the harbour and medieval castle in the old Pisan village of Lerici, on the eastern shore of the Gulf of La Spezia, and (facing page) tall, green-shuttered houses built into the steep slope at Riomaggiore, Liguria. The harbour of Portofino (overleaf left), which once served only the village's fishing craft, now gives precedence to the yachts of rich visitors. Overleaf: (right) strips of houses on the harbour in the fishing village of Portovenere.

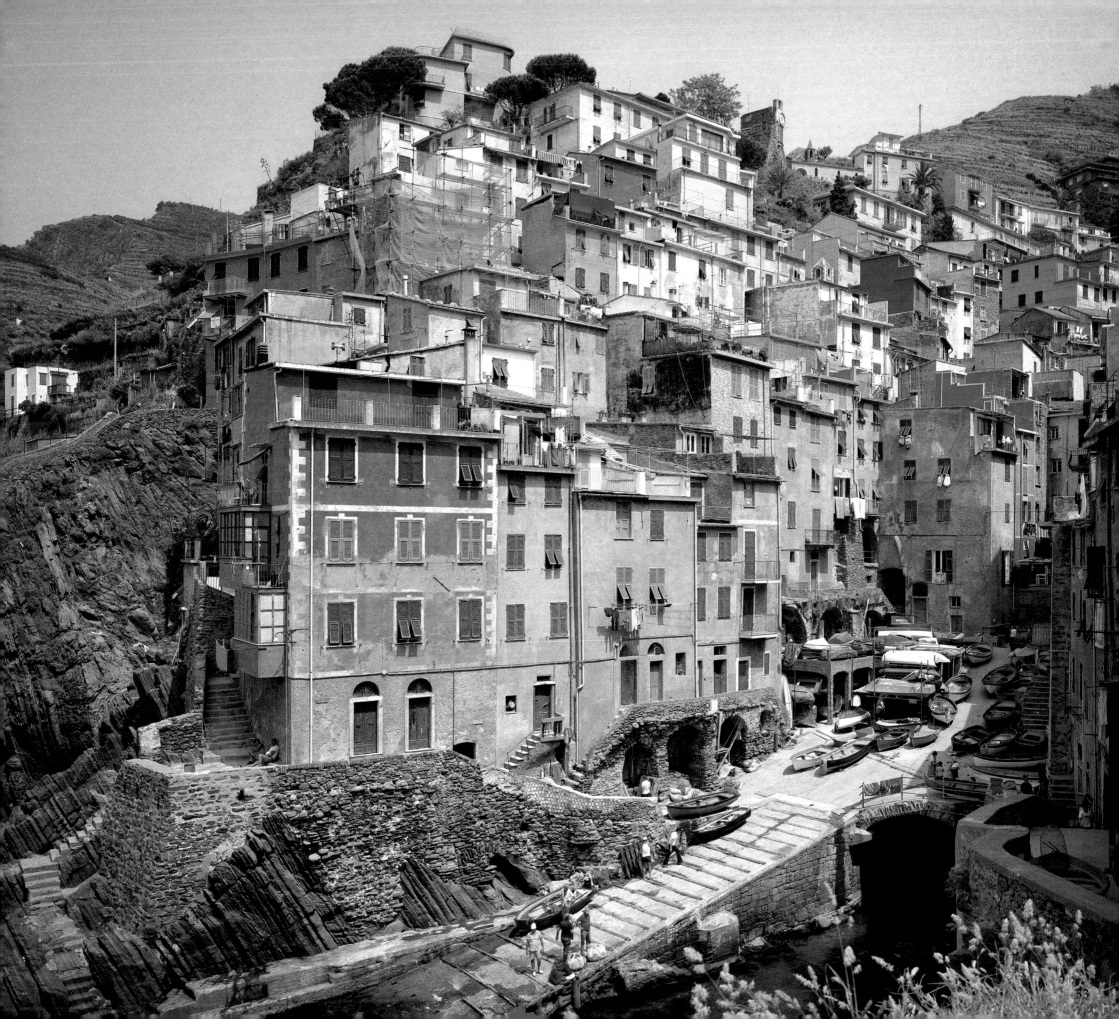

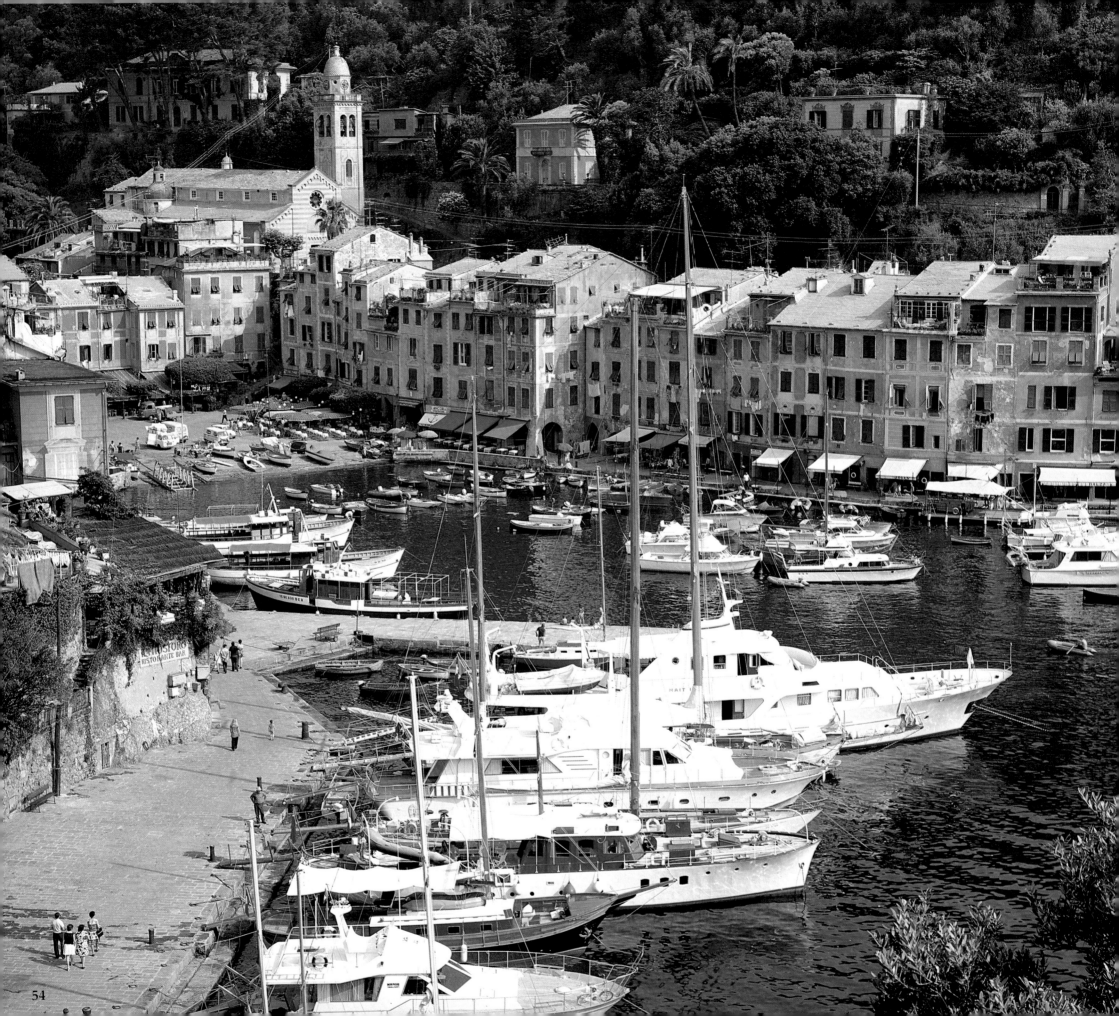

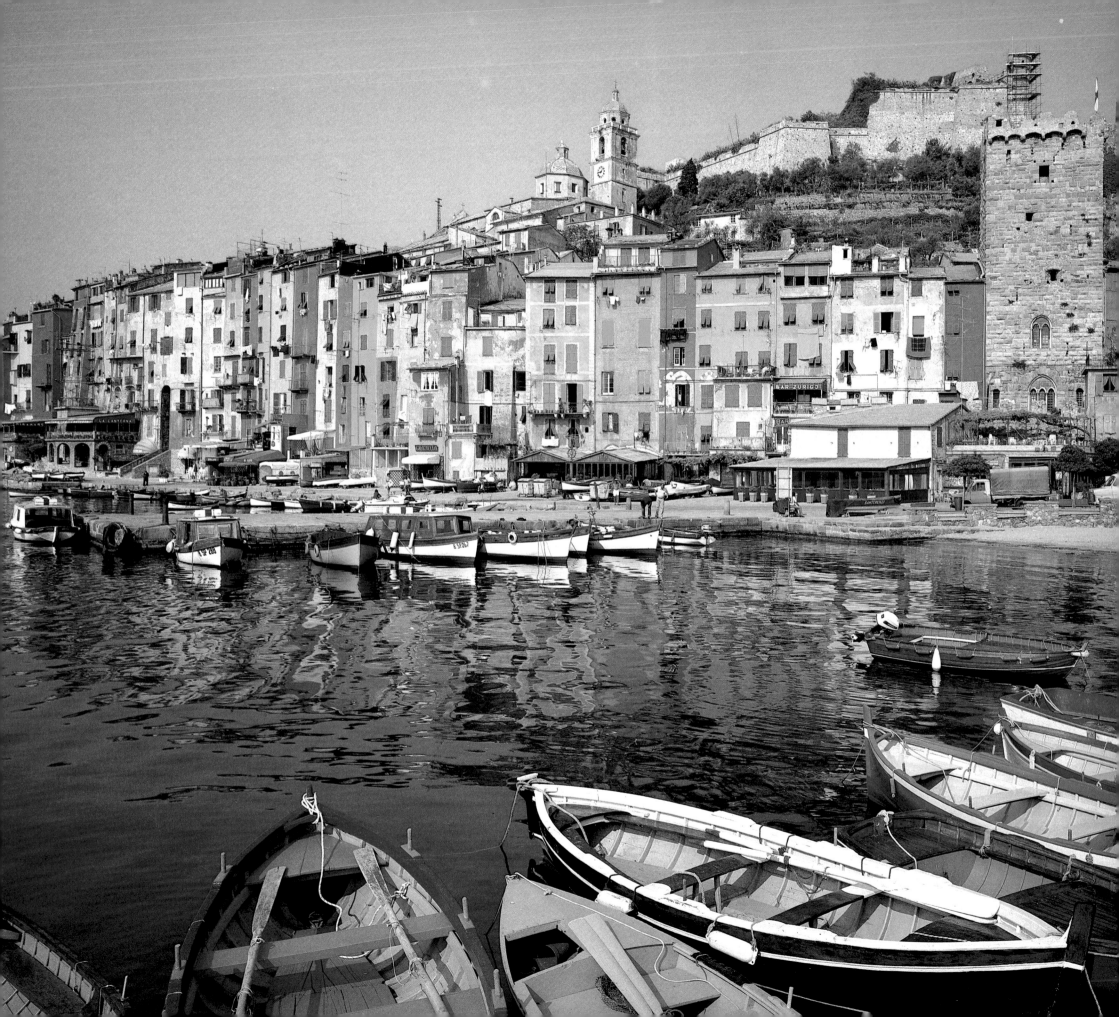

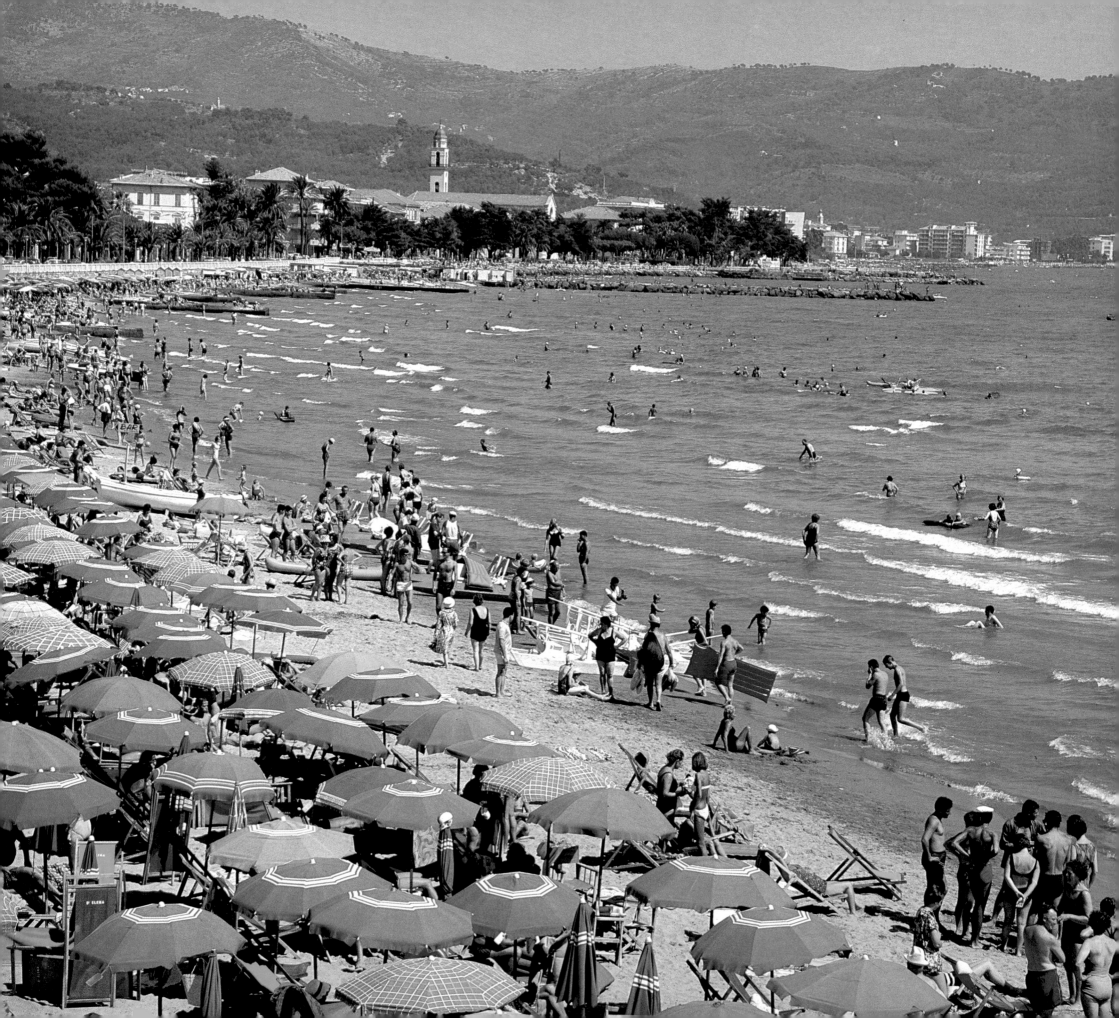

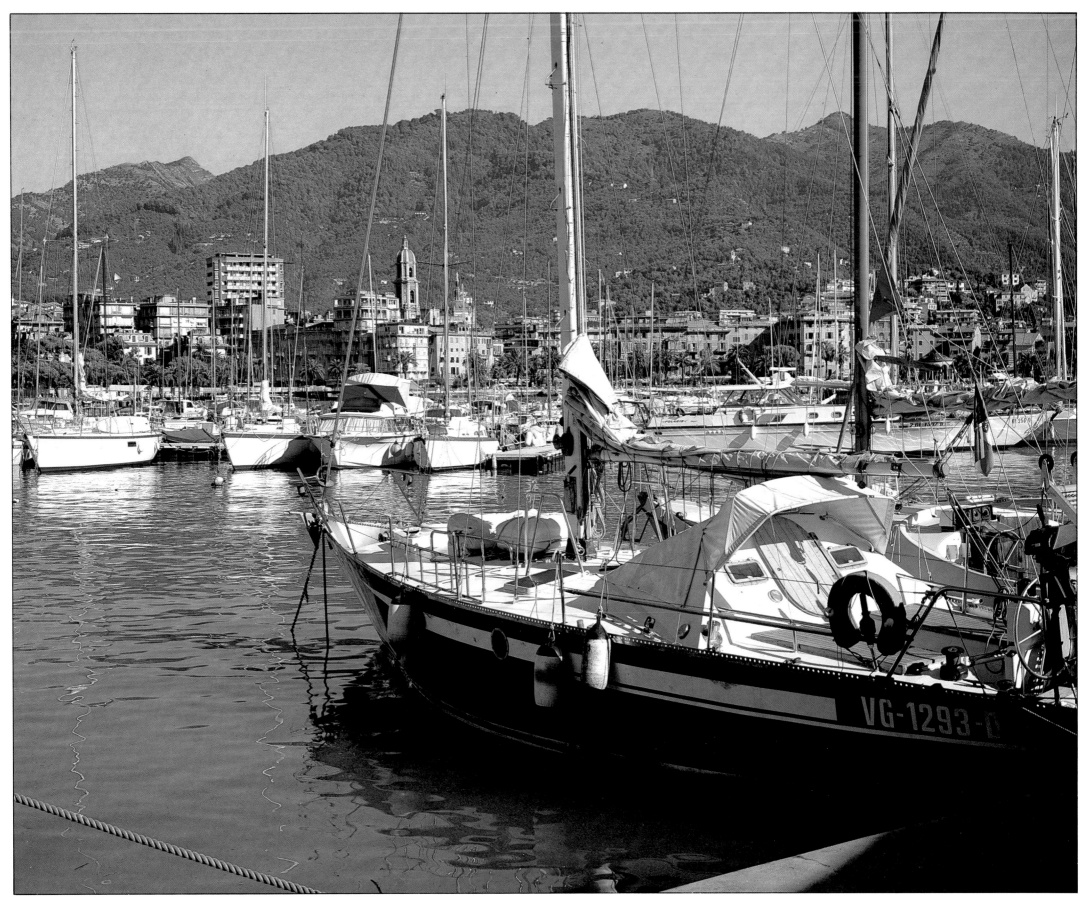

Situated on the Riviera di Levante, the little port town of Rapallo (above) became popular when frequented by the wealthy, the titled, and by the literary set, led at one time by Sir Max Beerbohm, who lived in the town for many years. Facing page: Diano Marina, a busy beach resort on the Ponente Riviera.

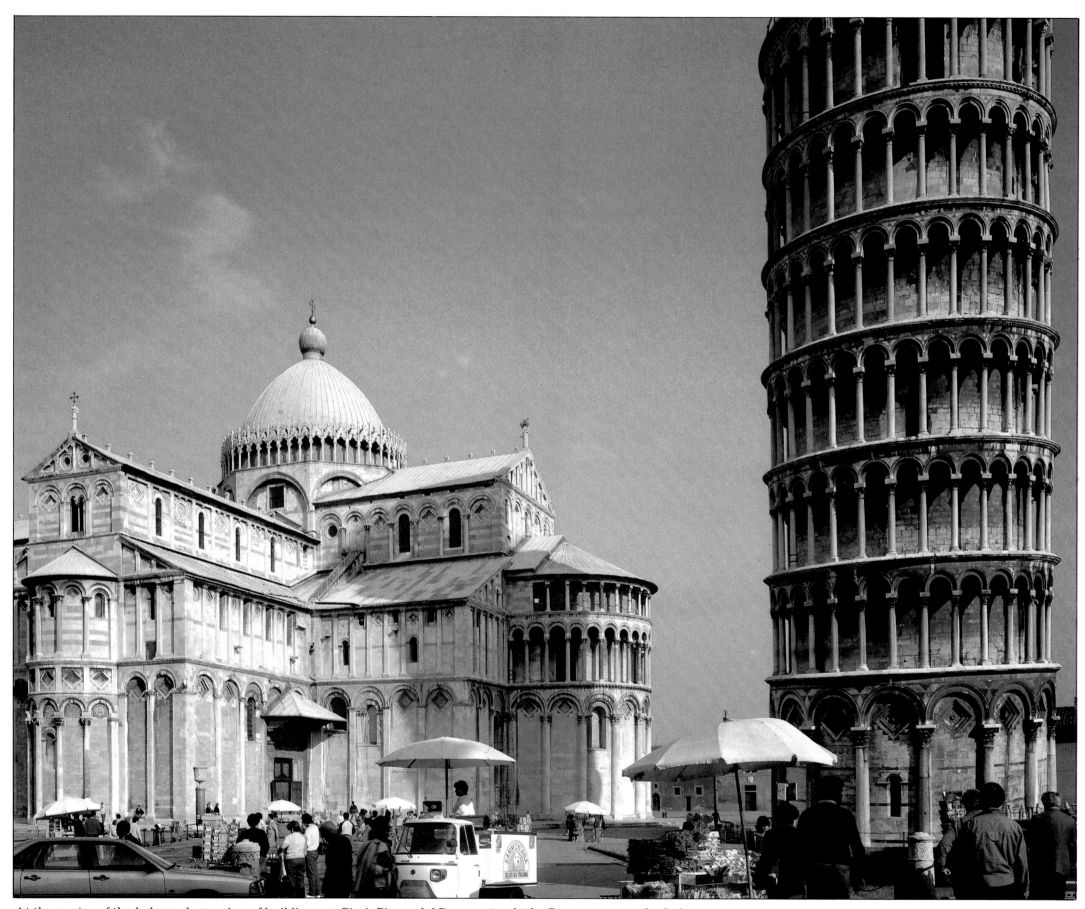

At the centre of the balanced grouping of buildings on Pisa's Piazza del Duomo stands the Romanesque cathedral (above and overleaf), begun in 1063 following a Pisan naval victory over the Saracens at Palermo. The cathedral was completed in the 13th century, and is built of white and warmer-shaded marble, with transepts, an elliptical dome over the cross, and a graceful, four-galleried facade (facing page). The approximately 14-foot tilt of the campanile or Leaning Tower (above and overleaf) was caused by a landslip during its construction in the 12th century. Overleaf: (right) the marble-clad, circular Baptistry.

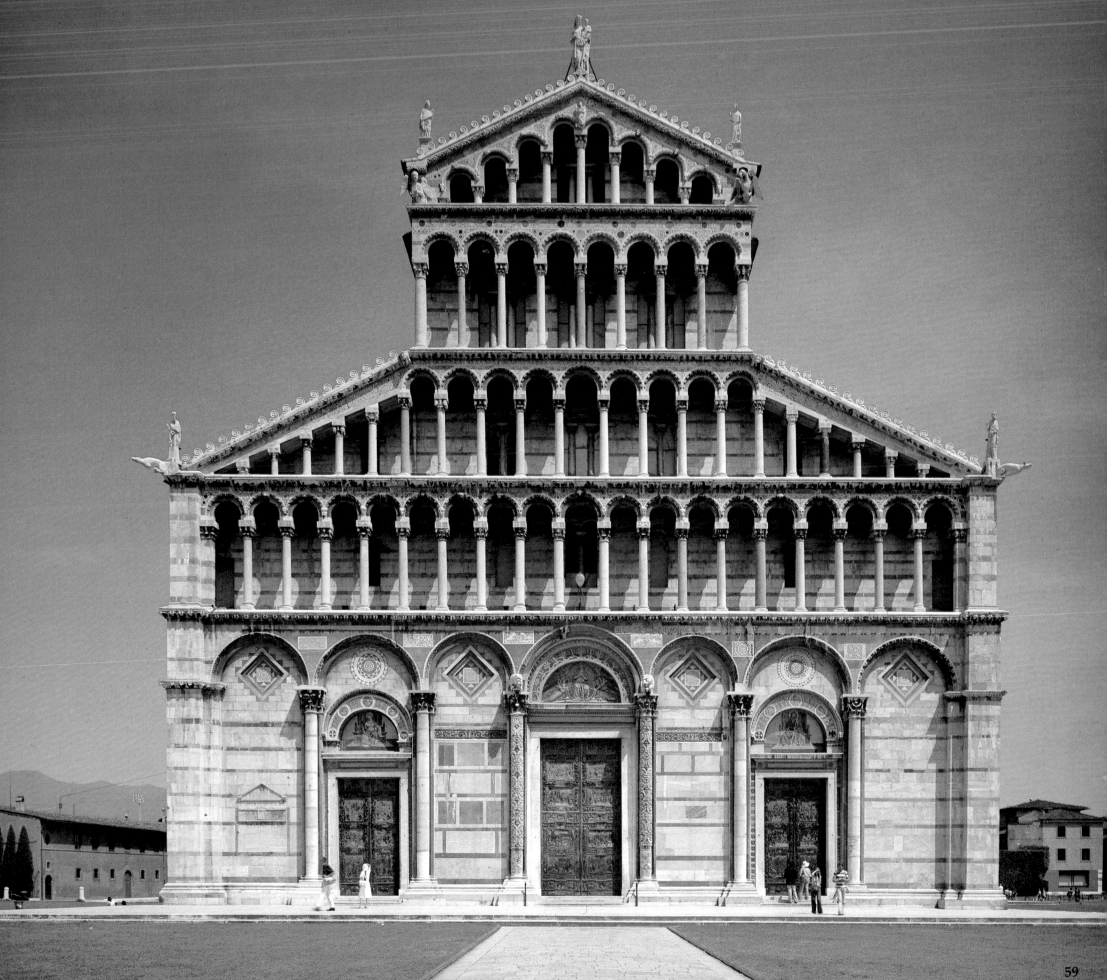

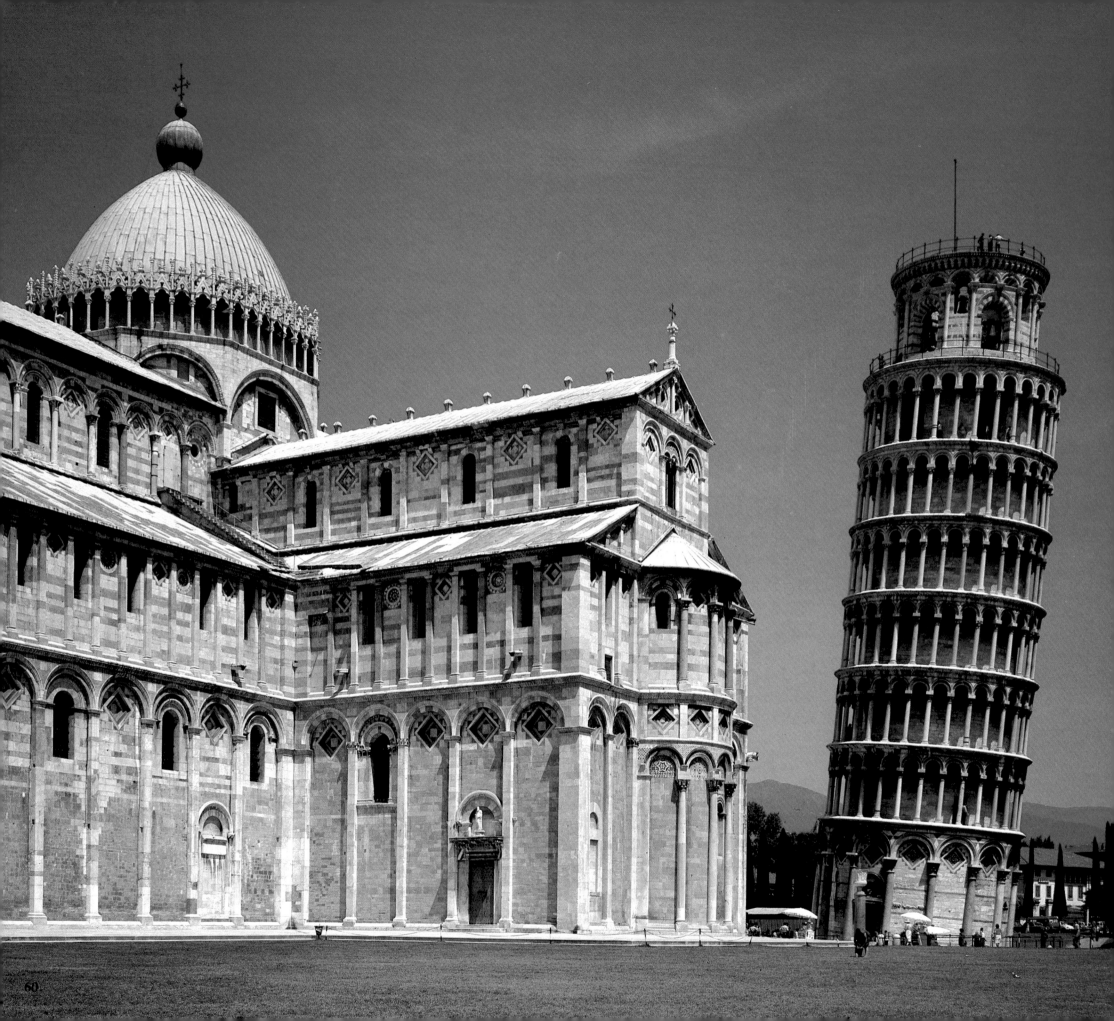

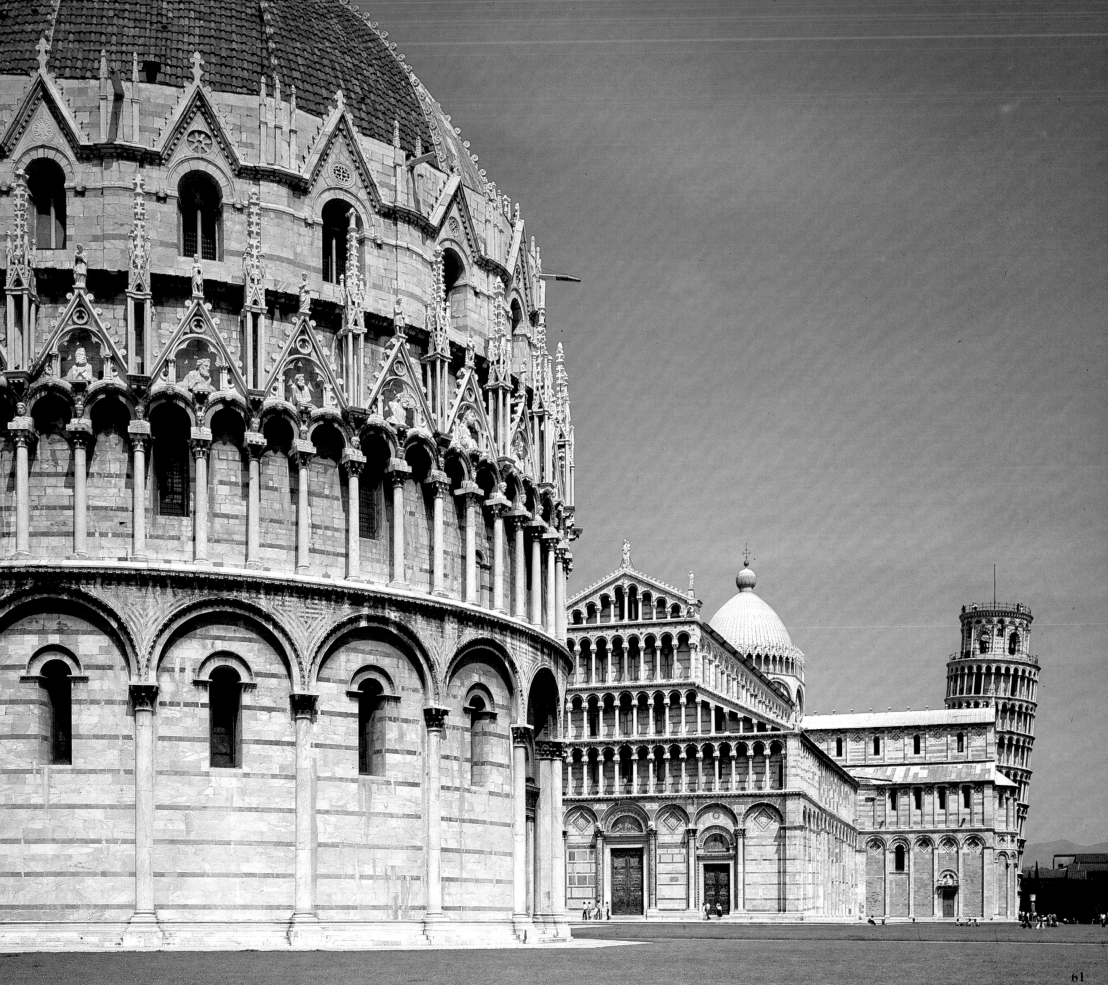

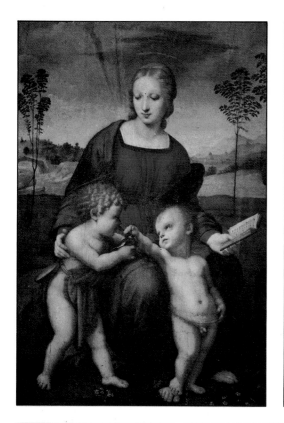

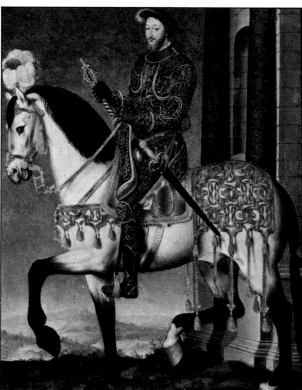

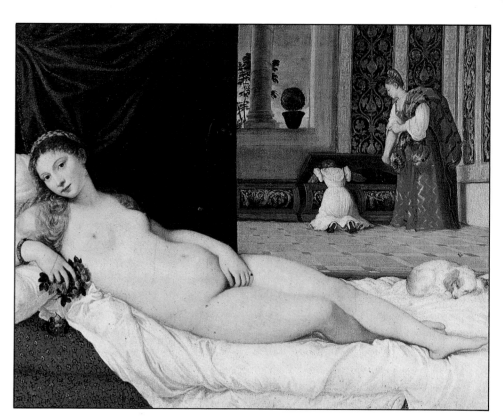

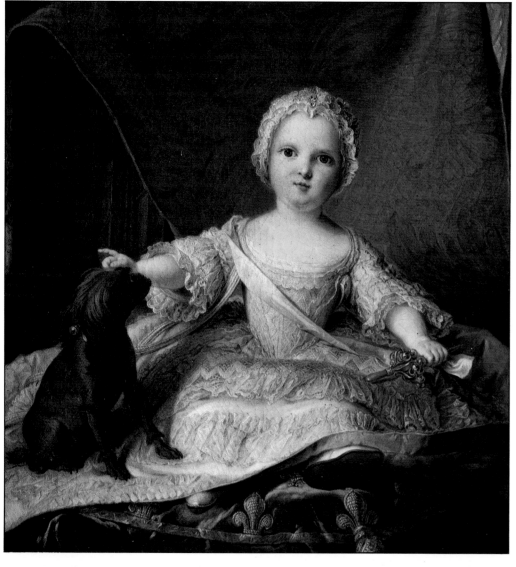

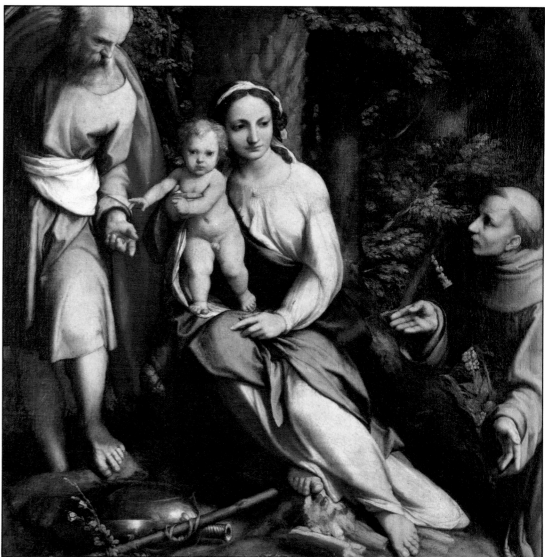

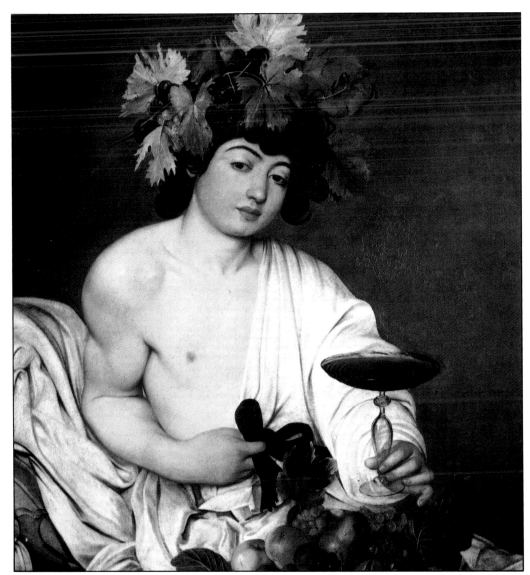

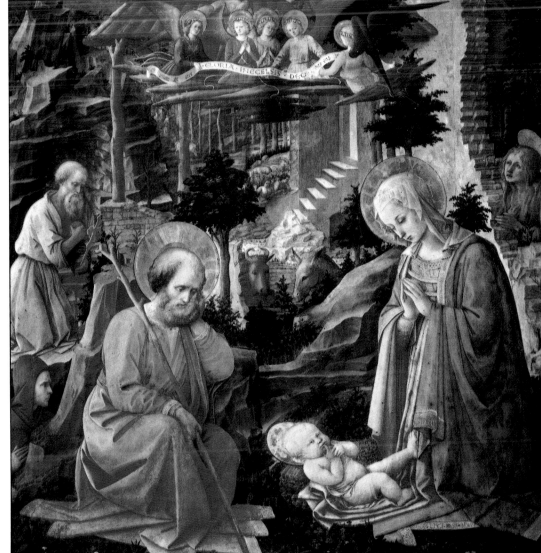

The 16th-century Uffizi Gallery in Florence, Tuscany, houses many of the treasures of Italy's artistic heritage. Facing page: (top, far left) 'The Madonna of the Goldfinch' (1506), one of the first of Raphael Santi's series of altarpieces. (Top centre) full-length portrait of 'Francois I of France' by Francois Clouet (c1515/20-1572). (Top right) Titian's 'The Urbino Venus', and (bottom left) 'Portrait of Marie Zefferina of France', daughter of Louis XV, by Jean-Marc Nattier (c1685-1766). (Bottom right) 'Rest on the Flight into Egypt', an early work of Corregio, a Renaissance painter of the Parma school. This page: (above) Caravaggio's 'The Youthful Bacchus'. Top right: 'Adoration of the Magi with St. Hilarius' by Fra. Filippo Lippi (c.1457-1504), and (right) 'The Annunciation', painted by a youthful Leonardo da Vinci (1452-1519) for the Church of San Bartolemeo di Monteoliveto, near Florence.

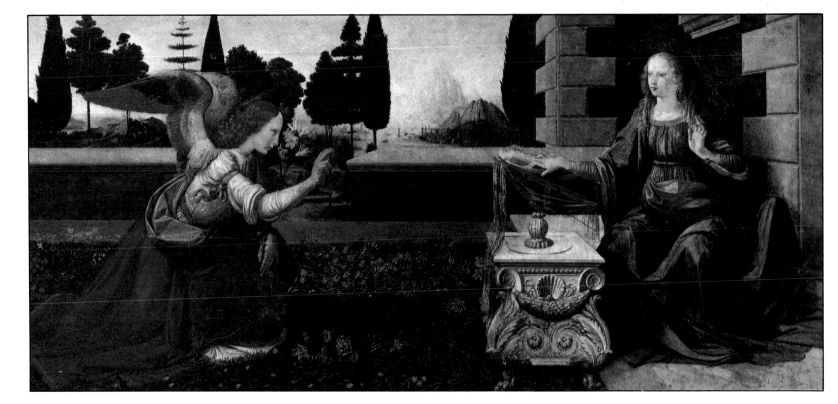

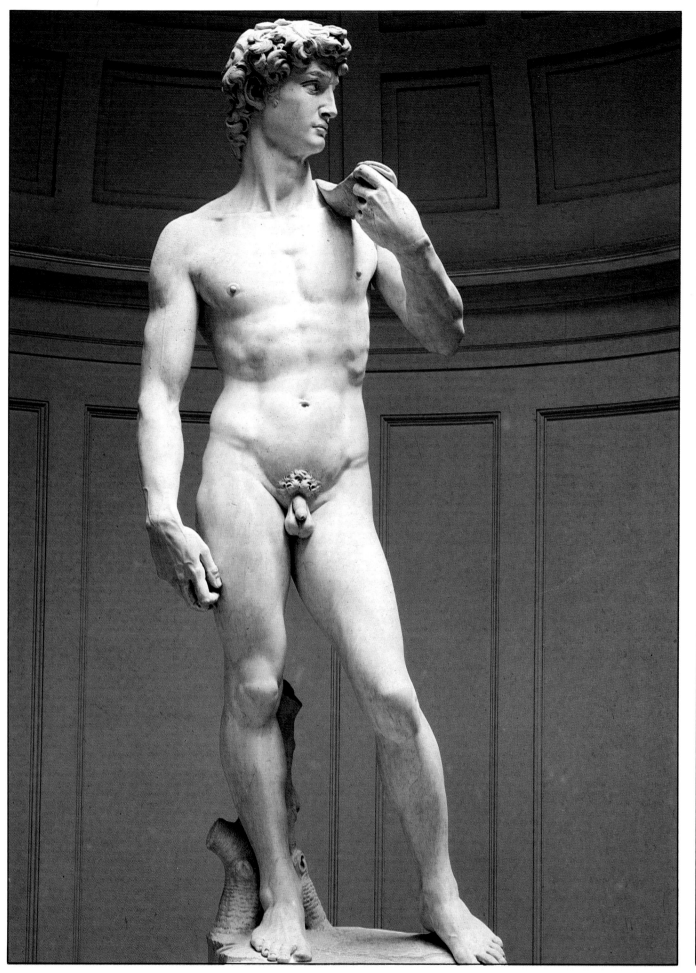

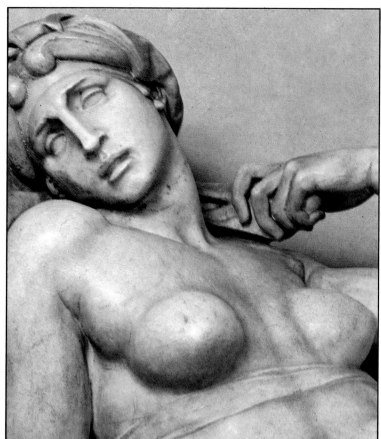

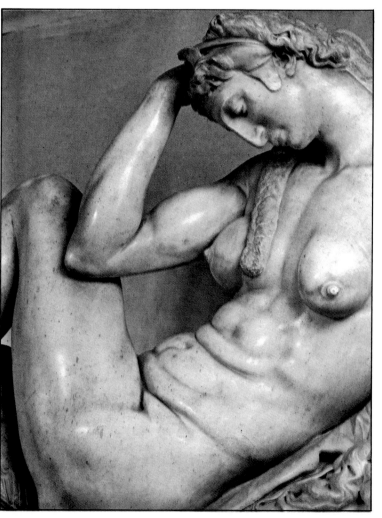

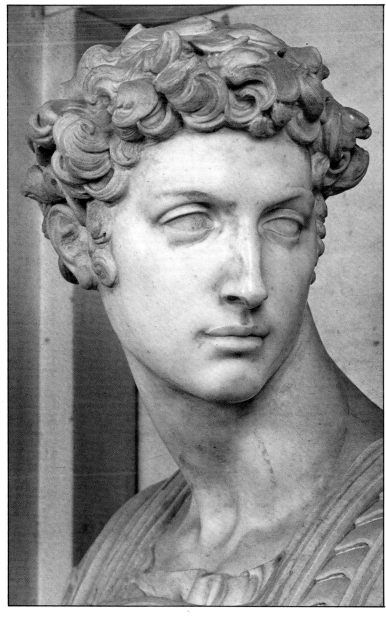

Michelangelo's statue of David (facing page, left), begun in 1501 and completed three years later, now stands in the Gallery of the Academy. The new Republic of Florence commissioned the statue as an allegory of the moral strength of the city, and it was carved from a huge block of marble reserved for the purpose since 1462. The New Sacristy in the Medici Chapels, begun by Michelangelo in 1520 and completed by Vasari in 1557, contains the tombs of the Medici princes, the great rulers of Florence. Facing page: (top) Michelangelo's figure of Dawn, which, together with his image of Dusk, adorns the tomb of Lorenzo, Duke of Urbino. The artist's representation of Night (facing page, bottom), with the complementary figure of Day, reclines on the sarcophagus beneath the seated figure of Giuliano, Duke of Nemours (above). Right: 'The Descent from the Cross' by Fra Angelico (c1400-1455), one of a series of frescoes depicting the suffering of Christ, in the Dominican monastery of San Marco, now a museum. Overleaf: (left) the Neptune Fountain in the Piazza della Signoria, and (right) the Arno and the city of Florence seen from Piazzale Michelangelo.

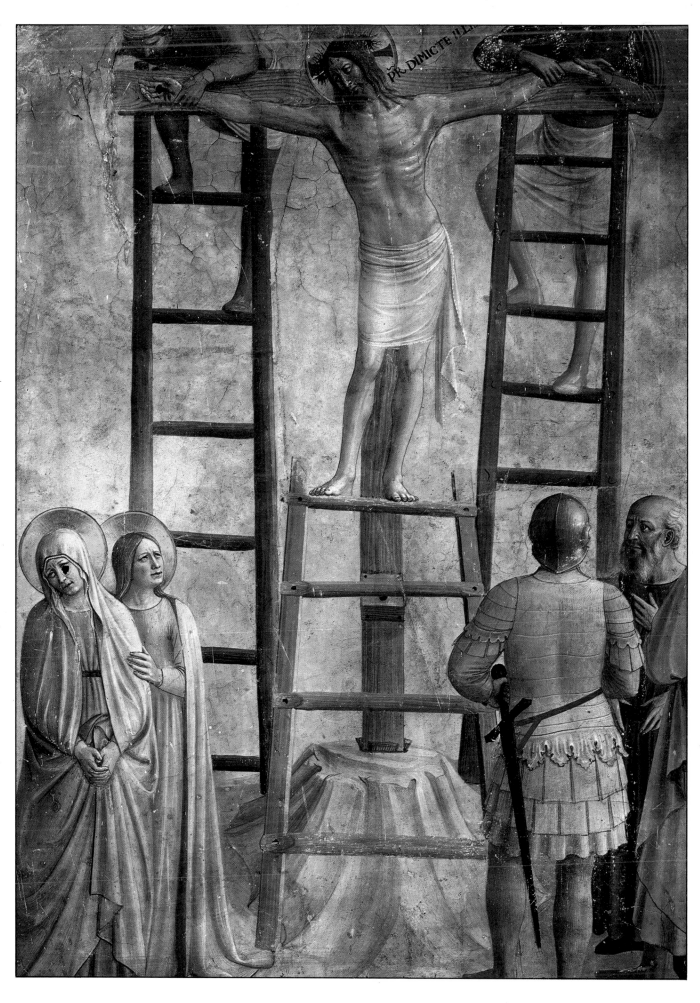

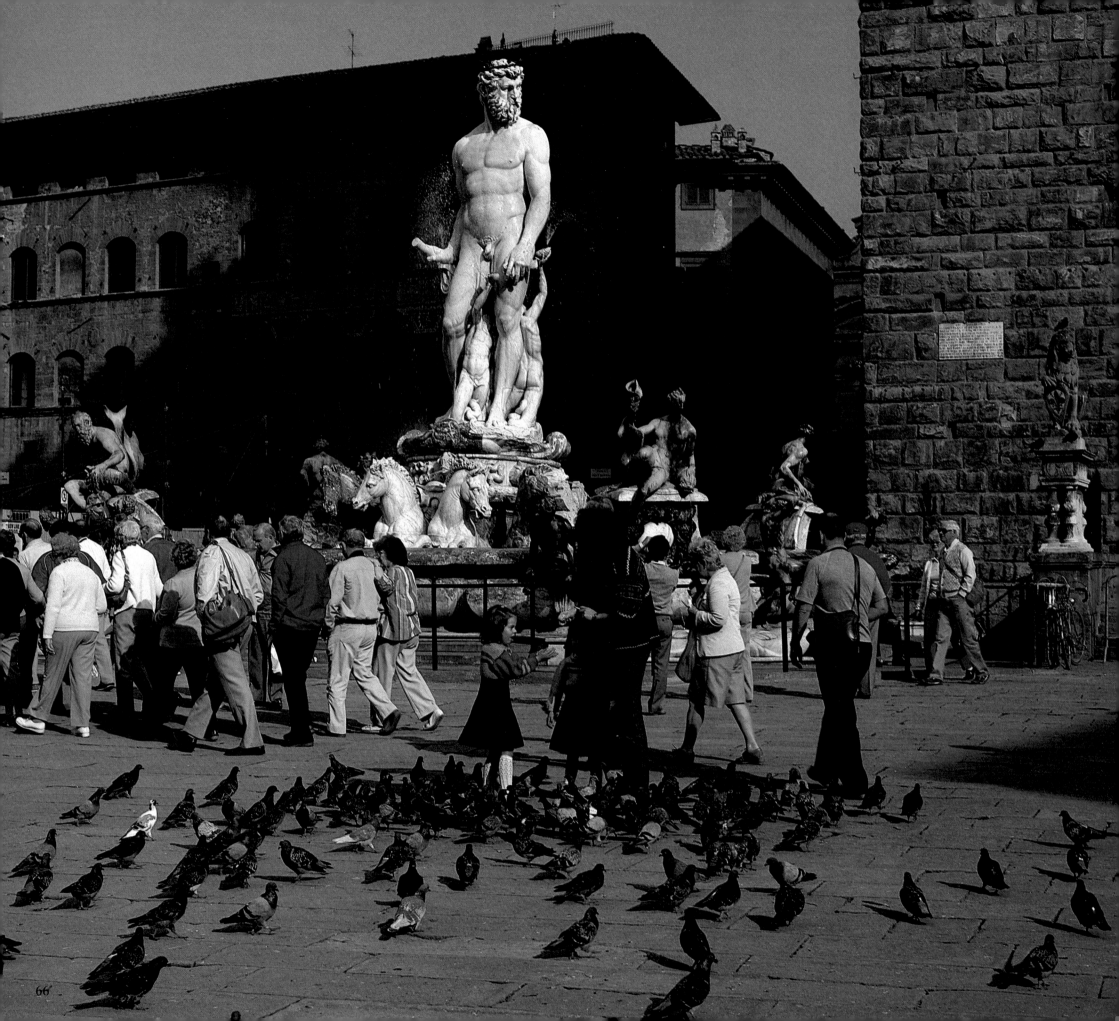

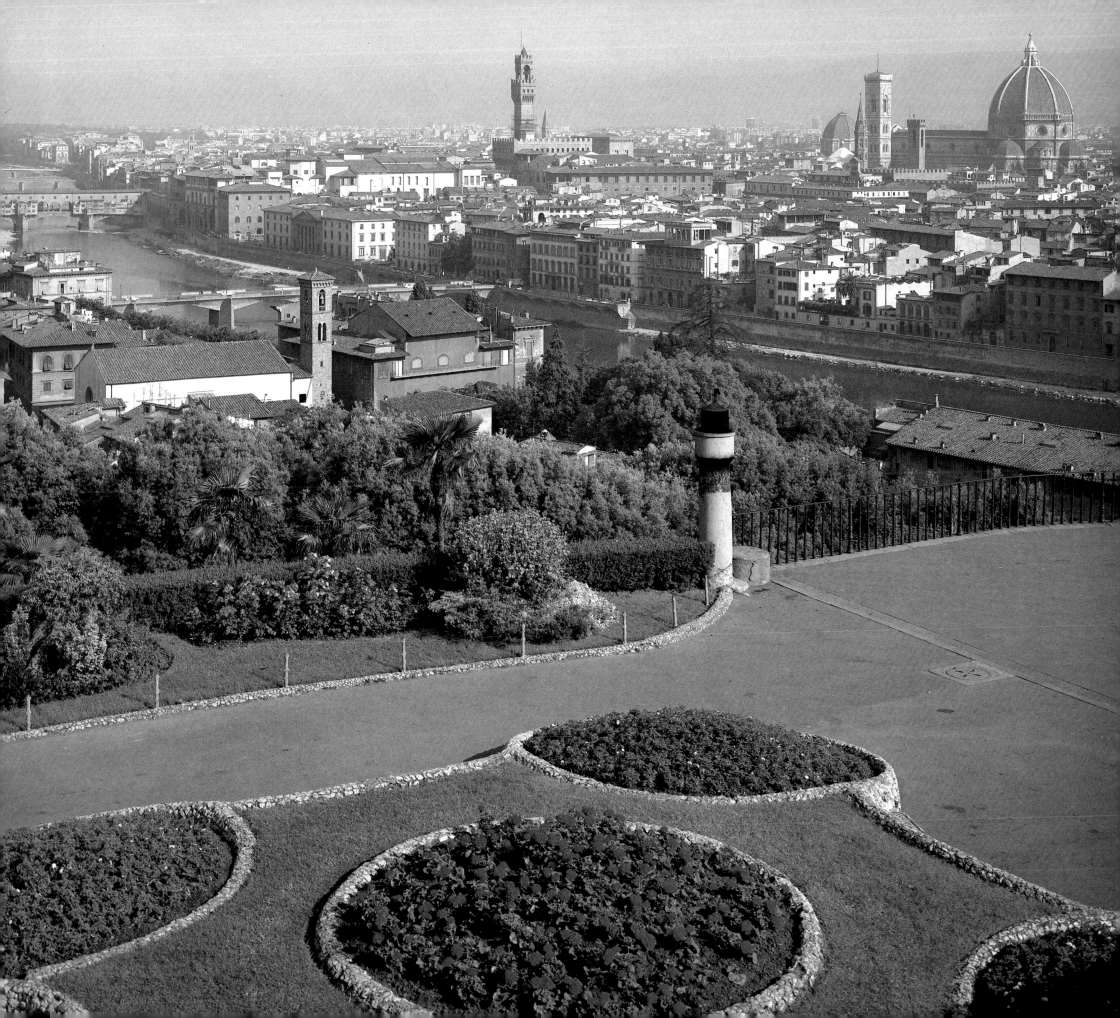

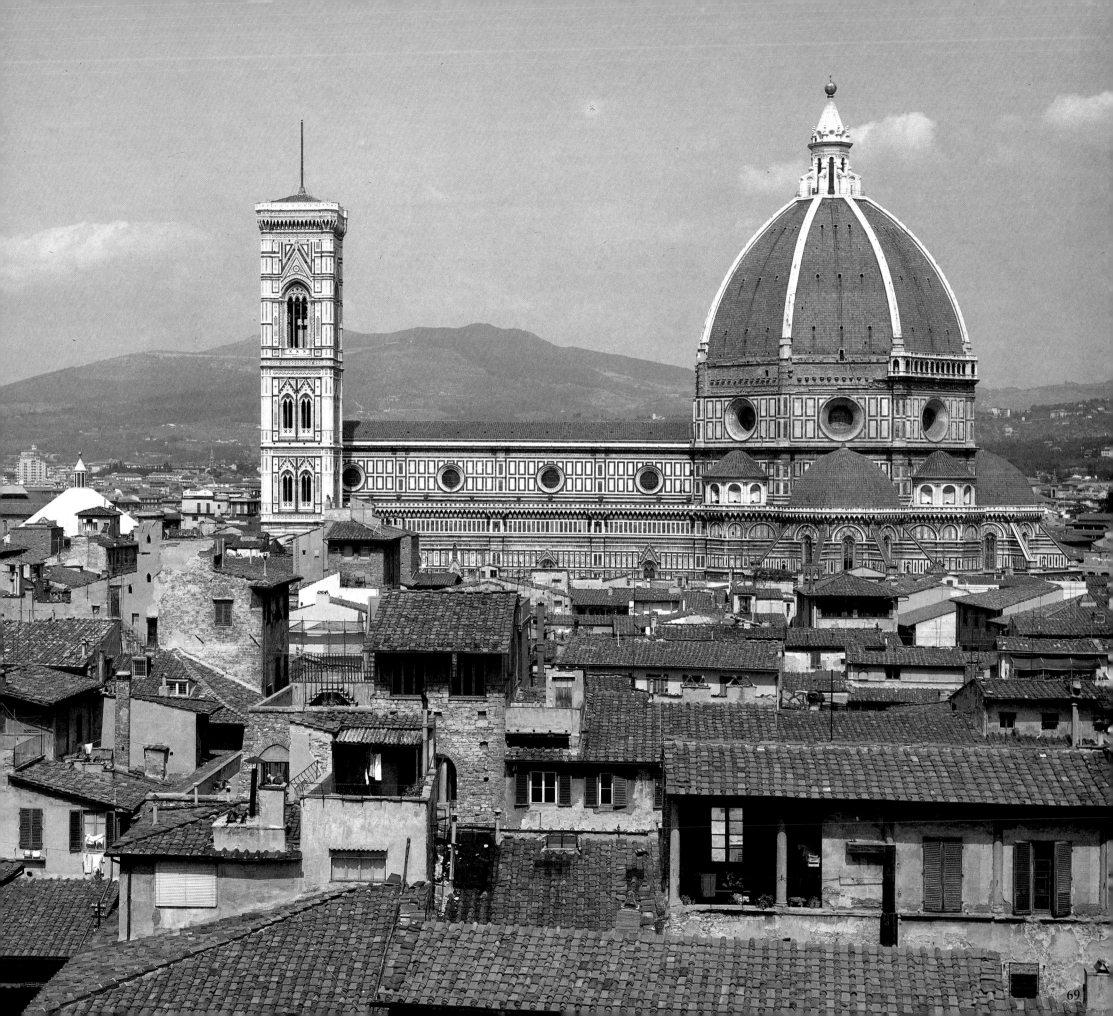

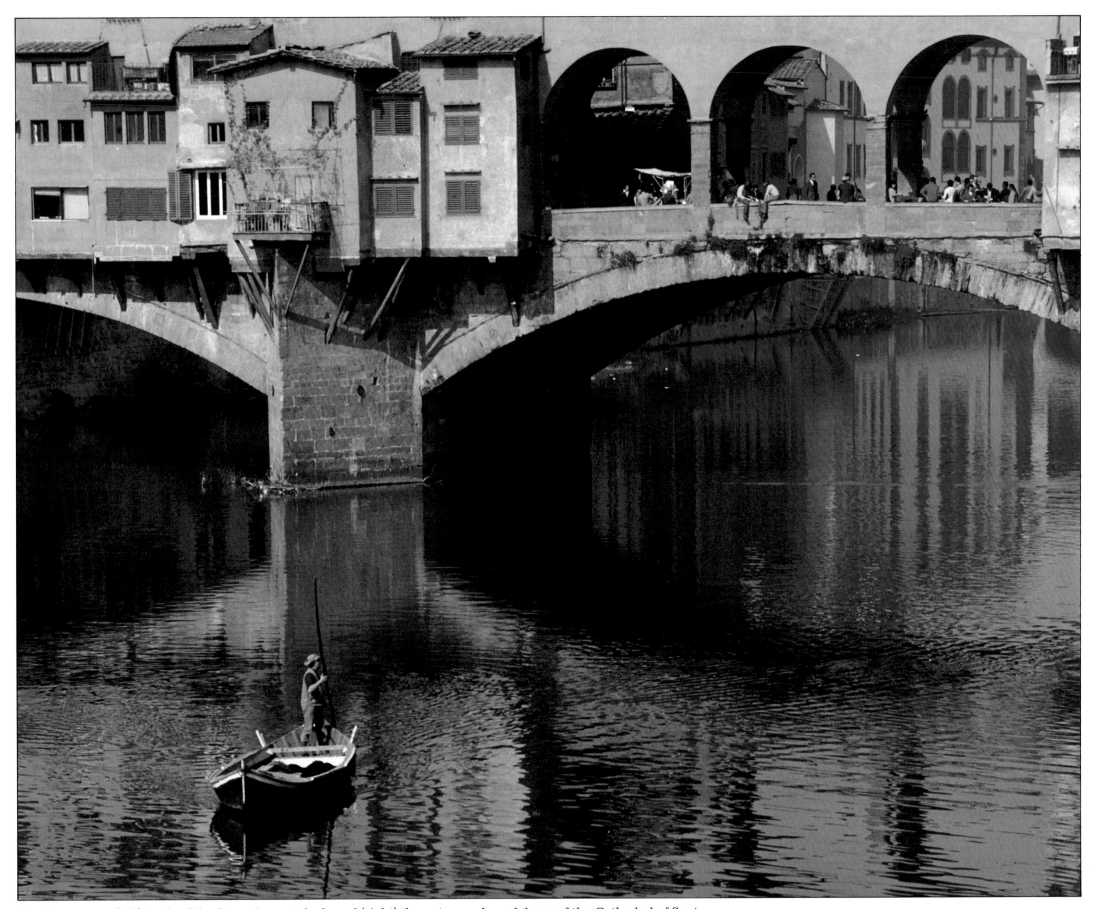

Previous pages: (left) bank of the River Arno at dusk, and (right) the octagon-shaped dome of the Cathedral of Santa Maria del Fiore and the Campanile. Work began on the predominantly Gothic cathedral in 1296 under the direction of the sculptor and architect Arnolfo di Cambio, and continued until 1436. The campanile was built in the 14th century to the design of Giotto, and is faced with bas-reliefs and panels of marble – red from Siena, white from Carrara, and green from Prato. The Ponte Vecchio (these pages), built around 1345 by Neri di Fioravante, is lined with small shops and topped by the Vasari Corridor, which once linked the Palazzo degli Uffizi with the Palazzo Pitti.

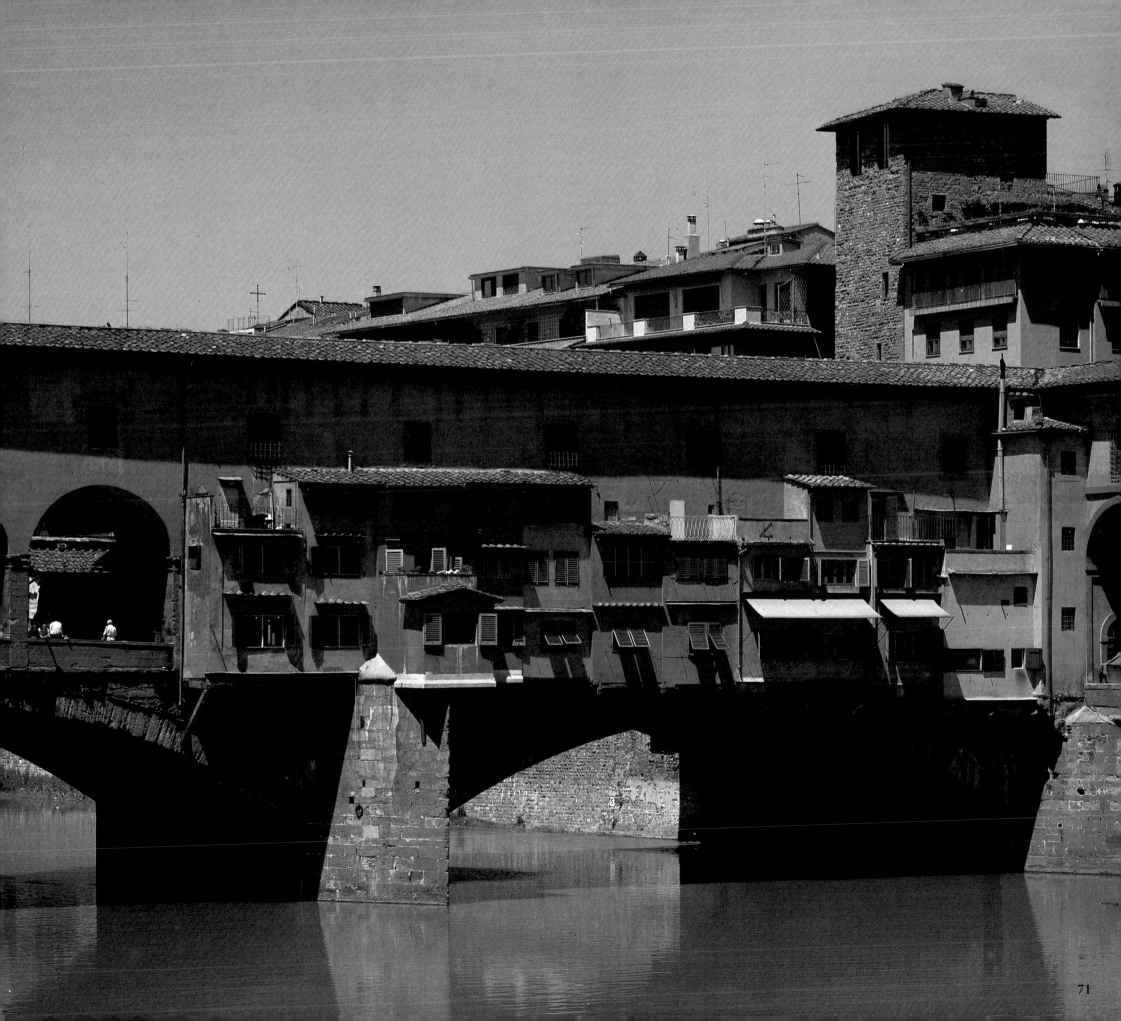

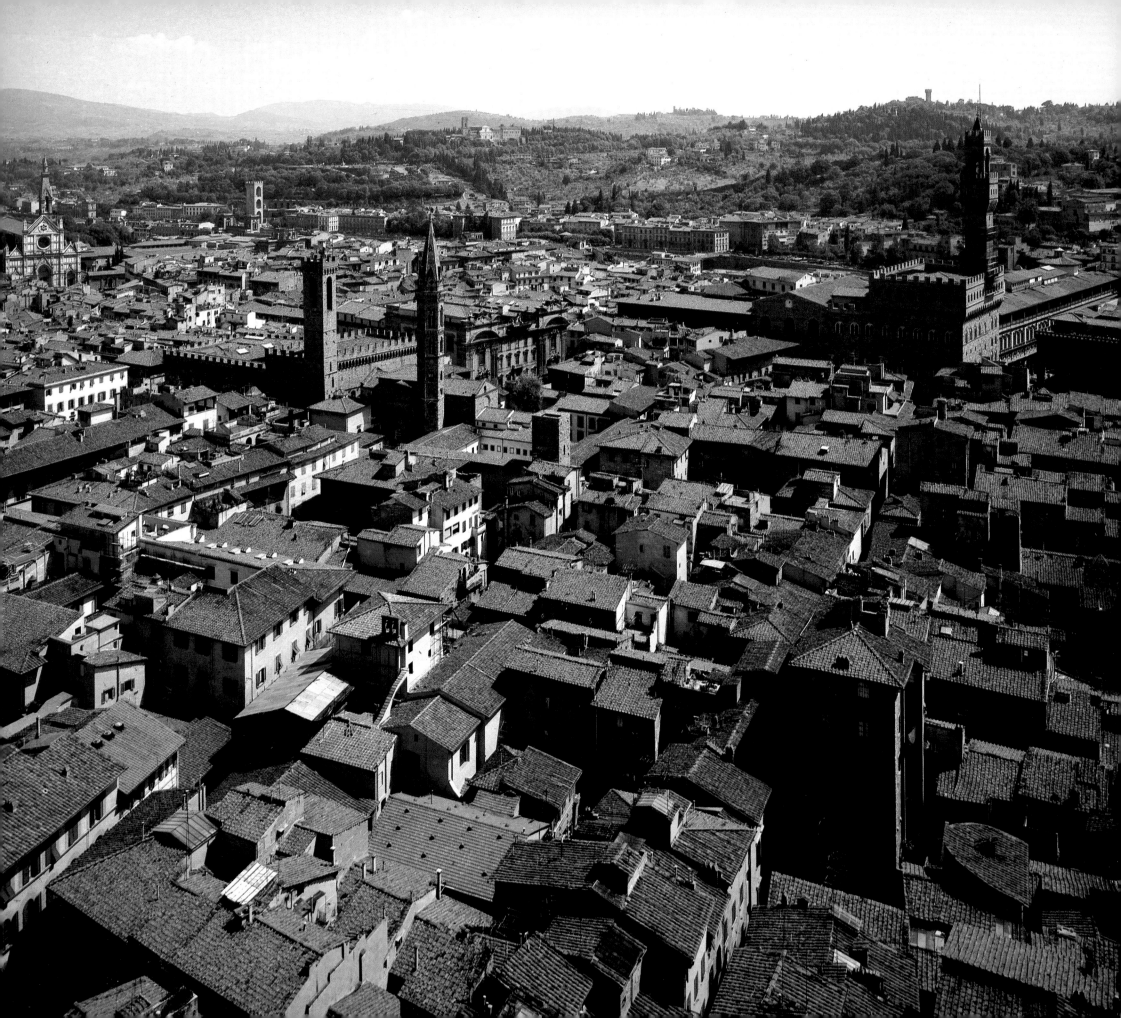

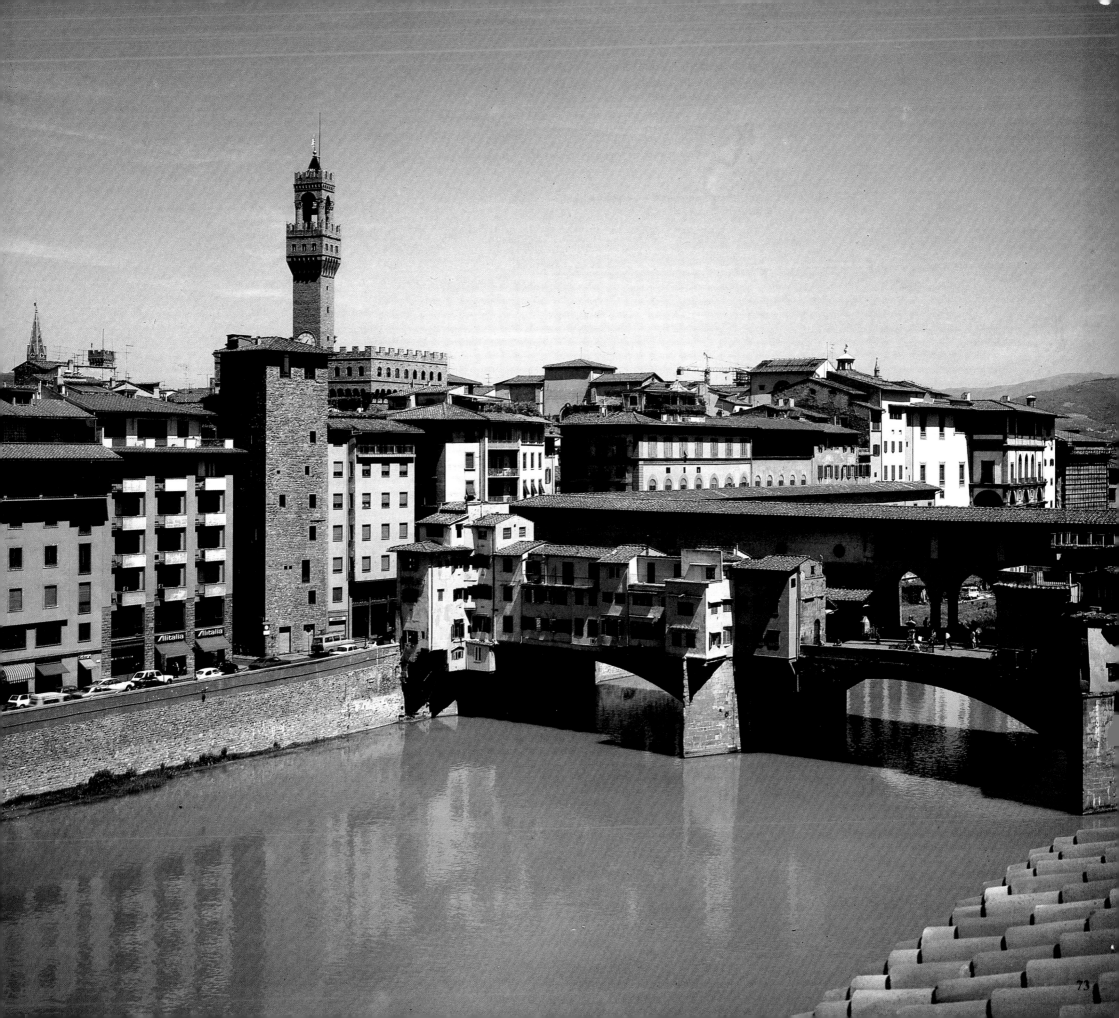

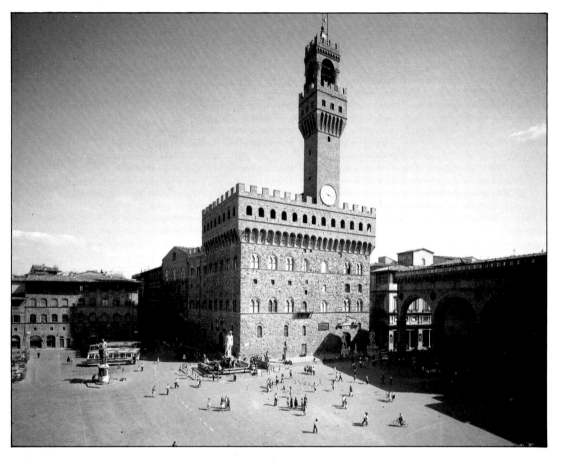

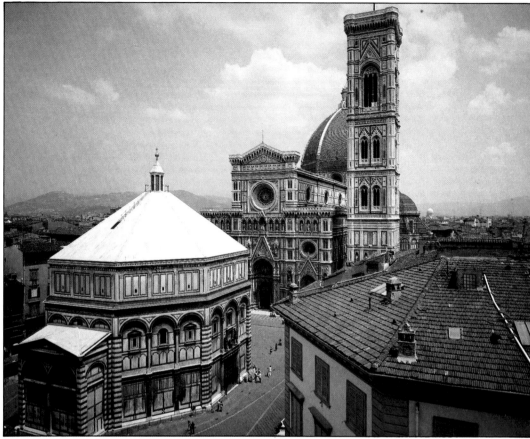

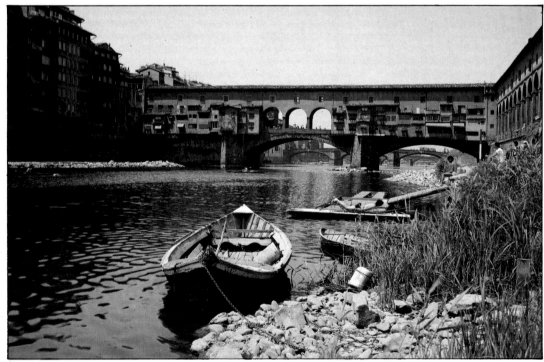

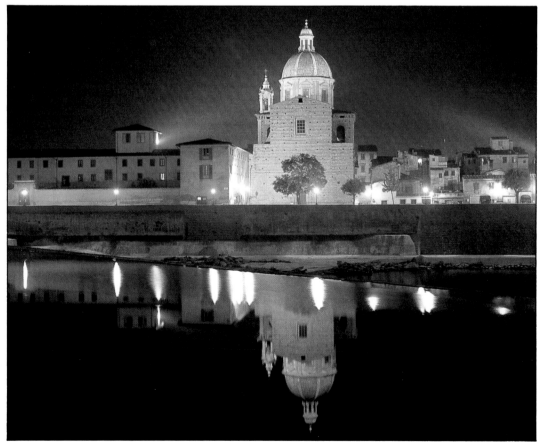

Previous pages: (left) Florence seen from Giotto's campanile. Above, facing page and previous pages, right: the Ponte Vecchio, and (top) Piazza Signoria and the 13th-century Palazzo Vecchio. Top right: 19th-century façade of the Cathedral and the octagonal, Romanesque Baptistry of San Giovanni, built in the 11th-12th centuries. Right: Church of San Frediano in Cestello. Overleaf: (left) Tuscan farm and (right) the Carthusian Monastery near Galluzzo.

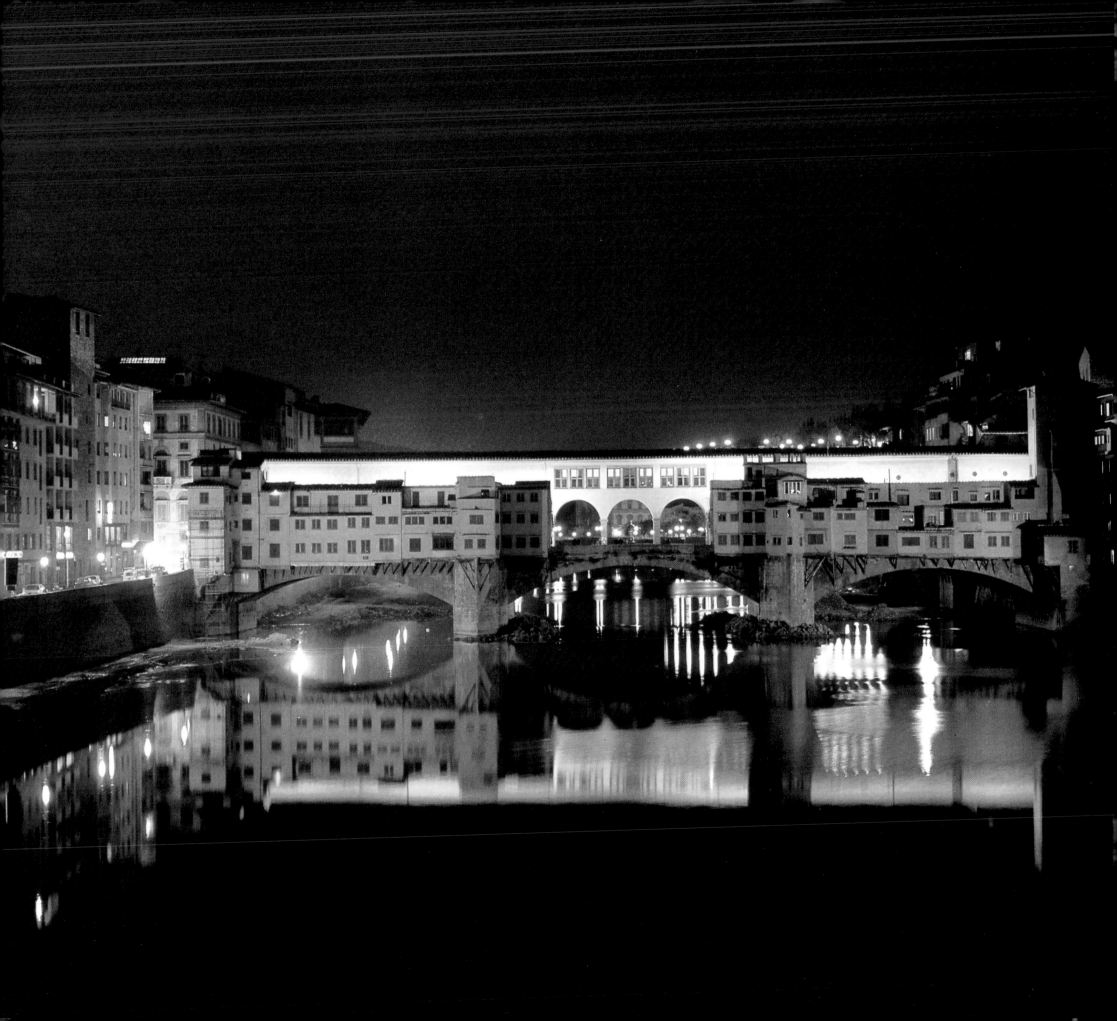

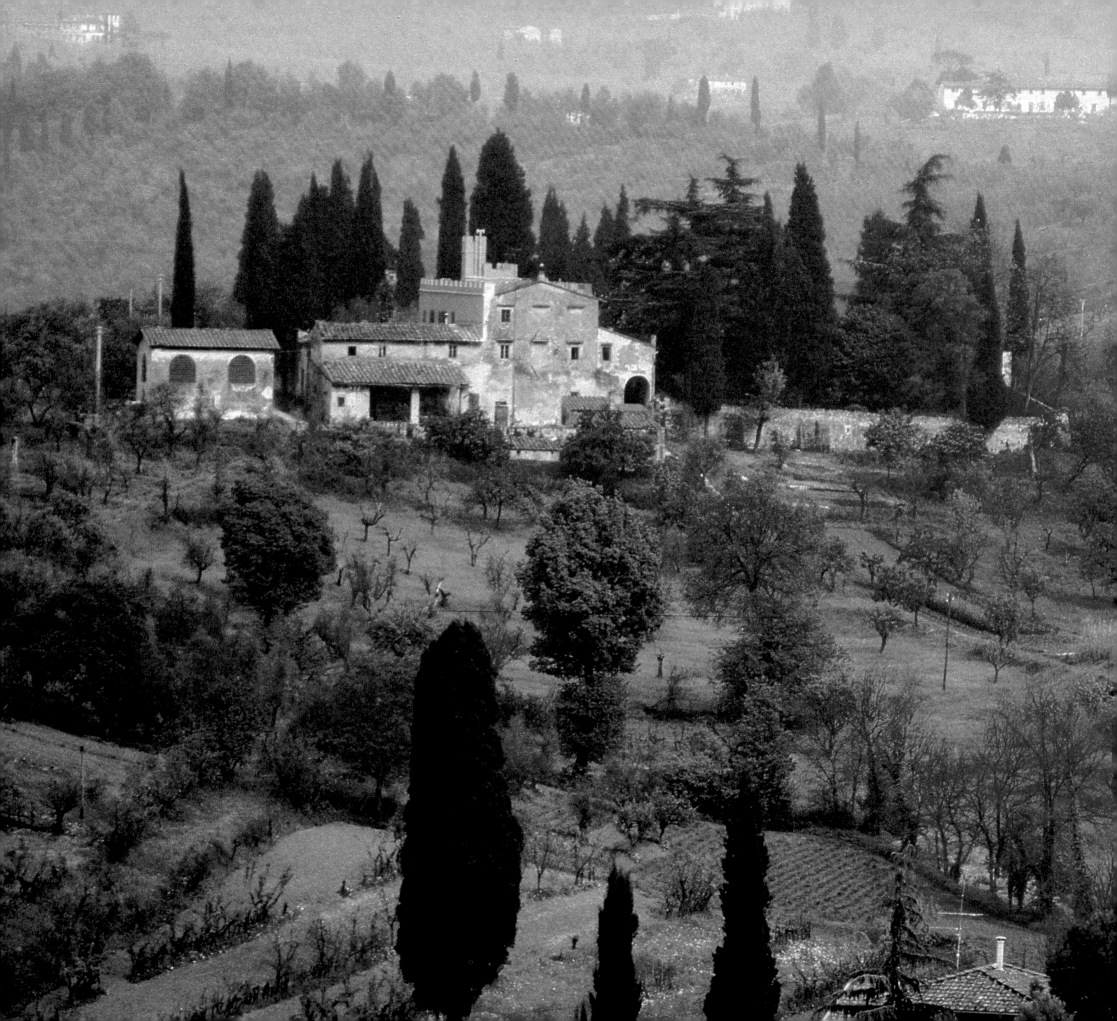

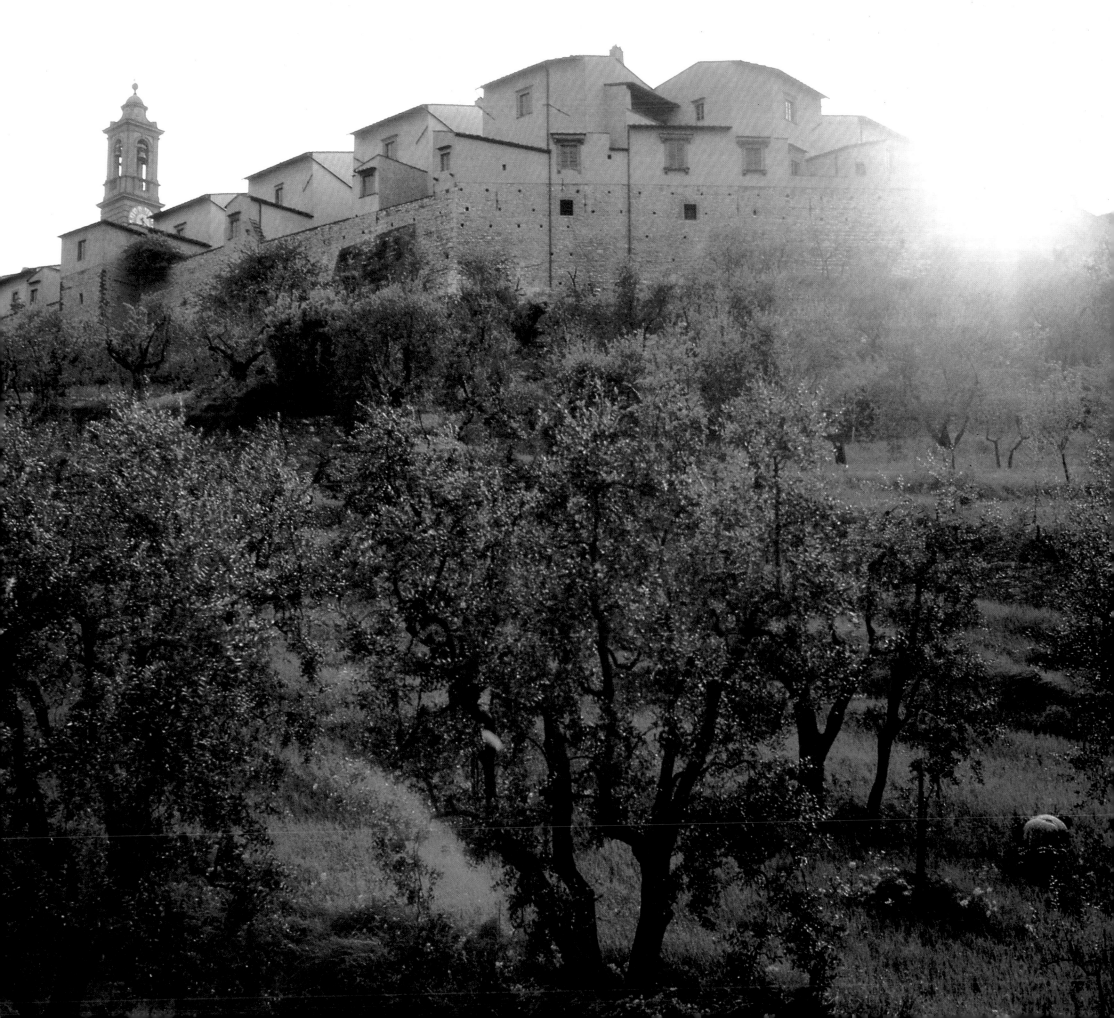

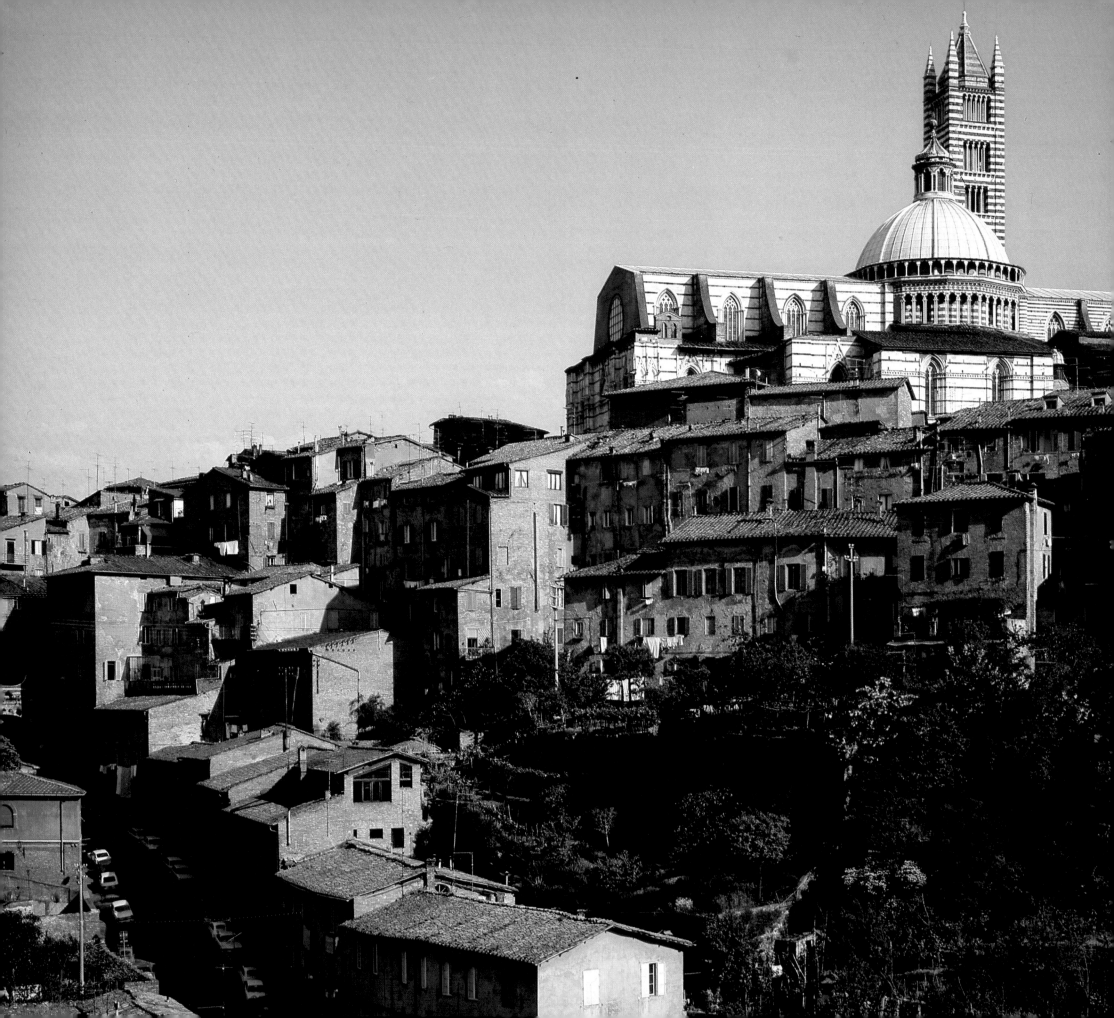

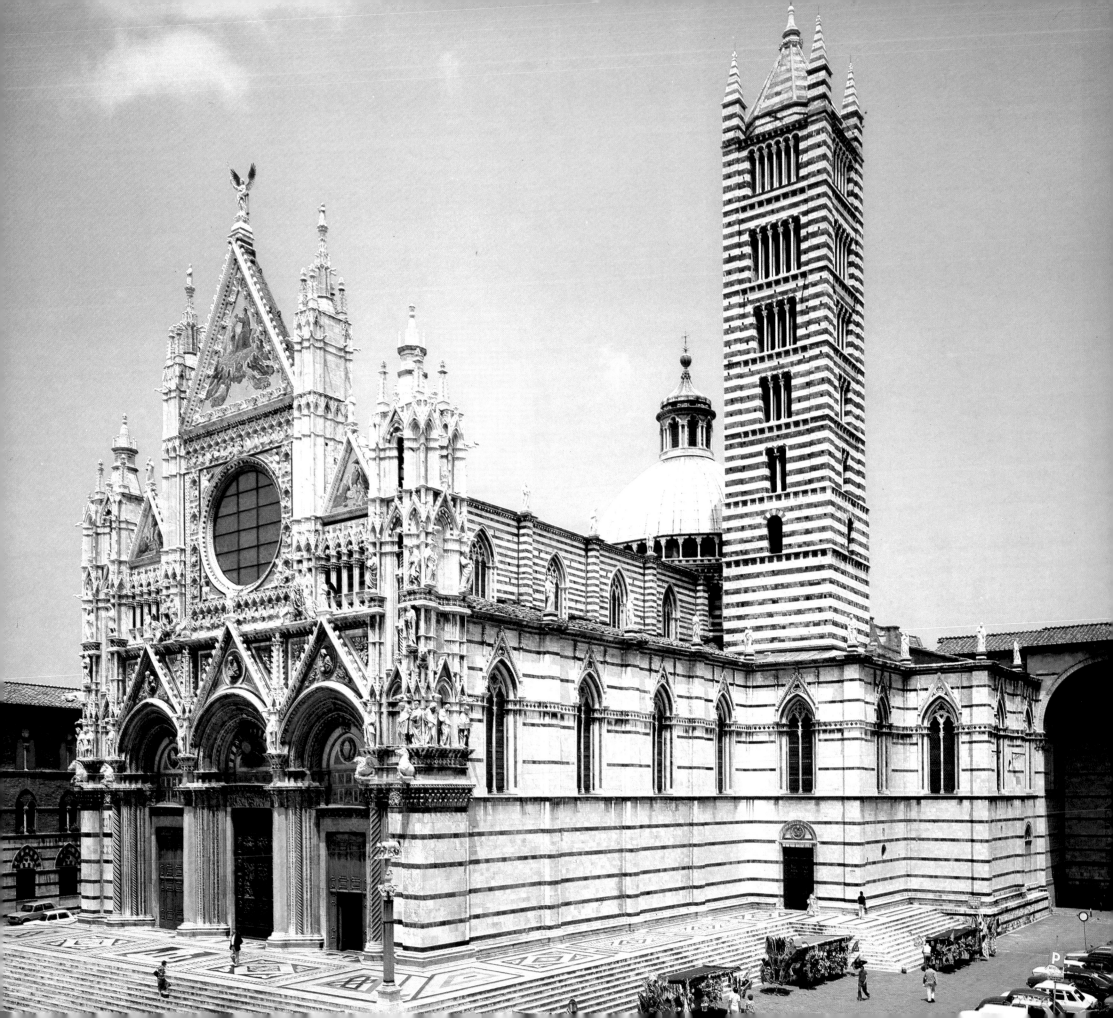

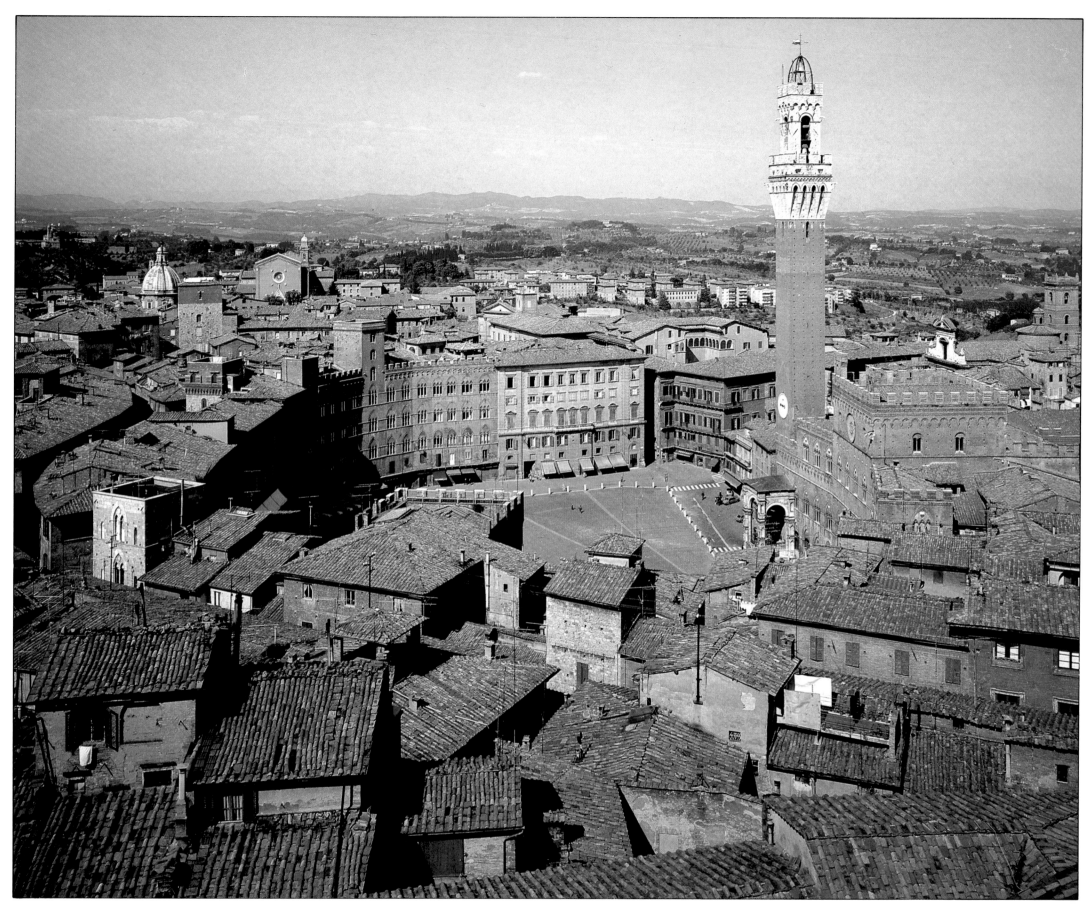

Siena, in the Tuscan hills due south of Florence, has for centuries been a centre of fine Italian art, architecture and learning. The black and white marble layered Cathedral (previous pages) was begun in 1229, and the facade completed in 1380, though the highly ornate carvings and mosaics date from a restoration in the 19th century. Above: Siena's Piazza del Campo and the Palazzo Pubblico. Facing page: a Gothic-style church in the hills near Spoleto. Overleaf: (left) silent cloisters in the monastery of San Domenico in Perugia, and (right) the hill-top town of Trevi, Umbria.

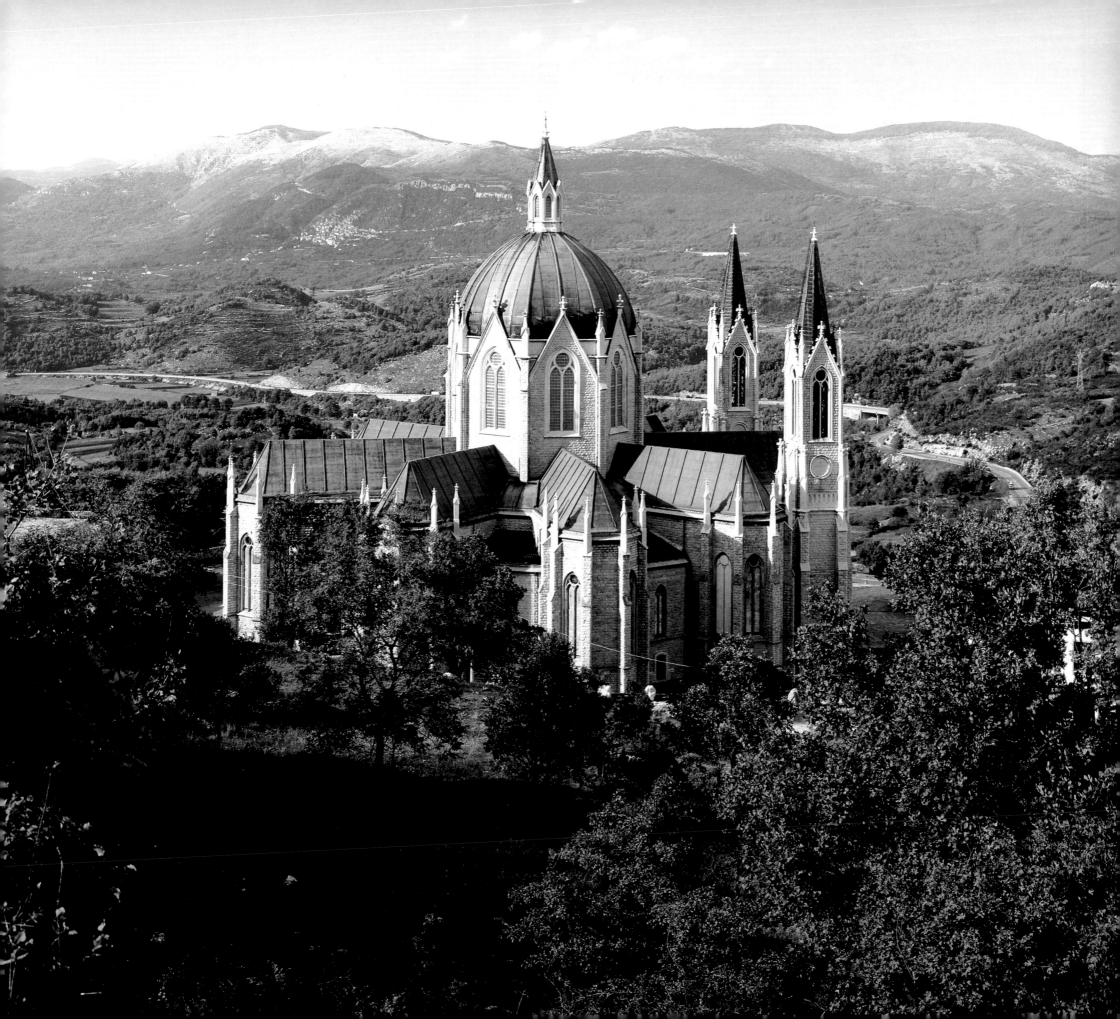

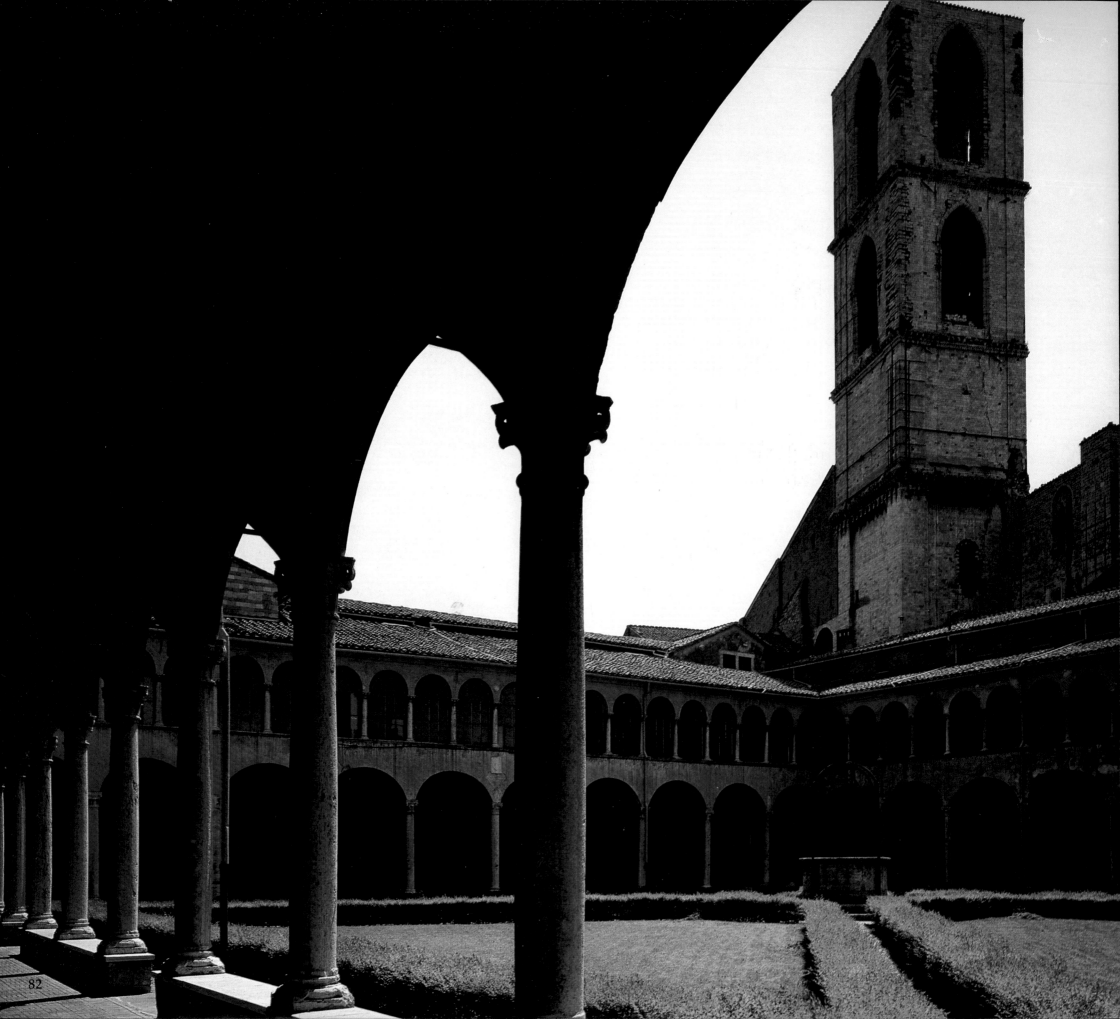

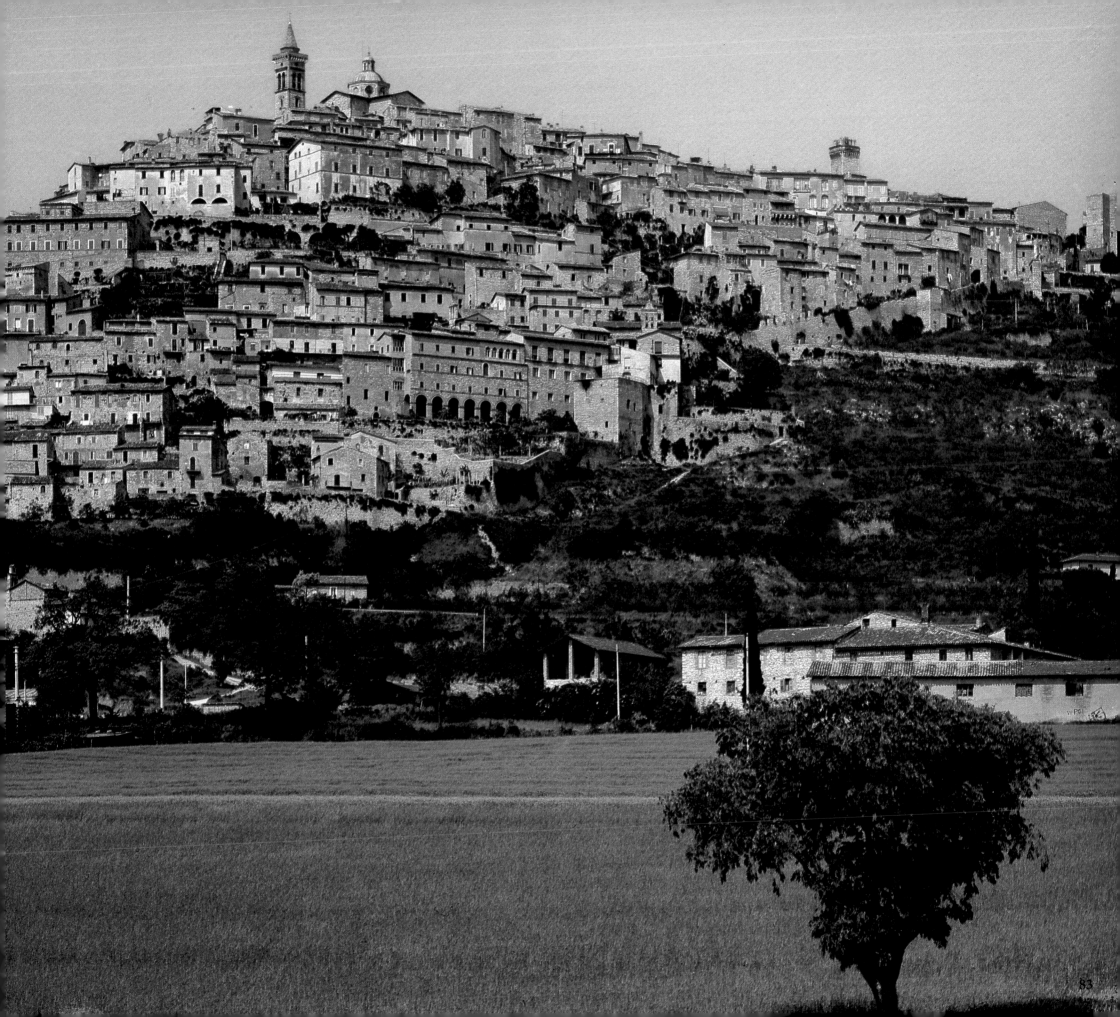

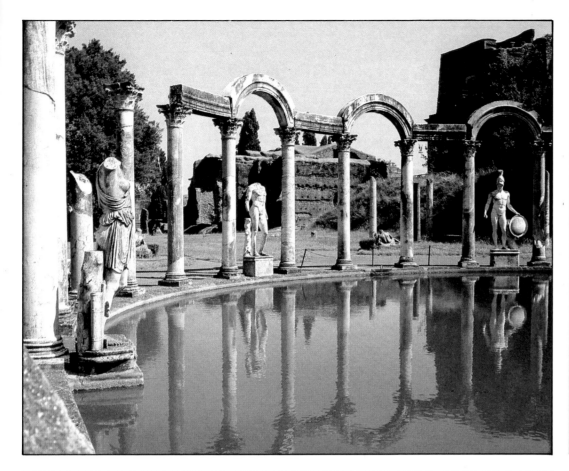

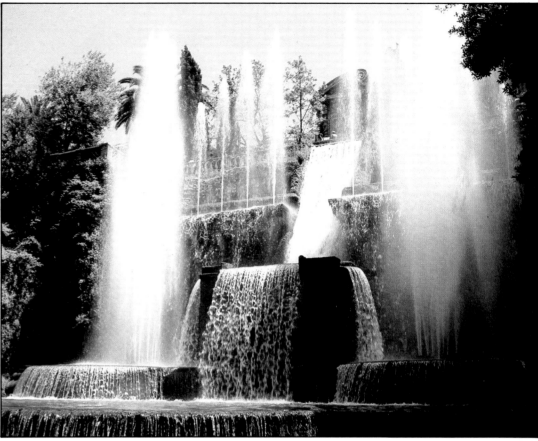

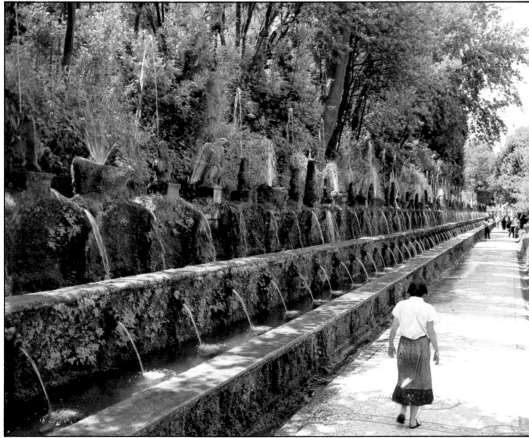

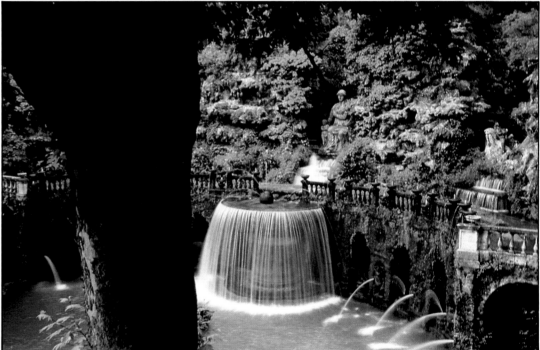

Grottoes and fountains, (top and left) in the gardens of the Villa D'Este, Tivoli, and (facing page) in Rome, at the Trevi Fountain. Top left: still water at Hadrian's Villa, Tivoli. Overleaf: (left) the Colosseum, begun by Vespasian in AD 75. The triple Arch of Septimius Severus (right) has survived almost intact among the ruins of the Roman Forum, backed by the Palazzo Senatorio and the white, Brescia marble National Monument to Victor Emmanuel II.

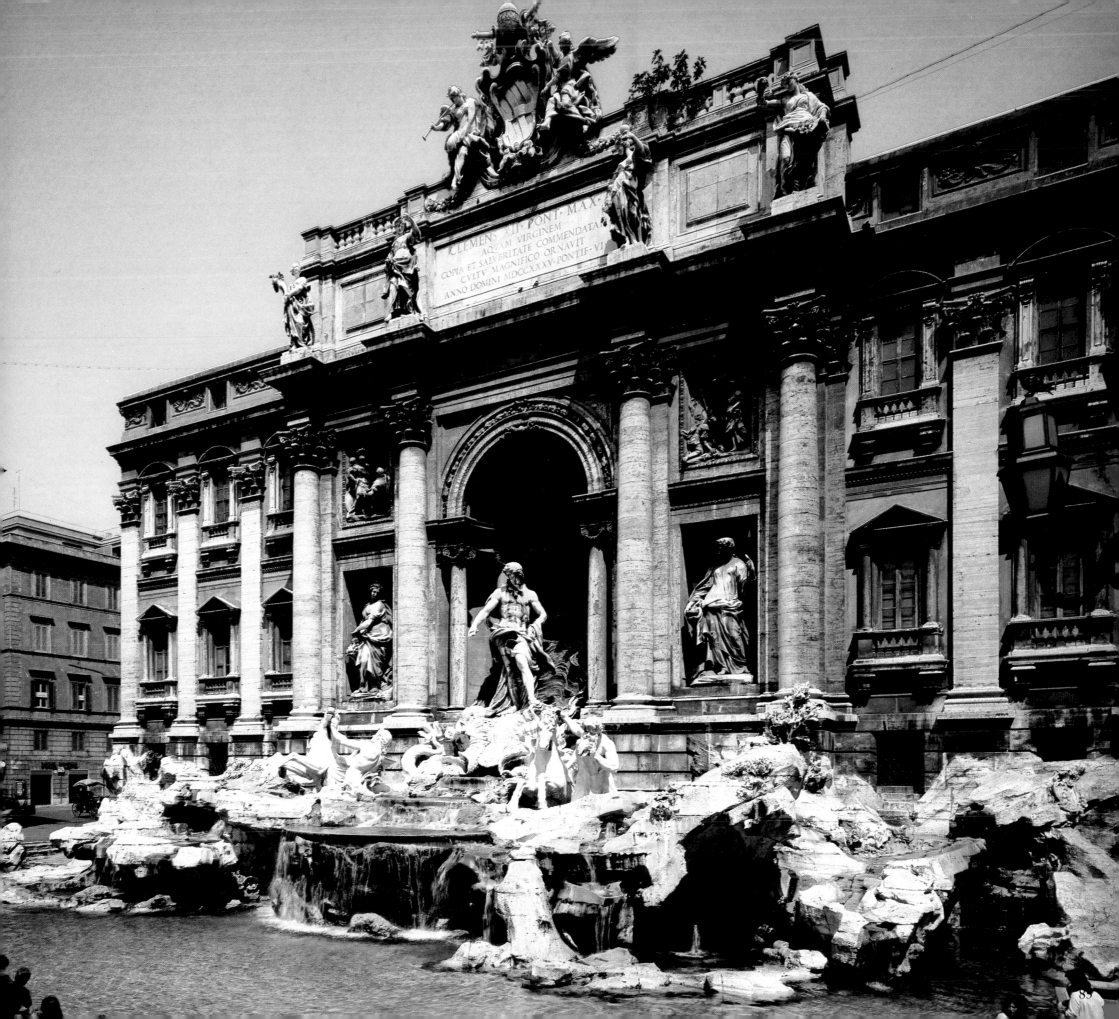

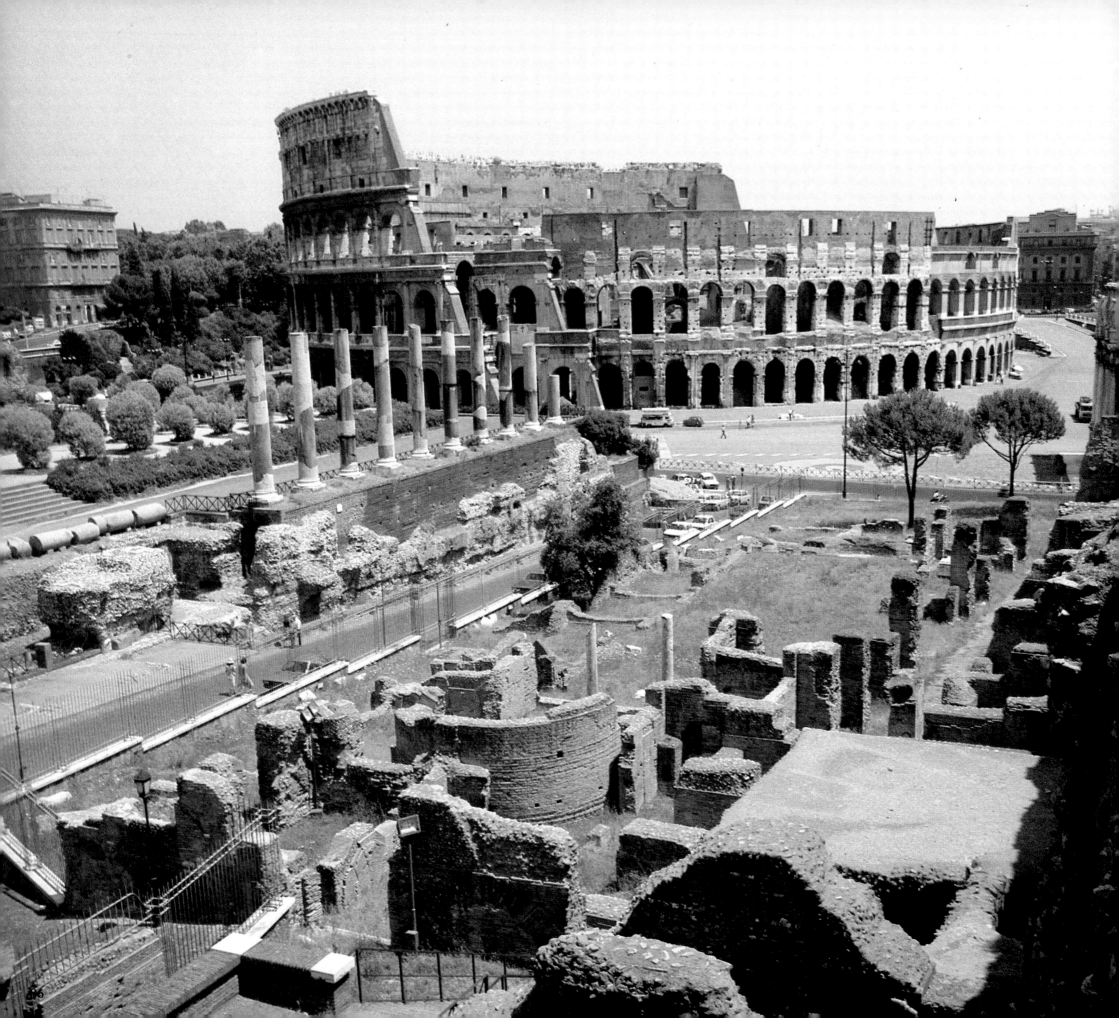

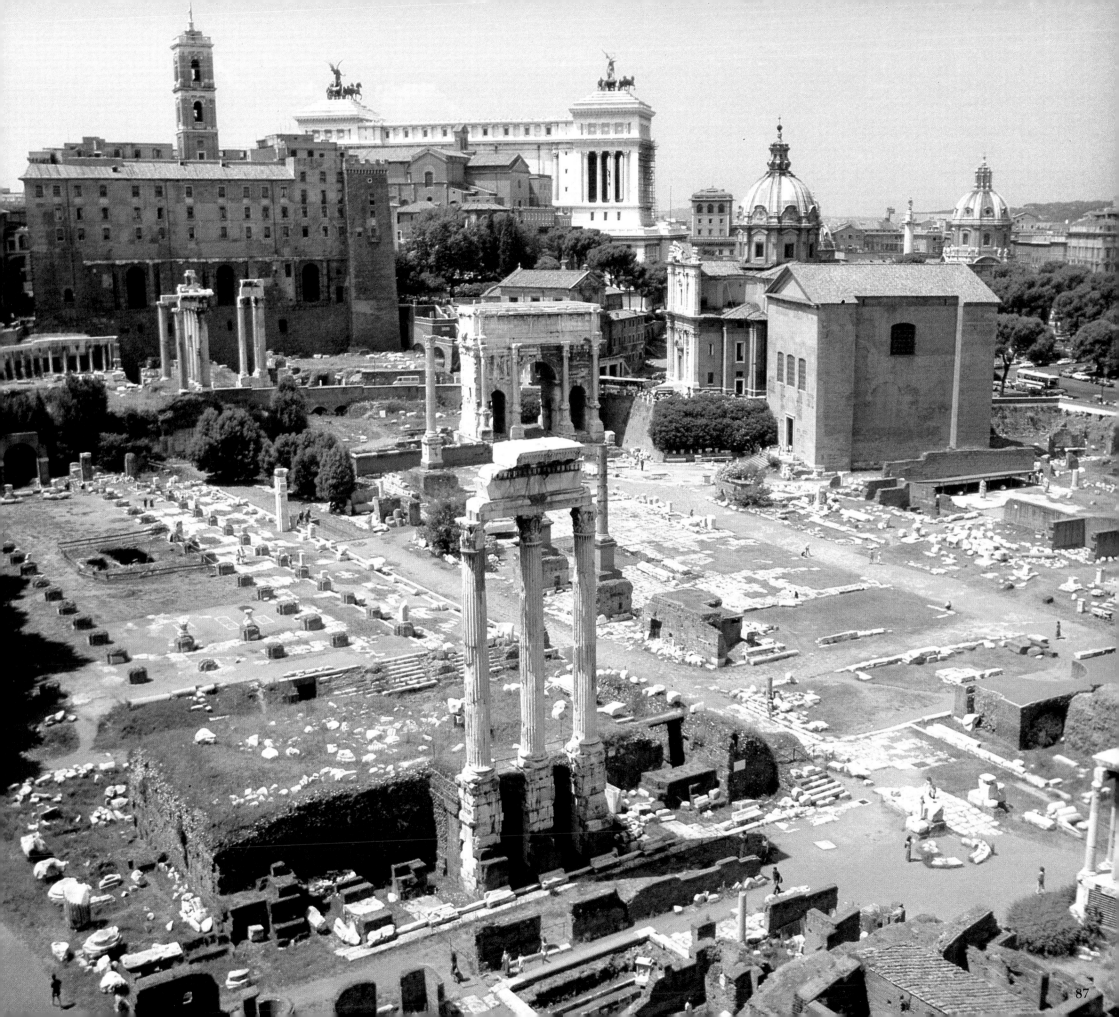

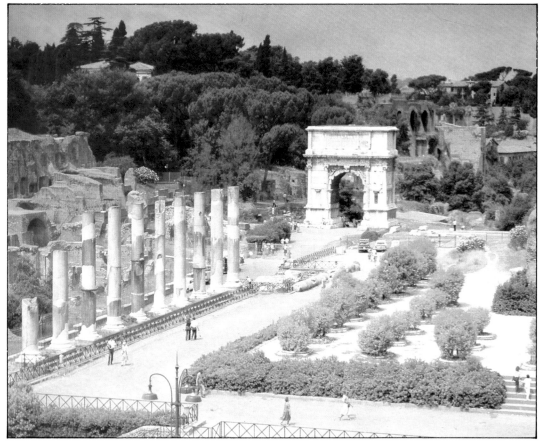

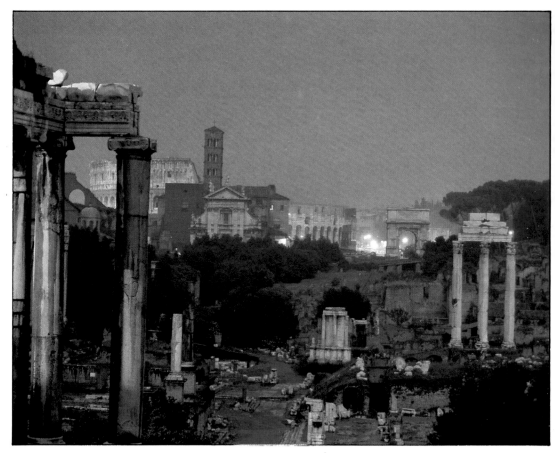

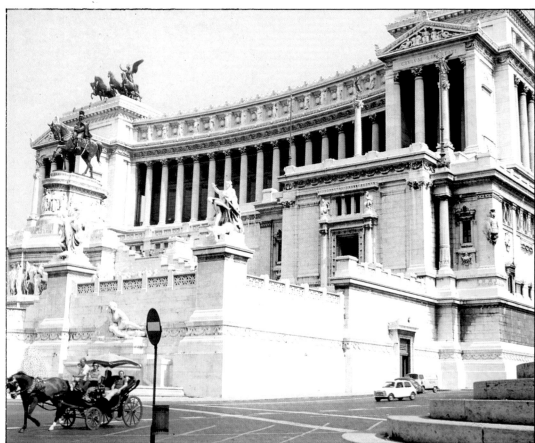

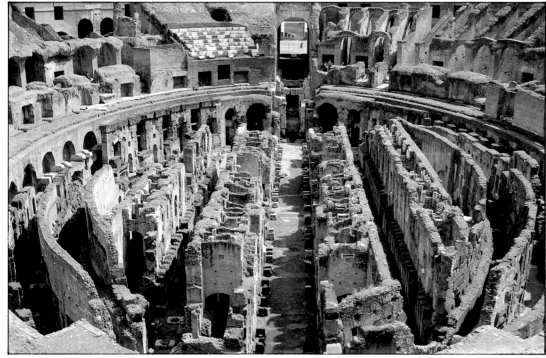

The Arch of Titus (top left), beyond the ruined temples of Vespasianus and Castor and Pollux (top), was erected to commemorate the capture of Jerusalem in AD 70. Left: the National Monument to Victor Emmanuel II, and (above) substructures beneath the Colosseum arena. Facing page: the triumphal Arch of Constantine, built in celebration of his victory over Maxentius at the Milvian Bridge, AD 312.

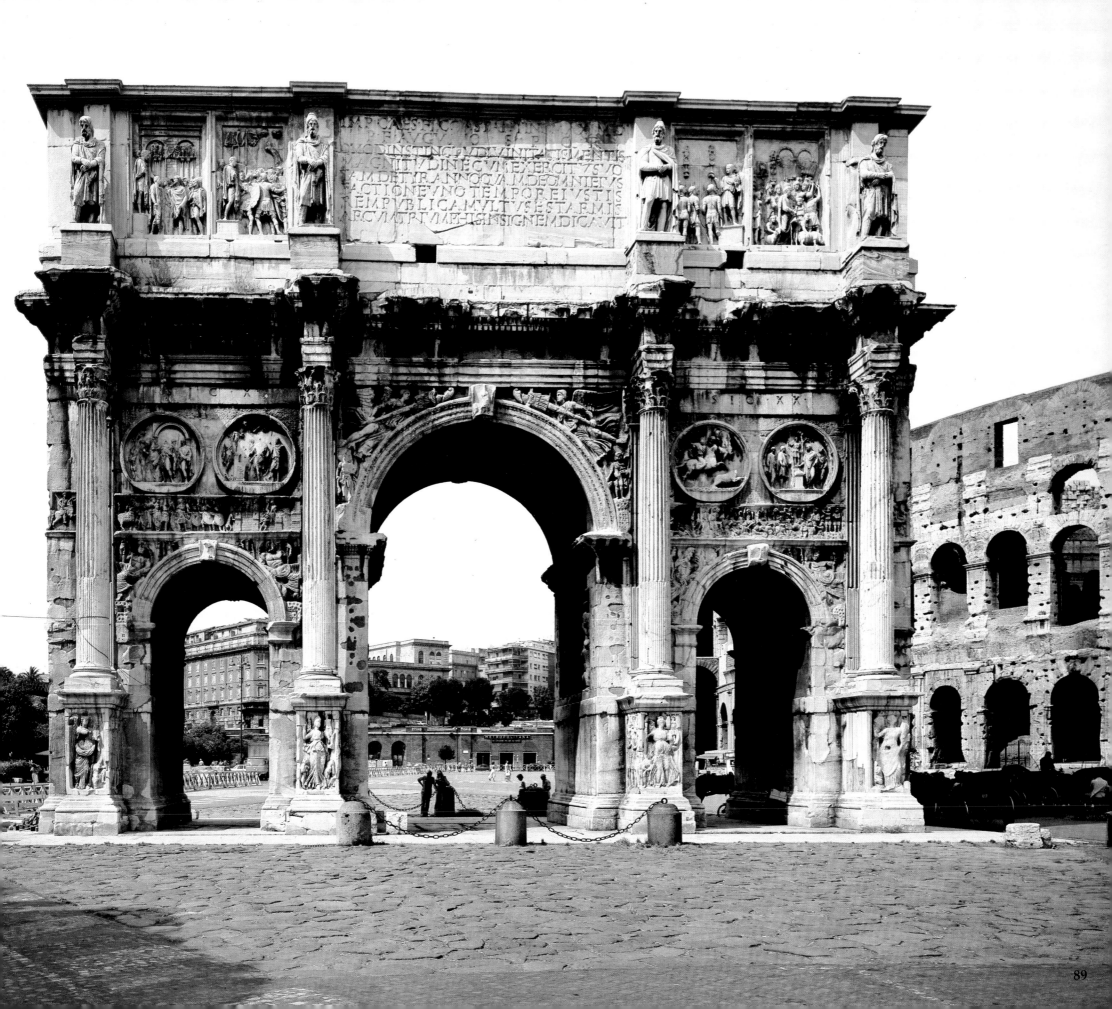

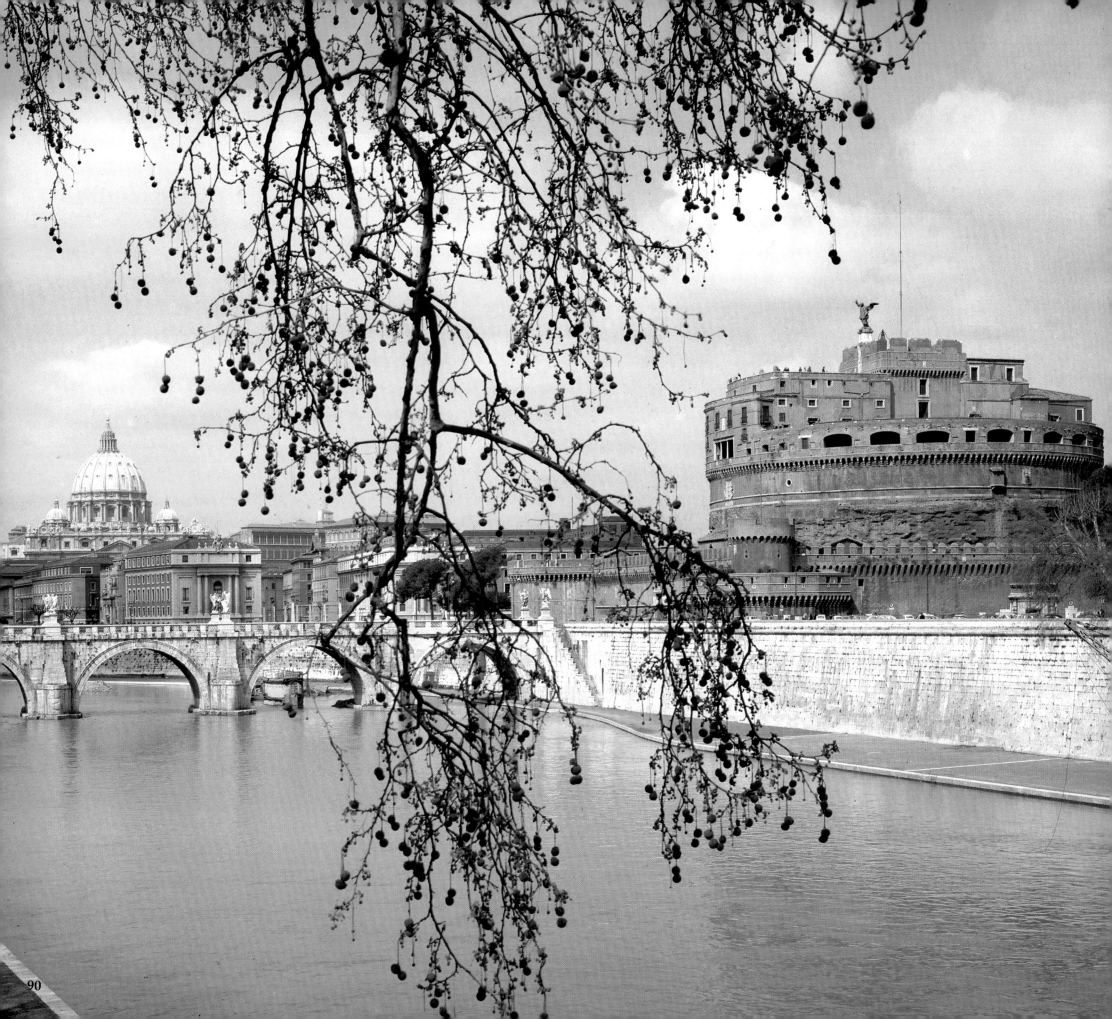

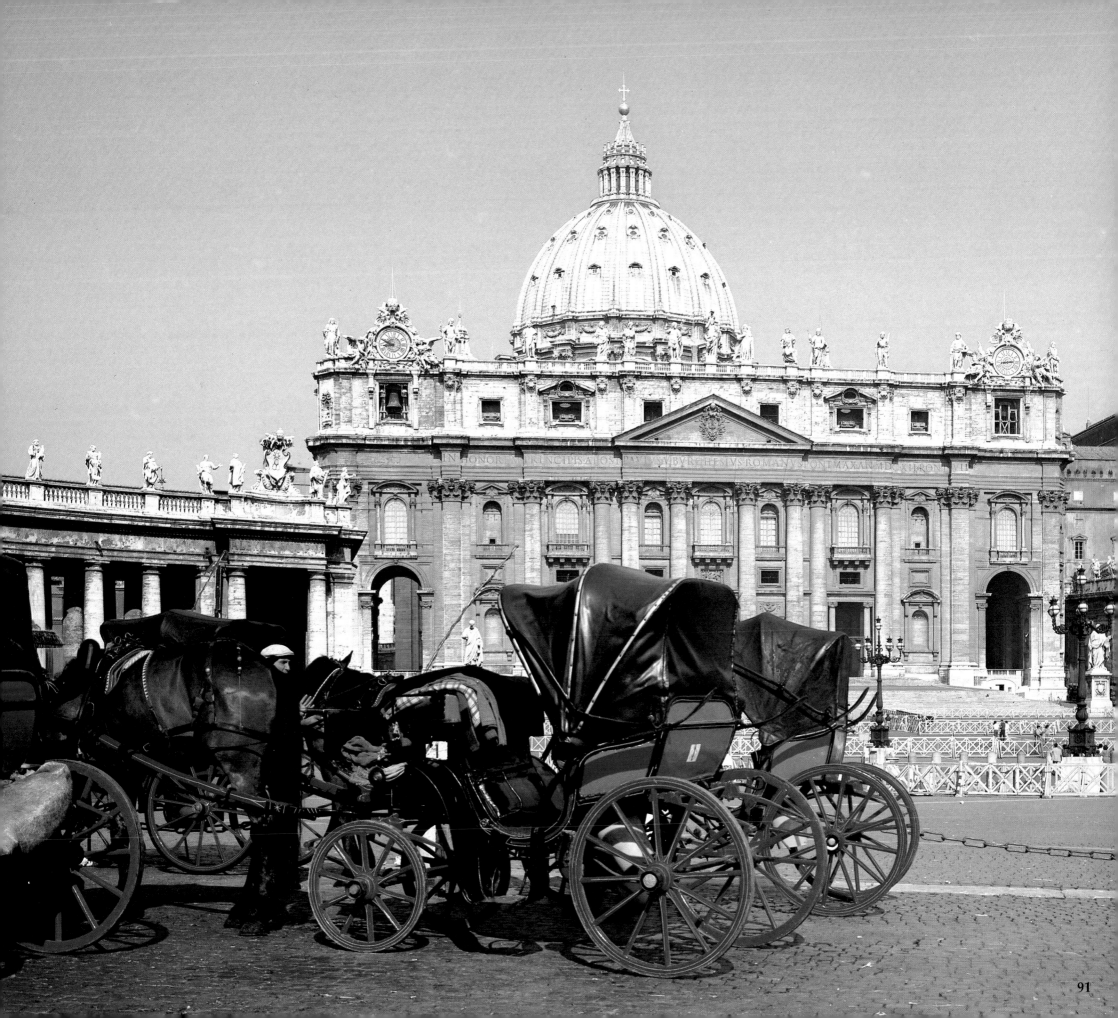

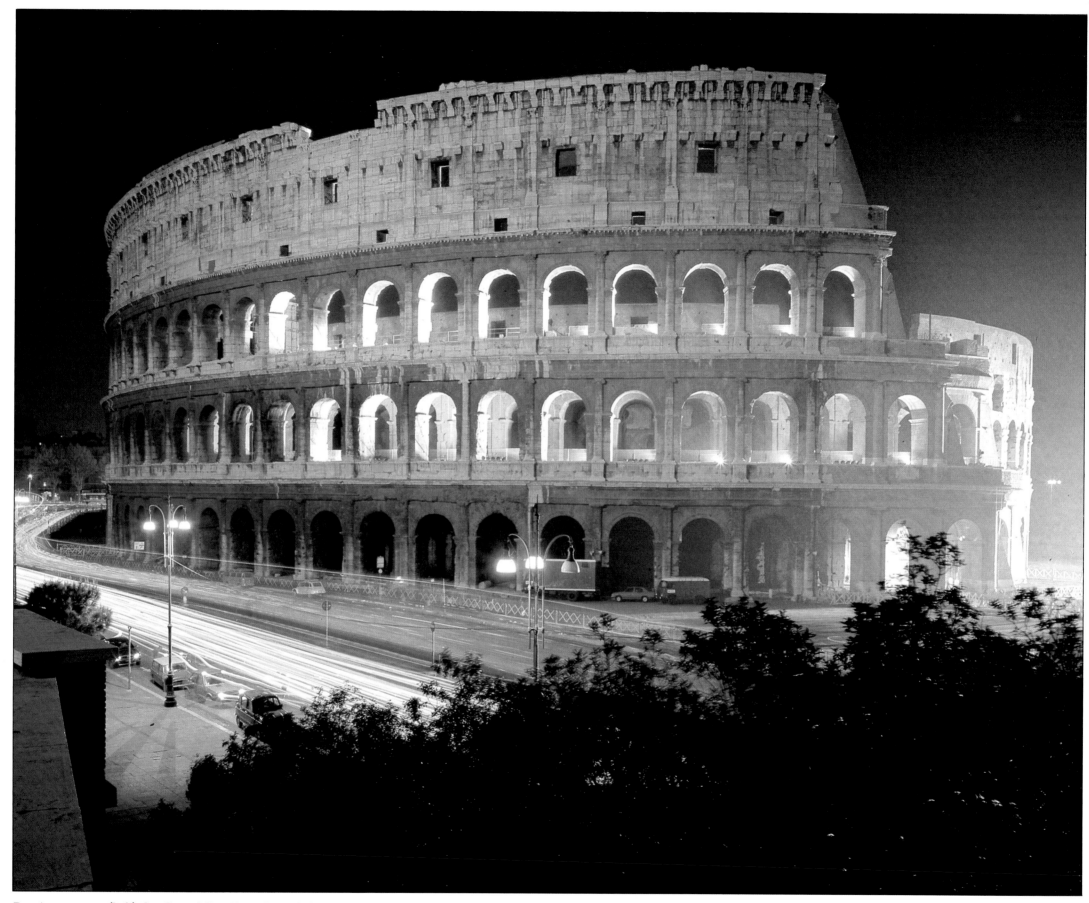

Previous pages: (left) the Castel Sant'Angelo and the Basilica of St Peter beyond the River Tiber and (right) the Baroque facade of St Peter's, which was completed in 1614. Above: the floodlit northeastern side of the Colosseum, which still retains all four storeys. Originally titled the Flavian Amphitheatre, the arena was inaugurated by Titus in AD 80 in celebrations lasting 100 days and involving 1,000 gladiators and 5,000 animals. Facing page: the three Corinthian columns of the Temple Vespasianus, and the well-preserved, Ionic Temple of Saturne.

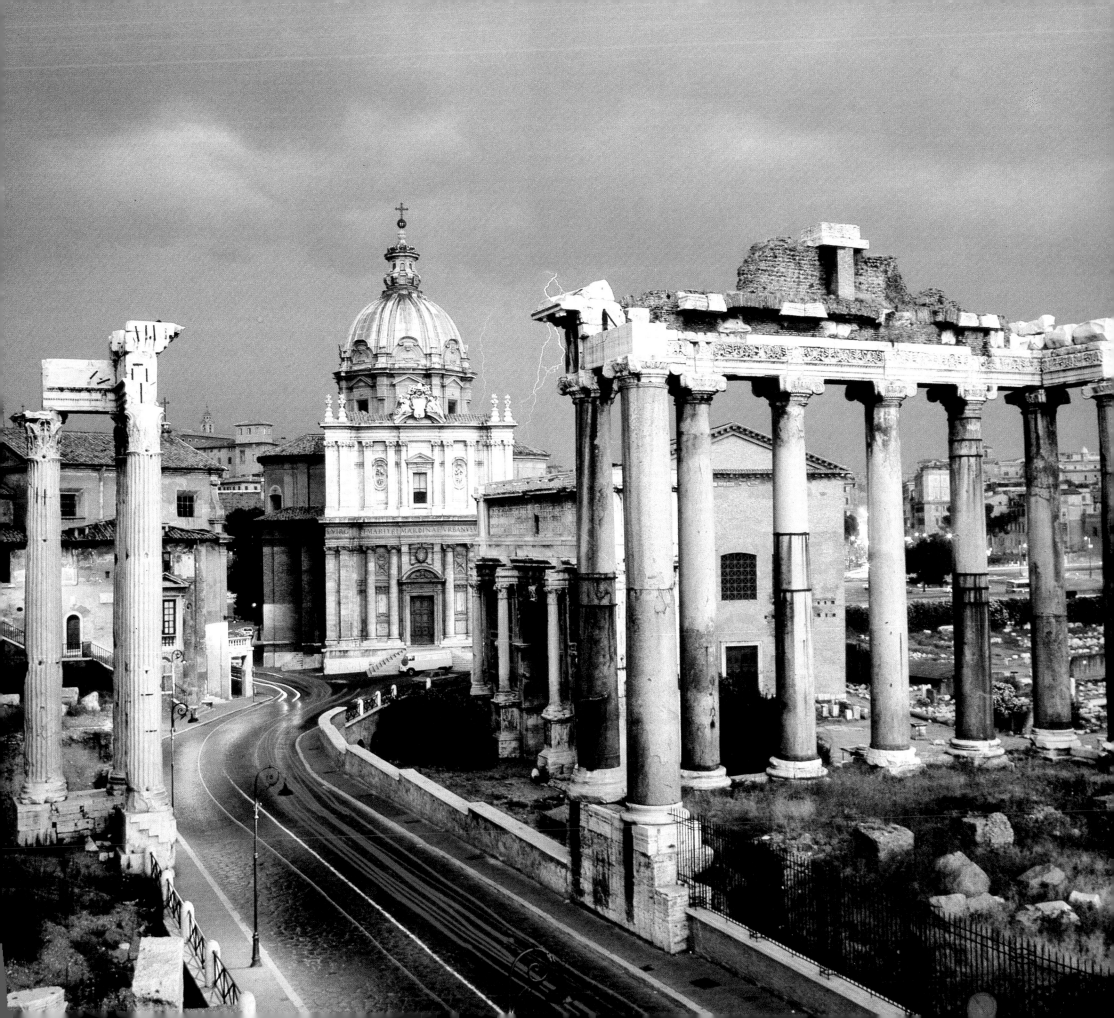

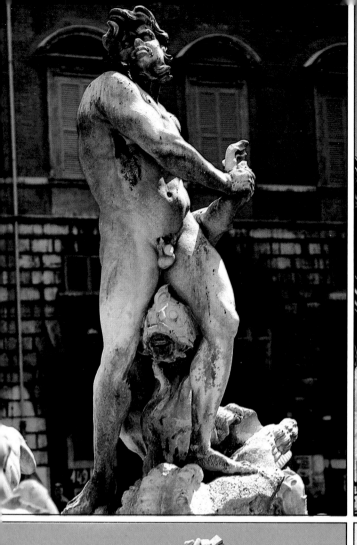
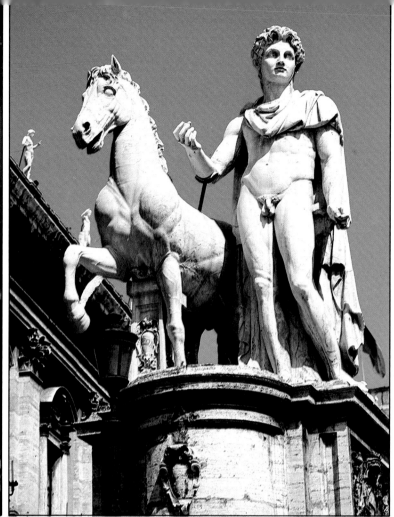
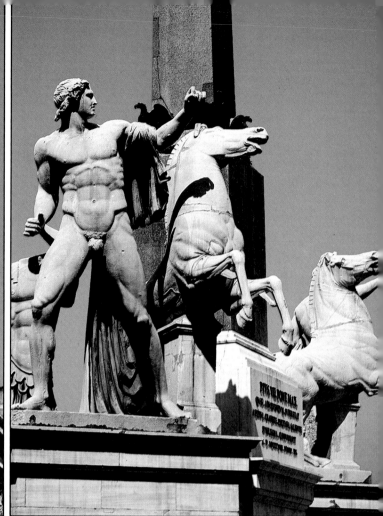
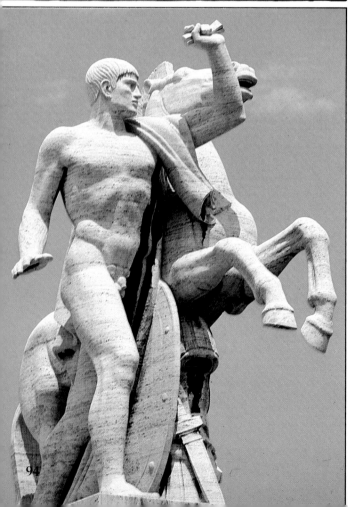
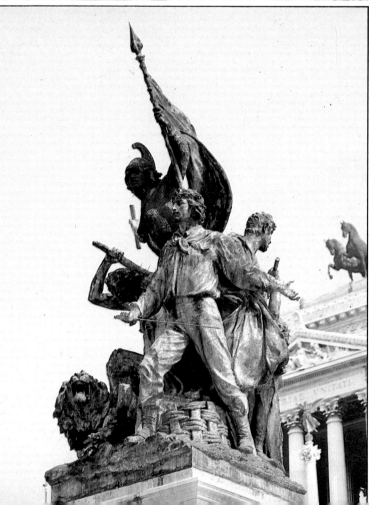
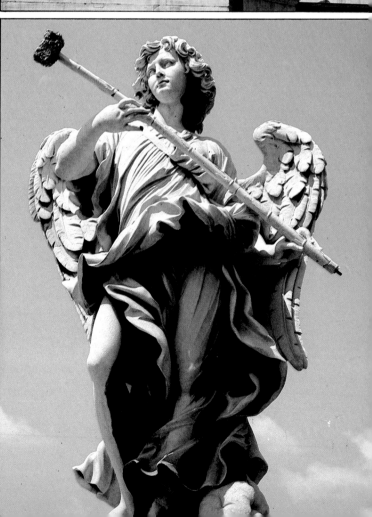

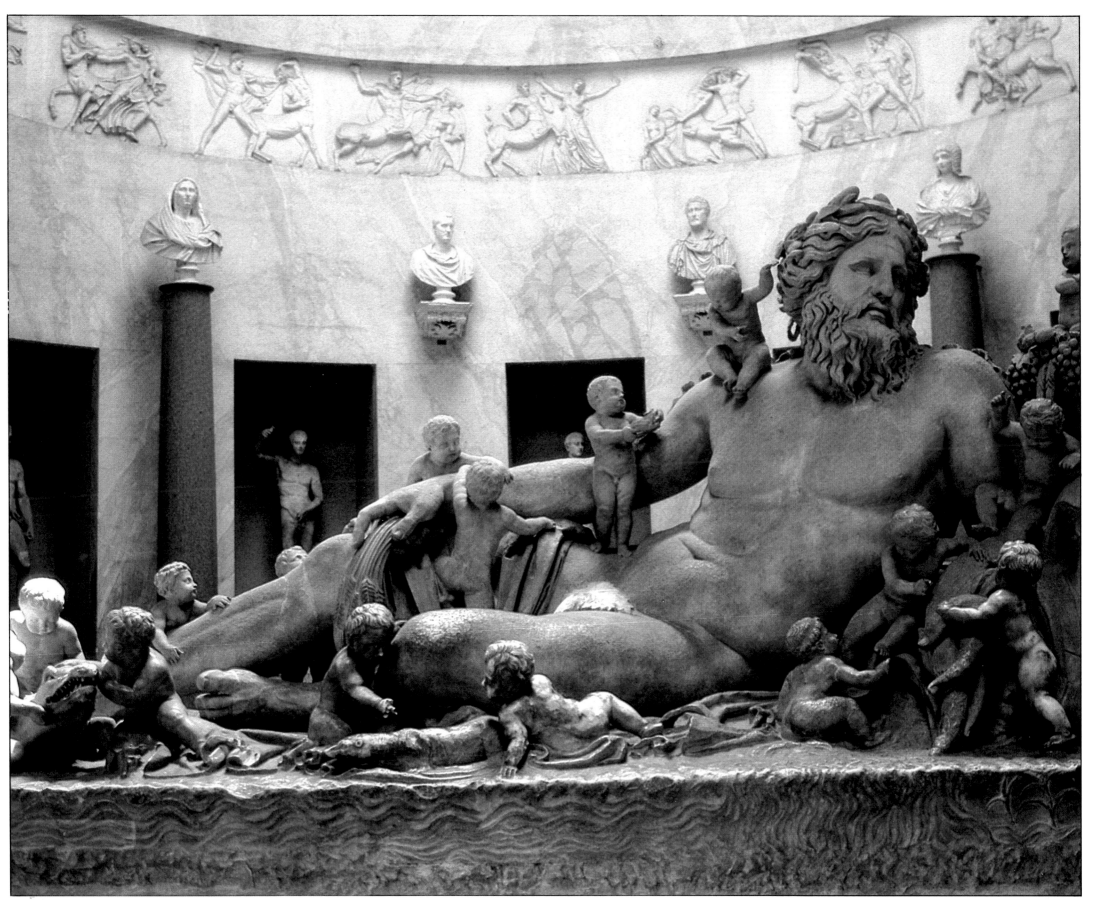

Facing page: (top left) the central figure of the Fountain of the Moor, in Navona Square. Centre top: one of the
colossal groups of the Dioscuri, the twin gods Castor and Pollux, which stand at the top of Michelangelo's
Cordonata. (Top right) monument erected in honour of Pope Pius VII, and (bottom right) one of ten angels adorning
the Ponte San Angelo. (Bottom centre) statue at the base of the National Monument to Victor Emmanuel II and (bottom
left) a statue in the Palazzo della Civilta dei Lavoro. Above: 'The Nile' in the Chiaramonti Musuem in the Vatican.
Overleaf: (left) St Peter's Square, Vatican City, and (right) the cupola of St Peter's.

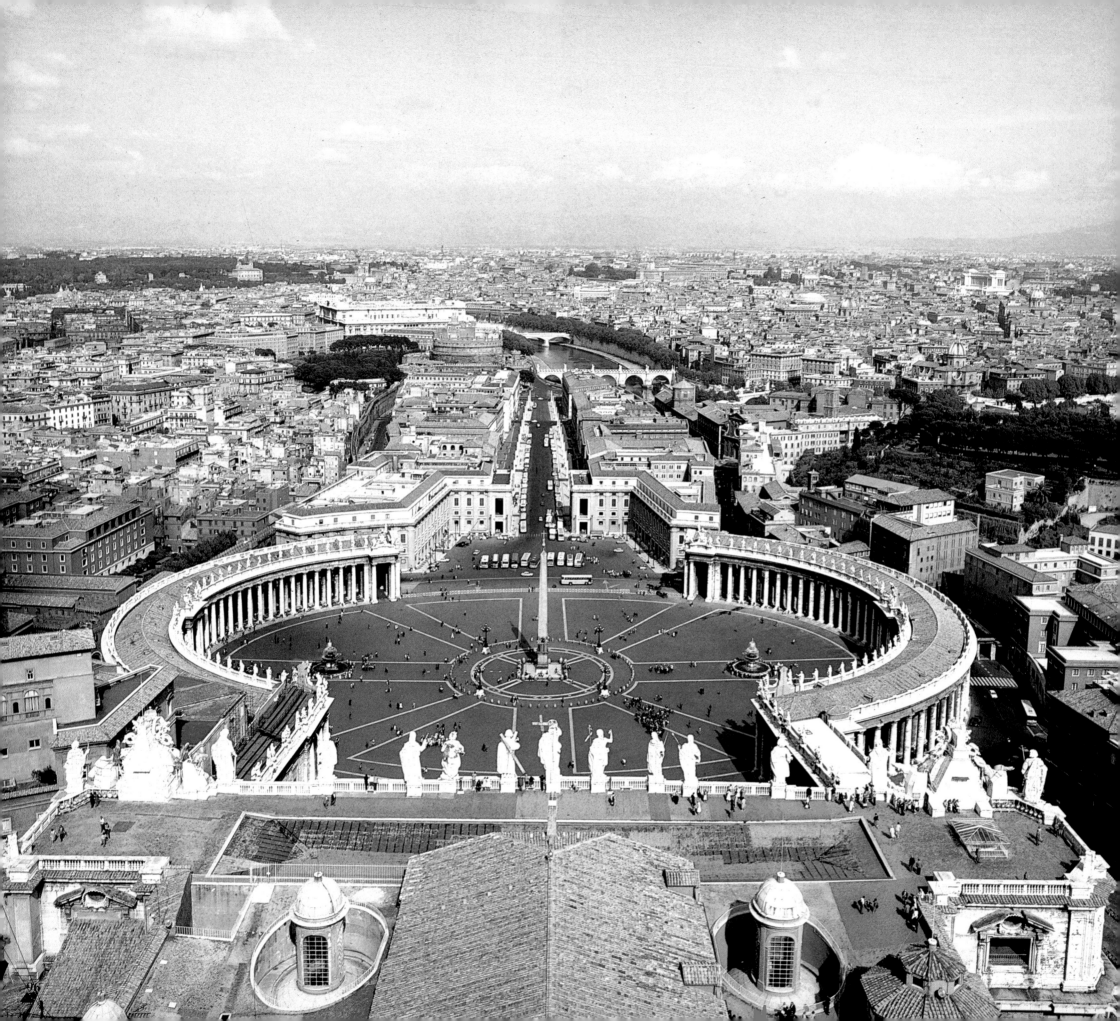

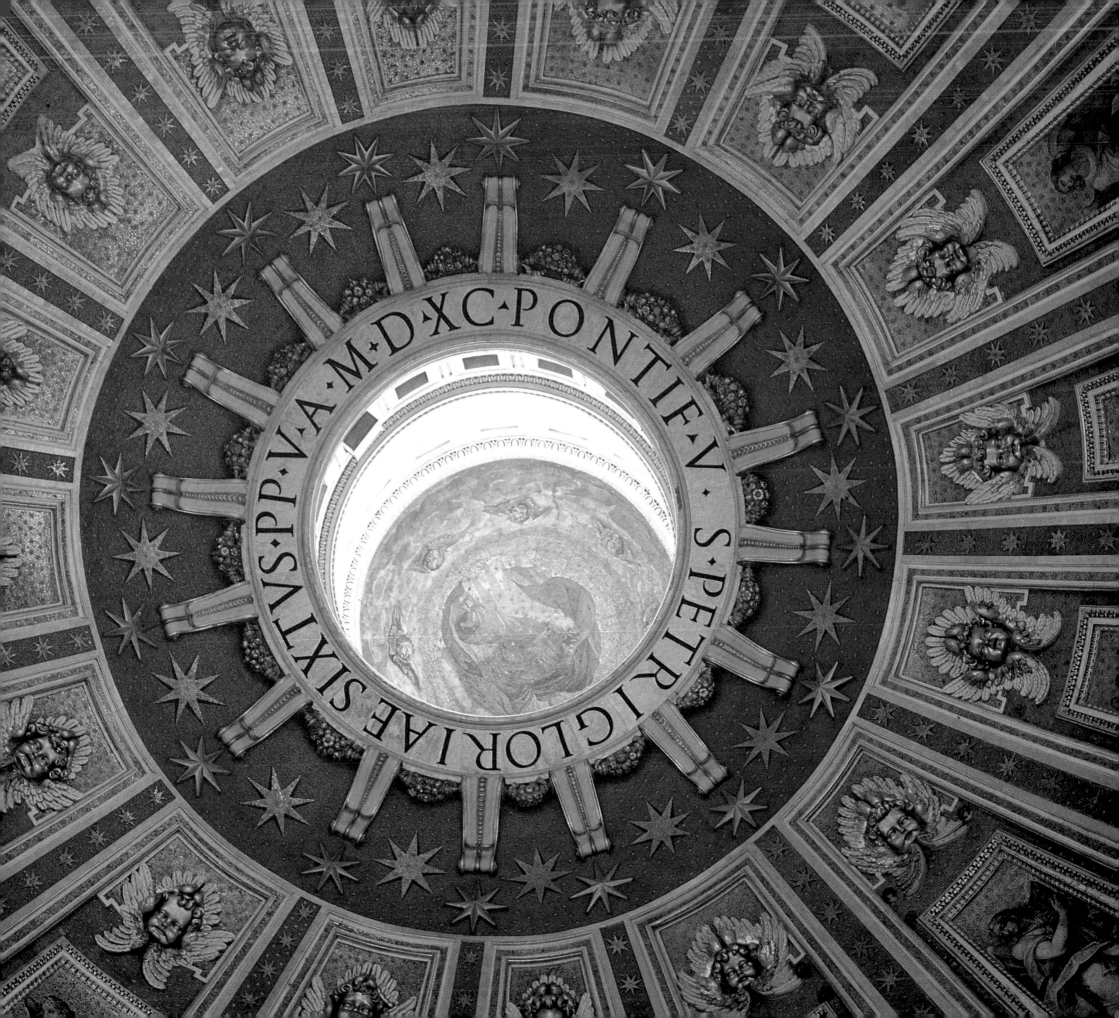

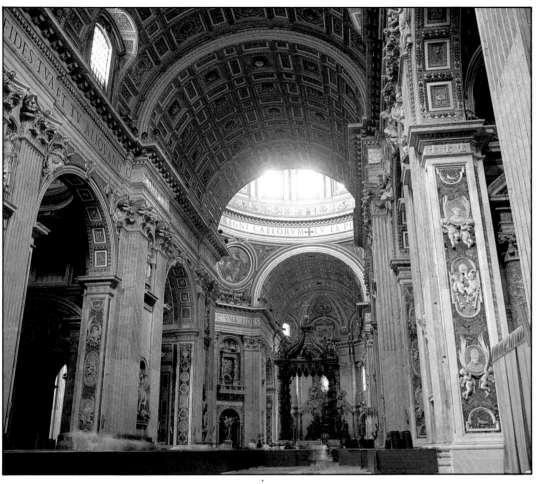

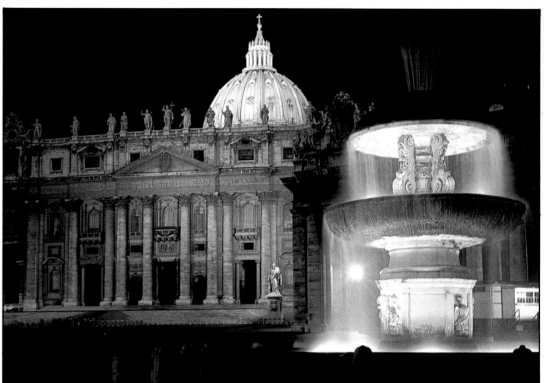

Left: the Bronze Canopy, seen through the nave of the St Peter's (below). Bottom and bottom left: Bernini's vast Colonnade, enclosing St Peter's Square and the facade of St Peter's (facing page). Overleaf: (left) Fountain of Neptune, and (right) the Fountain of the Moor, in the Piazza Navona.

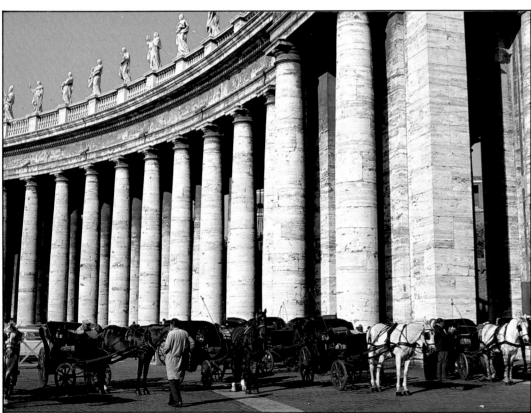

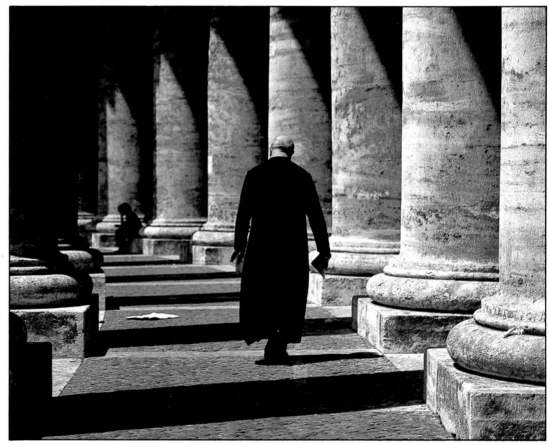

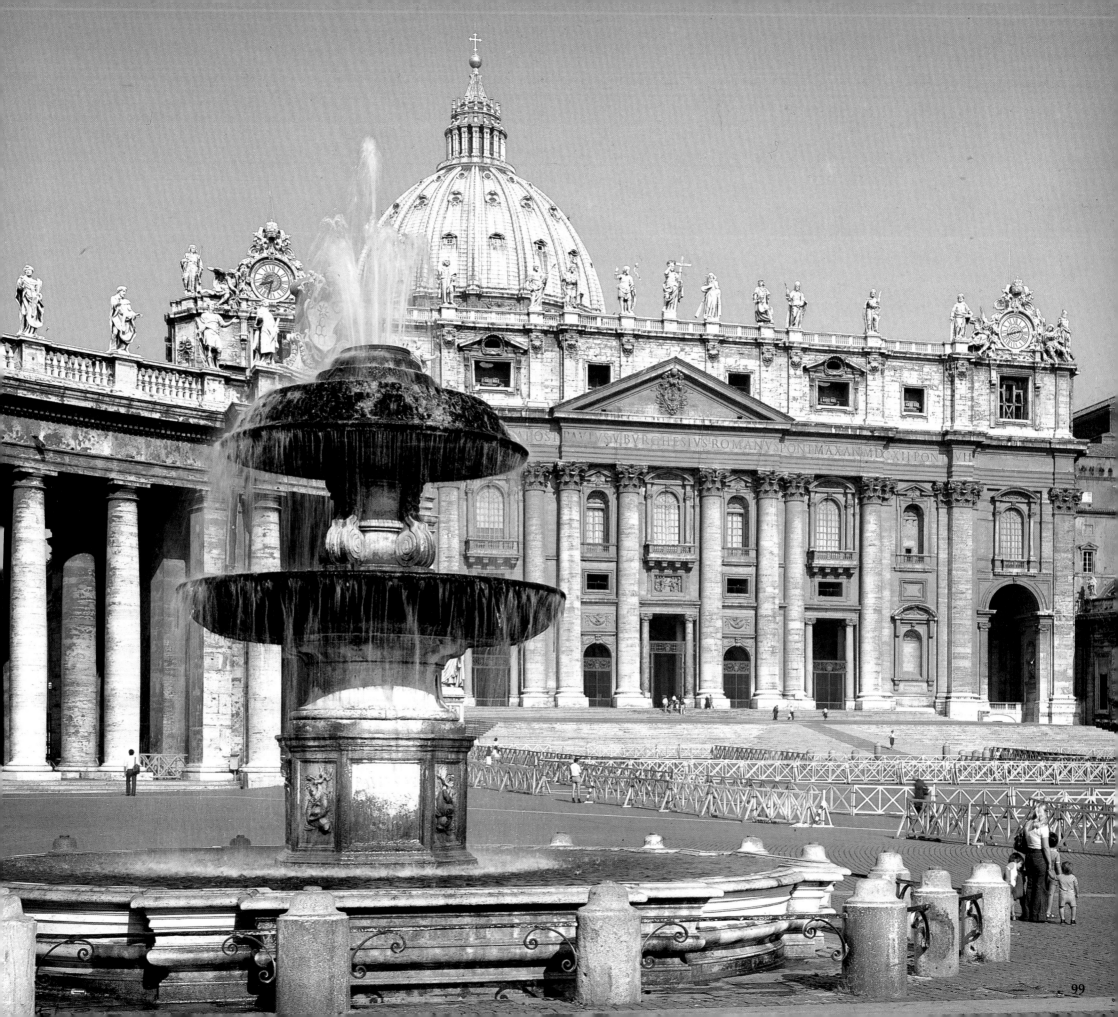

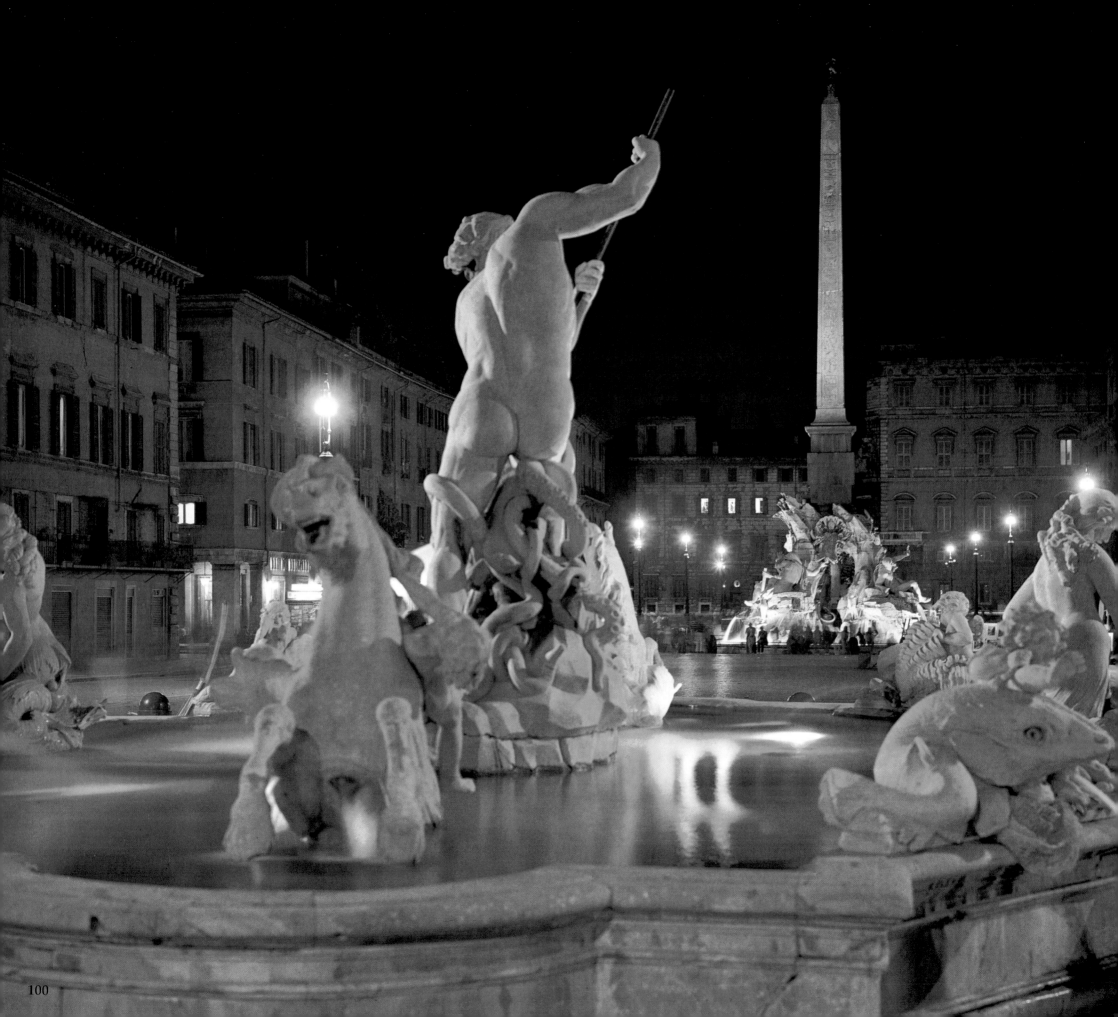

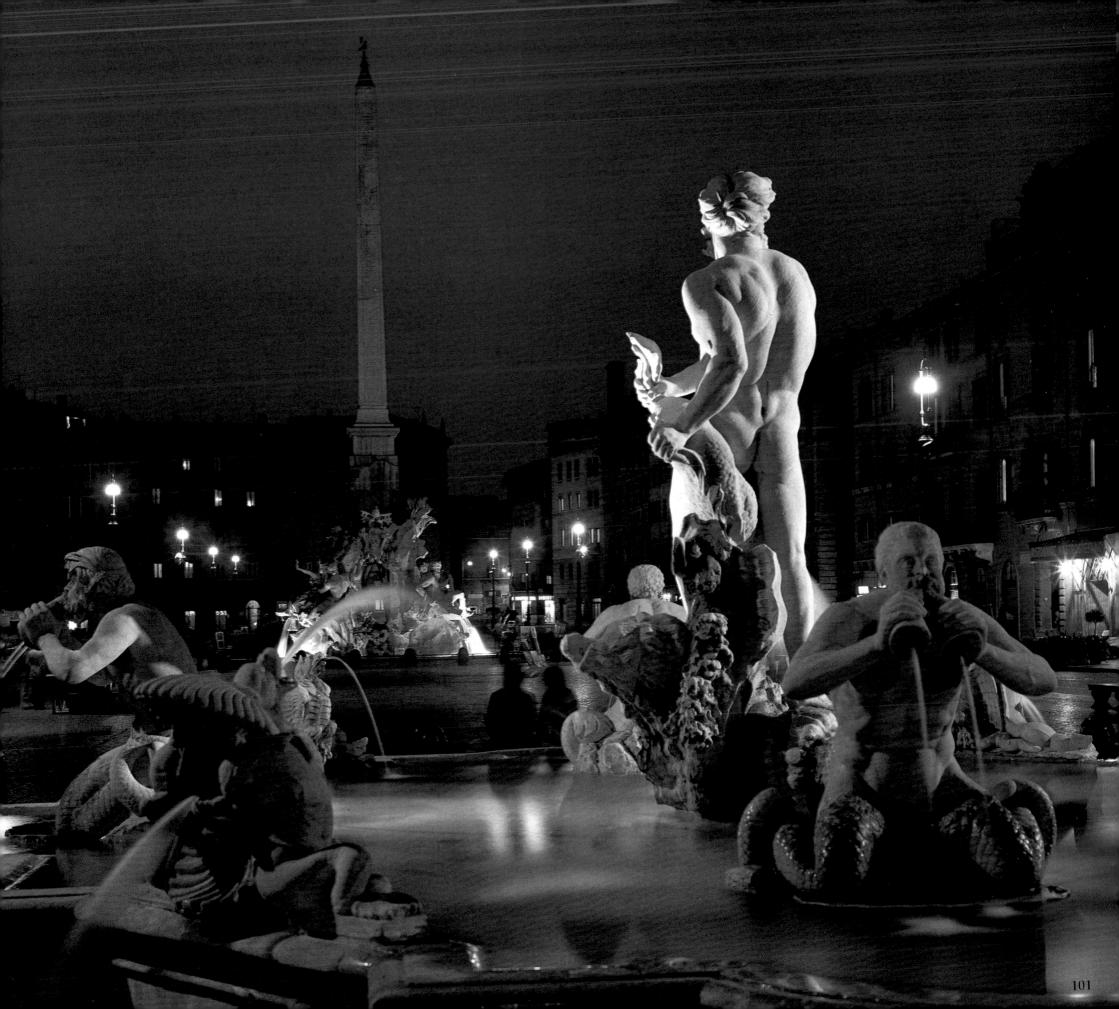

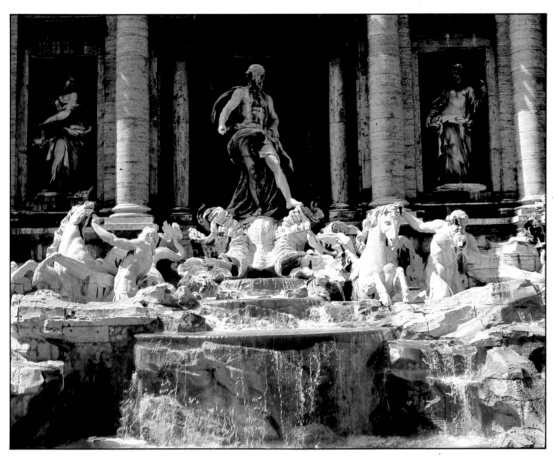

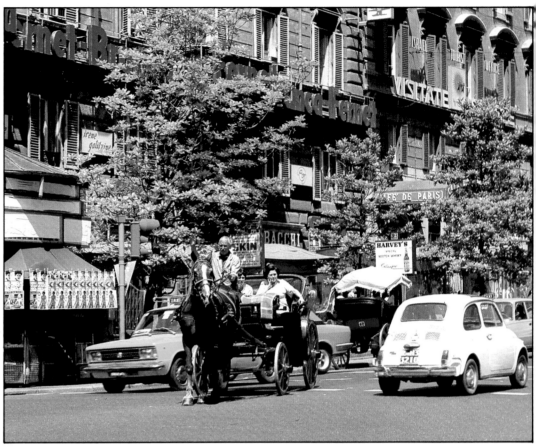

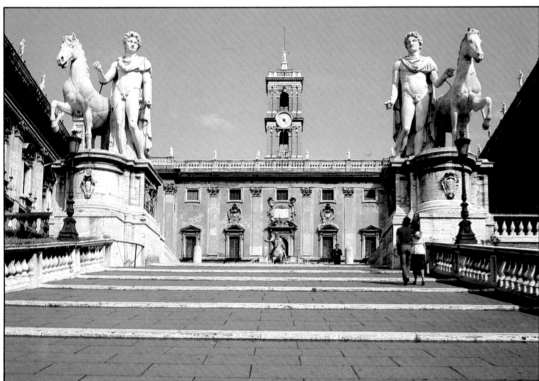

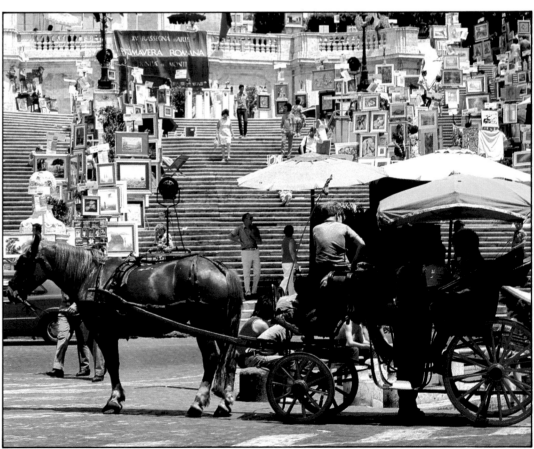

Above: the Dioscuri and Palazzo Senatorio on the Capitol, (top) the Fountain of Trevi, and (top right) the Via Veneto. Right and facing page: the Spanish Steps, leading from the Piazza di Spagna to the Church of Trinita dei Monti.

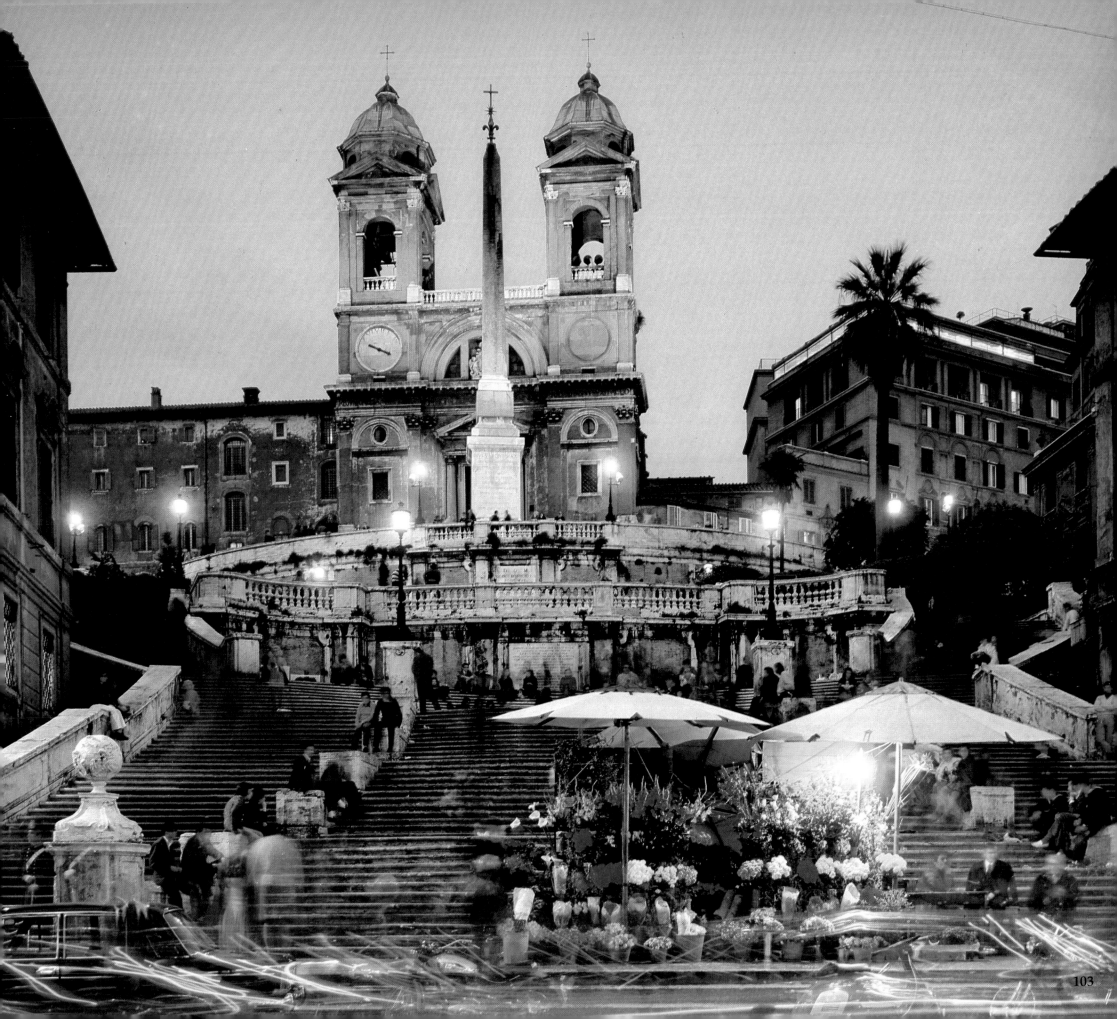

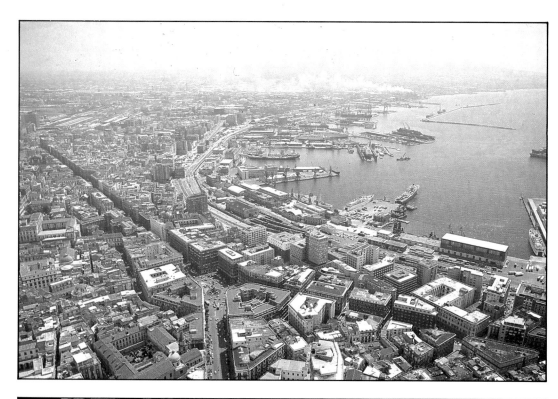

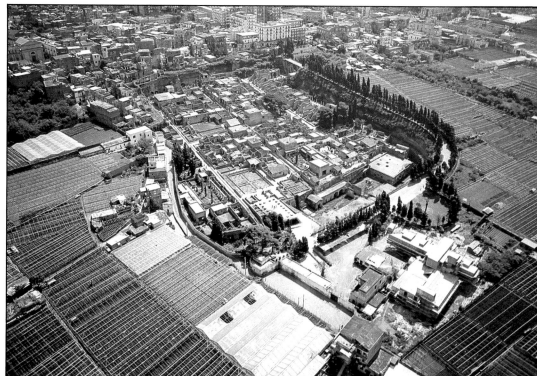

Left: Naples harbour and (bottom left) a narrow street off the Via Partenope, Naples. Bottom and facing page: Porto Sannazzaro at Mergillina, Naples, and (below) the remains of Roman Herculaneum. Overleaf: (left) the Temple of Genii Augusti, and (right) tombs in the Necropoli, Pompeii.

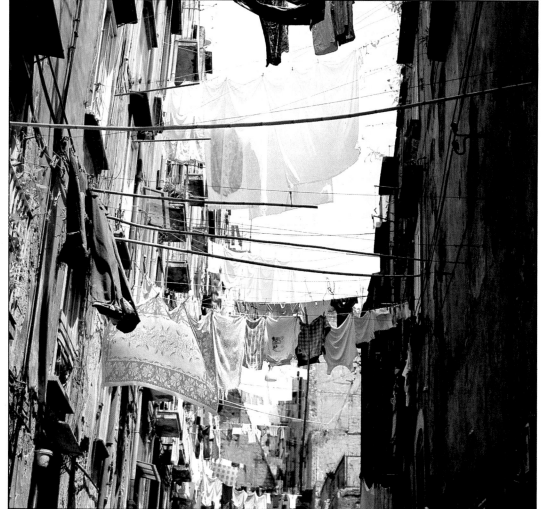

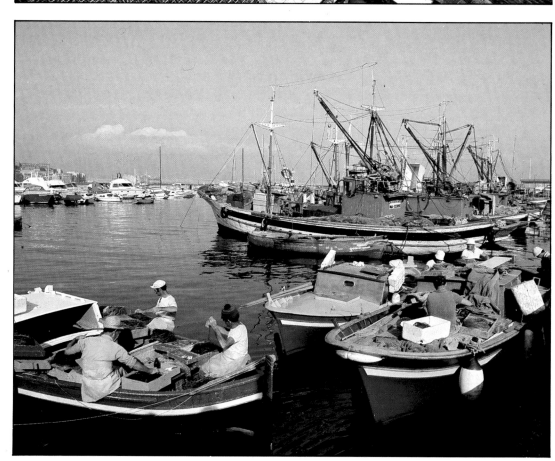

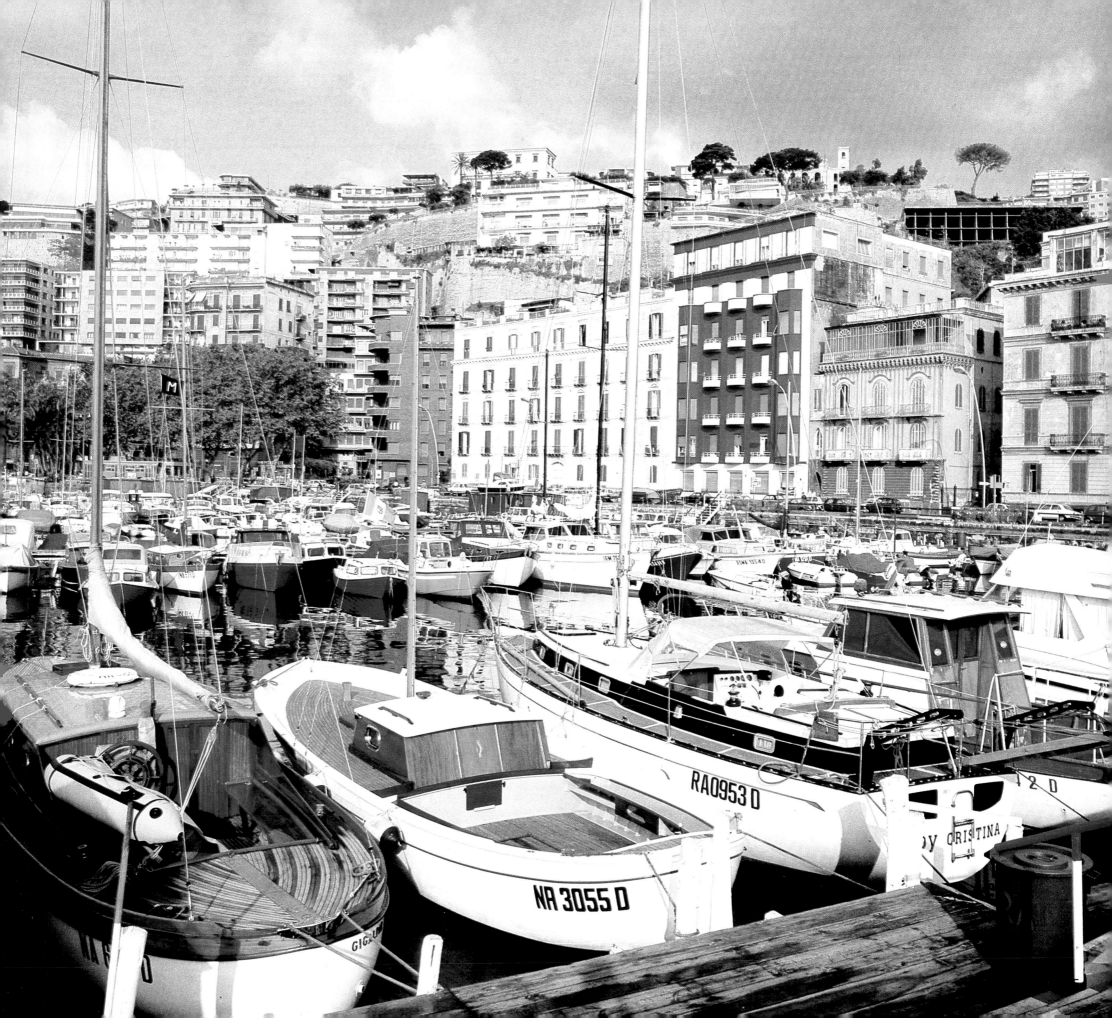

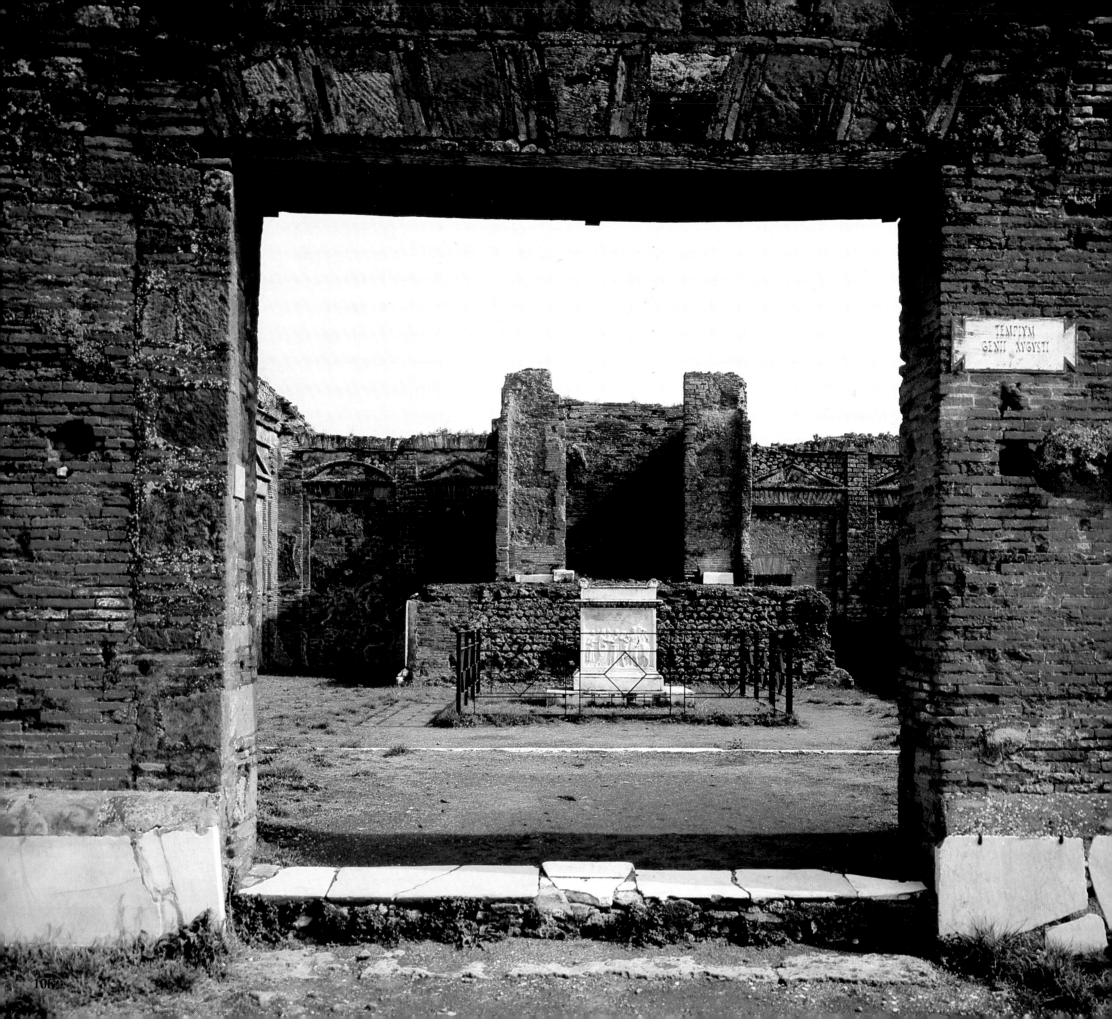

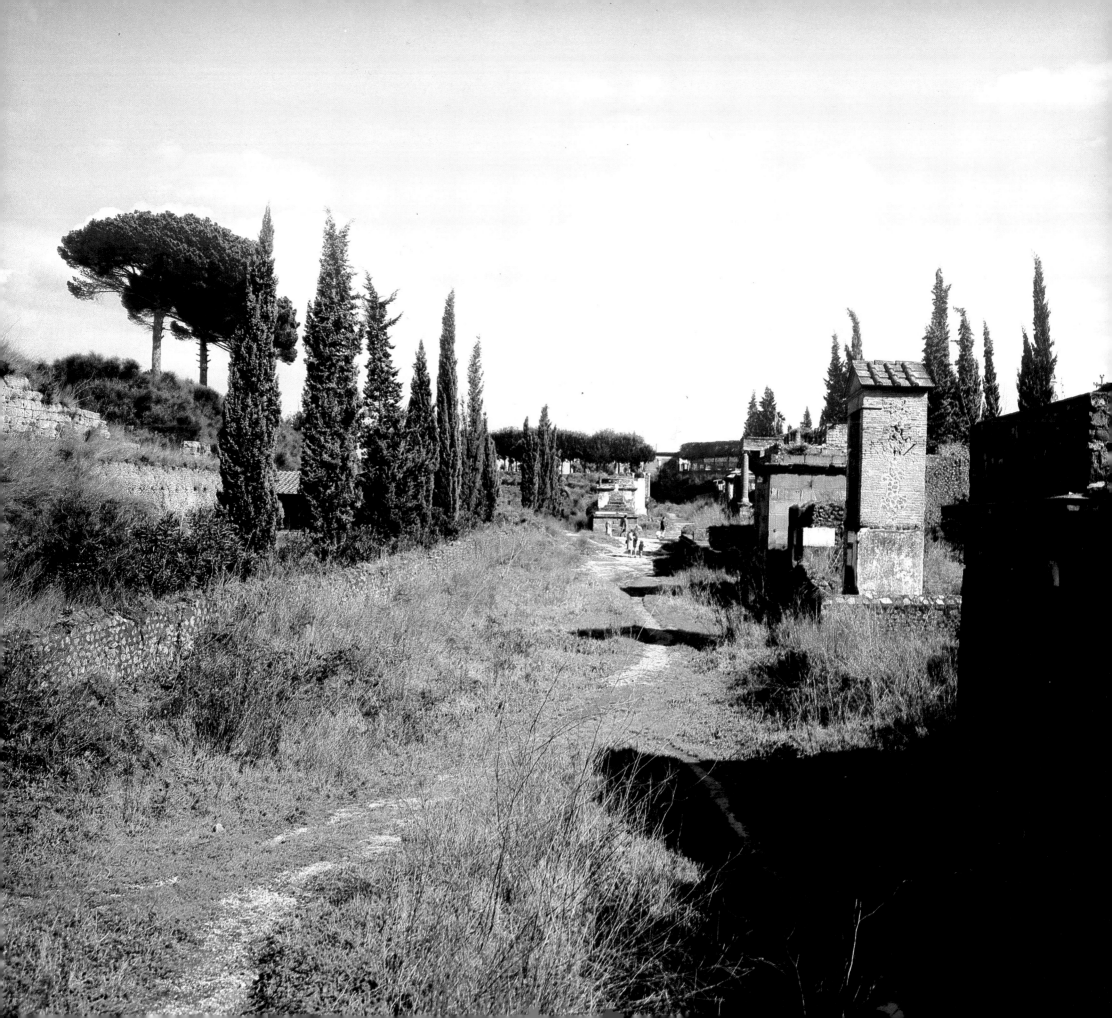

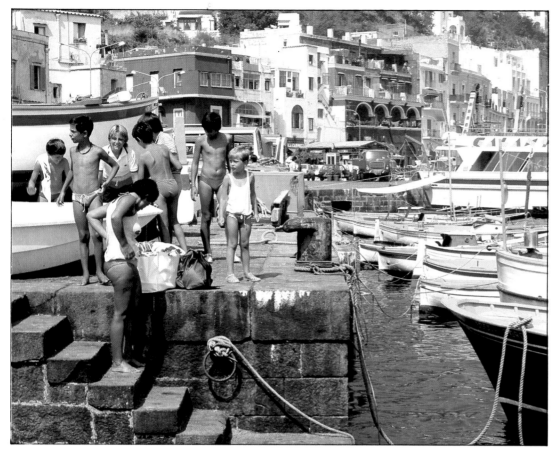

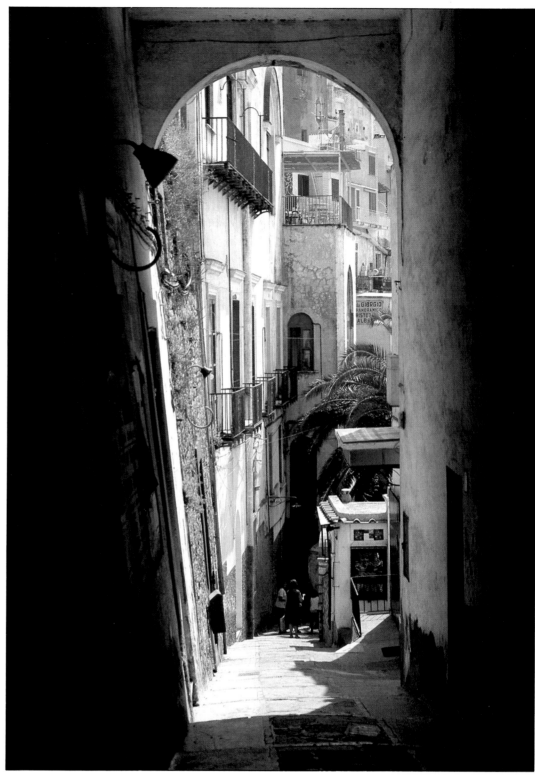

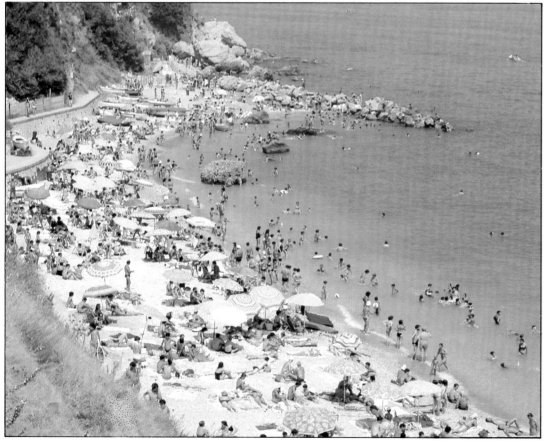

The small island of Capri (these pages) lies in the Tyrrhenian Sea, off the tip of the Sorrento peninsula. Regular boats carry passengers from the mainland to the port of Marina Grande (top left and left), from which the stepped footpath of the Strada Campo di Pisco leads up the cliff to the steep streets of Capri town (above). Once the pleasure retreat of the Roman emperors Augustus and Tiberius, Capri remains an island favoured by the rich. Facing page: the 12th-century Tower of Damecuta, on Capri's northwest coast. Overleaf: (left) the Marina Grande, and (right) sun-bathers, in Sorrento.

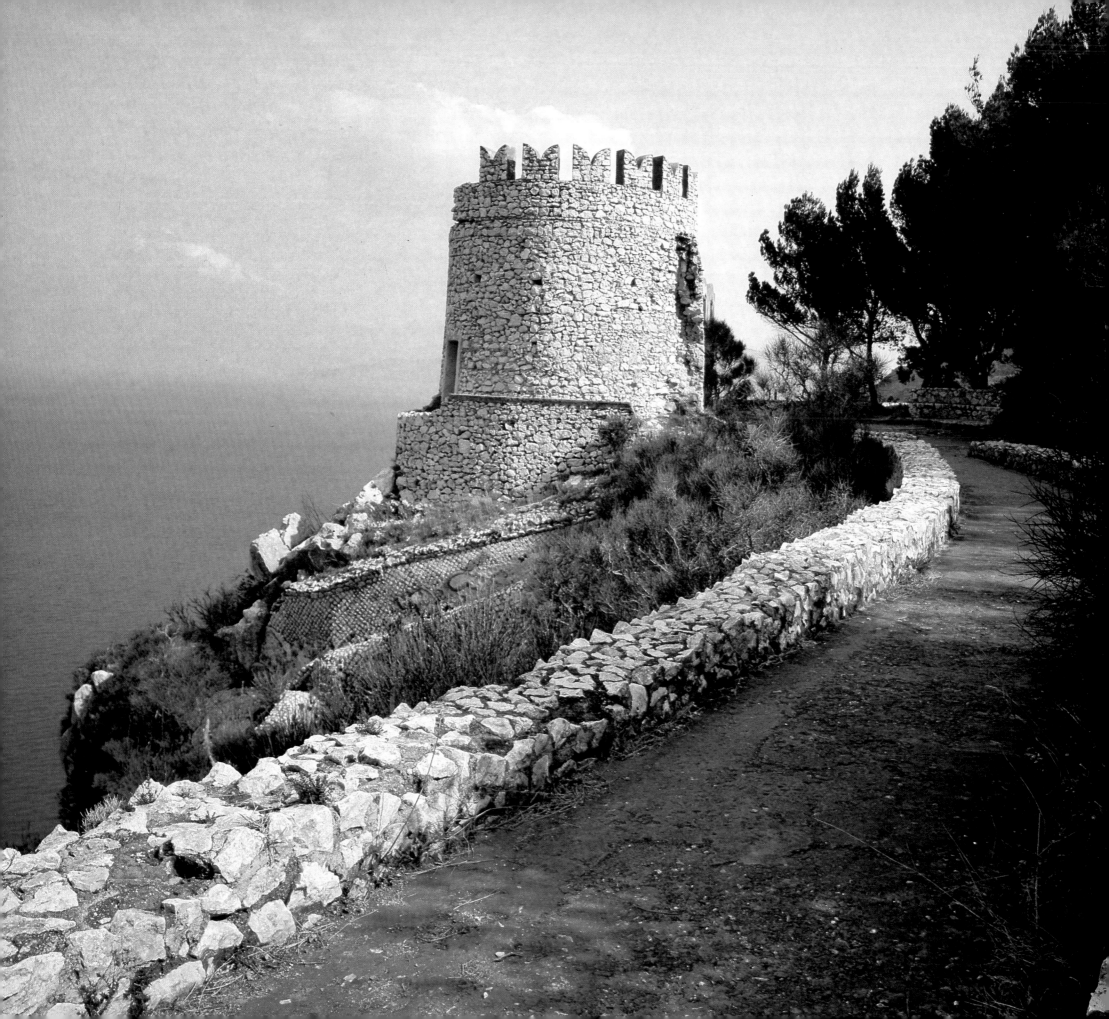

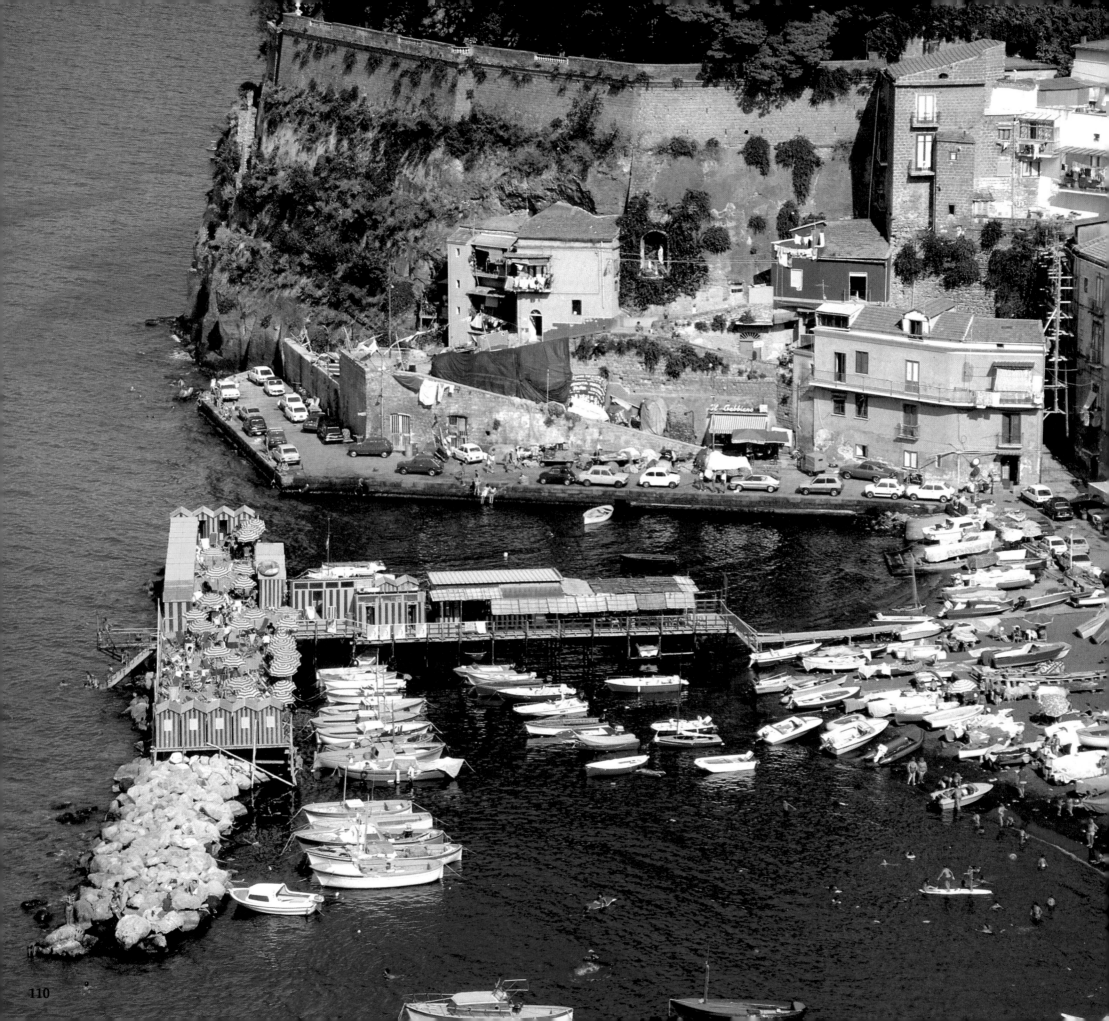

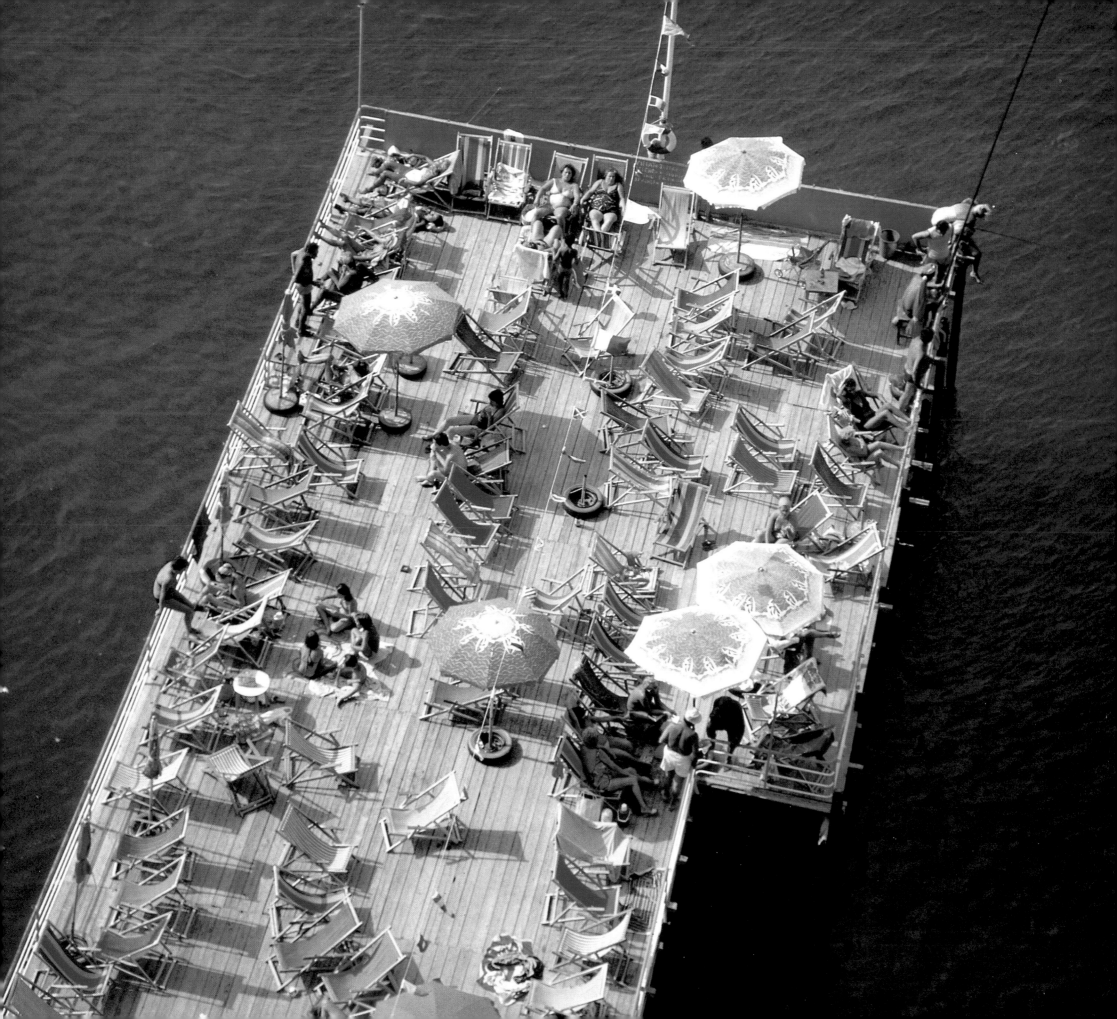

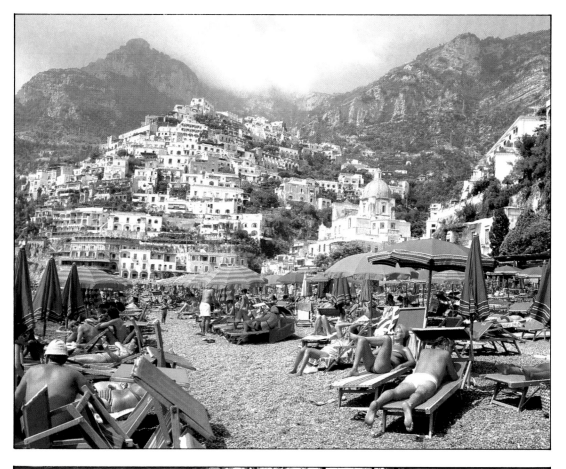

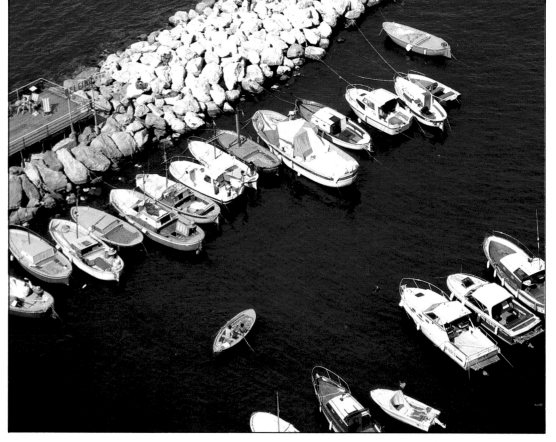

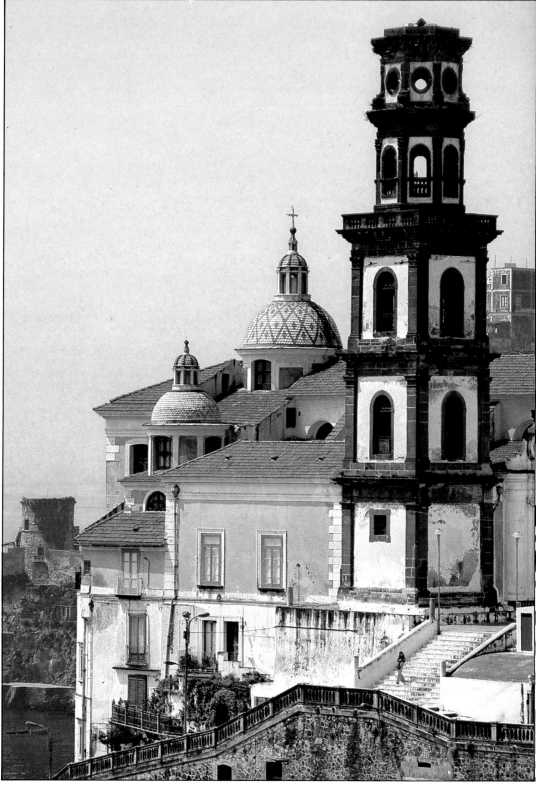

Top left: the piled houses of the fishing village of Positano, now thriving more on tourism than the sea, and (left) the harbour at Sorrento. Above: the tiled cupolas of the church of Atrani (facing page), on the rocky south coast of the Sorrento peninsula. Positano (overleaf), built on steep, terraced slopes along the same coastline, was first 'discovered' by writers, artists and sculptors with an appreciation of the dramatic.

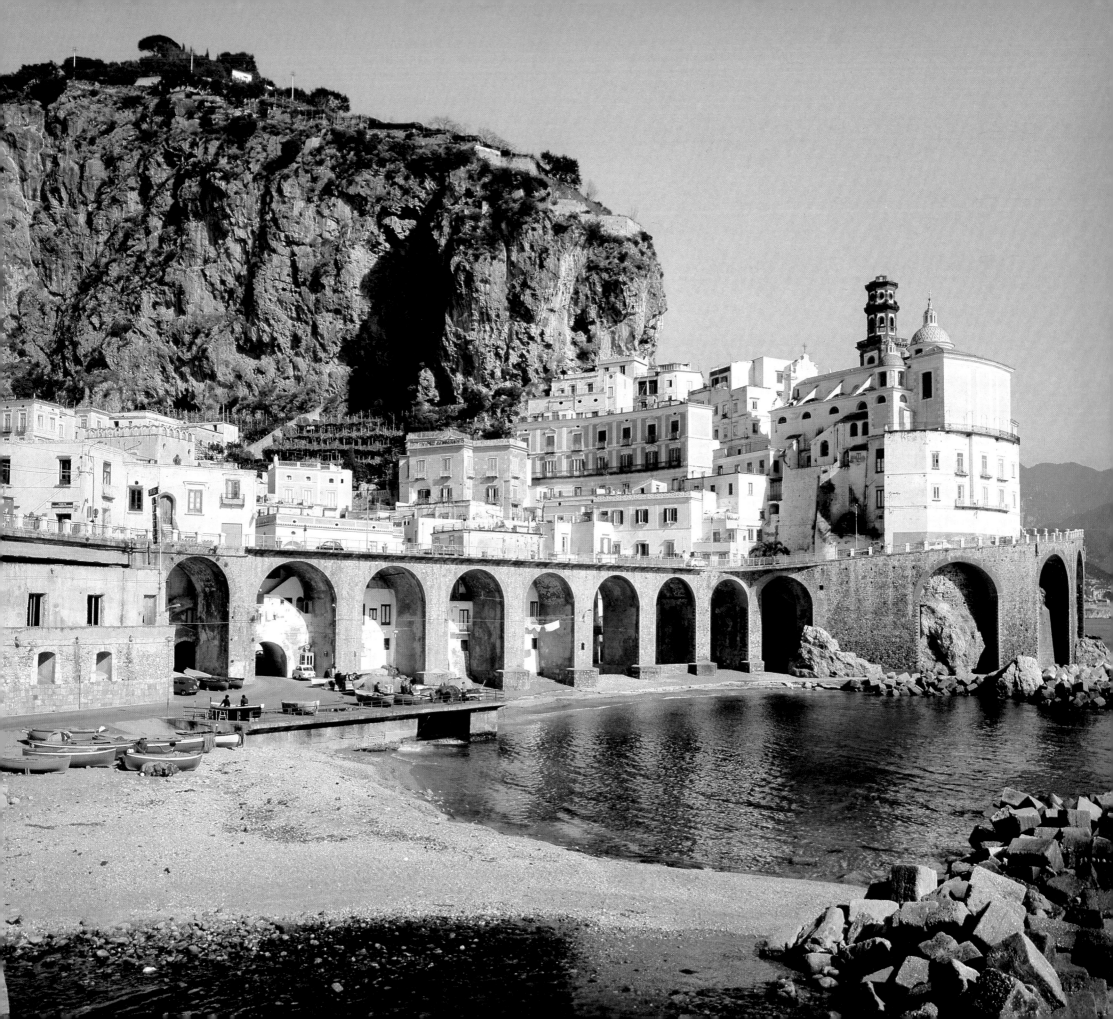

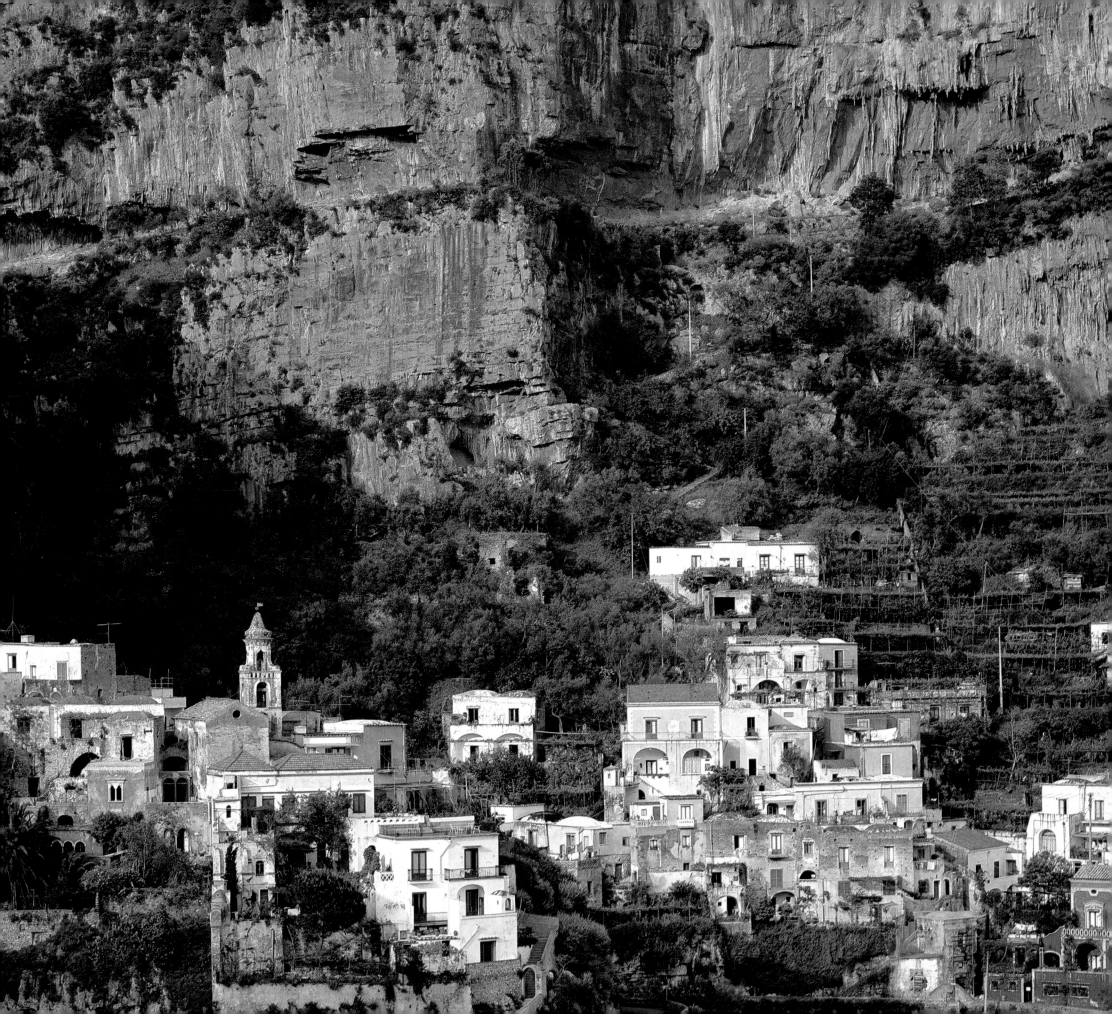

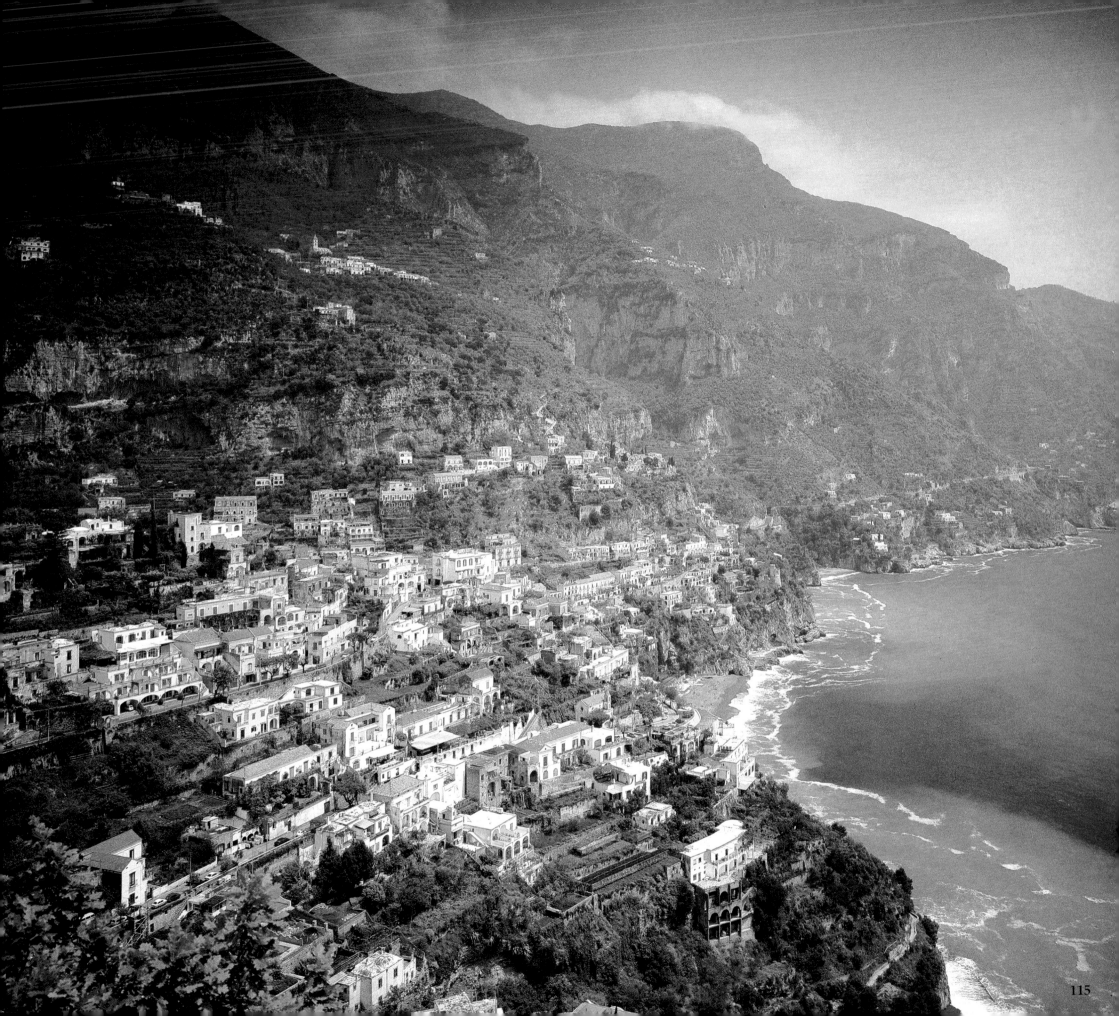

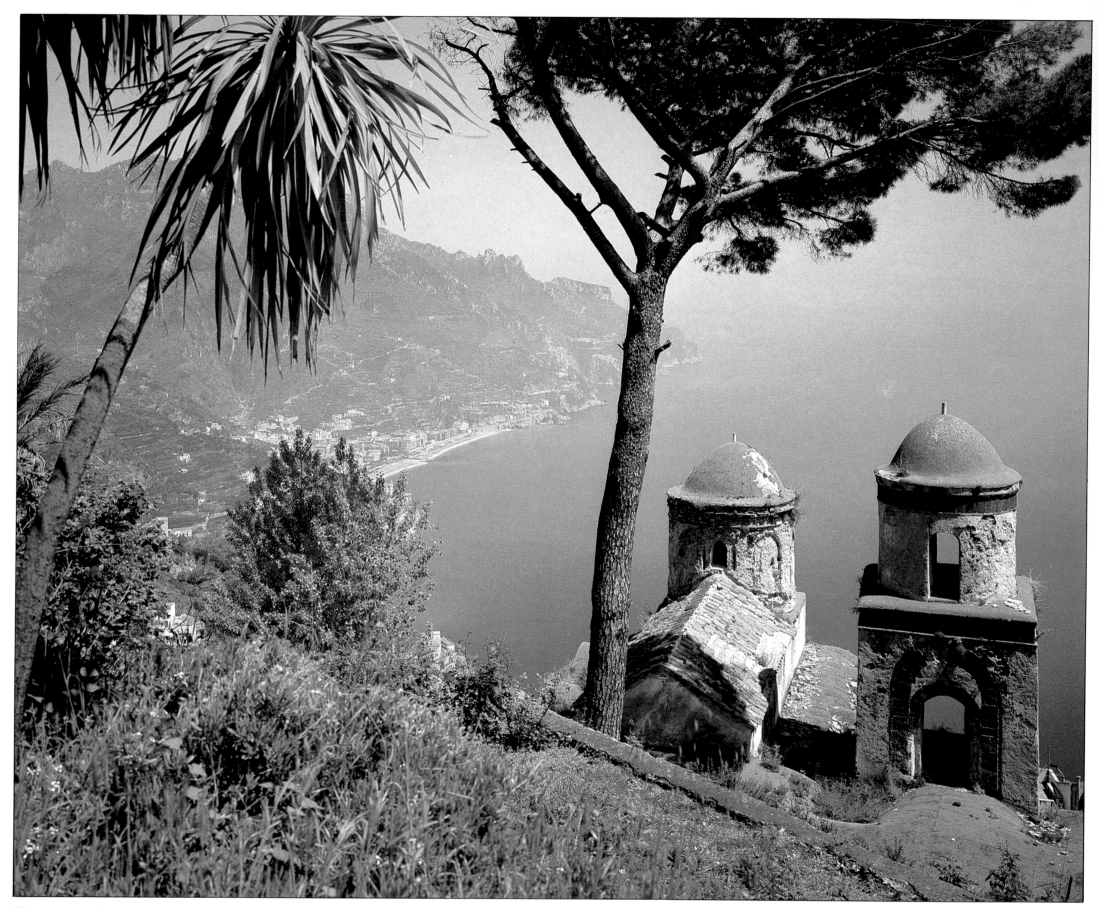

These pages: the Gulf of Salerno seen from the gardens of Palazzo Rufolo in Ravello, built by the Rufoli family during the 13th century. Overleaf: (left) the harbour of Vietri sul Mare on the Gulf of Salerno, and (right) the village of Rivello, in the arid mountains above the Gulf of Policastro.

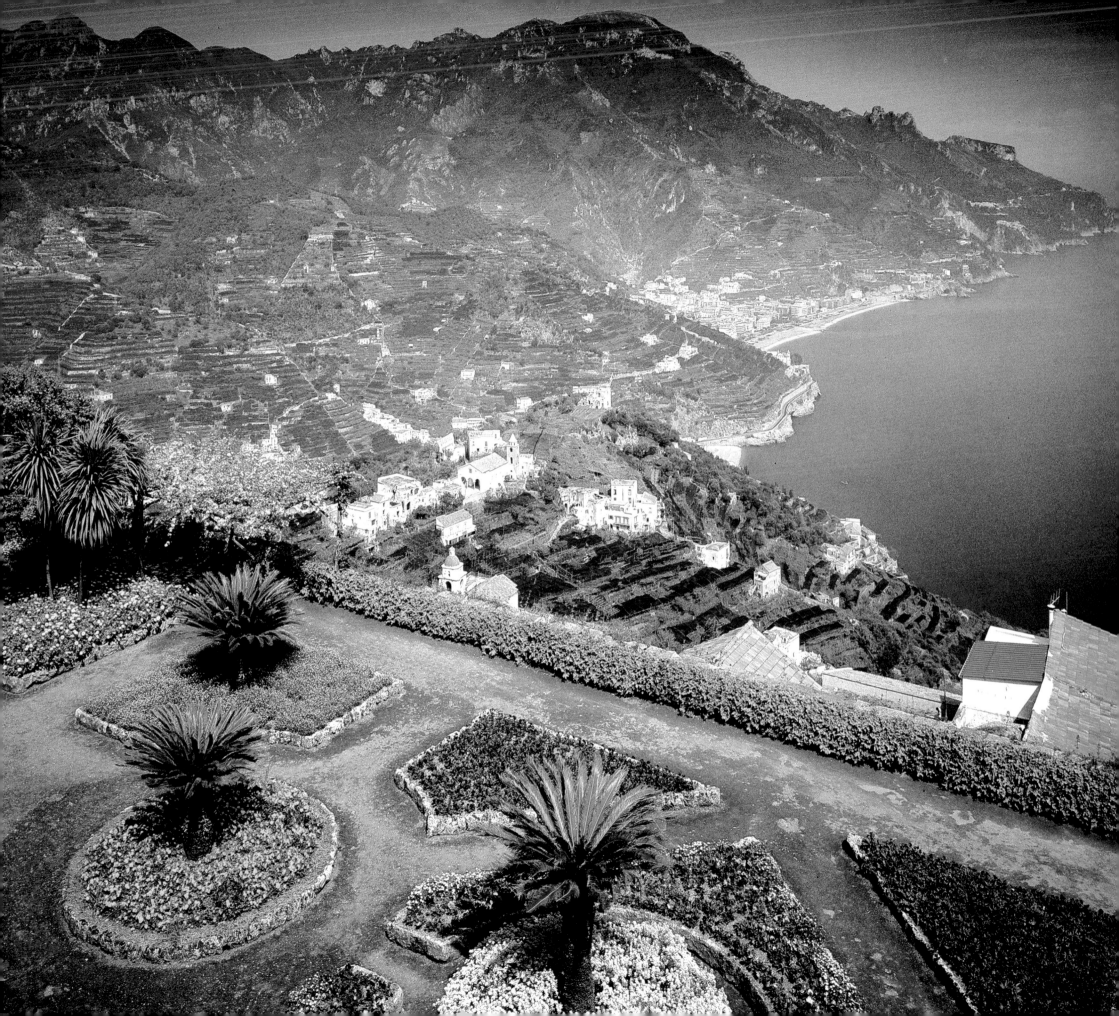

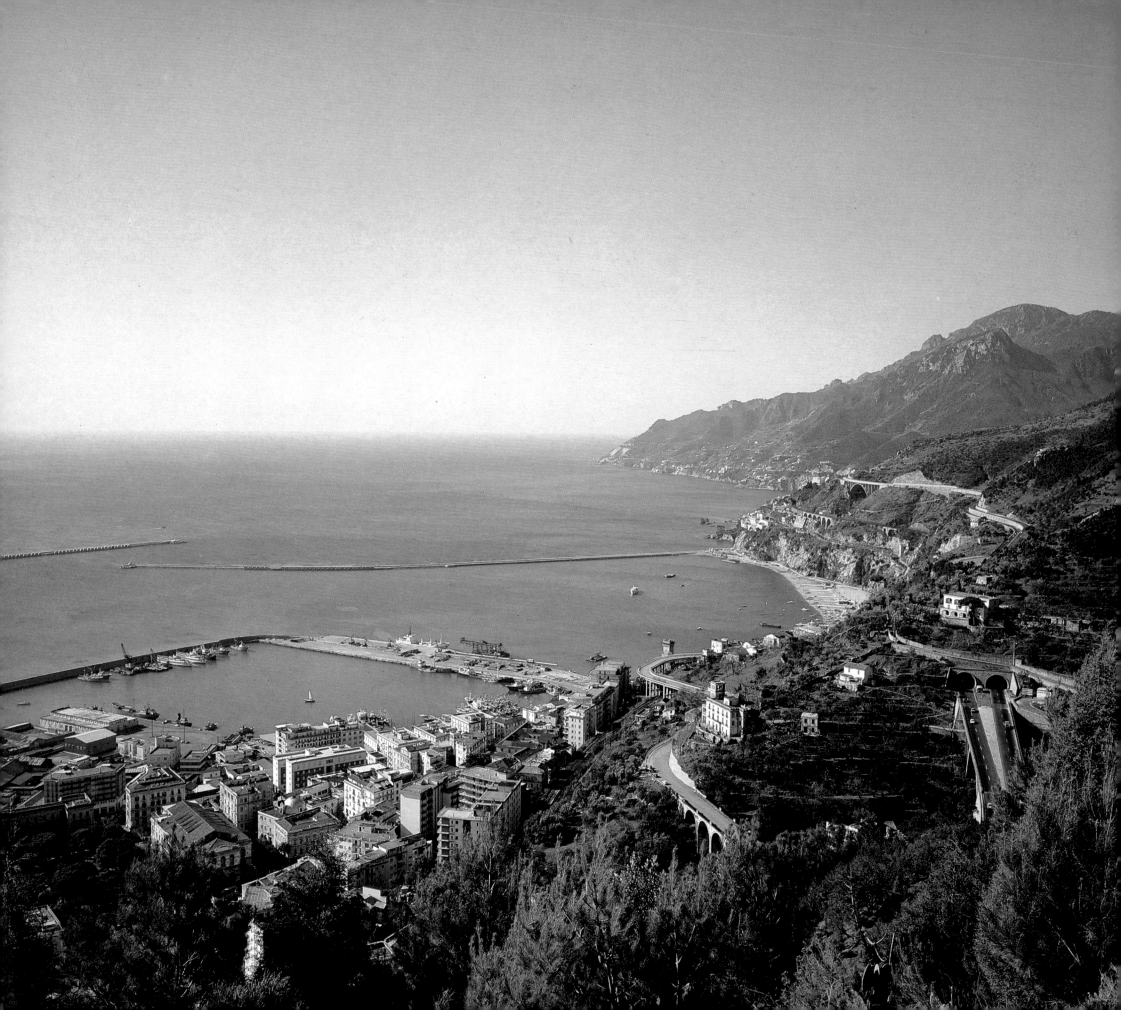

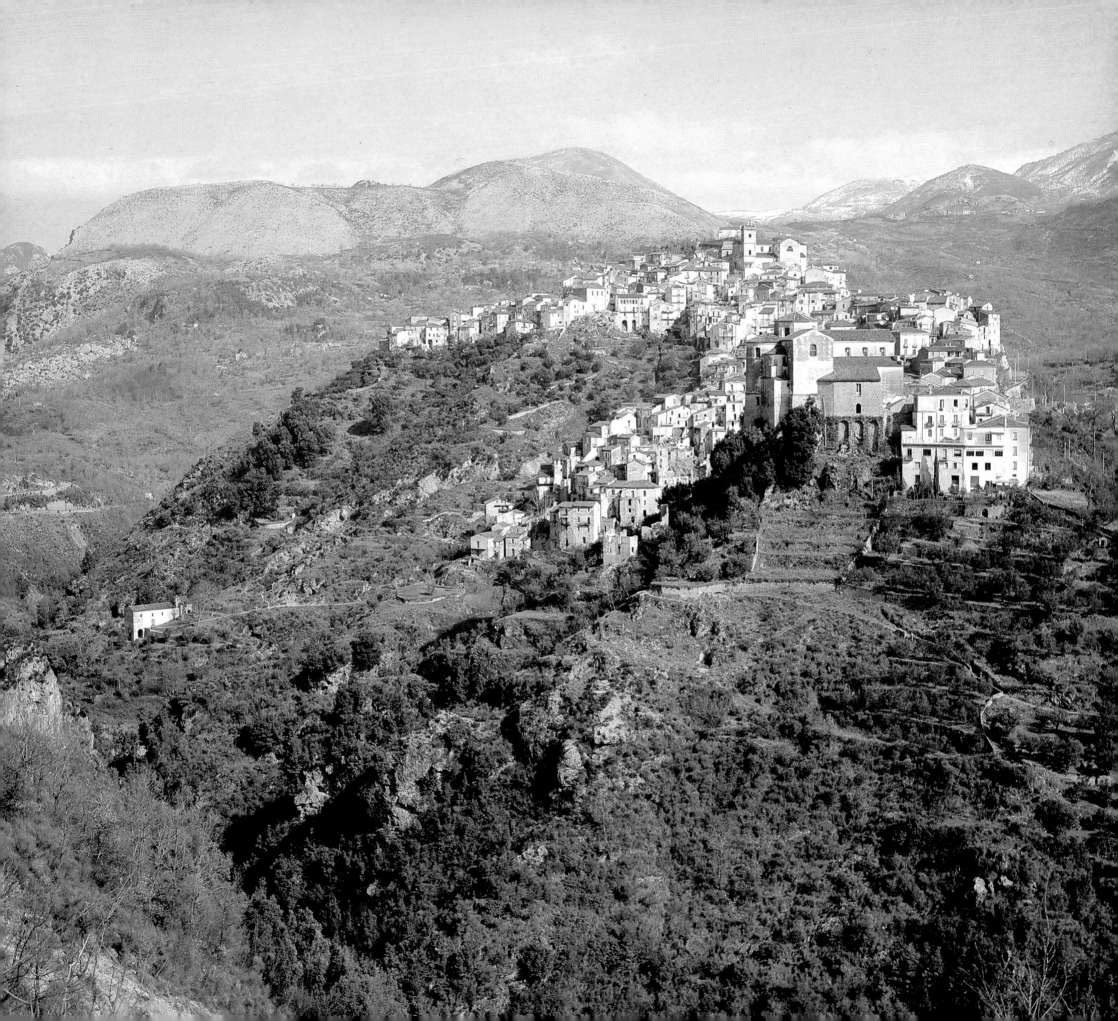

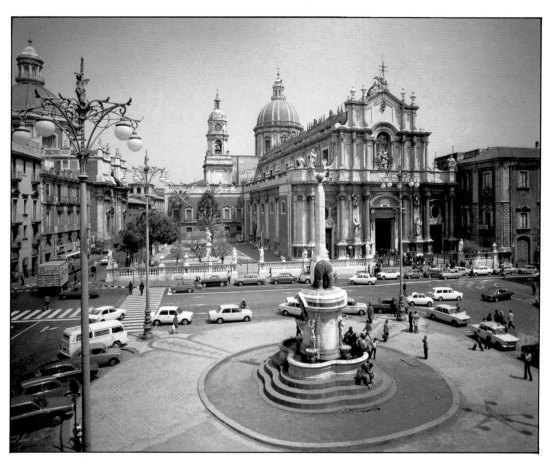

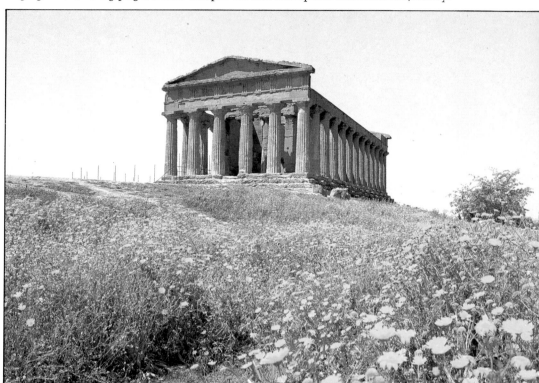

Left: the Elephant Fountain and the Cathedral in Catania, (bottom left) the Cathedral, Palermo, and (overleaf) the harbour and roofs of Messina, Sicily. Below: the Temple of Concord, and (bottom) the Temple of the Dioscuri, in Agrigento. Facing page: Doric temple on the Acropolis at Selinunte, Sicily.

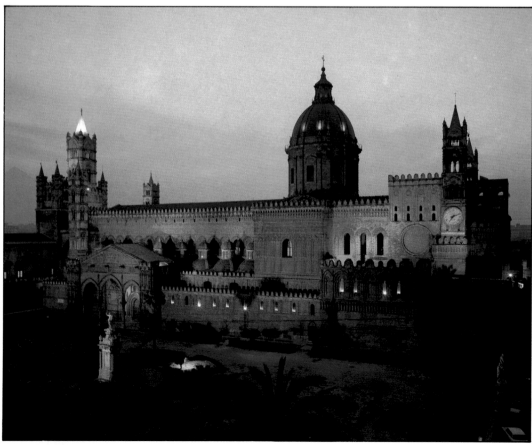

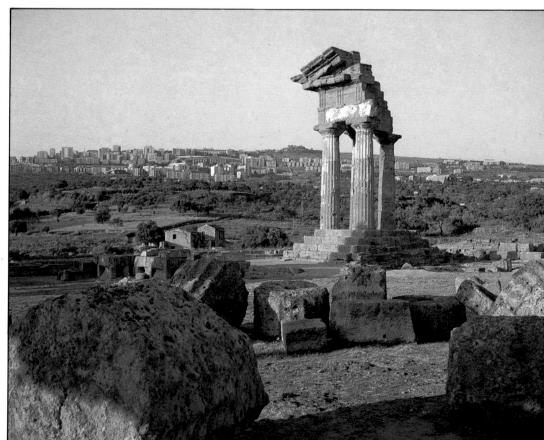

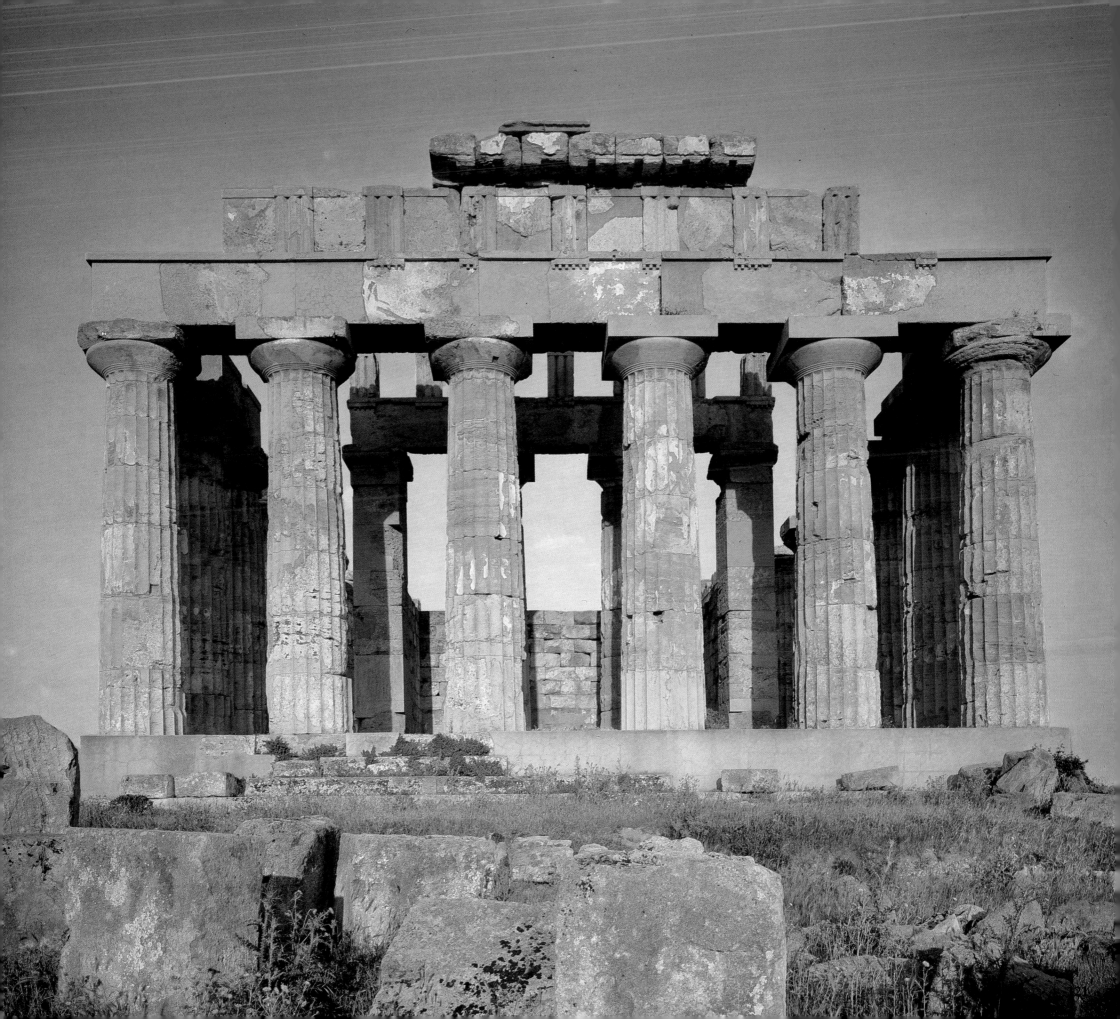

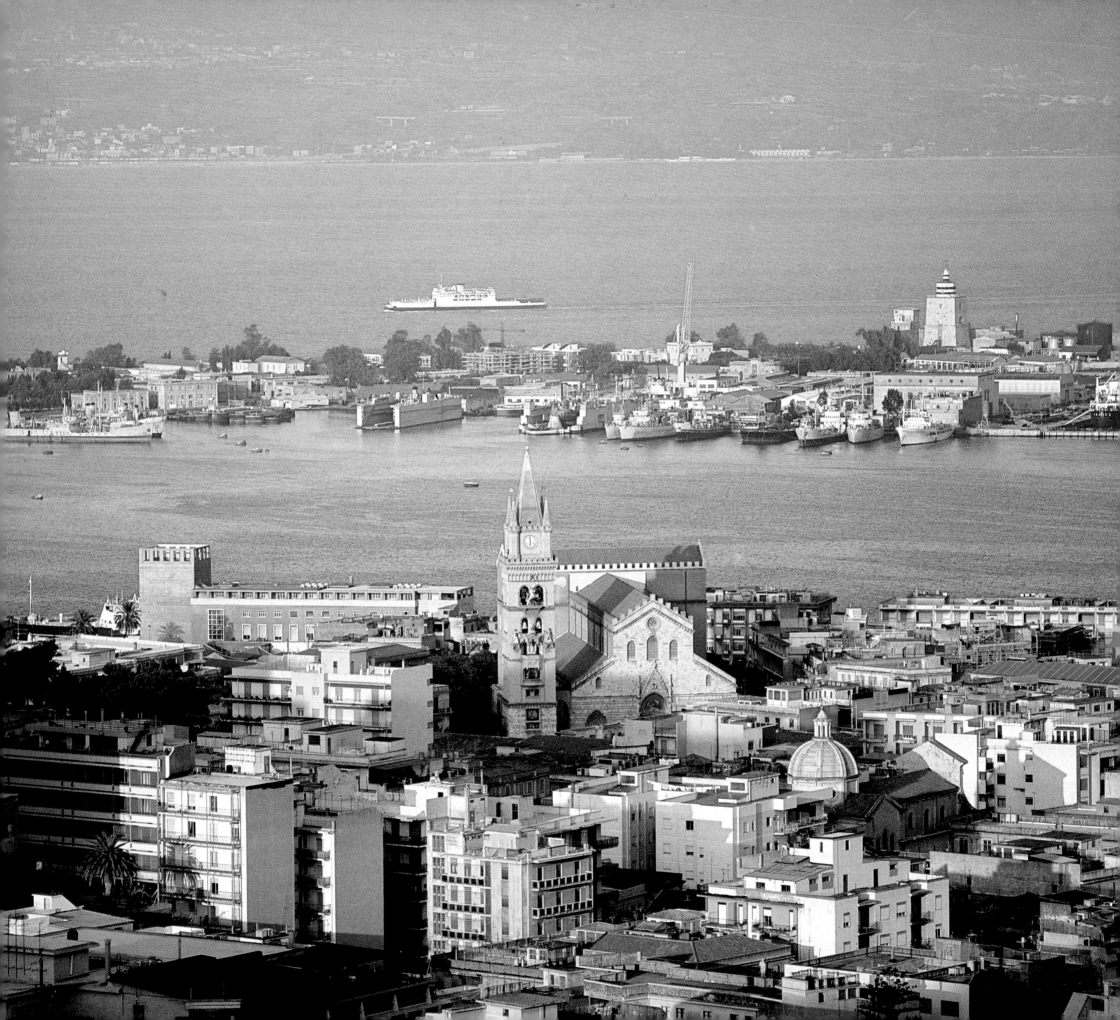

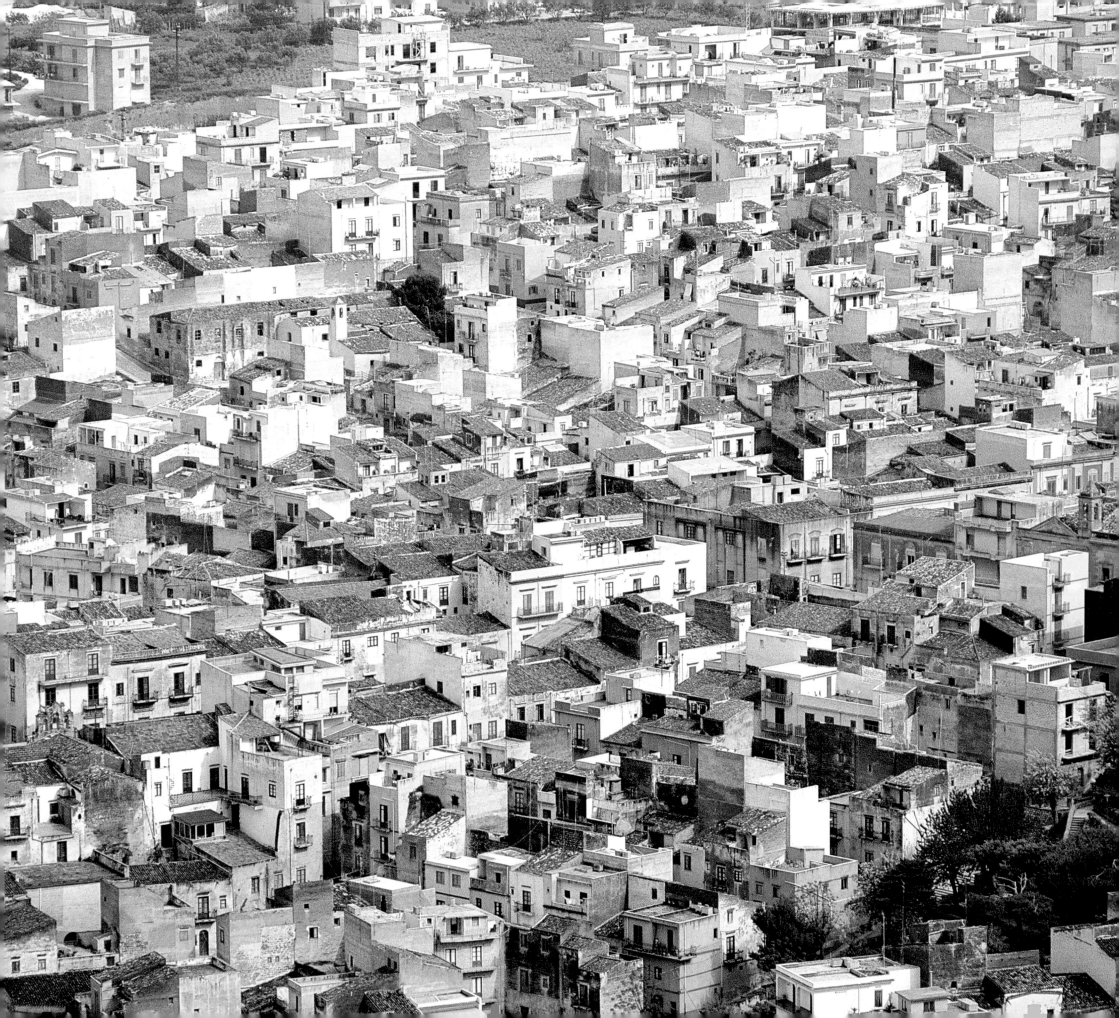

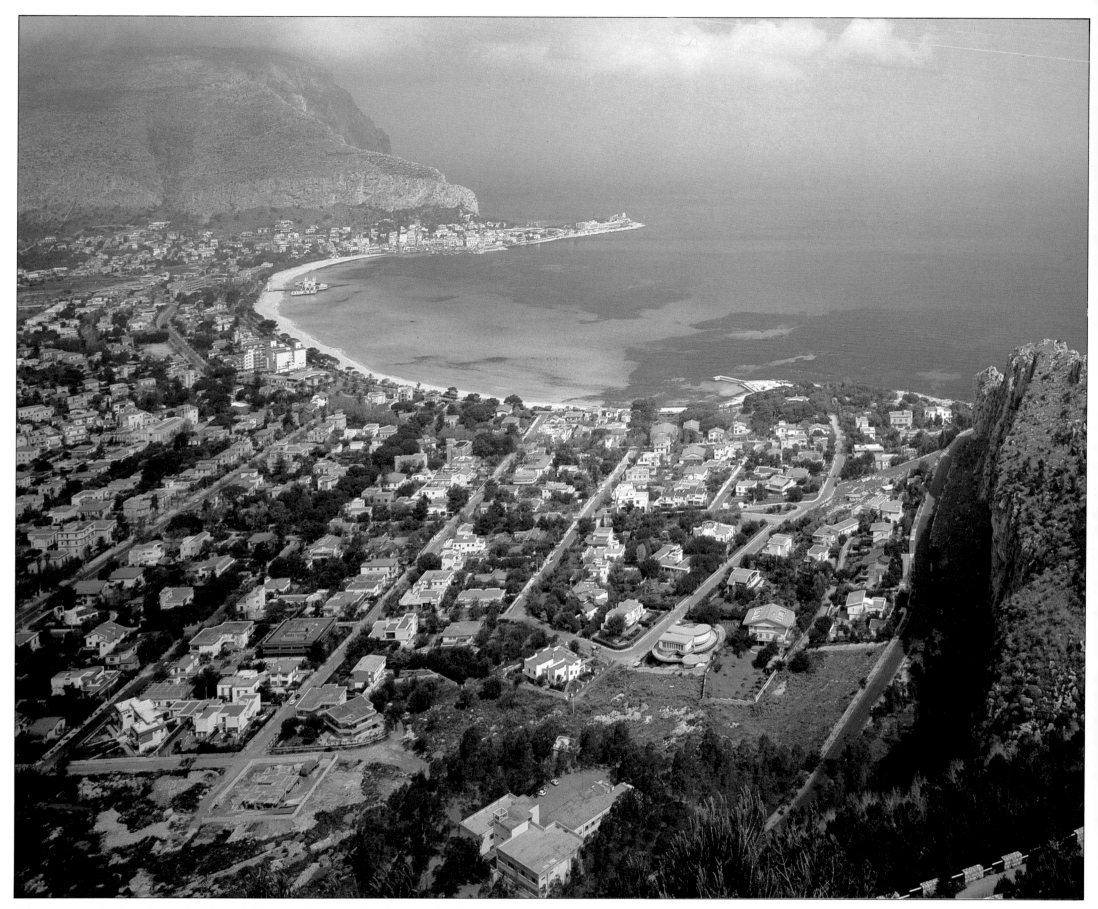

These pages: the beach resort of Mondello, near Palermo. Overleaf: (right) Ragusa Ibla, built into the mountainside, and (left) Taormina, high on a terrace above the Ionian Sea, and distant Mount Etna (following page) beyond.

124

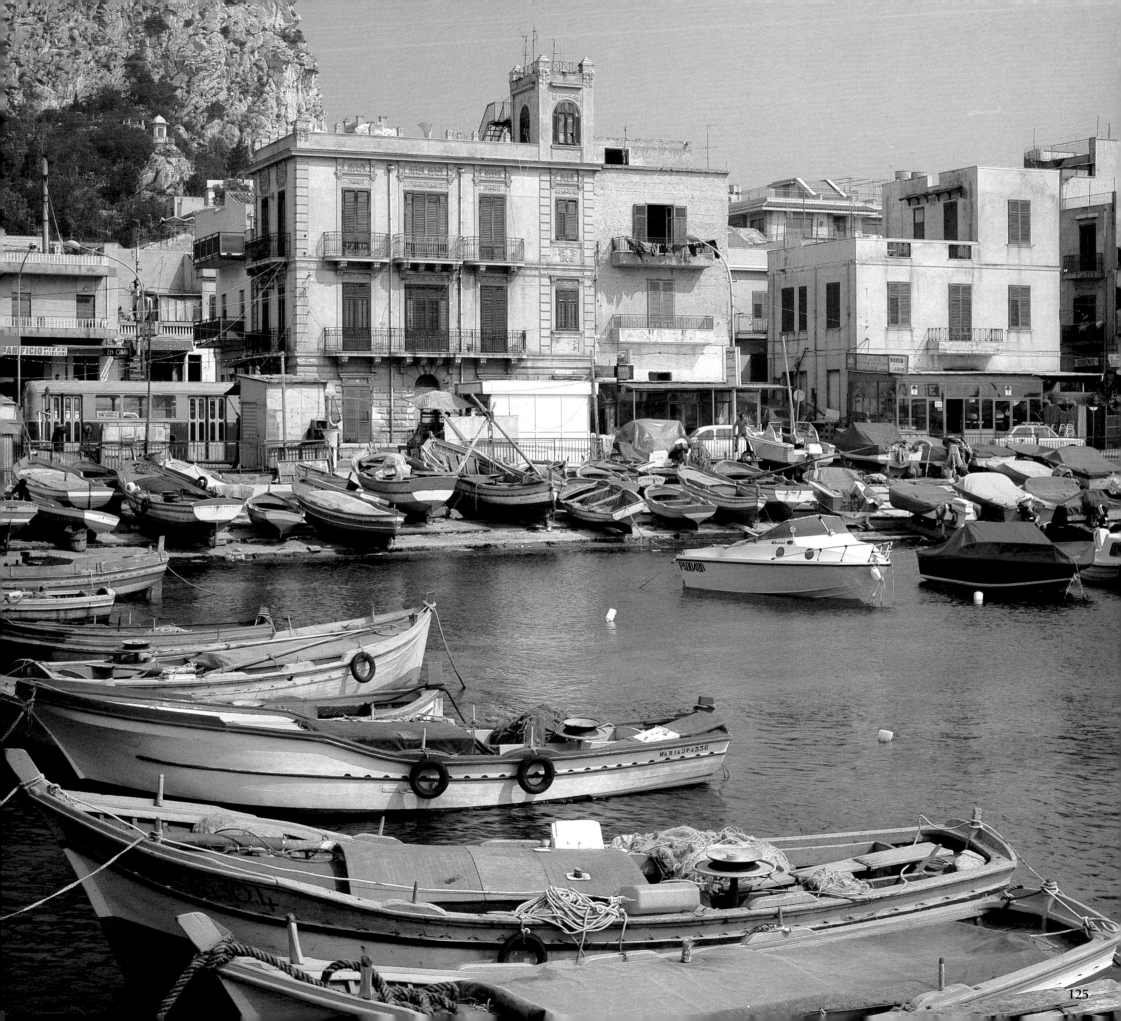

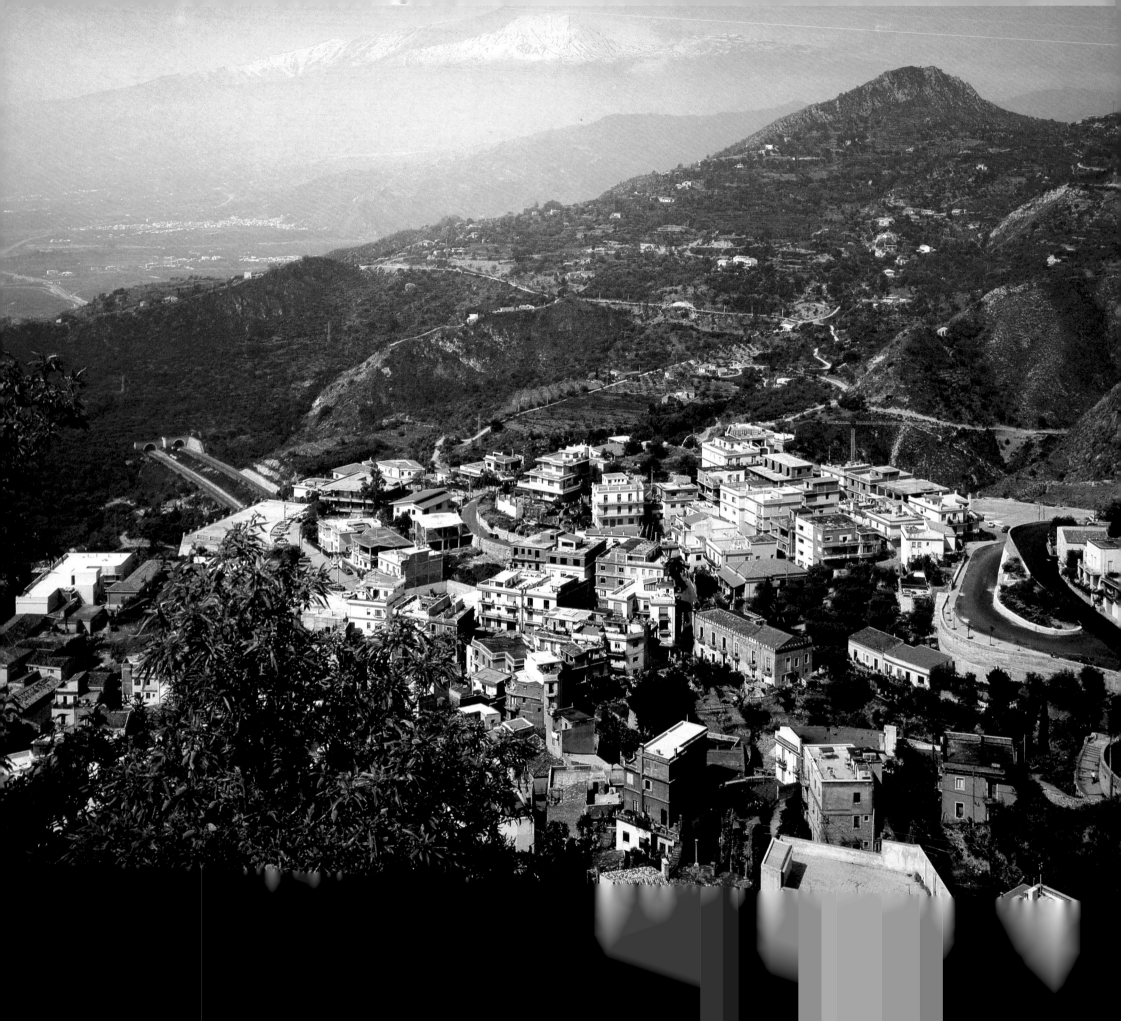

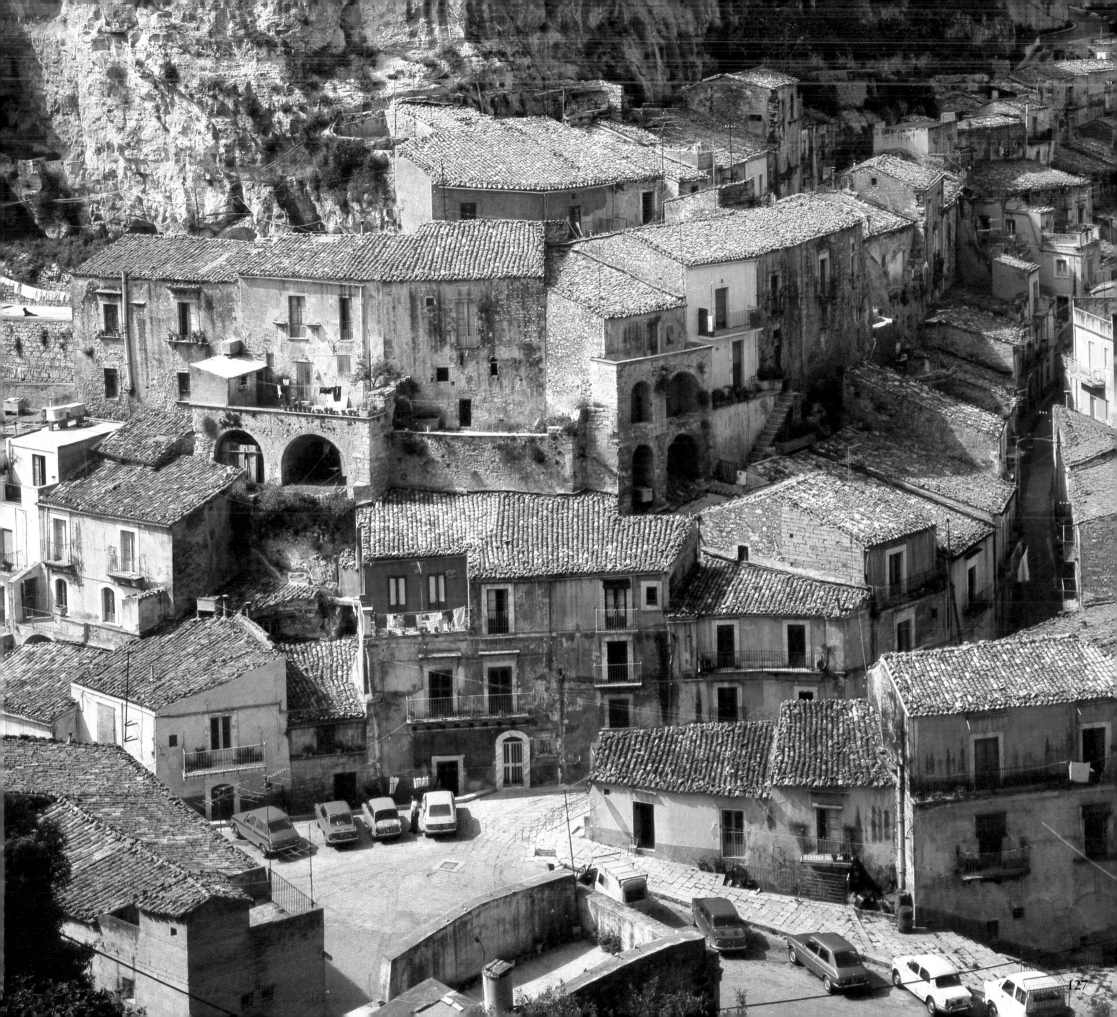

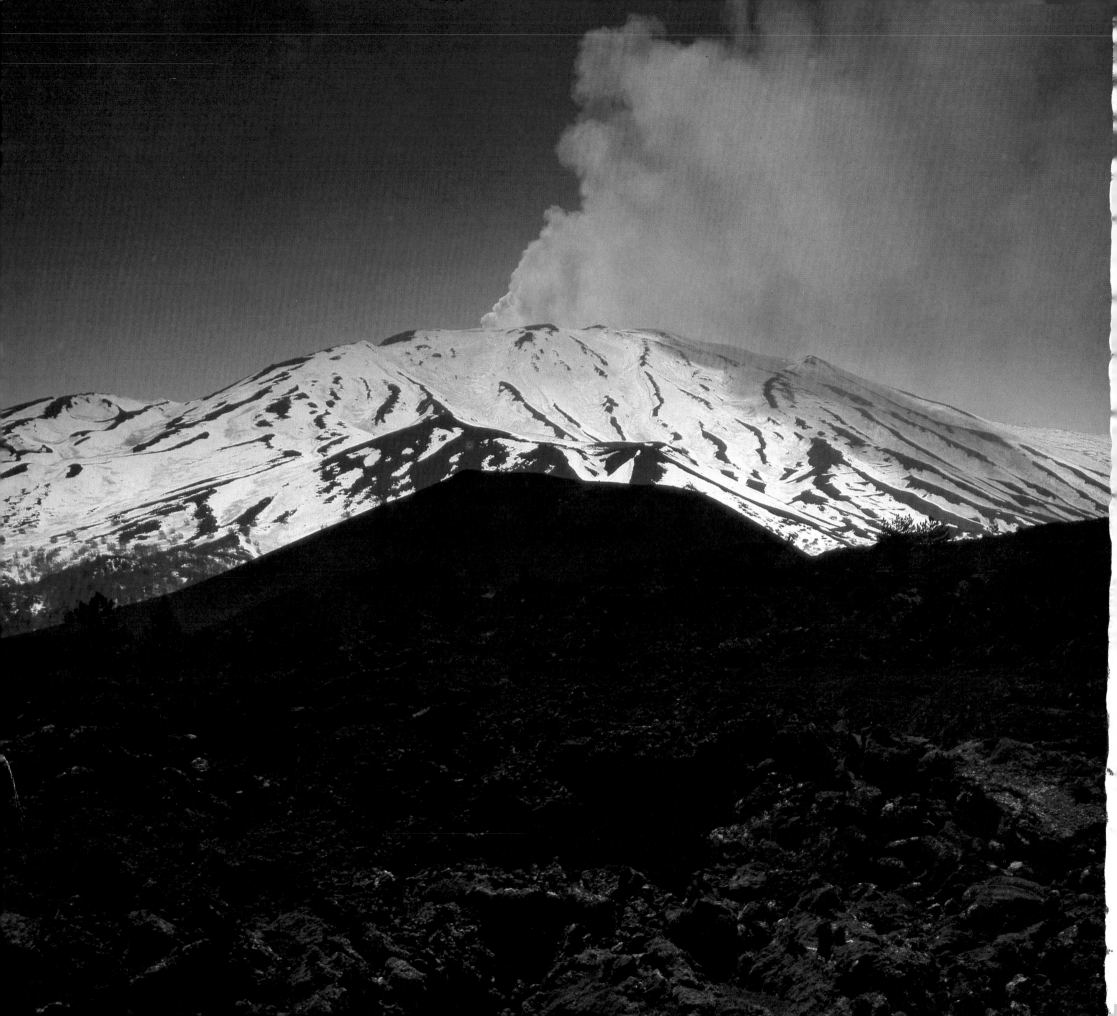